THIRD EDITION

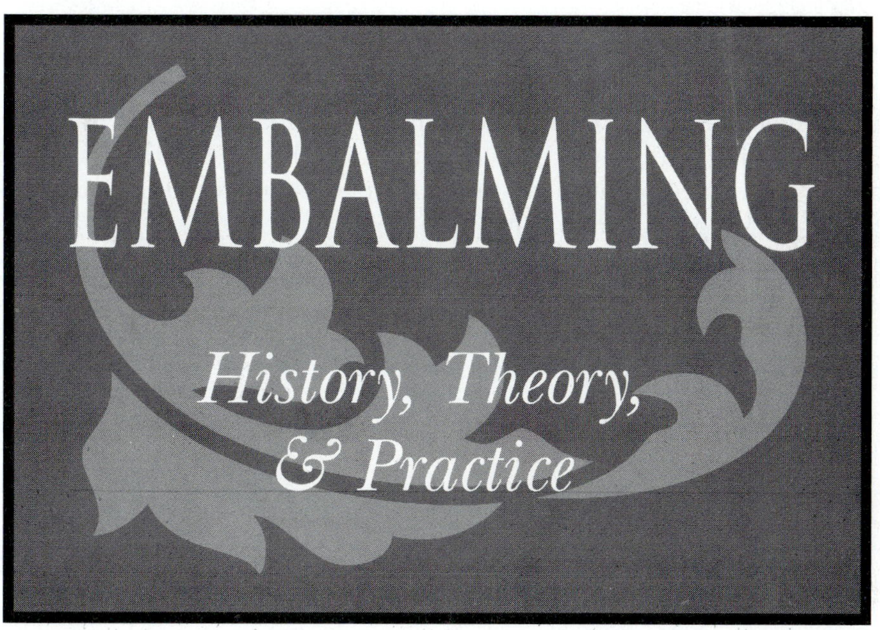

Robert G. Mayer
Licensed Embalmer and Funeral Director
Pittsburgh, Pennsylvania

Adjunct Professor
Pittsburgh Institute of Mortuary Science
Pittsburgh, Pennsylvania

With a Foreword by

Daniel E. Buchanan, MA
President
Gupton-Jones College of Funeral Service
Decatur, Georgia

Past-President
American Board of Funeral Service Education

McGraw-Hill
Health Professions Division

New York St. Louis San Francisco Auckland Bogotá Caracas Lisbon London
Madrid Mexico City Milan Montreal New Delhi San Juan
Singapore Sydney Tokyo Toronto

McGraw-Hill
A Division of The McGraw-Hill Companies

Embalming: History, Theory, and Practice, 3/e

1234567890 CCWCCW 99

ISBN 0-8385-2187-8

Notice

Medicine is an ever-changing science. As new research and clinical experience broaden our knowledge, changes in treatment and drug therapy are required. The author and the publisher of this work have checked with sources believed to be reliable in their efforts to provide information that is complete and generally in accord with the standards accepted at the time of publication. However, in view of the possibility of human error or changes in medical sciences, neither the author nor the publisher nor any other party who has been involved in the preparation or publication of this work warrants that the information contained herein is in every respect accurate or complete, and they are not responsible for any errors or omissions or for the results obtained from use of such information. Readers are encouraged to confirm the information contained herein with other sources. For example and in particular, readers are advised to check the product information sheet included in the package of each drug they plan to administer to be certain that the information contained in this book is accurate and that changes have not been made in the recommended dose or in the contraindications for administration. This recommendation is of particular importance in connection with new or infrequently used drugs.

This book was set in New Baskerville by TCSystems.
The editor was Sally J. Barhydt.
The production supervisor was Catherine Saggese.
The production service was Jennsin Services.
The interior designer was Elizabeth Schmitz.
The cover designer was Almee Nordin.
The index was prepared by Jerry Ralya.

Courier Corporation, Westford, was printer and binder.

This book is printed on acid-free paper.

Dedication

To our trusted, loved, and dedicated colleague;
A man deeply committed to the centrality of embalming
to Funeral Service,
And a staunch supporter of, and advocate for,
Funeral Service Education,

William H. Pierce

We, the members of the American Board of Funeral Service Education
are proud to dedicate this text, *Embalming: History, Theory, & Practice.*

Author's Dedication

The third edition is dedicated to those individuals
who have inspired, mentored, and encouraged
my career in funeral service and
the mortuary preparation arts:

Alfred H. Davis and Paul H. Velker, John T. Rebol,
William J. Neff, William J. Musmanno,
J. Sheridan and Dorothy D. Mayer,
Dr. Emory S. James, Edward C. and Gail R. Johnson,
Melissa Johnson, William A. Smith, and David G. Williams.

EDITORIAL CONSULTANTS

John M. Kroshus, PhD
Assistant Professor and Director
Program of Mortuary Science
University of Minnesota
Minneapolis, Minnesota

Melissa Johnson
Funeral Director/Embalmer
Chicago, Illinois

Michael Landon
Chairman, Department of Funeral Service Education
Fayetteville Technical Community College
Fayetteville, North Carolina

Louis Misantone
President, Funeral Institute of the North East
Westwood, Massachusetts

CONTRIBUTING AUTHORS

These authors' contributions appear essentially unchanged.

James M. Dorn, MS
Chairman, Embalming Sciences
Cincinnati College of Mortuary Science
Cincinnati, Ohio

Jerome F. Fredrick, PhD
Director of Chemical Research
Dodge Chemical Company
Bronx, New York

Barbara M. Hopkins, PhD
Associate Professor and Chair
Chemistry Department
Xavier University
Cincinnati, Ohio

Edward C. Johnson
Funeral Director—Instructor of Embalming
Chicago, Illinois

Gail R. Johnson
Funeral Director—Instructor of Clinical Embalming
Chicago, Illinois

Melissa Johnson
Funeral Director/Embalmer
Chicago, Illinois

John M. Kroshus, PhD
Assistant Professor and Director
Program of Mortuary Science
University of Minnesota
Minneapolis, Minnesota

Michael C. Mathews, MA
Assistant Professor
Program of Mortuary Science
University of Minnesota
Minneapolis, Minnesota

Robert G. Mayer
Licensed Embalmer and Funeral Director
Pittsburgh, Pennsylvania

Faculty
Pittsburgh Institute of Mortuary Science
Pittsburgh, Pennsylvania

Robert W. Ninker
Executive Director
Illinois Funeral Directors Association
Springfield, Illinois

John B. Pludeman
Instructor
Milwaukee Area Technical College
Milwaukee, Wisconsin

Leandro Rendon, MS
Director of Research and Educational Programs
The Champion Company
Williamsburg, Virginia

Gordon Rose, PhD
Former Professor and Chairman
Mortuary Science Department
Wayne State University
Detroit, Michigan

C. Richard Sanders
The Dodge Company
Largo, Florida

Todd W. VanBeck, MA
Director
New England Institute of Funeral Service Education
Mount Ida College
Newton Centre, Massachusetts

CONTRIBUTORS

John Alsobrookd, MS
Associate Professor, Funeral Service Program
Vincennes University Junior College
Vincennes, Indiana

R. Stanley Barnes
Funeral Director
Canton, Ohio

Daniel Buchanan, MA
President
Gupton-Jones College of Funeral Service
Decatur, Georgia

William Counce, PhD
Funeral Service Education Department
Jefferson State College
Birmingham, Alabama

Emmet Crahan
Dodge Chemical Company
Jay, New York

Kenneth Curl, PhD
Chairman
Funeral Service Education Department
University of Central Oklahoma
Edmond, Oklahoma

Donald E. Douthit, MS
Supervisor of Clinical Services
Cincinnati College of Mortuary Science
Cincinnati, Ohio

Dan Flory, PhD
President
Cincinnati College of Mortuary Science
Cincinnati, Ohio

Arthur Grabowski
Former Chairman
Mortuary Science Department
State University of New York College of Technology
Canton, New York

Marvin E. Grant, MEd
Former Chairman
Mortuary Science Department
East Mississippi Community College
Scooba, Mississippi

Ralph Klicker, MSEd
Director
Thanos Institute
Buffalo, New York

Daniel Lawlor
Embalmer and Funeral Director
Providence, Rhode Island

Terry McEnany, MA
Dean
Simmons Institute
Syracuse, New York

Stuart E. Moen, MA
Dean
Commonwealth Institute of Funeral Service
Houston, Texas

Frank P. Nagy, PhD
Associate Professor
Department of Anatomy
Wright State University Medical School
Dayton, Ohio

N. Thomas Rogness, MA
Former Instructor
Institute of Funeral Service
Houston, Texas

Shelly J. Roy
Funeral Director
York, Alabama

Donald W. Sawyer
Director of Embalming Education
Dodge Chemical Company
Castro Valley, California

Dale E. Stroud
Former Associate Professor
Mortuary Science Department
University of Minnesota
Minneapolis, Minnesota

Brenda L. Tersine MA
Former Instructor
Mortuary Science Department
Hudson Valley Community College
Troy, New York

John R. Trout
Funeral Service Education Department
Northampton Area Community College
Bethlehem, Pennsylvania

Larry Whitaker
The Dodge Company
Beaverton, Oregon

Kenneth R. Whittaker
Dean of Students
Dallas Institute of Funeral Service
Dallas, Texas

CONTENTS

PREFACE

As the last year of the twentieth century closes, the third edition of this textbook was prepared for publication. The practice of embalming in the United States was begun in the mid to late nineteenth century; however, its widespread acceptance and use by society, its educational curriculum, instrumentation, and chemicals have been a development of the past one hundred years. It was also during this last century that the threefold purpose of embalming—sanitation, temporary preservation, and restoration—was established.

Ron Hast, noted publisher of *Mortuary Management Magazine* and the *Funeral Monitor,* has written these words summarizing why this third edition was prepared:

> "Nothing is more certain than change. This third edition is updated with new knowledge, techniques, and information relative to the history, theory, and practice of embalming.
>
> Embalming is the best known method of presenting a deceased person throughout the memorial event. It is incumbent on us not to overstate the purpose and results of embalming as longer terms of preservation. Artistic value coupled with preservation is primary. In time, nature consumes all who die back unto itself.
>
> Many professionals devoted to high achievement in embalming are constantly practicing and learning. New students beginning their educational process pursuant to a career in funeral service and those who continue to master their technique will find this book a constant resource for information leading to the best results in the embalming process.
>
> Embalming is a choice. Those we are privileged to serve need to know the values of this process to make intelligent decisions. Consistent, masterful presentation of each decedent entrusted to our care builds positive reputations.
>
> Knowing of the peace of mind and comfort the art of embalming brings to the living, I hope this book will inspire you to continually enhance your interest and skill in this noble service to mankind."

As in the previous two editions, this third edition of *Embalming: History, Theory, & Practice,* is designed as a basic textbook for the mortuary science student and as a reference source for the practitioner. Incorporated throughout this work is the American Board of Funeral Service Education *Embalming Basic Course Content Curriculum and Glossary (1996)* and portions of the *Restorative Art Basic Course Content Curriculum and Glossary (1998).*

This edition includes for the first time in one text all the parameters for the preparation of the dead for funeralization as practiced at the close of the twentieth century in the United States. The three interdisciplinary mortuary arts and sciences of embalming, restorative art, and mortuary cosmetology are presented in this single volume. Restoration of the body as well as cosmetic treatments are interdependent with the embalming of the remains.

Stressed throughout the chapters of this edition is the original premise of the first edition, that the primary decisions as to selection of vessels for injection, choice of arterial fluid, the strength and volume of the arterial solution, the use of supplemental chemicals, and injection and drainage techniques, must depend on the embalming analysis for each individual preparation. It has been stated that the **art** of embalming is the raising of the vessel but the **science** of embalming is knowing which vessel to raise! For these reasons the chapter on minimum standards, which appeared in the second edition, has been removed; however the protocols of that chapter have been retained and placed in the Selected Readings Section for reference. We see such extreme conditions in many bodies embalmed today–effects of long term use of medications; delays brought about by the need to ask for the donation of organs and tissues, permission for autopsy examination, permission to embalm and restore the body, local coroner or medical examiner rules pertaining to pronouncement, manner and cause of death; effects of vascular surgery, organ and tissue donation, partial autopsy, delays in shipping and receiving remains; effects of drug resistant viral and bacterial infections; and the use of life support systems. Not only does the condition of the body make it difficult to establish a "minimum standard" but the variety of embalming products adds to the dilemma. A 20 index fluid produced by one company does not always have the same reactions as the same index fluid produced by another company. Thus, "minimum standards" can become too generalized and more of simply a "guideline." In the preparation of each body it becomes the responsibility of the embalmer to determine the thoroughness, effectiveness, and quality of the work.

Chapter 1 has been revised and includes an introduction placing emphasis on the psychosocial reasons why our society "cares for its dead." This material was prepared by Todd VanBeck. It is followed by a discussion, prepared by Robert W. Ninker, of the ethical demands and responsibilities placed on the licensed practitioner. Chapter 3 has been rewritten, incorporating in one chapter all the governmental regulatory rules pertaining to the safety and protection of the practitioner and the health concerns of the community. The reorganized and updated material in this chapter was prepared by Dr. John Kroshus.

A new chapter in this edition entitled, "Embalming for Delayed Viewing," prepared by Melissa Johnson, places emphasis on quality preparation work when there is to be a long delay between death and final disposition. It provides foundation material for the preparation of bodies to be shipped to distant points or to allow for viewing by relatives and friends when time is needed for them to travel long distances to attend the funeral rites and ceremonies. General shipping concerns are also addressed in the first chapter of this edition.

The section on restorative art places emphasis on the actual practices carried out by the embalmer. It is not intended to be a complete discussion of this subject. The history of this art and its relationship to embalming was introduced in the second edition and remains an important part of this discussion in the text. Necessary background material in this discipline and techniques such as modeling of the individual features have purposely been omitted. The material here shows the relationship between the disciplines of embalming and restoration of the viewable areas of the deceased. Edward Johnson has stated ". . . restorative art is an emotional occupation; it requires concentration and needs time . . . . There are two goals with respect to restorative art: one is to conceal all evidence of trauma and disease; the second is to obtain a reasonable resemblance of the deceased."

Accompanying the restorative art material is a new chapter on the subject of mortuary cosmetology. In the end the only picture the family and friends have of the deceased is the appearance of the body, in particular the face and hands. The restorative and cosmetic treatments are as much a part of the final appearance of the remains as the embalming process. The material presented here was developed by C. Richard Sanders, well known for his many years of writing and seminars on the topic of mortuary cosmetology.

Finally, a word needs to be said about environmental and health issues. With the advent of OSHA regulations, the consciousness of the funeral director was raised as to the working conditions of the embalmer. We began to put into use better personal and environmental work practices. Ventilation systems and work practice techniques with embalming chemicals have improved environmental working conditions as have the use of improved personal protection products, and improved chemicals for disinfection and their strict usage. Lifting devices have reduced bodily injury, and proper waste disposal has helped to protect the work and community environment. Sanitation has been a fundamental goal of the embalmer since the pandemic flu outbreak in the second decade of this twentieth century. This concern was carried through the years when a cure for polio was unknown. Within the closing two decades of this century the embalmer again prepared bodies dead from AIDS, a disease with first an unknown cause and to date an uncertain cure. Deadly flu, polio, AIDS, tuberculosis, and drug-resistant strains of virus, and bacteria have all challenged the embalmer to practice sanitary techniques to protect personal and community health. In spite of these diseases the embalmer continues to practice a skill that allows one last comforting look on the face of loved ones at their ceremony of farewell.

Robert G. Mayer
Pittsburgh, Pennsylvania
December 1999

ACKNOWLEDGMENTS

Financing for this edition has been made possible through the American Board of Funeral Service Education, Appleton & Lange publishers, The Dodge Company of Cambridge, Massachusetts, the Illinois Funeral Directors Association, and the Ohio Embalmers Association. Seed moneys and underwriting for this project have been made possible, since the inception of this textbook project, through The Heritage Club and the National Funeral Directors Association.

Special thanks and appreciation must be made to Dr. Gordon Bigelow, retired executive director of the American Board of Funeral Service Education, who has managed the contractual and administrative phases of this textbook and overseen this project since its inception in 1987.

This third edition recognizes with gratitude the contributions made by the following individuals in particular for their creative ideas and writing skills: Melissa Johnson for numerous editorial and content suggestions throughout the text, but in particular for the organization and writing of materials related to long-term preservation and shipping. Dr. John Kroshus has reorganized and rewritten major portions of this edition, in particular those chapters concerning the personal health and environmental concerns related to embalming, including all of the OSHA material. In addition, John has reorganized the material related to the postmortem changes and preparation of the organ and tissue donor. Michael Mathews, a veteran teacher of embalming chemistry, has reviewed and reorganized the two chapters on embalming chemicals. Todd VanBeck and Robert Ninker provided excellent materials for the introductory social and ethical concerns of the embalming practitioner. Finally, a great debt of gratitude is owed to C. Richard Sanders, who in retirement prepared an extraordinary text on the application of mortuary cosmetics.

A number of individuals contributed ideas and suggestions to the writing of Chapter 25, "Embalming for Delayed Viewing." For many of us this chapter has become a chapter on the philosophy of embalming. Melissa Johnson did the writing but contributions were made by Jan Hart, William Smith, Robert Buhrig, John McDonough, and the Electronic Funeral Service Association, John Pludeman, Kerry Peterson, and Richard Sanders.

Contributors and content review was provided by Jan Hart of the University of Pittsburgh School of Medicine and John B. Pludeman from The Milwaukee Institute in Wisconsin. Professor Edward C. Johnson reviewed and edited the new section on restorative art and changes made to his chapters on the history of embalming and modern restorative art. Thomas J. Soxman of Pittsburgh and Mark T. Higgins of Durham, North Carolina edited the introductory chapter and provided valuable support and encouragement. From The Dodge Company in Cambridge, Massachusetts, Arnold and John Dodge provided permissions and review of materials; within their organization Larry Whitaker and Dennis Daulton reviewed and commented on new and prior material. Original artwork for this text was prepared by Jeffrey C. Pierce of Pittsburgh; art review for this edition was provided by Jude Waples of Oakville, Ontario, whose parents Raymond C. and Shirley Waples of Pittsburgh encouraged my career in funeral service.

Finally, I am grateful to Daniel E. Buchanan, president of the Gupton-Jones College of Funeral Service in Decatur, Georgia, and past chairman of the American Board of Funeral Service Education, who wrote the Foreword to this third edition. A friend and colleague for over 30 years, no educator in funeral service is more dedicated to the teaching of the mortuary arts and sciences, and in particular the subject of embalming.

Robert G. Mayer
Pittsburgh, Pennsylvania
December 1999

FOREWORD

Show me the manner in which a nation cares for its dead, and I will measure with mathematical exactness the tender mercies of its people, their respect for the laws of the land and their loyalty to high ideals.

William Gladstone

Consider if you will the prophetic profoundness of the statement made over a century ago by the English political and religious leader, William E. Gladstone. Undoubtedly, there is no other event that has the impact and evokes the depth of emotion as does the death of someone close. The loss of a loved one strikes so deeply at the core of human feelings that even physical as well as emotional distress is often the result. Such a traumatic event in the lives of humankind requires a tender, kind, and decent response from society as those directly affected attempt to adjust to their new life with a vacant place at the table.

Funeral Service as a profession in America began through the friendly efforts on the part of neighbors and friends who came to the aid of those who suffered a loss through death. In other words, the vocation of funeral directing came about in the spirit of *service,* not merchandise. It is service that conceived and nurtured this awesome profession, and it is only service that shall sustain and maintain our vocational endeavor.

There is no service provided by the mortician more significant and more paramount than embalming. As significant as the operation is to the lives of family members and even the community at large, it is imperative that embalming be performed by one who understands and appreciates its value. Beyond having the proper attitude toward embalming, the successful embalmer must be properly and adequately trained in the art and science. Without such training, the operation would be merely a mechanical process with little understanding on the part of the operator.

The proper use and application of this or any good textbook on the subject of embalming should bring to the funeral service practitioner an extensive understanding of the true nature of the operation. Applying the information herein, certainly to include the extensive use of embalming analysis, will enable the professional to understand and anticipate those circumstances routinely or not so routinely encountered which could lead to disastrous results if not recognized and compensated for during treatment. As a result, the families and community at large will be better served, and the image of the profession enhanced.

Over the many years since embalming was brought to the American scene by Thomas Holmes during the Civil War, there have been many distinguished individuals who have been instrumental in bringing the art and science of embalming to the professional level it has reached today. Certainly there have been no two individuals more devoted to the cause of embalming and the value of it than the principal author of this text, Mr. Robert G. Mayer, and the one to whom this text is dedicated, Mr. William H. Pierce. Both of these distinguished gentlemen have devoted their entire professional careers to the advancement of embalming. They both believed in embalming, performed by men and women well trained and dedicated to this ministry we call funeral service, as paramount to the emotional and intellectual acceptance of death on the part of the many who go through the trauma of death in the family.

Surely if the principles of embalming as presented in *Embalming; History, Theory & Practice* are applied in the preparation room, the public and the profession will be well served. Truly, embalming is the very foundation, the cornerstone, of the funeral profession and the fundamental service we offer the public. I would encourage all to whom these pages come, to use this information, and use it well.

This book covers embalming as no other book ever has. It is useful as a teaching text and, in that regard, follows the American Board of Funeral Service Education curriculum guide on this subject. It is also useful as an historical or technical reference for the funeral service practitioner or the lay reader.

Gordon S. Bigelow, PhD
Executive Director
American Board of Funeral Service Education
March, 1996

You must express your grief at the death of a loved one, and then you must go on. The eyes of the dead must be gently closed, and the eyes of the living must be gently opened.

Jan Brugler, 1973

Daniel E. Buchanan, President
Gupton-Jones College of Funeral Service
Atlanta, Georgia

THIRD EDITION

EMBALMING

History, Theory, & Practice

THE THEORY AND PRACTICE OF EMBALMING

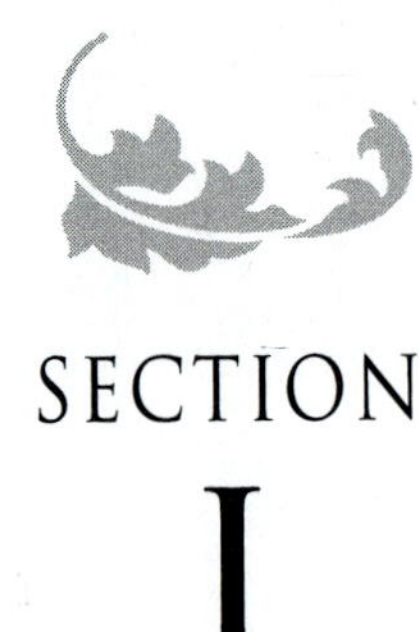

SECTION I

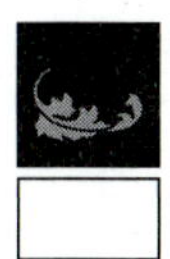

CHAPTER 1
EMBALMING: SOCIAL, PSYCHOLOGICAL, AND ETHICAL CONSIDERATIONS

In the United States, the practice of embalming is regulated primarily by the legislatures of the individual states. Two principal bodies may have control of the care and disposition of dead human remains: the board of health (or bureau of vital statistics) and the state board of embalmers and funeral directors (or similar governing body) that regulates funeral homes and licensing of funeral directors and embalmers. These two groups promulgate and enforce statutory law as well as rules and regulations governing the disposition of dead human bodies.

In recent years, in addition to state agencies, several federal agencies have come to play an important role in the activities of the funeral establishment, especially in the preparation room. These agencies include the Centers for Disease Control and Prevention (CDC), the Environmental Protection Agency (EPA), the Federal Trade Commission (FTC), and the Occupational Safety and Health Administration (OSHA). We will see later in this chapter the influence federal and state governments have on the preparation and disposition of dead human bodies. Chapter 3 will give detailed attention to OSHA standards affecting funeral service.

First, we will examine the psychosocial, religious, and philosophical reasons a culture continues the practice of embalming its dead and the role this scientific and artistic treatment of the dead plays in the final ceremonial rites of disposition, and the impact it can have on the adjustment and well-being of the survivors. This chapter also provides an overview of the governmental organizations (state, federal, and international) regulating the preparation and transportation of human remains—the movement or shipping of remains within a state, between states, and between countries.

▶ LEGISLATIVE INTENT

The law is said to be the minimum ethic of a community. Members of a society place their trust and confidence in certain persons, charging them to fulfill in a competent manner their wishes and desires over certain matters, one of them being the responsibility for disposition of the dead. Certain individuals within a community have been appointed by law, and by the trust of the members of the community, to oversee the disposition of the dead in a legal, ethical, reverent, and respectful manner. Certain standards of performance are not only expected but demanded from embalmers and funeral directors.

When a state issues an embalming license to a qualified practitioner, it is declaring that

> 1) Embalming is a practice affecting the public health, safety and welfare and is subject to regulation and control in the public interest. 2) That the preparation, care and final disposition of a deceased human body should be attended with appropriate observance and understanding, having due regard and respect for the reverent care of the human body and for those bereaved and the overall spiritual dignity of mankind. 3) As a matter of public interest, that the practice of embalming merits and receives the confidence of the public and that only qualified persons be authorized to practice embalming in their state. 4) The state codes should be liberally construed to best carry out these subjects and purposes.

These declarations form a foundation for the development of specific professional performance standards.

▶ SOCIAL PSYCHOLOGICAL PERFORMANCE STANDARD

Here, we describe the ethical, psychosocial, and practical values of embalming to provide its practitioners the opportunity to define and articulate to the community the great social value of their work, and why it is an important mainstay of the funeral service profession. This material helps the reader to develop a clear, balanced understanding of the social advantages of embalming and basic care for the dead, and the importance of having the body embalmed and present at death rituals.

Reverence for the dead is the basic ethical axiom of the funeral service profession. Preparation of the dead is humankind's means of ethically fulfilling our ingrained ancient, emotive instinct to care for the dead. As funeral service practitioners, we are charged with the maintenance of this moral and ethical responsibility, and it is important that students and practitioners actively embrace this concept.

Ethical Model

Every profession has a primary and supreme ethic of paramount importance in the disposition of its duties. Medicine, for example, bases its professional practice on the Hippocratic Oath, which articulates the ethic of healing. Law bases its practice on the ethic of justice. The supreme ethic for the funeral service profession has come to be known as reverence for the dead. The ethical question "What should be done with the dead?" can be controversial. Some people believe the dead should be buried; others believe the dead should be cremated. Still others endorse donating the dead to medical schools, and some people avoid the question altogether.

Human Nature

In Western culture, there is an attitude of denial and defiance toward death and dying. American culture in particular places tremendous value on things that are new, shiny, and healthy while devaluing things that are old, dull, and dead. Consequently, the value of a human corpse is often morally downgraded, because the dead human body symbolizes that which is abhorrent to our materialistically shallow culture—death—precisely what the culture is trying to avoid.

In addition, the dead human body represents a psychological and ethical paradox for people, stemming from the fact that the living are simultaneously attracted, yet sometimes repulsed, when viewing the dead. The dead represent defeat and despair, and because human beings do not deal well with defeat and despair, we have devised an elaborate system of barriers to help us cope with the situation.

Reverence for the dead, however, is deeply ingrained in human nature, no matter how much we profess our ignorance, apathy, or even disgust. What we call the ethical or reverential care of the dead has been discovered to exist as far back in our ancestry as Neanderthal man. Anthropological study shows that the burial of the human body is the oldest of all religious customs, and was practiced as far back as about 60,000 BC by *Homo sapiens neanderthalensis.* In the Shandiar cave in northern Iraq, researchers discovered corpses adorned with elk antlers and shoulder blades. Also found were pollen fragments from flowers that were probably used as gifts to the dead and to mask unpleasant odors during the burial ritual. Neanderthals exhibited the primal behaviors characteristic of our natural and instinctual drive to treat the dead with great reverence. That genetic and instinctive legacy continues today, tempered by our modern culture and intellect.

Consequences of the Act

When one examines the reasons behind the decline of the governmental and sociological order, historically, the neglect of reverence for the dead and its consequences is clearly a major contributing factor. History shows us that the ultimate destruction of many civilizations was heralded by a rise in a community's apathy about the care of their dead. Ancient Rome, Greece, and Nazi Germany are examples that fit this pattern. In examining the downfall of each of these powerful regimes, the lack of proper care for the dead was commonplace. Time and again, the annals of history show that the rites, rituals, and ceremonies mourning the dead serve as excellent barometers of the accomplishments of past cultures.

The ethical, moral, and sociological consequences of neglecting the importance of proper care for the dead was summed up concisely by the eminent William Evart Gladstone when he wrote:

> Show me the manner in which a nation or community cares for its dead and I will measure with mathematical exactness the tender sympathies of its people, their respect for the laws of the land, and their loyalty to high ideals.

Because this quote embodies a great ethical truth with power and eloquence, it has been cited many times by funeral service practitioners, and no matter how often these words are uttered, their impact on our profession, our society, and humanity as a whole never wanes.

▶ UNIVERSAL CONVICTIONS

All of the world's cultures attend to the proper care of the dead and each has developed its own rituals to implement this care. Anthropological, archaeological, and religious literature all describe the importance to a culture of its chosen forms of funeralization ceremonies, and the significance of the presence of the dead body in helping the community overcome the overwhelming experience of the death of one of its members.

Every civilization ever studied has been found to

maintain sacred locations where the bodies and the relics of the dead were placed, including cemeteries, mausoleums, and columbaria. All cultures commemorate their dead through the creation of art, music, and literature, including monuments and memorials; requiem masses and funeral hymns; and biographies and elegies. In fact, human customs and rituals concerning basic care for and commemoration of the dead are so diverse and widespread that no one publication could possibly document all of them in complete detail.

This universal ethic of reverence for the dead is ingrained in the human psyche, and though the ways different cultures manifest this reverence may vary widely, it is a basic thread binding together all of humanity.

Morality

The issue of morality in reference to reverential care of the dead is embodied in the conflict between logic and emotion. The logical mind might well dismiss the corpse as nothing more than a mass of dead tissue, but our emotional selves will not allow such easy dismissal of something so inherent to our humanity, and this leads to an internal conflict between our logical and our emotional selves. When we feel this clash of logic and emotion, we should realize that our deepest emotions are crying out for recognition. In other words, this conflict should serve to shock us into listening to our deepest emotions, as the Neanderthal did, to avoid falling into the trap of rationalization and denial.

An illustration of the power of the emotions associated with death was seen in 1963, a year of supreme importance for the funeral service profession. Jessica Mitford published *The American Way of Death*, a savage and relentless attack on the profession, causing a counterattack on Mitford herself by America's funeral directors. Then came November 22, 1963, and the shocking assassination and subsequent funeral of President John F. Kennedy, an act that rocked our entire nation's moral and emotional foundations. The public did not feel comfortable criticizing funeral directors, symbols of death and funerals, when the nation was in the throes of mourning a slain president. To describe President Kennedy's body merely as "dead tissue," and to dispose of it without ceremony would have been morally irresponsible and blasphemous. This same need for public mourning and ritual was evident again following the deaths of other celebrities, such as Martin Luther King, Jr., Princess Diana, and Mother Teresa.

These moral feelings representing our instinct to reverently care for the dead also emerge at other times. For example, if a body is missing due to war or a tragic accident, the community can be distraught beyond description. Thousands of taxpayers' dollars are spent on search and recovery efforts, and there is anxiety and remorse if these efforts fail. If we view this from a strictly logical viewpoint, and reduce the issue to one of the costs of such an effort, accepting the notion that the dead body has no value, then these magnanimous recovery efforts make little sense, and may be viewed as a waste of taxpayers' dollars. Without a body, an essential element to the grieving process is missing; an important piece of the bereavement puzzle missing.

The Neanderthals made memorials with elk antlers and shoulder blades; today we use granite or marble. The ethic is the same; only the materials are different. We have an innate ethical drive to care for the dead; it is simply part of our humanity.

Religion

Religious convictions are important to consider in this discussion, because for centuries the funeral has been an essentially religious ritual, is certainly so within the Judeo-Christian tradition, and is so within all of the world's religions. Specific reference to embalming is made twice in the Old Testament. Genesis 50:2–3 recounts the death of Jacob, who was also known as Israel: "And Joseph commanded his servants the physicians to embalm his father. So the physicians embalmed Israel." Genesis 50:26 also refers to embalming in connection with Joseph's death: "So Joseph died, being one hundred and ten years old and they embalmed him, and he was put in a coffin in Egypt." Of course, we should not confuse the embalming described in the Old Testament with the modern procedure, but the intent to care reverently for the dead is the same, regardless of current technology.

In addition, the New Testament contains references that reflect the Judeo-Christian tradition to care reverently for the dead. John 11:44 describes burial preparations for Lazarus similar to those in use today, including the use of grave straps to bind the arms, feet and chin, allowing the body to be manipulated into a normal appearance. The description of Jesus' funerary preparations mirror those used today in some cultures: his body was bound and dressed in fine white linens, and anointed with spices, fragrant oils, and myrrh.

So we see the tradition of treating the dead with great reverence and respect is an age-old custom, as old as humanity itself. Those of us in the funeral service profession must always be cognizant of and maintain this high level of dignity and veneration of the dead in all our practices. To put this basic tenet of funeral service succinctly: Reverence for the dead is expressed through the consistent application and practice of showing respect and honor for, as well as maintaining the dignity of, the dead.

Psychosocial Model

Human beings are basically social creatures. We talk, live, work, and play with other people. Our social interactions take on many different dimensions. We can have shallow or very deep interactions; we can act with indifference or with profound sympathy. In the course of a single day, we may exhibit these and a thousand other characteristics. It is through this complex web of daily interactions that we experience life and create attachments to others. The quality of these attachments varies from one relationship to another; some are deep, some shallow, others indifferent, joyful, or painful. Here we shall explore the role embalming plays in the process of helping us separate from these attached relationships.

Within the realm of attachments between people are the so-called "deep links." Here, our attachments are strong and profound interwoven psychological bonds that are extremely powerful. In these circumstances, our needs for security and devotion are satisfied, and virtually every part of the human psyche is involved. Through daily visual and interactive reinforcement of these deep attachments, our relationships with significant persons undergo a kind of layering process in our brains. The thoughts and feelings create perceptual patterns of recognition. These patterns of recognition that develop between people become so familiar that there are instances in which the individual involved is frequently unaware of the depth of these attachments until the relationship is terminated through separation by death or physical or emotional distance.

The how and why of attachments are baffling. Attachments are among our most rudimentary attributes, they flourish throughout our lives, and they can be so powerful as to continue even beyond the grave. The magnitude of these attachments is often unrealized by the person, and individuals are often unaware of how deeply their behaviors and attitudes are affected. Attachments arise from countless life experiences; from suckling at the mother's breast, to seeing someone every day, to sleeping with them every night. They are created by the sound of a voice, the color of someone's eyes, the texture of someone's hair, and in their style and manner of dress and movement. It is fortunate indeed that humans have the capacity to develop these attachments, because they often culminate in deeply cherished, singular relationships with others; feelings of *love.* It is from this type of deep relationship that we experience the joy of love, but it is equally true that from these same deep attachments, we also experience the inevitable anguish of separation and loss. As painful as it is at times, a fact of human existence is that attachments cannot exist without grief.

It is through continual life experiences shared with significant others that our attachments become rooted. As the theories of attachment demonstrate, our ability to connect with our fellow humans goes very deep. Through this process, familiarity with the characteristics of the significant other is *imprinted* on our minds. This imprinting is caused by constant exposure to the attached person, and a mental photograph develops in our hearts and minds. In funeral service, this mental photograph is referred to as the *body image.*

The body image that develops is reinforced unconsciously and consciously through our personal interactions with the attached person; we relate and respond to their created sensory image. The sightless are particularly talented at creating a body image using sensory data derived from the senses other than sight, and their verbal descriptions of what they imagine with their mind's eye are remarkably accurate.

We habitually relate to, recognize, and identify our significant others based on the familiar body image to which our perceptions have become attached. Due to this constant exposure to the body image and because our culture promotes death denial, people often form an unrealistic expectation of permanency in the attached relationship.

It becomes simple for individuals who are profoundly attached to one another to feel confident that the relationship will last forever, irrational as this may seem. Although we know subconsciously that such permanence in even the strongest relationship is simply not possible, many prefer to live under the blissful misconception that death will not end the attachment. Human relationships, however, are not limitless; they too must die, either through physical or psychological separation or through death.

It is crucial that the funeral service student appreciates the complex processes behind these human attachments and separations. It is these psychological processes on which the ethic of reverence for the dead is based, and which necessitate the need for funeralization. Without human attachments, there would be little, if any, need for funerals. A funeral is, in its most elementary form, a social function that reflects the reality of our capacity to form deep attachments, and that most human need to grieve and mourn our dead.

Death brings with it a finality that challenges our means to cope psychologically. With death comes the realization that what was once thought to be permanent and everlasting is in truth temporary and finite, and after death comes the long and often painful process of grief and mourning.

During the mourning process, the bereaved are challenged to divest themselves of their close attachments to the dead person and are asked to rechannel that emotional energy into relationships with other people. The process of mourning is vital and necessary for healthy grieving. Grieving begins in the bereaved psyche by sensory (visual and tactile) confrontation with the dead person's retained body image.

It is often said that it is better to remember the

dead as they were when they were alive. The comment, "I would rather remember them alive," is a form of death denial. For honest confrontation of the reality of death, it is necessary for the mourners to see the deceased person (or a symbol of the deceased person in cases where it is impossible to view the body) to bring home the reality of death. By seeing or touching the deceased, the mourners have the visual and physical opportunity that is crucial in verifying the stark reality of death. If the body of the deceased is lost forever and there is no chance to establish the reality of death, there is a risk of complicated bereavement, and mourners may feel a lack of resolution.

Viewing the Body

Honest confrontation of the reality of death requires the mourners to see the deceased or a symbol of the deceased. Viewing and touching a dead human body is the *best* way for the bereaved to overcome any death denial feelings. It is common in the study of grief to observe bereaved persons denying the significance of the death of someone to whom they were strongly attached. The process of denial takes many forms.

Denial is frequently manifest as an avoidance of contact with the reality of death—namely the dead person's body. At first glance, this avoidance may appear to reflect the fact that the bereaved is endeavoring to maintain his or her composure. Unfortunately, the bereaved are often rewarded for this type of rationalizing behavior. Bereavement is not a simple enough process to be adequately managed by rational thought alone; grief is an emotional, not a rational, process. It is important that the funeral service student recognize this attitude for what it truly is—the denial of the significance of death.

The comprehension of human separation can never fully be accomplished through intellectual rationalizations. Often the people who are the most aggrieved by the death, the same ones who most need to accept the reality of death, are precisely the people who take the path of least resistance, by avoiding visual and tactile confrontation of the dead body image. Establishing the reality of death is always an issue of need more than want.

Dr. Erich Lindemann, a pioneer in the study of grief management, has suggested that there is really no escaping the slow wisdom of grief. Lindemann postulates that avoidance of the dead body is always done at the psychological peril of the aggrieved, and that this avoidance may appear at first to be consoling in the initial phase of acute grief. But in truth, Lindemann says, this consolation is just an illusion. In time, the necessity to view the body becomes a major issue in postbereavement care.

Lindemann says that a common characteristic in persons experiencing complicated bereavement is an inability to recall a clear mental image of the body in death. Establishment of this mental image is an essential ingredient in creating a strong foundation for subsequent steps in the grieving process. An unclear image of the deceased person, or no image at all, fosters a lack of full acceptance of the reality of death.

Lindemann believed that the most significant benefit of funeralization and embalming is achieved at that moment when the finality of the death is fully comprehended by the bereaved person. It is this moment of truth, this awareness of the reality of death, that serves as the psychological framework for the validation of embalming.

Many believe, as does the Reverend Paul Irion, that the embalmer's task is to make the body "presentable" for viewing. This is similar to other life situations, such as when a person prepares for social activity by bathing and combing their hair before greeting people in public. The ethical concepts of reverence for the dead, decent disposition, and dignity in death all demand that the dead body be prepared for viewing so it will not be offensive to mourners during the process of funeralization.

The embalmed body image permits an open, realistic acceptance of death. In this type of stark confrontation, there is no denying the finality of death. Embalming the body permits time for family and friends to engage in the valuable process of leave-taking. The embalmed body image challenges the denial of death and promotes an atmosphere of emotional stability. By confronting the frightening, lonely feelings caused by the emotional conflict of death's denial, the embalmed body image acts as a catharsis for the strong emotions of panic, fear, frustration, and guilt. An embalmer's ultimate purpose, then, is to make the body presentable for viewing, and through the technical work of the embalmer, the realization of the finality of death takes place practically and tastefully.

▶ RITUALS AND CEREMONIES

Nowhere do we see the need to be social in order to live a happy, balanced life more than in the rituals and rites performed by human beings. So entrenched in the make-up of humankind is ritualistic behavior that a breakdown or corruption of these rituals may result in human cataclysm.

Dr. Carl Jung, a pioneer in psychology, saw human psychological life as a universal phenomenon whereby identification with what he termed the "collective unconscious" linked all humanity together. Although we may differ in ethnicity, religion, or social attitudes, some constants exist in our mentality that all of us can identify with and understand. An archetype of our collective unconscious is funeralization and its associated issues.

Psychological archetypal images commonly surface through dreams, and research shows that grieving individuals who do not view the body of a loved one may have frightening dreams about the deceased. However, people who view the dead human body have no such dreams. Their dreams are instead pleasant recollections of past experiences with the deceased. To be effective, the funeral requires the display of the dead body image for the essential psychological detachments to occur.

Practical Model

To fully implement the ethical, psychological, and sociological values of funeralization, *people need time.* People need time to organize funerals, think about them, participate in them, and make decisions about how they should be carried out. Time is also required for the bereaved to assimilate all that has happened, and acknowledge the ramifications in their own lives. Because of the diverse issues to be resolved involving the death of a loved one, the bereaved need the time to assimilate the reality of their death.

Embalming slows decomposition and thus affords the bereaved time to make important decisions. It also serves the practical purpose of rendering the body inoffensive and making it presentable for viewing. Embalming serves as an emotional buffer for the bereaved when the reality of traumatic death might be burdensome, because embalming restores the body image, not to mask reality, but to give the bereaved a body image they can more easily accept. The embalmed body affords the aggrieved the opportunity to accept the finality of death, and does so in a discreet and professional manner.

Embalming also serves a practical need when the body must be transported to another location, offering extended time for transport, and the assurance that the body will remain intact while arrangements are made and during final transportation.

Finally, modern embalming reflects the technology of the age. Today, instead of using herbs and spices as was done in antiquity, we use sophisticated chemicals. As licensed funeral directors and embalmers, we assume the primary responsibility for care of the dead, and that responsibility carries with it a valuable and impressive professional heritage.

▶ THE ETHICAL PERFORMANCE STANDARD

Embalmer Ethics

In the United States, where Judeo-Christian tradition has fostered respect for the human dead and considerations of public health require protection of the living against infection or contagion, the preparation of dead human bodies is entrusted to a specialized group: licensed embalmers.

Ethical Practice. Ethics is the science of rectitude and duty. Its subject is morality and its sphere is virtuous conduct. It is concerned with the various aspects of rights and obligations. In essence, ethics is a set of principles that governs conduct for the purpose of establishing harmony in all human relations. For practical purposes, ethics is fair play.

In the absence of a specific set of rules by which men and women are governed or through which they learn to govern themselves in their relations with others, they are dependent upon traditional customs and practices as rules of conduct. This chapter, therefore, is intended to suggest some desirable uniform rules of conduct by which any embalmer may be guided in the practice of embalming. No code can specify all the duties of the embalmer in every circumstance that confronts him or her. It can serve as a guide in promoting professional attitudes and insuring ethical conduct in many of the situations where neither custom nor tradition have provided a standard of practice that serves the best interests of the public and the profession.

Judicious Counsel. Experience qualifies embalmers to be of great value to those whom they serve and it is their professional obligation to give judicious counsel. In accordance with the wishes of the family, the embalmer should advise them concerning their expectations for a visitation, with viewing, when circumstances dictate the need for special attention such as restoration, any necessary invasive procedures, or the embalmer's need for available photos of the deceased to aid him or her in the embalming and feature setting, taking into account any of the deceased's cosmetic or hairdressing preferences.

Whenever the service is made challenging, because of the circumstances of death, the embalmer should communicate realistic expectations to the family directly or through the arranging funeral director. Representations concerning embalming and restoration should be full and factual. Misrepresentations are unethical and unprofessional and should be avoided at all times.

Body Donation, Organ Donation, and Autopsy

The embalmer should encourage an inquiring family wishing to donate organs or tissue of a deceased family member for the benefit of others. Even in the presence of expected delays, inconvenience in terms of having to deal with a remains where prosthesis may have to be used or extensive repair of the remains is necessary for a proper viewing or reconstruction of the individual for burial purposes, the embalmer and funeral director should always support the family's wishes. Such instances are opportunities for the embalmer to demonstrate his or her professionalism in serving not only the individual family but the public in general. It is not only ethical for an embalmer to take the time for cooperative efforts with organ procurement organizations, it is also a professional expression of their responsibilities as a licensee. Any attempt to dissuade a family from donating organs or tissue would be unprofessional.

The embalmer shares with all medical and hospital personnel the professional responsibility of cooperating with all groups and in supporting all measures that promote health, safety, and public welfare. Courtesy, tact, and discretion should characterize all of the embalmer's professional actions.

Misrepresentation

Embalmers should never aid or abet an unlicensed person, where licensure is required to represent himself as a licensed embalmer or to engage in practices reserved to the holder of an embalming license.

Confidentiality

The family must be able to rely on confidentiality between themselves, the funeral director, and the embalmer on all matters relating to cause and manner of death, surrounding circumstances, condition of the body, and any other issues raised. The embalmer may be privy to other matters shared with him or her by the family. All such confidences must be assured by the embalmer and funeral director.

Defamation of Others

Comments by one embalmer concerning another funeral director or embalmer should always be selected with care. Insinuations, nonfactual statements, or the overplay of facts that have the intent or effect of harming another professional should be avoided at all times.

Enticement of Another Embalmer

It is unethical for an embalmer to willfully entice the employees of another firm with the purpose of unduly hampering, injuring, or prejudicing that firm or professional.

Accommodation of the Family

Not every family may wish or be able to pay for a visitation with viewing, but may express an earnest desire to view the remains in the preparation room. To the extent possible, embalmers should attempt to accommodate families in this regard and should present the remains with features set and whatever other helpful preparations are feasible. Such accommodation may be considered the family's right to check the embalmer's performance.

Identification

The embalmer has responsibility to ascertain that he or she has a properly identified body and must manage the care and internal identification of the remains such that there can be no mistake, especially when viewing is not planned or cremation is the method of final disposition.

Observing Laws, Rules, and Regulations

The embalmer is duty bound and legally responsible to assure that he or she observes all legal and regulatory requirements of federal, state, or local government. The embalmer also has the responsibility of informing the funeral home owner of the resources or capital investments required to meet OSHA standards, any applicable EPA requirements, or other measures needed to be in compliance.

Maintaining Competence

The embalmer has a moral and ethical responsibility to assure that he or she receives whatever continuing education is necessary to maintain skills commensurate with professional practice. State-of-the-art practices and procedures should be known to and practiced by the embalmer at all times.

Health Protection and Sanitation

The embalmer is ethically responsible for protecting the health of any person allowed to enter the preparation room for any reason, and for restricting entry to any person not authorized to be there. That responsibility includes appropriate sanitation procedures to maintain a safe working area for any individual. The embalmer is responsible for safe sheltering so that no unauthorized persons have access to the human remains in his or her care.

Proper Care of the Deceased

The embalmer should deliver and document quality care of the deceased body. The embalming procedures used should be documented on an embalming report for possible future reference. A record of clothing or other personal articles or valuables received by the firm would be appropriate. In addition, written permission to embalm or a record of the expressed permission should be obtained.

Handling the Remains of the Deceased Human Body

Funeral practitioners are charged with the task of making a removal from the place of death and assuring that in the moving process the body receives the respect and care it would receive if the person was alive. The movement of the remains from a hospital, home, hospice or nursing home, or public morgue should be accomplished with the same degree of care as if the person was a patient being transferred. All equipment—cots, sheets, pillows, pouches, and so on—should be clean.

The remains should be protected by a wrap or appropriate covering that maintains the modesty of the deceased person. The remains should be handled as if the body were dead from a communicable disease; universal precautions should always be followed by those making the removal. This needs to be practiced only in the immediate wrapping and handling of the remains. After the body is placed in protective wrappings and cover, street wear is acceptable for those removing the body. Failure to observe universal precautions is unprofessional and violates the principle of acknowledging that the public welfare is affected by the acts of the funeral practitioner or his or her representatives. If the removal is in a home, soiled linen may also be removed for cleaning. In these situations the bedding should be made up so the room looks orderly.

The practitioner or their representative should be prompt in responding to a home call or a call from a nursing home, hospice, or hospital. In this respect the practitioner should realize that federal rules require a window of opportunity for organ procurement organizations to invite the family to consider organ or tissue donations where circumstances are appropriate for that request. The 1998 requirement has the worthy purpose of increasing the number of organs for transplant available to Americans and others who are in need of these human resources.

Once the remains are in the embalmer's facility, respect for the deceased human body takes on even more importance. The preparation of the remains should be viewed as a right of the deceased person to be cleansed, sanitized, groomed, restored, and embalmed with dignity. Special care should be taken in the presentation of the remains to the family. These efforts are ethically correct whether or not there will be a formal viewing. The embalmer should take into account information or photos from the family that would allow the embalmer to best present the remains in a natural way. Such efforts will benefit the viewers who knew the individual when he or she was alive.

In the care of remains, the embalmer should treat it as he would a member of his family. That means that every consideration is given to what would be appropriate. For example, putting instruments on the person of the deceased while embalming or otherwise would be disrespectful. Failure to thoroughly cleanse or care for the hair and physical appearance of the individual is unprofessional and should be grounds for discipline of the licensee.

When an embalmer takes responsibility for the body, he or she has a duty to see that the body is carefully handled and secure in its location. Negligent behavior, such as leaving the preparation room door open or accessible to nonlicensed persons, is unprofessional and should be avoided at all times. The protection of the deceased human body is as important as the embalming procedure itself. Photos of the deceased should never be taken without permission or direction of the persons in charge of arrangements. Doing so would be unprofessional and make the licensee and owner subject to suit or discipline. The embalmer should insist that the proprietor provide adequate means of security for the remains. Any act that would allow an unlicensed person to have access to the deceased human being, without the presence of an embalmer, must be avoided both by policy and practice.

There are many times when the embalmer knows or should anticipate that the final preparation of the remains may require other special handling. Determining what needs to be done and seeing that it *is* done is a professional obligation of the embalmer. For example, an obese person should, where possible, be moved with overhead lifts rather than engaging several persons to move the individual's remains. The ergonomics of lifting excessive or awkward weight should dictate appropriate procedures, while still handling the remains with respectful care.

Quality control in the removal, transportation, preparation, care, and security of the remains is a primary obligation of the embalmer for which he or she should take full responsibility. The embalmer should recognize that there is no act, provided by any member of the firm, that has a greater impact on consumer satisfaction than properly prepared and presented remains. Accordingly, the embalmer should demand and receive whatever resources are necessary to accommodate this professional responsibility. The owner, operator, or manager of the funeral home also has an obligation to search out what special needs the embalmer may have to allow him or her to maximize professional presentation of the remains for viewing. If the visitation is marred by embalming errors, the funeral itself can hardly be fully successful.

The ethical standing of the embalmer is maintained through the consistent demonstration that he or she understands and has incorporated these goals and obligations. Embalming is science, but it is also an art. The successful embalmer must have the occupational leeway to take additional time, whenever it is necessary, to adequately restore and present a professionally prepared remains for visitation, shipment, or burial. Owners, even licensed ones, who fail to authorize purchase of the necessary equipment, accessories, fluids, supplies, instruments, or protective procedures do, in effect, unethically inhibit the embalmer from delivering an optimum remains for funeralization. Such negligence shows disrespect for the deceased, marginalizes the embalmer's effectiveness, and fails the legislative intent test for appropriate care of the deceased.

Any licensee who fails to act in an ethical way should be accused by the observer, chastised by the licensing board and agency, and disciplined as a signal to others that unprofessional behavior is intolerable in funeral service. Embalming failures, for whatever reason, are injurious to the health and welfare of the public, create anguish for families, and unfairly expose the profession as a whole to criticism. Peer review, discipline, and cooperation for excellence are remedies that can insure public confidence.

These professional concerns are the reason the Funeral Ethics Association was formed in 1994 to assist the profession in elevating standards to the high levels increasingly being demanded of licensed embalmers and funeral directors by those they serve. If the embalmer or his or her funeral organization are unable or unwilling to practice embalming excellence, the profession should remove them from practice so that the public welfare is best served. The embalmer, by each of his acts of service, contributes to family satisfaction, serves the public, and contributes immeasurably to the future success of any firm.

▶ CORONER OR MEDICAL EXAMINER

In addition to state and federal rules pertaining to preparation of the body, the embalmer is also responsible for reporting any suspicious circumstances surrounding the death to the coroner or medical examiner. It is important that the funeral personnel in charge of arrangements ascertain who will sign the certificate of death if the nature of the death is such that the coroner or medical examiner must be notified to investigate. The following list (issued by the Ohio Department of Health) shows the types of deaths about which the coroner or medical examiner must be notified. *This list applies to only one state. It is important that the embalmer be familiar with the requirements of the state in which he or she is practicing.*

I. **Accidental deaths: all forms including death arising from employment**
  - A. Anesthetic accident (death on the operating table or prior to recovery from anesthesia)
  - B. Blows or other forms of mechanical violence
  - C. Burns and scalds
  - D. Crushed beneath falling objects
  - E. Cutting or stabbing
  - F. Drowning (actual or suspected)
  - G. Electric shock
  - H. Explosion
  - I. Exposure
  - J. Firearms
  - K. Fractures of bones, not pathological (such cases to be reported even when fracture is not primarily responsible for death)
  - L. Falls
  - M. Carbon monoxide poisoning (resulting from natural gas, automobile exhaust, or other)
  - N. Hanging
  - O. Heat exhaustion
  - P. Insolation (sunstroke)
  - Q. Poisoning (food, occupational, narcotic, sedative, and other)
  - R. Strangulation
  - S. Suffocation (foreign object in bronchi, by bed clothing or other means)
  - T. Vehicular accidents (automobile, street car, bus, railroad, motorcycle, bicycle, or other)

II. **Homicidal deaths: including those involving child abuse**

III. Suicidal deaths

IV. Abortions—criminal or self-induced: When the manner of death falls within the above classifications, such death must be reported to the coroner even though the survival period subsequent to onset is 12 months.

V. **Sudden deaths: When in apparent health or in any suspicious or unusual manner including**
  - A. Alcoholism
  - B. Sudden death on the street, at home, in a public place, at place of employment
  - C. Deaths in unknown circumstances, whenever there are no witnesses or where little or no information can be elicited concerning the deceased person (deaths of this type include those persons whose dead bodies are found in the open, in places of temporary shelter, or in their home under conditions that offer no clues as to the cause of death)
  - D. Deaths that follow injuries sustained at place of employment whenever the circumstances surrounding such injury may ultimately be the subject of investigation
    1. Industrial infections (anthrax, septicemia following wounds including gas bacillus infections, tetanus, etc.)
    2. Silicosis
    3. Industrial poisonings (acids, alkalies, aniline, benzene, carbon monoxide, carbon tetrachloride, cyanogen, lead, nitrous fumes, etc.)
    4. Contusions, abrasions, fractures, burns (flame, chemical, or electrical) received during employment which in the opinion

of the attending physician are of sufficient import, either as the cause or contributing factor to the cause of death, to warrant certifying them on the death certificate

E. All stillborn infants where there is suspicion of illegal interference

F. Death of persons where the attending physician cannot be found, or death of persons who have not been attended by a physician within 2 weeks prior to the date of death

G. All deaths occurring within 24 hours of admission to a hospital unless the patient has been under continuous care of a physician for a natural disease that is responsible for death

▶ FEDERAL REGULATORY AGENCIES

The FTC and OSHA have a direct connection with funeral service and preparation of the dead human body. Four divisions of OSHA affect the funeral home: (1) the General Rule, (2) the Hazard Communication Standard, (3) the Formaldehyde Rule, and (4) the Bloodborne Pathogen Rule. Chapter 3 of this text is devoted almost entirely to the regulations set by OSHA. The FTC mandates that permission (with several exceptions) must be obtained for the embalming of the dead human body. Several sample forms are provided for obtaining oral and written permission.

Forms

The form in Figure 1–1 provides information regarding the "First Call," authorization to take possession of the body to the funeral home and authorization for embalming of the body. Figure 1–2 is a combined release and permission to embalm form. The form in Figure 1–3 is a permission to embalm form which was designed for use when apprentices, mortuary students or trade embalmers may be involved in the preparation of the body. It also gives permission for preparation at a location other than the funeral home. Figure 1–4 is a form for when operative restoration work may be necessary in the preparation of the body. A sample inventory form for personal possessions obtained with the body is contained in Figure 1–5. Sample form 1–6 is included for obtaining permission for the donation of organs and/or tissues. Finally form 1–7 is an authorization for release of a body to a funeral home for disposition without embalming. The body should **always** be identified when there is to be a direct disposition; this form documents who identified the body. These are only sample forms; any forms used by a funeral home or embalming service should be approved by an attorney to be certain wording is in compliance with federal and state regulations.

Federal Trade Commission

In April 1984, the federal government through the FTC promulgated a rule governing the activities of funeral directors and embalmers. The rule, which is commonly referred to as the Funeral Rule, was amended by the FTC in 1994. It is most important that all embalmers be fully aware of the statutes and rules and regulations of the state in which they are practicing. These rules differ from state to state, but the Funeral Rule applies to *all* states. For this reason the following excerpts are reprinted from the *Federal Register:*

Misrepresentations

EMBALMING PROVISIONS—DECEPTIVE ACTS OR PRACTICES. In selling or offering to sell funeral goods or funeral services to the public, it is a deceptive act or practice for a funeral provider to:

1. Represent that state or local law requires that a deceased person be embalmed when such is not the case
2. Fail to disclose that embalming is not required by law except in certain special cases

PREVENTIVE REQUIREMENTS. To prevent these deceptive acts or practices as well as the unfair or deceptive acts or practices defined in §453.4(b) (1) and §453.5 (2) [of the Funeral Rule], funeral providers must:

1. Not represent that a deceased person is required to be embalmed for:
   A. Direct cremation;
   B. Immediate burial; or
   C. A closed casket funeral without viewing or visitation when refrigeration is available and when state or local law does not require embalming; and
2. Place the following disclosure on the general price list, required by §453.2 (b) (4) in immediate conjunction with the price shown for embalming: "Except in certain special cases, embalming is not required by law. Embalming may be necessary, however, if you select certain funeral arrangements, such as a funeral with viewing. If you do not want embalming, you usually have the right to choose an arrangement that does not require you to pay for it, such as direct cremation or immediate burial." The phrase "except in certain special cases" need not be included in this disclosure if

NECESSARY INFORMATION

1. Name of Deceased ______ Age ______
   Home address ______ City ______ State & Zip ______
2. Where is deceased ______
3. Is autopsy scheduled: ( ) Yes ( ) No - if yes Time ______ Date ______
   Can the body be embalmed before the autopsy ( ) Yes ( ) No
4. *Who called:* Name ______ *Phone No.* ______
   Relationship to deceased ______ Other ______
5. Who will be making arrangements: ______
   Address ______ Phone No. ______
   Relationship to deceased ______
6. When will arrangements be made: Date ______ Time ______ AM/PM
7. Other information: ______
8. When was call received: Date ______ Time ______ AM/PM
9. Signature of person taking call ______

AUTHORIZATION TO TAKE POSSESSION OF BODY

( ) ______ *(name)*, ______ *(relationship)*, a family member.

( ) ______ *(name)*, ______ *(capacity)*, a person acting upon instructions of the family.

( ) ______ *(name)*, ______ *(title)*, a legally authorized local official.

Requested that our firm, including our proper agents, take possession of the body of *(deceased)* ______ ______ This request received at *(time)* ______ AM/PM, on *(date)* ______ by the undersigned.

______ *(Firm Name)* ______ *(Signature of person receiving request)*

AUTHORIZATION FOR EMBALMING OF BODY

( ) ______ *(name)*, ______ *(relationship)*, a legally authorized family member.

( ) ______ *(name)*, ______ *(capacity)*, a legally authorized representative of the family.

( ) ______ *(name)*, ______ *(title)*, a legally authorized local official.

Read, or was read the following statement and granted the permission therein: "Permission is given for embalming the body of *(deceased)* ______ " This oral permission was granted at *(time)* ______ AM/PM *(date)* ______ and received by ______
(Firm Name) ______ *(Signature of person receiving permission)*
If person granting permission available sign here ______

CONCURRENCE WITH VERBAL AUTHORIZATIONS

The above verbal authorizations were given, to the best of my knowledge, as recorded

______ *(Signature of person authorized to arrange for service)* ______ *(Date)*

Figure 1–1. First call and authorization report. *(From Resource Manual, Brookfield, Wis: National Funeral Directors Association; 1979, with permission.)*

AUTHORIZATION FOR RELEASE AND EMBALMING

The undersigned hereby authorize

____

Name of Institution or Person

to release the body of ____

Deceased

to ____ and/or

Name of Funeral Home

its agents and authorize said funeral home and/or its agents to care for, embalm and otherwise prepare said body for burial and/or other disposition.

I (we) hereby represent that I am (we are) of the same and nearest degree of relationship to the deceased and/or are legally authorized or charged with the responsibility for such burial and/or other disposition.

____

Name Relationship

____

Name Relationship

____

Name Relationship

Witness ______________________________

Date ______________________________

Figure 1–2. Authorization form for release and embalming a body. *(From Resource Manual, Brookfield, Wis: National Funeral Directors Association; 1979, with permission.)*

AUTHORIZATION FOR EMBALMING

The undersigned represents to ______________________________

(name of the funeral home)

("Funeral Home") that the undersigned is the surviving spouse or the next of kin of ______________________________(the "Decedent"), or is the

(Name of the deceased)

legal representative of such person, and, as such, has the paramount right to direct the disposition of the body of the Decedent.

The undersigned authorizes and directs the Funeral Home, its employees, independent contractors, and agents (including apprentices, interns, and/or mortuary students under the direct supervision of a licensed embalmer), to care for, embalm, and prepare the body of the Decedent. The undersigned acknowledges that the authorization encompasses permission to embalm at the Funeral Home facility or at another facility equipped for embalming.

SIGNATURES **RELATIONSHIP TO DECEDENT**

____

____

____

Date: ______________________________

Figure 1–3. Authorization form to embalm body. *(From The National Funeral Directors Association; Brookfield, Wis, 1995, with permission.)*

AUTHORIZATION FOR RESTORATIVE AND COSMETIC CARE

I/we ______________________________, hereby authorize the ______________________________ Funeral Home to perform cosmetic and restorative work on the remains of ______________________________, who is related to me as ______________________. I/we hereby acknowledge full responsibility for results of same and do hold harmless, ______________________ Funeral Home, its owners, employees and agents for results herewith performed.

I/we hereby represent that I/we are of same and nearest degree of relationship to the deceased:

______________________________ (seal)

______________________________ (seal)

______________________________ (Witness)

______________________________ (Date)

______________________________ (Witness)

Figure 1–4. Authorization for restorative and cosmetic care. *(From Restorative and Cosmetic Care, permission by The Dodge Company, Cambridge, Mass, 1999.)*

Time Body Received at Funeral Home __________ Page No. _____

MEMO OF CLOTHING AND EFFECTS

NAME ______________________________ ______________________________ Date __________

Removed from ______________________________ By ______________________________

☐ BLOUSE	☐ HOUSECOAT	☐ P.Js.	☐ SLIPPERS	☐ UNDERWEAR
☐ BRA	☐ NECKTIE	☐ SHIRT	☐ SLIP	☐ VEST
☐ COAT	☐ NIGHTGOWN	☐ SHOES	☐ SKIRT	☐ OVERNIGHTER
☐ DRESS	☐ NIGHTSHIRT	☐ SOX	☐ SWEATER	☐ SUIT CASE
☐ GIRDLE	☐ PANTS	☐ STOCKINGS	☐ TOPCOAT	☐ CASH $_____
				☐ KEYS

Valuables and Jewelry ______________________________

Medical Devices (i.e., pacemaker) ______________________________

Disposition Authorized by ______________________________ Date __________

member of family

☐ Give to Family at once

☐ We dispose

Date ______________________________ ______________________________

Signature of Funeral Director

Figure 1–5. Example of the form used to inventory personal property of the deceased. *(From Resource Manual, Brookfield, Wis: National Funeral Directors Association; 1979, with permission.)*

CONSENT BY NEXT-OF-KIN FOR THE DONATION OF ORGANS AND TISSUES

I/WE ____ as next-
(name of next-of-kin)

of-kin and* ______________________ of ______________________
(relationship) (name of donor)

for humanitarian reasons hereby give consent for the donation of his/her

____ for the purposes
(specify donated organs or tissues)

of transplantation or research, if medically suitable, after the time of his/her death has been determined by the attending physician.

I/WE understand that these gifts are made to the Pittsburgh Transplant Foundation and that the recovery, distribution and determination of use of these gifts will be coordinated by the Foundation in accordance with medical and ethical standards. The Foundation will be responsible for the costs related to the organ and tissue recovery.

I/WE understand that death has been determined and its time recorded based on the fulfillment of brain death criteria. I/WE understand that artificial support of heartbeat and respiration will be continued during the recovery of vital organs and discontinued upon completion of the procedure. I/WE give consent for the recovery of the organs and tissues specified above under the circumstances described. I/WE also authorize the Pittsburgh Transplant Foundation to obtain complete medical history, autopsy findings (if performed), and tissue specimens for immunology studies necessary to insure the safety of the organs and tissues for transplantation.

______________________ ______________________
(signature of next-of-kin) (date) (signature of next-of-kin) (date)

______________________ ______________________
(signature of witness) (date) (signature of witness) (date

____
(Organ Procurement Coordinator)

*The Uniform Anatomical Gift Act establishes the following order of priority: (1) spouse; (2) adult son or daughter; (3) either parent; (4) adult brother or sister; (5) guardian of the person of the decedent; (6) any other person authorized or under obligation to dispose of the body.

Figure 1–6. Sample organ donor form. *(From Resource Manual, Brookfield, Wis: National Funeral Directors Association; 1979, with permission.)*

AUTHORIZATION FOR REMOVAL AND DISPOSITION WITHOUT EMBALMING

The undersigned hereby direct and authorize the ______________________
name of funeral home

and/or its agents, to remove and take possession of the body of ______________________
(deceased)

______________________ and to provide for the final disposition of said body by ( ) earth burial, ( ) entombment, ( ) cremation, ( ) burial at sea, ( ) other ______________________
We direct that there be no embalming or other preparation or care of the body. The undersigned also wish hereby to indicate the desire (not to have) (to have) rites/ceremonies with the casketed body present.

The undersigned do further state that they (have) (have not) identified the body of the above named decedent and assume all responsibility and/or liability of anyone whomsoever for mistaken identity.

The undersigned do hereby agree to indemnify and hold harmless the above-named funeral home, its officers, agents and employees from any claims or causes of action, including a reasonable attorney's fee for the defense thereof arising out of their act of identification or failure to identify, or arising out of their decision not to embalm, or arising out of any other decision indicated by this agreement which may result in mental or physical distress or anguish or harm or financial loss to themselves or to others.

______________________ ______________________
Name Relationship to deceased

______________________ ______________________
Name Relationship to deceased

______________________ ______________________
Name Relationship to deceased

Witness ______________________

Date ______________________

Figure 1–7. Authorization form for removal and disposition without embalming. *(From Resource Manual, Brookfield, Wis: National Funeral Directors Association; 1979, with permission.)*

state or local laws in the area(s) where the provider does business do not require embalming under any circumstances.

Services Provided Without Prior Approval

UNFAIR OR DECEPTIVE ACTS OR PRACTICES. In selling or offering to sell funeral goods or funeral services to the public, it is an unfair or deceptive act or practice for any provider to embalm a deceased body for a fee unless:

1. State or local law or regulation requires embalming in the particular circumstances regardless of any funeral choice which the family might make; or
2. Prior approval for embalming (expressly so described) from a family member or other authorized person; or
3. The funeral provider is unable to contact a family member or other authorized person after exercising due diligence, has no reason to believe the family does not want embalming performed, and obtains subsequent approval for embalming already performed (expressly so described). In seeking approval, the funeral provider must disclose that a fee will be charged if the family selects a funeral which requires embalming, such as a funeral with viewing, and that no fee will be charged if the family selects a service which does not require embalming, such as direct cremation or immediate burial.

PREVENTIVE REQUIREMENT. To prevent these unfair or deceptive acts or practices, funeral providers must include on the itemized statement of funeral goods and services selected, required by §453.2 (b) (5), the statement: "If you selected a funeral that may require embalming, such as a funeral with viewing, you may have to pay for embalming. You do not have to pay for embalming you did not approve if you selected arrangements such as direct cremation or immediate burial. If we charge for embalming, we will explain why below."*

▶ SHIPPING OF HUMAN REMAINS†

Terminology

Air tray—used for casketed remains, only the bottom is made of wood, top sides and ends are made of heavy grade cardboard

Burial-transit permit—a disposition permit which is a legal document issued by a governmental agency, authorizing transportation and/or disposition of a dead human body

Combination case—a transfer container consisting of a particleboard box with a cardboard cover used to ship a remains in place of a casket or airtray

Common carrier—any carrier required by law to convey passengers or freight without refusal if the approved fare of charge is paid; travels according to a set schedule (e.g., airlines, railroads)

Death certificate—a legal document containing vital statistics, disposition and final medical cause of death pertaining to a deceased human body

Hermetically sealed—airtight, impervious to external influence; completely sealed by fusion or soldering

Human remains—a dead human body or cremains

International—between countries

Interstate—between two or more states

Intrastate—within one state

Private carrier—an individual or company who transports only in particular instances and only for those they choose to contract with, for example, livery companies, private aircraft

Removal—(first call or transfer of remains) transfer of remains from the place of death to a funeral establishment

Ziegler case—(liner) a gasket-sealed container which can be used as an insert into a casket or a separate shipping container

Shipping is the transportation of human remains away from the place of death to another location for final disposition. Human remains can be defined as a dead human body or cremains. The shipping (transportation) may be via a private carrier (e.g., hearse, van, airplane, etc.) operated by a funeral home, livery company, or family of the deceased; or a common carrier (e.g., commercial airline, train, bus). There are no definitive data on the number of human remains transported in a given year, but a conservative estimate might be 20,000 by common carrier within the United States. Shipping can be divided into three categories based on the destination of the remains: (1) intrastate, between cities within a state; (2) interstate, between cities located in two different states; and (3) international, between countries. Intrastate shipping or transporting of a body is the least complicated of the three. Each of these divisions can have its own rules and reg-

*Review and update provided by Scott Gilligan, Esq., National Funeral Directors Association General Counsel.

†See Chapter 25 for details concerning the preparation of remains for shipping.

ulations for the transportation of human remains. A general rule is that all remains transported by common carrier *must* be accompanied by a burial-transit permit (or similar document). Some states issue a Provisional Transit Permit when a death certificate has not been signed by a physician or coroner; other states require that the medical examiner or coroner be notified and provided with the cause of death prior to consent being given for the transportation of the deceased. In some states the local jurisdiction at the place of death may impose additional requirements, such as that the death certificate must be signed by a doctor prior to removing the deceased from a hospital or place of death. From a legal standpoint, all the same criteria for release of the remains from the location of death must be met. This may include written authorization from the decedent's immediate next of kin or legal representative, an executor of the estate, or if no next of kin exists, the Public Administrator's Office at the place of death can authorize release of the remains. Several states (e.g., California) require written authorization for embalming beyond what is required by the FTC. The FTC regulations do not change when the death takes place away from the area where the purchaser of the goods and services resides. If a funeral home embalms remains and it was not authorized by the person in charge of disposition, no charge can be made for the embalming. A funeral home serving an out-of-town funeral director must also release the remains without receiving payment for its services, to another funeral home should there be a request to do so. A funeral home may not hold remains for payment.

Regardless of the type of shipment or carrier certain rules apply for the preparation of the body.

- Thoroughly cleanse and embalm the remains; thoroughly dry the body.
- Pack all external orifices.
- Place the remains in a plastic garment (pants, coveralls, or unionalls).
- Partially dress the remains using underclothing, pajamas, or a hospital gown, and envelop in a clean sheet.
- When shipping by common carrier place the shrouded body on a sheet of plastic which can envelop the body.
- Do *not* place one hand over another, as this might not be the desired position.
- When shipping casketed remains, place a very heavy layer of cotton around the head and face to protect the casket and clothing from any purge; be certain to turn the pillow over for shipping to prevent soilage from purge or cosmetics.
- Secure the body on a cot if shipping within the container; if casketed, place the bed of the casket in the lowest position and move the feet to the furthest end; secure the head end so the body will not slide.
- Document the condition of the body prior to, during, and after embalming. Send a copy of the embalming report with the remains.
- Notify the receiving funeral director of any unusual conditions (e.g., trauma, obesity, edema).

Intrastate and interstate shipping regulations will usually be set by a governmental agency in the state where the death occurs (certification of the death would be filed in the state or county of the state where the death occurred). One or more agencies may formulate the rules relative to the removal of a dead human remains from the place of death to another location within or outside of the state. Shipping regulatory agencies may include a local or state board of health, local or state bureau of vital statistics, state board of embalmers and funeral directors, local or state coroner or medical examiner's office, and transportation agencies (airline regulations, livery regulatory unions, etc.). There is no uniform, universal death certificate and vital statistics registry shared by all states and likewise there are no uniform regulations governing the transportation of dead human remains between states. For example, some states allow the transportation of dead human remains between cities within the state and outside of the state by private carrier without a burial-transit permit; other states allow the transport of a body by private carrier with a temporary transit permit or no permit at all. Some local municipalities may make requirements such as the need for a signed death certificate before a body can be removed from an institution such as a nursing home, hospice, or hospital. Intrastate transportation is the least complicated of the three types of shipping.

For intrastate and interstate shipping of cremains the United States Post Office is the only method available. Federal Express, UPS and other carrier services will not accept cremated remains for shipment. The majority of airlines will accept cremains for shipment within their small package cargo systems.

Regardless of the final destination—within the state, between states or to a foreign country—there are responsibilities for both the shipping and the receiving funeral establishments. The shipping facility must:

- Remove the remains from the place of death
- Embalm and thoroughly preserve the remains, the exception being if shipping is to Israel
- Secure the necessary documents for shipping and disposition
- Arrange for private or common carrier transportation and, if necessary, the required container

- Communicate to the receiving funeral establishment the condition of the remains and the time schedules of the carrier and provide the service as expediently as possible to relieve any anxiety on the part of the family and the receiving funeral establishment.

The receiving funeral establishment must:

- Avoid making promises to the family about the time and the date of the funeral services.
- Cooperate with the shipping funeral establishment in providing statistical information for the filing of the death certificate and disposition information.
- Be prepared for unexpected delays due to weather, flight cancellations, and problems with a local coroner, medical examiner, or organ retrieval teams.

There are two types of containers used when shipping a body by common carrier. The "combination air tray," which is a wood-based container that has sides, ends, and inside top all made of wood (plywood or fiber board) with an exterior covering of cardboard. The shrouded remains are placed directly in the wood bottom and the sides, ends, and top are closed around the body. The second container is referred to as an "air tray." This container is for casketed remains with only the bottom being made of wood and the sides, ends, and top being of heavy-grade cardboard. These two containers are used throughout the United States and some foreign countries such as Great Britain. They come in infant, child, adult, and oversized units and are meant to be used *once,* with most airlines stringently enforcing this rule. Because of cargo door size limitations, the airline should always be consulted when using an oversized container. When booking the flight advise the airline of the outside dimensions of the container. Many foreign countries still require an all wooden box (previously known as a railroad box). The airline needs to be advised of the dimensions of the wooden box because some cargo holds for international flights will only accommodate one all wooden box. Information on international shipping containers can be obtained from the consulate or shipping directory publications (e.g., American Funeral Director Blue Book).

International shipping is by far the most complicated type. The country where the body is to be buried has rules and regulations that must be followed before the transportation can take place. The funeral director at the place of death must notify the local consulate of the foreign country and obtain the regulations. In almost all countries today, permission must be granted for the deceased to enter the country. The foreign government where the remains are being shipped has an embassy in Washington D.C. The embassy then has smaller branch offices in various locations within the United States called "consulates." Smaller countries may offer only an embassy to deal with; other countries may have consulates in most major cities. The consulate of jurisdiction may handle the affairs for a specific geographic region of the United States. The local funeral director who is shipping the remains will generally deal with this office in obtaining the necessary requirements and documentation. It should be noted there are countries that have no diplomatic relations with the United States (e.g., Cuba), and shipping remains to these countries may not be possible or may need to be done through another foreign government. Remains cannot be shipped to countries where there is a declared war.

The consulate of jurisdiction will request documentation to be presented and will in turn provide documents that will allow entry of the remains into the country. Some consulates will accept faxing of the documents as originals. It is advised to check with the consulate to obtain its policy. Documents generally required can include:

- Certified copy of the death certificate
- Noncontagious disease letter issued by the local health department where the death occurred stating there are no contagious diseases or epidemics in the city or county of death
- Embalmer's affidavit saying the remains were embalmed in accordance with the laws of the state where the death occurred
- Noncontraband letter stating the casket contains only the body and clothing necessary for burial.

A fee is usually paid to the foreign consulate for processing of the documents.

When shipping overseas, some unusual requirements can be made by the foreign country. Examples include the following.

- Need for a sealing casket or a wood casket with a sealing ziegler case inside
- An all-wood shipping container possibly lined with zinc and soldered closed
- Exact dimensions for the outer shipping box and the material of composition
- Bottom of the casket be filled with sawdust (Egypt)
- Israel does not require embalming, but if embalmed, the remains must be embalmed by the gravity method and no drainage taken
- Require embalming using chemicals illegal in the United States such as bichloride of mercury (Italy).

Individual airlines may also impose regulations on foreign shipments. Puerto Rico airlines, for example, requires a noncertified copy of the death certificate to be presented to the airline officials when the body is delivered to the airport. Some airlines require that they have written permission from the foreign country to allow them to bring the remains into the country. There are also significant security precautions taken. Examples include a security endorsement stating the container has no explosive devices, requiring the person dropping off the shipment to have 2 picture IDs, and a letter of certification that the shipment meets all Federal Aviation Administration (FAA) rules and regulations. The shipment may need to be x-rayed, arrive in the cargo area at a certain time, and allow no additional items to be placed inside the container. Shipments sent *unembalmed* can either be packaged in dry ice or in freezer packs similar to the kind used for food. Many airlines charge a premium for the shipment of dry ice because it is considered a hazardous material. The freezer packs come in much larger sizes and do not carry the tariff that dry ice does. The cost of shipment is per pound (or kilogram) weight and the airlines all require that the shipment be paid for at the time it is dropped off at their cargo area. It cannot be charged to an airline account. The length of time involved to process an international shipment can take anywhere from 5 to 14 business days. Most foreign consulates observe American holidays and do not work on weekends. Additionally, some foreign consulates require that one of their officers inspect the casket, container, and seal the outer box with wax and the seal of their government. This may require that the shipment first go to another larger city (e.g., Chicago, New York, Los Angeles) to fulfill this obligation.

▶ TERMS AND CONCEPTS FOR STUDY AND DISCUSSION

1. Define the following terms:
   Air tray
   Combination case
   Common carrier
   Interstate
   Intrastate
   Ethics
   Profession
   Reverence for the dead
   Rule and regulation
   Statute
   Ziegler case
2. Discuss some of the causes of death which must be reported to the coroner or medical examiner.
3. Discuss the difference between the "cause of death" and the "manner of death."
4. Discuss the difference between "organ donation" and "tissue donation."
5. Discuss the statute, rule or regulation by your state as to obtaining permission for the embalming of a body.
6. Discuss the FTC rule for obtaining permission for the embalming of a body.
7. Under the FTC Rule, give the choices a family may have for disposition when they do not wish to give permission for embalming.
8. Under the statutes and rules and regulations of your state, when *must* a body be embalmed?
9. Why should a body be identified by a family representative prior to immediate burial or cremation?
10. What are "Universal Precautions"?

▶ BIBLIOGRAPHY

Duncan, L. Funerals Are for the Living, *Women's Health,* (March 1986), 28.

Gladstone, WE, *Dictionary of Thoughts,* Standard Books, Inc. 1974, 213.

Holy Bible, Revised Standard Version, Thomas Nelson and Sons, New York, 1952.

Irion, PE, *The Funeral Vestage or Value,* Nashville, TN: The Parthenon Press, 1966.

Lindemann, E. Psychological Aspects of Mourning, as cited in Edgar Jackson's, *For the Living,* The Channel Press, Des Moines, IA, 1963.

Organ and Tissue Procurement Manual, Pittsburgh, PA: Pittsburgh Transplant Foundation; 1987.

Resource Manual, Brookfield, WI: National Funeral Directors Association; 1979.

Rules and Regulations, *Federal Register.* 1982; 47 (no. 186):42301–42302.

Solecki, RS. Leroi-Gourhan, A. Paleoclimatology and Archeology in the Near East. *Annals of the New York Academy of Sciences,* Vol. XCV, Art. 1 (1961), 729–39.

Undertaking Ethics, Funeral Ethics Association; Springfield, IL, 1994.

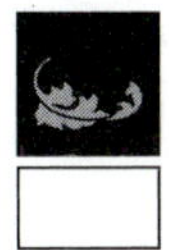

CHAPTER 2
FUNDAMENTALS OF EMBALMING

▶ TERMINOLOGY

- **Embalming***—process of chemically treating the dead human body to reduce the presence and growth of microorganisms, retard organic decomposition, and restore an acceptable physical appearance.
- **Embalm**—(14c)* 1: to treat (a dead body) so as to protect from decay 2: to fill with sweet odors: PERFUME 3: to protect from decay or oblivion: PRESERVE 4: to fix in a static condition—**embalmer** n—embalmment n
- **Decay**—(15c) 1: to undergo destructive dissolution; implies a slow change from a state of soundness
- **Decay***—decomposition of proteins by enzymes of aerobic bacteria
- **Decompose**—(ca 1751) 1: to separate into constituent parts or elements or into simpler compounds 2: to break up into constituent parts or as if by a chemical process: decay—**decomposition** n
- **Decomposition***—separation of compounds into simpler substances by the action of microbial and/or autolytic enzymes
- **Preserve**—(14c) 1: to keep safe from injury, harm, or destruction: PROTECT 2 a: to keep intact, or free from decay b: MAINTAIN 3: to keep or save from decomposition—**preservation** n
- **Preservation***—The science of treating the dead human body chemically so as to temporarily inhibit decomposition
- **Preservative**—(15c): something that preserves or has the power of preserving; an additive used to protect against decay, discoloration or spoilage
- **Preservative***—chemicals which inactivate saprophytic bacteria, render unsuitable for nutrition the media upon which such bacteria thrive, and which will arrest decomposition by altering enzymes and lysins of the body as well as converting the decomposable tissue to a form less susceptible to decomposition
- **Putrefaction**—(14c) 1: the decomposition of organic matter; the typically anaerobic splitting of proteins by bacteria and fungi with the formation of foul-smelling incompletely oxidized products
- **Putrefaction**†—decomposition of proteins by the action of enzymes from anaerobic bacteria

Embalming is an applied chemical process used to bring about the preservation and sanitizing of the dead human body. The terms *embalming* and *preservation* indicate an indefinite perpetuity of the body, and there are such documented results. However, embalming as practiced in funeral service today provides a temporary preservation of the human dead, allowing society time to perform secular and religious rites and ceremonies. Embalming permits the presence of the human dead at the funeral.

Preservation can occur naturally under special conditions, depending on such elements as temperature, climate, and the surrounding environment. Documentation shows the art and science of embalming has been performed, in one form or another, for well over 5500 years. Certain forms of preservation for anatomic or museum study can maintain the integrity of the body for many years. These bodies, while in a state of excellent preservation, do not always maintain the recognizable condition they had in life.

The definition adopted by the American Board of Funeral Service Education summarizes the term "embalming" as it is used in our society today as "the process of chemically treating the dead human body to reduce the presence and growth of microorganisms, to retard organic decomposition, and to restore an acceptable physical appearance." As practiced in the United States and other developed countries, its results purport more than simply the preservation of the vis-

* From the American Board of Funeral Service embalming syllabus.

† Date of earliest recorded use in English: *Merriam Webster's Collegiate Dictionary*, 10th ed, 1993.

age of the deceased. Embalming allows time for the mourners to travel long distances to attend funeral ceremonies with the body present. The embalmed body is in such a state of preservation that it is not offensive to the senses. The deceased should appear natural and recognizable to friends and relatives who want to view him or her. Embalming allows the deceased to be moved long distances. The return of a body from a foreign country to his or her native land for funeral ceremonies with a viewing of the deceased, if desired, is made possible by embalming.

"Decomposition, the separation of compounds into simpler substances by the action of microbial and/or autolytic enzymes," begins at death. Embalming slows this process. Indefinite preservation, by standard embalming techniques, is not possible. The length of preservation by embalming depends on a variety of intrinsic and extrinsic factors. Intrinsic factors include the pathologic processes within the body, circulatory conditions, level of body moisture, distribution of the preservative chemicals, and so on. Extrinsic factors include the type of preservatives used, strength and volume of embalming chemicals, climate and environment within the burial chamber, environmental molds and bacteria, and other factors. Under the correct conditions, bodies may be preserved for a reasonable period of time, and some for many years; however, with sufficiently unfavorable factors, the preservation may be as brief as several days. There is no way to determine the degree or length of time preservation can be maintained.

▶ PRESERVATION AND SANITATION

Embalming preservatives and germicides act primarily on body proteins. The colloidal nature of the protein changes by establishing many cross-linkages that were not formerly present between adjacent proteins. This forms a latticework of inert firm material—the *embalmed tissue*—that can no longer be easily broken down by bacterial or autolytic body enzymes.

Proteins have many reactive centers and a great affinity to hold water. Embalming destroys these reactive centers, and the new protein-like substance no longer has the ability to retain water. As a result these new (embalmed) protein structures are more stable and longer lasting. Thus, the tissues are temporarily preserved. The inability of embalmed tissue to hold water results in a dryness to the embalmed tissue.

Enzymes have the ability to react with body proteins, fats and carbohydrates and break down (decompose) these body substrates. Embalming preservatives also inactivate enzymes; an enzyme is protein. The enzymes originate from body cells (autolytic enzymes) or bacteria (bacterial enzymes). Embalming chemicals also destroy bacteria (pathogenic and nonpathogenic), through reactions with the proteins which are a part of these organisms. Thus the body, to a certain extent, becomes sanitized. The likelihood of the body remaining a source of disease-producing microbes or their products is greatly reduced. Through conversion or inactivation (embalming) of (1) protein of the tissues, (2) protein of enzymes, and (3) protein of microbes, the body is sanitized and temporarily preserved. The length of time of preservation will depend on the number of contacts made between the preservative chemicals and the millions and millions of body and bacterial proteins.

▶ RESTORATION

Restoration of the deceased to a natural form and color is the third purpose of embalming. The goal of restoration of the dead human body is not so much to make the deceased look lifelike, but rather to try and remove from the body the evidence of devastation caused by long-term disease and illness, visible surgery, visible trauma, disfigurements brought about by the long-term use of therapeutic drugs, visible postmortem changes, and undesirable embalming results (e.g., swelling, discolorations). Injection of the proper embalming chemicals can (1) raise sunken facial tissues, (2) decrease facial swellings from edema and gases, (3) remove postmortem intravascular discolorations, (4) bleach extravascular blood discolorations, and (5) restore natural facial coloring. Embalming manual operations such as the posing and closure of the eyes and mouth help to establish a natural restored appearance.

▶ CLASSIFICATIONS OF EMBALMING

There are four embalming treatment classifications: arterial (or vascular), cavity, hypodermic, and surface. It is possible that one or all four types of treatments can be used in the embalming of an autopsied or unautopsied body.

Arterial embalming can be used to prepare general or localized body regions. **Cavity embalming** is limited to treatments of the walls, organs, organ contents, excretions and secretions within body cavities. **Surface** and **hypodermic embalming** (supplemental embalming techniques) are generally used for localized treatments for areas not reached by arterial embalming. Exceptions for localized use of hypodermic and surface embalming can be found in, for example, autopsied bodies, where hypodermic embalming will be used to prepare very large body regions.

Arterial and Cavity Embalming

Through use of arterial and cavity embalming treatments, complete preservation of the "normal" unautopsied body can be accomplished. Arterial (vascular) embalming makes use of the blood vascular system. A preservative chemical solution is injected into a major artery(s) and blood is drained simultaneously from a vein. Cavity embalming, performed after arterial embalming, is the direct treatment of the contents of the body cavities (abdominal, thoracic, and pelvic) and the materials in the lumen of the hollow viscera. This is carried out by first aspirating the cavities followed by the injection of concentrated chemicals into the cavities. Both processes use a trocar.

A working description might state that embalming of the unautopsied body is performed in two stages; stage one is the arterial injection (infusion) and stage two is cavity embalming. Arterial embalming consists of the injection of 3 to 4 gallons of preservative solution, under pressure, into the circulatory system of the deceased through a large artery (e.g., carotid, femoral). Blood and a portion of the injected solution is concurrently removed from a large (e.g., internal jugular, femoral) vein to provide room for the preservatives. The preservative solution flows through the arterial, capillary, and venous routes in basically the same course followed by blood in the living body, a basic difference being that the embalming solution does not pass through the heart. The solution travels to the ascending aorta where it places pressure on the aortic semilunar valves and forces them closed. After the valves are tightly shut, the ascending, arch, and entire aorta fill with the solution and the preservative begins to flow into the various branches.

The structural mediator of the delivery of the injection chemicals to receptive tissue sites is the fundamental and simplest division of the blood vascular system, the capillary. In this sense, arterial embalming might be referred to as *capillary embalming*. These simple endothelial tubes with an average diameter of 7 to 9 micrometers connect the terminal arterioles and the venules. The surface area of the capillary network in the human body approaches 6000 square meters or 64,585 square feet. This vast membrane of over 1.5 acres is the permeable barrier that controls the delivery of preserving and disinfecting chemicals to deep and superficial body tissues. The circulatory system of humans normally contains 5 to 6 quarts of blood, or 8% of the body weight, 85% of which is contained within the capillaries. Obviously, thorough profusion of the soft tissue sites with appropriate concentrations of injection chemicals involves far more than filling the aorta and its primary branches. A portion of the embalming solution passes through the capillaries and enters the tissue spaces. Finally, it is here that it will make contact with the cells of the tissues and the body protein.

Cavity embalming is the treatment of the contents of the abdominal and thoracic cavities. Many of the contained organs are hollow and their contents are not reached by the preservative solution. The contents of these hollow organs along with any liquids or gases that may have accumulated in the body cavities are suctioned out by a process called *aspiration*. A long hollow needle called a trocar is inserted through the abdominal wall. An attempt is made to pierce each organ and all cavity areas. After removal of accumulated liquids, gases, and semisolids, a very concentrated preservative called cavity fluid is injected through the trocar. Approximately 32 to 48 ounces of cavity fluid is introduced into the cavities through the trocar by gravity pressure. In some situations, several hours later the embalmer will re-aspirate and possibly reinject the cavities.

Hypodermic and Surface Embalming

Hypodermic embalming is the subcuticular injection of a suitable preservative chemical directly into the tissues. The chemical may be injected by a syringe and needle, infant or standard trocar. The area of treatment may be localized, such as a finger or area of the cheek, or it may be quite large, as in the hypodermic treatment of the abdominal and chest walls in the autopsied body, or an entire lower extremity when gangrene is present.

Surface embalming is the application of an embalming chemical directly to the surface of the tissues. The chemicals can be applied as a preservative spray in aerosol form, painted on the surface by brush in the form of a liquid or gel, or applied on cotton as a surface compress. The outside skin surface or under the skin in areas such as the eyelids and the mouth can be treated, and with autopsied remains surface chemicals can be applied to the inner surfaces of the cavity walls and the undersurface of the cranial scalp.

Summary and Expectations of the Embalming Process

In 1928, Professor Charles O. Dhonau, dean of the Cincinnati College of Embalming, defined an embalming fluid. He did not define the fluid itself but defined the functions of the fluid and the process by which the fluid reaches the cells of the body. He further explained how the fluid functions to achieve sanitation, preservation and a restoration to the body tissues. This definition is as relevant today as it was more than 70 years ago and it serves well to explain the entire embalming process:

> An **embalming fluid** is a chemical substance which when given physical application (or injection)

at the right time
at the right temperature
in the right quantity
of the right quality, strength dilution, concentration
so as to receive a complete distribution in arteries, capillaries and veins
will diffuse (spread) from the capillaries
to the lymph spaces and to the intercellular spaces
and to the cellular tissues
to unite with the cellular substances
so as to normalize their water content
restore their colors
and so to fix and preserve them that they will be preserved against organized (bacterial)
and unorganized (enzymatic) decompositions
and will be preserved against other kinds of changes
such as in water content; oxidation; from soil chemicals
just so long as the after-care provides the necessary means to protect
what has been embalmed.
A part which has been embalmed will not discolor
from any cause within several weeks; it will not become
blood discolored; or show dehydration changes;
or show greenish colors from protein decompositions;
or become malodorous from protein decompositions;
by proteolytic bacterial enzymes by which spore forming
anaerobes, seeking (bound) oxygen, break up compounds
containing it and release odorous gasses such as hydrogen sulfide;
or become gas distended from the gaseous decomposition of proteins
or carbohydrates (tissue gas); nor will the tissues soften and finally liquefy
through the work of organized or unorganized ferments;
nor will the tissues of the body pass through the cycle of changes
which at the end converts the hundred or more body compounds into
water, nitrogen, methane and carbon dioxide, as a result of all the
oxidations through which decompositions proceed. A part which has
not been properly embalmed should be thought of by the embalmer
as an unsolved embalming problem, to which he or she has
contributed either by lack of understanding, by carelessness or by both.

Cincinnati College of Mortuary Science, 1928, with permission.

From Dhonau C.O., Defining Embalming Fluid. File 100. Cincinnati, OH.

▶ EMBALMING CASE REPORT

An embalming case report should be completed for each body. This should be done for each body brought into the embalming room or embalming facility. Applicable portions of the report should be completed if the body is not embalmed or minimal preparation was performed for identification, if the body is embalmed for local disposition, or shipped to another funeral facility. The embalming report is of significant value in trauma cases if testimony as to the condition of the body by the embalmer is necessary in a court proceeding. When the body is being prepared for shipping to another funeral facility, a copy of the report should accompany the remains. Case reports should be filled out in detail and kept as a permanent record. The report should be complete enough that accurate descriptions could be given of (1) the body before preparation, (2) manner and methods of the preparation, and (3) any postembalming treatments. A sample Embalming Report is shown in Figure 2–1.

▶ EMBALMING SEQUENCE

The following embalming chronologies provide an overview of the entire embalming procedure from start to finish. The first suggested chronology gives the step-by-step procedure for embalming the adult *unautopsied* body; the second chronology gives the sequence of treatments for preparation of the *autopsied* adult body.

Suggested Chronology for Embalming the Unautopsied Adult Body

The steps that follow are the general order for embalming the unautopsied adult body. Note that the steps need not be taken in this recommended order. For example, features can be set before, during, or even after arterial embalming; many embalmers prefer to suture incisions after cavity embalming; aspiration of the organs relieves the pressure on the vascular system and reduces the chance of incision leakage. The embalmer should be appropriately attired and gloved when handling the dead human body. The embalming report should be prepared throughout the embalming of the body.

After the body has been placed on the embalming table the following steps are suggested:

1. Remove all clothing from the body. Be certain to examine for any valuables. If rings or jewelry are present, make a list. Some embalmers prefer to tape rings to fingers or affix them with a string. Jewelry such as necklaces, religious articles, and watches should be removed and carefully stored.

EMBALMING REPORT
(Confidential)

Embalmer ______________________ **Master No.:** ______________

Assisted by ______________________

FUNERAL HOME ______ IN-HOUSE ______ SHIP-IN ______ SHIP-OUT ______

DATE ______ TIME ______ PERMISSION TO EMBALM ______

PROTECTIVE ATTIRE WORN ______ COMMUNICABLE DISEASE ______

NAME ______ DATE OF DEATH ______ TIME OF DEATH ______

CAUSE OF DEATH ______ DOCTOR/MEDICAL-EXAMINER ______

PERSONAL EFFECTS ON BODY ______

AGE ______ SEX ______ RACE ______ HEIGHT ______ WEIGHT ______ FACIAL HAIR ______

NATURAL TEETH ______ DENTURES ______ NO DENTURES ______ OTHER ______

DESCRIBE HAIR ______ DISTINGUISHING MARKS ______

CONDITIONS PRIOR TO EMBALMING

GENERAL: CLEAN ______ REFRIGERATED ______ RIGOR MORTIS ______ SURGERY ______

EVIDENCE OF DISEASE ______ EVIDENCE OF TRAUMA ______ TRACHEOTOMY ______ PACEMAKER ______

I.V. PUNCTURE(S) ______ STOMACH FEEDING TUBE ______ COLOSTOMY ______ GAS IN TISSUES ______

SKIN SLIP ______ CATHETER (URINARY) ______ DISCOLORATION(S) ______ PURGE ______

OTHER ______

FACE: NORMAL ______ EMACIATED ______ SWOLLEN ______ TRAUMA ______ EDEMA ______ GAS IN TISSUES ______ LESIONS ______

SKIN-SLIP ______ TUBE MARKS ______ DISCOLORATION(S) ______

OTHER ______

AUTOPSEY: CRANIAL ______ THORACIC ______ ABDOMINAL ______ PELVIC ______ SPINAL ______

NECK ORGANS REMOVED ______ TONGUE REMOVED ______ PARTIAL AUTOPSY ______ EYES DRAINED ______ EYE(S) REMOVED ______

VISCERA RETURNED WITH BODY ______ PLACEMENT OF VISCERA (AFTER EMBALMING) ______

TISSUES SAMPLES TAKEN (IF NO AUTOPSY PERFORMED) ______

ORGAN DONOR: ______ DESCRIBE ______

______

ENUCLEATION (WHOLE EYE) ______ CORNEA ONLY ______

PREPARATION OF THE BODY

SURFACE DISINFECTION ______ BODY WASHED ______ HAIR WASHED ______ NAILS CLEANED ______

NOSTRILS TRIMMED ______ FACE SHAVED ______ METHOD OF EYE CLOSURE ______

MOUTH SUPPORT IF USED ______ METHOD OF MOUTH CLOSURE ______

ALL ORIFICES DISINFECTED AND PACKED ______

Figure 2–1. Sample embalming report.

PRESERVATIVE TREATMENTS

I. PRIMARY INJECTION PLAN [ARTERY(S)]:

a. One-point injection ______________________

b. Restricted cervical injection ______________________

c. Six-point injection ______________________

d. Other (describe) ______________________

TOTAL VOLUME OF SOLUTION INJECTED ______________

SOLUTION MIXTURES USED ______________ (indicate Solution Gallon #)

DRAINAGE SITE ______________________

DRAINAGE METHOD ______________________

II. IF THE HEAD IS SEPARATELY EMBALMED (RESTRICTED CERVICAL OR AUTOPSY): ______________

SOLUTION MIXTURE USED ______________________

VOLUME INJECTED ______________________

III. AREA(S) RECEIVING AN INADEQUATE AMOUNT OF ARTERIAL SOLUTION: ______________________

IV. SUPPLEMENTAL ARTERY(S) INJECTED: ______________________

TOTAL VOLUME OF SOLUTION INJECTED ______________

SOLUTION MIXTURES USED ______________ (indicate Solution Gallon #)

V. SUPPLEMENTAL EMBALMING TREATMENTS (HYPODERMIC, COMPRESSES, GELS, ETC.) ______________

VI. CAVITY TREATMENT (UNAUTOPSIED): IMMEDIATE ASPIRATION ______________; DELAYED ASPIRATION ______________

NAME OF FLUID INJECTED ______________________ VOLUME INJECTED ______________

ARTERIAL FLUIDS AND SOLUTIONS

FLUID COMPANY AND NAME:

A. WATER

B. PRE-INJECTION ______________________

C. ARTERIAL #1 ______________________

D. ARTERIAL #2 ______________________

E. CO-INJECTION ______________________

F. WATER SOFTENER ______________________

G. HUMECTANT ______________________

H. DYE ______________________

I. OTHER ______________________

ARTERIAL SOLUTIONS (MEASURED IN OUNCES PER GALLON; 1 GALLON = 128 FLUID OUNCES) PLACE THE LETTER OF THE FLUID FROM THE LIST ABOVE IN THE LEFT COLUMN; IN THE RIGHT COLUMN PUT THE NUMBER OF OUNCES USED.

GALLON #1	GALLON #2	GALLON #3	GALLON #4	GALLON #5
A ___ ___ (oz)	A ___ ___ (oz)	A ___ ___ (oz)	A ___ ___ (oz)	A ___ ___ (oz)
___ ___	___ ___	___ ___	___ ___	___ ___
___ ___	___ ___	___ ___	___ ___	___ ___
___ ___	___ ___	___ ___	___ ___	___ ___
___ ___	___ ___	___ ___	___ ___	___ ___

COMPLETION

AREA(S) OF DISTENSION RESULTING FROM ARTERIAL INJECTION ______________________

PURGE DURING ARTERIAL INJECTION [DESCRIBE] ______________________

PURGE TREATMENT ______________________

EYELIDS GLUED ________ LIPS GLUED ________ INCISION SEAL POWDER ________ INCISIONS GLUED ________

PLASTICS USED: ______________________; EMBALMING POWDER IN PLASTICS ______________

Figure 2–1. (Continued)

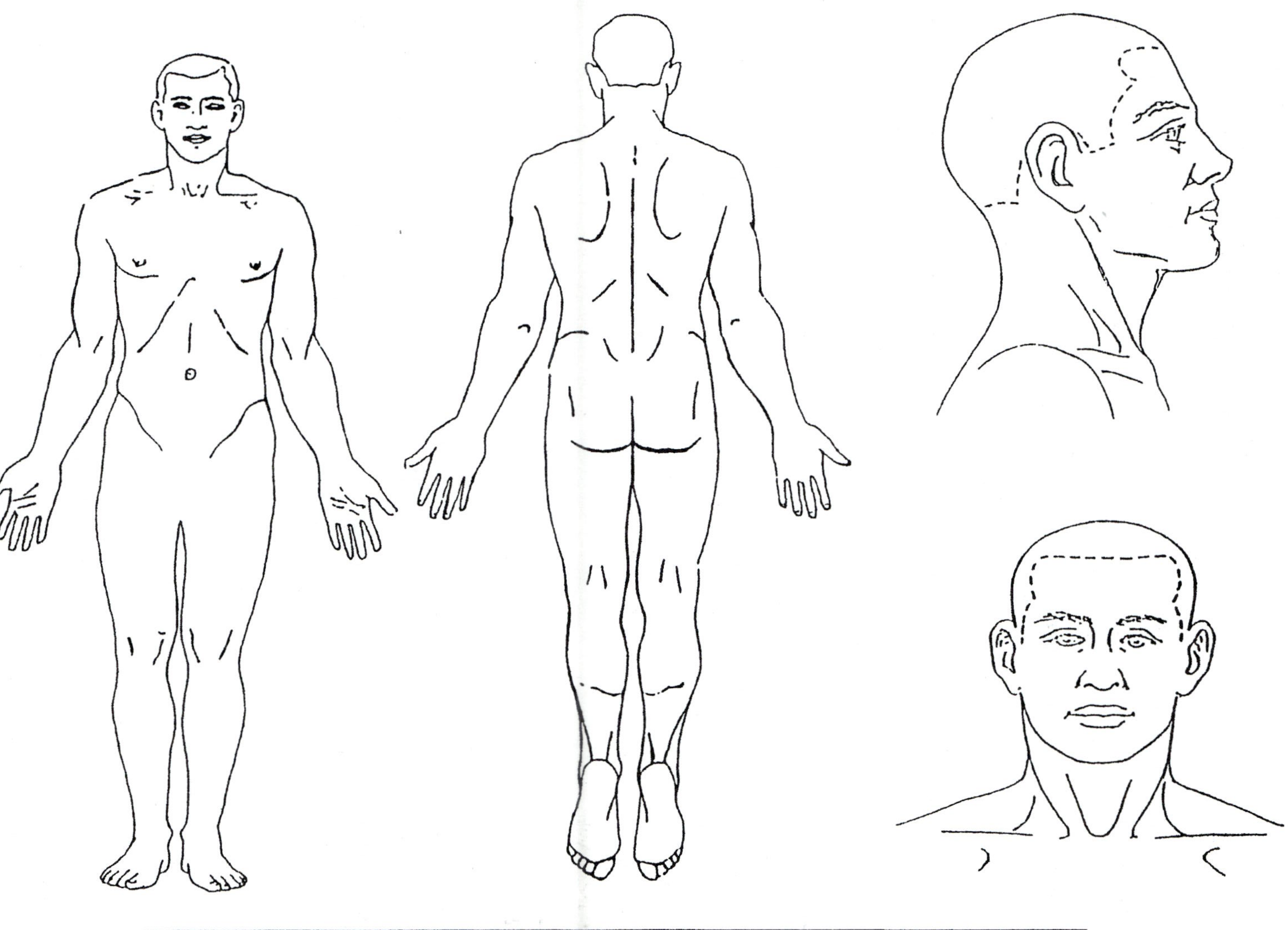

MARK POINTS OF INTEREST &
PLACE COMMENTS ON THE BACK PAGE

Figure 2–1. (Continued)

DESCRIPTION OF RESTORATIVE TREATMENTS

DESCRIPTION OF COSMETIC TREATMENTS

SHIP-IN CONDITIONS AND CORRECTIONS

Body received from: ______________________ City/State ______________________

Describe problem conditions and their correction:

COMMENTS

____

____

____

____

____

____

____

____

____

____

____

____

____

____

Figure 2–1. (Continued)

   A. Soiled clothing should either be destroyed or cleaned.
   B. All contaminated bedding (such as sheets and hospital gowns) should be destroyed or properly laundered.
2. Disinfect the body with a droplet spray or with a disinfectant solution that is sponged onto the body. Allow the disinfectant time to work. Disinfect all body orifices and swab these orifices with cotton. Remove all material from the mouth and throat. A nasal tube aspirator can also be used to remove material from the mouth, throat, and nasal passages.
3. Position the body. Rigor mortis should be relieved at this time. Limbs can be flexed and exercised and hands extended and manipulated. The head should be elevated above the chest and the chest elevated above the abdomen. Slightly tilt the head to the right. The hands can remain at the sides or even down over the table at this point. This allows the blood to gravitate into the hands and helps to expand the vessels. Once arterial injection has begun and the hands show signs of fluid distribution, they can be placed in the correct position. Special blocking is necessary for arthritic conditions or where limbs have atrophied. Attempt to straighten the limbs by wrapping them with cloth strips. It is not recommended that any tissue be cut to extend limbs.
4. Wash the body surface with a germicidal warm-water soapy solution. Give particular attention to face and hands. The hair should be washed. At this time the fingernails can be cleaned. It is much easier to get any dirt out from under the nails at this time than after arterial embalming. Clean using a brush; an instrument may tear the skin under the nail and a discoloration will result. Use solvents to remove any surface stains. Thoroughly dry the body.
5. Shave the facial hair. Any facial hair remaining may interfere with the later cosmetic application. Be certain to check if a mustache or beard is to be removed or merely trimmed. If there is any doubt, the beard or mustache can be shaved after embalming once the family has been consulted. Removal of facial hair is much simpler than reconstruction of a mustache or beard. Facial hair should be removed from all bodies, including women and children.
6. Close the mouth using an appropriate method such as the needle injector method or suturing. If dentures are available, they should be properly cleaned and disinfected. If dentures or teeth are absent a replacement of cotton or a "mouth former" can be substituted. The eyes should be cleaned and closed using cotton or an "eyecap." If fever blisters are present on the lips or if there is crusted material along the eyelashes, using a soft rag or gauze moistened with warm water will easily remove these items. A solvent such as trichloroethylene or the "dry hair washes" also serve as a good cleaner. Care should be taken at this point to straighten the nostrils with cotton and to carefully clip any nostril hairs that may be visible. Some embalmers prefer at this time to place a light coating of massage cream over the face, hands, and neck. This cream should not be placed over discolored areas where opaque cosmetics will later be applied. Surface compresses of bleach (phenol or formaldehyde) can be placed on blood or pathologic discolorations at this time.
7. Select the artery that will be used for injection and the vein that will be used for drainage. This choice is based on the embalming analysis.
8. Select the arterial fluid and prepare the embalming solution.
9. Inject the embalming solution. The pressure and rate of flow of the injection are determined by the embalming analysis. Look for signs of arterial solution distribution. Where fluid is lacking, manipulate the injection methods to encourage even distribution of the fluid throughout the body. Four questions need to be asked at this stage of embalming: (i) How much solution is needed? (ii) What should the strength of the solution be? (iii) Which areas of the body *are* and which *are not* receiving solution? (iv) When has the body or body areas received sufficient arterial solution?
10. After arterial injection, make an analysis of the body to determine if all areas have been perfused with sufficient arterial solution. If areas lack fluid, secondary points of injection can be injected. In addition, areas that cannot be reached by arterial injection can be embalmed using hypodermic injection and surface preservative techniques at this time.
11. Remove arterial tubes and drainage devices. Dry and tightly suture incisions.
12. You can now aspirate the body. Some embalmers prefer to delay this process for several hours. Condition of the body helps to dictate whether cavity embalming should be done immediately after arterial injection or several hours later.

13. After aspiration, inject the cavities via the trocar with an undiluted cavity fluid. Size and condition of the body determine the amount of fluid to inject. For the average body, 32 to 48 ounces is generally satisfactory. After cavity fluid injection, close the openings(s) in the abdominal wall with a trocar button or by suture.
14. Remove any surgical drains and close the openings by suture. Remove all intravenous lines or products of other invasive procedures into the vascular system and seal any punctures. Remove a pacemaker if the body is to be cremated. Disinfect colostomy openings with a phenol solution and close by suture. Open, drain, disinfect, and suture any unhealed surgical incisions.
15. Rewash the hair and the body. Dry the body thoroughly, being certain to roll the body to one side so the back, shoulders, and buttocks can be dried. After washing and drying, apply surface glue to all sutured areas. At this time, check the mouth to be certain it is dry and free from any purge material. If there has been purge or blood in the oral cavity, this cotton should be replaced with dry cotton. Now, the mouth and the eyes can be glued. The anal orifice can be packed with cotton saturated with cavity fluid or autopsy gel. By delaying this treatment until this time, fecal matter will have had time to exit during the cavity embalming process.
16. If reaspiration of the cavities is to be performed it is usually done several hours after completion of the embalming.
17. Clean and fill the embalming machine with clean water. By filling the machine now, gases such as chlorine have time to escape prior to the next use of the machine. Instruments can be cleaned and all waste properly disposed of.
18. Dress the body in plastic garments (pants, coveralls, stockings, or a unionall) and place some embalming powder within the garment. If necessary, plastic stockings can also be used.
19. Cosmetic treatment will now follow.

Suggested Chronology for Embalming the Autopsied Adult Body

Employing Universal Precautions, the embalmer should be properly attired prior to any handling of the deceased. The embalming process needs to be documented using an embalming report. Notation in the report should be made of the type of autopsy performed; organs and tissues removed; and organs, tissues, and personal effects that are returned with the body.

1. Place the autopsied body on the center of the preparation table. Spray with a droplet surface disinfectant. Wash the body with a good liquid soap using warm water. Take care to remove blood stains from the autopsy. Pay particular attention to the hands and cleaning of the fingernails. The hair can be rinsed; however; because of the cranial autopsy, the hair will need rewashing after embalming.
2. Open the autopsy temporary sutures and aspirate any liquids that have accumulated within the cavities. Spray the inside walls of the cavities with a droplet disinfectant spray.
3. Examine the extent of the autopsy. If a partial autopsy has been performed, the extent should be evaluated. If the eyes have been removed the procedure for treatment can begin at this time. Rigor morris can be relieved by flexing, bending, and massaging the limbs. This allows for a temporary positioning of the body.
4. Shave the facial hair.
5. Clean the oral cavity and replace dentures or, if they are not available, replace missing teeth or dentures with cotton or a "mouth former." The mouth can be held closed by needle injector wires or sutures. If the tongue has been removed, the oral cavity can be swabbed with a phenol cautery agent on cotton. The area can also be painted with autopsy gel.
6. Clean areas around the eyes. The eyes can be closed using cotton or an "eyecap."
7. Prepare the arterial solution. Strength and quantity depend on conditions of the body.
8. Raise the arteries that will be used to inject the legs. Place the arterial tubes into the arteries. Drainage will be taken by letting the drainage collect in the body cavities. Control over drainage may be obtained by using a hemostat clamped to the vein.
9. Inject the legs. Give attention to the distribution of the fluid. Increase pressure or rate of flow to establish uniform distribution. Areas not reached can be treated by hypodermic injection later.
10. Prepare the arteries that will be used to inject the arms—the subclavian arteries or the right and left axillary arteries. Drainage can be con-

trolled by the use of a hemostat applied to the accompanying veins.

11. Inject the arms. Be certain good distribution is achieved through all the fingers. If distribution is not complete the radial or ulnar arteries can be raised and injected at this time.
12. Isolate and place arterial tubes into the right and left common carotid arteries. Inject the left side of the head *first*, then inject the right side of the face. Leakage from the internal carotid arteries in the base of the skull can be controlled with hemostats.
13. Prepare a strong solution. Diluted cavity fluid or a strong arterial solution can be used. With a small trocar inject the buttocks, trunk walls, shoulders, and back of the neck (any trunk areas where arterial fluid is absent or insufficient). All this can be done from within the cavities.
14. Aspirate and dry the cranial, abdominal, thoracic, and pelvic cavities. Coat the inside walls of the cavities with an autopsy gel. This gel should also be placed on the reflected scalp.
15. Fill the cavities with an absorbent sheeting that can also be soaked with cavity fluid. The neck areas can be filled with cotton or kapoc to achieve a natural look. If the viscera is being returned to the cavities the neck will have to be filled out with cotton or kapoc. Likewise, the pelvic cavity should be filled with cotton or kapoc. Place the bag containing the viscera into the cavities. A minimum of two bottles of concentrated cavity fluid should be poured into the bag over the viscera.*
16. Suture the abdominal and thoracic cavities closed. Use a strong linen thread. The baseball suture provides an airtight suture.
17. Anchor the calvarium into position. Suture the scalp closed beginning on the right side of the head and ending on the left. A worm suture helps to stretch the scalp tissue.
18. Wash the body and hair. The body and hair should be thoroughly dried and the body should be turned and dried underneath.
19. Apply a surface sealer to the autopsy sutures of the thorax and abdomen.
20. Glue the mouth and eyes.
21. Place the body in plastic garments. Place some embalming powder into the garments.
22. The body is now ready for cosmetic application and dressing.

*There are several types of visceral treatments.

▶ PREPARATION OF THE BODY FOR IDENTIFICATION AND/OR STORAGE

Permission is necessary for embalming of the body. This permission can be oral, faxed, or in writing. If verbal permission has been given, it should later be confirmed in written form whenever possible. There may be a long or short delay by a funeral establishment between obtaining the body and receiving permission to embalm it. The body can be placed in storage until permission to embalm is obtained and/or details of disposition can be arranged. Many funeral establishments and almost all embalming centers have storage coolers. The proper topical sanitation and preparation of the body for storage will allow the body to later be (1) identified by the person or persons in charge of disposition, or (2) embalmed (when permission is given) for identification only, viewing, presence at funeral ceremonies without viewing, immediate disposition, or shipping to another location. Bodies placed in storage where embalming is a possibility should be stored with the head and shoulders elevated; this will lessen blood discolorations in the face and neck (Figure 2–2). If the body is only to be identified by the family or family representative for immediate cremation or burial, and the proper permission is obtained for cavity embalming only, this will lessen the degree of blood discolorations in the face and neck; lessen gas distention of the cavities; and lessen the possibility of purge. If there is a possibility that permission will be obtained for arterial embalming, no cavity treatment should be performed for this would later interfere with the arterial embalming of the body. Autopsied bodies can follow the same storage protocol.

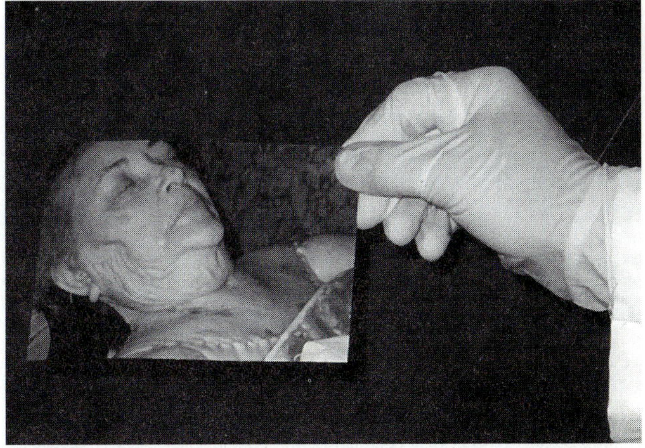

Figure 2–2. Use of Poloroid photo for cremation or burial identification.

Refrigeration Storage and Identification

1. Remove all clothing and personal effects from the deceased.
2. Do not remove identification tags or bracelets.
3. Disinfect and pack all orifices; disinfect the body surface.
4. Remove oropharyngeal tubes, gastric tubes, medical apparatus, bandages, and dressings. If the body is to only be identified for cremation or burial, and permission has been given, cavity aspiration and injection can be done at this time.
5. Do not remove circulatory invasive devices such as IV tubes; these can be taped in place, lessening exposure to blood. The body is easier to embalm with these in place; after arterial embalming they can be removed.
6. Remove the pacemaker if present (with permission).
7. Bathe the remains; wash hair and groom nails.
8. Shave and set the features.
9. Glue features. Place a light coating of massage cream on the face, neck, and hands.
10. Tape, bandage, superglue, or suture any leakage sites.
11. Place plastic pants or coveralls on the body with some embalming powder in them.
12. Place a clean gown on the body and attach an ID tag to the arm or foot.
13. Place a plastic sheet over a cloth sheet (a clean body bag can also be used).
14. Place the body on the plastic and cloth sheets and wrap the remains.
15. Tie the body with cloth strips at the feet, waist, and above the head; *do not tie* around neck. Keep sheets *loose* around the face.
16. Attach an ID tag to the wrapped remains and a biohazard tag if the body is not embalmed. Identify the body as "unembalmed" and "caution blood/body infectious material" (Figure 2–3).

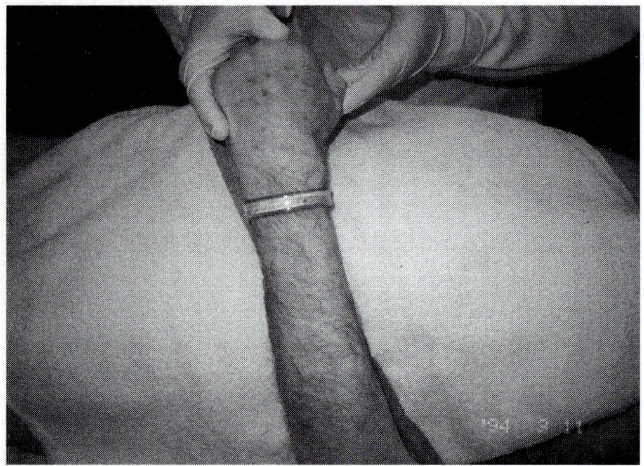
A

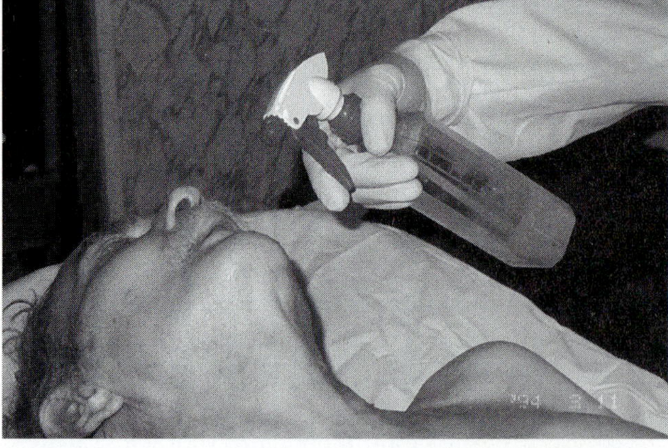
B

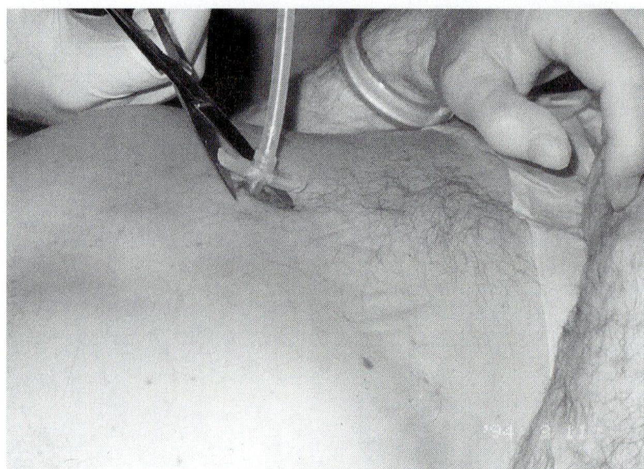
C

Figure 2–3. A. Identification band remains on the body. **B.** Topical disinfection. **C.** Removal of gastric tube.

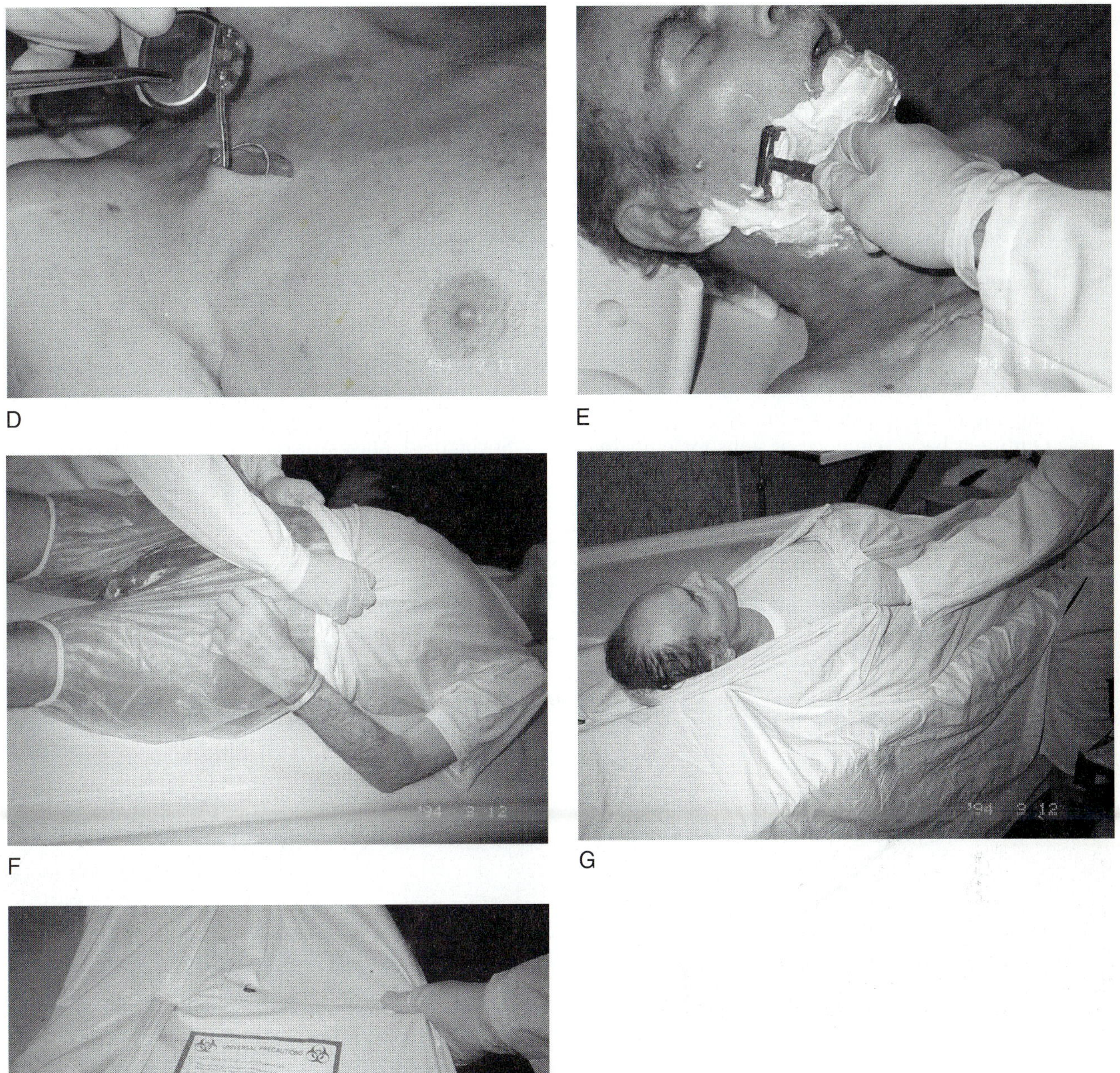

H

Figure 2–3. (*Continued*) **D.** Removal of pacemaker. **E.** Shaving and setting features. **F.** Partial dressing using plastic pants. **G.** Cotton sheet placed around body enveloped in a body storage bag. **H.** Biohazard and identification label for storage.

▶ KEY TERMS AND CONCEPTS FOR STUDY AND DISCUSSION

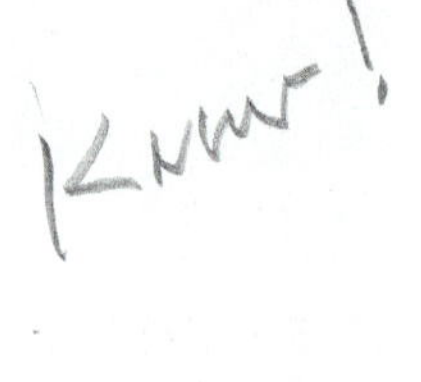

1. Define the following terms.
   - Arterial embalming
   - Cavity embalming
   - Embalming
   - Hypodermic embalming
   - Preservation
   - Supplemental embalming
   - Surface embalming
2. List and define the three primary objectives accomplished by embalming.
3. Outline a basic sequence of steps for the embalming of the unautopsied body.
4. Outline a basic sequence of steps for embalming the autopsied body.
5. Outline a basic sequence of steps for the preparation of a body for identification for immediate cremation; and when no permission for any type of embalming has been granted.

▶ BIBLIOGRAPHY

Dorn J, Hopkins B. Thanatochemistry, 2 ed. Upper Saddle River, NJ: Prentice Hall; 1998.

Dhonau CO. Manual of Case Analysis. Cincinnati, Oh: 1924.

Embalming Course Content Syllabus. Brunswick, Me: American Board of Funeral Service Education; 1996.

Merriam Webster's Collegiate Dictionary, 10th ed. Springfield, Mass: Merriam-Webster; 1993.

Pervier NC. Textbook of Chemistry for Embalmers. Minneapolis: University of Minnesota; 1961.

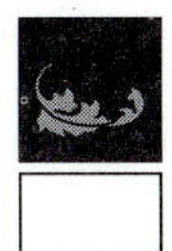

CHAPTER 3
PERSONAL AND PUBLIC HEALTH CONSIDERATIONS

Embalming has historically encompassed principles and practices that are part of public health. The process of disinfecting and preserving dead human bodies raises a number of health issues for individuals engaged in embalming and for public health in general.

The embalmer is professionally responsible for a two-tiered spectrum: (1) public health safety, (2) personal health safety. Both levels of responsibility involve the maintenance of a work environment that is hygienically clean and safe. Through efforts to create and maintain such an environment, the embalmer protects both public and personal health. The "at risk" nature of preparing human remains for disposition has been documented in the medical and public health literature.

▶ OCCUPATIONAL RISKS

Exposure to Biological Hazards

A 1996 Centers for Disease Control and Prevention (CDC) study reported that there is ample reason for concern about the exposure embalmers have to bloodborne and airborne pathogens (McKenna and coworkers, 1996). The CDC analyzed the risk for tuberculosis by determining potential exposure within certain occupational groups, based on historical observation, and the impact that infection within a group could have on public health. The occupational groups were first categorized by their level of risk. The researchers then applied a statistical formula to estimate the number of tuberculosis cases that could be expected within each occupation group. A comparison of the number of cases predicted by statistical formula for an occupational group, and the number of actual cases that were reported for each occupational group showed a strong relationship between occupation and the risk of contracting tuberculosis.

> A notable exception to the association between occupational SES (socioeconomic status) and tuberculosis was the occupation of 'Funeral director.' Even though this occupation was included in the highest SES category of 'Executives, administrative and managerial occupations,' 16 cases were allocated to this occupation where only 4.1 were expected (McKenna and associates, 1996, p. 590).

The CDC concluded that funeral directors had an elevated risk of contracting tuberculosis as a result of their contact with dead human bodies.

Gershon and colleagues (1998) reported the results in a Johns Hopkins University study which concluded that funeral home employees who worked as embalmers had a greater exposure to tuberculosis than funeral home employees who did not embalm bodies. The study found that 101 out of 864 (11.7%) funeral home employees who volunteered to be tested reacted to a tuberculin skin test. It was determined that funeral home employees who engaged in embalming were twice as likely to have a positive tuberculin skin test when compared to funeral home employees who did not embalm bodies.

Beck-Sague and co-workers (1991) also addressed the potential for occupationally acquired infections among embalmers. In particular, this study suggested that embalmers were at potential risk of acquiring infection as a result of their frequent contact with blood (Figure 3–1). This study reported that 89 of 539 (17%) morticians who responded to a survey reported contracting infectious diseases attributed to their occupation. Among the most frequently reported diseases in the study were hepatitis, staphylococcal and other skin infections, and pulmonary and skin tuberculosis. The most commonly reported exposure was by skin contact with blood (393 out of 539, or 73%). Needle sticks were far more common than cuts. Of the 539 morticians who responded to the survey, 212 (39%) reported a needle stick within the 12 months prior to the survey, while 61 (11%) morticians reported having been cut.

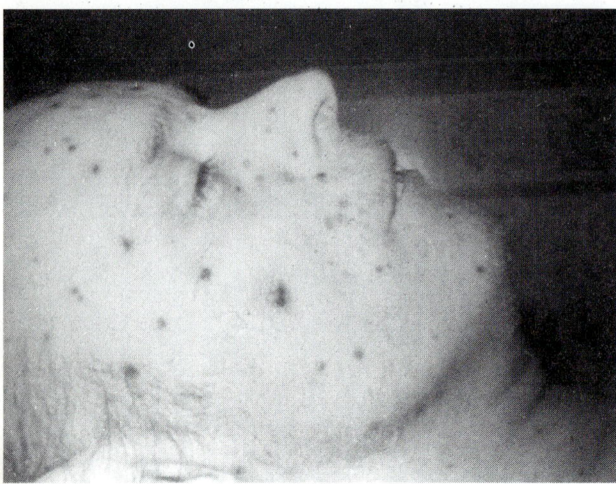

Figure 3–1. Secondary infection. Cause of death was listed as leukemia; however, the individual also exhibits the secondary infection of chicken pox.

Turner and colleagues (1989) reported that embalmers in the Boston area were about two times more likely to test positive for hepatitis B (HBV) infection than a blood donor comparison group. The study also reported that the length of time a person had been working as an embalmer elevated the risk of contracting an HBV infection.

McDonald (1989) published an editorial which stated that embalmers face much the same risk of exposure to infectious diseases as clinical pathologists. The basis of this finding was the common exposure to blood and body fluids for both pathologists and embalmers.

Exposure to Chemical Hazards

The objectives of the embalming process are to disinfect, preserve, and sanitize the body. These objectives are accomplished by the application of chemicals. Many of the chemicals used in embalming and related processes have been categorized, or contain components that have been categorized, as hazardous substances. Hazards associated with using these substances have been well documented in the health and medical literature.

A study conducted by Williams and associates (1984) stated that exposure to formaldehyde, particularly formaldehyde vapor, is probably the most significant of the chemical exposures to which embalmers are subjected. Over the years, a number of other studies have reported on the adverse effects of chronic exposure to formaldehyde (Kerfoot, 1972; Kerfoot & Mooney, 1975; Bender et al, 1983).

Nethercott and Holness (1988) noted that Canadian funeral service workers were more likely to complain about irritations of the nose and eyes than were members of a control group. The study went on to say that those funeral service employees who were in contact with formaldehyde were likely to experience skin and mucous membrane irritation.

Many of the chemicals used in embalming are regulated by state and Federal Occupational Safety and Health Administration (OSHA) standards. Hazardous substance standards adopted in Minnesota, for example, contain a list of nearly 1100 substances controlled because of the hazards that result from their use (State of Minnesota, 1995). Many of the substances on that list are used in the embalming process, or are components of products used in the embalming process. Most notable among the health problems that can result from chemicals in the preparation room are contact dermatitis, eye and nose irritations, and upper respiratory irritations.

Exposure to Other Hazards of Embalming

In addition to the hazards associated with biological and chemical agents, embalmers are exposed to hazards including: heat, ionizing radiation, and non-ionizing radiation. Although these hazards may not be as prevalent as chemical or biological hazards, they are worth noting, and may necessitate action by a funeral home.

Heat. Funeral homes must give consideration to the ventilation and temperature in the embalming room. If the temperature of a room is high, an embalmer wearing a full set of personal protective equipment (PPE) may have difficulty ventilating body heat. This can result in an elevation of core body temperature. Some PPEs can trap body heat within them and that, coupled with any combination of high room temperature, inadequate ventilation, and high humidity can cause some embalmers to feel discomfort, or even lead to fainting.

Ionizing Radiation. There is the possibility that an embalmer might come into contact with a body that has undergone radiation therapy. Hospitals and clinics that administer radiation treatments are supposed to monitor radiation levels. Bodies that have undergone radiation treatment should not be released until such time that they no longer pose a hazard. If embalmers have questions or concerns about radiation exposure, they should contact the radiation officer at a local hospital, clinic, or contact government agencies that have authority in matters related to radiation exposure.

Non-ionizing Radiation. The possibility of adverse exposure to non-ionizing radiation is remote. Exposure could result from electromagnetic radiation given off by microwave ovens or computer monitors. Although it is unlikely that either of these sources would cause a major health concern for embalmers, it is still appropriate for funeral homes to consider exposures of this nature.

▶ DEALING WITH EXPOSURE TO EMBALMING HAZARDS

Biological Hazards

Health and safety issues associated with embalming are addressed by compliance with *The Bloodborne Pathogen Rule.* The Bloodborne Pathogen Rule is administered by the United States Department of Labor through OSHA. The rule is directly applicable to occupations and professions, including funeral service, where employees are exposed to infectious agents. In addition, many individual states have enacted *employee right-to-know* laws that support or expand the scope of federal OSHA regulations. Embalmers must be aware of the duties and responsibilities that are imposed on them by the laws and rules of the various jurisdictions within which they practice. Compliance with the Bloodborne Pathogen Rule, and any state regulations that support or expand it, is required.

Under the Bloodborne Pathogen Rule, employers are required to conduct an evaluation of their workplace(s) to determine if employees have occupational exposure to infectious agents regulated by OSHA. If such exposure exists, a written *Exposure Control Plan* must be developed to control, minimize, or eliminate employee exposure. Exposure control plans, which by law must be accessible to employees, are to be reviewed and updated at least once per year so that changes in personnel, procedure, and/or work assignments can be documented. The minimum documentation required for an Exposure Control Plan includes exposure determination, methods of compliance, hepatitis B vaccination and postexposure evaluation and follow up, hazard communication, and record keeping.

Exposure Determination. Employers are required to examine workplace(s) to determine (1) if occupational exposure to bloodborne pathogens exists, and (2) what types of duties are being performed when occupational exposure to bloodborne pathogens occurs. If occupational exposure to bloodborne pathogens is identified, employers must then list all job titles or classifications which have exposure. In a funeral home setting this might include, but not be limited to, embalmers, intern/apprentice embalmers, removal personnel, and any other person having direct contact with unembalmed human remains, or with any regulated infectious waste materials. Employers must also identify those employees who have "some" occupational exposure to infectious agents. This might include, but not be limited to, hairdressers, housekeepers, maintenance personnel, funeral directors, drivers, and clerical staff. Employers must identify and list duties that involve exposure to infectious agents. Examples of duties that might appear on such a list include removal of human remains, embalming, hairdressing, cosmetizing, and laundry.

Methods of Compliance. Compliance with the Bloodborne Pathogen Rule is accomplished by the application of (1) universal precautions, (2) engineering controls, and (3) work practice controls. The basic premise of *universal precautions* is for the embalmer to treat all human remains as if they were infected with HIV, HBV, or other pathogens. In other words, the embalmer should treat all bodies with the same caution that would be applied for extremely hazardous, potentially fatal infections. By the implementation of this extreme caution the embalmer attempts "To prevent parenteral, mucous membrane, and non-intact skin exposure" (Code of Federal Regulations, 1992). In other words, the embalmer will avoid needle sticks or cuts, which create parenteral exposure by breaking the protective barrier provided by the skin. The embalmer will also avoid other situations that might result in ingestion of contaminated material through the nose or mouth. The embalmer must take care to avoid allowing infectious agents to invade through the eyes, or be absorbed through or otherwise penetrate the skin. Care must also be taken to prevent infectious agents from invading the host by means of an existing break in the skin, such as cuts, scratches, and so on. To seek protection from possible infection, the embalmer will (1) utilize personal protective equipment, (2) properly decontaminate infected surfaces, (3) properly handle and dispose of infectious wastes, (4) apply appropriate measures to control leaks, drips, and spills of infectious materials, (5) apply proper work practice skills, and (6) properly handle contaminated laundry.

Engineering controls are those mechanical systems and devices engineered into the architecture of a building. Engineering controls that are used to provide personal and public health protection should be examined and maintained or replaced on a regular schedule. Doing so will insure that the systems and devices are offering the most effective means to reduce exposure. The two primary areas of consideration are *adequate ventilation*, and *proper plumbing.*

During embalming there is a possibility that infectious agents can become aerosolized or in some other way become airborne. The purpose of adequate ventilation is to remove contaminated air from the work area and replace it with fresh air. The most important factor in the ventilation system is the location of the exhaust. It should be at the foot of the embalming table and below the level of the tabletop. The air replacement or intake should ideally be high on the opposite wall. Thus, fresh air is being blown toward the embalmer while potentially contaminated air is being drawn down and away from the embalmer's breathing zone (Figure 3–2).

The number of air exchanges per hour may be determined by (1) the contents of the room, (2) whether more than one embalming will be in progress at the same time, (3) the shape of the room, and (4) other factors, such as hot or cold weather or the preference of the embalmer. As a rough rule of thumb, for a single-table room, the number of air changes ranges from 12 to 20 per hour. The Public Health Guidelines have recommended that a ventilation system create a minimum of six air changes per hour, and preferably more in the preparation room environment.

Proper plumbing plays an important role in insuring that infectious substances and materials commonly associated with embalming do not find their way into the public water supply. Examples of engineering controls that could reduce the possibility of water contamination might include (1) vacuum breakers on the main water line leading into the building, (2) vacuum breakers on hydroaspirators, (3) discharge basins/flush sinks that are in good working order, (4) having a suitable water source for the preparation table, (5) having a proper eye wash station, (6) having a proper drench shower, (7) having a proper hand washing station, and (8) having proper shower room facilities for embalmers to use after the embalming is completed.

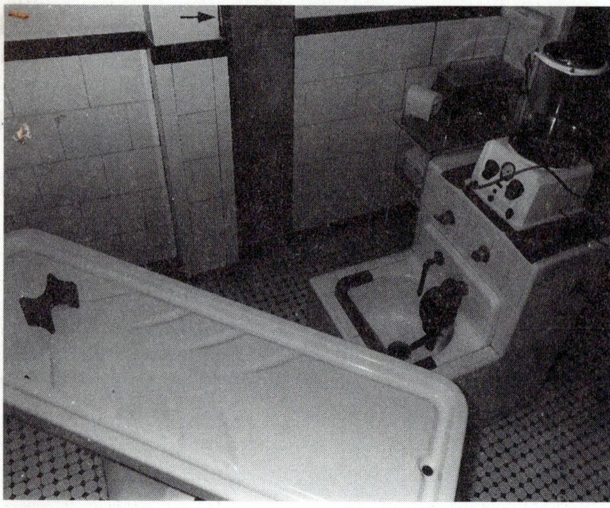

Figure 3–2. Note the exhaust duct against the back wall. It exhausts fumes from the floor level.

Devices such as vacuum breakers on aspiration equipment and on water lines leading into the funeral home help to contain the threat that any contaminated material could be back-syphoned from the preparation room to other water lines. In many instances, funeral homes may find that local and state authorities have extensive plumbing codes that must be satisfied for the protection of public health.

In addition to providing protection for building or public water supplies, plumbing considerations can also assist embalmers in keeping their work areas as clean and hygienic as possible. Adequate water service to preparation room equipment and embalming tables, and suitable sinks or flush basins can offer important aids to sanitation and hygiene.

Work Practice Controls. Work practice controls are common sense steps taken to avoid unnecessary or excessive exposure to infectious agents. Common work practices that contribute to a hygienic environment include (1) hand washing, (2) proper handling and disposal of contaminated waste and contaminated sharps, (3) avoiding splashing, spraying, or splattering when working with potentially infectious agents, (4) consistent and proper use of personal protective equipment, and (5) adequate housekeeping, including a written record of housekeeping provisions. Work practice controls must be spelled out and enforced. Such controls would include immediate hand washing after removal of gloves. Employees must receive training and instruction on the use and accessibility of PPE, cleaning and laundering procedures, repair and replacement procedures, procedures to follow when personal protective equipment is contaminated or damaged while in use, and procedures for the proper storage of personal protective equipment.

Employers are required to provide appropriate PPE suitable in terms of size, use, and application. Personal protective equipment is considered to be appropriate only if it prevents blood or other potentially infectious substances from passing through, or otherwise reaching, the employee's work clothes, street clothes, undergarments, skin, eyes, mouth, or other mucous membranes under normal conditions of time and use. Further, employers are required to see that employees who are performing duties where there is exposure wear the provided PPE. Personal protective equipment should literally cover the embalmer from head to toe. During embalming, the embalmer should wear a surgical cap, hood, or other suitable head covering. All hair should be tucked up underneath the head covering. The mouth, nose, and chin should be covered by a surgical mask. The embalmer's forehead, cheeks, and neck should be protected by a face shield. The eyes should be protected by goggles. The arms, torso, and

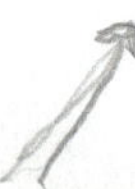

legs should be protected by a garment or combination of garments that provide suitable coverage. The feet should be covered by suitable foot coverings. A rule of thumb for protective garments is to have *no* exposed skin. Employers must make arrangements for cleaning, laundering, or otherwise disposing of contaminated PPE. In addition, employers must make arrangements for damaged PPE to be repaired or replaced (Figure 3–3).

All PPE must be removed immediately on leaving the work area and placed in a designated area or container for storage, washing, decontamination, or disposal. Used needles and other sharps should not be sheared, bent, broken, recapped, or resheathed by hand. Sharps are to disposed in closable, puncture-resistant, disposable containers that are leakproof on the sides and bottom and that bear proper warning labels or are color coded (red). Eating, drinking, smoking, application of personal beauty products, and handling of contact lenses are prohibited in work areas. No food or drink should be stored in refrigerators where blood is stored or in other areas of possible contamination. All procedures involving blood or other potentially infectious body fluids should be performed in such a manner as to minimize splashing, spraying, and aerosolization.

Employers must ensure that work areas are maintained in a clean and sanitary condition, in accordance with a written schedule for cleaning and disinfection. This could be on completion of embalming or at the end of the work shift. All instruments, equipment, and environmental and working surfaces must be property cleaned and disinfected after contact with blood or other potentially infectious materials. All pails, containers, and receptacles intended for reuse that have a potential for becoming contaminated with blood or other potentially infectious materials should be inspected, cleaned, and disinfected on a regular basis or as soon as possible on visible contamination.

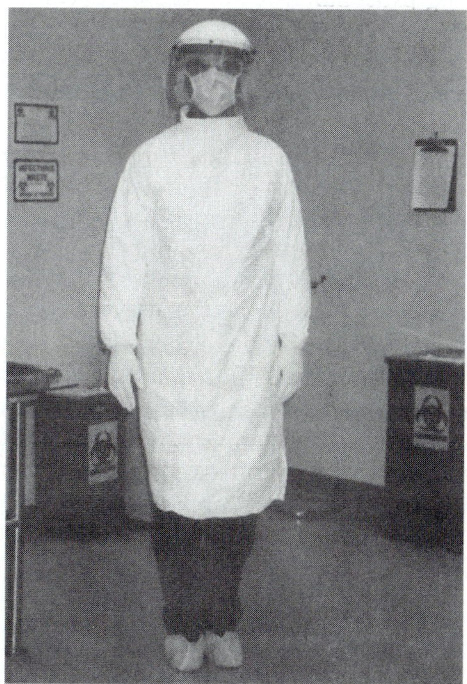

Figure 3–3. Attired embalmer.

Hepatitis B Vaccination. Hepatitis B vaccination must be made available to all employees who have occupational exposure. The vaccination program must be (1) offered at no cost to the employee, (2) offered at a reasonable time and place, (3) performed by or under the supervision of a licensed physician, or by or under the supervision of another licensed healthcare professional, and (4) provided according to the recommendations of the U.S. Public Health Service. Employees have the option of accepting or declining the vaccination. If the employee is offered vaccination but declines, a special declination statement should be signed by the employee to document the offer and the choice to decline. If an employee first declines hepatitis B vaccination, but later decides to accept, the declination document is discarded, and the employee must be given the vaccination.

Postexposure Evaluation and Follow Up. In the event an exposure incident occurs, employers must immediately implement procedures for postexposure evaluation and follow up. The postexposure evaluation and follow up will include (1) a detailed explanation of the events and circumstances of the exposure, (2) identification and documentation of the source individual, unless doing so is impossible or prohibited by law, (3) collecting and testing of blood for HBV and HIV, (4) taking steps necessary to assist in the prevention of infection or disease, (5) offering counseling, and (6) conducting an evaluation of any reported illnesses.

Hazard Communication. The following can be used to label or distinguish containers used to store, transport or ship blood or other potentially infectious agents: (1) fluorescent orange labels, (2) orange and red labels, (3) predominantly orange and red warning labels, (4) labels with lettering and symbols in contrasting colors, or (5) other suitable substitutes for labels, such as red bags or red containers. The labels used to mark infectious hazards must include the legend shown in Figure 3–4.

In addition to the labeling provisions required by the Bloodborne Pathogen Rule, employers must also provide information and training to those employees who are exposed to infectious hazards in the workplace. Employers will ensure that all employees with occupational exposure receive training related to bloodborne pathogens, and training on methods for dealing with

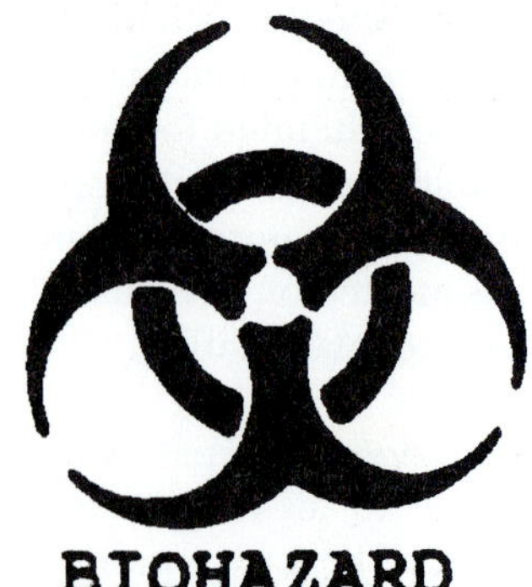

Figure 3–4. BioHazzard symbol.

infectious agents. The training must be given at or before the time the employee is assigned a task where exposure exists. Training updates must be repeated at least once per year.

The training program must contain the following components.

1. A copy of the regulatory text must be readily available and accessible to employees.
2. A general explanation of the epidemiology and symptoms of bloodborne diseases must be provided.
3. An explanation of the modes of transmission of bloodborne pathogens must be provided. To satisfy the need for information about epidemiology, symptoms and modes of transmission, books such as *Control of Communicable Diseases Manual* (Benenson, 1995) have become commonplace in funeral homes as resources that satisfy OSHA compliance standards. This type of reference material provides ready access to information helpful in the identification of infectious agents, as well as information related to the occurrence; reservoir; mode of transmission; incubation period; period of communicability, susceptibility and resistance; and methods of control.
4. An explanation of the employer's exposure control plan and the means by which the employee can obtain a copy of the written plan must be provided.
5. An explanation of the appropriate methods for recognizing tasks and other activities that may involve exposure to blood and other potentially infectious materials must be provided.
6. An explanation of the use and limitations of methods that will prevent or reduce exposure, including appropriate use of engineering controls, work practice controls, and universal precautions must be provided.
7. Information on the types, proper use, location, removal, handling, decontamination, and disposal of PPE.
8. An explanation of the basis for selection of PPE.
9. Information on the hepatitis B vaccine, including information on its efficacy, safety, method of administration, the benefits of being vaccinated, and that the vaccine and vaccination will be offered free of charge.
10. Information on the appropriate actions to take and persons to contact in an emergency involving blood or other potentially infectious materials.
11. An explanation of the procedure to follow if an exposure incident occurs, including the method of reporting the incident and the medical follow up that will be made available.
12. Information on the postexposure evaluation and follow up required after an exposure incident.
13. An explanation of the signs, labels, and color coding used to mark biohazardous materials and containers.
14. An opportunity for interactive questions and answers with the person conducting the training session.

Record Keeping. Employers are responsible for establishing and maintaining accurate records for each employee with occupational exposure to bloodborne pathogens. The record must contain (1) the name and social security number of the employee, (2) a copy of the employee's hepatitis B vaccination, (3) results of any examinations, medical testing, and follow up procedures that occurred as a result of an exposure incident, (4) employer's copy of any healthcare professional's written opinion regarding examinations, medical testing or follow up in the aftermath of an exposure incident, and (5) a copy of the healthcare professional's report of any examinations, medical testing, or follow up in the aftermath of an exposure incident.

Employers must maintain records of each training session. Training records are to be kept for a period of 3 years from the date the training occurred. The record must include (1) the date of each training session, (2) a summary of each training session, (3) the name(s) and qualification(s) of trainer(s), and (4) the names and job titles of all persons attending each training session. Employers are required to make all records available to the employees or their representatives. If employment is terminated or if the employee transfers to another location or employer, the training records must be made available to the new location or employer. If an employer ceases to operate and has no successor, OSHA must be notified so that records can

TABLE 3–1. BREAKING THE CYCLE OF TRANSMISSION OF INFECTIOUS AGENTS IN THE PREPARATION ROOM: PUBLIC HEALTH GUIDELINES FOR THE AT-RISK EMBALMER "HOST"

Portal of "Host" Entry	Infectious Agent
Skin or mucous membrane respiratory tract, alimentary tract, body openings—natural and/ or artificial (abrasions, cuts, lacerations, wounds)	Bacteria, fungi (molds and yeasts), viruses, rickettsia, protozoa
Proper "barrier" attire	Personal health practices
Aseptic technique(s)	Personnel health policies
Handwashing, gloves	Environmental sanitation
Disinfection and decontamination	Disinfection and decontamination
Modes of Transmitting the Infectious Agent	**Reservoirs of Infectious Agents in the Preparation Room**
Direct contact (aerosol or droplet infection) and indirect contact (air, contaminated surfaces) and objects or fomites, body fluids and exudates, insects	Remains, equipment (e.g., hydroaspirators, trocars, razors), instruments, adjacent hard surfaces, air contaminated linens, bandages and dressings, solid and liquid wastes
Proper "barrier" attire Handwashing, gloves Proper disposition of wastes Effective air handling system Concurrent and terminal disinfection	

Note: Proper "barrier" attire may include whole-body covering, head cover, shoe covers, gloves, oral–nasal mask, and eye protection (safety glasses).

be transferred to an appropriate place and filed for future use.

Embalmers have to make judgements about exposure to potentially infectious agents. Information is vital to the decision making process, and embalmers should have access to as much information as possible.

The assumption in the embalming process is that all bodies contain infectious agents and, therefore, represent reservoirs in which infectious agents can be found. Inasmuch as the embalming procedure is invasive, it is a given that infectious agents will escape from the body during embalming. The embalmer represents a potential host for the escaped infectious agents because the embalmer will be in direct contact with any infectious agents that are released from the body. In spite of the exposure, infectious agents can be pre-

TABLE 3–2. ACTIVITY LEVELS OF SELECTED MICROBICIDES

Liquid Microbicide[a]	Use Concentration	Activity Level
Glutaraldehyde, aqueous, e.g., Cidex, Sonacide, Sporicidin	2.0%	High
Formaldehyde + alcohol	8.0% + 70.0%	High
Stabilized hydrogen peroxide	6.0–10.0%	High
Formaldehyde, aqueous	3.0–8.0%	High to intermediate
Iodophors, e.g., Betadine, Wescodyne, HiSine, Iosan	75–200 ppm	Intermediate
Iodine + alcohol	0.5% + 70.0%	Intermediate
Chlorine compounds, e.g., sodium hypochlorite as in chlorine bleach	1000–5000 ppm	Intermediate
Phenolic compounds, aqueous, e.g., Amphyl Staphene, O-Syl	0.5–3.0%	Intermediate to low
Quaternary ammonium compounds, e.g., Phemoral, Zepharin Chloride, Diaparine Chloride	0.1–0.2% aqueous	Low
Mercurial compounds, organic and inorganic, e.g., Merthiolate, Mercurochrome, Metaphen	0.1–0.2%	Low

[a] Trade names of certain microbicides are given.
From Block SS: Disinfection, Sterilization, and Preservation. 3rd ed. Philadelphia: Lea & Febiger; 1983, with permission.

TABLE 3–3. ACCEPTABLE ANTIMICROBIAL PROCEDURES/EXPOSURE INTERVALS

	Vegetative Bacteria and Fungi, Influenza Viruses	Tubercle Bacilli, Enteroviruses Except Hepatitis Viruses, Vegetative Bacteria and Fungi, Influenza Viruses	Bacterial and Fungal Spores, Hepatitis Viruses, Tubercle Bacilli, Enteroviruses, Vegetative Bacteria and Fungi, Influenza Viruses
Objects	*Disinfection*	*Disinfection*	*Sterilization*
Smooth, hard surface objects	A—10 min D—5 min E—10 min F—10 min H—10 min L—5 min M—5 min	B—10 min D—10 min G—10 min H—10 min L—10 min M—10 min	D—18 h J K L—9 h M—10 h
Rubber tubing, rubber catheters	E—10 min F—10 min H—10 min	G—10 min H—10 min	J[a] K
Polyethylene tubing, polyethylene catheters	A—10 min E—10 min F—10 min H—10 min	B—10 min G—10 min H—10 min	D—18 h J[a] K L—9 h M—10 h
Lensed instruments	E—10 min F—10 min H—10 min K M—10 min	K M—10 min	K
Hypodermic needles	Sterilization only	Sterilization only	J
Thermometers[b]	C—10 min K	C—10 min K	D—18 h L—9 h M—10 h
Hinged instruments	A—20 min D—10 min E—20 min F—20 min H—20 min L—10 min M—10 min	B—30 min D—20 min G—30 min H—30 min L—20 min M—20 min	J K L—9 h M—10 h
Floors, furniture, other appropriate room surfaces	E—5 min F—5 min H—5 min I—5 min	G—5 min H—5 min	Not necessary or practical

Key

A. Isopropyl alcohol (70–90%) plus 0.2% sodium nitrite to prevent corrosion
B. Ethyl alcohol (70–90%)
C. Isopropyl or ethyl alcohol plus 0.2% iodine
D. Formaldehyde (8%)—alchol solution plus 0.2% sodium nitrite to prevent corrosion
E. Quaternary ammonium solutions (1:500 aq.) plus 0.2% sodium nitrite to prevent corrosion
F. Iodophor—75 ppm available iodine plus 0.2% sodium nitrite to prevent corrosion
G. Iodophor—450 ppm available iodine plus 0.2% sodium nitrite to prevent corrosion
H. Phenolic solutions (2% aq.) plus 0.5% sodium bicarbonate to prevent corrosion
I. Sodium hypochlorite (1:500 aq.—approx. 100 ppm)[a]
J. Heat sterilization } see manufacturers' recommendations
K. Ethylene oxide gas } or technical literature
L. Aqueous formalin (40%)
M. Activated glutaraldehyde (2% aq.)

[a] Investigate thermostability when indicated.

[b] Must be thoroughly wiped, preferably with tincture of soap, before disinfection or sterilization. Alcohol–iodine solution will remove markings on poor-grade thermometers.

Note: 1000 ppm of available chlorine is recommended for inactivation of hepatitis B virus and 5000 ppm for inactivation of HIV (AIDS). Thoroughly rinse all inanimate surfaces of any excess formalin prior to application of the hypochlorite disinfectant. Keene (1973) cautions that when formaldehyde reacts with hydrochloric acid, the compound bischloromethyl ether (BCME) may be formed. BCME is a highly toxic, carcinogenic compound.

vented from entering the embalmer with the proper application of work practice controls, engineering controls, and universal precautions. In addition to the controls and physical barriers that can be utilized to protect the embalmer, it is important for the embalmer to maintain good personal health to maintain resistance to infection.

Decontamination of instruments, equipment, the work area, and the body are important weapons in the fight against infectious diseases. In preparation room settings where exposure levels are high, decontamination is accomplished by using physical or chemical means (Table 3–1).

Good work practices and universal precautions would dictate that the body, instruments, equipment, counter tops, table tops, walls, floors, sinks, cabinets, and waste receptacles be sanitized and disinfected. Disinfection and decontamination activity should occur as necessary during an embalming procedure, concurrent disinfection and decontamination, and then be done thoroughly at the completion of the embalming process, terminal disinfection and decontamination.

The human remains should be thoroughly cleaned and bathed with disinfectant soap and topical disinfectant in the initial steps of the embalming process. Concurrent cleaning and bathing should occur during the embalming process, followed by another thorough bathing with disinfectant soap and another application of topical disinfectant at the conclusion of the embalming process.

Embalmers could consider steam sterilization, or *autoclaving*, for contaminated instruments, *or* immersion of instruments in a suitable cold chemical sterilant. Embalmers will find a number of commercially prepared cold chemical sterilants on the market (e.g., Cidex, Sonacide). These cold chemical sterilants have formulations containing acid glutaraldehyde, or alkalinized glutaraldehyde, or formaldehyde in ethanol or isopropanol as their active ingredients (Table 3–2). All other contaminated surfaces should be cleaned, sanitized, disinfected, and decontaminated with a suitable disinfectant solution or topical disinfectant (Table 3–3).

The following terms are commonly associated with methods of disinfection and sterilization (Table 3–4).

Asepsis—freedom from infection and from any form of life; sterility.

Bactericidal—destructive to bacteria.

Bacteriostatic—inhibiting the growth or multiplication of bacteria (no destruction of viability implied).

Cleaning—removal of infectious agents by scrubbing and washing, as with hot water, soap, or a suitable detergent.

TABLE 3–4. CHEMICAL AND PHYSICAL METHODS FOR CONTROLLING MICROBIAL CONTAMINATION

Method of Decontamination	Temperature Requirement	Minimum Interval of Exposure (min): 0 2 10 12 15 20 90 120 150 180
Sterilization: Complete destruction of all forms of microbial life	285°F (140°C)	(instant)
Saturated steam under pressure (autoclaving)	270°F (132°C)	
	250°F (121°C)	30 min for hepatitis viruses
Ethylene oxide gas	130°F (54°C)	2 to 12 h
Hot air, e.g., oven	320°F (160°C)	2 h or more
Chemical sporicide solution, e.g., 8.0% formaldehyde plus 70% isopropanol, glutaraldehyde[a]	Room temperature	3 to 12 h … or more
Disinfection: killing of disease-producing microbial agents, but not resistant spores		
Boiling water or free-flowing steam	212°F (100°C)	or more, 30 min for hepatitis viruses
Chemical germicide solutions, e.g., iodophors, phenylphenols, quarternary ammonium compounds	Room temperature	or more
Sanitization: Chemicals aided by physical methods of soil removal	Maximum of 200°F (93°C)	

[a]Recommended for high-level disinfection.
Modified from a chart copyrighted in 1967, Research and Development Section, American Sterilizer Co., Erie, PA.

Disinfectant—an agent, usually chemical, applied to inanimate objects/surfaces for the purpose of destroying disease causing microbial agents, but usually not bacterial spores.

Germicide—an agent, usually chemical, applied either to inanimate objects/surfaces or living tissue for the purpose of destroying disease-causing microbial agents, but usually not bacterial spores.

Sanitizer—an agent, usually chemical, that possesses disinfecting properties when applied to a pre-cleaned object/surface.

Sterilization—a process that renders a substance free of all microorganisms.

▶ HAZARD COMMUNICATION

Chemical Hazards

The Federal government has mandated that business and industry, including funeral service, comply with regulations related to the safe handling and use of hazardous substances and materials. The Federal *Hazard Communication Rule* requires that employers communicate to employees the dangers that exist in the workplace as a result of hazardous substances or materials, and directs employers to train employees in the safe use and handling of hazardous substances or materials (Code of Federal Regulations, 1988). Under the Hazard Communication Rule, any chemical or mixture of chemicals that expose employees to a health or physical risk are considered to be hazardous. Mixtures of chemicals with a composition of 0.1% or more of an ingredient(s) classified as a carcinogen, teratogen, or mutagen are considered to present a physical or health hazard. Mixtures of chemicals with a composition of 1.0% of an ingredient(s) which, although not being classified as a carcinogen, teratogen, or mutagen, are classified as hazardous substances are considered to present a physical or health hazard. Information about the hazards of using certain materials or substances is provided by *Material Safety Data Sheets* (MSDS), labeling, and training.

Material Safety Data Sheets. The Hazard Communication Rule requires manufacturers or suppliers of hazardous materials or substances to include an MSDS with each shipment. The MSDS contains critical information related to the hazards, exposure levels, and symptoms associated with the material or substance. An MSDS must be kept on file for each hazardous substance or material present in the work area, and must be accessible to employees (Figure 3–5).

Labeling. Under the Hazard Communication Rule, all containers that hold hazardous substances or materials must be properly marked with the name of the product as it appears on the MSDS. To be in compliance, the case would be appropriately labeled on the exterior of the box making it clear what the case contained. An MSDS would be found in the case. Because it is likely that each individual bottle of chemical would be removed from the case and stored separately, each bottle would also need to be clearly labeled.

Training. The Hazard Communication Rule mandates that employers develop a training program that meets the following criteria.

1. The employer must identify hazardous substances found in the workplace by their generic, chemical, trade, and/or common names. This information must then be made known to employees who may potentially have contact with the identified substances.
2. The employer must identify hazardous substances exposure levels that trigger restrictions. There are standards that mandate that protective procedures and safeguards be put in place when exposure to hazardous substances approaches, reaches, or exceeds a level that has been determined to be harmful or injurious.
3. The employer must identify the routes of entry, and acute or chronic effects of exposure to hazardous substances. For example, fumes from hazardous substances may be inhaled during normal breathing. Other hazardous substances may be absorbed if they come into direct contact with an employee's skin.
4. The employer must explain the symptoms that accompany exposure. In the case of formaldehyde, the employer might caution the employee to be aware of skin sensitization or irritations of the eyes, nose, and throat.
5. The employer must identify and explain other dangers associated with hazardous substances to which the employee is exposed. Some chemicals, for example, may be flammable or caustic and require special care when being used.
6. The employer must explain emergency treatments that will be employed if there is an exposure incident. If, for example, embalming chemicals get sprayed into the eyes of employees, or onto employees' bodies, training will have already been provided on the proper utilization of an eyewash station or a drench shower.
7. The employer must explain to employees the proper use and handling of hazardous sub-

Material Safety Data Sheet
May be used to comply with
OSHA's Hazard Communication Standard,
29 CFR 1910.1200. Standard must be
Consulted for specific requirements.

U.S. Department of Labor
Occupational Safety and Health Administration
(Non-Mandatory Form)
Form Approved
OMB No. 1218-0072

IDENTITY *(As Used on Label and List)*	*Note: Blank spaces are not permitted. If any item is not applicable, or no information is available, the space must be marked to indicate that.*

Section I

Manufacturer's Name	Emergency Telephone Number
Address *(Number, Street, City, State, and ZIP Code)*	Telephone Number for Information
	Date Prepared
	Signature of Preparer *(optional)*

Section II — Hazardous Ingredients/Identity Information

Hazardous Components (Specific Chemical Identity; Common Name(s))	OSHA PEL	ACGIH TLV	Other Limits Recommended	% *(optional)*

Section III — Physical/Chemical Characteristics

Boiling Point		Specific Gravity (H_2O = 1)	
Vapor Pressure (mm Hg.)		Melting Point	
Vapor Density (AIR = 1)		Evaporation Rate (Butyl Acetate = 1)	
Solubility in Water			
Appearance and Odor			

Section IV — Fire and Explosion Hazard Data

Flash Point (Method Used)	Flammable Limits	LEL	UEL
Extinguishing Media			
Special Fire Fighting Procedures			
Unusual Fire and Explosion Hazards			

(Reproduce locally) OSHA 174, Sept. 1985

Figure 3–5. Sample MSDS sheet.

Section V — Reactivity Data

Stability	Unstable		Conditions to Avoid
	Stable		

Incompatibility (*Materials to Avoid*)

Hazardous Decomposition or Byproducts

Hazardous Polymerization	May Occur		Conditions to Avoid
	Will Not Occur		

Section VI — Health Hazard Data

Route(s) of Entry:	Inhalation?	Skin?	Ingestion?

Health Hazards (*Acute and Chronic*)

Carcinogenicity:	NTP?	IARC Monographs?	OSHA Regulated?

Signs and Symptoms of Exposure

Medical Conditions
Generally Aggravated by Exposure

Emergency and First Aid Procedures

Section VII — Precautions for Safe Handling and Use

Steps to Be Taken in Case Material Is Released or Spilled

Waste Disposal Method

Precautions to Be Taken in Handling and Storing

Other Precautions

Section VIII — Control Measures

Respiratory Protection (*Specify Type*)

Ventilation	Local Exhaust	Special
	Mechanical (*General*)	Other

Protective Gloves	Eye Protection

Other Protective Clothing or Equipment

Work/Hygienic Practices

* USGPO 1986-491-529/45775

Figure 3-5. (Continued)

stances. Employees, for example, should be taught methods by which they can protect themselves from the dangers of hazardous substances, such as wearing protective equipment, and avoiding careless or unsafe use of chemicals.

8. The employer must explain cleanup procedures for leaks and spills. An employer, for example, may require that any spill of embalming chemical on the floor of the preparation room be immediately cleaned up with a paper towel, which is then placed in a container that is used to handle contaminated materials.
9. The employer must provide information on the name, telephone number, and address of the companies that supply to the work place chemicals that are considered hazardous. The employer can easily satisfy this requirement by referring to the manufacturer information section of an MSDS included with chemicals.
10. The employer must inform employees of the existence and location of written materials related to hazardous substances that are found in the work place. In addition, the employer upon request, must provide access to employees, representatives of employees, or regulators, copies of training materials.

The Formaldehyde Standard. This standard, which is also part of Federal OSHA requirements, is aimed specifically at addressing hazards associated with exposure to formaldehyde, formaldehyde gas, its solutions, and materials that release formaldehyde. Under the provisions of the Formaldehyde Standard, employers must monitor employees to determine how much exposure exists in the workplace. Studies have shown that exposure to formaldehyde at certain levels will likely cause employees to experience eye, nose, throat, and upper respiratory tract irritation.

Exposure monitoring is accomplished by sampling the air in work spaces where formaldehyde is used. Employers can purchase sampling kits from chemical supply companies and other vendors. Exposure monitoring is intended to determine if the level of exposure to airborne concentrations of formaldehyde in a work area is at or below a specified concentration. The Formaldehyde Standard establishes specific limits on the amount of exposure that is allowed. The specific point at which exposure is unsafe is called the *action level.* If sampling reveals that exposure has reached or exceeded the action level, employers are required to take steps to reduce the exposure. The purpose of requiring exposure reduction at the action level is to insure that exposure does not reach the *permissible exposure limit* (PEL). The permissible exposure limit sets the maximum exposure that is allowed by OSHA.

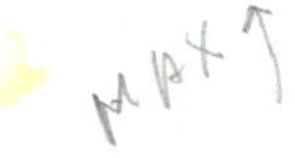

A funeral home has two monitoring options to determine exposure levels for employees. It can either monitor individual employees to determine exposure levels, or use a representative sample of air quality to make a general determination of air quality for all employees (Burnside, 1997, p. 18). Because of the expense involved in individual monitoring, James Burnside, (1997, p. 20) has stated that, "In funeral homes, it is almost always best to conduct a representative sampling." Representative sampling requires (1) sampling for each job classification where exposure exists, (2) sampling for each work area where exposure might occur, and (3) sampling for each work shift, unless employers can document that exposure levels would be the same for all shifts. (Burnside, 1997, p. 20).

There are two types of tests that must occur in every funeral home where any formaldehyde is used, (1) the *time-weighted average* (over 8 hours) (TWA), and (2) the *short-term exposure level* (over 15 minutes) (STEL). These tests are to be conducted in a "worst case" environment. For example, the time-weighted average testing should be done at a time when there is embalming taking place in the preparation room. It is recommended that short-term exposure level testing be done during an autopsy embalming. When test results document worst case situations that are within limits specified by OSHA, it is reasonable to conclude that the air quality of the preparation room at all other times is also acceptable.

TIME-WEIGHTED AVERAGE. Employers are required to take steps necessary to assure that no employee is exposed to unsafe concentrations of airborne formaldehyde. If the results of sampling for formaldehyde indicate that the exposure is below 0.5 ppm over an 8-hour period, the action level has not been reached, no additional time-weighted average testing is needed, *except* if (1) an employee makes a complaint about formaldehyde concentrations, or (2) there are any changes in procedure, equipment, chemicals, personnel, or other circumstances that affect the work area.

If time-weighted average sampling reveals exposure that falls between 0.5 ppm and .7499999 ppm, the action level has been reached. Employers are then compelled to implement steps to reduce the exposure by (1) placing formaldehyde warning signs on areas where the concentration of formaldehyde has exceeded the action level, and (2) beginning medical surveillance of employees who work in areas where the concentration of formaldehyde has exceeded the action level. The formaldehyde warning signs must bear the following information:

Danger
Formaldehyde
Irritant and potential cancer hazard
Authorized personnel only

Medical Surveillance requires that employers take a series of steps aimed at protecting employees. Those steps include having the employees complete a medical questionnaire, which is then reviewed by a physician who can make recommendations based on the employees' responses. The physician can recommend that the employees are having no ill effects and should return to work, or that sufficient cause exists to order that employees be given a medical examination. If the employees are given a medical examination the physician can recommend that there is no health problem present and employees should return to work, or that a health problem is present and *medical removal* will be ordered.

If medical removal is ordered, the affected employee may not be given preparation duties for up to 6 months. If there is improvement in the physical condition of the employee, the physician may release the employee to return to preparation room duties. If the medical condition of the employee does not improve, (1) the employee may be permanently re-assigned to duties other than in the preparation room, or (2) the employee may be terminated. If employers elect to terminate employees who are medically unable to perform the tasks and duties for which they were hired, there may well be issues related to disability coverage and Worker's Compensation to be addressed.

TIME-WEIGHTED AVERAGE SAMPLING AT OR ABOVE .75 PPM. In those cases where time-weighted average sampling reveals airborne concentrations of formaldehyde at or above .75 ppm the permissible exposure limit has been reached. Employers are then required to (1) post formaldehyde warning signs in and around the work area(s), (2) begin medical surveillance, and (3) provide respirators for employees who are assigned to work in the posted area(s).

RESPIRATORS. There are employers who think that respirators are an easy solution to any problems that arise from formaldehyde concentrations in the preparation area. This is not true! Employers and employees should be aware that OSHA has a respirator standard that must be followed when respirators are put into use in the preparation room. Two of the major provisions of the Respirator Standard are that (1) employees must be tested to see if a respirator is appropriate for them, and (2) a personal respirator must be fitted to each individual employee.

THE SHORT-TERM EXPOSURE LEVEL. In addition to the time-weighted average (which is sampled over 8 hours) employers are required to sample for airborne concentrations of formaldehyde over a 15-minute period. If the sampling reveals a concentration of airborne formaldehyde that is *below* 2 ppm, the permissible exposure limit has not been reached and no further short-term exposure limit testing is required, unless (1) an employee makes a complaint about formaldehyde concentrations, or (2) there are any changes in procedure, equipment, chemicals, personnel, or other circumstances that affect the work area.

If short-term exposure level sampling reveals airborne concentrations of formaldehyde *at or above* 2 ppm the permissible exposure limit has been reached and the employer is required to (1) use formaldehyde warning signs, (2) begin medical surveillance, and (3) require employees assigned to duties in the preparation room to wear respirators.

If the initial testing shows airborne concentrations of formaldehyde above either the action level for the time-weighted average, or the permissible limit for the short-term exposure level, employers must begin periodic testing of the employees. Periodic testing means that employers must retest the work area at least every 6 months. If employers have two consecutive retests, conducted at least 7 days apart, that show concentrations below the action level for the time-weighted average, and below the permissible exposure limit for the short-term exposure level, the periodic monitoring of employees can be stopped.

Methods of Compliance with the Formaldehyde Standard.

WORK PRACTICE CONTROLS. Examples of work practice controls for compliance with the formaldehyde standard include

1. Wearing appropriate protective equipment when handling chemicals to avoid exposure by contact with the skin.
2. Exercising care when handling and pouring chemicals to avoid spills.
3. Handling and pouring chemicals in a way that prevents vapors from escaping into the room.
4. Keeping instruments and equipment in good working condition to prevents spills and vaporization.
5. Keeping the lid on the embalming machine when embalming solution is in the tank.
6. Recapping fluid bottles.
7. Properly rinsing fluid bottles.
8. Continuously aspirating body cavities during autopsy embalming.
9. Controlling drainage and leakage from the body.
10. Utilizing a continuous flow of water over the embalming table to rinse and dilute chemicals.
11. Keeping the lid on hazardous waste containers.

ENGINEERING CONTROLS. Examples of engineering controls for compliance with the formaldehyde standard are essentially the same as for biological hazards. They can be considered in terms of proper plumbing and adequate ventilation. Plumbing considerations include

1. Vacuum breakers on the main water line leading into the building.
2. Vacuum breakers on hydroaspirators.
3. Maintaining discharge basins/flush skins in good working order.
4. Having a suitable water source for the preparation table.
5. Having a proper eye wash station.
6. Having a proper drench shower.
7. Having a proper hand washing station.
8. Having proper shower room facilities.

Ventilation considerations include having an exhaust for the room located at the foot of the embalming table, *below* the level of the table top. As previously stated, the air replacement vent for the room should ideally be high on the opposite wall. The idea is to introduce fresh air blown toward the embalmer, while the contaminated air is being drawn away from the embalmer. As a rough rule of thumb for a single-table room, the number of air changes ranges from 12 to 20 per hour. The number may vary depending on the contents of the room, the number of bodies that will be embalmed in the room at one time, the shape of the room, weather-related factors, and the preference of the embalmer. Again, the Public Health Guidelines have recommended that a ventilation system create a minimum of 6 air changes per hour, and preferably more in a preparation room.

The formaldehyde standard also requires employee information and training. Employers must introduce employees who have occupational exposure to Material Safety Data Sheets, and identify methods by which employees will have access to the information. Initial training must be provided to employees prior to their being exposed to hazardous substances. In addition, employees must receive additional training if a change in work assignment results in exposure to hazardous substances. Employees must also receive annual updates at intervals of not greater than 1 year. The purpose of the training is to provide employees with information, procedures, and techniques necessary to safely handle substances that contain formaldehyde.

▶ CONCLUSION

The dictates of logic, reason, and research all demand that the dead human body be considered a source of pathogenic microorganisms. Embalmers are charged by the same dictates and by law with the responsibility to implement protective and thorough procedures to ensure that the potential for contagion through exposure to the body is minimized.

▶ KEY TERMS AND CONCEPTS FOR STUDY AND DISCUSSION

1. Define the following terms
   Action level
   Additional training
   Airborne pathogen
   Annual training updates
   Aerosolization
   Asepsis
   Autoclaving
   Bactericidal
   Bacteriostatic
   Biological hazard
   Bloodborne pathogen
   Bloodborne Pathogen Rule
   Cleaning
   Cold chemical sterilant
   Concurrent disinfection/decontamination
   Disinfect
   Employee Right-To-Know laws
   Engineering controls
   Exposure control plan
   Formaldehyde standard
   Germicide
   Hazard Communication Rule
   HBV
   Initial training
   Ionizing radiation
   Medical removal
   Medical surveillance
   MSDS
   Non-ionizing radiation
   OSHA
   PEL
   Respirator standard
   Sanitizer
   STEL
   Sterilization
   Terminal disinfection/decontamination
   TWA
   Universal precautions
   Work practice controls
2. Describe the research findings documenting the occupational risk faced by embalmers as a result of their exposure to biological hazards.
3. Describe the research findings documenting the occupational risks faced by embalmers as a result of their exposure to chemical hazards.
4. In addition to biological and chemical hazards, what other occupational hazards do embalmers face?

5. What is the minimum documentation required for a Bloodborne Pathogen Exposure Control Plan?
6. Describe the basic premise of universal precautions.
7. What are the two primary areas of consideration for engineering controls.
8. Name five common work practice controls that would contribute to a hygienic environment in the embalming room.
9. List the six areas of training and instruction required for Personal Protective Equipment.
10. Describe the provisions of hepatitis B vaccination and postexposure evaluation and follow up.
11. List the four types of labeling provisions that can be used to communicate the hazards of potentially infectious agents.
12. With regard to hazardous chemicals, what are the two main requirements of the Hazard Communication Rule?
13. At what concentration does formaldehyde vapors in a room constitute a potential health hazard to the embalmer?
14. Describe the provisions that make up medical surveillance of employees who are exposed to formaldehyde vapors in the embalming room?
15. Describe the three categories of training required under the formaldehyde standard.

▶ REFERENCES

Beck-Sague C, Jarvis W, Fruehling J, et al. Universal precautions and mortuary practitioners: Influence on practices and risk of occupationally acquired infection. *J. Occup Med,* 33, 1991; 874–878.

Bender JR, Mullin LS, Grapel GJ, Wilson WE. Eye irritation response in humans to formaldehyde. *Am Indust Hygiene Assoc J,* 44, 1983; 463–465.

Benenson, Abram S., Editor. Control of Communicable Diseases Manual, 16 ed., American Public Health Association, 1995.

Burnside, James F. "Formaldehyde: Who, What, When, Where, Why & How of Monitoring" *The Director,* May 1997, p. 18.

The Bloodborne Pathogen Rule. Code of Federal Regulations. Title 29 CFR Part 1910, Occupational Safety and Health Administration, Department of Labor, Toxic and Hazardous Substances. The Bloodborne Pathogen Rule, 1910.1030, 1992.

Code of Federal Regulations. Title 29: Subtitle B- Regulations Relating to Labor: Chapter XVII- Occupational Safety and Health Administration, Department of Labor; Part 1910, Hazard Communication-1910.1200, 1988.

Gershon R, Vlahov D, Escamilla-Cejudo J, et al. Tuberculosis risk in funeral home employees. *J Occup Environ Med,* May 1998; 497–503.

Kerfoot EJ. Formaldehyde Vapor Emission Study in Embalming Rooms. *The Director,* 42, 1972.

Kerfoot EJ, Mooney TF. Formaldehyde and paraformaldehyde study in funeral homes. *Am Indust Hygiene Assoc J,* 36, 1975, 533–537.

McDonald L. Blood exposure and protection in funeral homes. *Am J Infect Control,* August 1989; 193–195.

McKenna MT, Hutton M, Cauthen G, Onorato IM. The association between occupation and tuberculosis. *Am J Resp Crit Care Med,* 154, 1996; 587–596.

Nethercott JR, Holness DL. Contact dermatitis in funeral service workers. *Contact Dermatitis,* 18, 1988; 263–267.

State of Minnesota. Minnesota Rule Chapter 5206.0400, Subpart 5. *Employee Right-To-Know Standards,* Minneapolis: Department of Labor and Industry, 1995.

Turner S, Kunches L, Gordon K, et al. Occupational exposure to human immunodeficiency virus (HIV) and hepatitis B virus (HBV) among embalmers: A pilot seroprevalence study. *Am J Public Health,* October 1989; 1425–1426.

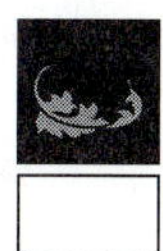

CHAPTER 4
TECHNICAL ORIENTATION OF EMBALMING

Today's progressive, professional funeral home owner realizes that embalming is a vital, important part of the total service and that the preparation room is as important as any area in the building. Therefore, the room is given its fair and generous share of the operating and building budgets. Each funeral establishment may have a preparation room or funeral homes with several branch operations may have the embalming done at one location. A newer concept is the independent centralized embalming facility. Many states have licensed such facilities. These centralized embalming centers are shared by several funeral homes in a community. Where central facilities are used most funeral establishments maintain a preparation room for cosmetizing, dressing, and casketing the bodies after they have been delivered from the embalming center. Many states require that each funeral facility maintain a preparation room even if a central embalming facility is used.

▶ OBJECTIVES

The primary purpose of a well-designed and organized preparation room is to provide a safe and comfortable workplace. It should also be available to serve as a public relations tool if a community group wishes to tour the funeral establishment. Informational visitations need not stop with the opening of a new funeral home. Many organizations such as church groups and service clubs visit the funeral home and are gratified by the response and reactions they receive. A tour that does not include the preparation room can only serve to heighten unfounded suspicions and misconceptions concerning the embalming process.

In planning remodeling or new construction, emphasis should be placed on making the area functional and efficient. A layout that saves a few steps here and there can save many working hours in the course of a year. A door planned just barely wide enough to accommodate the removal cot can be a source of annoyance, inconvenience, and irritation long after the small extra cost of a slightly wider door is forgotten. Whether the owner/manager does his or her own embalming or hires a large staff, he or she naturally wants to provide a clean, comfortable, cheerful, and efficient workplace. If the workplace is unpleasant, unattractive, or inefficient, best efforts are not put forth in spite of good intentions. This psychology has been demonstrated repeatedly in classrooms, industrial plants, offices, and other work places.

▶ PREPARATION ROOM CONSIDERATIONS

General Rules

1. Preparation room is kept strictly private during body preparation. Persons admitted should be limited to:
   a. Licensees and registered trainees.
   b. Those authorized by the family.
   c. Those authorized by state statute or rules and regulations.
2. Limited authorized persons can be in the room when preparation work is not being performed:
   a. Maintenance employees.
   b. Hairdresser, cosmetologist, barber, persons with other responsibilities.
   c. Staff members for dressing and casketing remains.
3. Identify the room by signage:
   a. Strictly private area
   b. OSHA warnings
4. Secure the preparation room.
   a. State regulations may require security locks.
   b. Establish a security plan for the handling of the remains of high-profile persons.
   c. Inventory and label personal effects.
   d. Preparation room should not be located so that it becomes a passage to other building areas.
5. Maintain the dignity of the remains. Be sure that
   a. The body is properly identified.
   b. The remains are covered.
   c. A modesty cloth is used during preparation.

6. Maintain highest moral standards.
   a. Keep body covered as practical.
   b. Guard loose talk and remarks.
   c. Repeat nothing outside of preparation room.
   d. Disclose no confidential facts as to age, condition of the body, deformities, or diseases causing death.
7. Maintain a clean and healthy environment.
   a. Properly dispose of clothing of the deceased:
      i. launder and return to the family or
      ii. destroy after proper authorization.
   b. Proper disposition of all waste (see chapter 3)
      i. Statutes, rules, and regulations vary for individual states.
   c. Be sure ventilation, heating, and cooling systems work properly.
   d. Maintain all mechanical apparatus so no leakage occurs.
   e. Perform regular maintenance and cleaning of the preparation room.
8. Maintain an adequate supply of chemicals and sundries necessary for preparation work, restorative, and cosmetology treatments.
9. Maintain an adequate number of tables and positioning devices; this will help to keep movement of bodies minimal.
10. Document through the **embalming report** each preparation.

▶ HEALTH AND SAFETY STANDARDS

Today, with the abundance of scientific evidence on the infectious nature of the dead human body, and with the importance of embalming to protection of the public health, sanitation and ease of housekeeping should be major concerns in planning a preparation room. At one time, the simple installation of a sterilizer was all that was thought to be necessary. **A means of sterilizing instruments after each embalming is still essential in every preparation room,** but is far from the total answer. To fulfill professional obligations in this regard the embalmer must take other factors into account.

Funeral home facilities are governed by a variety of laws and regulations from federal, state, and local agencies because they are public places of business and employ workers in a workplace. A brief review of the major sources of regulations governing the preparation room environment follows, and throughout this chapter reference is made generally to standard requirements. Funeral service students learn many of the regulations governing employer/employee duties, responsibilities, and rights during the course of their funeral service education. Funeral home owners are advised to consult experts in the legal and construction fields to be certain that their facilities, planned or existing, conform to all local requirements.

▶ SOURCES OF REGULATIONS

OSHA Requirements

The federal Occupational Safety and Health Administration (OSHA) prescribes in detail the physical and environmental requirements that employers must meet to provide a safe workplace. These requirements are enforced through workplace inspections, warnings, and citations. In the event of failure to correct continual noncompliance or serious violations, substantial fines are levied. A well-known example is the Hazard Communication Standard.

Lesser known requirements have to do with the necessity for an adjacent shower and locker facility, electrical grounding, ramp and stair-step angles and heights, and a host of other areas of concern to the worker. Caution should be exercised to be certain that **all** OSHA requirements are being met in the workplace.

Four areas of OSHA directly impact the funeral service practitioner: (1) OSHA General Rule, (2) Hazard Communication Standard, (3) Formaldehyde Standard, and (4) Bloodborne Pathogen Standard.

"Right to Know" Laws

An emerging area of legislation on the local and state levels is "right to know" legislation. This is directed at employers and requires them to post information warning employees of chemicals that may be hazardous or harmful to their health and well-being. Firms in locales that have enacted such legislation may have to meet these requirements as well as those of OSHA.

Building Permits

All construction of any magnitude requires that a building permit be obtained from local authorities. The application procedures usually require that detailed plans and specifications be submitted regarding plumbing, electrical, and other construction materials to ensure that all materials and construction meet certain minimum standards. Although the materials and methods recommended in this chapter generally conform to most building code requirements, a competent architect, contractor, or both should be consulted prior to permit application in a particular locale.

State Codes and Local Ordinances

State boards of health and mortuary science have enacted regulations governing the minimum standards for preparation rooms. *Two examples demonstrate such minimum standards.* The State Board of Funeral Directors of Pennsylvania and the Board of Embalmers and Funeral Directors of Ohio have published the following rules and regulations dealing with the facilities and equipment requirements for the preparation or embalming room.

Pennsylvania

The preparation room shall be constructed solely for the purpose of scientifically preparing human remains and shall contain the following facilities and equipment for the purpose of preventing disease and properly disposing of waste material arising out of the embalming process:

1. A sink with running water and sewage connections and possessing a two-inch capacity drain pipe.
2. A metal or porcelain-covered operating or embalming table.
3. A metal cabinet or metal or glass shelves or a material impervious to water and stain.
4. A waste container with cover.
5. A first-aid kit placed in a conspicuous place.
6. Surgical instruments and apparatus for the preparation of embalming of a body. Aspirator must be a nonbackflow type or have a nonbackflow valve in the line.
7. Walls which are airtight and covered in their entirety by tile, plaster, composition board, or similar material. With the exception of tile, all of those materials must be finished with enamel or some other smooth, hard, waterproof material.
8. Airtight ceiling.
9. A floor which must be entirely of concrete with glazed surface or tile or wood flooring covered with linoleum or material of similar composition so as to be impervious to water.
10. Outside ventilation which may be provided by screened windows or transoms or, in lieu thereof, by an eight-inch pipe leading to the exterior of the building and otherwise constructed so as to conform to the highest health standards.
11. Solid doors which are painted or enameled and windows which are screened.
12. Sterilizer, chemical or otherwise.
13. Flushing facilities to flush injurious corrosive materials from the eyes or body
    (a) The facilities, which must be accessible, operable, and near the work area, are to be either:
        (1) An eye bubble or eye shower, or both, available from safety equipment suppliers; or
        (2) A four-foot length of $\frac{3}{4}$-inch hose attached to simple quick opening valve.
    (b) Clean cold water must be available for either of the facilities listed in subparagraph (i) of this paragraph and must not exceed 25 pounds pressure.
    (c) Portable eye washers are permitted if of a type approved by OSHA.
14. Protective wearing apparel as follows:
    (a) Rubber gloves or other type impervious to the chemical being handled.
    (b) Goggles.
    (c) Suitable clothing or apron, rubber or other material impervious to the chemicals being handled.

Ohio

The minimal requirements for the preparation or embalming room shall be as follows:

1. Sanitary floor (cement or tile preferred).
2. All instruments and appliances used in the embalming of a dead human body shall be thoroughly cleansed and sterilized by boiling or immersion for ten minutes in a one percent solution of chlorinated soda or an equivalent disinfectant immediately at the conclusion of each individual case.
3. Running hot and cold water with a lavatory sink for personal hygiene.
4. Exhaust fan and intake vent, permanently installed and operable with the capacity to change the air in the room four times each hour.
5. Sanitary plumbing connected with sewer, cesspool, septic tank, or other department of health approved system.
6. Porcelain, stainless steel, metal-lined or fiberglass operating table.
7. All opening windows and outside doors shall be adequately screened and shielded from outside viewing.
8. All hydroaspirators shall be equipped with at least one air breaker.
9. Containers for refuse, trash and soiled linens shall be adequately covered or sealed at all times.
10. First-aid kit and eyewash.
11. The embalming or preparation room shall be strictly private. A "private" sign shall be posted on the door(s) entering the preparation room. No one shall be allowed therein while the body is being embalmed except the licensed embalmers, apprentices and other authorized persons and officials in discharge of their duties.
12. All waste materials, refuse, used bandages and cotton shall be destroyed by reducing to ashes by incineration, or shall be buried in a licensed landfill.
13. Every person, while engaged in actually embalming a dead human body, shall be attired in a clean and sanitary smock or gown covering the person from the neck to below the knees and shall, while so engaged, wear impervious rubber gloves.
14. All bodies in the preparation room should be treated with proper care and dignity and should be properly covered at all times.

Extensive planning and consultation are required in advance of any construction in the funeral home in general and the preparation room in particular. Funeral home owners, as business people serving the public and employing people in the workplace, have special obligations that must be met. Add to these the public health aspects of the embalming operation and environment, and it should be clear that extraordinary care in construction and design in the embalming laboratory are in the best interests of all concerned.

▶ LOCATIONS

Basement

The basement is often where space is most readily available, although frequently this is not the most desirable site. Ceiling height is the most common difficulty in this area because of overhead pipes as well as heating and air conditioning ducts. Often there is little that can be done to remedy the situation with reasonable cost. Sometimes, pipes and ducts may be diverted, run between floor joists, or sometimes concealed in wall cabinets. Lighting fixtures may also be kept from lessening head room if they are recessed between floor joists.

Plumbing can present vexing questions if sewer drains are substantially above floor level. A sump pump in this circumstance may be the only answer, but it should be remembered that a sump pump becomes inoperative during a power failure. There are other plumbing considerations, too, which will be discussed later. Ventilation and air conditioning are more costly in basement areas. Stairs can be a considerable inconvenience—even a hazard. An elevator, lift, or ramp may offer a solution here.

A wet basement might be the greatest single deterrent to using this area. One should be certain beyond all doubt that the water problem can be completely corrected by interior or exterior waterproofing of the walls, relocation of dry wells, grading away from the building, or some other means before any construction is begun and especially before any flooring is laid. Normal dampness is rather easily handled by a dehumidifier, and it is essential that this be done.

First or Second Floor

The first floor is usually the most logical and least costly location of a preparation room if ample space is available. Most of the basement problems are eliminated and certain advantages accrue automatically. Climbing stairs, building a ramp, or installing an elevator becomes unnecessary. Natural daylight is normally available to create more pleasant working conditions; however, other considerations now arise. Access to the room should be from a nonpublic area. If the room is adjacent to a public area such as the selection room, adequate soundproofing is extremely important. If this is impractical or impossible, a flashing light should be installed in the preparation room to alert staff members that a family is in the next room. Odor control and proper exhaust venting must be provided. Those who work in a funeral home become accustomed to certain odors that would be obvious and objectionable to a visitor.

If the installation of an elevator is feasible in a two-story building, the second floor may well be the best of the several alternatives. More natural light is available, and ventilation is less expensive and more effective. Normally, a second floor room is completely removed from the public areas. Here again, sound levels must be considered. Plumbing may be nonexistent in the immediate area, but totally new plumbing may be reasonable considering the other advantages to be gained.

▶ PREPARATION ROOM SIZE

The size requirement of the preparation room is also of critical importance in determining the location. A room that is too large can necessitate extra steps and encourage use of the surplus space for storage. Many problems can be forestalled by partitioning a part of the area for planned storage. Allow adequate work space but keep all equipment, instruments, and supplies readily accessible.

The firm that conducts as many as 100 funerals annually should find one permanent table ample. A folding table that may be stored in a closet when not in use will serve in an emergency and can double as a dressing table when required. An area 120 to 150 square feet for this room should be considered a minimum. This should allow for ample cabinets and counter space, assuming the room is not an unusual shape and that it does not have more than one or two doors opening into it. When locating plumbing for the table, keep in mind the need to allow ample passage for the removal cot and for a casket, if casketing is to be done in the preparation room. Doors and corridors leading to the room must also be of ample width, especially if turning corners is required.

A firm anticipating 100 to 150 funerals per year should try to provide a bit larger area if at all possible. One table would normally still be adequate, but the extra folding table is essential.

A firm contemplating 150 to 350 funerals annually should provide a minimum area of approximately 400 square feet and two completely equipped tables. A firm doing a larger volume should seriously consider a separate dressing room where hairdressing and cosmetizing may be done.

Some considerations when remodeling or building new might include:

- Once volume of use is determined, keep the space where the embalming operation will be performed as small as is practical.
- Minimum operating spaces saves steps.
- Minimum operating spaces are easier to keep sanitary.

- Minimum operating spaces are easier to ventilate, heat, and cool.
- Keep instruments, fluids, and sundries in convenient locations within the area of operation; storage spaces should be placed so bending is not necessary.
- Lifting devices should be used for moving bodies.
- Adequate tables will decrease the necessity to move bodies; ideally, once the body is placed on a preparation table it should not have to be moved until it is placed in a casket, shipping container, or on a cot.
- Floors, countertops, and all flat surfaces should be constructed of materials that can easily be sanitized.

The "station" or "booth" concept in embalming room design uses one or more fully equipped small operating areas (within a large preparation room) where the embalming is performed. The room space adjacent to the embalming stations is where restorative work, cosmetizing, hairdressing, dressing, and casketing of the remains are performed. The small operating stations are more private and, because of their size, easily sanitized and cleaned. The number of preparations performed per year determines the number of stations that should be constructed. One station for each 200 preparations has been suggested. The following floor plans #1 (Figure 4–1A) and #2 (Figure 4–1B) show the use of the "station concept." Floor plan number 3 (Figure 4–1C) is suggested for a central embalming facility or an embalming facility within a large funeral estab-

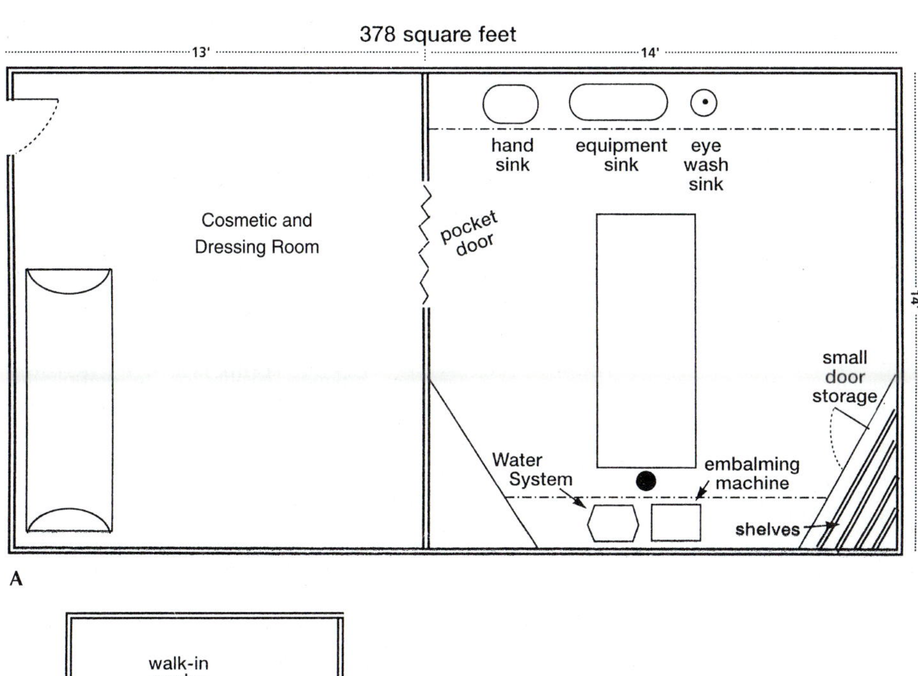

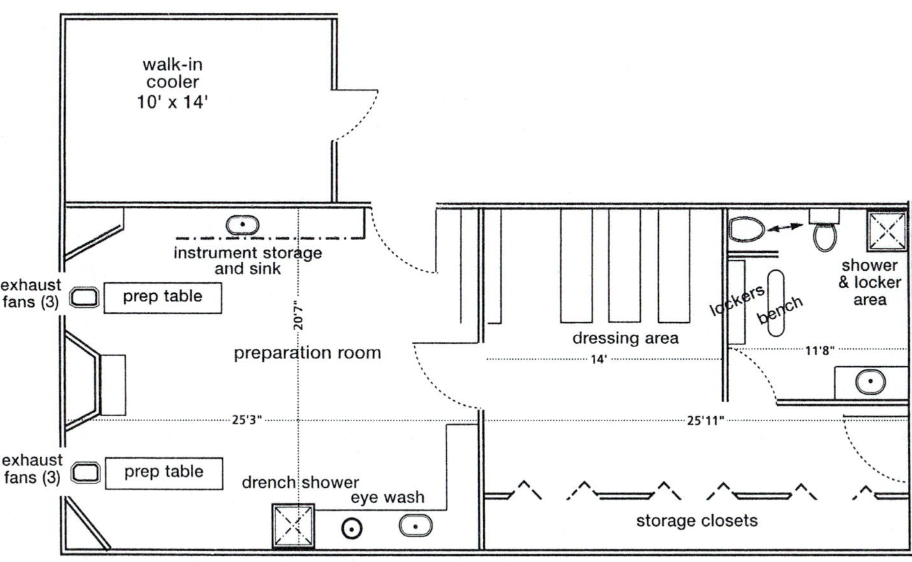

Figure 4–1AB. Flooring plans showing use of the "station or booth concept." (*Continued.*)

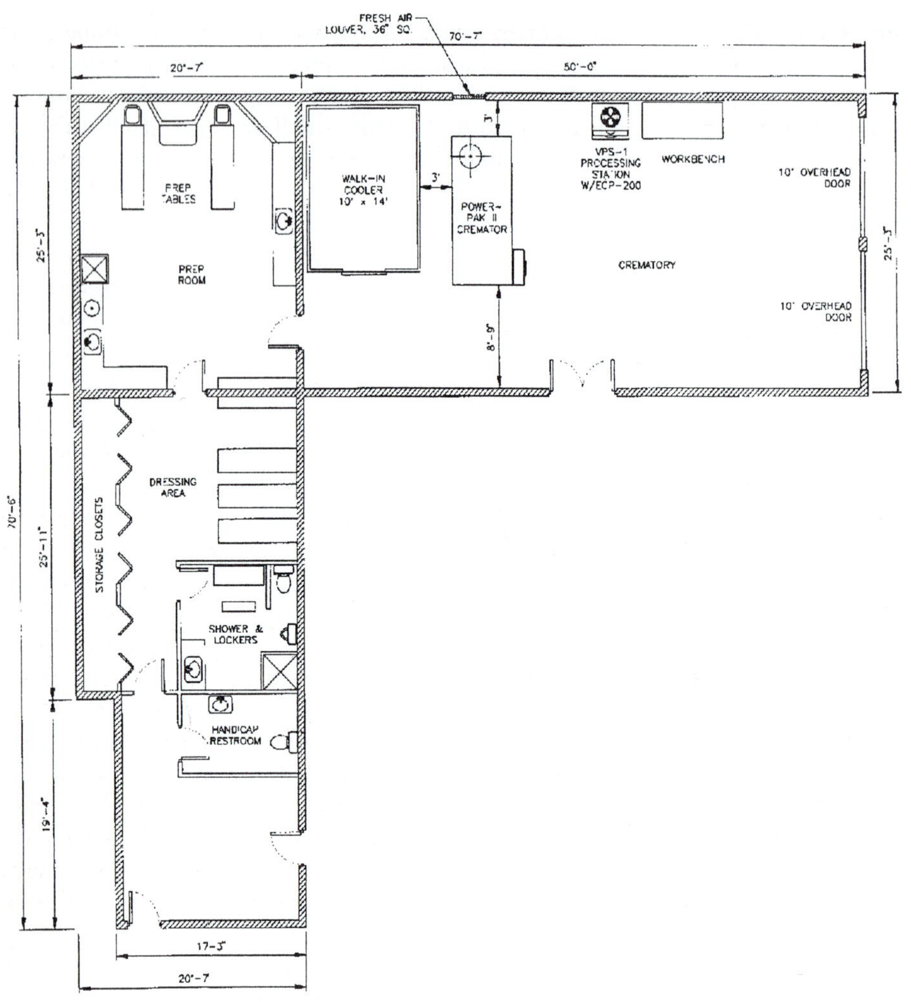

Figure 4–1 (*Continued*). **C.** Flooring plan suggested for central embalming facility or an embalming facility within a large funeral establishment.

lishment. Note that this plan includes a covered delivery and receiving area, walk-in cooler for storage, crematory facility, "station" preparation area, dressing and casketing areas, and an employee restroom, shower, and changing area.

▶ PHYSICAL DESIGN

Discuss the requirements with an architect on a new building or when remodeling. Show the architect the existing equipment and describe the movement made in the room. Consider plumbing needs. Plumbing costs should not always be the overriding determining factor.

Maneuverability within the finished room is tremendously important. When the tentative location for the table(s) is set, mentally go through the motions of getting the removal cot and the casket into the room. Once the general plan seems satisfactory, draw the room to scale with all equipment in place and think again about all the movements that must take place in the finished room.

Storage Cabinets and Countertops

Next, consider storage cabinets. Although space should be provided for working quantities of supplies, the preparation room should not double as a storeroom. Ready-made base cabinets are generally 24 inches deep. Obviously, these would normally be the least costly. Depending on the size and shape of the room, however, custom cabinets may be a necessity. They could be 18 or 12 inches deep, if space is very limited. If the space is such that cabinet depth is not a problem but counter length is limited, it might be desirable to use a stock 24-inch cabinet and hold it out from the wall to permit a 30-inch deep countertop. The vacant space behind the cabinets might be used for water pipes or electrical wiring.

The Doorway

Unless an architect is made aware that caskets will be taken through the door, she or he might well specify a conventional 30-inch door. **A 3-foot opening should be an absolute minimum. The narrower the corridor or passageway from which the room is to be entered, the**

wider the door should be to permit turning. In addition to width, the direction in which the door opens is very significant. If a normally hung door might create problems, perhaps a "pocket" or recessed sliding door might be the answer. Should there be a structural reason that this is not practical, double-hinged doors folding to the right or left may be required.

Table Arrangements

There are virtually as many table arrangements as there are sizes and shapes of rooms; however, two are the most common and popular.

Conventional Parallel Table Plan. The conventional parallel table plan is a perfectly functional layout, although it may not be the best choice because the exhaust system, depending on where it is placed, may draw odors past the embalmers. With this plan, caution must be taken against making the waste sink a part of the cabinet line. This makes the sink and surrounding areas more difficult to clean. Instead, mount the sink on the face of the base cabinets or on the floor, leaving some clearance between the sink and cabinet.

Better yet is the "island" cabinet (Figure 4–2), which gives the embalmer freedom to pass completely around the table without stepping over hoses and electric cords. No part of the wall storage cabinets is obstructed. In fact, a drum of hardening compound or similar item may be stored in the base of the "island." All plumbing connections are within the cabinet and readily accessible if a problem should arise.

Two-Table Room Arrangement. If a sufficiently large square or rectangular room is available, the two-table room arrangement is preferred. It provides two completely separate work areas, allows maximum flexibility in movement within the room, and generally does not interfere with doors (see preceeding "station" discussion).

▶ FLOORING

Now that the location of the preparation room in the building and the layout of the room itself have been considered, perhaps the first specific aspect of the room that should be discussed is the floor.

The floor must withstand very heavy traffic and considerable static weight. If selected carelessly it can harbor infectious organisms, cause anything on wheels to roll toward low spots, cause glare, and create difficult working conditions or perhaps require recovering or even structural repair sooner than it should. The architect must be made fully aware of the weights this floor will hold and, therefore, the amount of structural support necessary. Flooring should be scuff mark and stain resistant. Dyes in embalming fluids should be easily removed. Fluid dyes can be used for testing new flooring materials for their ease of cleaning. Light colored flooring puts more brightness in the work area. A matte finish to the floor is more desireable than a glossy finish. The matte finish produces less glare, shows fewer scuff marks, and is easier to maintain than a glossy finish.

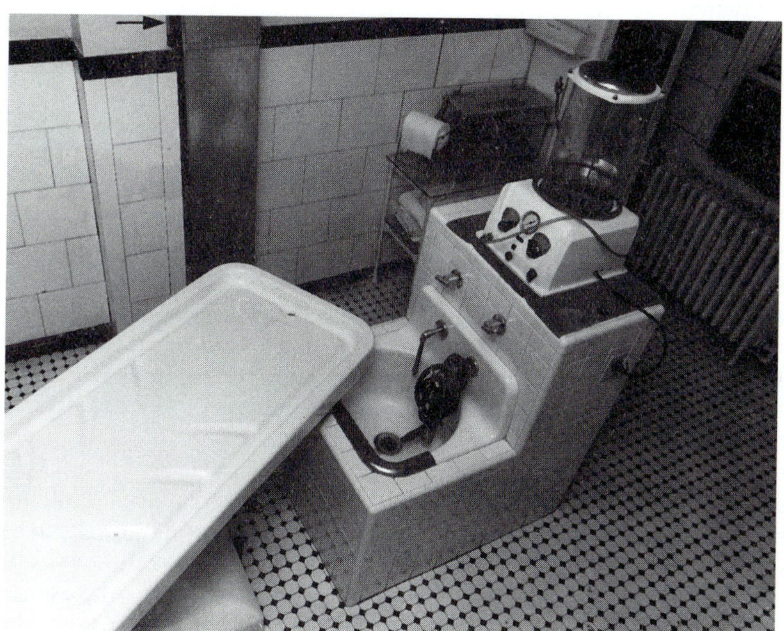

Figure 4–2. Island preparation design. Note the duct for exhaust that pulls fumes to the floor, away from the embalmer.

Basement Preparation Room

It is essential that the proper base be laid for any cement floor. There should be a thick stone bed covered by vinyl vapor barrier sheeting underneath the cement. A small ditch should be constructed around the outside, with ample leach lines to feed into the ditch in case water does start to collect. The cost of a small sump pump might well be worthwhile. Located in an out-of-the-way spot, it would pick up and discharge any water accumulation. Building codes should be consulted.

If the new floor is to be tiled, be sure to consider the curing time. The alkalines in uncured cement will affect the tile adhesive. When tiling an old cement floor, hollows and cracks in the cement must be filled and the floor leveled before proceeding. There are cementing compounds on the market that have four times the compressive strength of ordinary concrete. These compounds cure rapidly, are highly resistant to chemicals, and are impervious to moisture and temperature extremes. They are applied with a trowel in any thickness desired and adhere to wood, concrete, brick, steel, and aluminum.

If the preparation room is located in a basement with a cement floor, it is best to cover it with something; standing on cement is uncomfortable. Building a wood floor over the cement is a common answer to this problem. If the wood floor were built directly on top of the concrete, moisture would cause it to rot. Therefore, various methods are used to raise the wood floor and leave an air space between it and the concrete. In addition to preventing rot, the space acts as an excellent sound absorber.

It is also important to have enough floor joists and a thick enough wood subfloor to support the heavy concentrated weight the floor will bear. Try to anticipate locations for desired electrical and plumbing lines before closing up the floor.

First or Second Floor Preparation Room

When building a preparation room on the first or second floor, the architect should again be cautioned about the loads that the floor must support. An embalming table can weigh 300 or 400 pounds and that, plus the weight of a subject, could create a low spot on an insufficiently supported floor. The floor's sinking, in turn, can cause cracking of tiles or other floor coverings. Over a span of 12 feet a normal floor (without a bearing wall) could use 2 × 10-inch timbers on 16-inch centers for floor joists; however, a preparation room with 2 × 12-inch timbers on 12-inch centers is preferred. Alternatively, to keep timber height uniform with that of adjoining rooms, the 2 × 10-inch timbers on 16-inch centers should be doubled.

▶ FLOOR COVERING

Terrazo Floor

A terrazo floor is one sort that might be considered for this application. It is a natural polished floor that is very durable and easy to maintain. Terrazo is very hard and, therefore, tiring to stand on for extended periods. Also, it is slippery when wet. This problem can be overcome with the use of rubber mats.

Clay and Ceramic Tile

Clay and ceramic tile are both excellent choices. The size of such tiles makes a very important difference. The large 4 × 4-inch tiles with a slight roundness on the top make a natural recess or ditch for the grout fill as well as for dirt and accumulated wax. Some 1 × 1-inch tiles are also rounded and create the same difficulties. There are, however, flat 1 × 1-inch tiles and these are good. Any cleaning implement, from a hand sponge to an electric scrub brush machine, will make contact at all points and leave the floor completely clean. Remember that liquids will be spilled occasionally. A floor of glazed ceramic tiles would become slippery and such tiles should be avoided.

Vinyl Tile

Vinyl tile is, for good reason, probably the type of flooring most commonly chosen. It is very resilient so it is comfortable to stand on for several hours. It is attractive and sold in many colors and patterns so it can easily be color coordinated with any room. The three basic types of vinyl flooring are no-waxing sheet vinyl, homogeneous vinyl tile, and vinyl-asbestos tile.

Vinyl flooring is intended for home use and if it is selected for a preparation room it is very necessary to purchase tile rated to withstand a load limit in excess of 100 pounds per square inch. When using sheet vinyl, have the flooring cut so it can extend several inches up the walls, this seals the seams where the wall and floor come together.

Asphalt Tile

Asphalt tile has been around for a long time. Made of resin asphalt compounds and asbestos fibers, it is very hard and brittle. Asbestos fibers are no longer used in these products. Of all tile floors it is the least expensive per square foot. It is easy to install, too! However, it must be used on cement or on an exceptionally strong floor that will not "work" (move) at all. Asphalt tile becomes increasingly brittle with age and new tiles will not have the aged appearance of those around them, making repaired areas very visible. This type of floor needs to be well waxed to ensure long life in the preparation room.

Epoxy

Another kind of floor covering is epoxy. It is usually used directly over a cement floor. A layer of epoxy is spread over the floor and then chips of color (supplied with the epoxy) are often sprinkled onto it. The epoxy flooring should be finished in a rough coat fashion to prevent slippage. When the epoxy sets, several coats of clear plastic are applied. The number of coats (and the quality of the particular brand chosen) determine the durability of the floor. There are several types on the market. Epoxy coverings can also be used over old tile, wood, and other types of floors, but preparation of the old surface must be extremely thorough. Finally, these preparations can also be used on all surfaces. Epoxy floors are seamless so it is an easy surface to disinfect.

Paint

Paint, of course, is the least expensive floor covering of all. But it will not stand up under wear and it is especially susceptible to damage from chemicals, so spillage is a real problem. If a floor is to be tiled, all the paint must be sanded off to obtain good bond for the tile. An oil-based enamel paint is recommended.

▶ WINDOWS, DOORS, AND CEILINGS

Windows, doors, and ceilings all function to some degree to control sound, light (Figure 4–3), and odors.

Windows

The first factor influencing the selection of a window is the location of the preparation room in the building. Local climate and the direction of prevailing winds should also be considered. If the preparation room is built in the basement there will probably be a need to augment the natural ventilation available with some system of forced air. Aside from the obvious odor problems, the natural summer dampness in most parts of the country is a problem in a basement. Windows can be an available source for fresh incoming air when mechanical exhaust systems are running.

Privacy must always be ensured in the preparation room. In a basement location, frosted glass is usually necessary. Wire reinforcement in the glass is often essential in city areas because of vandalism. Frosted jalousie windows afford privacy while permitting air

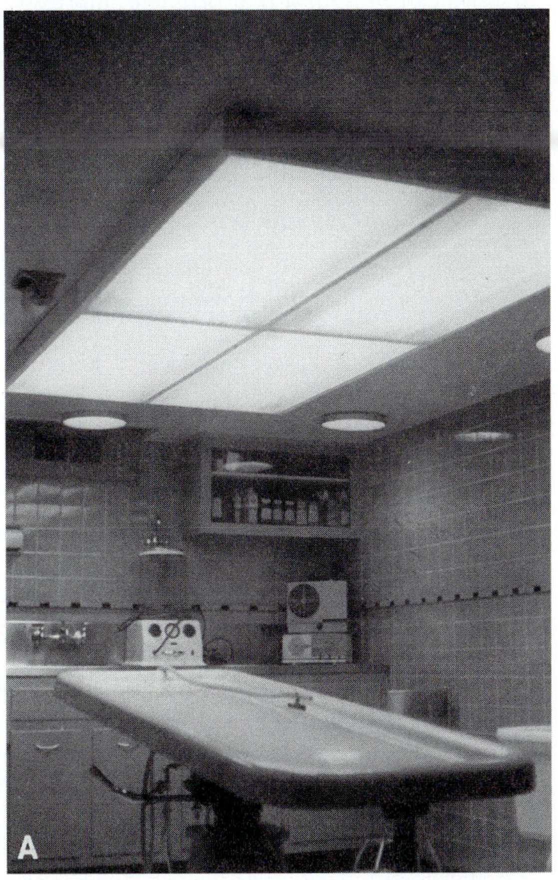

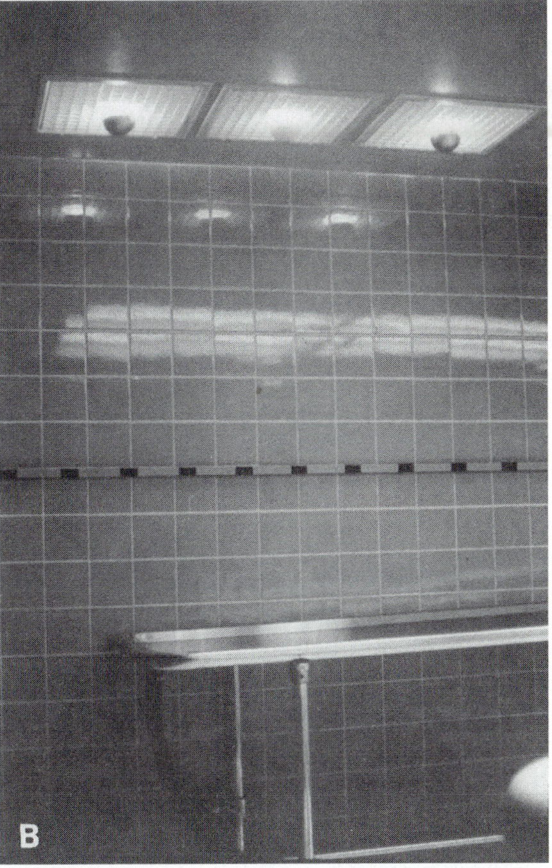

Figure 4–3. Preparation room lights. **A.** Adequate lighting. Note the number of electrical outlets available. **B.** Adjustable cosmetic lights.

flow and can be a good choice. The inverted awning-type window ensures privacy when the window is open.

Look for windows associated with the fewest maintenance problems. Below (or even just above) ground level, a wooden sash is likely to swell in dampness and create opening and closing problems. Keeping paint on damp wood (to prevent rot) also requires frequent attention; steel, aluminum, or vinyl sashes should be used here instead. If a basement window is below grade and drainage around the window is poor, a well can be dug and a plexiglass bubble placed over the window and well to keep snow or rain from accumulating.

There are other considerations in selecting windows for first and upper floors. Movements within the room should not be visible as silhouettes or shadows on the window. When work must be done at night, heavy drapes are suggested as well as rolling floor screens or folding screens. At street level, windows can be protected from view by shrubbery or a louvered fence. Use inside or outside the building of materials that substantially decrease the volume of air flow possible through the windows should be avoided. Access to fresh air is important.

Select windows for quality. There is a little maintenance with good windows but cheaper ones can be very irritating. They warp, bind, rattle, and leak. Unlike poor-grade windows, good-quality wood, metal, and vinyl frames are dimensionally stable. Good windows also prevent heat loss.

One of the best sources of light if architecture permits is the glass block wall; however, additional windows then become necessary for ventilation. If the preparation room is located on the top floor and is wedged between other buildings, restricting light and air flow from regular windows, plastic dome skylights should be considered. This sort of window also allows full use of wall space. Ventilation is aided as warm air rises rapidly to the ceiling and through the skylight under most weather conditions.

Doors

Some state rules now require that preparation room doors be locked. This would be a good rule for all establishments to follow. Many funeral establishments use touchpad locking devices. This eliminates the need for keys, and the codes can be periodically changed.

The doors in the preparation room should be of the same high quality as the windows. These doors will get a heavy flow of traffic and must not warp, bind, catch poorly, or need to be slammed shut. Prehung doors are an excellent choice because they are of good quality and also save time in installation. To some extent the size of the entrance and the area to which that entrance leads determine the type of door needed. If the door leads to an adjoining garage, the insurance company or building code will probably call for a metal-covered door. In selection of an interior door, choices include doors with solid cores, hollow cores, solid fresco cores, solid wood staved cores, solid wood flake cores, or lead shield cores. All are available with different odor and sound control properties. Be sure that the door selected is able to stand up to heat, moisture, scuffs, and stains.

Busy doors should always have push plates and kick plates to save on wear and tear. Flat-surface doors are best with regard to sanitation. Ridges and crevices in old-style doors are hard to clean well and are, therefore, bacterial breeding grounds. Old doors may be renovated and flush-surfaced by simply laminating them with any of the variety of materials available for this purpose. Advise the architect that all doors must be wide enough so that a stretcher or casket can easily pass through, and that the stretcher or casket may need to be turned at various angles to move it into or from a hallway or around some wall or other obstacle on one side of the door or the other. This warning has been previously mentioned but bears repeating. **Improper door size is one of the most common errors in preparation room planning.** The minimum width of the door should be at least 36 to 40 inches.

Ceilings

Ceilings can present a real problem, more so in renovation than in new construction, and, in particular, if the preparation room is in the basement. Frequently, the basement location means a low ceiling made lower by water pipes, heating ducts, and electrical lines. If consideration is being given to renovate such a ceiling to better insulate for sound, for the sake of appearance or for sanitation reasons, it must first be determined if there is sufficient height below the pipes, ducts, and electrical lines to construct a ceiling. If there is not enough height in the room or a room is being designed for a new building, be sure that at least 4 inches of sound insulation material is used, and the contractor allows complete and easy access to all pipes, valves, and electrical connections.

New "hung" or suspended ceilings can be an excellent choice if sufficient height is available. The large tiles provide easy access to everything above. These tiles are available in many materials. Repainting or even replacing old ceiling tiles is a fairly inexpensive way to brighten up the room every few years.

Many suspended ceilings are available as complete systems, incorporating light fixtures and ventilation systems as well as the tile. Such systems, which disperse air through large areas of the ceiling, are especially suited to delivering large quantities of air at considerable temperature differentials with minimal draft and noise. Most of these systems require at least 15½ inches of hanging height.

Johns–Manville offers acoustical tile specially treated with antibacterial finish and bacteriostatic core.

Tests have shown that the finish reduces bacterial population on the surface by 90% in 6 hours, and the bacteriostatic core does not support bacterial proliferation.

For ceilings full of pipes or ducts, remember to clean the tops of these regularly with a good disinfectant. Infectious organisms often rest on such areas, and a breeze from a door or window can dislodge these organisms. If they fall on a host who provides the proper conditions, the organisms may proliferate.

Many funeral homes are created from old residences, and this usually means plaster ceilings. If the ceiling is in good condition a coat of paint will make it look excellent again. If the plaster is at all loose, do not add ceiling material to it. Pull off the old ceiling, or at least all that is loose. Fur out the old base to align the new ceiling correctly.

The material of the various suspended ceilings should be checked for fire-retardant qualities. Ratings are given by most manufacturers in their data booklets.

Simple painting may not be sufficient to save an old ceiling, but the "hung" ceiling may not be a good choice because of height limitations. The assortment of ceiling material is large, and the selection depends on the amount of money available for the project. A new ceiling of $\frac{3}{8}$-inch plasterboard properly nailed with the new, better-gripping plasterboard nails and correctly taped can give years of service. Use of the new acrylic enamel paint would make it an easy ceiling to wash. **A white ceiling is a must. It gives the advantage of reflected light, and as accumulation of dirt is readily apparent on white, it is easy to make sure the ceiling is kept clean and sanitary.**

Another good ceiling material is one of the high-gloss finish hardboards. Marlite is a good example. These are usually available in 12 × 12- and 12 × 16-inch blocks. They also come in 4 × 8-feet sheets. The thickness is usually only about $\frac{1}{4}$ inch. The small squares are easy to install and have tongue-and-groove edges for easy alignment. These boards can be glued in place. Try to avoid unnecessarily deep grooves between sections in the ceiling because they can collect dirt and serve as a possible breeding ground for bacteria. The 4 × 8-feet Marlite hardboards come with matching joint moldings. Good-quality chrome finish moldings stand up well. Poor-quality chrome moldings will "pit" (form small spots of rust) as a result of temperature variations and moisture.

Walls

As with ceilings, walls hould be selected with careful concern for the ease with which they can be kept sanitary (Figure 4–4). Late in 1974, California enacted new regulations specifying sanitary requirements not only for preparation rooms but also for storage rooms (where bodies are held awaiting disposition). If a new wall is to be created, the material and method of construction are, in part, determined by the sort of room that will be on the other side. If that room is to be used by the public (as an arrangement or smoking room), then the wall must be insulated against noise and odor. Planning for a series of cabinets along such a wall is ideal in that they can serve as the needed insulation. If there must be electrical or plumbing lines in this wall, perhaps cabinets can be built out in front of these. Never plan an employee bedroom or kitchen next to a preparation room. Control of odor and bacteria is a constant worry. There are plans for setups such as this, but they should not be seriously considered.

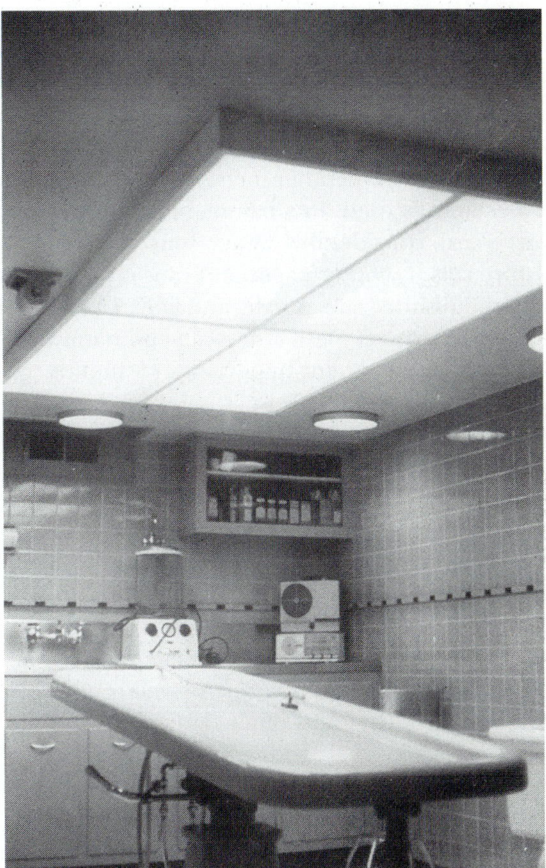

Figure 4–4. Walls tiled from the floor to the ceiling. The ceiling is soundproof.

A possible covering or finish for any wall of concrete is glazed masonry block. This comes in many sizes, styles, and colors and is easy to keep clean. The contractor must see to it that the mason keeps the grout joints smooth and close to flush with the tile surfaces for ease of cleaning. A poured concrete wall can be spray-painted after imperfections are plastered. Many plain and multicolored epoxy paints are available for use over any concrete surface. These surfaces should be finished with a clear glaze.

Modern adhesives make it possible to use ceramic tile on wallboard, which creates an excellent looking, durable wall. When dry wallboard is used by itself it should be taped and surfaced carefully and sealed with good washable enamel. Plasterboard will absorb moisture, so it must be kept an inch or two from the floor and a cove base used. In a basement or damp area, set plasterboard considerably away from the outer wall. Moisture rots the outer paper and causes the plaster to soften and disintegrate. Acrylic and latex enamel paints will seal and protect plaster, drywall, and natural wood. It will also render them impervious to liquids, gasses and microbes.

Marlite wallboard is used extensively and is available in many colors with matching moldings. Marlite is one of the easiest walls to maintain, as are formica surfaced cabinets. Formica has to be glued to a solid base like plywood or particle board. The thickness of the board is dependent on stud spacing and anchoring techniques used. Reinforced fiberglass panels are available, which are a highly sanitary material. It is always good to make panels in this type of wall removable for easy access to wiring and other equipment located inside the wall.

Many choose to use tile of some sort only part of the way up the wall and paint or wallpaper above that. This is fine provided that good, washable paint or paper is used. A flexible vinyl floor covering can also be used on a wall if there is a solid base surface to which it may be glued. In short, as long as the selection is durable and able to be cleaned thoroughly, the wall is a question of taste and budget.

Sound Insulation

Sound insulation should not be overlooked. If the room is below, above, or adjacent to public areas the sounds of instruments dropping or machines in operation will certainly be unwelcome in those areas. Many companies make special-density cellulose fiber structural board that can be used in ceilings, walls, and floors to deaden sound. The use of such material in preparation room construction is highly recommended.

▶ PLUMBING

As with all facets of preparation room planning, to avoid later difficulties with plumbing, work closely with the architect and describe all the work that goes on in the area so that all fixtures, waste lines, and other equipment can be properly located. In case of blockages, all cleanout points in waste lines should be conveniently accessible. After the room is constructed, changes are often difficult. For example, feed lines are generally buried in floors and walls (Figure 4–5). Addition of a fixture not initially planned will probably not be easy.

Water pipe is like electrical service wire in that the larger the diameter of the pipe or wire, the more water or current will flow through it. Today, copper is usually used for water pipe because it does not easily corrode or rust. The size of pipe used to bring the water in from the street is determined by the size and use of the building. Another very convenient material to work with is polyvinyl chloride (PVC) for both supply and drain. It is approved by many communities for residential use, but restrictions may be enforced for commercial applications. To avoid excessive commercial water rates when a residence is planned in the building, it might be well to have a separate water meter installed to measure the water consumption in the residence.

The feed line after the water meter is normally $\frac{3}{4}$ to 1 inch in diameter. It then decreases to $\frac{1}{2}$ inch as it feeds into the individual fixtures in the building. The supply lines to the preparation room should be at least $\frac{3}{4}$ inch in diameter. This size allows enough volume to operate waste sink flushometers properly and creates a good vacuum in a hydroaspirator. Some embalmers find that the vacuum is not great enough in their aspirators un-

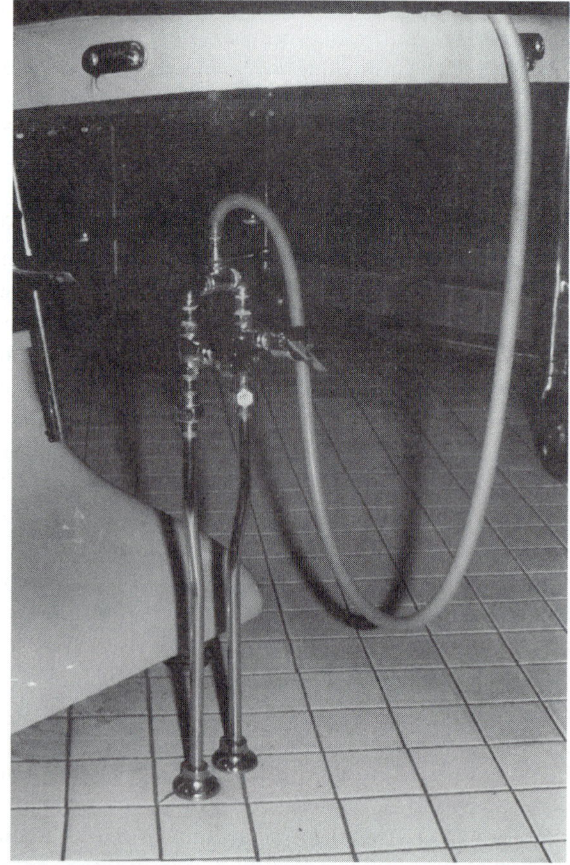

Figure 4–5. A floor water supply for the preparation table.

less they run both hot and cold water through a dual mixing faucet. This lack of suction could be the result of very small feed pipes or old, galvanized pipes. These pipes corrode and the buildup on their internal walls restricts flow and, therefore, reduces vacuum.

A good reason to have removable panels and ceiling tiles in strategic areas (so that access to plumbing and electrical wiring is convenient) is that of changing municipal codes. If there is a question of compliance with a plumbing code, it will be possible to make changes without ripping out the walls.

The second major plumbing consideration deals with codes. Having discussed bringing in an adequate water supply, the subject of disposal of waste water must be considered. How wastes are handled is a major concern. Codes and regulations change as knowledge of good sanitation procedures increases. In some areas the water table is very high and good filtration is needed or life is endangered by feeding harmful bacteria back into the drinking water.

Backflow

Backflow is the unwanted reverse flow of liquids in a piping system. It can be caused by back-siphonage, back-pressure, or a combination of both. Back-siphonage is due to a vacuum or partial vacuum in the water supply system. It is caused by *ordinary gravity*—when water supply is lost and a fixture that is elevated is opened, allowing air into the system, water will (by gravity) reverse flow; *undersized piping*—high-velocity water traveling through undersized piping can cause an aspirator effect and draw water out of branch pipes causing a partial vacuum and a reverse flow; and *vacuum*—pumping water from the supply system creates a pressure drop or a negative pressure in the system, or a break in the main or excessive usage at a lower level in the system can also be a cause.

Many water departments now require a backflow prevention (one-way) valve at the point at which the water enters the funeral home from the street. Several types are available. The installation of these devices is favored where the water enters the preparation room (not just the funeral home) on both hot and cold lines. In this way the public within the funeral home, as well as the community, are protected from accidentally contaminated water.

Incredible concentrations of bacteria of various types exist on and within every subject brought into the preparation room, so the need for precautionary measures is obvious. In early 1970, the state of Connecticut started a program requiring the use of blackflow prevention devices. Since then, additions to these regulations now require special faucets to be used with hydroaspirators, which must be equipped with vacuum breakers. These faucets are made for industrial use as in commercial laundries. The fixture is dull in finish and has a vacuum breaker built into the top of the spout.

Electric Aspirator. The trocar is attached via the hose on the right side of the impeller casing. The hose coming off the left side leads directly to the top of the flush sink. The small tube off the top of the impeller casing draws water from the bulb that is attached to the water faucet. The water faucet attachment has two water supplies—one to the bulb to keep the impeller lubricated when no aspirant is flowing through the trocar, and one off the opposite side (with an attached hose) for water to be supplied for other purposes. The impeller casing has three screws that allow for removal of the impeller for replacement or drying (Figure 4–6A).

Hydroaspirator. The hydroaspirator is attached to a water faucet over a flush sink. A clear plastic hose connects the aspirator and trocar. The level near the bottom of the aspirator allows for clean water flow from the hose or for aspiration (suction) if the lever is vertically aligned with the aspirator (Figure 4–6B).

Vacuum Breakers. Two vacuum breakers are shown at two levels: The lower one is the top half of the aspiration unit and is directly attached to the water faucet. The second one is higher and is seen behind the clear plastic hose in line with the plumbing pipes. The hydroaspirator is a part of a counter installation of aspirator and two water lines. The larger open pipe nearest the counter is the aspirator unit. The vacuum breaker is shown to the right side and at a higher level than the hose attachment. The hose is attached in line via a hydraulic connector and can easily be removed for cleaning and disinfection. The handle on the right side controls the water flow; it is the water flowing through the unit that creates the suction (Figure 4–7; also see Figure 4–9A).

One consideration is to put vacuum breakers into the hot and cold supply lines for the preparation room rather than on each faucet. A siphon-breaking device or backflow preventer is a rather simple mechanism that is attached to a threaded faucet before the hydroaspirator is mounted. It combines a check valve and air vents. When water forces open the check valve, the air vents are automatically closed. If water pressure drops, the check valve closes automatically and the air vents are opened, preventing any backflow into the supply line. The air vents break any built up vacuum. This

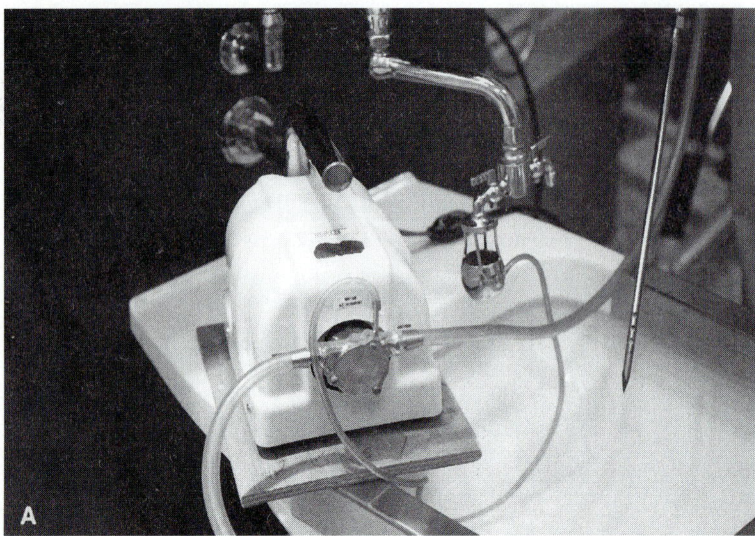

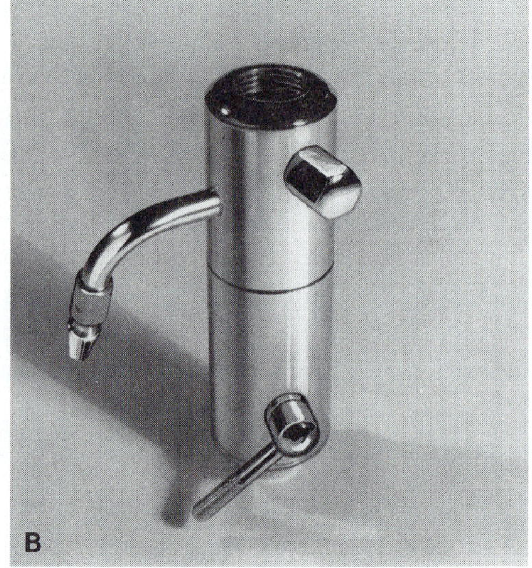

Figure 4–6. A. Electric aspirator. **B.** Hydroaspirator.

inexpensive but effective device is available through most preparation room suppliers.

Backflow and siphonage are very real hazards in funeral homes, especially if the volume and pressure of the water entering the building are not great enough to adequately supply all outlets in the building. For example, if the pressure is barely adequate for aspiration, flushing a toilet or starting a washing machine can cause such a drop in pressure at the aspirator faucet that a vacuum results, drawing waste materials into the waterline.

Because of the serious nature of backflow problems, OSHA has addressed the problem nationally, whereas many states have yet to do so. Subpart J of the Occupational Safety and Health Act pertains to general environmental controls. Paragraph 1910.141(b)(2)(ii) contains the following statement: "Construction of nonpotable water systems carrying any other nonpotable substance shall be such as to prevent backflow or back siphonage into a potable water system.*

Some manufacturers claim that their backflow valves work when installed in the drain line at a point lower than the level at which that drain pipe ultimately empties. This sort of installation is very undesirable, however, and is most often not in compliance with sanitary codes.

In discussing placement of hydroaspirators, it is im-

*This revision was published in *Fed Regist.* 1973;38:10930.

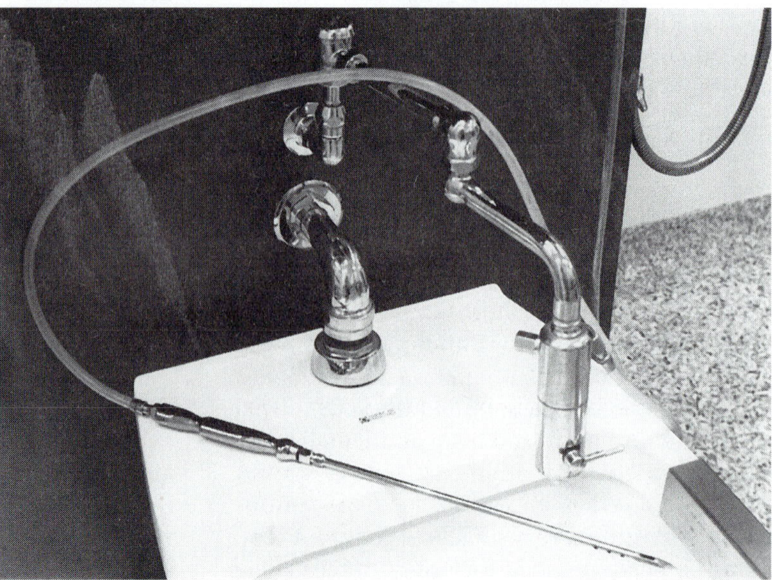

Figure 4–7. Vacuum breakers.

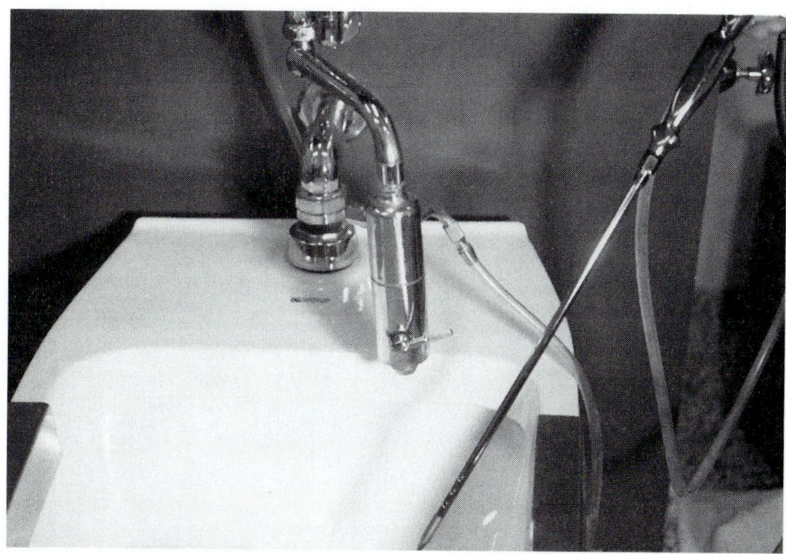

Figure 4–8. Hydroaspiration in a visible position.

portant to remember that the aspirator should not be attached to a faucet in a sink in such a way that it is below the top of the sink walls (Figure 4–8). This means that the operator cannot see the aspirator. The sink drain's runoff may not be as fast as the inflow of water from the faucet. With the aspirator deep in the sink or below the rim, the vents will be covered with water. If, for example a toilet is flushed elsewhere in the system, backflow will result. The aspirator, therefore, should be at least 2 inches above the rim of the sink. Another problem with hydroaspirators can occur during aspiration of tissue particles. These can become lodged in the aspirator throat and block it, causing the operator to inject water into the body via the trocar.

Drains

No discussion of preparation room plumbing needs would be complete without a thorough discussion of drains. In planning the location of drains, remember that the drain pipe must have a downward slope of $\frac{1}{4}$ inch over every foot of length from point of entry into the room to the point of exit. Commercial sealed sump pumps can be installed to lift wastes. Also, where codes allow, flush-up toilets may be used (Figure 4–9A). Such toilets need a minimum of 40 pounds psi of pressure sustained at 4 gallons per minute for a 10-foot lift. Many basement preparation rooms use small electric pumps to lift drainage water. Any unit of this type should be checked frequently to make sure the collecting pot is being thoroughly rinsed.

A central floor drain surrounded by a slope is inconvenient. Church trucks and cots can wobble, roll, and cause damage. A floor drain in an out-of-the-way corner surrounded by a small area of slope avoids these problems (Figure 4–9B). Waste drains must be vented to flow properly. A drain in a basement floor, in an area with a high water table, must have a one-way flap installed to prevent backup. Also, in areas where sewers are not available and septic tanks are used, remember to check codes to determine minimum distances between septic tank systems and wells for water.

Water Supply

Most codes require hot as well as cold water in the preparation room. Certain states even set a minimum temperature requirement of 130° or 145°. The need for hot water in the preparation room is easy to understand. OSHA requires that all steam and hot water pipes be insulated when it is possible for an employee to come in contact with the pipes. It is not always convenient to insulate. One possible alternative for pipes leading to freestanding sinks is to enclose them in a cabinet.

Convenient water service to the embalming table, the embalming machine, and the sinks can save much time and many steps. The table is the work center. Water can be fed to it either from an overhead supply or directly from service sinks. If the table is permanently located, a supply line can be placed under the head area, coming up from the floor or dropping from the ceiling. The overhead service is really handy for washing the remains and shampooing and rinsing the hair.

Sinks

There are many alternatives from which to choose in selecting a waste sink for the embalming table (Figures 4–8 and 4–9A). Room size and expense are two factors to be weighed. A sink that permits good floor maintenance should be selected. Flushable sinks, whether floorstanding or wall-hung, are the most sanitary. The flush valve incorporates a vacuum breaker. A minimum of 20 pounds psi is required at the valve while flushing.

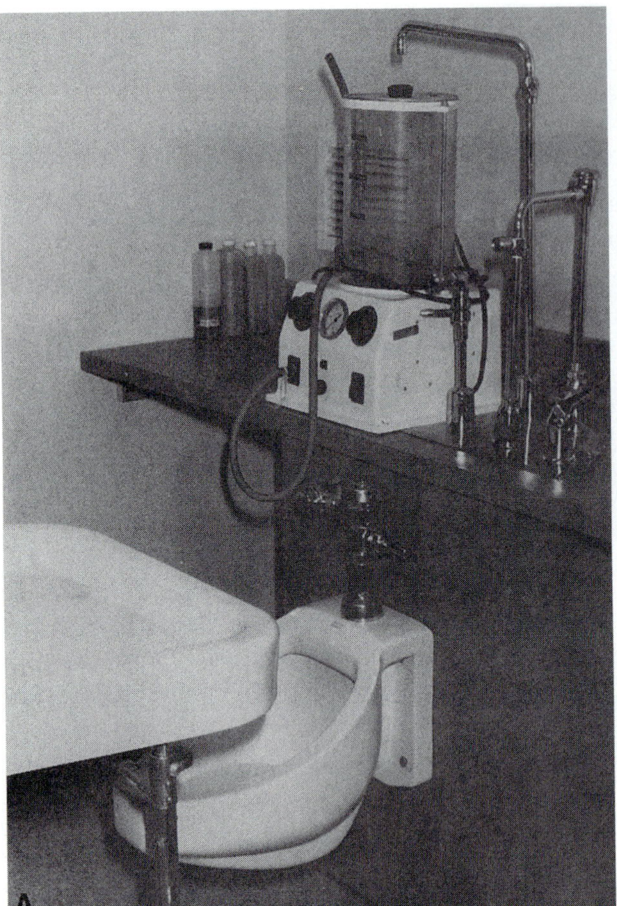

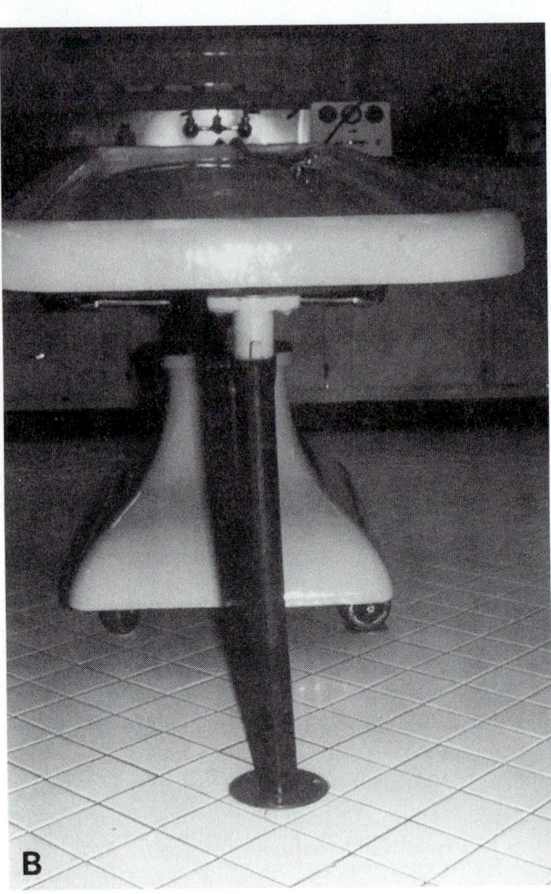

Figure 4–9. A. Flush drain. **B.** Floor drain.

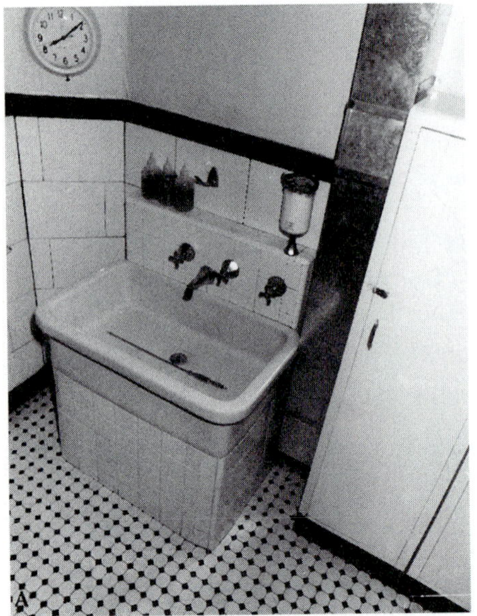

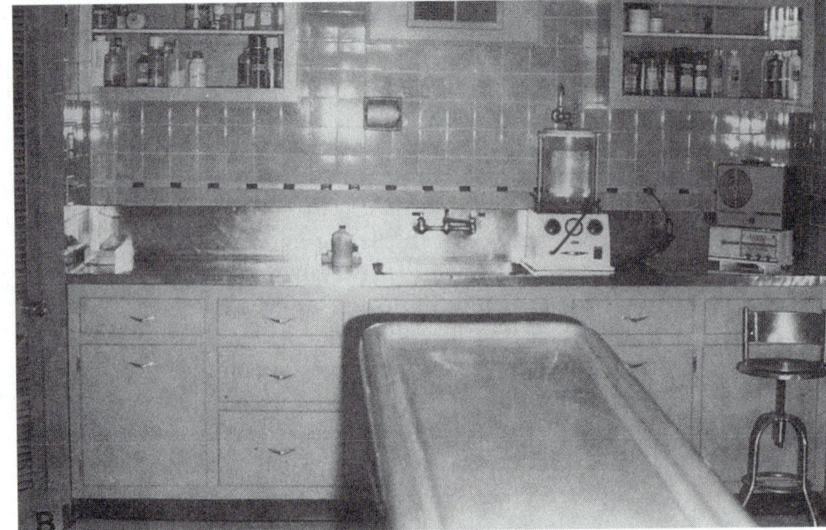

Figure 4–10. A. Wide porcelain utility sink. **B.** Stainless-steel utility sink.

Hand sinks should be located conveniently for the operator and need not be too large. Remembering the need for sanitation, controls should be selected that do not require handling of faucets, which will collect untold numbers of bacteria. There are controls for knee operation, foot operation, and elbow or forearm operation. A gooseneck faucet facilitates the filling of large bottles and pails (Figure 4–10A).

Sinks can have surfaces of china, enamel on pressed steel, or stainless steel. Enamel on pressed steel chips easily but is least expensive to replace. Stainless steel is popular but harder to keep clean looking. A bottle or instrument dropped in a stainless sink makes an awful racket! Flush-surface hand sinks in countertops are even easier to maintain than wall-mounted ones. If plans call for a separate dressing room, the cosmetician and hairdresser should have their own sink.

▶ VENTILATION

The subjects of ventilation and operator exposure to airborne microbes are often relegated from the position of potential health hazard to a position secondary to the threat of direct physical contact with pathogens from the body itself. Because of this, teaching and funeral home management policy directives often emphasize the need for protective gloves, garb, and cleaning, while ignoring the necessity to monitor and limit the inhalation of disease organisms in the preparation room. No discussion of the embalming environment is complete without a thorough and cautionary discourse on the subject of ventilation and the necessity to protect the embalmer. Adequate ventilation is essential. A preparation room should have 12 to 20 air exchanges per hour.

Formaldehyde

There are two very real problems with formaldehyde. First, it is irritating to work with if encountered in levels above the 1 ppm currently allowed by OSHA. For this reason alone, proper ventilation is an absolute necessity.

The second problem is that formaldehyde gas may cause severe irritation to the mucous membrane of the respiratory tract and eyes. Morrill reported sensory irritation (itching of eyes, dry and sore throat, increased thirst, and disturbed sleep) in paper process workers at 0.9–1.6 ppm formaldehyde. Bourne and Seferian reported from another occupational setting intense irritation of eyes, nose, and throat at levels ranging from 0.13 to 0.45 ppm. More recent studies by Kerfoot and Mooney and Moore and Ogrodnik* conducted in funeral homes indicate that concentrations from 0.25 to 1.39 ppm evoke numerous complaints of upper respiratory tract and eye irritation and headache among embalmers. Schoenber and Mitchell report that acute exposure to formaldehyde phenolic resin vapors at levels around 0.4 to 0.8 ppm causes lacrimation and irritation of the upper as well as the lower respiratory tract.

Taking this into account, NIOSH has recommended a 30-minute ceiling of 1.0 ppm. The levels at which serious inflammation of the bronchi and lower respiratory tract would occur in humans are unknown; inhalation of high levels, however, has caused chemical pneumonitis, pulmonary edema, and death.

In humans, concentrations of 2 to 3 ppm have caused mild tingling sensations in the eyes, nose, and posterior pharnyx. At 4 to 5 ppm, the discomfort increases rapidly, and some mild lacrimation occurs in most people. This level can be tolerated for perhaps 10 to 30 minutes by some persons. After 30 minutes, discomfort becomes quite pronounced. Concentrations of 10 ppm can be withstood only a few minutes, and profuse lacrimation occurs in all subjects, even those acclimated to lower levels.

Very little is known about the effects of long-term exposure to low levels of formaldehyde; however, several instances of "occupational asthma" caused by formalin have been reported, even in persons who were not known to be atopic. Although there remains the question of whether the illness represents a true hypersensitivity reaction or an acute chemical pneumonitis provoked by formalin, progressive dyspnea and chest tightness accompanied by attacks of wheezing and productive cough seem to be the common features. All these symptoms return to normal within hours or days of withdrawal, depending on the exposure dose.

Emerging technology and thought in the design and construction of preparation rooms reflect the recognition that because formaldehyde is heavier than air, exhaust systems located at or near floor level, when combined with the introduction of uncontaminated air from the ceiling level, are an efficient method of ventilation. In addition, such systems have the added advantage of drawing fumes and contaminants down and away from the operator's face during the embalming procedure. There are, nevertheless, several alternate and more conventional methods of ventilating a preparation room that are satisfactory. **The key to the creation of an embalming environment protective of the embalmer's health and comfort is air flow and adequacy of ventilation.**

Anything so crucial to the comfort and safety of those working in the preparation room warrants careful consideration. The number and location of windows and doors are obviously components of the total ventilation system. Cross-ventilation (which requires windows

*See Selected Readings for complete Kerfoot-Mooney Study and Moore–Ogrodnik study.

on opposite walls) is highly desirable and should be designed into every preparation room if at all possible.

If there is sufficient height in the room to install a hung ceiling, install one that will dispense air through large areas in the ceilings. These have the ability to deliver large quantities of air at considerable temperature differentials with minimal draft and noise.

Many preparation rooms are equipped with the familiar kitchen exhaust hood. When it is installed over the waste sink at a height of about 4 feet, air is drawn out slightly above table level. Because the hood is located over the waste sink, unpleasant odors are kept away from the operator. In many places, the embalmer must stand between the exhaust fan and the source of the odor. This is uncomfortable as these odors pass by the face; it is also dangerously unsanitary. In choosing the location of the exhaust, care should always be taken so that air flows *away* from the operator. Calculations should also be obtained from a ventilation engineer to determine the number of room air changes per hour created by the system. See Figure 4–2; the ventilation duct opens at floor level.

The grill on the exhaust fan, and on all other grills in the room, should be easily removable for cleaning. Grills are often loaded with dust "kitties," and this environment is a perfect site for proliferation of bacteria. Be careful when planning an exhaust vent that goes directly from the preparation room to the roof. The architect may not realize that such a vent, located too near a roof-mounted air conditioner, could cause foul odors and pathogens to return through the air conditioner's intake vent.

Basement preparation rooms are the toughest to ventilate properly. One major problem in some areas of the country is the stagnant, humid air that can make a basement very unpleasant during the summer. Mold can start developing unless a dehumidifier is installed. Then, the water from the machine must be emptied periodically, unless it can be linked directly to a drain. Without a dehumidifier other problems can occur. Any of the various types of absorbent embalming powders can become thick and lumpy or harden completely if left uncovered. Linens, too, can absorb moisture and feel clammy.

The possibility of drafts creating dehydration should be considered carefully in laying out the preparation room. Several new preparation rooms have required expensive redesign and reinstallation of ventilation systems because the first few cases embalmed were so seriously dehydrated by drafts.

Air Conditioning

Today, most people planning a new preparation room will air condition it. Although there are many different air conditioning units to choose from, the size of the room in cubic feet and the desired number of room air changes per hour determine the size of the unit needed. If the entire funeral home is air conditioned by the same unit, there must be independent controls for the preparation room. Odors must not reach the main air flow serving the funeral home. Many times, a separate preparation room "zone," controlled manually, is recommended.

The wall or window unit is also adaptable for cooling the preparation room. Such units pull in cool fresh air from outdoors. If properly balanced with the exhaust system, a "once through" ventilation system can be created and used during the embalming operation.

In summary, ventilation experts can use the guidelines recommended to create a system of ventilation, either ongoing or manually controlled, that will provide for adequate ventilation of the embalming environment.

▶ PREPARATION ROOM EQUIPMENT

Tables

Embalming tables are available with stainless-steel or porcelain tops and cast iron, steel, or aluminum bases. These bases may have a hydraulic or ratchet-type raising, lowering, or tilting mechanism. They all have a drain channel around each side, with a drain hole at the foot end. Most stainless-steel tables have wheels, whereas the porcelain tables have a swivel-action base (Figure 4–11). Porcelain tables may be undercoated to reduce the noise of instruments laid on the table surface.

At the completion of the embalming, the body may be transferred from the embalming table to a dressing table. Dressing tables usually have a laminated plastic top and an aluminum frame. The frame usually has wheels, is adjustable in height, and perhaps can fold in the middle. There is no drain channel or hole in a dressing table as in the embalming table.

Injection Apparatus

Today, almost all arterial embalming is done using electric machines for the injection of arterial solution. To be complete, however, several older mechanical methods are considered in this discussion. These devices are generally used today when the electronic machines are not working or when there is an electrical failure. Basically, six devices can be used to inject arterial solution: (1) gravity, (2) bulb syringe, (3) combination of gravity and bulb syringe, (4) hand pump, (5) air pressure machine, and (6) centrifugal pump.

Gravity Injection (Historical). Of the six methods of injection the simplest is the use of the gravity perco-

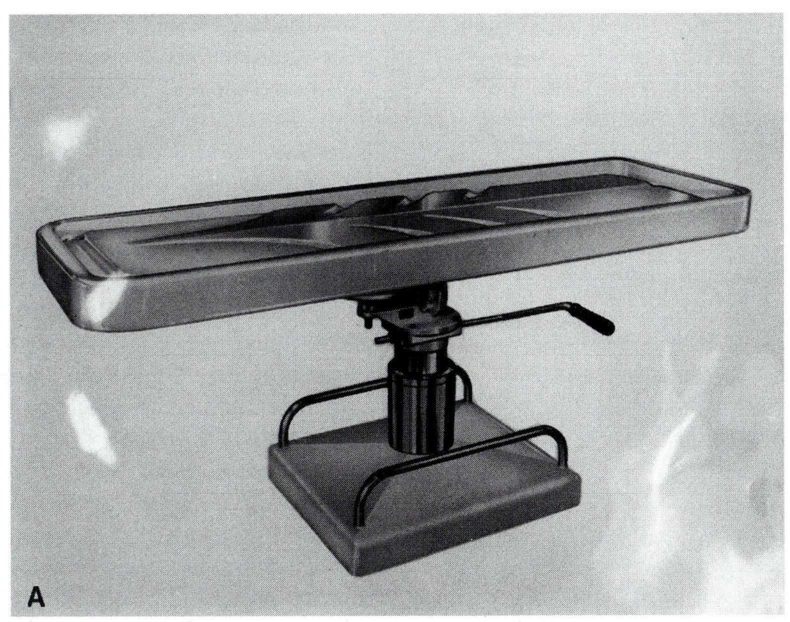

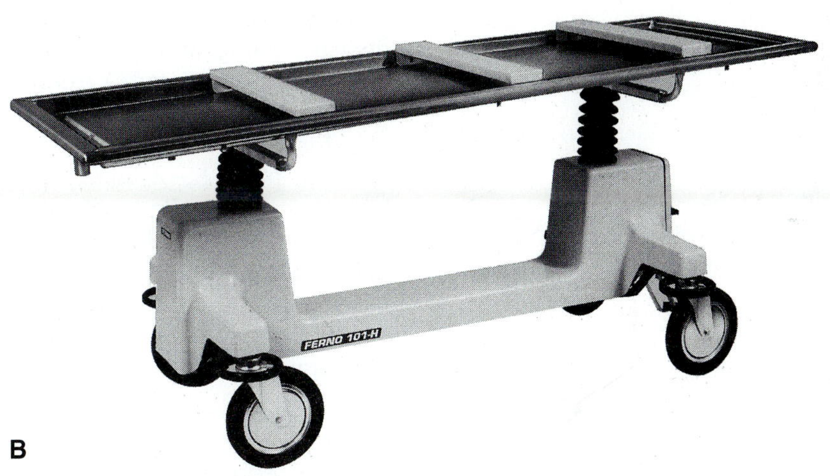

Figure 4–11. A. Hydraulic, porcelain preparation table. Note the elevated central portion and ribs to drain fluids away from the body. **B.** Hydraulic, stainless steel embalming table shown with body "bridges." (*Courtesy of Ferno-Washington, Inc., Wilmington, Ohio.*)

lator (Figure 4–12). Fluid is simply poured into a large glass percolator which has a delivery hose attached to the bottom of the bowl. The device is then elevated above the body and the fluid flows into the arterial system. Approximately one-half (0.43) pound of pressure is developed for each foot of height the device is raised above the injection point (for every 28 inches of height, one pound of pressure is created). Years ago, when this method of injection was popular, the percolators held several gallons of fluid. The percolators sold today generally hold a gallon or less of fluid. This creates a need for constant refilling. Because of height restrictions in most preparation rooms pressure is limited with gravity injection. The most frequent uses for this form of injection are as a substitute for mechanical injectors when they are not working or when there is an electrical power failure and in the embalming of bodies for dissection in medical schools. The advantage of this method of embalming is that it provides a slow, steady method of injection that allows the body to accept the embalming solution at a slower but much more thorough rate. Too often, mechanical injectors rapidly force fluid into the body, and much of the fluid rushes through the vascular system

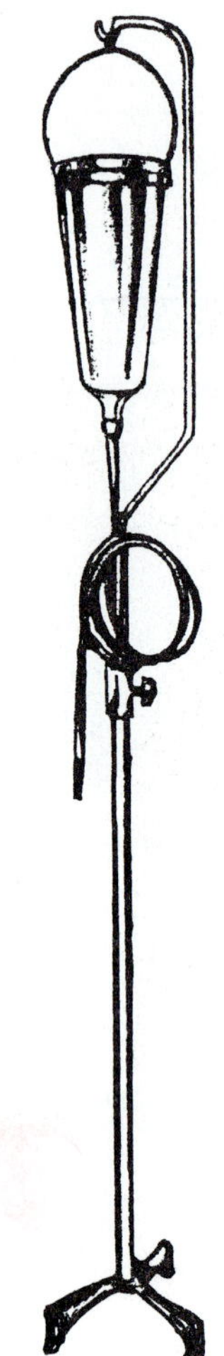

Figure 4–12. Gravity injector.

with little time for absorption and is lost in the form of drainage.

Bulb Syringe (Historical). This hand-held and -operated device consists of a rubber bulb with hoses attached to either end. A one-way valve in the device allows for this pump to operate. One hose is dropped into a container of embalming solution. Fluid flows into the bulb when the device is squeezed and continues out through the second delivery hose and into the body. It is important to remember that fluid actually passes through the bulb syringe. A body can be injected quite rapidly with this device when it is combined with the gravity percolator. Pressures created are unknown and the operator, when working alone, must use one hand constantly to operate the device. This method of injection can be used today, like the gravity percolator, when mechanical equipment fails. The tank of the mechanical embalming machine can be used as the source for the mixing and storage of the embalming solution. In this manner the embalmer can be aware of the volume of fluid injected. As pressures build in the body during injection the operator finds the bulb syringe more and more difficult to squeeze (Figure 4–13A).

Combination Gravity and Bulb Syringe (Historical). In this method of injection the delivery hose from the gravity percolator connects to the bulb syringe. The body can be embalmed by the gravity method, but pressures and rate of flow can be increased periodically by squeezing on the bulb syringe. The reason for adding the bulb syringe to the gravity device is to overcome the limited ceiling height that can limit the pressure created by the gravity system.

Hand Pump (Historical). This hand-held device is a pump that not only creates pressure but can also be adopted to create a vacuum for aspiration. Unlike the bulb syringe, arterial fluid does *not* flow through the hand pump. Fluid is placed in a jar and the lid is sealed into position. Air pumped by the hand pump enters through the hose leading from the hand pump to the jar. A delivery hose, which drops to the bottom of the jar, then carries the fluid out of the jar and into the body. By attaching the air hose to the other nozzle of the hand pump, air can be withdrawn from the jar and, thus, a vacuum created. A trocar can be attached to the delivery hose and the system of hand pump and jar used for aspiration (Figure 4–13BC).

The pressure of injection is unknown. The containers are generally small (about a half gallon) and must be constantly refilled. As with the bulb syringe, the operator must constantly use one hand to operate the hand pump. Also, like the bulb syringe, any resistance to the flow of fluid in the body will be noticed by the difficulty in operating the hand pump. There always ex-

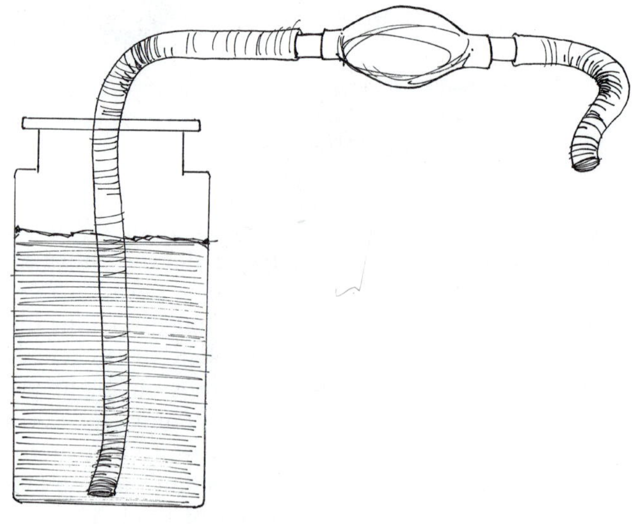

Figure 4–13. A. Bulb syringe. *(Continued.)*

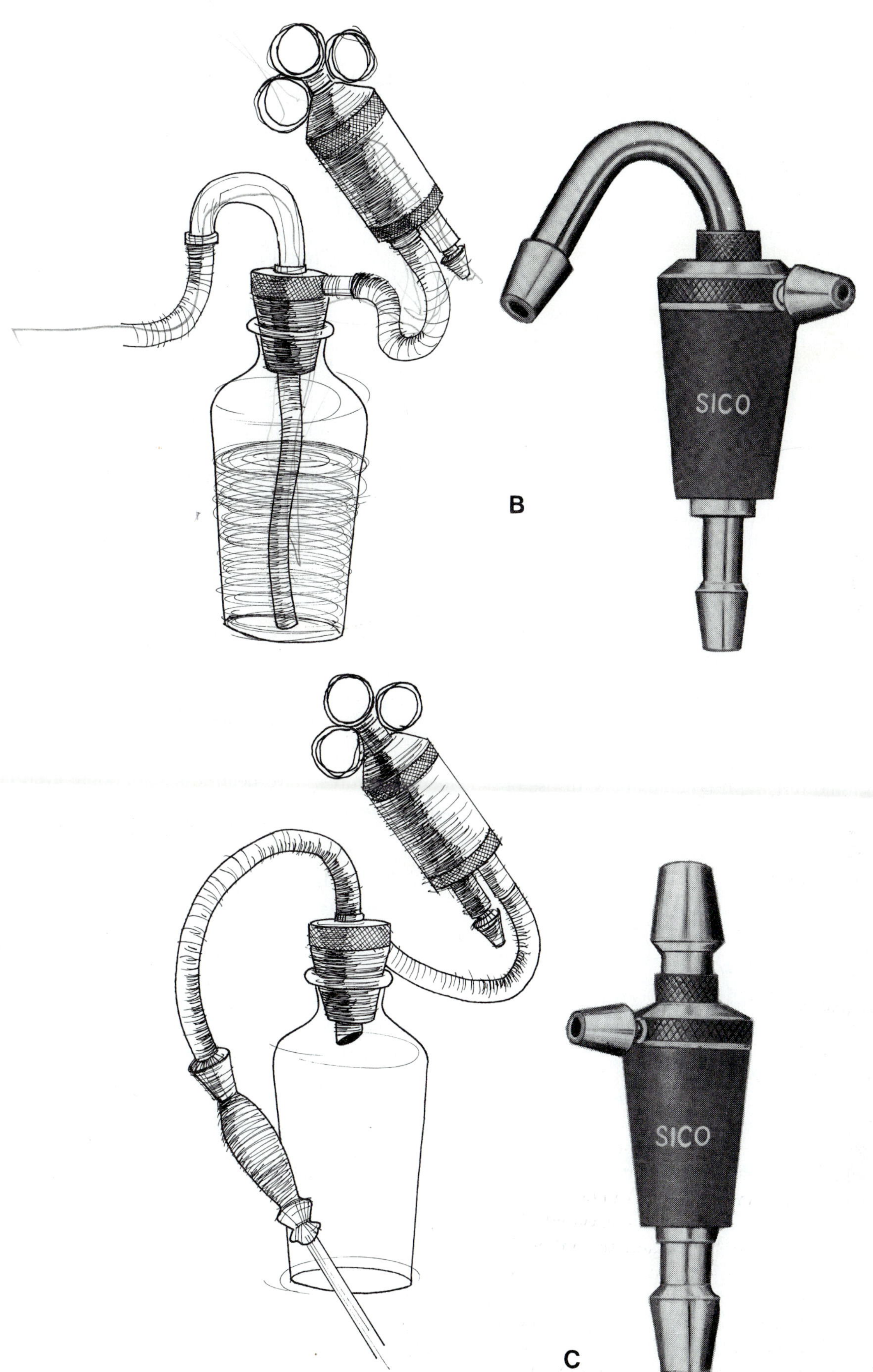

Figure 4–13 (*Continued*). **B1.** Hand pump used for injection. **B2.** Gooseneck stopper used for injection. **C1.** Hand pump used for aspiration. **C2.** Gooseneck stopper used for aspiration.

ists the possibility that the glass jar may explode or implode. It is easy, if a careful check is not kept on this operation, to inject air into the body. Like the devices previously described, this is used when the mechanical apparatus is inoperable.

Air Pressure Machine. The air pressure machine (Figure 4–14) operates just like the hand pump, but because it is motorized, it relieves the embalmer from having to physically operate the device. The air pressure machine, like the hand pump, can be adapted to aspiration. Embalming solution and aspirated materials *do not* flow through the machine. The machine provides only air pressure or a vacuum. The delivery hose from the machine is attached to a glass jar or metal pressure tank. The jar is the source of arterial solution, the container into which aspirated materials will collect. This device can be very dangerous and pressures must be carefully observed. With the mechanical air pump the bottles can easily explode.

When these machines were popular as injection devices, special metal shields could be purchased that were placed around the bottles to protect the operator. Care must be taken to observe when arterial solution has about run out of the bottle, for air can easily be injected into the body. These machines do provide a steady pressure and one that can be regulated. Because of the small volume of the bottles a great amount of time can be wasted refilling fluid containers. In use of this type of machine, note the following:

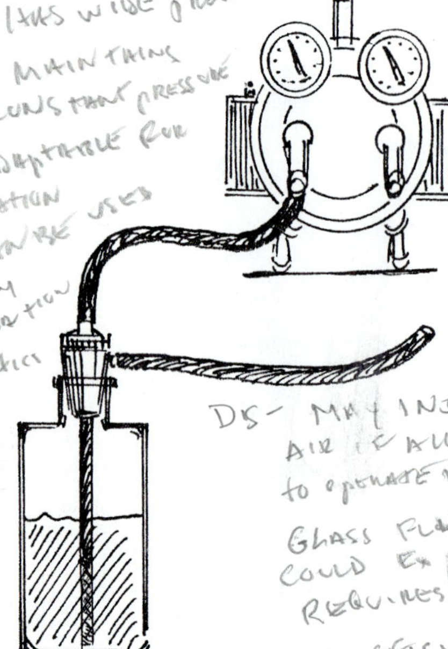

Figure 4–14. Air pressure machines may be used for injection (as illustrated) or aspiration.

1. Fill the glass bottle with the solution to be injected.
2. Place the rubber gooseneck adaptor in the bottle.
3. Connect the flexible tube from the injection control on the motor to the gooseneck.
4. Connect a second flexible tube from the gooseneck to the arterial tube. When the motor is turned on and the pressure is set, the motor forces air into the bottle through one connection on the gooseneck and forces fluid through the gooseneck and out the other connection.

In use of the air pressure machine for aspiration, the flexible tube from the gooseneck to the motor is attached to the suction valve rather than the injection valve, and the other connection in the gooseneck is attached to a flexible tube connected to the trocar. When the machine is turned on it creates a vacuum in the bottle. This vacuum causes a suction to be created in the trocar, allowing the body to be aspirated.

Centrifugal Pump. Because the centrifugal pump is the most widely accepted method of injecting arterial solution today, a more extensive explanation is given for this mechanical pump (Fig. 4–15). The centrifugal pump embalming machine is a self-contained device. Over the years a wide variety of machines, each with special features, have been available. Some even contain a separate system similar to an air pressure machine for aspiration. Most of these machines have large-volume tanks, a few of which hold as much as $3\frac{1}{2}$ gallons of fluid. With the motorized force pump a constant preset pressure can be maintained in addition to the preset rate of flow of arterial fluid into the body. It is always recommended that pressure be adjusted prior to injection of arterial fluid into the body. The rate of flow can be determined as the arterial injection begins.

During the embalming it may become necessary to reset pressure and rate of flow to establish a good distribution of the embalming solution. The pressure ranges in the motorized force pump can be very great. Some machines are capable of producing up to 200 pounds of pressure. In some machines the motorized centrifugal pump runs at a constant speed. In others, the speed can be varied, and in yet other machines two separate motors operating at different speeds are available. Many of these machines can produce a pulsating injection of fluid into the body.

Several terms must be explained at this point. ***Pressure*** is the force required to distribute the embalming solution throughout the body. The ***rate of flow*** is the amount of embalming solution that enters the body in a given period and is measured in ounces per minute. ***Potential pressure*** is the pressure reading on the gauge in

"15" - *Potential Pressure* - Rate of Flow Closed

"10" - *Actual Pressure* - Rate of Flow Open

"5" - *Differential Pressure* - The Rate of Flow

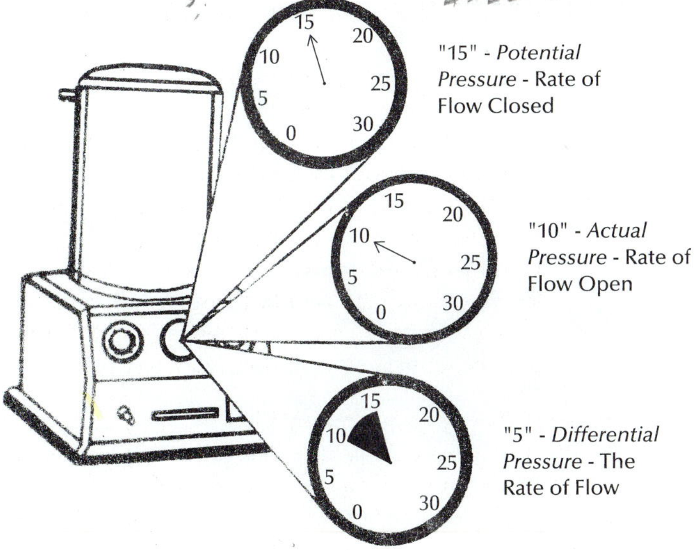

Figure 4–15. Centrifugal pump. **A.** Potential pressure (15), rate of flow closed. **B.** Actual pressure (10) rate of flow open. **C.** Differential pressure (5) or rate of flow.

the centrifugal machine, indicating the pressure in the delivery line of the machine with the rate-of-flow valve closed or the arterial tubing clamped shut. ***Differential pressure*** is the difference between the potential pressure reading and the actual pressure reading; this is an indicator of the *rate of flow.* ***Actual pressure*** is the reading on the pressure gauge on the centrifugal pump when the rate-of-flow valve is open and the arterial solution is entering the body.

In the example described in Figure 4–15, with the rate-of-flow valve *closed,* the potential pressure is 15 pounds psi. The differential pressure is 5 and the actual pressure when the rate of flow valve is open is 10. If it were open until the gauge dropped to 5 actual pounds, the differential would be 10, or it can be said that the rate of flow would be twice as fast as the previous setting. The differential reading indicates the amount of resistance in the body, in the arterial cannula, and in the tube running from the machine to the cannula. The differential is also an important indicator of the rate of flow. Flow-rate gauges may also be added to the centrifugal machine.

There has been much misunderstanding in regard to the pressure that may exist inside the body as a result of the injection of solution. The mere fact that a pressure gauge reading on the device used for injection indicates a given pressure at which the fluid is leaving the machine does not necessarily mean that this pressure exists within the body. To determine what the pressure reading on the gauge really means, take a look at the schematic diagrams (Figures 4–16 and 4–17) showing the internal structure of an embalming machine, with four different flow paths shown as "filled" tubes (solid black) numbered from 1 to 4.

Liquid flows from the "well" beneath the tank to

EMBALMING MACHINE TANK

PUMP

FLOW GAGE

FLOW CONTROL VALVE

PRESSURE GAGE

PRESSURE VALVE

Path No. 1

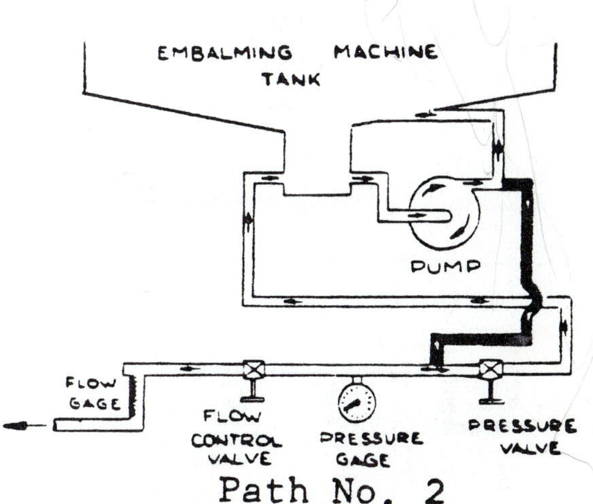

Figure 4–16. Pressure paths 1 and 2.

the pump from which it follows either path 1 or 2 or both paths (Figure 4–16). Path 1 represents the bypass flow from the pump back to the tank. As the pump functions at a steady and continuous capacity, it is necessary to provide such bypass when injection of fluid at a slow rate is desired. Otherwise, the full force of the pump pressure could not be controlled to permit such low injection rates. Path 2 is the flow from the pump to the intermediate line just prior to the outlet line.

The intermediate line contains the rate-of-flow control valve and the pressure control valve. As may be surmised, the pressure control valve determines how much fluid will be returned to the tank via path 3 (Figure 4–17), which constitutes a second bypass in the system. If, for example, a maximum pressure is set at the pressure valve control, very little, if any, liquid will flow through path 3. The needle valve in the pressure control valve actually cuts off fluid flow to that bypass and so the fluid is forced, then, to flow on to the outlet.

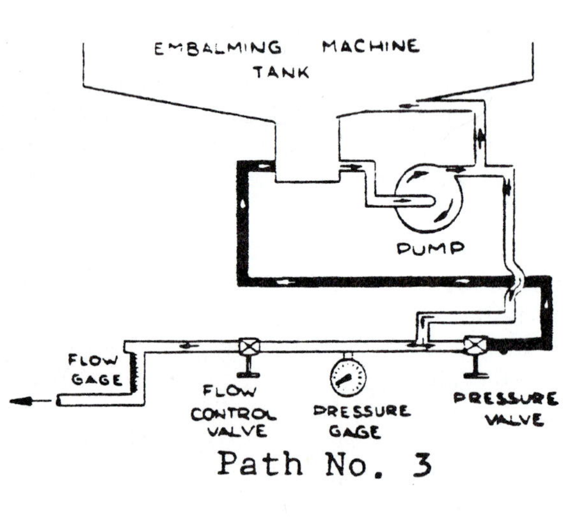

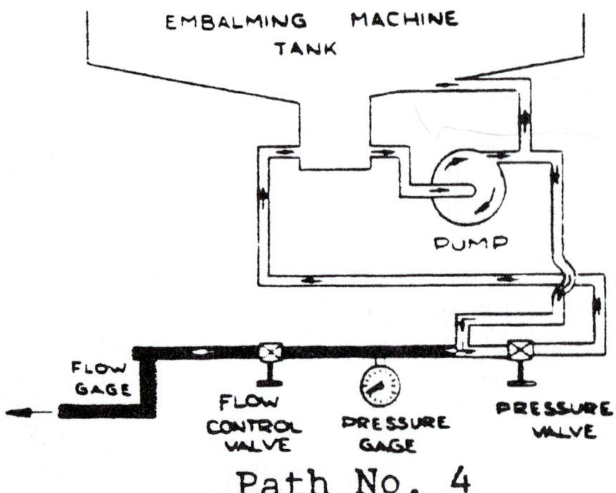

Figure 4–17. Pressure paths 3 and 4.

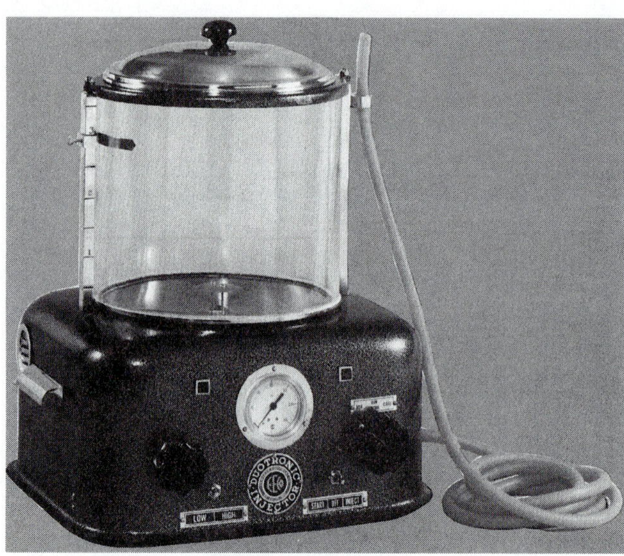

Figure 4–18. Centrifugal embalming machine. These machines are available with or without pulsation.

As the fluid proceeds to the outlet, the rate-of-flow control valve will determine how much will be delivered to the arterial tube outlet indicated by path 4. When the rate-of-flow control valve is drastically reduced so that only a small trickle of fluid is delivered, then high pressures can readily be registered on the pressure gauge. This does not mean, as can be readily realized, that the fluid is leaving the arterial tube under *that* much pressure!

In other words, with liquid flow paths 3 and 4 cut off by reducing the rate of flow and cutting off the bypass of fluid beyond the pressure control valve (causing high pressures to be registered), fluid can then leave the pump in large quantities only through path 1, which is the bypass back to the tank. It should be remembered that regardless of the amount of pressure being used or how fast the rate of flow might be, the pump *always* operates at the same speed and its output is *always* the same. With this knowledge in mind, safety features in the nature of the bypass are included in pressure machines. The pressure reading on the gauge merely indicates the amount of resistance being offered to the flow of the liquid *within* the confines of the machine. Continual use of "high" pressure places a heavy load on the motor and pump and, most often, this is not necessary (Figure 4–18).

▶ INSTRUMENTATION

An embalming chemical supply catalog lists several hundred instruments, most of which come in a variety of sizes and modifications. For this reason the list seems

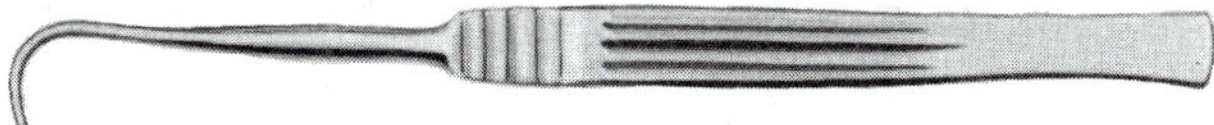

Figure 4–19. Aneurysm needle.

so long. Actually, very few instruments are needed in the preparation of the unautopsied or autopsied body. Most instruments have several uses and this helps to limit the number needed. Unlike a surgical procedure, embalming is not performed under sterile conditions, so instruments can be reused during the embalming process. Most instruments are constructed of steel and plated with nickel or chrome for protection against rust or chemical agents. They are chemically treated to be heat resistant and durable.

General instruments

Aneurysm Needle. A blunt instrument (Figure 4–19), the aneurysm needle is used for tissue dissection for the location and elevation of arteries and veins. The aneurysm needle has an "eye" in the hook portion of the instrument, which could be used for passing ligatures around a vessel. An *aneurysm hook* is similar but has a sharp pointed tip. Most embalmers prefer to work with the blunt instrument.

Bistoury Knife. The bistoury knife is a curved cutting instrument that cuts from the inside outward (Figure 4–20). Some embalmers prefer this type of instrument for opening arteries and veins. It can also be used for the excision of tissues.

Hemostat (Locking Forceps). A wide variety of hemostats are available. The hemostat can be used to clamp leaking vessels. A modification is the arterial hemostat, which is used to hold the arterial tube in an artery. The ends of hemostats may be curved or straight, serrated or smooth, or plain or rat-toothed. *Dressing forceps* are very long hemostats. They can be used for packing orifices or handling contaminated bandage dressings (Figures 4–21 to 4–23).

Scalpel. The scalpel is a sharp cutting instrument used for making incisions (Figure 4–24). It can be purchased with a permanent blade, or the handles can be purchased and disposable blades used.

Figure 4–20. Bistoury knife.

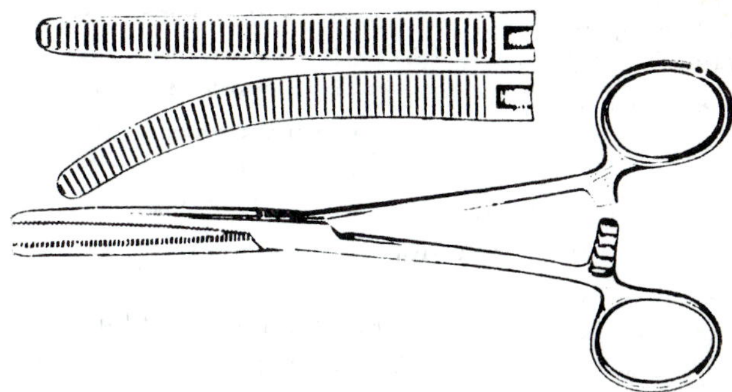

Figure 4–21. Serrated edges.

Scissors. Scissors are used for cutting. Like the bistoury knife and scalpel, scissors can also be used to open arteries and veins (Figure 4–25). There is an *arterial scissor* (Figure 4–25D) manufactured for opening vessels. Scissors vary in length, and their tips may be straight or curved, or pointed or blunt. The blunt side should be used against the skin surface of the body. *Bandage scissors* (Figure 4–25E) have a very large blunt end to help protect the skin from being cut.

Separator. The separator is used to keep vessels elevated above the incision. This instrument can be made of hard rubber, bone, or metal. Often, the handle of an aneurysm needle is designed to function as a separator (Figure 4–26).

Suture Needles. A variety of suture needles are available (Figure 4–27). The large *postmortem needles* (Figure 4–27AB) are used to close autopsy incisions as well as incisions made to raise vessels for injection. These needles are curved or double curved. The $\frac{3}{8}$-inch *circle needle* is used for more delicate suturing. The needle eye may be the patented type called a "spring eye" for "self"-threading. The edges can be smooth or cutting (Figure 4–27C). The half-curved *Loopuypt needle* (Figure 4–27E) is designed to better grip the instrument.

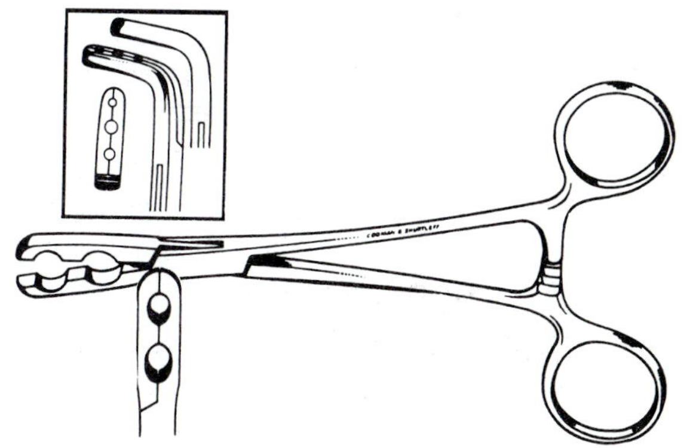

Figure 4–22. Arterial hemostat.

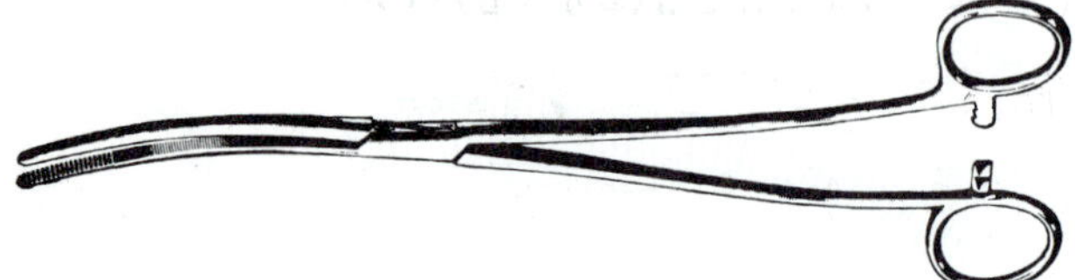

Figure 4–23. Dressing forceps.

Figure 4–24. Scalpel.

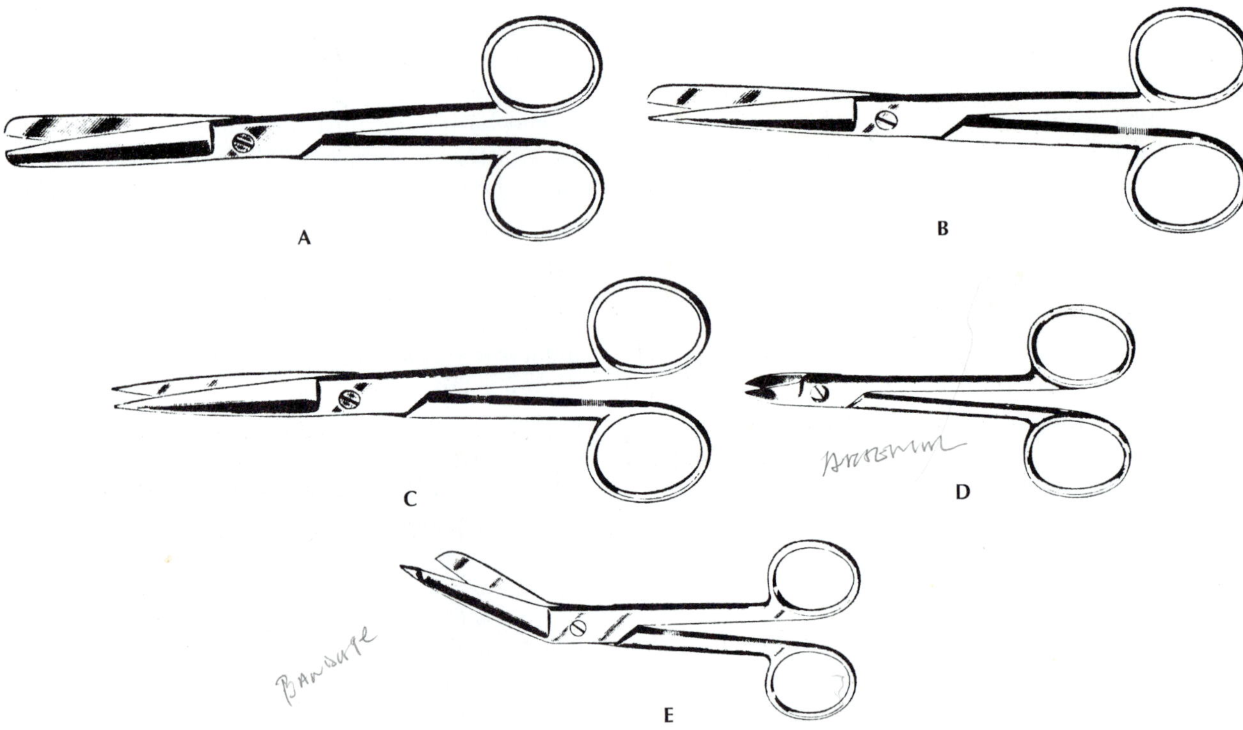

Figure 4–25 A–E. Various types of scissors.

Figure 4–26. Separator.

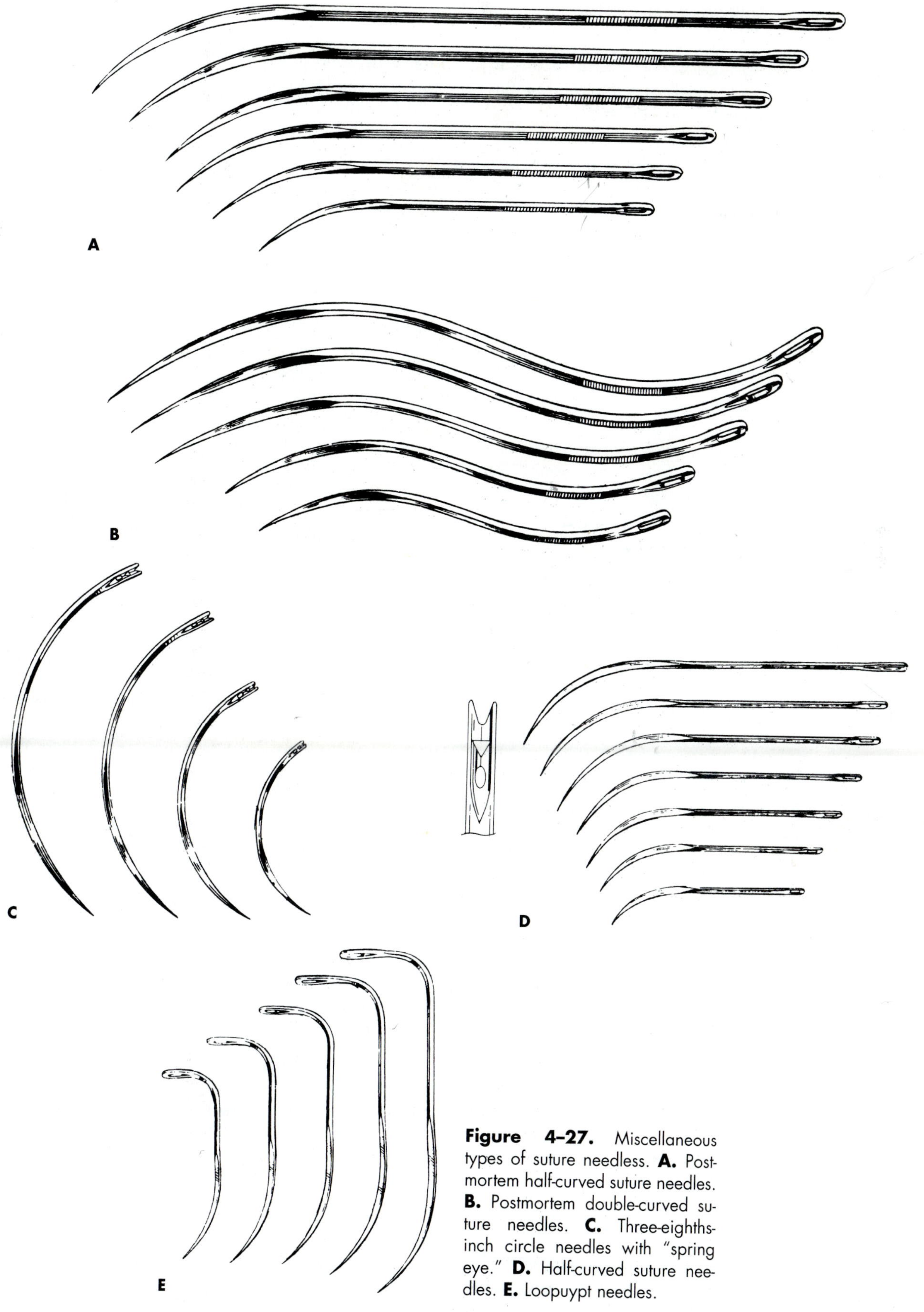

Figure 4–27. Miscellaneous types of suture needless. **A.** Postmortem half-curved suture needles. **B.** Postmortem double-curved suture needles. **C.** Three-eighths-inch circle needles with "spring eye." **D.** Half-curved suture needles. **E.** Loopuypt needles.

Spring Forceps. The spring forceps is an instrument used for grasping and holding tissues. The limbs may be straight, curved, or angular (Figure 4–28). Angular spring forceps are used as a drainage instrument, generally in the internal jugular vein. The tips of forceps may be serrated, smooth, or rat-toothed. Most embalmers use several types and lengths of spring forceps. This instrument is available in a large variety of lengths.

Suture Thread. Suture thread is sold by the twist or cord, 3 cord being thinner than 5 or 7 cord. Suture thread is available in nylon, cotton, and linen. Some embalmers prefer that it be waxed. Dental floss can also be used for suturing.

Injection Instruments

Arterial Tubes. There are many types, lengths, and sizes of arterial injection tubes: those small enough for injection of infants and distal arteries, such as the radial and ulnar arteries in the adult, and those large enough for injection of the large carotid arteries. Carotid tubes are short and very large in diameter. The hub of an arterial tube can be *threaded* (Figure 4–29A), to which a stopcock can be attached, or a *slip-type,* to which the delivery hose from the machine can be directly attached. The tube itself can be curved or straight. Luer-Lok (Figure 4–29C) arterial tubes were developed for high-pressure injection. These tubes attach to a connector on the delivery hose much the same as a hypodermic needle attaches to a syringe.

Stopcock. The stopcock is used to attach the delivery hose from the injection device to the arterial tube (Figure 4–30A). Luer-Lok stopcocks are used for arterial tubes with Luer-Lok attachments (Figure 4–30B). The stopcock can be used to maintain and stop the flow of fluid into the arterial tube.

Y Tube. The Y tube was developed for the embalming of autopsied bodies. It allows the embalmer to embalm both legs or arms or sides of the head at the same time (Figure 4–31). Double "Y" tubes have been developed that allow for injection of four body regions at the same time.

Drainage Instruments

Drain Tube. The drain tube is a metal cylinder with a cleaning rod designed to be inserted into a vein (Figure 4–32). Drain tubes are always inserted *toward* the heart. They help to keep the vein expanded and can be closed to build circulatory pressure. The stirring rod can be used to fragment large clots. There are many sizes. Jugular drain tubes are generally very large in diameter and short; axillary drain tubes are often slightly curved; infant drain tubes can be used for small vessels such as the femoral and iliac in the infant. A hose can easily be attached to the drainage outlet so the blood drained can easily be controlled or collected and disinfected.

Iliac Drain Tube. The iliac drain tube is a long drain tube designed to be inserted into the external iliac vein and the tip is directed into the right atrium of the heart (Figure 4–33). These tubes may be soft rubber, plastic, or metal.

Grooved Director. The grooved director is used to expand a vein to help guide a drain tube or drainage de-

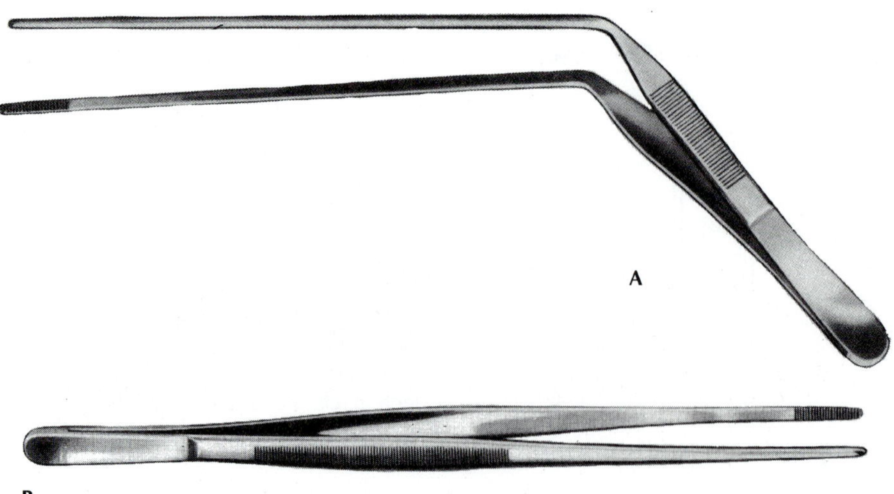

Figure 4–28. Forceps. **A.** Angular springs. **B.** Straight spring.

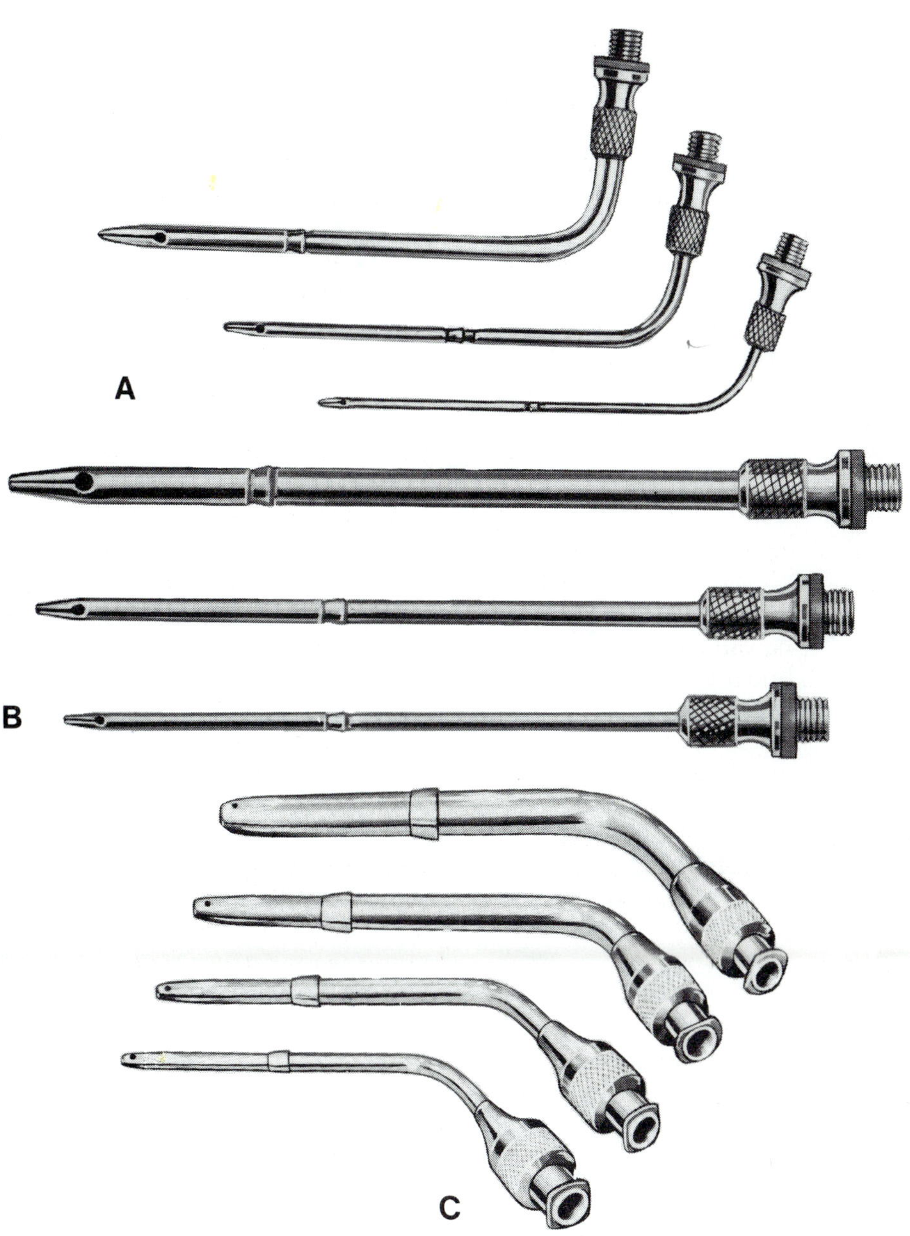

A

B

C

Figure 4–29. A. Curved threaded arterial tubes. **B.** Straight threaded arterial tubes. **C.** Luer-Lok.

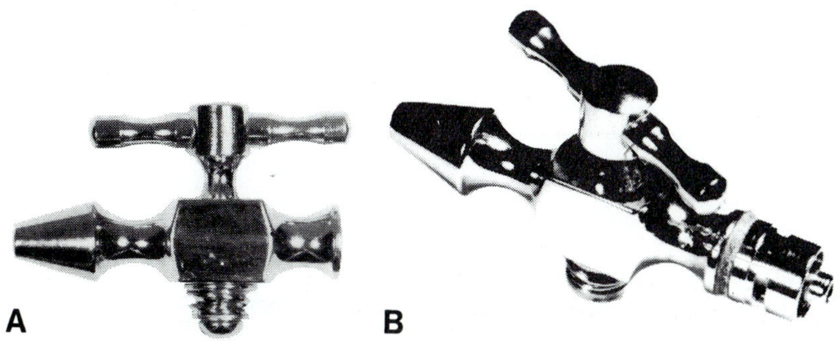

Figure 4–30. Stopcocks. **A.** Stopcock used to attach the delivery hose from the injection device to the arterial tube. **B.** Luer-Lok stopcock used for arterial tubes with Luer-Lok attachments.

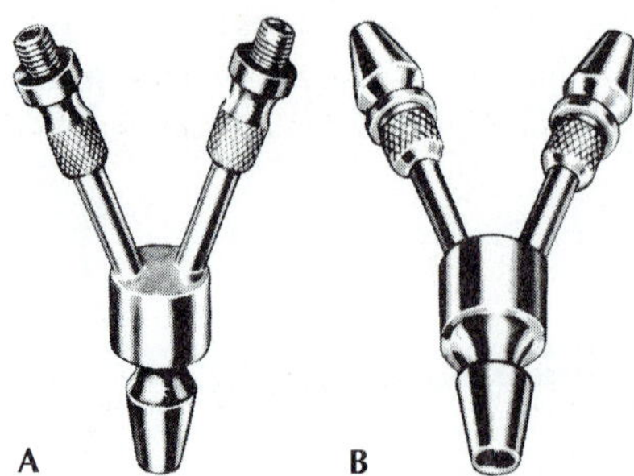

Figure 4–31. A Y tube used for embalming autopsied bodies.

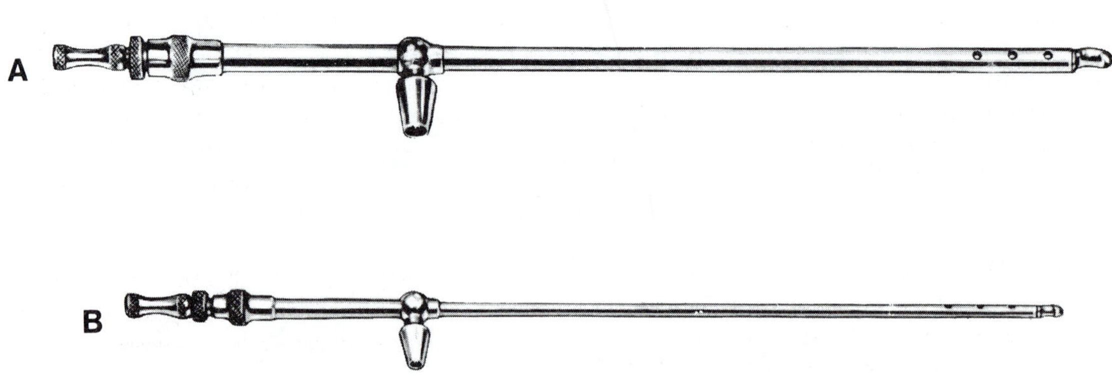

Figure 4–32. Drain tubes can be used to build circulatory pressure.

Figure 4–33. Iliac drain tube. This long tube is designed to be inserted into the external iliac vein.

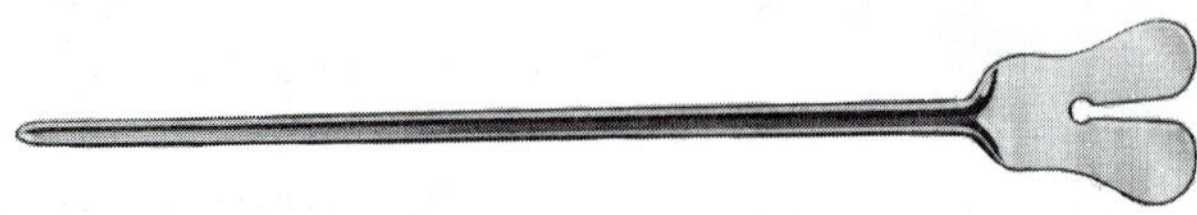

Figure 4–34. Groove director. Used to expand a vein to help guide a drain tube or drainage device into the vein.

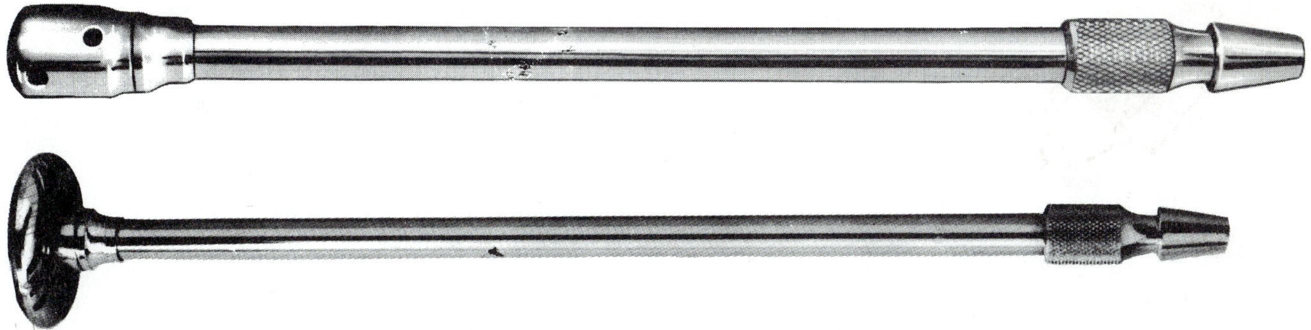

Figure 4–35. Autopsy aspirator. The many openings guard against clogging during aspiration of either blood or arterial fluid from the cavities of autopsied bodies.

vice such as angular spring forceps into a vein for a drainage (Figure 4–34).

Aspirating Instruments

Autopsy Aspirator. An autopsy aspirator has many openings so as to be "nonclogging." It is used to aspirate blood and arterial fluid from the cavities of autopsied bodies (Figure 4–35).

Hydroaspirator. The hydroaspirator is an aspirating device that creates a vacuum when water is run through the mechanism (Figure 4–36). Most are equipped with a vacuum breaker so aspirated material flowing through the device does not enter the water supply should there occur a sudden drop in water pressure.

Nasal Tube Aspirator. The nasal tube aspirator attaches to the aspirating hose. It is designed to be inserted into the nostril or throat for limited aspiration of the nasal passage or the throat (Figure 4–37).

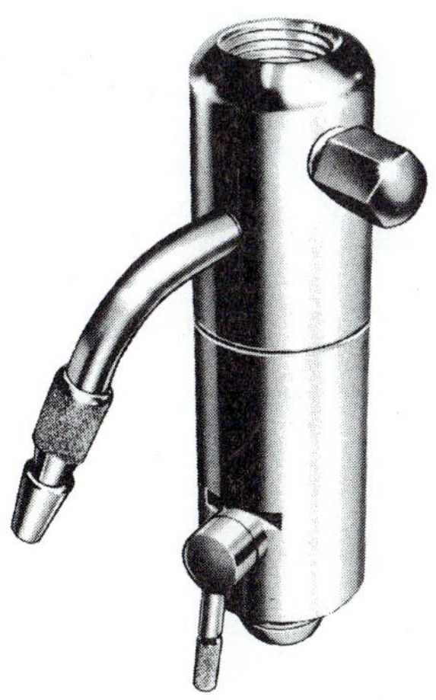

Figure 4–36. Hydroaspirator. This aspirating device creates a vacuum when water is run through the mechanism.

Trocar. The trocar is a long hollow needle. The length and the diameter of this instrument are quite variable (Figure 4–38). The points are threaded so they may be changed when dull. The handle may be threaded or have a slip hub. Infant trocars are short and small in diameter. They may also be used for hypodermic injection treatments. The standard trocar is used to aspirate and inject body cavities.

Hypovalve Trocar. The hypovalve trocar is designed for hypodermic treatments (Figure 4–39). It is *not* used for aspiration but rather for injection.

Cavity Fluid Injector. The cavity fluid injector screws onto the cavity fluid bottles. When the device is inverted, cavity fluid flows through the trocar into the body cavities (Figure 4–40).

Trocar Button. A threaded plastic screw used for closing trocar punctures, the trocar button may also be used to close small punctures, surgical drain openings, and intravenous line punctures (Figure 4–41).

Trocar Button Applicator. The trocar button applicator is used to insert the trocar button (Figure 4–42).

Feature Setting Devices

Eyecaps. Eyecaps are plastic disks inserted under the eyelids. They keep the eyelids closed and prevent the eyes from sinking into the orbit (Figure 4–43).

Mouth Formers. Mouth formers are plastic or metal devices used to replace the teeth when the natural teeth or dentures are absent (Figure 4–44).

Needle Injector. A needle injector is used to insert a "barb" into the mandible and maxilla to hold the lower jaw in a closed position (Figure 4–45).

Figure 4–37. Nasal tube aspirator. Attaches to the aspirating hose. Designed for nasal insertion.

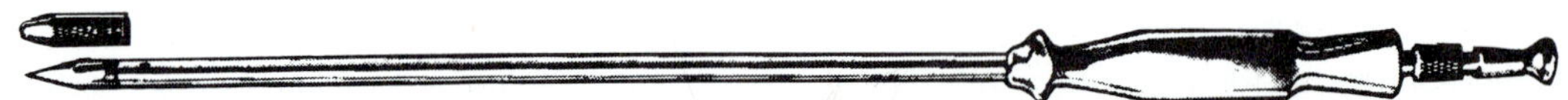

Figure 4–38. Trocar. A long hollow needle with threaded points that can be changed.

Figure 4–39. Hypovalve trocar. Designed for hypodermic treatments. Used for injection, not aspiration.

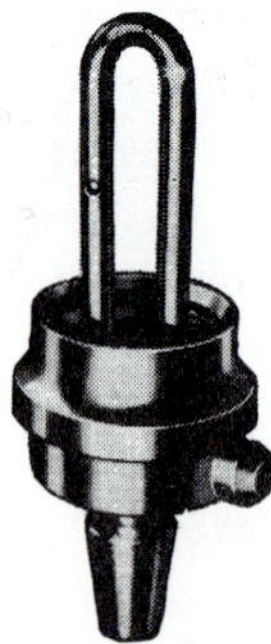

Figure 4–40. Cavity fluid injector. Screws onto cavity fluid bottles.

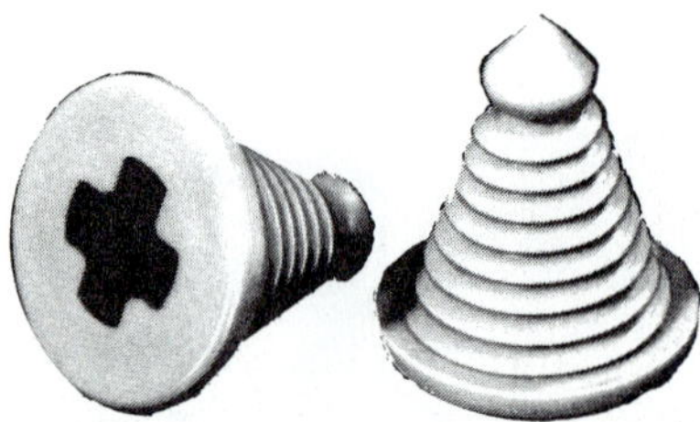

Figure 4–41. Trocar button. Threaded plastic screw used for closing trocar punctures.

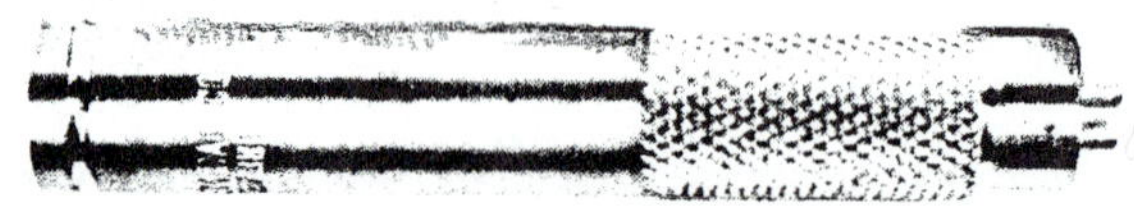

Figure 4–42. Trocar button applicator. Used to insert the trocar button.

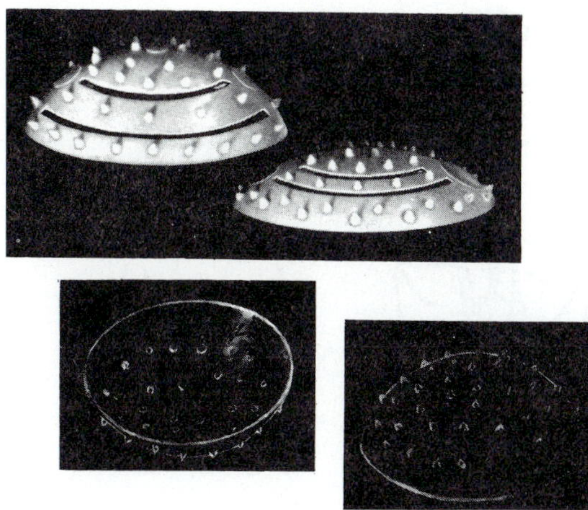

Figure 4–43. Eyecaps.

Positioning Devices

Positioning devices enable the embalmer to properly position the head, arms, hands, and feet of the deceased. Most are constructed of metal, hard rubber, or plastic. Embalmers often employ specially cut blocks of wood to elevate shoulders, arms, and feet. These devices should be properly painted with a water-resistant paint so they can be cleaned after each use.

Head Rests. Head rests can be used to elevate the head and neck. They can be used to support the arms and raise the feet. A head rest can also be placed under the thigh area to help steady bodies with severe spinal curvature or an arthritic condition (Figure 4–46).

Arm and Hand Rests. Arm and hand rests consist of two curved metal arm holders attached by an adjustable strap. The strap rests across the body while the arms are secured in the arm holder. It is designed to fit bodies of different size and retain both arms and hands in a desirable position.

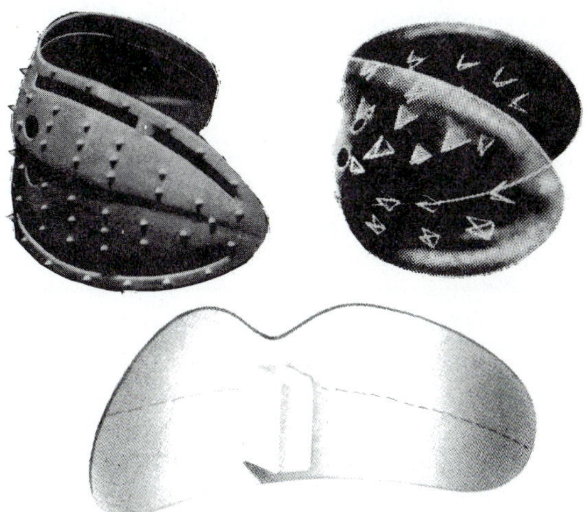

Figure 4–44. Mouth formers.

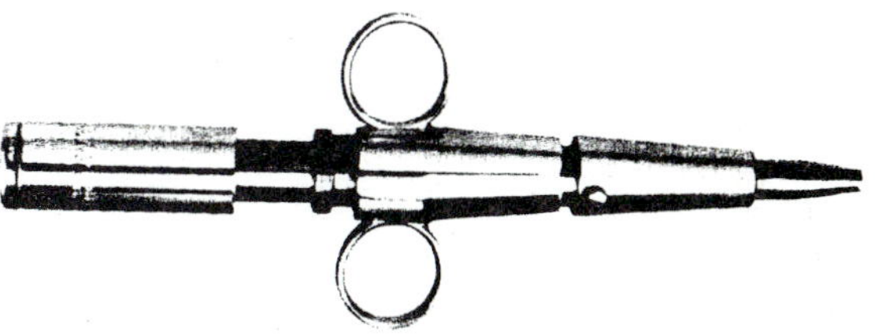

Figure 4–45. Needle injector.

Shoulder, Body, and Foot Rests. Rests of plastic or metal blocks are used to raise shoulders, feet, or buttocks off the table.

▶ PLASTIC UNDERGARMENTS

Plastic undergarments are a necessity. These garments can be used to protect clothing from conditions such as ulcerations, gangrene, or burnt tissue. Plastic garments help to control leakage from the autopsied body or the condition of edema. Powdered deodorants and preser-

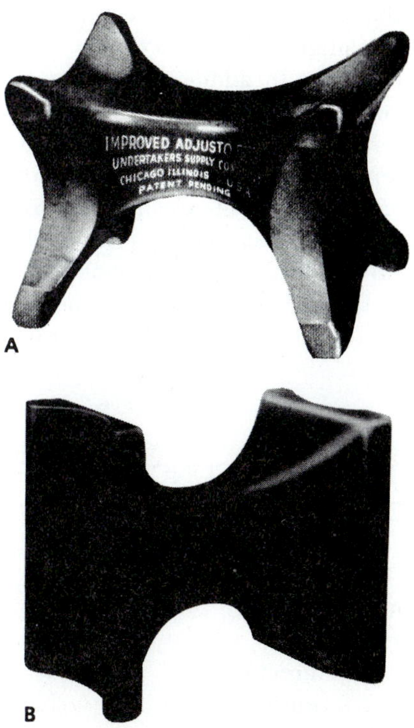

Figure 4–46. Headrests.

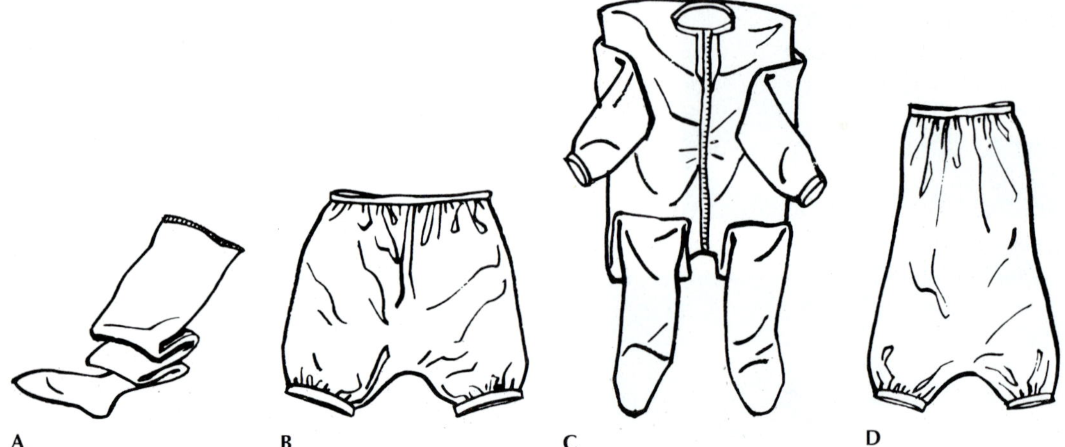

Figure 4–47. A. Plastic stockings. **B.** Plastic pants. **C.** Plastic unionall. **D.** Plastic coveralls.

vatives may be placed within the garment to help control these conditions. The coverall covers the trunk of the body from the upper thigh to the armpit. The unionall covers the entire body except for the hands, neck, and head areas (Figure 4–47).

▶ CONCLUSION

This chapter has emphasized that the preparation room is an essential part of the physical facility known as the "funeral home." It has evolved with technology and with the recognition of the central role that embalming and public health concerns play in American funerary behavior. In addition, an attempt has been made to provide advice and counsel that might be helpful to funeral service practitioners and architects in planning renovations or new construction of the preparation environment. Finally, the necessity to design and construct a facility that facilitates rather than hinders achievement of the objectives of embalming, not the least of which is the personal health and protection of embalming personnel and the general public, is stressed.

▶ KEY TERMS AND CONCEPTS FOR STUDY AND DISCUSSION

1. Define the following terms:
   autopsy aspirator
   bistoury
   grooved director
   hydroaspirator
   pressure
   rate of flow
   serrated edge/smooth edge
   slip hub/threaded hub
   unionall
   vacuum breaker
2. Discuss the disadvantages of a basement preparation room.
3. Discuss the proper locations for an exhaust system in the preparation room.
4. How does the hand pump differ from the bulb syringe.
5. With reference to the centrifugal injection machine explain the terms potential pressure, actual pressure, and differential pressure.
6. Review the statutes, rules, and regulations your state has concerning the preparation room.

▶ BIBLIOGRAPHY

Bourne H, Seferian S. Formaldehyde in wrinkle-proof apparel processes: Tears for my lady. *Ind Med Surg* 1959;28:232.

Hendrick DJ, Lane DJ. Occupational formalin asthma. *Br J Ind Med* 1977;34:11.

Johnson P. NIOSH Health Hazard Evaluation Determination Report HE 79-146-670, March 1980.

Kerfoot E, Mooney T. Formaldehyde and paraformaldehyde study in funeral homes. *Am Ind Hyg Assoc J* 1975;36:533.

Moore LL, Ogrodnik EC. Occupational exposure to formaldehyde in mortuaries. *J Environ Health* 1986;49(1):32–35.

Morrill E. Formaldehyde exposure from paper process solved by air sampling and current studies. *Air Cond Heat Vent* 1961;58:94.

Porter JAH. Acute respiratory distress following formalin inhalation. *Lancet* 1975;2:876.

Proctor NH, Hughes JP. *Chemical Hazards of the Workplace.* Philadelphia: JB Lippincott; 1978:272.

Riccobono PX. *Current Report: Bureau of National Affairs.* October 1979:471.

Sakula A. Formalin asthma in hospital laboratory staff. *Lancet* 1975;2:876.

Schoenber J, Mitchell C. Airway disease caused by phenolic (phenol–formaldehyde) resin exposure. *Arch Environ Health* 1975;30:575.

U.S. Department of Labor. *Occupational Safety and Health Standards (OSHA) for General Industry.* January 1978.

USDHEW/PHS/HRA. *Minimum Requirements of Construction and Equipment for Hospitals and Medical Facilities.* National Technical Information Service, DHEW Publication No. (HRA) 74-4000, September 1974.

Whitaker L. The Preparation Room. *Dodge Mag* 1997–1998; 89(2)–90(3).

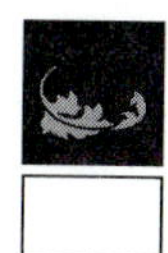

CHAPTER 5
DEATH—AGONAL AND PREEMBALMING CHANGES

> Death is a process and not a moment in time. During the process there is a series of physical and chemical changes, starting before the medico-legal time of death and continuing afterward. . . . In the sequence of death there is a point of irreversibility that can generally be diagnosed by physicians. When this point is reached nothing more can be done to restore intelligent life.

Because most deaths in the United States occur in an institutional setting, the pronouncement of death is typically the responsibility of persons who have the legal certification and authority to make a determination that death has, in fact, occurred. There are those times, however, where death may occur someplace other than an institution. In such cases, funeral home personnel may be among the first to arrive at a death scene. As such, it is important that they understand and honor the medical-legal relationships that exist in the jurisdiction where the death has occurred.

From a layperson's perspective, death might be thought of as the point at which an individual "draws his last breath." In reality, there is a sequence of steps leading up to that point, and a series of changes associated with the steps. In higher biological organisms, such as humans, these changes result in a cessation of integrated tissue and organ functions. As a result, there is a loss of heartbeat, cessation of spontaneous breathing, and absence of brain activity.* The process takes place in a sequence of steps which can be described as an expanding inability of the body to sustain the physiologic and metabolic processes that are necessary for life. The period of time over which the steps occur is known as the **agonal period**.

The agonal period might be quite short, as would be the case in an accident where death resulted from sudden, fatal injuries. Or, the process might take place over an extended period of time, as would be the case in a death caused by chronic illness. Whether the agonal period is long or short, at a given point in the process, the body can no longer function as a whole organism.

TIME LINE FOR THE PROCESS OF DEATH

Agonal period	Clinical death	Brain death	Biological death	Cellular death

Progression of somatic death

Agonal refers to death or agony.† During the agonal period the body is said to be **moribund**, a dying condition, or dying.‡ Physical observations that can be made during the dying process include such things as **death rattle** and **death struggle**. Death rattle is a respiratory gurgling or rattling in the throat of a dying person, caused by the loss of the cough reflex and accumulation of mucous.¶ Death struggle is the semiconvulsive twitches that often occur before death.

The agonal period occurs prior to the point in the process where the body loses its ability to sustain vital physiologic and metabolic activities. Once the body loses its ability to sustain physiologic and metabolic activity, **somatic death** occurs. Somatic death is defined as the death of the entire body.* It proceeds in an orderly progression from clinical death to brain death, then to

**Stedman's Medical Dictionary;* 26th ed. Baltimore: Williams & Wilkins; 1995:443.

†*Taber's Cyclopedic Medical Dictionary,* 15th ed. Philadelphia: Davis; 1985:49.

‡*Taber's Cyclopedic Medical Dictionary,* p. 1067.

¶*Stedman's Medical Dictionary,* p. 444.

**Stedman's Medical Dictionary,* p. 444.

biological death and, finally to postmortem cellular death.

Clinical death occurs when spontaneous respiration and heartbeat cease. It is during this time that the person can be resuscitated and, therefore, this is the reversible phase of the somatic death process. If respiration and heartbeat are not re-established, **brain death** will result. **Biological death** refers to the period in the process where simple life processes of the various organs and tissues of the body begin to cease. When biological death occurs, respiration and circulation cannot be restored.

Even after the process of dying has begun, however, there may still be a store of oxygen, nutrients, and other vital elements at the cellular level. Individual cells can sustain metabolic activity by utilizing available stores of essential elements. At some point, individual cells will use up stored elements, or will be overcome by autolytic processes, and die. This is **postmortem cellular death**. Cells that are more specialized and/or active will react more quickly to the decrease of oxygen or nutrients. The progression of cellular death can thus continue for a number of hours after somatic death, as shown in these examples:

Brain and nervous system cells	5 minutes
Muscle cells	3 hours
Cornea cells	6 hours
Blood cells	6 hours

It is worth noting that cellular death also occurs in the body as part of normal biological processes and as a result of disease processes.

ANTEMORTEM PERIOD

Cellular Death
- Necrobiosis
- Necrosis

STAGES OF DEATH

Agonal Period
Somatic Death
- Clinical death
- Brain death
- Biological death
- Postmortem cellular death

The accompanying chart presents an order of occurrence for changes that take place in the body before death (**antemortem period**), and as death is progressing. The terms are defined as follows:

- **Necrobiosis** refers to the physiologic, or natural, death of cells as they complete their life cycles.
- **Necrosis** refers to the pathologic death of body cells as a result of disease processes (e.g., gangrene or decubitus ulcers).
- **Clinical death** occurs when spontaneous respiration and heartbeat irreversibly cease.
- **Brain death** occurs in a sequence of events that are a function of time without oxygen. The first part of the brain to die, usually in 5 or 6 minutes, is the cerebral cortex. Next the midbrain dies, followed by the brain stem.
- **Biological death** is the irreversible phase of somatic death, and represents the cessation of simple body processes. The organs no longer function.
- **Postmortem cellular death** is the process during which individual cells die. It may take a matter of hours depending on numerous variables.

▶ CHANGES DURING THE AGONAL PERIOD

As the process of death progresses, there are changes that take place in the body. These changes are of great importance to embalmers because, in their variations, they contribute to multiple complications that must be addressed by embalming procedures and techniques. The changes that occur in the death process will, to an extent, dictate what procedures and techniques are appropriate for a given case. Therefore, it is important that embalmers recognize and understand death as a process.

As medical science has brought new therapies and treatments to medicine, the potential for an extended agonal period has been increased. As a result, the embalmer is more likely to encounter cases where: (1) disease processes have had longer to work on the body, (2) secondary infections have increased in the body, and (3) drug therapies have dramatically affected tissue conditions and the chemical balance of the body.

Agonal period changes can be categorized according to their effect on the: (1) temperature of the body, (2) ability of the body to circulate blood, (3) moisture content of the tissues, and (4) translocation of microorganisms within the body.

Temperature Changes

Two thermal changes can occur during the agonal period. **Agonal algor** is a cooling or lowering of the body temperature just prior to death. This is often seen in the death of elderly patients, especially when death occurs slowly. The metabolism has slowed in these individuals and, no doubt, the circulatory system has slowed. **Agonal fever** is an increase of the body temperature just prior to death. This is often seen in persons with infection, toxemia, or certain types of poisoning. Frequently, elevated temperature can stimulate microbial growth.

Circulatory Changes

Three circulatory changes are possible in the agonal period. **Agonal hypostasis** is the settling of blood into the dependent tissues of the body. It occurs as a result of the slowing of circulation just prior to death, which allows the force of gravity to overcome the force of circulation. **Agonal coagulation** occurs as the circulation of blood slows and the formed elements of the blood begin to clot and congeal. **Agonal capillary expansion** is the opening of the pores in the walls of the capillaries. It occurs as the body attempts to get more oxygen to the tissues and cells.

SIGNS OF DEATH

The presence of death might be manifested by changes that have taken place in the body. The signs of death might include:

1. Cessation of respiration.
2. Cessation of circulation.
3. Muscular flaccidity.
4. Pallor of the skin.
5. Changes in the eye, including
   A. Clouding of the cornea.
   B. Loss of luster of the conjunctiva.
   C. Flattening of the eyeball.
   D. Dilated and unresponsive pupils.
6. Postmortem lividity.
7. Rigor mortis.
8. Algor mortis.
9. Decomposition.

Moisture Changes

Two changes in tissue moisture are possible during the agonal period. **Agonal edema** is an increase in the amount of moisture, or fluids, in the tissues and body cavities. It may result from disease processes or from agonal capillary expansion. **Agonal dehydration** is a decrease in the amount of moisture, or fluids, in the tissues and body cavities. It may result from disease processes or from agonal capillary expansion.

The relationship between agonal edema and agonal dehydration can be thought of in terms of shifts in the balance and location of body moisture. The tissue fluids that flow or gravitate to other places in the body will create a shift in the moisture balance. Thus, one area may become edematous because of moisture that has left, or dehydrated, another area. In agonal capillary expansion, the increased size of the openings in the capillary wall, while intended to allow more oxygen into the tissues, also allows fluids to flow out of the capillaries and into the intercellular spaces. This movement of fluids constitutes a shift in the moisture balance by which the greater amounts of moisture flow to the intercellular spaces while the moisture within the capillary will be reduced.

Translocation of Microorganisms

Translocation is the movement of microorganisms from one area of the body to another. It occurs as organisms normally confined to a specific area of the body by natural body defenses are able to move as the body loses its ability to keep them in check. The movement may be the result of the organism: (1) having natural motility, (2) entering the blood stream and circulating to other parts of the body, or (3) gravitating to other parts of the body during hypostasis or shifts in tissue moisture.

▶ POSTMORTEM CHANGES

In the period between death and embalming the composition and condition of the body continues to change (Table 5–1). Generally, unless there are some intervening variables, the nature and extent of the changes will be greater if the time between death and embalming is longer. The embalming process is intended to retard, interrupt, or reverse the changes. For that reason embalmers tend to prefer having all legal and professional requirements satisfied in a timely fashion so that they can begin the embalming process as soon after death as possible. If the time lapse between death and embalming is too long, there may be complications severe enough to affect the successful outcome of the embalming process. These postmortem changes are classified as physical changes and chemical changes.

Physical changes are brought about by forces of nature. The forces of nature act on the body in such as way as to create changes in the physical state of the body or body tissues. These physical changes, however, do not create chemical byproducts or change the chemical composition of the body. The force of gravity, for example, may move blood from one place to another in the body. No new products are formed by this movement. The blood merely changes physical location.

TABLE 5–1. POSTMORTEM PHYSICAL AND CHEMICAL CHANGES

Change	Classification	Description
Algor mortis	Physical	Cooling of the body to the temperature of the surrounding environment.
Dehydration	Physical	Loss of moisture from the surface of the body to the surrounding atmosphere.
Hypostasis	Physical	Gravitation of blood and body fluids to dependent areas of the body.
Livor mortis	Physical	Postmortem intravascular blood discoloration brought about by the presence of blood in the dependent surface vessels of the body.
Increase in blood viscosity	Physical	Thickening of the blood after death caused primarily by loss of the liquid portion of the blood to the tissue spaces.
Endogenous invasion of microorganisms	Physical	Relocation of microorganisms in the body as a result of the cessation of natural and metabolic activities which, in life, keep the organisms in check.
Postmortem caloricity	Chemical	Temporary rise in body temperature after death.
Change in body pH	Chemical	Change in body tissues from slightly alkaline in life (pH 7.38–7.40) to acid (pH 6.0–5.5) during rigor, then a return to alkaline in decomposition.
Rigor mortis	Chemical	Temporary postmortem stiffening of body muscles by natural body processes.
Postmortem stain	Chemical	Extravascular color change brought about by hemolysis where liberated hematin seeps through the capillary walls and into the body tissues; this type of stain cannot be removed by arterial injection and venous drainage.
Decomposition	Chemical	Separation of compounds into simpler substances by the action of bacterial and/or autolytic enzymes.

A **chemical change** is brought about by chemical activity. As a result, new substances are formed. For example, there are autolytic processes taking place in the body during the postmortem period. These processes are largely dependent on autolytic enzymes, which break tissues down by stimulating chemical reactions between substances found in the tissues. As existing substances react chemically with one another, new chemical compositions are formed (Figure 5–1).

Postmortem Physical Changes

Included among the postmortem physical changes are (1) algor mortis, (2) hypostasis, (3) livor mortis, (4) dehydration, (5) increased viscosity of the blood, and (6) endogenous invasion of microorganisms (Table 5–2). These changes are brought about by the stoppage of blood circulation, gravity, and surface evaporations.

Algor Mortis. Algor mortis is the postmortem cooling of the body. Generally, the temperature of the surrounding environment is cooler than the temperature of the body and, over time, the temperature of the body will cool to the temperature of the surrounding environment. The rate at which a body will cool depends on a number of variables. Factors within the body itself are called **intrinsic factors** and those in the surrounding environment are called **extrinsic factors** (Figure 5–2).

Intrinsic factors include (1) the ratio surface area of the body to body mass, (2) body temperature at the time of death, and (3) combinations of the effects of the ratio of surface area to body mass, and body temperature at the time of death.

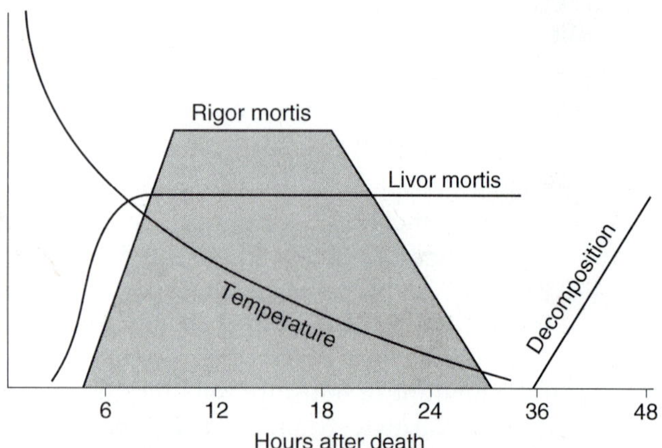

Figure 5–1. Principal postmortem changes.

TABLE 5–2. EMBALMING SIGNIFICANCE OF POSTMORTEM PHYSICAL CHANGES

Algor Mortis	Slows the onset of rigor mortis and decomposition. Helps to keep blood in a liquid state. Can increase the degree of livor mortis and postmortem stain.
Hypostasis	Responsible for livor mortis. Hemolysis can later cause postmortem stain. Increases tissue moisture in dependent tissues.
Livor Mortis	Discoloration can vary from slight reddish hue to almost black, depending on blood volume and viscosity. Intravascular so it can be cleared. Can be "set" as a stain if excessively strong uncoordinated embalming solution is injected. Can help to expand the capillaries. If it clears during arterial injection it can be used as a sign of fluid distribution. May be gravitated or massaged from an area.
Dehydration	Accompanied by increased blood viscosity. Can create a "temporary" postmortem edema in the tissues. Darkens skin surface and cannot be bleached. Causes wrinkling and shriveling of features. If extreme enough, can retard decomposition. If extreme enough, can preserve the body.
Increase in blood viscosity	Thickened blood and coagulation. Increased resistance of arterial injections. Hampers drainage.
Endogenous invasion of microorganisms	Pathologic danger to the embalmer. Promotes and aids decomposition.

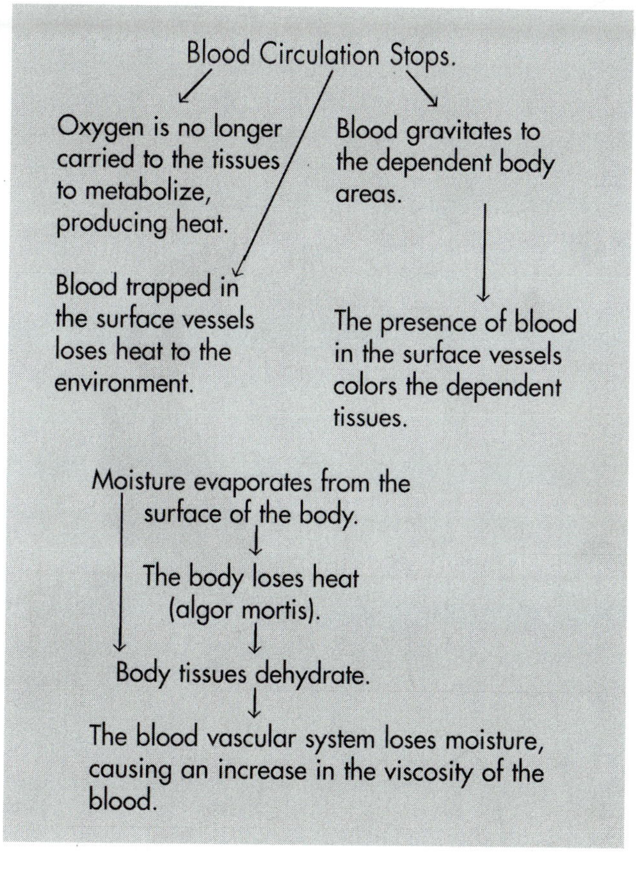

Blood Circulation Stops.

Oxygen is no longer carried to the tissues to metabolize, producing heat.

Blood gravitates to the dependent body areas.

Blood trapped in the surface vessels loses heat to the environment.

The presence of blood in the surface vessels colors the dependent tissues.

Moisture evaporates from the surface of the body.

↓

The body loses heat (algor mortis).

↓

Body tissues dehydrate.

↓

The blood vascular system loses moisture, causing an increase in the viscosity of the blood.

In life, a portion of body heat is lost to conduction, radiation, and convection as the blood circulates through the superficial vessels of the skin. The blood is warmed again as it circulates back through the body's internal organs. A larger person will have more surface area from which to lose body heat, but that potential to lose heat can be offset by body mass. A smaller person will have less surface area from which to lose body heat, and would therefore require less body mass to offset the loss of heat. In death, there is no opportunity for the blood to regain lost heat because there is no circulation. Therefore, if a body has a larger surface area from which heat can be lost, its temperature will decrease more rapidly, unless there is something to offset the potential to lose heat. Here again, heat loss can be offset by body mass. In short, a body with more mass will be better insulated against heat loss and will, therefore, cool at a slower rate. Infants, for example, are more likely to cool faster because, among other factors, they have a higher ratio of surface area as compared with their body mass.*

*Walter J. B. *Pathology of Human Disease.* Philadelphia: Lea & Febiger; 1989:327.

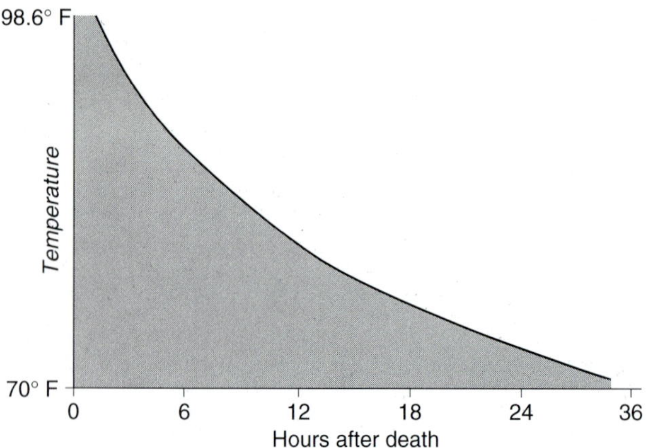

Figure 5–2. Algor mortis versus time.

If body temperature is elevated at the time of death, it will take longer for the body to cool to the temperature of the surrounding environment because the temperature will simply have farther to drop. Body temperature can become elevated because of increased metabolic activity, the presence of fever, or an inability of the body to regulate its temperature. Likewise, low body temperature at the time of death will influence the length of time it takes for the body to cool to a point of equilibrium with the surrounding environment. Body temperature can become low as a result of exposure to cold or an inability of the body to regulate its temperature.

Rapid cooling of the body by refrigeration or natural means helps to slow the onset of rigor mortis, slow the onset of decomposition, and keep the blood in a liquid state. These are all advantageous for embalming. A body that has been cooled rapidly will, however, be more likely to have discoloration from livor mortis and postmortem staining.

Extrinsic factors that affect postmortem cooling of the body include (1) body coverings and (2) the surrounding environment. Body coverings include clothing or other coverings that protect the skin from direct exposure to the environment. In addition to providing added insulation, an external covering will also retard or prevent heat loss that results from conduction, radiation, and convection.

The surrounding environment itself will affect the rate at which a body loses heat. A body submerged in 70° water, for example, would lose heat more rapidly than in 70° air temperature, because water would conduct heat away from the body more quickly than air.

Hypostasis. Hypostasis is a process by which blood settles, as a result of gravitational movement within the vessels, to the dependent, or lowest parts of the body. The dependent part(s) of the body would be those parts closest to the ground. The designation of dependent part(s) would change depending on the position of the body. For example, if a body lay on its back, the tissues of the back of the body (trunk, neck, legs, etc.) would be the areas where blood settled. If a person were sitting upright, blood would gravitate to the hips, legs, and feet.

It is also important to note that the gravitational movement of the blood can be effected by constrictions, ligatures, or other factors that would impede free movement of the blood within the vessels. **Contact pallor** refers to areas where blood movement has been inhibited. It is most obvious in areas where the body has been in contact with a surface. The weight of the body pressing against the capillary beds prevents blood from settling into the area. Although the surrounding area may be discolored, the area in contact with the surface will stay quite pale (Figure 5–3).

Thinner, or less viscous, blood will tend to flow with less resistance, and will thus gravitate to dependent parts of the body more readily. Factors which effect the viscosity of the blood will therefore influence the speed at which postmortem hypostasis takes place. Possible factors include refrigeration, medication, and disease processes. Conversely, factors which thicken, or increase viscosity, will slow rate at which postmortem hypostasis takes place. Possible factors include heat, medication, and disease processes.

The embalming significance of hypostasis lies in the postmortem discolorations that potentially result from the gravitational movement of blood. In embalming terminology, hypostasis describes the process by which blood gravitates to dependent parts of the body.

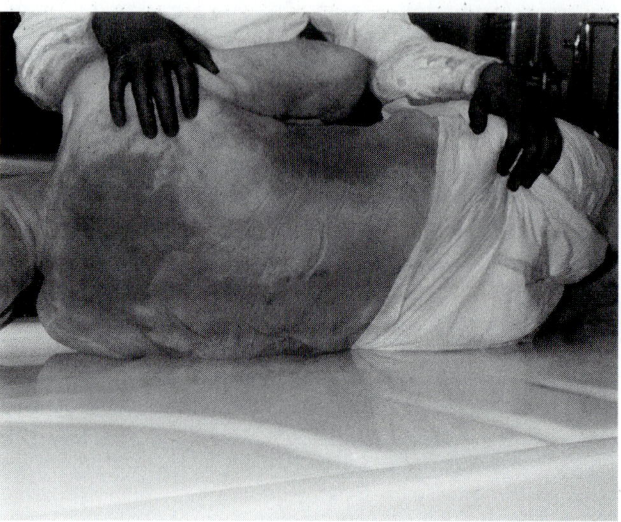

Figure 5–3. Dark areas show livor mortis and postmortem stain. The light-colored area on the back shows contact pallor where the body rested against the table.

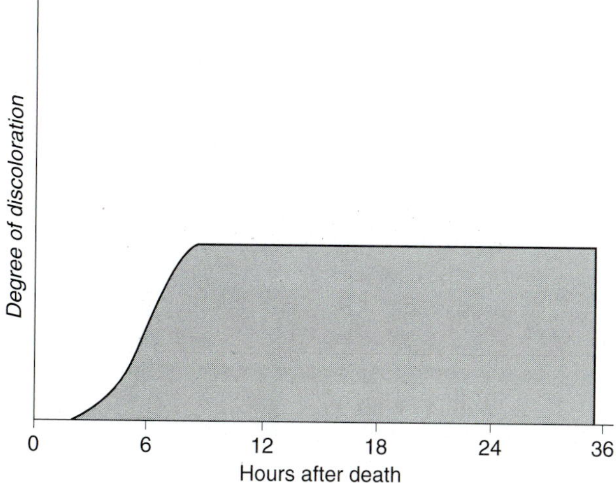

Figure 5–4. Livor mortis.

Hypostasis is the term for the process, not for the discoloration.

Livor Mortis. The settling of blood brings about a discoloration that appears within $\frac{1}{2}$ to 2 hours after death.* In embalming terminology, this discoloration is called livor mortis. Livor mortis is a postmortem intravascular blood discoloration that occurs as a result of hypostasis. It is also known as **postmortem lividity** or **cadaveric lividity.** The discoloration may first be noticed as dull reddish patches. As it becomes more established it can take on a deep reddish-blue appearance. Livor mortis is categorized as an intravascular discoloration, meaning that it occurs within the blood vascular system and can be reduced or removed during the embalming process as embalming solution flushes the pooled blood from the area (Figure 5–4).

Two factors play an important role in the degree of intensity of livor mortis: blood volume and blood viscosity. In cases where excessive bleeding has taken place, either internally or externally, there will be less blood available to pool. This may reduce the instance or intensity of livor mortis. Likewise, if blood is thicker and not readily subject to gravitation, the appearance of livor mortis may be effected (Table 5–3).

Dehydration. The loss of water from body tissues and fluids by surface evaporation is called dehydration. There are two basic factors at work in postmortem loss of body moisture: **surface evaporation** and **gravitation or hypostasis** of blood and body fluids.

Surface evaporation results from the passage of air or air currents over the surface of the body. It is to the embalmer's advantage to have the body covered or in some way protected against the effects of the air currents.

Gravitation or hypostasis of the blood and body fluids is the physical movement of body fluids to dependent regions of the body. The higher areas where the liquids move from are likely to become dehydrated. Conversely, the lower areas where the liquids are flowing to may become engorged, a condition called **postmortem edema.**

A third factor also works in conjunction with the gravitation of liquids, **imbibition.** Imbibition is the ability of cells to draw moisture from the surrounding area into themselves. The areas where the liquids move to can become edematous (e.g., postmortem edema).

As dehydration occurs, the blood will become increasingly viscous. Eventually the formed elements of the blood will stick together in clumps, a process that creates what is referred to as **sludge.** Obviously, sludge does not lend itself to establishing good drainage during arterial embalming.

Dehydration will bring about surface discolorations ranging from a yellow into the browns and, finally, black. In addition to being very hard to the touch and discolored, dehydrated tissue is also shriveled and wrinkled. Dehydration is a postmortem physical change that occurs before embalming, but can also be increased by embalming and can continue after embalming (Figure 5–5).

Increase in Blood. Viscosity. Viscosity refers to the thickness of a liquid. The blood is composed of two portions: (1) a "solid" portion made up of the various groups of blood cells, and (2) a "liquid" portion in which the cells are suspended. After death, blood has a tendency to increase in viscosity and thicken. This thickening is brought about by the dehydration of the body. As the tissues lose moisture to the surrounding air, the liquid portion of the blood begins to move through the capillary walls into the tissue spaces. Given enough time and the proper conditions, this liquid could leave the body by surface evaporation. The remaining blood begins to thicken as a result of a gradual loss of the liquid or serum portion of the blood.

As a result of this thickening, the blood cells begin to stick together, and if this occurs in the arterial system, the agglutinated blood will eventually clog small arteries during arterial injection. On the venous side, blood drainage will be difficult. Not only is dehydration responsible for the thickening of blood, but gravity alone tends to "drain off" the liquid portion of the blood, leaving behind a more viscous blood.

**Stedman's Medical Dictionary*, p. 990.

TABLE 5–3. EMBALMING CONSIDERATIONS AND BLOOD DISCOLORATIONS

Antemortem Hypostasis	Postmortem Hypostasis	Time → Livor Mortis Time →	Postmortem Stain Embalming →	Formaldehyde Gray
Occurs prior to death or during the agonal period	Begins at death	Seen as soon as blood fills superficial vessels; begins approximately 20 minutes after death; depends on p.m./a.m. hypostasis	Normally occurs about 6 hours after death; cause of death and blood chemistry vary rate	Occurs after embalming
Intravascular	Intravascular	Intravascular	Extravascular	Intravascular or extravascular
Movement of blood to dependent tissues[a]	Movement of blood to dependent tisues[a]	p.m. blood discoloration as a result of p.m./a.m. hypostasis	p.m. blood discoloration as a result of hemolysis	Embalming discoloration
a.m. physical change	p.m. physical change	p.m. physical change	p.m. chemical change	—
	Speed depends on blood viscosity	Color varies with blood volume and viscosity and amount of O_2 in blood	May occur prior to, during, or after arterial fluid injection	Seen after arterial fluid injection
Antemortem	Postmortem	Postmortem	Postmortem	Postmortem
—	—	Pressed on skin clears	Pressed on skin does NOT clear	Seen as a gray stain
—	—	Removed by blood drainage	Not removed by blood drainage	Methemoglobin HCHO + blood
—	Arterial injection stops progress	Arterial injection (mild) clears/with drainage	Strong solutions bleach and "set" livor as stain	—
	Speeded by cooling of body, low blood viscosity	Speeded by cooling, blood "thinners," low blood viscosity, CO deaths	Speeded by cooling, rapid red blood cell hemolysis, CO deaths	Speeded by poor drainage

p.m. postmortem; a.m. antemortem.
[a] Dependent body area varies with body position.

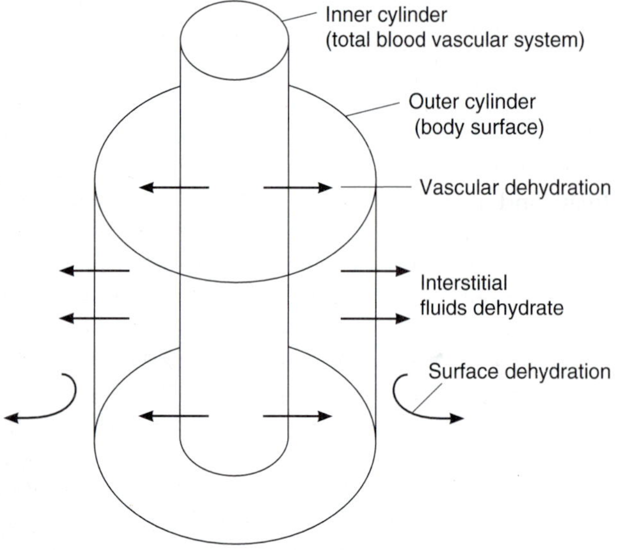

Figure 5–5. Total vascular system and the effects of dehydration.

If this thickening occurs fast enough it will diminish the degree of discoloration created by livor mortis, because the blood will not move as fast into the dependent tissues. What generally happens is the blood settles into the dependent tissues first; then the blood increases in viscosity.

Endogenous Invasion of Microorganisms. Endogenous invasion of cerebrospinal fluid by bacterial agents associated with the colon occurs within 4 to 6 hours of death. *The colon, designated as the postmortem origin of "indicator" organisms recovered from extraintestinal sampling sites, seems to be the primary source of many of the translocated microbial agents.* The isolation of "indicator" organisms as well as nonindicator organisms from such sampling sites as the left ventricle of the heart, the lungs, the urinary bladder, and the cisterna cerebellomedullaris indicates the extent to which microbial agents of low, moderate, and high virulence can translocate within a relatively brief postmortem interval of 4 to 8 hours.

TABLE 5–4. EMBALMING SIGNIFICANCE OF POSTMORTEM CHEMICAL CHANGES

Rigor Mortis	Creates extravascular resistance. Makes positioning the body more difficult. Makes posing features more difficult. May contribute to tissue distention during arterial injection. Increases demand for preservative. Reduces the absorption of preservative. pH change affects chemical reaction of embalming solution. May contribute to uneven (splotchy) coloration if arterial dye is used. May create a false sign of preservation.
Postmortem Stain	Extravascular discoloration that generally cannot be removed by arterial injection alone. May result in gray discoloration when reacting with embalming chemicals. Sign of delay between death and embalming. Indicates an increased demand for preservative.
Postmortem Caloricity	Speeds the rigor mortis cycle. Speeds decomposition.
Shifts in pH	Interferes with arterial solution reactions. May result in "splotching" of dye on the skin surface.
Decomposition	May cause poor distribution of embalming solution. Tissues may easily distend during arterial injection. Increased demand for preservatives. May be manifested by discoloration, odor, skin-slip, gases in cavities and tissues, purge.

The postmortem multiplication of systemic and translocated recoverable microbial agents may begin within 4 hours of somatic death and reach peak densities of 3.0 to 3.5 $\times 10^6$ organism per milliliter of body fluid or per gram of body tissue within a 24 to 30 hour postmortem interval.*

Postmortem factors contributing to the translocation of endogenous microflora include (1) chemical and physical changes, (2) movement and positional changes of the body, (3) passive recirculation of blood from contaminated body sites, (4) thrombus fragmentation and relocation, and (5) the inherent true mobility of many of the intestinal bacilli. The relocated organisms may exit from body openings, natural and other, and contaminate adjacent animate and inanimate surfaces. They may also become airborne particulates in the form of aerosols (droplet infection particle) or dried particles (droplet nuclei), expanding the potential spread of biological hazards.

For the embalmer, the most troublesome organism that could translocate and cause very definite postmortem problems is *Clostridium perfringens.* This tissue gas–producing anaerobic bacillus is responsible for true tissue gas. Its presence throughout the body after death can bring about immediate embalming and preservation problems. Within just 1 or 2 hours of death, if this organism is present in the tissues, it can produce gases that distend the tissues to the point where viewing the body might be impossible. Of all the agonal changes, the problems that can arise from the translocation of *C. perfringens* are most critical to the embalmer.

* See the Selected Readings section for the complete Rose and Hockett reprint.

Postmortem Chemical Changes

The postmortem chemical changes include postmortem caloricity, postmortem stain, shift in pH, rigor mortis, decomposition, and hydrolysis (Table 5–4).

Postmortem Caloricity. Metabolism is defined as the sum of all the chemical reactions that occur within a cell. It is dependent on oxygen. There are two phases to metabolism: 1) **anabolism** the building phase and 2) **catabolism** the breakdown phase that releases heat and energy. After death occurs, the cells may still have a supply of oxygen and, therefore, metabolism will continue. The continuation of metabolism after death will create heat, and may be responsible for the elevated postmortem temperature known as postmortem caloricity.

Postmortem Stain. Postmortem stain is the extravascular blood discoloration brought about by the hemolysis of blood. After death, the blood gravitates into the vessels of the dependent areas of the body. The pooling of blood in the dependent areas of the body results in an intravascular discoloration called livor mortis. Over time, the red blood cells of the pooled blood begin to break down. The breakdown or hemolysis of red blood cells begins approximately 6 to 10 hours after death. The onset of hemolysis occurs faster in some bodies, most frequently in persons who died from carbon

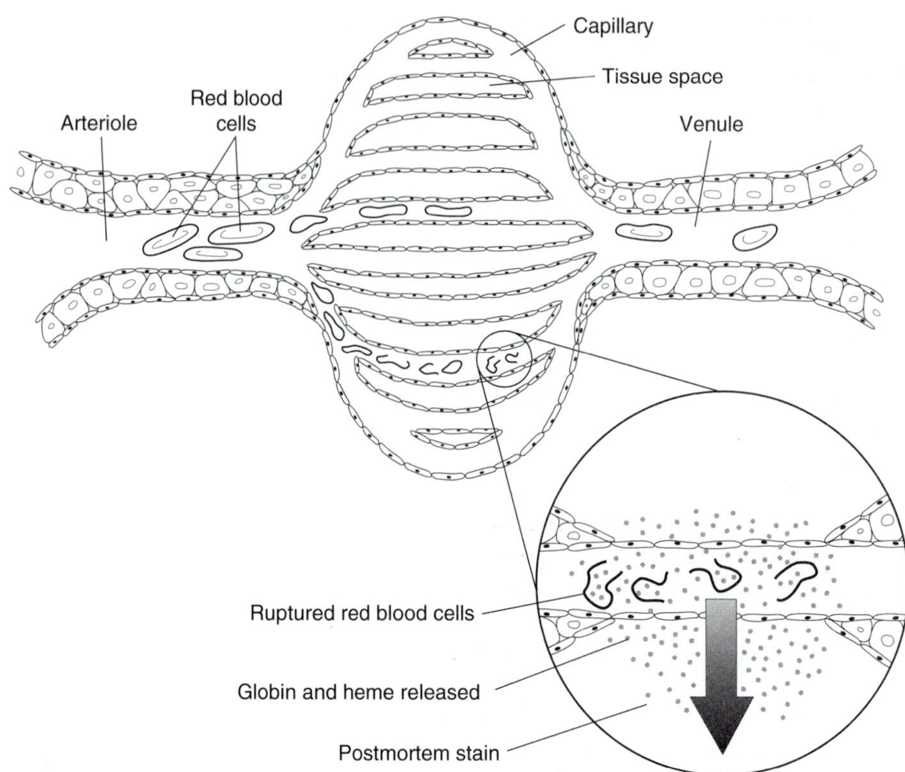

Figure 5–6. Release of globin and heme.

monoxide poisoning or in bodies that have been refrigerated (Figure 5–6).

Each red blood cell contains several million hemoglobin molecules. Hemolysis releases the hemoglobin, which rapidly decomposes into globin and heme. The heme then passes through the walls and pores of the capillaries and moves into the tissue spaces where it stains the tissues a reddish color. This reddish stain is permanently fixed, because it is now extravascular.

Shift in Body pH. In chemistry, degrees of acidity or alkalinity of a substance are expressed in pH values. The neutral point, where a solution would be neither acid or alkaline, is pH 7. Increasing acidity is expressed as a number less than 7 and increasing alkalinity as a number greater than 7. Maximum acidity is pH 0 and maximum alkalinity is pH 14. Because each unit on the scale represents a logarithm, there is a 10-fold difference between each unit.*

Normal pH for a body is about 7.4. After death there is a drop in pH of the blood and tissue fluid into the acid range (about 3 hours after death). The body remains acidic during rigor mortis and then gradually, as the decomposition process advances, the body becomes increasingly alkaline.

* *Taber's Cyclopedic Medical Dictionary,* p. 1277.

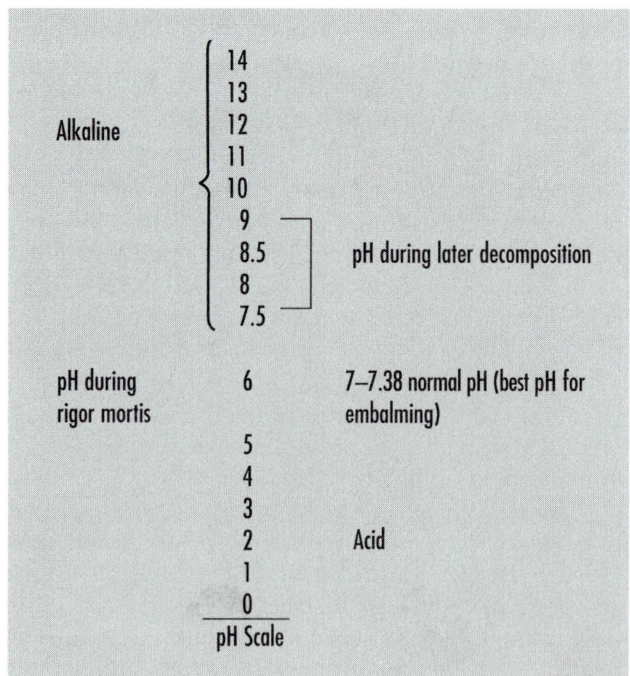

During life the carbohydrates (glycogen) stored in the liver and muscles are broken down to pyruvic and lactic acid by the oxygen present. Normally, this pyruvic acid is oxidized to carbon dioxide, water, and energy. The energy, in turn, is used to build up the adenosine triphosphate of the body by converting adenosine diphosphate and adenosine monophosphate to adenosine triphosphate. The oxygen present in life prevents the buildup of lactic acid by oxidizing it to carbon dioxide and water. After death occurs, the oxygen is gradually used up, and the lactic acid is no longer inhibited and begins to accumulate in the muscle tissues. This buildup of acid occurs during the first hours after death (approximately the first 3 hours). This cycle is closely and directly related to the cycle of rigor mortis. The pH will drop to an acid level of approximately 6.0 and has been recorded as low as 5.5.

As a result of the acid buildup in the tissues, conditions become right for the breakdown of the soft proteins of the body. Later, as the protein breaks down, there is a gradual buildup in the tissues of nitrogen products such as ammonia and amines. The ammonia, which is basic, neutralizes the acids present in the tissues from carbohydrate breakdown. As the body contains much more protein than carbohydrates, the ammonia products gradually begin to build to a point where the pH of the tissues becomes basic (or alkaline). During decomposition the tissues are found to have an alkaline pH.

Rigor Mortis. Rigor mortis is the postmortem stiffening of muscles by natural processes. This condition affects only the muscles, and usually all of the muscles of the body are affected. Once the condition passes it does not recur. Usually, the muscles are relaxed as death occurs. This is called **primary flaccidity.** If the body is embalmed while the muscles are flaccid the proteins will react well with the preservative and tissue fixation will occur. If the body is embalmed while rigor is fully developed, the stiffness of the muscles will impede distribution. The proteins of the muscles are tightly bound together so they are less reactive. Within 36 to 72 hours, rigor mortis passes naturally from an unembalmed body. This is called **secondary flaccidity.** In this phase, there will be a greater demand for preservative because muscle protein has been broken down to some extent. Rigor results from the body's inability to resynthesize ATP that causes the muscle proteins to lock together and form an insoluble protein. Rigor marks the end of muscle cell life, and is generally observed in the average body 2 to 4 hours after death (Figure 5–7).

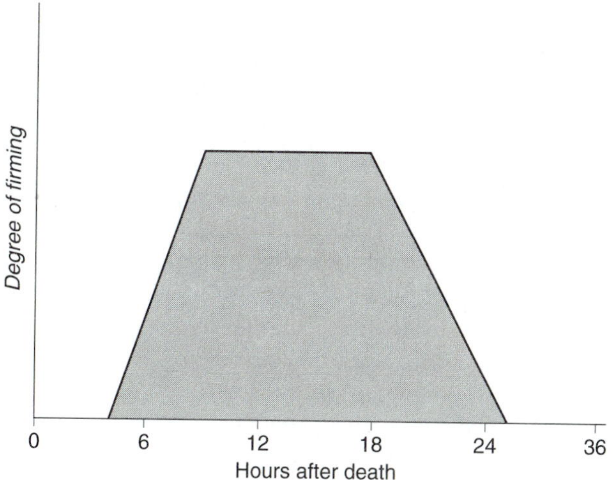

Figure 5–7. Rigor mortis.

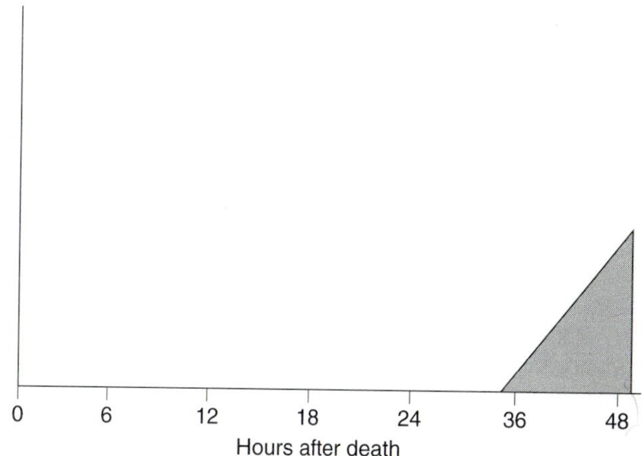

Figure 5–8. Decomposition.

Rigor appears to begin in the involuntary muscles of the eye, then moves to the face, neck, upper extremities, trunk, and lower extremities. It can be forcibly broken by flexing, bending, rotating, and massaging the joints and muscles. Once broken, rigor does not redevelop.

Cadaveric spasm, which is a sudden involuntary movement or convulsion brought about by involuntary muscular contractions, may also be associated with rigor mortis.* If rigor mortis occurs irregularly in the different muscles, it can cause movements in the limbs, which are known as cadaveric spasms.†

Decomposition. The three major biochemicals in the body are proteins, carbohydrates, and lipids. Of the three, proteins are most important from the standpoint of structure and function. Proteins are the principle component in connective tissue, tendons, cartilage, ligaments, skin, hair, and nails. They are responsible for body movements by the action of contractile proteins found in the muscles. They play a number of other roles in body function, and can be described as essential elements to the living body (Figure 5–8).

**Taber's Cyclopedic Medical Dictionary*, p. 1589.
†*Stedman's Medical Dictionary*, p. 1640.

Proteins are also an essential element from the standpoint of embalming because successful embalming is achieved by establishing crosslinkages between proteins of the body and proteins of microorganisms. Proteins are large molecules that contain elements of carbon, hydrogen, oxygen, and nitrogen. The chemical bond that links two proteins together is called a **peptide bond** or **peptide linkage.** It is possible for many proteins to link together. During decomposition, the protein chains break down. If the breakdown is caused by catalytic enzymes, the enzymes are called **proteases.**

AUTOLYSIS

In human remains the enzymes of decomposition have two different sources: saprophytic bacteria, and lysosomes. These bacteria are normal residents of the human digestive tract. After death, they translocate and increase in number by using dead organic matter for their nutrition. Aerobic bacteria may also enter the body through the respiratory tract. They deplete the tissues of oxygen, producing chemical conditions favorable for anaerobic organisms, most of which originate in the intestinal tract.

In addition to bacterially caused decompositions, living cells have their own self-destruct mechanisms. During life, organelles called lysosomes contain the digestive enzymes of a cell. As the pH changes from alkaline to acidic, the membranes surrounding the lysosomes rupture. As the cells' own digestive enzymes are released, they digest the surrounding cellular material. This process is called *autolysis,* which means cell self-decomposition. The products of autolysis are amino acids, sugars, fatty acids, and glycerol. These substances are sources of food and energy for microorganisms. Therefore, autolysis also favors microbial destructive action on human remains.

Hydrolysis has been called the single most important factor in the initiation of decomposition. It is a chemical reaction in which the chemical bonds of a substance are split by the addition or taking up of water.* The result of this reaction is the formation of simpler compounds which have water's hydrogen ion (H^+) and hydroxyl ion (^-OH) on either side of the chemical bond.† When hydrolysis occurs, water is broken apart, another compound is broken apart, and new products are formed. The process requires (1) water, (2) catalysts, and (3) compounds with which to react. Hydrolysis is the first chemical reaction in the putrefactive process. During hydrolysis large protein molecules are broken down into smaller fragments called **proteoses, peptones**, and **polypeptides.** These intermediates are a good food source for bacteria, which increase dramatically during putrefaction. As degradation continues, the final products are amino acids.

These amino acids undergo further chemical changes. Amines, carbon dioxide, and water are some of the products. **Amines** are organic compounds that are considered to be derivatives of ammonia. Two of these amines, **putrescine** and **cadaverine**, are alkaline substances that have a foul odor. They are commonly called **ptomaines.**

Protein decomposition is known as **putrefaction.** Some authorities restrict the term putrefaction to the decomposition of proteins by **anaerobic bacteria** (those able to live without oxygen), and use the term **decay** for the decomposition of proteins by **aerobic bacteria** (those that need oxygen to live).

Water is abundant in the human body, and is therefore present and available for hydrolysis during life and after death. Hydrolysis requires the presence of a **catalyst**, which is a substance that influences the rate of a chemical reaction, without itself becoming part of the products of the reaction. Enzymes found within cells act as catalysts. After death, tissues become slightly acid. This shift in pH causes the lysosomes within the cells to rupture. Lysosomes are cell inclusions that contain digestive enzymes. In the presence of water, the released enzymes begin to digest the carbohydrates, fats, and proteins of the cell. The end products of the hydrolysis of the proteins are amino acids. As proteins hydrolyze, the resulting products make more and more sites available for union with the preservative. It can be stated then that hydrolytic processes greatly increase the preservative demand of the body tissues. The presence of amino acids increases formaldehyde demand because there are more sites available for a union with formaldehyde. Carbohydrates are reduced to monosaccides (simple sugars) and fats are reduced to fatty acids and glycerine.

The rate at which hydrolysis occurs is speeded by heat and slowed by a cold environment. A mild acid pH can also stimulate hydrolysis. As the process continues, more and more nitrogen end products are produced. This causes the pH to shift to an alkaline condition. The alkaline (or basic) condition now provides an excellent medium for bacterial growth. With this growth of bacteria the process of putrefaction greatly increases.

* *Taber's Cyclopedic Medical Dictionary*, p. 788.
†*Stedman's Medical Dictionary*, p. 817.

CATALYSTS

In the previous discussion of the types of decomposition reactions, it was shown that catalysts were needed for chemical reactions to take place. A catalyst is a substance that speeds up the rate of a chemical reaction without itself being permanently altered in the reaction. Inasmuch as decomposition is a chemical change, the presence of catalysts are needed in addition to the reactants. In every chemical reaction there is a *transition state,* where chemical bonds of reactants are broken and new chemical bonds are formed. At this point in a reaction, there is a higher level of energy needed. That boost of energy is provided by the catalyst. Enzymes serve as catalysts. Enzymes are also proteins, and are therefore influenced by such things as temperature and pH.

It is known that there are temperature fluctuations related to the agonal period and to the period between cellular death and embalming. It is also known that after death, the pH of the body changes from its normal 7.4 to a more acidic pH. As the body becomes somewhat acidic, it also becomes a favorable environment for microorganisms to multiply and contribute to decomposition. As the process continues, the pH of the body shifts back to alkaline, which is an excellent environment for enzymes to accelerate decomposition.

Decomposition of Carbohydrates. The breakdown of carbohydrates does not have any significant effect on embalming. Carbohydrates are stored in the body as glycogen (a polymer of glucose). The process by which glucose breaks down is called *fermentation.* We say, therefore, that fermentation is the bacterial decomposition of carbohydrates under aerobic conditions. The products of this breakdown of carbohydrates are organic acids, but they are not produced in sufficient quantity or strength to alter the overall alkaline environment that exists in a decomposing body and do not produce any foul odors. The final products of the breakdown are carbon dioxide and water.

Decomposition of Lipids. Body fats are broken down by hydrolysis that occurs in the presence of enzymes called lipase. The products of this breakdown are glycerol and fatty acids. These byproducts do not significantly affect the embalming operations because they do not change the alkaline environment, nor do they give off any bad odors.

Of note to embalmers is the formation of a compound called **adipocere**, commonly known as "grave wax." Adipocere is thought to be composed of fatty acids and appears in bodies that have been dead for an extended period of time (3 months or longer).

▶ SIGNS OF DECOMPOSITION

There are five signs of decomposition. It should be pointed out that not all of these signs may be present even though decomposition is occurring. Decomposition proceeds at different rates in various body areas. The following orders of decomposition demonstrate this fact:

1. Order of body decomposition
   A. Cells
   B. Tissues
   C. Organs

Cells, tissues, and organs that contain high levels of moisture and autolytic and bacterial enzymes break down before similar structures that contain less water and autolytic and bacterial enzymes.

2. Order of tissue decomposition
   A. Soft tissues
   B. Firm tissues
   C. Hard tissues

The vascular system is one of the last organ systems to decompose. Even in advanced decomposition it would be possible to inject some preservative chemicals in an attempt to slow decomposition and control odor.

When the body is considered as a whole there are five cardinal signs of decomposition. They include color changes, odor, skin-slip, gases, and purge.

Color Change

The first external color change that occurs in the unembalmed body is a greenish discoloration over the right lower quadrant of the abdomen. This discoloration is caused by the combination of hydrogen sulfide (a product of putrefaction) with hemoglobin from the blood (Figure 5–9). In many bodies this discol-

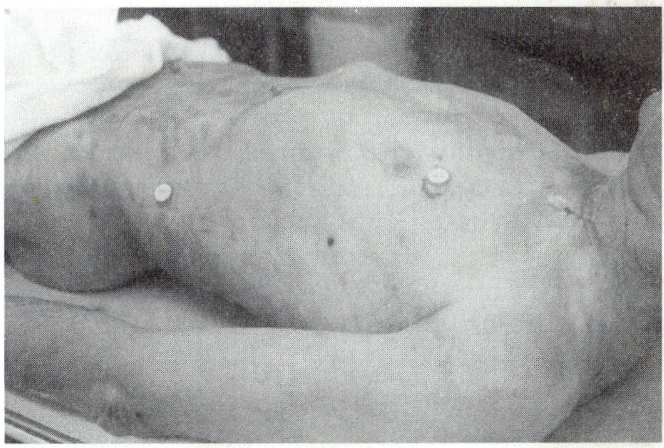

Figure 5–9. Partial decomposition. Both hypodermic and arterial embalming treatments were used. Note the discolorations.

oration follows the surface outline of the large intestine, which is located just beneath the abdominal wall. The abdomen as a whole gradually discolors and the chest, neck, and upper thighs are affected in time.

The blood trapped in the superficial vessels gradually breaks down, staining the surrounding tissues. The outline of the veins on the surface of the skin is easily detected. This purplish-brown discoloration of the superficial veins is most pronounced in the veins of the shoulder, upper chest, lower abdomen, and groin. An early discoloration that occurs as a result of the hemolysis or breakdown of red blood cells is postmortem stain.

Odor

As the proteins of the body decompose, putrefactive odors become apparent. This odor is caused by foul-smelling amines, mercaptans, and hydrogen sulfide.

Desquamation (Skin Slip)

The outer layers of the skin weaken because the deeper skin layers are undergoing autolysis. Hydrolysis of collagen and elastin causes the superficial skin to be pulled away easily from the deeper skin layers. As decomposition progresses, accumulations of gases and liquids can separate layers of skin, forming blisters. The blisters, which can become quite large, contain a putrid-smelling, gassy, watery, blood-stained fluid. If the blisters are touched or disturbed, the skin easily slips away; thus the term "skin-slip." When the skin is pulled away a shiny, pink, moist surface is exposed. Gradually, this moist area dehydrates, turns brown, and becomes slightly firm to the touch.

Gases

As decomposition progresses, gases begin to form in the viscera. This formation of gas generally starts in the stomach and intestines. Later, gases form in the body tissues. The gas causes the abdominal cavity to swell, and later the body tissues become distended. Gases in the tissues can actually be moved by the application of pressure. This movement is called **crepitation.** As the gas moves through the tissues it can be felt, and may actually make a crackling sound. Weakened areas such as the eyelids, scrotum, and breasts easily distend with gases. In time, eyelids, cheek, and lips distend and the tongue protrudes.

Purge

Purge is defined as the evacuation of gases, liquids, and semisolids from a natural body orifice. In decomposition, purge is generally caused by the build up of pressure from gas formed in the abdomen. The pressure forces gases, liquids, and semisolids along the path of least resistance, which is usually toward a natural body orifice. The purge from the stomach is generally a foul-smelling liquid that resembles the appearance of coffee grounds. Purge from the lungs is generally described as frothy, and if blood appears in this purge it may retain its red color. Stomach and lung purge will usually exit from the mouth and nose.

▶ TESTS OF DEATH

Although generally not the professional or legal responsibility of the embalmer, there are circumstances where an embalmer might benefit from knowledge of how medical personnel make a determination that death has occurred. Inasmuch as the legal requirements of death certification call for medical verification from a physician, it follows that tests for death would be conducted by a physician. However, it is also true that a physician may not necessarily view the body before certifying the medical cause of death, and therefore, the tests for death can also be performed by a properly trained individual.

Expert Tests

Expert tests require certain training and skills of the person who administers the test. Any procedure used to prove a sign of death that is conducted by a person or persons who are legally certified and authorized to do so, would be categorized as an expert test. Expert tests will, as a rule, be conducted or reviewed by a physician. Examples include:

- **Stethoscope**—an instrument used to mediate sounds produced in the body. This instrument would be used to listen for sounds of respiration or cardiac activity.*
- **Ophthalmoscope**—an instrument used to examine the interior of the eye, especially the retina. This instrument would be used to examine the blood vessels in the retina for signs of circulating blood. Because it is a light source, it could also be used to detect responses in the pupils of the eyes.†
- **Electroencephalogram (EEG)**—a record of the electrical activity of the brain.‡
- **Electrocardiogram (ECG, EKG)**—a record of the electrical activity of the heart.§

---

* *Taber's Cyclopedic Medical Dictionary,* p. 1682.
† *Taber's Cyclopedic Medical Dictionary,* p. 1167.
‡ *Taber's Cyclopedic Medical Dictionary,* p. 524.
§ *Taber's Cyclopedic Medical Dictionary,* p. 522.

- **Evoked response**—Method of testing the function of certain sense organs, even if the subject is unconscious or uncooperative.|| For example, in a living patient, an **auditory evoked response** will appear on an electroencephalograph if sound reaches the brain.# If there is no evoked response, the technician may conclude that sound did not reach the brain. Brain death would be one reason for the absence of an evoked response.

Inexpert Tests

There are situations where individuals may want to check to see if death has occurred where the equipment or expertise required for expert tests is not available. When such a test is used, it is called an **inexpert test.** Inexpert tests include:

- **Ligature test**—a finger is ligated with string or a rubber band. If the ligation causes swelling or discoloration, that indicates that circulation of blood is still occurring.
- **Ammonia injection test**—a small amount of ammonia is injected subcutaneously. If there is a reddish reaction in the skin, it indicates that life is present.
- **Pulse**—digital pressure to check for pulse beat.
- **Listening for respiration or heart beat** by placing your ear over the chest of the individual.

▶ KEY TERMS AND CONCEPTS FOR STUDY AND DISCUSSION

1. Define the following terms:
   Adipocere
   Agonal
   Agonal algor
   Agonal coagulation
   Agonal dehydration
   Agonal edema
   Agonal fever
   Agonal hypostasis
   Agonal period
   Algor mortis
   Anaerobic bacteria
   Biological Death
   Brain Death
   Cadaveric spasm
   Cadaverine
   Catalyst
   Clinical Death
   Crepitation
   Death rattle
   Death struggle
   Desquamation
   Endogenous invasion
   Extrinsic factors
   Fermentation
   Hydrolysis
   Hypostasis
   Imbibition
   Intrinsic factors
   Livor mortis
   Moribund
   Necrobiosis
   Necrosis
   Peptide bond
   pH
   Postmortem caloricity
   Postmortem cellular death
   Postmortem chemical change
   Postmortem edema
   Postmortem physical change
   Postmortem stain
   Primary flaccidity
   Protease
   Ptomaines
   Purge
   Putrefaction
   Putrescine
   Rigor mortis
   Secondary flaccidity
   Somatic death
   Translocation
2. Discuss agonal changes and how they change the physical and chemical makeup of the body.
3. What factors can speed or slow the establishment of livor mortis?
4. Discuss the signs of decomposition.
5. Discuss the process of hypostasis and explain how the progression of events leads to livor mortis and postmortem stain.
6. Discuss the pH changes that occur in the dead human body after death.
7. Discuss postmortem physical and chemical changes and how they change the makeup and condition of the body.

|| *Taber's Cyclopedic Medical Dictionary*, p. 581.
The Merck Manual of Diagnosis and Therapy. Rahway, NJ: Merck, Sharp & Dohme; 1982:1941.

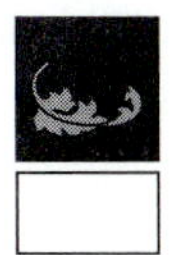

CHAPTER 6
EMBALMING CHEMICALS

This chapter looks at the eight groups of chemicals and their ingredients that are used to compose the various embalming fluids:*

1. Preservatives
2. Disinfectants (germicides)
3. Modifying agents (including buffers, humectants, and inorganic salts)
4. Anticoagulants (water conditioners or water softeners)
5. Surfactants (wetting agents, surface tension reducers, penetrating agents, or surface active agents)
6. Dyes (coloring agents)
7. Perfuming agents (masking agents)
8. Vehicles

These groups of chemicals are combined in various concentrations to produce vascular (preservative) embalming fluids, cavity fluids, supplemental embalming fluids and some accessory chemicals, used in the preparation of the dead human body:

- **Vascular fluids**
  - Arterial preservative fluid
  - High preservation demand fluid
  - Jaundice fluid
- **Cavity fluids**
- **Supplemental fluids**
  - Preinjection (primary injection) fluids
  - Coinjection fluids
  - Humectant (antidehydrant) fluids
  - Restorative fluids
  - Edema corrective fluids
  - Water corrective fluids
  - Fluid dyes
- **Accessory chemicals**
  - Autopsy gels
  - Surface preservatives
  - Cautery agents

* Much of this chapter was prepared by Leandro Rendon, Director of Chemical Research and Educational Programs, The Champion Company, Springfield, Ohio.

Seven of the previously listed eight groups of chemicals are designed to overcome the adverse effects of the preservative group, formaldehyde in particular. The seven groups of chemicals added to the standard bottle of fluid concentrate are there to control the adverse effects of formaldehyde, to maintain stability of the fluid, and to lengthen its shelf life.

Terms associated with embalming chemicals and fluids include the following:

- **Arterial (embalming, vascular, or preservative) fluid**—the concentrated, preservative embalming chemical that will be diluted with water to form the arterial solution for injection into the arterial system during vascular embalming.
- **Arterial solution (embalming solution, primary dilution)**—the in-use solution composed of embalming fluid diluted with water and other additive (supplemental) chemicals for injection into the body.
- **Cavity fluid**—concentrated embalming chemicals, which are injected into the cavities of the body following aspiration in cavity embalming. This chemical can also be used for surface and hypodermic embalming.
- **Supplemental fluid**—fluid injected for purposes other than preservation and disinfection. Some are injected before the preservative solution, others are injected with the preservative solution.
- **Accessory chemicals**—a group of chemicals used in addition to vascular and cavity embalming fluids; most are applied to the body surface.

▶ ESTABLISHMENT OF MINIMUM STANDARDS

After the turn of the century (approximately 1906), when formaldehyde became a widely used ingredient in embalming fluids, various state health departments required that a minimum standard of formaldehyde be used to embalm bodies to render them sanitized. This established a standard amount of formaldehyde to incorporate into the formulations. At that time a minimum amount of embalming solution was to be used in the preparation of bodies dead from noninfectious diseases as well as those dead from infectious and contagious diseases. The minimum standard established was not less than the following: 1 gallon of 14% of a 40% solution of formaldehyde (5.60%) for every 100 pounds of body weight for "normal cases" and 1 gallon of this same strength for every 75 pounds of body weight for infectious and contagious disease cases.

In these early years the manufacturers of embalming fluid sold it with the water already added. (The fluid was sold by the half-gallon ready for injection.) Later, because of the costs involved in bottling, packing, and shipping, it was decided to omit as much of the water as possible and sell the concentrated solution in pint bottles. To maintain the required minimum standards established by state laws, each pint bottle had to contain at least 8.96 ounces of 40% formaldehyde and the same proportion of other chemical ingredients. It must be kept in mind that formaldehyde acts harshly on body tissues, does not distribute or diffuse well, dehydrates, and darkens and grays body tissues. The use of strong embalming solutions (approximately 5.75%) was enforced in the years immediately following the influenza pandemics of 1918 and 1919. To overcome the adverse effects of formaldehyde on the body, a variety of supplemental fluids, such as blood solvents (later known as preinjection solutions), were developed; coinjection and jaundice fluids were developed and in use as early as 1910. It would not be until the development of penetrating agents and machine injection in the mid- to late 1930s that milder arterial solutions would be employed; the standard until the early 1970s would be 1 to 1.5% solution strength. This was quite sufficient to produce firming. The suggested in-use standard using these milder solutions since the mid 1930s has been to use 1 gallon of arterial solution for every 50 pounds of body weight. It was not until the early 1970s that research demonstrated that a minimum of at least a 2% formaldehyde-based arterial solution was necessary to sanitize body tissues effectively. In the near future it is expected that formaldehyde and phenol-based preservative fluids will be replaced with fluids containing preservatives and sanitizing elements that do not have the adverse effects of the preservatives currently in use. The "50 pound rule" is of little value today as a standard, for so often extreme conditions are seen, with edema, delayed preparation, decomposition, systemic infections, low protein levels, liver and kidney failure, using a 1.0% solution at a volume of 1 gallon for every 50 pounds of body weight may certainly be inadequate. The conditions of the body, the degree of firmness desired by the embalmer, and the length of time between death and disposition must be the determining factors in selecting an arterial fluid and the strength and volume at which it must be injected.

▶ GENERAL CHEMICAL PRINCIPLES OF EMBALMING FLUIDS

Commercial embalming fluids are composed of various chemicals and the same chemicals, when used in different concentrations, may produce different effects. This means each individual chemical ingredient has a specific function to perform and it reacts according to its own concentration, distribution, diffusion, and individual activity.

Among the main chemicals common to almost all embalming preservative solutions are formaldehyde and methyl alcohol. The remaining ingredients used in embalming solutions vary immensely.

Just as important as the need to replace equipment at frequent intervals and to maintain the proper facilities with which to manufacture and compound chemical solutions is the need to improve on and make changes in the general nature of formulations. These changes are occasioned by developments in the technical fields. Suppliers make use of such developments and adapt them into existing products or design new products containing them. This factor makes it unlikely that two different "brands" of fluid will have a similar composition. The continuing investigations and studies conducted by the technical staffs of fluid manufacturers who maintain research laboratories also often result in attention being devoted to some particular compound that produces an innovative effect when blended with special ingredients.

Years ago, because of the similar chemical makeup of the fluids, it was possible in many instances to take the label off one firm's product and place it on another. The user could not readily distinguish the difference in the fluids from the embalming results obtained! Today, the many commercially available chemical preservative solutions differ with respect to the following factors: pH of the solution; type of buffer materials used to maintain pH; grade of formalin used; type of alcohol; surfactants (anionic, nonionic, or cationic); anticoagulants; modifiers; physical features such as specific gravity and surface tension; and so on.

In brief, the "20-index" fluid made by one manufacturer today can be expected to be chemically different in composition and even to produce different embalming results from that produced by another firm.

There is no general agreement on what constitutes a "standard" embalming fluid. Embalmers show varying preferences in the type of results they desire. Some require a fast-acting fluid with little or no internal cosmetic effect, whereas other desire such a fluid to produce an internal cosmetic effect. In other instances, a mild to moderately firming fluid that produces a noticeable coloring is preferred. An important factor for consideration is the effect of pathologic conditions on the fluid injected and vice versa. Finally, the chemical preservation solution may produce different results when applied to different cases.

▶ BRIEF SUMMARY OF CHEMICAL COMPONENTS

The ingredients that might be found in the majority of embalming fluids can be classified according to the specific purposes for which they are used (Figure 6–1).

Preservatives

Preservatives, which inactivate saprophytic bacteria, render the medium on which such bacteria thrive unsuitable for nutrition. They arrest decomposition by altering enzymes and lysins of the body as well as convert the decomposable tissues into a form much less susceptible to decomposition. Formalin, as the commercial source of formaldehyde, is the most commonly used chemical for this purpose. Other examples are paraformaldehyde, formaldehyde polymerization products or formaldehyde "donors," "light" aldehydes, glyoxal, glutaraldehyde, phenol, phenolic derivatives, and lower alcohols (see p. 121).

Germicides

Germicides are employed in embalming fluids to kill microorganisms or to render them inactive. This can be accomplished in two ways: (1) the chemical acts directly on the protein of which the microbe is composed or (2) the chemical acts on the protein material from which it derives its nourishment.

These chemicals kill or render incapable of reproduction the disease-causing microorganisms. As these microbes are made of proteins and the enzymes that they make are protein in nature, most of the preservative chemicals act as germicides. Formaldehyde, phenol, and phenolic derivatives are germicidal. Glutaraldehyde in an alkaline pH is particularly effective. Quaternary ammonium compounds such as Roccal and Zephiran Chloride are good examples of germicides incorporated into cavity fluids.

An important purpose of embalming is the sanitizing of the tissues of the body. Germicides are incorporated into **arterial fluid, some coinjection fluids, cavity fluids, and surface disinfectants.** The embalmer uses the surface disinfectants to sanitize the nasal and oral cavities as well as the surface of the body and, in the case of an autopsied body, the surface walls of the abdominal, thoracic, pelvic, and cranial cavities (see pp. 122–129).

Modifying Agents

Modifying agents influence the chemical reactions produced by the preservative solution and function in embalming fluids to control the action of the main preservative agents. Modifying agents are chemicals for which there may be greatly varying demands predicated on the type of embalming, the environment, and the embalming fluid to be used. Because of special needs, embalmers may wish to greatly increase the concentration of one or more ingredients in a given embalming fluid (see pp. 122–129).

Humectants. A humectant can be used to moisturize tissues as well as to dehydrate tissues. These chemicals

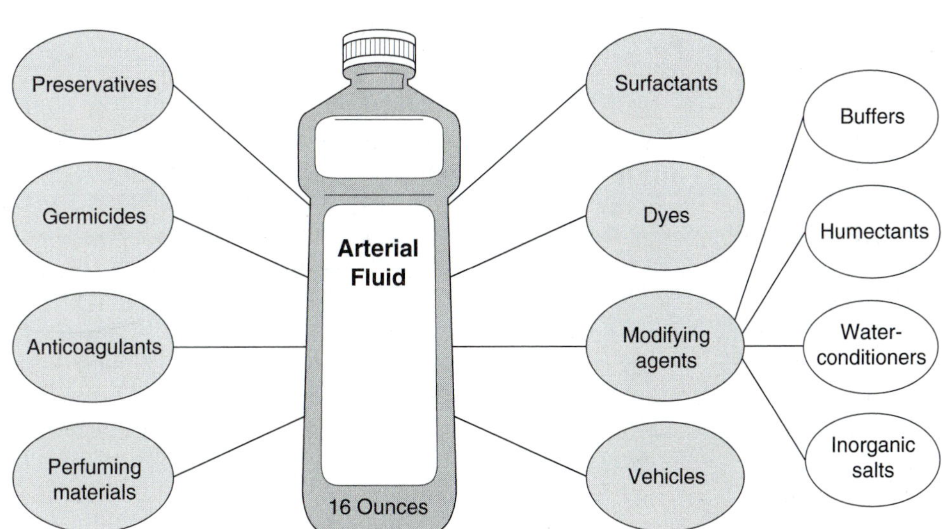

Figure 6–1. Ingredients that may be found in the majority of embalming fluids.

increase the capability of embalmed tissues to retain moisture. These would be added to dilute solutions when the body predisposes to dehydration. They also function to control and delay the firming and/or drying action of the preservative ingredients. Examples include glycerin, sorbitol, emulsifiable oils, and lanolin.

Buffers. Buffers effect the stabilization of the acid–base balance within embalming solutions and embalmed tissues. Many of the chemicals used as anticoagulants serve as buffer pairs to control the pH. Examples include borates, citrates, carbonates, monodisodium phosphate, and ethylenediaminetetraacetic acid (EDTA) salts (see pp. 122–129).

Inorganic Salts. Inorganic salts should be included under the heading of "modifying agents." These salts are actually found in a number of the other categories of the chemicals that constitute an arterial fluid. They can be found in buffers, preservatives, germicides, water conditioners, and anticoagulants. The salts play an important role in determining the osmotic qualities of the embalming solution. The osmotic force of the solution is responsible for its diffusing qualities (see pp. 122–129).

Anticoagulants

Anticoagulants retard the tendency of blood to become more viscous by natural postmortem processes or prevent adverse reactions between blood and other embalming chemicals. The anticoagulants may be the principal ingredients of a nonpreservative, preinjection fluid, or coinjection fluid. They maintain blood in a liquid state and, thus, facilitate the removal of blood from the circulatory system. The chemicals employed for this purpose can also function as water softeners or water conditioners. Water conditioners are added to the water used to dilute arterial embalming fluids when it is known that the water contains such minerals that it would be classified as "hard" water. When added in sufficient concentration, they will reduce the water used in preparing the embalming solution to zero hardness (or nearly so). Water conditioners contain high concentrations of sequestering or chelating chemicals that might not be compatible with the other ingredients in embalming fluids over a long shelf life and so *must be packaged in separate formulations.* The amount of this type of chemical incorporated into regular arterial formulations is insufficient for "water conditioning" purposes. Examples of anticoagulants are citrates, phosphates, oxalates, borates, and EDTA (see pp. 122–129).

Surfactants

Wetting agents, surface tension reducers, penetrating agents, surface-active agents, and emulsifying agents—all surfactants—reduce the molecular cohesion of a liquid and thereby enable it to flow through smaller apertures. This class of compounds is used to promote diffusion of the preservative elements through the capillary walls to saturate the tissues uniformly. They also help to distribute the coloring agents uniformly for internal cosmetic purposes. The presence of surfactants in the chemical solution aids in the displacement of body liquids from body tissue so that the injected preservative chemical elements may readily replace the volume previously occupied by body liquids (blood and tissue fluids). Examples include sulfonated oils (alkyl sulfonates), polyethylene glycol ethers, alkyl aryl polyether alcohols, alkyl aryl polyether sulfonates, alkyl aryl polyethyl sulfates, alkyl diethyl benzylammonium chloride, and sodium lauryl sulfate (see pp. 122–129).

Dyes

Dyes are substances that on being dissolved, impart a definite color to the solvent. They are classified with respect to their capacity to impart permanent color to the tissues of the body into which they are injected as *active* (staining) and *inactive* (nonstaining). Active dyes are usually a blend of dyes, mainly coal-tar derivatives, and they have an internal cosmetic effect. Red dyes of various shades and degrees of intensity are usually blended in an attempt to restore a natural color to the tissues. The coloring materials blended for the purpose specified may range from those that impart a straw or amber color to those that emit a brilliant shade of red. The coloring materials selected for use in any given embalming fluid formulation depend to a great extent on the pH of the solution. Examples include eosin, erythrosine, ponceau, fluorescein, amaranth, and carmine (see pp. 122–129).

Reodorants (Perfuming and Masking Agents)

Reodorants have the ability to displace an unpleasant odor or to convert an unpleasant odor into a more pleasant one. Their primary function is to enhance the odor of the embalming solution. This class of chemicals is usually selected not only for its power in covering harsh chemicals, but also because of its pleasant odor and antiseptic value. Actually, the use of these chemicals in embalming fluid is not intended to cover the harshness of formaldehyde. It is, rather, to give the product a more pleasing odor. The materials generally used are those that are water soluble and are derived from essential oils. Most of the reodorants used are floral compounds, which have been found to more successfully mitigate the irritating fumes associated with embalming formulations. Examples include methyl salicylate (oil of wintergreen), benzaldehyde, and many related higher aldehydes (see pp. 122–129).

Vehicles

Vehicles serve as the solvents for the many ingredients incorporated into an embalming fluid. Most embalming formulations consist of a mixture of alcohols, glycerine-like materials, water, and possibly glycols, which function to keep the ingredients of the formulation in proper chemical and physical balance. It is necessary that vehicles also provide some stability to the formulation. In specially designed formulations it is possible that a special solvent may be added as a part of the innovation to dissolve or keep in solution any special additive materials in the product. Later, the concentrated chemical is further diluted by the solvent water.

▶ PRESERVATIVES

Generally speaking, the chemical compounds classified under "preservative ingredients" are the agents in the chemical preservative solution that cause the proteins to change in nature. Such compounds change a protein from a state in which it is easily decomposed to a state in which it will endure and not undergo putrefaction. In June 1988, *The New York Times* reported that it is now felt that it is the "unfolding of the proteins by formaldehyde with the result that the long strings of protein then intertwine into a network that hardens. This result is the *fixed protein.*" The type of action may be described as a "cooking" action in which the nature of the protein is changed, as occurs when a raw egg is fried. In that particular instance, the heat causes the albumin to change from a water white to a dull white.

What are some of the materials that are regarded as the main active preservative ingredients in modern-day embalming fluid preparations? The chemical compound employed is selected because of its chemical reactive properties that change the basic nature of the protein molecule.

Aldehydes, for example, react with the amino radicals of the protein structure to form a new compound in which the aldehyde radical adds on to the protein structure and water is released. The formula below represents a simple explanation of the action of the aldehyde on the amido part of the amino acid.

The amount of aldehyde that is taken up by the protein structures depends on such factors as initial concentration of aldehydes, pH value of the solution, effect of certain chemical compounds on aldehyde uptake, temperature, and conditions of tissue.

Formaldehyde and Formaldehyde-Type Preservatives

Formalin. Formalin is the commercial source of formaldehyde. Formaldehyde solutions containing 37% by weight formaldehyde gas absorbed in water, or in water and methyl alcohol, are known as formalin. The solution has a density slightly above that of water and contains approximately 40 grams of formaldehyde per 100 cubic centimeters. Therefore, commercial formaldehyde solution (i.e., "formalin") is described as containing "40% formaldehyde by volume." The NF (formerly USP) grade of formalin contains an average of 7% methyl alcohol, 37% minimum–37.3% maximum formaldehyde, and the remainder water. The alcohol present in the solution helps to stabilize the formaldehyde so that it will not precipitate and settle to the bottom as a powdery sediment (paraformaldehyde) at ordinary temperatures.

The regular product of commerce is a 37% by weight (40% by volume) formaldehyde gas in water solution. There are available, however, certain solutions that contain 40, 55, and even 70% formaldehyde in alcohol. The last two concentrations mentioned are subject to precipitation, and at cool temperatures the formaldehyde tends to fall out of solution very readily and form a fine powdery sediment at the bottom of the container. The sediment that settles to the bottom is actually **paraformaldehyde,** a solid form of formaldehyde. The formaldehyde that drops out of solution to the bottom of the container is not available for chemical reaction and results in a weaker concentration of formaldehyde in the top layers of the solution than at the bottom. In other words, the concentration of formaldehyde throughout the solution is not uniform.

$$\mathrm{HO{-}\overset{\overset{O}{\|}}{C}{-}\overset{\overset{R}{|}}{CH}{-}\overset{\overset{H}{|}}{N}{-}H + H{-}\overset{\overset{O}{\|}}{C}{-}H \longrightarrow HO{-}\overset{\overset{O}{\|}}{C}{-}\overset{\overset{R}{|}}{CH}{-}N = \overset{\overset{H}{|}}{C}{-}H + H_2O}$$

Amino acid + Formaldehyde ⟶ Fixed amino acid + Water

OR

$$\mathrm{HO{-}\overset{\overset{O}{\|}}{C}{-}\overset{\overset{R}{|}}{CH}{-}\overset{\overset{H}{|}}{N}{-}H + 2OH{-}CH_2{-}OH \longrightarrow HO{-}\overset{\overset{O}{\|}}{C}{-}\overset{\overset{R}{|}}{CH}{-}\overset{\overset{CH_2-OH}{|}}{N}{-}CH_2{-}OH + 2H_2O}$$

Amino acid + Formalin ⟶ Fixed amino acid + Water

A "formaldehyde solution" is any solution that contains formaldehyde. The NF or USP grade of formalin, on the other hand, is a formaldehyde solution consisting of 40% formaldehyde gas by volume or 37% formaldehyde gas by weight. In view of the various grades and types of formalin solutions now commercially available, it is important to designate the grade of formalin being used to state the percentage of formaldehyde gas present.

For many years the word *index* was generally understood to be the percentage strength of concentrated embalming fluid, and referred to the amount of absolute formaldehyde gas by volume present. It should be understood that the reference was to formaldehyde gas and not to formalin, which is the 40% (by volume) solution of formaldehyde. The Embalming Chemical Manufacturers Association and the schools and colleges of mortuary science have generally agreed on the following definition of index: "An embalming fluid will be said to have formaldehyde index, *N*, when 100 milliliters of fluid, at normal room temperature, contain *N* grams of formaldehyde gas." Thus, a 20-index product contains 20 grams of formaldehyde gas per 100 milliliters of concentrated fluid. The word *index*, therefore, identifies only the absolute formaldehyde gas present in any given product. It is not a measure of the total aldehyde concentration present. *Index refers only to the amount of formaldehyde gas present.*

Formaldehyde is a colorless gas at ordinary temperatures and has a strong, irritating pungent odor. **It is very soluble in water and is extremely reactive.** Because of its chemical nature, which makes it highly reactive, formaldehyde cannot be properly masked without affecting its chemical structure. In other words, to mask the odor of formaldehyde completely, it is necessary to neutralize it, and in such cases, the formaldehyde could not be available for preservation in embalming.

The chemistry of formaldehyde is a very specialized and complicated field of study, and F. J. Walker (1964) of DuPont published a book on the subject. This compound has been studied quite extensively and has been found to be **a very powerful germicide.** It destroys putrefactive organisms when carried by a proper vehicle that permits it to penetrate these organisms. It preserves tissues by forming new chemical compounds with the tissues. The new compounds that are formed are stable and unfit as food for organisms. An interesting comparison has been used effectively:

> The buttons on your coat, the barrel of your fountain pen, the comb on your dresser, and many other things you may commonly use are made of formaldehyde and phenol or carbolic acid, as it is commonly known. Either formaldehyde or carbolic acid would injure you severely if taken into your mouth. You may, however, with impunity hold a button from your coat in your mouth because it differs definitely from either of its component ingredients. In other words, it is a resin.

This statement describes exactly the action of formaldehyde on albuminous materials. New resins are formed that are neither formaldehyde nor albumin. These resins may be hard resins, soft resins, or semihard resins, depending on the control chemicals (modifying or plasticizing materials) used in combination with the formaldehyde.

Formaldehyde acts quickly on the particular area with which it is in contact. The more formaldehyde there is in a certain area, the greater the action on the tissues in that area. The closer the tissue to the formaldehyde, the greater the action on it. This action takes up more formaldehyde than may be needed for preservation, possibly leaving little or no formaldehyde for the more remote tissue areas.

To use an analogy, the preceding action of formaldehyde on tissue may be compared with the action of a sponge in water. The sponge absorbs or takes up water depending on how much water there is to begin with and also depending on how long the sponge is permitted to remain in contact with the water.

If an embalming solution is hurried through the circulatory system as the result of too much pressure and excessive drainage, some tissue area will receive little or no formaldehyde. This, in turn, causes "soft spots" to develop. Such areas result when tissue does not receive a sufficient amount of formaldehyde to preserve them. There is also the possibility that a localized tissue area, because of some pathologic condition, may be undergoing decomposition. Thus, the free amines may absorb more than their usual share of formaldehyde so that little formaldehyde is left for remote parts. This situation is further exacerbated when an average of only 2 gallons of solution is injected. In such a case it is possible that an insufficient amount of formaldehyde is used to achieve thorough preservation of the body tissues.

There are disadvantages to the use of formaldehyde as a preservative in embalming fluids; it rapidly coagulates the blood, converts the tissues to a gray hue when it mixes with blood not removed from the body, fixes discolorations, dehydrates tissues, constricts capillaries, and deteriorates with age, can be oxidized to formic acid, and can be decomposed to alcohol and formic acid in a strong alkaline pH, unpleasant odor, and irritant to the embalmer. It may also be carcinogenic.

However, the advantages of formaldehyde as a preservative in embalming fluids outweigh the disadvantages. The advantages include the following. Formaldehyde is inexpensive, bactericidal, and inhibits the growth of yeast and mold. It can rapidly destroy autolytic enzymes, and rapidly acts on the body proteins and converts them to insoluble resins that stop tissue decomposition. Only a small percentage of formaldehyde is needed to act on a large amount of protein; it produces rapid fixation, which aids in positioning the dead human body and also indicates that preservation is taking place. Finally, formaldehyde deodorizes the body amines formed during putrefaction.

Paraformaldehyde. Paraformaldehyde is described as a polymer of formaldehyde. It is a white, powdery solid containing from 85 to 99% formaldehyde. The NF grade of paraformaldehyde contains 95% formaldehyde. Paraformaldehyde is generally prepared from water solutions of formaldehyde by processes involving evaporation and distillation until concentration to a point at which solidification or precipitation take place. This form of formaldehyde is used where powdered preparations are involved, such as in hardening compounds or other powdered preparations used for "dusting" the body walls and viscera.

Trioxane. Another polymer of formaldehyde is trioxane, a colorless crystalline material with a rather pleasant odor resembling that of chloroform. This material is sometimes incorporated into formulations to act as an accessory preservative along with formates. It is rather costly when compared with other forms of formaldehyde and, therefore, is too expensive to warrant its extensive use for embalming purposes.

Other Aldehydes. Some of the other lower or "light" aldehydes have been proposed for use in embalming preparations and some are occasionally found in modern embalming fluids. Examples of these are acetaldehyde, propionaldehyde, and pyruvic aldehyde. Among the higher aldehydes, furfural and benzaldehyde may be listed. The important requirement of an aldehyde is that it possess denaturing and crosslinking properties that enable it to produce a firm tissue.

Condensation Products (Formaldehyde "Donor" Compounds, Formaldehyde Reaction Products). Aliphatic nitrohydroxy compounds are formed as the result of a condensation reaction between nitroparaffins (nitromethane, nitroethane, etc.) and certain aldehydes. Compounds of this type, in the presence of the proper catalyst (such as potassium carbonate), give off formaldehyde at a slow rate. When in solution, such formaldehyde condensation products exhibit an acid pH and need the alkali catalyst to release the formaldehyde.

Other types of formaldehyde "donor" compound are the methylol derivatives of hydantoin. These also liberate formaldehyde at a slow rate. Both types are used in low-odor or "fumeless" products. These complex organic substances make it possible to formulate fluids that are pleasant to use, because they do not give off noxious, irritating fumes. The formaldehyde is released after being distributed to all soft tissue areas where the usual preservative action is exerted. The disadvantage in using such materials is twofold: they have a slow reaction rate and are very expensive.

Dialdehydes

Another group of chemicals that are also aldehydes is the dialdehyde (two functional aldehyde groups in the molecule) class of chemical compounds. As far back as 1941, several firms in this industry investigated the possibility of using the then-known dialdehyde compounds available on a commercial scale. The principal dialdehyde and probably the only one available at that time in large commercial quantities and at an economical price that made its use in embalming formulations feasible was glyoxal, the lowest member of the dialdehydes. On November 2, 1943, a patent was granted relating to the use of glyoxal in embalming fluid formulations.

Glyoxal. Glyoxal is available commercially as a 30% yellowish, aqueous solution containing small amounts of ethylene glycol, glycolic acid, formic acid, and formaldehyde. It is also available as a special 40% clear solution. Because it contains a chromophore group, glyoxal solution tends to stain tissue yellow. This feature limits the use of glyoxal mainly to cavity fluid formulations, especially because its optimal pH range of activity is about 9 to 10.

Glutaraldehyde. In the early 1950s, a method was developed that made it possible to manufacture the five-carbon, straight-chain dialdehyde glutaraldehyde in commercial quantities. Glutaraldehyde was first employed as an embalming and fixative agent in early 1955 and was subsequently patented for use in embalming preparations. Commercially, it is supplied as a stable 25% aqueous solution that has a mild odor and a light color. Glutaraldehyde reacts through crosslinking to insolubilize both protein and polyhydroxy compounds. The pH of the commercial solution is 3.0 to 4.0 and the specific gravity is 1.058 to 1.068.

An interesting feature of glutaraldehyde is that, unlike other aldehydes, it is capable of reacting with protein structures over a wide pH range. This is an important advantage for an aldehyde in embalming, because after death, tissue pH varies in different parts of the body and as time elapses between death and embalming.

Both glyoxal and glutaraldehyde are liquids, whereas formaldehyde is a gas. The following structural formulas serve to acquaint the reader with some of the aldehydes that have been mentioned:

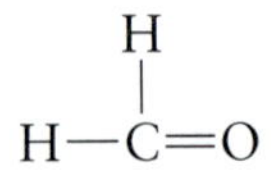

```
                                                        O
                                                        ‖
                                                      H—C
                                                        |
                                                      H—C—H
                                                        |
                                                      H—C—H
                           O              H             |
                         /   \            |           H—C—H
      H                 C     C——C=O                    |
      |                 \\   //                       H—C
   H—C=O               H—C——C—H                         ‖
                                                        O
Formaldehyde    Furfural, 2-Furaldehyde        Glutaraldehyde

      H  H          H  H
      |  |          |  |
   H—C—C=O       O=C—C=O
      |
      H
  Acetaldehyde      Glyoxal
```

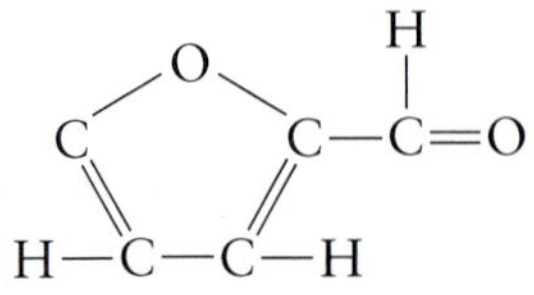

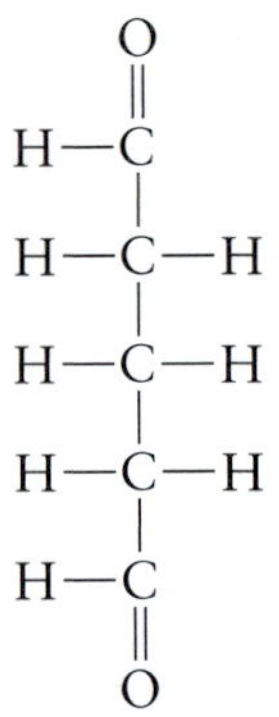

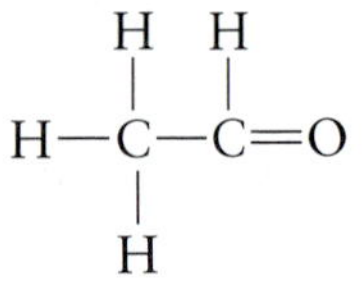

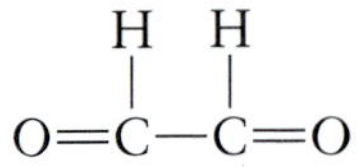

In combining with proteins and tissue, glutaraldehyde changes the nature of the proteins, makes them unsuitable as food for bacteria, and makes them resistant to decomposition changes. At the same time less moisture is removed from the tissues as the result of the chemical reaction between glutaraldehyde and proteins than when formaldehyde is used. In addition, glutaraldehyde has been found to be many times more effective as a disinfectant than formaldehyde.

Other Preservative Agents

Other preservative agents generally used in combination with formaldehyde include the lower alcohols and the phenol (carbolic acid) compounds. The latter materials are usually selected on the basis of solubility, penetrability, compatibility, and stability. Some of the newer preservative ingredients include certain aromatic esters and formaldehyde reaction products. They react with proteins in a similar manner as formaldehyde to form insoluble resins, the main difference being in the rate of reaction. Formaldehyde firms tissue at a faster rate.

Methanol (Methyl Alcohol, CH_3OH). Generally, the synthetic grade of methanol is used and it is 99.85% pure. Methanol is used in embalming formulations for six reasons:

1. It is an outstanding preservative that destroys many organisms and precipitates albumins.
2. It is a good solvent for other chemicals not readily soluble in water alone, for example, derivatives of phenol.
3. It is an excellent penetrator of the tissues and it also exerts some bleaching action.
4. Methanol is a stabilizer of formaldehyde. It prevents the formaldehyde from changing to the powdered form.
5. Methanol serves as a diluent or vehicle for other ingredients of the formulation.
6. Investigations have indicated that methanol is more toxic to bacteria than ethanol or ethyl alcohol.

Methanol and the lower alcohols have a dehydrating effect on protein structure. As methanol has the greatest precipitating effect of the lower alcohols and aids in removing body liquids, it is used more extensively in embalming fluids than either ethyl or isopropyl alcohol.

Phenol (Carbolic Acid, C_6H_5OH). Phenol is one of the most commonly found ingredients in both arterial and cavity fluids manufactured in the "early" days of the fluid industry. Today, it is used chiefly in cavity fluid formulations. Phenol is a coal-tar derivative that is a colorless crystalline solid. On exposure to strong light and metallic contamination, it darkens and assumes a dark amber or reddish brown appearance when in solution. Such change in color is due mainly to oxidation. The potency of phenol is not impaired to any great extent when such change occurs.

Phenol is very rapidly absorbed by protein structures and penetrates the skin very readily. Phenol and phenolic derivatives are good germicides. In addition, they assist formaldehyde in forming insoluble resins with albumins. Generally, their use in embalming fluids is confined to cavity fluids because they tend to produce a "putty gray" tissue. Formulations containing these compounds are often used as bleaching agents to lighten discolorations on the skin surface. The solution either is applied as an external pack or is injected subcutaneously with a hypodermic syringe.

USES FOR CONCENTRATED PHENOL SOLUTIONS IN EMBALMING

- Preservative
- Germicide and fungicide
- Bleaching agent
- Cautery agent
- Reducing agent
- Drying agent

(Care should always be taken when working with phenol to protect skin and eyes.)

It is unfortunate that the most powerful germicides among the phenols are not water soluble. Some of the halogenated phenols found in embalming formulations include orthophenyl phenol, *para*-chlormetacresol, dichloro-*ortho*-phenyl phenol, tribromothymol, and other sodium salts of these and other phenol-related chemicals.

Sometimes the expression *triple-base fluid* is heard. This refers to a fluid containing phenol, alcohol, and formaldehyde. A "double-base" fluid presumably is one containing formaldehyde and alcohol, or formaldehyde and phenol, or alcohol and phenol. Commercial fluids almost always contain phenols in combination with formaldehyde and alcohol. The presence of the latter two compounds improves the bacteria-killing power of phenols. Phenols generally do not produce readily detectable firmness of tissue such as that produced by aldehydes.

Quaternary Ammonium Compounds. These materials are used chiefly for their germicidal and deodorizing qualities. They consist of mixtures of alkyl radicals from C_8H_{17} to $C_{18}H_{37}$, that is, high-molecular-weight alkyl dimethyl benzylammonium chlorides. Aqueous solutions are usually neutral (pH 7). These compounds are not compatible with the wetting agents used in arterial fluids nor with many of the coloring materials incorporated into such fluids. Consequently, their use is restricted to cavity fluids and specialty formulations used for cold sterilization of instruments, linens, gowns, clothing, and other items; cleaning agents for mold-proofing remains; deodorant sprays; and so on. Two of the best known "quats" are Roccal and Zephiran Chloride.

Salts. Various salts have been used in embalming products since the early days of embalming. Among the more commonly used compounds are potassium acetate, sodium nitrate and nitrate, and some salts of aluminum. The salts of the heavy metals are not used, as after 1906, many states prohibited their use in embalming compositions.

Germicides

Obviously, the ingredients used as preservatives also function as germicides. In addition, chemicals such as phenol, the quaternary ammonium compounds (chloride), and glutaraldehyde are used as surface disinfectants and in embalming fluid solutions.

▶ MODIFYING AGENTS

Modifying agents control the rate of action of the main preservative ingredients of embalming formulations. Many preservative ingredients, when used alone, exert adverse effects that interfere with good embalming results. For example, formaldehyde (when used alone) is so harsh an astringent that it sears the walls of the small capillaries and prevents diffusion of the preservation solution to remote soft tissue areas. It is necessary to control the rate of fixation so that the firming action is delayed long enough to permit thorough saturation of tissue cells. When the hardening effect of the aldehyde is delayed, the more uniform distribution of the coloring or staining agent is made possible. Buffers, antidehydrants, water conditioners, and inorganic salts usually control the rate of chemical action, modify the adverse color reaction produced by the preservative ingredient in the tissues, and control capillary restriction or other undesirable results produced by the preservative materials.

1. *Buffers:* agents that serve to control the acid–base balance of fluid and tissues
2. *Humectants* (antidehydrants): agents that help to control tissue moisture balance
3. *Inorganic salts:* agents that help control the osmotic qualities of the embalming solution

It should be pointed out that many chemicals in the preceding list serve similar functions. Many buffers can also act as water conditioners and anticoagulants. In addition, some of these chemicals are also inorganic salts and contribute to the osmotic qualities of the embalming solution. Even humectants can play a role in the osmotic quality of an embalming solution. Because certain chemicals have multiple uses in embalming solutions, specific chemicals appear under different headings. For example, in a discussion of the anticoagulants, buffers are also reviewed.

Buffers

Buffers are employed in embalming fluids to stabilize the acid–base balance of the fluid. These pH stabilizers not only help to maintain the acid–base balance of the fluid, but, in addition, assist in stabilizing the pH of the tissues where the embalming fluid reacts with the cellular proteins. **Keep in mind that the tissues of the body after death contain varying levels of acids or bases.** Normal body pH is about 7.38 to 7.4 after death, and through the rigor mortis cycle the tissues will have an acid pH as a result of carbohydrate breakdown. After the rigor cycle the tissues become basic as a result of protein breakdown. These reactions are not uniform throughout the body, so tissues will vary in pH depending on rigor mortis and decomposition cycles. In addition, the cause of death can influence tissue pH. Buffers play a very important role in providing good pH medium for the reaction of preservative with body proteins.

Alkaline Compounds

Certain alkalines are commonly employed to modify the action of formaldehyde. They "neutralize" the formalin used in making the fluid.

Borates. In a report released by the Public Health Service in 1915, it was found that **borax** (sodium borate) was a good, efficient neutralizer of formalin, providing a desired degree of alkalinity that rendered formalin stable for long periods. It has been found to reduce the hardening and graying actions of formaldehyde. Depending on the specific type of formulation and other ingredients present, boric acid may also be employed in embalming formulations. Formulations containing a well-balanced mixture of borates have been found to keep formaldehyde fairly stable beyond 2 years. The loss in formaldehyde strength in such instances is insignificant.

Carbonates. Sodium carbonate is used alone or in combination with borates to modify the action of formaldehyde on tissue. Magnesium carbonate is also used sometimes and may be added to the formalin prior to combination with the other ingredients in a formulation. This procedure is said to neutralize formalin and maintain it at pH 7. From all indications it would appear that carbonates are not as efficient as borates in preventing deterioration of formalin over long periods.

In a *Report and Review of Research in Embalming and Embalming Fluids* by the Minnesota State Department of Health, N. C. Pervier and F. Lloyd Hansen of the University of Minnesota studied the tissue reaction to injections of formaldehyde at various pH values. These investigators found that addition of a strong base, such as sodium hydroxide, improved tissue coloring; however, the high concentration of sodium hydroxide used caused deterioration of the preservative. When they injected formaldehyde solutions containing 1, 2, and 3% acid (HCl), the tissue tended to assume a putty-gray coloration.

The investigations of these two workers confirmed the findings of the U.S. Hygienic Laboratories reported some 50 years ago. Today, most arterial fluids are found to be slightly alkaline (with a pH of 7.2–7.4), whereas cavity fluids tend to be acidic in nature.

Humectants (Antidehydrants/ Polyhydric Compounds)

Humectants are described as having a coating action; they wrap around the formaldehyde molecule and thus keep the formaldehyde from making direct contact with albuminous material until the tissues are thoroughly saturated and bathed with the preservative solution. The formaldehyde is under shackles for a time, and as it travels through the capillaries and to the tissue cells it gradually sheds its shackles and, on release, acts on the albuminous material. The addition of polyhydric compounds to embalming fluids assists in making the tissue more flexible and rubbery. In some instances such materials are also called plasticizing agents because of their pliable effects. These compounds include glycerin, sorbitol, glycols, and other polyhydric alcohols. Cosmetic oils, lanolin, and its derivatives are also used for their emollient properties.

Glycerine. A by-product of the manufacture of soap, glycerine is a member of the large family of alcohols. It has been produced synthetically from petroleum products. Although glycerine is not itself a germicide and has no preservative qualities, it does increase the germ-killing power of other chemicals, probably because it is an excellent solvent for disinfecting chemicals; its good solubility makes it an efficient carrier for the chemicals. Glycerine is a good lubricator, is a good solvent for other compounds, and is hygroscopic, which means it has affinity for moisture. If retained in the tissues, it helps to prevent overdrying.

Sorbitol and the Glycols. Sorbitol is probably used more extensively today in embalming fluids than is glycerine. Chemically, it has a straight chain of six carbon atoms and six hydroxyl groups, whereas glycerine has three carbon atoms and three hydroxyl groups in its structure. Commercially, sorbitol is generally available as a 70% aqueous solution. An important characteristic of sorbitol is that it loses water at a slower rate than glycerine, and consequently, for controlling the rate of moisture loss, it is more efficient than glycerine. One disadvantage of sorbitol solutions is that at very low temperatures, sorbitol tends to drop out of solution. Different types of glycols (mainly propylene, ethylene, and diethylene) are also found in embalming preparations. Sometimes, these materials are used alone with formaldehyde; in other instances, they may be incorporated into a formulation already containing either glycerine, sorbitol, or both.

Ethylene glycol is a colorless, syrupy liquid with very little odor. It is quite readily soluble in water. Because of its hygroscopic properties it is used as a moisture-retaining and softening material.

Propylene glycol is reported to be superior to glycerine as a general solvent and inhibitor of mold growth. Like ethylene glycol, it is colorless, odorless, and completely soluble in water.

Emulsified Oils. Many materials have been investigated for their emollient characteristics. Materials such as lanolin and silicon are not in themselves water soluble, but certain fractions or derivatives are used that can easily be dispersed in aqueous solutions. It is the purpose of these materials in embalming fluid to mitigate the drying effect of the preservative agents. Highly penetrative oils of the oleate and palmitate types are also employed to help reduce the drying effect of aldehydes. Use of such materials requires an emulsion system that is able to maintain the formulation in a stable and uniform state over a long period.

Gums—Vegetable and Synthetic

The use of vegetable and synthetic gums is generally prompted by the need to restore moisture to tissue or to maintain the normal appearance of tissue when the subject is to be held for a period prior to burial. These materials, when added to water, swell and retain the moisture as the gum molecule is distributed to the soft tissue areas. Because of their molecular size, the gums, on taking up moisture, are actually trapped in the capillary bed and aid both in restoring moisture to the area and in filling out the tissues to overcome the emaciated appearance.

As these materials are large molecular entities they are generally added to the arterial embalming solution after the initial injection has been made and all surface discolorations have been cleared. Use of such compounds prior to complete removal of blood from the tissues may interfere with proper distribution of the injected preservative solution.

Examples of vegetable gums include **karaya** and **tragacanth.** The synthetic gums are generally cellulosic compounds of varying composition.

Inorganic Salts

The inorganic salts used in embalming fluids serve a variety of functions. They can act as buffers, anticoagulants, preservatives, germicides, and water conditioners. Their use is quite simple in that they can be dissolved in the limited space of the 16-ounce standard bottle of concentrated embalming fluid. By controlling the amount of inorganic salts used, the fluid remains balanced, as some of the salts do not "settle out" of the concentrated fluid. An obvious role for salts in any solution is their ability to control the osmotic qualities. This is true in embalming fluid. Once the embalming solution reaches the capillary beds it is very important that the solution be able to pass through the microscopic pores of the capillaries and thus enter the tissue spaces. It is a role of the inorganic salts to maintain an osmotic quality of the embalming solution that helps to draw fluid from the capillaries into the tissue spaces. Likewise, special fluids are used on bodies whose tissues are saturated with edema. These "special-purpose" fluids, when mixed according to the manufacturer's directions, actually draw the excess tissue moisture (edema) from the tissues back into the capillaries, from which it can then be removed by the drainage process. It is the osmotic qualities of those "special-purpose" fluids that bring about the dehydration of these bodies (see Chapter 21).

▶ ANTICOAGULANTS (WATER CONDITIONERS OR SOFTENERS)

Anticoagulants are an important component of embalming fluids, especially arterial fluids, because they are used to maintain blood in a liquid state and thereby make it easy to remove from the circulatory system.

When blood collects in the capillary bed in the dependent parts of the body after death, it has a tendency to thicken and clot very easily. In some cases, as in death from pneumonia, the blood tends to clot more readily. The volume of circulating blood tends to decrease when high fever precedes death, and the blood becomes more viscous and clots more readily after circulation stops.

It is therefore necessary to include, in an embalming fluid, chemicals that maintain blood in a liquid state so that it is easily displaced from the body. Such chemicals inhibit or stop the clotting of blood. Claims are often made that such materials also "liquefy" clotted blood, but it is not likely that this happens.

The ingredients that are used for this purpose must be chemically compatible with, or inert toward, other intimately blended ingredients of the formulation. The materials that are employed as anticoagulants also function as "water softeners" or "water conditioners"; however, products specially designed for that purpose are commercially available and are sold for use as additives or supplemental chemicals with the arterial solution.

The products known as water "softeners" or water "conditioners" are used for one or all of four reasons.

First, such products are intended to be used as aids to improve drainage by keeping blood in a liquid state during the embalming operation and softening the framework of clotted material so that it readily breaks up into smaller pieces.

Second, by reducing "hard" water to zero hardness, such materials make it possible for the arterial fluid to function under better conditions. The interfering "hardness" chemicals such as calcium and iron actually prevent the preservative chemicals present in arterial fluids from performing their intended function of penetrating soft tissues to achieve preservation.

Third, experience and experimental work have indicated that the dyes used in embalming fluids produce the best internal cosmetic effect under slightly alkaline conditions. The arterial fluids cannot be compounded to stay on the alkaline side of the pH scale because aldehydes, especially formaldehyde, undergo breakdown and lose strength when kept under alkaline conditions for long periods. Consequently, the alkaline conditions must be created at the time the solution is going to be used. During such short periods, alkaline pH does not adversely affect the preservative chemicals. Addition of water softeners ("clot-dispersing products") to the embalming solution prepared for injection produces a most desirable alkaline condition. Such materials enhance the coloring properties and action of dyes by increasing their intensity.

Fourth, recent investigations have definitely shown that most aldehydes (and formaldehyde in particular) function better as fixative or firming agents under slightly alkaline conditions. But, as pointed out in the preceding paragraph, aldehydes cannot remain under alkaline conditions more than a couple of weeks (even less) without losing their effectiveness. Therefore, the alkaline conditions must be created more or less "on the spot" at the time the fluid is used. This is where the specially designed additive products come into play. Greater firmness is attained by progressive action where such materials are used along with the arterial fluid.

Often, it is claimed that a certain arterial fluid contains all of the materials necessary to reduce to zero hardness the water used in preparing the embalming solution. Because of the preservative materials that must be incorporated into the arterial fluid formulation (in addition to wetting agents, modifiers, coloring agents, perfuming materials, etc.), however, there is a limit to the amount of anticlotting and water-softening compounds that can be added to the formula. If sufficient amounts of such compounds were to be added to the regular arterial fluids to achieve the results expected from and produced by "water softeners," the chemical and physical balance of the formulation would be adversely affected. And what happens when the chemical and physical balance of the arterial fluid is adversely affected?

- There may be interference with proper penetration and diffusion of the preservative solution.
- There may be interference with the drainage qualities of the embalming solution.
- By disruption of the chemical balance of the solution, addition of the extra amounts of anticlotting and water-softening chemicals to the arterial fluid formula could cause a gradual reduction of the formaldehyde strength of the fluid.

Consequently, embalming fluid manufacturers supply, as separate supplemental products, "water softeners and conditioners" that are added to the embalming solution prepared for injection. This procedure enables the embalmer to use as much material as the case may require for proper and effective water- and clot-softening action.

The compounds in this class of embalming chemicals include those usually found in buffer systems. As has been pointed out previously, the degree of acidity or alkalinity of the medium in which a chemical reaction takes place influences, to a great extent, the chemical reaction that takes place between compounds and substances. During life, blood and body tissues have a pH of 7.4. After death, however, tissue pH varies greatly. Also, the pH of the body tissues at the time of embalming depends on the time that has lapsed since death. An embalming formulation containing the proper buffer mixture will perform uniformly because the buffer mixture will neutralize excess acidity or alkalinity and, thus, facilitate the action in a given pH range.

It is also necessary to maintain an embalming formulation at a given pH if it is to be retained for a long shelf life. Some chemicals that are used are stable only in certain pH ranges and so buffer agents must be employed to keep constant the acid–base balance of the solution. This ensures against deterioration and breakdown of the chemical compounds. For example, earlier it was stated that formaldehyde is not stable at high pH, that is, under alkaline conditions, over long periods. When embalming fluid is compounded, the manufacturer must try to anticipate the shelf life of the product so that the fluid is as effective the day it is used as the day it was compounded. A formaldehyde index on a fluid bottle label is maintained only through the proper chemical balance of the formulation, which also includes proper acid–base control of the solution.

Another important factor to keep in mind is that as the prepared embalming solution diffuses through the circulatory system, it comes into contact with tissues that may well be at different pH values. The acid–base balance of the tissues should also be so controlled and maintained by the buffer so that the fluid performs under the best pH conditions.

Many preservative chemicals when used alone exert bad effects that interfere with the achievement of good embalming results. For example, formaldehyde when used alone is so harsh and astringent that it sears the walls of the small capillaries and prevents diffusion of the preservative solution to remote soft tissue areas. Consequently, it is necessary to control the action of the formaldehyde so that the fixation of tissue (firming action) is delayed sufficiently to permit thorough bathing of tissue cells. By delaying the hardening action of formaldehyde, uniform distribution of the coloring or staining agent is also possible. It can be said that these modifying agents also enhance the internal cosmetic effect.

Many years ago, the U.S. Hygienic Laboratories found that formaldehyde, when present in an acid solution or used at acid pH, tends to promote rapid bleaching of muscular tissue to an ashen gray. This observation suggested the use of alkaline materials in combination with formaldehyde for embalming formulations. Many alkalines, however, have a deteriorating effect on formaldehyde, especially over prolonged periods (longer than 2 weeks).

Citrates

Sodium citrate, a white, odorless, crystalline or granular material, is often used for its anticoagulant as well as its water conditioning properties in embalming fluid. This compound inactivates calcium in the blood as well as in the water supply. Without calcium, blood coagulation does not occur.

Oxalates

Another calcium precipitant, sodium oxalate, a white crystalline powder, is sometimes used, but not as extensively as the citrates.

Borates

Borates are the compounds most extensively found in embalming formulations. In addition to its function as a stabilizer of formaldehyde, sodium borate also serves to prevent or reduce coagulation. Sodium borate (borax, sodium tetraborate, or pyroborate) is a white crystalline powder that is readily soluble in a mixture of water and glycerine. Boric acid is a white powder that is often used in combination with borax.

Ethylenediaminetetraacetic Acid

The sodium salts of EDTA are very effective sequestering or chelating agents, which means that they very readily combine with calcium ions to prevent blood coagulation and also to remove hardness chemicals from the water supply. Generally, these materials are not found in arterial fluids. These agents are quite alkaline and are not compatible with the other ingredients in embalming fluids over a long shelf life. Such materials are used most advantageously as separate formulations; that is, in the form of supplemental or accessory chemicals that are added to the embalming solution at the time of use.

Other Materials

Among the other compounds often used as anticlotting materials are magnesium sulfate (Epsom salts), sodium chloride, sodium sulfate, and sodium phosphates. At one time or another these compounds have been recommended for use in capillary wash solutions, and some are still used in arterial fluid formulations. This class of chemicals also contains some of the materials employed in buffer systems to maintain a constant pH in a fluid formulation. These are used in combination with those mentioned earlier.

▶ SURFACTANTS (WETTING AGENTS)

Probably one of the greatest developments that has occurred in the chemistry and physics of embalming since the discovery of formaldehyde is the principle of removing body liquids by lowering their surface tension. It is necessary, before complete circulation may take place in the body, to remove the liquid that is held in the capillaries. Capillary attraction, or the force that attracts and holds liquid in the capillary tubes, is the result of surface tension. If the surface tension of the liquid in these tiny tubes is lowered, the liquid easily loosens and flows out.

Much has been said and written about the important role and use of surfactants (*surface-active agents, tension breakers, tension reducers*) in embalming formulations. Actually, there is no industry that has not investigated these compounds and found them adaptable for a variety of uses. The chemical structure of surfactants is rather complex: one part of the molecule has a strong attraction or affinity for water, whereas the other part of the molecule dislikes water. This latter part of the molecule has an affinity for nonaqueous liquids. Such a complicated molecular makeup functions to lower or reduce the surface tension of the solution to which the surfactant is added. In a water-and-oil mixture the surfactant destroys the surface tension of the components so that the oily mixture is more easily dispersible in water. Other materials are made "water soluble" in a similar manner.

It should also be called to mind that each cell in the soft tissues of the body is surrounded by a film of body liquid mostly water in composition. For easy, rapid penetration of the cell, this surface film must be dispersed. Such chemical substances, then, are used in embalming fluids for three reasons.

First, by lowering the surface tension of the preservative solution (the embalming solution), surfactants aid or cause the embalming solution to flow more readily and rapidly through the capillaries so that *all* of the millions of tissue cells are literally bathed by the embalming solution and, thus, thoroughly preserved. Naturally, the technique of injecting the solution and draining employed by the embalmer can assist or handicap the function of the surfactant. The process of moving the solution through the body being embalmed is a technique that should be planned and controlled by the embalmer to ensure that a sufficient amount of preservative chemicals is uniformly distributed throughout the body. It is also important that some of the normal moisture lost during embalming be replaced to safeguard against overdehydration.

Second, by reducing the capillary attraction (which is a phenomenon of surface tension) of blood and body liquids, surfactants cause the almost immediate clearing of blood from the capillaries. Surface tension is reduced, and the liquid more readily moves and flows out the capillary bed and through the venous drainage system. **Because two things cannot occupy the same space at the same time, the capillaries must be emptied of blood before injected solution can flow through them to reach the tissues of the body.** Only the solutions that pass by osmosis through the capillary walls into the intercellular spaces have any chance of being absorbed by the tissue cells. The embalmer must help the solution reach the tissues by employing the necessary physical manipulation such as massage and intermittent or restricted type of drainage.

Third, by increasing the ability of the solution to filter through the semipermeable capillary walls in a uniform manner, it is possible to incorporate coloring agents into the solution and obtain a normal appearance internally (Figure 6–2).

The preceding concepts have been incorporated into the manufacture of embalming fluids since the early 1930s. Industrial investigators have found that the uniform penetration of the tissues by the embalming solution is necessary to obtain positive, long-lasting preservation.

Surface Tension and Embalming Solutions

Solids, liquids, and gases are all made up of molecules arranged in characteristic patterns depending on the material being studied. These molecules have an affinity or attraction for one another. Again, depending on the materials under study, this degree of molecular attraction differs. For example, the attractive force is greater between water molecules than it is between alcohol molecules. At 20°C, the surface tension of water is 72.75

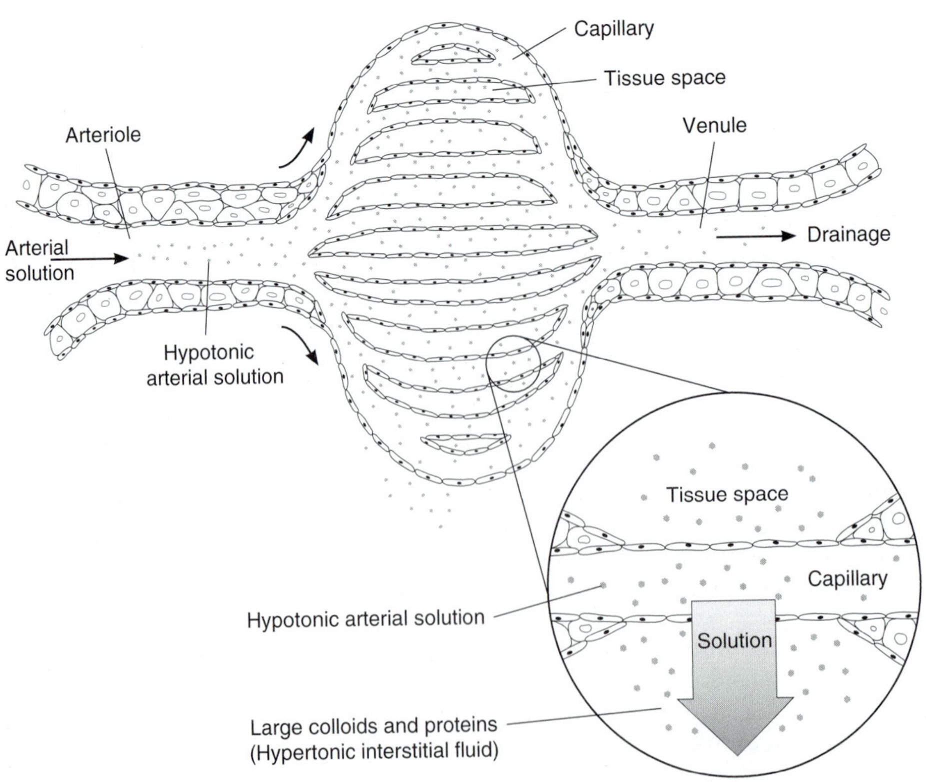

Figure 6–2. Movement of arterial solution from the capillaries into the tissue spaces.

dynes per centimeter, and for methyl alcohol it is 22.61 dynes per centimeter. (*Note: a dyne is the force required to accelerate a 1-gram mass 1 centimeter per second.*) Thus, water has a surface tension value more than three times that of methyl alcohol and penetrates much more slowly. In other words, **the lower the surface tension value, the faster the rate of penetration by the liquid substance.**

The surface tension of water is lowered by the addition of surfactants. Wetting or penetrating chemicals tend to destroy the bonds or attractive forces that normally exist between water molecules so that they seemingly break away from each other. The net effect of such physiochemical action is to cause liquids to diffuse and penetrate more readily through cellular tissue.

Surface tension is also defined as the contractive forces that causes liquids to assume the shape in which they have the least surface, that is, a sphere. Wetting agents reduce or destroy this contractive force so that the liquid film becomes "wetter."

In embalming solutions, the addition of surfactants in proper concentrations produces better penetration of the preservative chemicals in a more uniform manner. This enables the preservative solution to more readily displace the body fluids from all cellular tissue and replace them to achieve the embalming function. Also, coloring agents are uniformly distributed through the use of surfactants. The even diffusion of such agents throughout the soft tissues results in a more lifelike color and appearance.

Surface tension changes with variations in temperature. As the temperature rises, the surface tension value of a solution decreases. In embalming, this means that if warm water is used to prepare the solutions for injection, the resultant solution may be expected to penetrate more rapidly because of the lowered surface tension value. Also keep in mind that the chemical reaction between the preservative chemicals and the tissues will take place more rapidly as the result of using warm water. The fixative or firming action will also occur faster than usual.

Surfactants also increase the germicidal activity of chemical solutions. It is believed that this is due to an increased speed of penetration into the bacterial cells as a result of the lowering of the surface tension of the solution.

Surfactants and Surface Tension

From the preceding discussion it might appear that the embalmer could easily make his or her embalming technique more efficient by simply adding an extra surfactant to the embalming solution. This is not true. This class of chemical compounds is extremely temperamental and sensitive. Surfactants function best in very low concentrations and must be carefully selected by experienced chemists with respect to the other ingredients present in the formulation. It is necessary to determine compatibilities between all the components of an embalming fluid and the surfactant, and the amount of surfactant to use to produce a properly well-balanced chemical formula. Addition of extra surfactant to an embalming solution may result in excessive drainage as well as oversaturation of tissue.

The following considerations, which must be thoroughly explored by the chemist in evaluating specific applications for any given surfactant, serve to illustrate the complex nature of such chemicals. The discussion is by no means complete.

Surface-active agents are generally classified into three groups: anionic, cationic, and nonionic. In brief, **if the surfactant molecule tends to ionize, then it is either anionic or cationic. If it does not ionize in solution, it is nonionic.**

Surfactants such as soap, alkyl sulfonates, alkyl aryl sulfonates, salts of sulfated alcohols, and oils are *anionic.* These compounds are compatible with other anionic and nonionic agents. They are not normally compatible with and are frequently precipitated from solutions by cationic materials and by certain inorganic cations such as aluminum, calcium, and magnesium.

Nonionic surfactants do not ionize in solution, but owe their surface activity and water solubility or dispersibility to nonionized polar groups within the molecule, such as hydroxyl or ether linkages. Ethylene oxide condensation products with amides and fatty acids belong in this group (specific examples are the Atlas "Tweens" and "Spans").

In actual chemical formulating practice, the result to be achieved by the end product must be kept in mind in deciding the type of surfactant to employ. Most generally, a blend of such materials is incorporated into embalming fluids to achieve the results mentioned at the beginning of this discussion.

Preliminary selection of the proper surfactant or blend of surfactants is usually based on the following factors: specific application, pH of solution to which it is added (acid, alkaline, or neutral), physical form of surfactant (liquid, gel, flake, or powder), nature of other ingredients in the formulation, and concentration to use. The surfactant that works most satisfactorily in one brand of products may function poorly or not at all in another brand. As most of the water used in preparing embalming solutions tends to be "hard," it is customary among embalming fluid manufacturers to select surfactants that are not readily affected by "hardness" chemicals in the water.

▶ DYES (COLORING AGENTS)

The coloring materials used in modern embalming fluids generally are employed for the purpose of producing an internal cosmetic effect that closely simulates the natural coloring of tissues. Such materials have high staining qualities and as they diffuse to the superficial tissue areas from the circulatory system, they impart color to the tissue. Usually, a blend of coloring materials, ranging from straw or amber to brilliant red, is used. The type of dye used depends to great extent on the pH of the arterial fluid. Dyes that color tissues are called **active dyes**. Those that merely lend color to the fluid in the bottle are **inactive dyes**.

Types of Coloring Agents

Coloring materials may be placed into two classes.

Natural coloring agents are vegetable colors such as cudbear, carmine, and cochineal. **Cudbear** is a purplish-red powder prepared from lichens by maceration in dilute ammonia and caustic soda and fermentation. **Carmine** is an aluminum lake of the pigment from cochineal. **Cochineal** is a red-coloring matter consisting of the dried bodies of the female insects of *Coccus cacti*. The coloring principle is carminic acid, $C_{17}H_{18}O_{10}$. This class of dyes is not generally incorporated into modern solutions.

Synthetic coloring agents are the coloring materials used in modern fluids and are mainly coal-tar derivatives. They are economical to use and are the most permanent if they are chemically compatible with the other ingredients in the fluid. Many different types and shades are available under rather confusing diversified commercial names and chemical nomenclature. For better solubility, most of the coal-tar dyes are supplied in sodium or potassium salts of the synthetic coloring matter. These materials then may be said to be dyes of alkali metal salts that have been reacted with coal-tar compounds. Several dyes are available.

- Eosin: known as tetrabromofluorescein, $C_{20}H_8Br_4O_5$; red crystalline powder
- Erythrosine: brown powder that forms cherry red solutions in water; known chemically as the sodium salt of iodeosin, $C_{20}H_6I_4Na_2O_5$
- Ponceau: dark red powder that is soluble in water and acid solutions; forms a cherry red solution and is a naphthol disulfonate compound
- Amaranth: coal-tar azo dye that forms a dark red-brown color in water but is only slightly soluble in alcohol.

Other synthetic dyes include croceine scarlet, rhodamine, rose bengal, acid fuchsin, and toluidine red.

Coloring Materials in Embalming Fluids

Coloring materials in use today in embalming fluids belong to a group known as biological stains, as such materials are used in clinical laboratories to stain different types of tissue for study under the microscope. The coloring agents used in fluids must be stable in the presence of formaldehyde, must be water soluble, should impart a natural flesh color to the tissues, and should have high tinctorial or staining qualities so that small amounts can produce the desired color. This last requirement is important because arterial fluids are diluted before use.

The coal-tar dyes possess the requirements of a coloring agent for use in embalming fluids. Molecularly they are fine enough to diffuse evenly and uniformly through tissue cells. As soon as surfactants (wetting agents) began to be used in embalming solutions, it was found possible to add staining materials to the formulations because wetting agents diffused the dye very effectively. The specific material that is to be used in any given formulation must be carefully selected, as some dyes produce different coloring effects at different pH values and different extents of dilution.

Natural-color materials such as the vegetable dyes are considered too unstable for use in embalming fluids. Some have good color-fast features but do not diffuse evenly because of their large molecular structures.

The "older" embalming fluids contained coloring materials mainly for the purpose of identification. They did not produce staining effects as do those in use today. Such old fluids did contain salts known as nitrates, which caused a localized breakdown of red blood cells. As the contents of such cells spilled out, the hemoglobin, which is the coloring matter of blood, remained in the intracellular spaces and produced a color effect. One chemical theory states that the nitrate salts are converted to nitroso compounds which combine with a portion of the hemoglobin molecule, resulting in a permanent color.

Such salts are not generally used today because newer chemicals have replaced them and also because they required a slow type of action. The high-drainage-type chemical solutions in use now are made possible by replacing the older chemical compounds with modern ones that are faster acting and that produce even, uniform embalming results.

▶ PERFUMING MATERIALS (MASKING AGENTS, DEODORANTS)

Generally, reodorants or perfuming agents are selected not only for their power in covering harsh chemicals but also for the pleasant odor they impart to a solution. By blending special synthetic essential oils with the harsh preservative chemicals in a formulation, the harshness or "raw" odor of the solution is reduced and replaced to some extent by a more pleasing scent. No attempt is made, however, to mask completely the fumes of formaldehyde. Any attempt to mask formaldehyde generally results in neutralization or destruction of the active chemical.

Floral compounds such as wisteria, rose, and lilac types, along with nondescript essential oils and aromatic esters, are used quite extensively in embalming formulations because their "heavy" note. This property makes it possible to cover objectionable fumes during brief exposures. Such materials are made water soluble through the medium of nonionic-type surfactants.

If the formulation does not contain a high concentration of formaldehyde or other irritating chemicals, it is possible to use synthetic compounds that give off odors resembling spices (clove, cinnamon), fruit (strawberry, peach, etc.), mint (spearmint, peppermint, menthol), and many other "notes" designed by the essential oil chemist. Sassafras, oil of wintergreen (methyl salicylate), and benzaldehyde have been among some of the more commonly used materials for this purpose.

Occasionally, use is made of high concentrations of perfuming and masking agents in chemical solutions in an attempt to hide high concentrations of formaldehyde, especially in so-called fumeless fluids. Usually, the scent of the perfuming agent is immediately detected, while the presence of the formaldehyde remains in the background. The individual finally becomes aware of the formaldehyde as a result of a pinching sensation in the nose; the delayed awareness manifests in the form of an explosive effect with a resultant shortness of breath. The individual does not realize how much fumes are present until too late! Unfortunately, there are products still advertised as "fumeless" or "odorless" when, in reality, they are not. The true low-odor type of product is based on the use of "donor" compounds that release the aldehyde when contact is made with tissue so that a minimum amount of gas is released to bother the user.

The essential oils used in embalming fluids are selected on the basis of their stability in the presence of preservative chemicals and their ability to remain in solution when water is added. Some essential oils possess antiseptic properties but this usually is not why they are used in embalming formulations.

▶ VEHICLES (DILUENTS)

The active preservatives and other ingredients in the formulation must be dissolved in a common solvent. As water is an essential component of tissue, its use in embalming solutions facilitates the diffusion and penetration of the active preservative constituents of fluids. The vehicle (sometimes called "carrier") must be a solvent or mixture of solvents that keeps the active ingredients in a stable and uniform state during transport through the circulatory system to all parts of the body.

To maintain the proper density and osmotic activity, that is, the proper chemical and physical balance of the formula, the vehicle or diluent may include glycerine, sorbitol, glycols, or alcohols in addition to water. Quite often, a special solvent may be used as part of an innovation to dissolve or keep in solution any special "new" ingredient in the product.

▶ KEY TERMS AND CONCEPTS FOR DISCUSSION

1. Define the following terms:
   - Accessory chemical
   - Anticoagulant
   - Arterial fluid
   - Arterial solution
   - Buffer
   - Cavity fluid
   - Cosmetic fluid
   - Dye
   - Germicide
   - Humectant
   - Index
   - Noncosmetic fluid
   - Penetrating agent
   - Perfuming agent
   - Preservative
   - Primary dilution
   - Secondary dilution
   - Supplemental chemical
   - Surfactant
   - Vehicle
   - Water conditioner
2. List the uses for methanol in arterial fluids.
3. Describe embalming treatments using phenol.

▶ BIBLIOGRAPHY

Dorn JM, Hopkins BM. *Thanatochemistry, A Survey of General, Organic, and Biochemistry for Funeral Service Professionals.* Upper Saddle River, NJ: Prentice Hall; 1985.

Eckles College of Mortuary Science Inc. *Modern Mortuary Science.* 4th ed. Philadelphia: Westbrook; 1958:206.

Encyclopedia of Industrial Chemical Analysis. Vol. 12: *Embalming Chemicals.* New York: Wiley; 1971.

General chemical principles of embalming fluids. In: *Expanding Encyclopedia of Mortuary Practice,* Nos. 365–371. Springfield, OH: Champion Co.; 1966.

Walker J. *Formaldehyde,* 3rd ed. ACS Monograph No. 159. New York: Reinhold; 1964.

Hazardous Chemicals

The following three examples represent chemicals commonly used in the preparation room. Synonyms, dilution limits, and health effects come from a material safety data sheet (MSDS) directory available to the public on the Internet at the University of California, one of many sites that offer MSDSs. The term "MSDS" or the specific chemical name should be used when doing a search. A complete list of hazardous chemicals may be obtained by contacting the National Funeral Directors Association, 13625 Bishop's Drive, Brookfield, WI, 53005 for its publication, *Hazard Communication Program.* It is important to understand that the severity of the health effects listed for the chemicals will depend on the amount of material in the product, the frequency and duration of your exposure, and your individual susceptibility. Some states with their own OSHA programs have replaced the Federal Hazard Communication Rule with an Employee Right-to-Know Rule. For example, the State of Minnesota recognizes 1025 hazardous chemicals and provides a list of these chemicals in its Employee Right-to-Know Rule.

▶ EXAMPLES OF HAZARDOUS CHEMICALS

FORMALDEHYDE (formic aldehyde; paraform; formol; formalin (methanol-free); fyde; formalith; methanal; methyl aldehyde; methylene glycol; methylene oxide; tetraoxymethalene; oxomethane; oxymethylene; when in aqueous solution, the term formalin is often used.)

OSHA Action Level: 0.5 ppm	OSHA TWA (PEL): 0.75 ppm	OSHA STEL: 2 ppm

Health Effects: Ingestion. Acute Exposure—Liquids containing 10 to 40 percent formaldehyde cause severe irritation and inflammation of the mouth, throat, and stomach. Severe stomach pains will follow ingestion with possible loss of consciousness and death. Ingestion of dilute formaldehyde solutions (0.03–0.04 percent) may cause discomfort in the stomach and pharynx.

Health Effects: Eye Contact. Acute Exposure—Formaldehyde solutions splashed in the eye can cause injuries ranging from transient discomfort to severe, permanent corneal clouding and loss of vision. The severity of the effect depends on the concentration of formaldehyde in the solution and whether or not the eyes are flushed with water immediately after exposure.

Note: The perception of formaldehyde by odor and eye irritation becomes less sensitive with time as one adapts its use. This can lead to overexposure if a worker is relying on formaldehyde's warning properties to alert him or her to potential overexposure.
Chronic Exposure—Permanent corneal clouding and loss of vision.

Health Effects: Skin Contact. Acute Exposure—Formalin is a severe skin irritant and a sensitizer. Contact with formalin causes white discoloration, smarting, drying, cracking, and scaling. Prolonged and repeated contact can cause numbness and a hardening or tanning of the skin. Previously exposed persons may react to future exposure with an allergic eczematous dermatitis or hives.
Chronic Exposure—A hardening and tanning of the skin. Sensitive persons can develop an allergic eczematous dermatitis and hives.

Health Effects: Inhalation. Acute Exposure—Formaldehyde is highly irritating to the upper respiratory tract and eyes. Concentrations of 0.5 to 2.0 ppm may irritate the eyes, nose, and throat of some individuals. Concentrations of 3 to 5 ppm also cause tearing of the eyes and are intolerable to some persons. Concentrations of 10 to 20 ppm cause difficulty in breathing, burning of the nose and throat, cough, and heavy tearing of the eyes, and 25 to 30 ppm causes severe respiratory tract injury leading to pulmonary edema and pneumonitis. A concentration of 100 ppm is immediately dangerous to life and health. Deaths from accidental exposure to high concentrations of formaldehyde have been reported.
Chronic Exposure—Formaldehyde exposure has been associated with cancers of the lung, nasopharynx and oropharynx, and nasal passages. Prolonged or repeated exposure to formaldehyde may result in respiratory impairment. Rats exposed to formaldehyde at 2 ppm developed benign nasal tumors and changes of the cell structure in the nose as well as inflamed mucous membranes of the nose. Structural changes in the epithelial cells in the human nose have also been observed. Some persons have developed asthma or bronchitis following exposure to formaldehyde, most often as the result of an accidental spill involving a single exposure to a high concentration of formaldehyde.
Incompatibilities: Strong oxidizing agents, caustics, strong alkalies, isocyanates, anhydrides, oxides, and in-

organic acids. Formaldehyde reacts with hydrochloric acid to form the potent carcinogen, bis-chloromethyl ether. Formaldehyde reacts with nitrogen dioxide, nitromethane, perchloric acid and aniline, or peroxyformic acid to yield explosive compounds. A violent reaction occurs when formaldehyde is mixed with strong oxidizers. Oxygen from the air can oxidize formaldehyde to formic acid, especially when heated. Formic acid is corrosive.

Found in: Embalming adhesive gel, feature builder, embalming spray, sanitizing embalming spray, preservative cream, arterial embalming chemicals, preservative/disinfectant gel, supplemental embalming gel, accessory embalming chemical, incision sealer, pre-injection chemicals, bleaching agents, cavity embalming fluid/gel.

PHENOL (benzenol; carbolic acid; hydroxybenzene; monohydroxybenzene; monophenol; oxybenzene; phenic acid; phenyl alcohol; phenyl hydrate; phenyl hydroxide; phenylic acid; phenylic alcohol)

OSHA TWA (PEL) for skin: 5 ppm
ACGIH TWA (PEL) for skin: 5 ppm
NIOSH recommended TWA (PEL): 5 ppm
NIOSH recommended ceiling: 15.6 ppm

Health Effects: Ingestion. Acute Exposure—Inhalation may cause severe irritation of the mucous membranes, profuse sweating, headache, intense thirst, nausea and vomiting, abdominal pain, diarrhea, salivation, cyanosis, tinnitus, twitching, tremors, and convulsions. The central nervous system may initially be stimulated followed by severe, profound depression progressing to coma. The heart rate may increase then become slow and irregular. The blood pressure may increase slightly and then fall markedly with dyspnea and fall in body temperature. Stertorous breathing, mucous rales, and frothing at the mouth and nose may indicate the presence of pulmonary edema, which may be followed by pneumonia. Methemoglobinemia and hemolysis have been reported occasionally. Death may occur from respiratory, circulatory, or cardiac failure. If death is not immediate, jaundice and oliguria or anuria may occur. Ingestion of 250 ppm is immediately dangerous to life or health.

Chronic Exposure—Symptoms of chronic phenol poisoning may include vomiting, difficulty swallowing, ptyalism, diarrhea, anorexia, headache, vertigo, muscle weakness and pain, mental disturbances, dark or smoky urine, and possibly skin eruptions. Extensive damage to the liver and kidneys may be fatal. Hind limb paralysis has been reported in animals. Pathologic findings in animals repeatedly exposed to phenol vapors include extensive necrosis of the myocardium, acute lobular pneumonia, vascular damage, and liver and kidney damage.

Health Effects: Skin Contact. Acute Exposure—Contact with 0.5% solutions may cause local anesthesia, 1% solutions sometimes cause skin necrosis, and 10% solutions may cause burns. Phenol burns may be severe, but painless due to damage to nerve endings. The skin may turn white, and later yellowish-brown and may be deeply eroded and scarred. Gangrene may occur at the site of contact. Vapors and liquid may be readily absorbed through the skin to cause systemic effects as detailed in acute inhalation exposure. There have been several reports of cardiac arrhythmias associated with application of solutions of phenol, hexachlorophene, and croton oil to the skin. Profound coma and death have been reported to occur within 10 minutes following skin contact. Pathologic findings included congestion of the lungs, liver, spleen, and kidneys.

Chronic Exposure—Prolonged exposure may cause a blue or brownish discoloration of the tendons over the knuckles of the hands, dermatitis, vitiligo, and rarely, skin sensitization. Symptoms of chronic phenol poisoning may occur as detailed as under chronic inhalation exposure. Evaluated by RTECS as producing carcinogenic and neoplastic tumors in mice.

Health Effects: Eye Contact. Acute Exposure—Vapors have caused marked irritation from brief, intermittent industrial exposure to 48 ppm. Concentrated liquid or solid may cause severe irritation with redness, pain, and blurred vision. Concentrated phenol in human eyes has caused chemotic conjunctiva, hypesthetic, white cornea, edematous eyelids, and severe iritis. In some cases, the eyelids have been so severely damaged that they required plastic surgery. The final visual results have varied from complete recovery, to partial recovery, to blindness and loss of the eye. Crystalline or concentrated aqueous phenol on rabbit eyes causes almost instantaneous white opacification of the corneal epithelium. Eight hours later, the cornea was anesthetic, the surface ulcerated, and the stroma opaque. Five weeks later, entropion, scarring of the conjunctiva and opacity of the cornea occurred.

Chronic Exposure—Repeated or prolonged exposure to phenol vapors may cause conjunctivitis and has caused gray discoloration of the sclera with brown spots near the insertion of the rectus muscle tendon.

Health Effects: Ingestion. Acute Exposure—Ingestion may cause immediate intense burning of the mouth and throat, white or brownish stains and areas of necrosis on the lips and in the mouth and esophagus, marked abdominal pain, pale face, and contracted or dilated pupils. Systemic effects may occur as detailed under acute inhalation exposure. The approximate lethal dose in humans is 140 mg/kg.

Chronic Exposure—Persons ingesting phenol-contaminated well water experienced diarrhea, dark urine, and sores and burning in the mouth. Other symptoms of chronic phenol poisoning may occur as detailed under chronic inhalation exposure. Administration of phenol in drinking water to rats for three generations produced stunted growth at 7000 ppm over 2 generations; offspring of rats given 10,000 ppm died; at 12,000 ppm animals did not reproduce. Other reproductive effects have also been reported in animals.
Incompatibilities: Alkalies; acetaldehyde; aluminum and alloys; aluminum chloride plus nitrobenzene; 1,3-butadiene; boron trifluoride; diethyletherate; calcium hypochlorite; formaldehyde; lead and alloys; magnesium and alloys; metals and alloys; oxidizers (strong); peroxodisulfuric acid; peroxomonosulfuric acid; plastics; rubber; sodium nitrate; trifluoroacetic acid; sodium nitrite; zinc and alloys.
Found in: Embalming cauterant; embalming chemical disinfectant; cavity embalming fluid/gel, preservative/disinfectant gel; accessory embalming chemical.

GLUTARALDEHYDE (1,5-pentanedial)

OSHA PEL: 0.2 PPM ACGIH TLV: 0.2 PPM

Health Effects: Inhalation. Acute Exposure—Irritation, headaches, may cause nose and throat irritation and burning, difficulty in breathing.
Chronic Exposure—None known.

Health Effects: Ingestion. Acute Exposure—May cause nausea, vomiting and systemic illness.
Chronic Exposure—None Known.

Health Effects: Skin Contact. Acute Exposure—Sensitization dematitis.
Chronic Exposure—None known.

Health Effects: Eye Contact. Acute Exposure—Loss of vision.
Chronic Exposure—None known.
Incompatibilities: Strong oxidizing agent.
Found In: Arterial, cavity, and accessory embalming fluids; humectant; tissue filler; disinfectant and preservative gels.

▶ OTHER DANGEROUS CHEMICALS USED IN THE FUNERAL PROFESSION

The following is a sample listing of commonly used chemicals found in the compounding of products used in the preparation room. Each of these toxic chemicals is explained in more detail on the MSDS that accompanies the product.

Acetone (2-propanone; dimethylformaldehyde; dimethyl ketone; beta-ketopropane; methyl ketone; propanone; pyroacetic ether)—A narcotic in high concentrations which can cause skin irritation. Prolonged inhalation can cause headache, dryness, and throat irritation. A dangerous fire risk when exposed to heat, flame, or oxidizers. Found in: accessory embalming chemicals, external sealing composition, lip tint, solvents, sealants.

Alkyl dimethylbenzyl ammonium chloride—This material belongs to the chemical family quaternary ammonium compounds. It is a skin and eye irritant, has moderate to high oral toxicity, and is moderately toxic via skin absorption. Found in: cold disinfectant, embalming spray, and embalming cauterants.

Amaranth (trisodium salt of 1-[4-sulfo-1-naphthylazo]-2-naphthol-3,6-disulfonic acid)—Formerly known as red dye #2, this member of the azo dye family is a suspected human carcinogen. It is no longer acceptable in food, drugs, or cosmetics. Found in: coloring powder for arterial fluids.

Amitrole (2-amino-1,2,4-triazole)—Moderate to low oral toxicity. Listed by IARC and NTP as a possible carcinogen. Found in: cavity fluid.

Ammonia—Causes nose and throat irritation; may cause bronchial spasm, chest pain, pulmonary edema, and skin burns. Incompatible with hypochlorite (household bleach) which is often used to disinfect the preparation area after embalming. Found in: cleaning agents used to neutralize formaldehyde.

2-Butoxyethanol (butyl cellosolve, ethylene glycol monobutyl ether)—Mildly irritating to skin, and can be absorbed through contact. It is a strong respiratory and eye irritant, and exposure may result in transient corneal clouding; repeated overexposure can cause fatigue, headache, nausea, and tremors. It is a moderate fire risk which will react with oxidizers. Found in: arterial embalming chemicals.

Camphor—High to moderate ingestion hazard. Local exposure may cause irritation. Found in: embalming fluid.

Carbon tetrachloride (tetrachloromethane)—Can cause depression, nausea, vomiting, and local skin irritation; prolonged exposure and absorption through the skin could produce liver and kidney failure. Found in: organic solvents.

Chlorine Salts (hypochlorites)—Chlorine salts produce chlorinated vapor causing moderate to severe skin and eye irritations, tissue damage, and moderate to severe respiratory irritation. They are strong oxidizers and are highly reactive, and can be a serious fire risk when exposed to reducing agents (acids) or petroleum derivatives. Found in: embalming deodorant, bleach, and disinfectants.

Chloroform (trichloromethane)—Formerly used as an anesthetic, chloroform causes depression and skin and eye irritation; prolonged exposure can lead to cardiac and respiratory arrest or paralysis; chronic exposure may cause liver damage. Listed in IARC and NTP as a possible carcinogen. Found in: accessory embalming chemical sealant.

Cresol (2-hydroxy-4-methylphenol)—The health effects are similar to those of phenol, but not as severe. It is corrosive to skin, eyes, and mucous membranes; capable of causing burns at point of contact; and can be absorbed through the skin. Chronic low level exposure can cause skin rash and discoloration, gastrointestinal disturbances, nervous system disturbances, and kidney and liver damage. It is a moderate fire hazard that can react vigorously with oxidizing materials. Found in: disinfectant and accessory embalming chemicals.

Diethanolamine—A severe eye irritant and mild skin irritant which is moderately toxic through ingestion. It can react with oxidizers. Found in: humectant and arterial embalming fluid.

Diethylene glycol—A skin and eye irritant which is highly toxic through inhalation. It can react with oxidizers. Found in: arterial and cavity embalming fluids.

Dimethylformamide—A strong irritant to skin and other tissues, it is readily absorbed through the skin. Inhalation or skin contact can cause gastrointestinal disturbances, facial flushing, elevated blood pressure, CNS disorders, and liver and kidney damage. It is a moderate fire risk which can be an explosion hazard when exposed to flame. Dimethylformamide is reactive with a variety of halogenated materials and organics. Found in: solvents.

Ethyl acetate—Irritates the eyes, gums, skin, and respiratory tract. Repeated overexposure can cause conjunctivitis and corneal clouding; high concentrations can result in congestion of the liver and kidneys. Ethyl acetate is a dangerous fire risk. Found in: embalming cosmetic spray, cavity fluid, sanitizing spray, and sealing lacquer.

Ethyl alcohol (denatured ethanol, SD alcohol)—Ethyl alcohol is generally not considered an occupational health hazard, but its flammability makes it a safety hazard. The terms "SDA," or "SD alcohol," mean "specially denatured alcohol." SDA is ethyl alcohol to which another substance, such as tert-butyl alcohol, has been added to make it unfit for human consumption. Found in: cavity fluid, cosmetics.

EDTA (ethylenediaminetetraacetic acid)—EDTA is found in a variety of products as either tetrasodium or disodium salt. Both react chemically to bind calcium, which inhibits the blood clotting mechanism. EDTA is a skin irritant, causing dryness and cracking. Found in: arterial fluids, preinjection fluids, co-injection fluids, cavity fluids.

Ethylene dichloride (1,2-dichloroethene or 1,1-dichloroethene)—A strong irritant to skin and eyes which is toxic via inhalation and skin absorption. Ethylene dichloride is listed in IARC as a possible carcinogen. It is a dangerous fire risk. Found in: embalming fluid, cavity fluid.

Ethylene glycol (1,2-ethanediol)—Moderately irritating to skin, eyes, and mucous membranes; very toxic through inhalation, producing depression and damage to blood-forming organs. Ethylene glycol does not readily vaporize at room temperature, and inhalation would be likely only by heating or mechanical action (aerosolization). Ingestion can lead to respiratory, renal, and cardiac failure. Brain damage may also result. Chronic exposure can cause anorexia, decreased urinary output, and involuntary rapid eye movement. Ethylene glycol is combustible and can react violently with certain acids and oxidizers. Found in: arterial and cavity embalming chemicals, external embalming seal, tissue surface embalming seal, anticoagulant/clot remover, and water correctives.

Ethylene glycol-monomethyl ether (methyl cellosolve)—Moderately toxic via inhalation, ingestion, and skin absorption. May cause conjunctivitis, transient corneal clouding, and upper respiratory tract irritation. Found in: cosmetics.

Formic acid (methanoic acid)—Corrosive to skin, eyes, and mucous membranes. Formic acid has a moderate to high oral toxicity, and can be absorbed through the skin. It is a moderate fire risk. Found in: supplemental embalming chemicals and bleaching agents.

Hexylene glycol (2,4-hexanediol)—An eye, skin, and mucous membrane irritant which is moderately toxic through inhalation and ingestion. Large oral doses can have a narcotic effect. A low fire risk, hexylene glycol can react with oxidizers. Found in: arterial embalming fluid.

Isobutane (2-methylpropane)—While otherwise practically non-toxic, the inhalation of isobutane can cause suffocation. A dangerous fire risk when exposed to heat, flame, or oxidizers. Found in: aerosol propellants, cosmetics, insecticides, and deodorants.

Isopropyl alcohol (2-propanol)—An eye, nose, and throat irritant producing, in high concentration: mild narcotic effects, corneal burn, and eye damage. Drying to the skin; isopropyl alcohol is moderately toxic via ingestion. Ingestion or inhalation of heavy vapor concentrations can cause flushing and CNS depression. As little as 100 ml can be fatal if ingested. It is a dangerous fire risk and moderate explosion risk when exposed to heat, flame, or oxidizers. Found in: cavity and accessory embalming fluids, feature builder, cosmetics, color concentrate, fungal inhibitors, preinjection chemicals, liquid embalming cosmetics and sprays, tissue filler, supplemental embalming gels, aerosol deodorant, sealing lacquers, and solvent thinners.

Methyl alcohol (wood alcohol, methanol)—A skin, eye, and respiratory tract irritant which is moderately toxic via inhalation, and moderately to highly toxic through ingestion. The main target is the CNS, but it also affects the eyes, optic nerve, and possibly the retina. Overexposure can cause depression, sight impairment, weakness, and gastrointestinal disturbances. Severe overexposure can result in cardiac depression. Because methyl alcohol is metabolized slowly, sufficient daily intake can lead to cumulative exposure symptoms. Methyl alcohol is a dangerous fire and explosion risk when exposed to heat, flame, and oxidizers. Found in: arterial, cavity, and accessory embalming fluids and gels; cleaning and disinfecting fluids, gels, and solvents; tissue fillers; embalming cauterants; bleaching agents; cosmetics; and color concentrates.

Methyl ethyl ketone (2-butanone)—Repeated exposure can cause skin irritation and inflammation; vapors can produce eye, nose, and throat irritation. Methyl ethyl ketone is highly volatile and a narcotic by inhalation, affecting both the CNS and peripheral nerves. Methyl ethyl ketone can react violently with aldehydes and acids. It is a dangerous fire risk and moderate explosion risk when exposed to heat, spark, or flame. Found in: embalming cosmetic spray, sealing lacquer, thinners.

Methylene chloride (dichloromethane)—High oral toxicity, very dangerous to the eyes, causing corrosion of eye tissue. Because it vaporizes readily, inhalation is an important hazard, resulting in CNS depression, headache, dizziness, nausea, vomiting, and a feeling of intoxication. The material can also irritate the respiratory tract, cause liver damage, and exacerbate coronary artery disease. Chronic exposure can cause skin, CNS, and liver damage. The material is a suspected human carcinogen. The body metabolizes methylene chloride into carbon monoxide, lowering the blood's ability to carry oxygen. The problem is intensified for smokers and those with anemia or related conditions. Found in: external embalming sealants, aerosol insecticides and deodorizers, cosmetic sprays, and solvents.

Mineral spirits (naphtha, hexane and heptane distillates)—Moderately toxic via ingestion and moderately irritating to skin, eyes, and mucous membranes, the mist is highly irritating to the respiratory tract. Symptoms of overexposure often resemble drunkenness. Chronic overexposure can lead to photosensitivity, headache, nausea, dizziness, indigestion, and lack of appetite. Mineral spirits are incompatible with strong oxidizers and are a highly dangerous fire risk when exposed to heat, flame, or spark. Found in: liquid embalming cosmetics and sprays, and organic solvents.

Molding plaster (calcium sulfate, gypsum, plaster of Paris)—Generally considered a nuisance dust, although prolonged or repeated exposures can induce lung disease. Found in: cavity desiccant and embalming powders.

Nitrocellulose—A dangerous fire and explosion hazard when in dry form. Less flammable when wet. Found in: feature builder and sealing lacquer.

Orthodichlorobenzene (1,2-dichlorobenzene)—Moderately toxic via inhalation and ingestion; irritating to skin, eyes, and upper respiratory tract. Acute exposure can induce narcotic symptoms. Repeated or prolonged skin contact with liquid can cause burns. Chronic exposure may cause lung, liver, and kidney damage. It is a moderate fire risk when exposed to heat or flame and can react violently with oxidizing materials. Found in: cavity and supplemental embalming chemicals and gels, and bleaching agents.

Oxalic acid (ethanedioic acid)—Highly irritating and caustic to skin. Damage is characterized by cracks, fissures, slow healing ulcerations, blue skin, and yellowish, brittle nails. Highly irritating to tissues via ingestion. Can cause corrosion of mucous membranes, severe gastrointestinal disturbances, and acute poisoning. The major effects of inhalation of dusts and mists are corrosion and ulceration of the nose and throat, severe eye irritation, nosebleed, headache, and nervousness. Chronic exposure can cause upper respiratory and gastrointestinal disturbances, urinary disorders, gradual weight loss, and nervous system disturbances. Found in: embalming adhesive gels.

Paradichlorobenzene (1,4-dichlorobenzene)—Moderately toxic via inhalation; symptoms include irritation of skin, eyes, and upper respiratory tract. Prolonged or chronic skin exposure can cause burns. In liquid form, it can be absorbed through the skin. Chronic exposure can cause liver, kidney, and lung damage. It is a moderate fire risk, and incompatible with oxidizers. Found in: deodorizing powders.

Paraformaldehyde—Can produce formaldehyde when heated. Paraformaldehyde has moderate oral toxicity and low dermal toxicity. It is a moderate fire risk and can react with oxidizers. Found in: embalming/deodorizing powders, sealing powders, cavity desiccants, and hardening compounds.

Paratertiary Pentyl Phenol (p-tert-amyl phenol)—A skin and eye irritant, it is moderately toxic through skin contact and ingestion, and is slightly flammable. Found in: cavity embalming solutions, disinfectant sprays, antiseptic soaps, and bleaching agents.

Propane—Propane can cause suffocation and at very high concentrations can cause CNS depression. It is a dangerous fire and explosion risk when exposed to heat, flame, or oxidizers. Found in: propellants, aerosol embalming sealants, cosmetic sprays, and insecticide/miticide sprays.

Propylene Glycol (1,2-propanetriol, 1,3-propanetriol)—A skin and eye irritant. Found in: cavity embalming fluid.

Quartz (crystalline silicon dioxide)—Prolonged, repeated exposure to quartz can lead to lung disease characterized by shortness of breath and a troublesome, unproductive cough. Quartz can react violently with certain fluorine-containing compounds. Found in: finishing powder.

Quaternary ammonium compounds—Skin and eye irritants, a common cause of skin inflammation. Highly toxic via ingestion; symptoms include nausea, vomiting, possible convulsions, and collapse. Found in: disinfectants, cavity and accessory embalming fluids.

Sodium hypochlorite—Strongly irritating and corrosive to tissues. A strong oxidizing agent that will react violently with organic acids and formaldehyde. It is moderately toxic via inhalation and ingestion. Found in: household bleach and other bleaching agents.

Sodium pentachlorophenate—Widely used as a fungicide and disinfectant, the material has high toxicity via inhalation and ingestion and is highly irritating to the skin. Found in: arterial embalming chemicals.

Talc—Mainly regarded as a nuisance dust, prolonged or repeated exposure may lead to lung disease although the mechanism of inducement is unclear. Found in: drying powder.

Toluene (1,2-dimethylbenzene)—Skin, eye, and respiratory tract irritant. Prolonged or repeated contact can cause drying of skin. Overexposure can produce narcotic effects, depression, headache, dizziness, nausea, fatigue, lack of coordination, and a burning sensation of the skin. Acute poisoning, however, is rare. It is a dangerous fire risk when exposed to heat, spark, or flame. Found in: external embalming sealers, lip cosmetics and cosmetic sprays, sealing lacquer, solvents, and thinners.

Trichloroethane (1,1,2-trichloroethane)—A moderate skin and eye irritant causing inflammation and producing CNS depression, dizziness, drowsiness, incoordination, and psychological disturbances. Trichloroethane can also cause gastrointestinal disturbances and irregular heartbeat. High doses can have a narcotic effect and cause heart failure. Found in: cleaning solvents, sanitizing embalming sprays, aerosol lanolin skin creams, and cosmetics.

Trichloroethylene—A strong eye and skin irritant which can be absorbed through contact. Overexposure can cause CNS depression, headache, dizziness, tremors, nausea, vomiting, fatigue, and irregular heartbeat. Symptoms may resemble those of alcohol intoxication. Addiction and weakness in the extremities have been reported. Chronic exposure can damage the liver and other organs. Found in: cleaning solvents.

▶ MATERIAL SAFETY DATA SHEET TERMINOLOGY

Action level—That level at which certain actions must occur. In the formaldehyde standard, the level at which periodic monitoring for formaldehyde becomes necessary and at which medical surveillance becomes necessary.

Acute effect—Adverse effect on a human or animal which has severe symptoms developing rapidly and coming quickly to a crisis. Also see "chronic effect."

ACGIH—American Conference of Governmental Industrial Hygienists is an organization of professional personnel in governmental agencies or educational institutions who are employed in occupational safety and health programs.

Chronic effect—An adverse effect on a human or animal body, with symptoms which develop slowly over a long period of time or which recur frequently. Also see "acute effect."

Hazardous chemical—Any chemical whose presence or use is a physical hazard or a health hazard.

HCS—Hazard Communication Standard is an OSHA regulation issued under 29 CFR Part 1910.1200.

Health hazard—A chemical for which there is significant evidence, based on at least one study conducted in accordance with established scientific principles, that acute or chronic health effects may occur in exposed employees. The term "health hazard" includes chemicals which are carcinogens, slightly or highly toxic agents, reproductive toxins, irritants, corrosives, sensitizers, hepatotoxins, nephrotoxins, neurotoxins, agents which act on the hematopoietic system, and agents which damage the lungs, skin, eyes, or mucous membranes.

MSDS (Material Safety Data Sheet)—Any data sheet which contains information required under many state regulations and Federal Regulations, Title 29, Part 1910.1200 (g), regarding the physical, chemical, and hazardous properties of a substance or mixture.

NIOSH—National Institute for Occupational Safety and Health, U.S. Public Health Service, U.S. Department of Health and Human Services (DHHS). Among other activities, NIOSH tests and certifies respiratory protective devices and air sampling detector tubes, recommends occupational exposure limits for various substances, and assists OSHA and MSHA in occupational safety and health investigations and research.

PEL—Permissible Exposure Limit is an exposure limit established by OSHA's regulatory authority. It may be a time weighted average (TWA) limit or a maximum concentration exposure limit.

STEL—Short Term Exposure Limit (ACGIH terminology).

TWA—Time Weighted Average exposure is the airborne concentration of a material to which a person is exposed, averaged over the total exposure time, generally the total workday (8 to 12 hours).

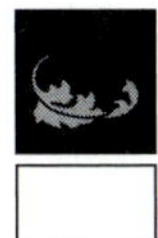

CHAPTER 7
USE OF EMBALMING CHEMICALS

The preceding chapter looked at the ingredients that constitute embalming fluids. This chapter examines the use of the various embalming fluids, including arterial fluids, coinjection fluids, preinjection (primary injection) fluids, water-corrective fluids, dyes, humectants, cavity fluids, autopsy gels, and cautery chemicals. The various factors that must be considered in selection and preparation of an arterial fluid are discussed. It is shown that many types of these fluids are available. *The embalmer selects the various chemicals he or she wishes to employ in the preparation room.*

Almost every funeral home will purchase at least one preservative arterial fluid and one type of cavity fluid. From that starting point, many types of fluids can be added to the shelf. There are a variety of arterial and coinjection fluids. **It is possible to embalm a body using preservative arterial fluid for injection and a cavity fluid for treatment of the cavities. All other fluids, such as preinjection and coinjection fluids, humectants, water conditioners, and fluid dyes, can be used to complement and enhance the embalming operation**. The selection and use of these chemicals become the personal preference of the embalmer.

In addition to a basic preservative arterial fluid, many embalmers prefer to keep on hand some of the special-purpose arterial fluids. Many funeral homes purchase a high-index arterial fluid for use when there has been a delay between death and preparation or when pathologic conditions make firming of the body difficult. In addition, many funeral homes like to have available a jaundice fluid for preparation of those bodies exhibiting this discoloration.

▶ DILUTIONS

The success of an embalming process relies to a great extent on the embalmer's ability to identify the problems and complications that are presented by the body. Because embalming problems present themselves in multiple combinations and variations, it is very difficult to make specific recommendations that have universal application. For that reason, it is essential that an embalmer possess the ability to analyze the complications and problems that exist, make judgements about what chemicals can be used to deal with the situation, and then properly apply the chemical or chemicals. The application of the chemicals will be influenced by: (1) the results the embalmer hopes to produce (e.g., tissue firmness, bleaching, etc.), (2) variations that exist among the chemical manufacturers' product lines, and (3) how the available chemicals react with the tissues. From this point of view, it is more accurate to say that embalming is more about critical thinking and problem solving than following "recipes."

▶ WORK PRACTICE CONTROLS IN THE USE OF CHEMICALS

The embalmer handles a variety of chemicals, disinfectants, and sanitizing agents during preparation of the body and the terminal disinfection after embalming. Care should be taken in the handling of all these chemicals, even such seemingly harmless products as talcum and drying powder used in cosmetic treatment of the body. Some general guidelines that apply to the handling of embalming chemicals include the following.

1. *Wear gloves when working with embalming chemicals.* Some individuals can develop a sensitivity to the chemical agents in embalming fluids. These sensitivities can cause skin irritations and eruptions similar to allergic reactions. Formaldehyde has a tendency to dry the hands of the embalmer. This drying (after several days) can lead to cracking of the skin. Broken skin is an avenue for the entrance of pathogenic microbial agents. Formaldehyde is also an irritant to the skin and, if concentrated enough such as in cavity fluids, can cause an inflammation of the skin.
2. *If chemicals are splashed or spilled onto the skin, flush the areas with cold running water.*

3. *Wear eye protection when handling embalming chemicals.* Eyeglasses, a face shield, or some type of protective eye covering should be used at all times. Formaldehyde, if splashed into the eye, is a severe irritant. Flush immediately with cool running water. An embalmer working with a chemical containing phenol (carbolic acid) or with concentrated phenol should be certain that his or her eyes and skin are protected. Phenol can cause severe burns. Whenever this chemical is accidentally splashed into the open eye, seek medical help immediately.
4. *Wear protective clothing during embalming.* Many embalming fluids contain dyes that leave permanent stains on clothing.
5. *When using chemicals, be certain that ventilation systems are in operation and, if necessary, wear a mask.* Formaldehyde fumes can be quite irritating and exposure to these fumes should be kept to a minimum. Care should also be taken in the handling of solvents used in mortuary cosmetology. Whenever embalming powders or cosmetic powders are in use, be certain rooms are well ventilated. Particulate matter from these powders is respirable and many of the small particulates in these powders are not exhaled, but retained in the lungs.
6. *Dilute any spillage immediately with cool water and clean.* Formaldehyde can be neutralized by applying a small amount of household ammonia to the spill. Any sponges or rags used in cleaning these spills should be flushed with cold water. If necessary, leave the room until the fumes decrease to a level at which working in the room to clean up the spill can be tolerated.
7. *Do NOT use formaldehyde-based chemicals as an antiseptic.* These chemicals are *not* for use on living tissue.
8. *Keep chemical material safety data sheets (MSDS) available as well as chemical manufacturers' first-aid information.*
9. *Be certain bottles that are destroyed have first been flushed out with water.*
10. *Keep machine tanks and fluid bottles covered and capped at all times to help reduce fumes.*
11. *Be certain formaldehyde is removed as much as possible before working with disinfectants such as sodium hypochlorite (laundry bleach).* Combination of formaldehyde with these chemicals create gases that have proven to be dangerous.
12. *Pour fluid into a filled tank rather than filling after fluid is in the tank (Figure 7–1).*

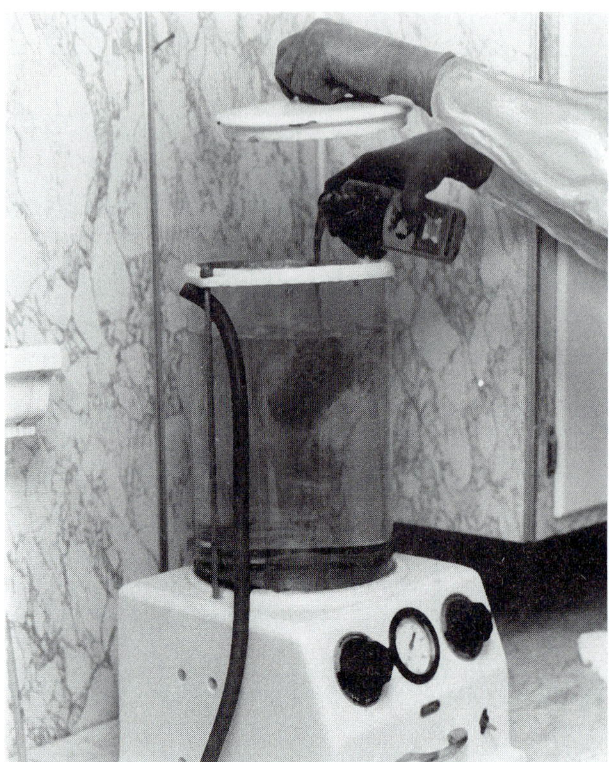

Figure 7–1. Pouring the arterial fluid into the machine tank after it has been filled with water reduces formaldehyde exposure. Keep the machines covered by using the lid.

▶ PRESERVATIVE VASCULAR FLUIDS

Preservative vascular fluid is the concentrated embalming fluid that contains the eight groups of chemicals: preservatives, germicides, anticoagulants, vehicles, surfactants, dyes, perfuming agents, and modifying agents. The vehicle water is used to dilute these fluids. It is added by the embalmer to create the embalming solution. In addition, supplemental fluids may be added to boost one or more of the chemicals.

1. Index
   A. *Strong:* those fluids with a formaldehyde index in the range 28 to 36.
   B. *Medium:* those fluids with a formaldehyde index in the range 19 to 27.
   C. *Weak:* those fluids with a formaldehyde index in the range 10 to 18.
2. Color
   A. *Noncosmetic:* those fluids that contain little or no active dye and do not color the tissues.
   B. *Cosmetic:* those fluids that contain an active dye that colors the tissues.

3. Firming speed
   A. *Fast-acting:* those fluids buffered to firm tissues rapidly.
   B. *Slow-firming:* those fluids buffered to firm body tissues slowly.
4. Degree of firmness
   A. *Soft:* those fluids that are buffered and contain chemicals to control the preservative reaction to produce very little firming of the tissues.
   B. *Mild:* those fluids that are buffered and contain chemicals to control the preservative reaction to produce a medium firming of the tissues.
   C. *Hard:* those fluids that are buffered and contain chemicals to control the preservative reaction to produce very definite and hard firming of the tissues.
5. Moisturizing qualities
   A. *Humectants:* those fluids that contain large amounts of chemicals that act to add and retain tissue moisture.
   B. *Nonhumectants:* those fluids that do not contain antidehydrant chemicals.
6. Special-purpose arterial fluids
   A. *Jaundice fluids:* those fluids compounded to cover or remove the discoloration of jaundice.
   B. *High-index special-purpose fluids:* a group of chemicals with indexes usually greater than 30, used in the preparation of extreme cases, such as bodies with edema, those dead from renal failure, and bodies dead for a long time.
      a. *Dehydrating:* fluids compounded to bring about dehydration of the body tissues.
      b. *Nondehydrating:* fluids compounded to contain large amounts of preservatives but controlled so as not to dehydrate tissues.
   C. *Tissue gas fluids:* fluids designed to arrest and control the causative agent of tissue gas.
   D. *Fluids for infants and children:* fluids designed for the delicate tissues of infants and babies.

All the chemicals in this classification are designed to preserve and sanitize the body. Eight major chemical manufacturers manufacture 86 different types of preservative arterial fluids. A look at other arterial fluids shows that these are used for specific reasons and, in and of themselves, do not embalm the body.

▶ SUPPLEMENTAL FLUIDS

Preinjection (Primary Injection) Fluids

Preinjection fluids are injected before the preservative arterial solution. They aid in blood removal and prepare the tissues for the preservative arterial solution.

Coinjection Fluids

Coinjection fluids are added to preservative vascular solutions to boost most of the arterial fluid chemicals, with the exception of dyes and preservatives. They are designed to increase the penetrating and distributing qualities of the vascular fluid and to help to modify and control the reaction of the preservatives.

Internal Bleach and Stain Removers

Internal bleach and stain removers are designed to bleach such blood discolorations as ecchymoses and postmortem stains.

Tissue Gas Coinjection Fluids

Tissue gas coinjection fluids are germicidal and act on the microbes responsible for tissue gas formation.

Edema-Corrective Coinjection Fluids

Edema-corrective coinjection fluids enhance the dehydrating effect of the arterial fluid and aid in drying tissues that are edematous.

Germicide Boosters

Germicide boosters increase the germicidal effects of the arterial fluid and are used in routine embalming as well as in the treatment of bodies dead from infectious and contagious disease.

Humectants

Humectants, antidehydrants, or restorative fluids, when correctly used, aid in preventing dehydration and maintaining tissue moisture.

Water (Conditioning)-Corrective Fluids

These supplemental fluids are added to the vascular solutions to overcome the adverse effects of various chemicals that might be contained in the water.

Dyes

Active dyes are added to vascular solution. Some companies require only a few drops of these dyes. Other manufacturers require addition of several ounces to bring about the desired color in the tissue. Both pink and suntan tints are available (Table 7–1).

▶ ARTERIAL FLUID DILUTION

The dilution of arterial fluid prepared by the embalmer is called the **primary dilution**. Arterial fluid dilutions can be highly variable. The many companies that produce fluids generally make dilution recommendations. Some of these recommendations are placed on the bottle label, others print a technical

TABLE 7–1. VARIOUS ARTERIAL CHEMICALS USED IN EMBALMING

Aldehyde-based Vascular Fluid (Preservative)	Supplemental Fluid
Index	Preinjection
Strong	Coinjection (standard)
Medium	Internal bleach
Weak	Tissue gas
Nonformaldehyde	Edema corrective
Color	Germicide booster
Noncosmetic	Humectant (restorative)
Cosmetic	Water corrective
Reds	Dyes
Suntan	Pink tints
Firming speed	Suntan tints
Fast	
Slow	
Firmness	
Low	
Medium	
Strong	
Antidehydrant	
Humectant	
Nonhumectant	
Special Purpose	
Jaundice	
High Index	
Dehydrating	
Nondehydrating	
Tissue gas	
Infants	

manual. For the experienced embalmer, the proper use of any embalming chemical comes with its use over time. Through the use of the chemical the embalmer observes its reaction on body conditions and at what strengths the chemical can be used to achieve the results desired by the embalmer. Most manufacturers also state that, if desired results are not being achieved, the judgment of the embalmer determines how the formulation should be changed.

The basic factor that should determine the starting fluid dilution is the **condition of the body** (embalming analysis). Subsequent dilutions will be determined by the reaction produced by the chemicals injected and the results desired by the embalmer. It may be very necessary to make changes, for example, to increase the strength of subsequent solutions, once the reaction of the body is observed following the initial injection. This is most important in the preparation of the unautopsied body. With the unautopsied body general conditions of the body are being treated, and an attempt is made at evenly distributing the chemical solution throughout the body. Localized conditions may require sectional arterial injection using a specific chemical dilution (e.g., facial trauma, burns to hand, gangrene of a leg, etc).

Labels often contain information pertaining to one general body condition, such as moisture content. Others may include a specific condition (e.g., recommended dilutions for decomposing bodies, frozen bodies, bodies dead from renal failure, or infants). Some may contain a minimum dilution at which to begin injection. Speaking in general terms, in the preparation of the unautopsied, "average body" milder solutions are used to begin the embalming because this will assist in the clearing of intravascular blood discolorations. Subsequent injections can be increased in strength to achieve desired firmness and sanitation of the tissues. Contrast that with a body where a condition such as renal failure, generalized edema, or early signs of decomposition may be present, and there is a necessity to begin and continue with a very strong arterial solution. **The analogy of arterial fluid could be likened to the prescribing of medicine in which not every type or dosage of a drug will react on each patient and each condition in the same manner.**

Fluid labels may contain an **index** number. Index is defined as *the amount of formaldehyde, measured in grams, dissolved in 100 milliliters of water.* Some manufacturers do not use "index" as a measurement of the overall capability of a fluid to preserve a body. One reason is that index is only a measure of formaldehyde. Often a combination of preservatives will be used in an arterial fluid formulation, therefore other preservative factors are present in the formulation. To determine the strength of a primary dilution using the index factor a very simple linear equation can be employed. This formula has four factors:

$$\text{Index} \times \text{amount of fluid} = \text{strength of solution} \times \text{total volume}$$
$$c \times v = c' \times v'$$

To prepare a 2.0% arterial solution using the 25-index fluid discussed, it is necessary to know how much fluid is needed to make 1-gallon solution of 2% strength:

$$25 \times x = 2.0\% \times 128 \text{ ounces of total } \textit{solution}$$
$$25x = 256$$
$$x = \frac{256}{25}$$
$$x = 10.2 \text{ ounces of arterial fluid}$$

Approximately 10 ounces of arterial fluid and 118 ounces of water would be needed to make 1 gallon of 2.0% strength arterial solution.

Using the label directions, determine the strength of the arterial solution when 7 ounces of fluid and 1 full gallon of water are used (Table 7–2).

TABLE 7–2. PREPARATION OF VARIOUS PERCENTAGE ALDEHYDE "IN USE" SOLUTIONS[a]

Concentrate per Gallon (oz)	% Aldehyde in Concentrate (Index)				
	15	*20*	*25*	*30*	*35*
4	0.47	0.625	0.78	0.94	1.10
5	0.59	0.18	0.98	1.17	1.38
6	0.70	0.94	1.17	1.41	1.64
7	0.82	1.10	1.37	1.64	1.91
8	0.93	1.25	1.56	1.88	2.19
9	1.05	1.41	1.76	2.11	2.46
10	1.17	1.56	1.95	2.34	2.73
11	1.29	1.72	2.15	2.59	3.01
12	1.41	1.86	2.34	2.81	3.28
13	1.52	2.03	2.54	3.05	3.55
14	1.64	2.19	2.73	3.28	3.83
15	1.76	2.34	2.93	3.52	4.10
16	1.88	2.50	3.13	3.75	4.38
17	1.99	2.66	3.32	3.98	4.65
18	2.11	2.81	3.52	4.22	4.92
19	2.23	2.97	3.71	4.45	5.20
20	2.34	3.13	3.91	4.69	5.47
21	2.46	3.18	4.10	4.92	5.74
22	2.58	3.44	4.30	5.16	6.02
23	2.70	3.59	4.49	5.39	6.29
24	2.81	3.15	4.69	5.63	6.56
25	2.93	3.91	4.88	5.86	6.84
26	3.05	4.06	5.01	6.09	7.11
27	3.16	4.22	5.27	6.33	7.38
28	3.28	4.38	5.47	6.56	7.66
29	3.40	4.53	5.66	6.80	7.92
30	3.52	4.69	5.86	7.03	8.20

[a] Ounces 3 index divided by 128 (oz/gal) equals % aldehyde in solution.
Courtesy of Champion Co., Sprinfield, Ohio.

$$25 \times 7 = x \times 135 \text{ (128 ounces of water and 7 ounces of fluid)}$$

$$175 = 135x$$

$$x = \frac{175}{135} \text{ or } x = 1.29\%$$

Arterial Solution pH

The pH of the arterial solution is determined by the fluid manufacturer. This is not an element of the fluid that the embalmer determines. Most arterial fluids are buffered to be slightly alkaline in pH, approximately 7.2 to 7.4. At this pH the fluid reaction is stable, dyes in the fluid work well, and the tissues do not exhibit a tendency to turn gray.

If the embalmer selects an arterial fluid buffered at acid pH, these fluids are usually labeled as "fast-acting" fluids. In addition to the fast reaction of the fluid with body tissues, the bodies tend to become slightly grayed several hours after arterial injection.

One word of caution concerning fast-acting arterial fluids: The embalmer must be certain that a sufficient volume of fluid has been injected. Because these fluids cause rapid firming of the body, there is a tendency to run an insufficient amount of solution. After surface blood discoloration has been cleared, it would be wise to use intermittent drainage. Running a sufficient quantity of fluid and making every effort to **retain** as much fluid as possible within the body should help ensure that a sufficient amount of arterial solution is needed.

Arterial Fluid Temperature

The best instructions to follow in diluting arterial fluids are the manufacturer's recommendations. Most companies state on the label what temperature of water to employ. The majority of fluids are diluted with room temperature water. Only in special cases, such as in the treatment of tissue gas or decomposition, is it recommended that fluids be diluted with warm water. When in doubt, use water at room temperature to dilute the fluid.

▶ SOME PROPERTIES OF CHEMICAL SOLUTIONS: EFFECTS ON EMBALMING

Certain physical factors influence the results produced by any chemical. These factors play a role in governing the reactions between the tissues and the preservative chemical ingredients. As the type and amount of chemical substances in a solution are changed, a number of properties of the solution can be controlled.

Density/Specific Gravity

Certain solid chemical substances commonly known as "salts" play an important role in determining the characteristics of the different embalming fluids and in controlling, to a large extent, the reactions between the cellular tissues and the chemical solution. If a "salt" is added to a liquid, a solution results. For example, common table salt is the "solute" and water the "solvent" when these are combined. After the salt has completely dissolved in the water and is thoroughly mixed by agitation, the results is a "true" solution. Naturally, if the solute does not dissolve completely in the solvent, a true solution does not exist. The more solute added to the solvent, the more concentrated the solution becomes. In other words, the strength of the solution actually indicates how much solute is present. The amount of solute in a solution has a direct effect on the density of the solution.

Density is defined as weight per unit volume and is expressed in such terms as grams per cubic centimeter or pounds per cubic foot. Thus, it can be seen how density relates to the concentration of the solute in the solution. Often it is desirable to compare the weight of a given volume of a substance with an equal volume of water. This ratio is called **specific gravity**. If a substance is said to have a specific gravity of 1.5, it means that compared with an equal volume of water, the substance weighs 1.5 times the weight of water. Again, as with density, the specific gravity of a solution varies with concentration.

In solutions used in medicine, the density or salt concentration of a solution is frequently compared with that of blood. If a solution contains less of a dissolved substance than is found in blood, it is said to be **hypotonic.** If it contains a greater quantity of a dissolved substance than is found in the blood, it is said to be **hypertonic.**

During embalming, blood and other body liquids are being displaced and replaced with the chemical preservative solution, which eventually changes the nature of tissue. Such change resists decomposition. The penetration of such solution into all soft tissue areas should be thorough to achieve complete preservation and produce the best results.

It has been found that a solution that is slightly hypotonic to blood and body fluids produces the best embalming results. A review of the scientific principle involved will show why this is so.

In the accompanying diagram, **A** is a membranous bag such as from a section of animal intestine that is

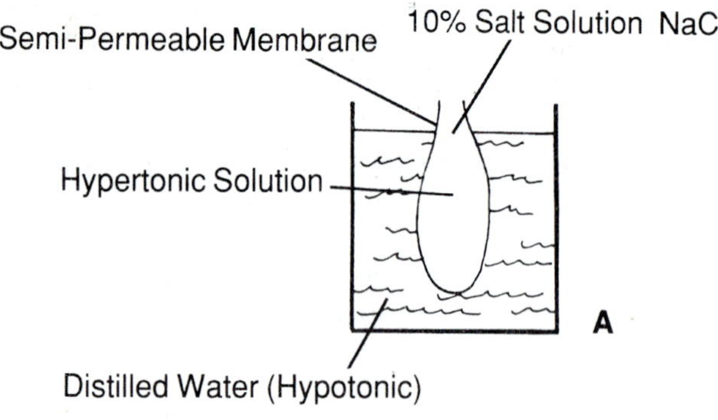

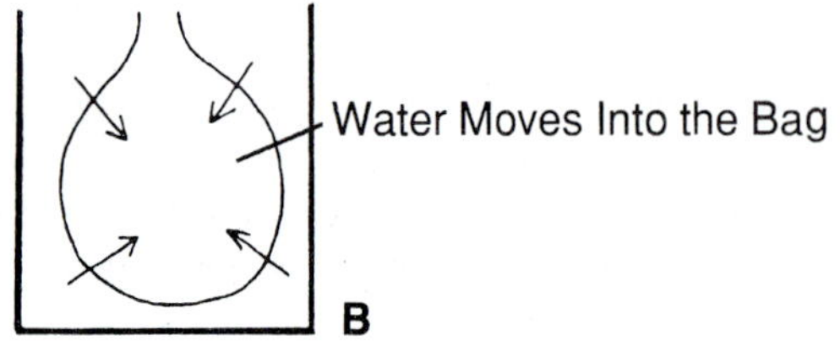

"semipermeable," that is, permeable to some materials but not to others. The bag contains a 10% salt solution. If the bag is immersed in a container, **B** is observed to increase. This proves that water has passed into the bag. Now, it will be interesting to reduce this observation to a simple explanation.

The distilled water, being "hypotonic" (i.e., of *less* density), passes to the inside of the bag, which contains the more highly concentrated solution (i.e., of *higher* density). The solution in bag **A**, then, is hypertonic to the distilled water. What is the importance of all this to the embalming operation and to embalming fluids?

It is known that a solution will penetrate to the side or region containing the more dense solution; this fact is used in compounding fluids and in establishing the proper concentrations to use in embalming. When diluted according to the recommended usage, the resultant solution is slightly hypotonic to blood and body liquids. If less of the concentrated fluid is used, then the resultant solution may be more hypotonic than desired for proper embalming results. The tissues tend to become "waterlogged," which eventually results in skin-slip because of the lack of sufficient preservative material.

On the other hand, if too much concentrated fluid is used, according to the preceding principle, a hypertonic solution results, and it will have the effect of removing too much moisture. This, of course, causes excessive dehydration. In some instances, the embalmer may want to make use of this principle to remove excess moisture from tissue areas, such as in dropsical or edematous cases. The "special" fluids designed for such purposes incorporate this principle.

Briefly, then, an embalming solution that is less dense (i.e., hypotonic) than the tissue liquids will flow rapidly through the capillary walls into the soft tissue areas. If the solution is designed so that it has a greater density (i.e., hypertonic) than the tissue liquids, it will draw tissue liquid through the capillary wall into the circulatory system and away from the soft tissue areas.

Osmotic Qualities

For the average or "normal" body, in which there is no edema or dehydration, the arterial solution should be hypotonic in its osmotic composition. This is generally achieved by following the manufacturers' dilution instructions. When the solution is hypotonic to the body tissues, the fluid moves from the capillary vessels into the tissue spaces. If these solutions were hypertonic, tissue fluids would move from the tissue space into the capillary vessels, thus causing dehydration and lack of arterial fluid in the tissues.

There are instances when hypertonic solutions are desired. This type of solution is generally used when embalming bodies with skeletal edema. These solutions help to move the excess water from the tissue into the capillary vessels by increasing the osmotic permeability of the cell walls. From there the water can be removed through drainage. Some embalmers add Epsom salts to the arterial solutions to create these hypertonic dehydrating solutions. The high-index special-purpose fluids, when diluted in a certain manner, create dehydrating hypertonic solutions.

Quantity

Consider this example of different bodies that required special attention:

> Two bodies weighing 110 pounds—one a healthy teenager killed in an automobile accident, the other a 65-year-old adult who died of a wasting disease (e.g., cancer; in good health the individual weighed 190 pounds). Should the embalmer proceed to embalm the two in the same manner using the same chemicals, same concentrations, same total solution volume, and so forth? This situation might be used to introduce the concept of "preembalming" considerations.

The total volume of arterial fluid injected is determined by a number of factors. These factors should be noted in making the embalming analysis. The embalmer must always determine if a sufficient quantity of fluid has been injected and if the fluid has been injected at a proper strength. Autopsied bodies have been prepared in which up to 3 or more gallons of solution have been injected into one leg! It is always wise to embalm the body on the assumption that the disposition will be delayed. Medications used over a long period of time may have had effects which increase the demand for fluid. Examples include:

- The effect of the drug on the preservative solution.
- The damage the drug has done to the body proteins.
- The damage done to specific organs such as the liver and the kidneys, causing retention of wastes such as ammonia and urea in the tissues.
- The damage done to the cell membrane—a possible condition in which it is difficult for fluids to pass through the cell membranes.

Consider these points in determining the strength and amount of fluid to inject.

- Time between death and preparation
- Time between preparation and disposition
- Moisture content of the body
- Renal failure and the buildup of nitrogenous **wastes** in the body
- Liver failure and the buildup of toxic wastes in the body tissues
- Weight of the body
- Amount of adipose tissue versus muscular tissues accounting for body weight
- Protein levels of the body
- Progress of the postmortem physical and chemical changes, especially the stages of decomposition and rigor mortis
- Nature of death—sudden heart attack versus wasting disease; use of life-support systems for many weeks
- Chemotherapy and medications given to the individual

▶ SPECIAL-PURPOSE ARTERIAL FLUIDS

High-Index Fluids

The preservative arterial fluids have a formaldehyde index of 30 to 35 or slightly above. These fluids are designed for use in the preparation of difficult-to-embalm bodies. In addition to these difficult preparations, these fluids have two other uses. First, some embalmers use these fluids for routine preparations. Second, these fluids can be used to fortify or increase the firming and preservative qualities of regular arterial solutions.

Example. An embalmer mixes a solution of arterial fluid using a 22-index fluid and uses 8 ounces to the gallon for the solution. If firming of the body seems not to be happening, in the second and subsequent gallons, several ounces of the high-index fluid will be added to the solution to help boost the preservative strength of the solution.

Keep in mind that solutions are always mixed from mild to strong, not the reverse. If there is to be a change in solution strength, embalming solutions are always increased in strength.

The following statement from the Dodge Chemical Company regarding one of their special-purpose high-index fluids explains well the use of this chemical:

> The more severe the conditions of the body, the stronger the primary solution should be. When little drainage is anticipated, stronger concentrations and less total volume of solution should be used. When normal drainage is achieved, the volume of solution to be used will be governed by the size, weight, and conditions of the body. In general, in treating bodies of "difficult" types, a good rule to follow is: more rather than less chemical—and less rather than more water. Water will not preserve nor will it arrest putrefaction—but it will create swelling and distension.

There are situations in which use of high-index fluid is advised:

- Bodies dead for extended periods (24 hours or longer)
- Bodies that have been refrigerated
- Bodies that have been frozen
- Bodies that have undergone extensive treatments with drugs
- Institutional bodies
- Bodies with traumatic injuries for which restorative treatments will be needed
- Bodies with evidence of decomposition
- Bodies with gangrenous limbs
- Bodies that are difficult to firm
- Bodies with skeletal edema
- Bodies dead from renal failure
- Bodies with bloodstream infections

Some companies produce two types of high-index fluids: **dehydrating** and **nondehydrating**. The nondehydrating fluid is designed to deliver a strong formaldehyde and preservative action with a minimum of dehydration. As with other arterial fluids, it is best to follow the dilutions recommended by the manufacturer. Most of the high-index fluids, when used as a "booster" fluid, work well with standard arterial fluids of other companies. Because of the problems encountered with delayed embalming and the wide use of drug therapy today, *this arterial fluid should always be kept on hand in the preparation room.*

Jaundice Fluids

A second special-purpose preservative arterial fluid is jaundice fluid. Jaundice fluids are used not only to preserve the body but to hide or rid the body of mild yellow jaundice or to prevent yellow jaundice from changing to green jaundice. These fluids are most effective on the body that has only a mild jaundice discoloration as opposed to bodies with the deep jaundice discoloration. These fluids do little to remove deep discoloration.

The conversion of yellow jaundice to green jaundice is an oxidation reaction and formaldehyde is a strong reducing agent. What appears to happen when excess formaldehyde is injected into jaundiced bodies is establishment of an acid condition. This condition now brings about the oxidation that converts the yellow to green. For this reason, most jaundice fluids have a low index, and because of this low index it is important to follow the manufacturer's instructions with respect to dilutions and quantity of fluid. Keep in mind that in treating the jaundiced body, preservation of the body must have precedence over the clearing of the jaundice discoloration. Never use a dilution *less* than that recommended by the particular jaundice fluid manufacturer. There are four types of jaundice fluids.

Bleaching Fluids. Bleaching fluids bleach the discoloration. The chemicals employed in the formulations include peroxides, oxalic or critic acid, and phenols. These chemicals are usually employed in an alcohol medium.

Buffer System Fluids. Buffer systems are used to control the pH so that an acid condition does not develop in the tissues. According to Leandro Rendon of the Champion Company,

> When aldehydes react with proteins, one of the chemical reactions that occurs has been said to be that of a release of hydrogen ions which, of course, results in low pH, which is acid in nature. A given amount of formaldehyde or aldehyde can unite with a given amount of protein to form a given aldehyde condensation resin. Once the proteins have received the necessary amount of aldehyde to form these condensation resins, any excess aldehyde tends to become more acid in character and, therefore, to cause oxidation changes.

The oxidation converts yellow jaundice to green jaundice. From another point of view, aldehydes, in combining with proteins or amino acids, increase the local acidity in the tissues by releasing proteins. The hydrogen ions that produce the acid condition result from the chemical reaction between the protein and the aldehyde. The yellow-orange pigment (bilirubin) is converted to the green pigment (biliverdin). It is not the formaldehyde that causes the oxidation (formaldehyde is a reducing agent). Rather, it is the chemical reaction (oxidation) that occurs as a result of acid present.

Coupling Compound System. The coupling compound system combines a chemical with the bile pigment to decolorize the pigment. A preinjection coupling compound, (e.g., a diazo agent in a nonacetic medium) is injected first. The aldehyde arterial injection follows. The system is complex, time consuming, and not always reliable.

Chemical Adduct System. In the chemical adduct system, a chemical is combined with formaldehyde; later, the formaldehyde is slowly released "on the spot," thus preventing an excessive buildup of hydrogen ions.

A final caution with regard to jaundice fluids: When using a jaundice fluid do *not* mix this fluid with other arterial fluids or preinjection fluids, unless the directions accompanying the jaundice fluid call for the use of a preinjection fluid. If a preinjection fluid is recommended, it would, no doubt, be best to use the preinjection fluid manufactured by the same company that made the jaundice fluid.

Tissue Gas Fluid

A variety of fluids have been manufactured by chemical companies to treat the condition known as tissue gas. This condition is caused by *Clostridium perfringens.* It is important that the directions for these fluids be carefully followed.

Infants and Children

Some chemical companies have produced fluids specifically for the embalming of infants and children. These arterial fluids generally have a low index and are very viscous. Care should be taken to follow the directions on the label.

▶ WATERLESS EMBALMING

Waterless embalming is a concept that has been discussed among embalmers and in funeral service literature for the past several years. It is usually not recommended for "normal" bodies, but for the more difficult cases. "Waterless embalming" is something of a misnomer. Many times water is a vehicle or dilutant in many arterial and specialty formulations, so no embalming can be truly "waterless." The concept is more specifically "no added, or very little added water embalming." This simply means that the arterial chemical is not diluted by tap water, but by a supplemental chemical. This may also mean that 20 to 24 bottles of fluid are used per body and can be somewhat expensive. Drainage may also be minimal, so there is a decrease of waste material taken from the body.

Waterless embalming has been recommended for the elderly, dehydrated or emaciated bodies, persons dead several days, refrigerated bodies, traumatic cases, decomposed bodies, or any case where pathologic conditions such as gangrene, tissue gas, or extreme edema might exist.

▶ USE OF PREINJECTION FLUID

A preinjection fluid is injected into the body before the preservative arterial solution is injected. These fluids were first used because the early arterial fluids were so strong and harsh that they caused difficulty in clearing the blood from the capillaries and veins. The preinjection fluid (also called a primary injection fluid or capillary wash) was designed to clear the blood vascular system of the blood prior to injection of the preservative solution.

Today, arterial fluids contain a number of modifying agents that allow the arterial solutions to distribute and diffuse uniformly. Many embalmers, however, still feel the necessity to flush the vascular system with a preinjection solution. This helps to clear blood discolorations, adjusts the pH of the tissues, reduces blood coagulation, and, thus, improves draining. Two factors are necessary to obtain the best results with this chemical: (1) a sufficient quantity should be injected and (2) some time should be allowed for the chemical to work properly.

It has been suggested that at least 1 gallon should be injected and that the chemical should be allowed to sit 20 to 30 minutes before the preservative solution is injected. Most embalmers, however, inject approximately one-quarter to one-half gallon of solution and immediately inject the preservative solution. In theory, any amount of preinjection fluid would enter the vessels *before* the preservative arterial solution. One-quarter to one-half gallon of this solution would, no doubt, fill the empty arterial system in the average-size body. Instructions will give dilutions for the use of the chemical and should be followed, for these fluids have little or no preservative and it is possible to waterlog the tissues and cells.

Some preinjection fluids contain small amounts of preservatives. For this reason, some embalmers use these chemicals to embalm infants and children. *This author feels that these fluids should NOT be used to embalm children; rather, standard preservative arterial fluid should be used for the preparation of infants and children.* The embalmer may wish to use a preinjection solution only to assist in preparing the circulatory system for the preservative arterial solution.

Preinjection treatment is generally used only on unautopsied bodies, not for treatment on autopsied bodies in which each body area is separately injected. Note also that preinjection fluids contain little or no active dye to color the tissues. Many embalmers also prefer to inject this solution with the drainage kept open.

In embalming bodies where there has been any great time delay between death and embalming or where the embalmer feels circulation may be difficult to establish, preinjection fluids should be avoided, or, if used, the embalmer should inject a minimal amount. A preinjection fluid loosens clots in the venous system and, thus, makes them easier to remove. This, in turn, improves blood drainage. If there is any clotting in the arterial system, preinjection fluids can loosen these clots as well. They will be carried by the fluid to smaller arteries where they can easily block circulation channels.

Preinjection fluid works best when it is used on bodies that are still warm and when the embalmer feels circulation will be very good. An embalmer who feels circulation may be difficult to establish and arterial clotting may be present should avoid the use of a preinjection fluid. Because embalming is usually delayed with bodies dying in large hospitals, less preinjection fluid is being used today.

The following sample has been compiled from several different fluid company catalogs and contains descriptions of different preinjection fluids. It will help the student, in particular, to understand the purpose of these fluids.

Preinjection Fluids

KLM promotes drainage and capillary circulation. *Many bodies present the challenge of a highly complex residual body chemistry. The extent and identification of this chemistry are not always known.* KLM is proven to be the embalmer's best and most direct approach to the control of adverse residual body chemistry. KLM is unmatched in its scope for body conditioning, and its use prevents complications.

PQR is a very fine primary injection fluid. It conditions the arterial system and expands the small arterioles and venules to make the subsequent arterial injections more effective and complete. Research has shown that an alkaline condition of the tissues is desirable to retain their natural color (acid brings on an ashen gray appearance), and yet, a strongly alkaline solution tends to waterlog the body.

The bonus feature of PQR is a *touch of preservative* effect. It has been found that a low index of formaldehyde in a *slightly alkaline* primary injection fluid is the complete answer, actually making the tissues more receptive to later contact with preservative chemicals. *One of PQR's most important functions is to establish the proper pH in the circulatory system and adjacent tissues to promote constantly uniform results in all cases.*

XYZ is a positive and dependable aid in *keeping the blood liquid and free flowing.* Its heavy specific gravity provides the driving force to keep the blood moving, while at the same time *strengthening and lubricating the capillary walls.* It is excellent for clearing discolorations caused by bruising and other injuries.

TUV acts with trigger-fast speed to dilute thick heavy blood and relieve the vascular congestion that acts as a barrier to arterial and capillary circulation. Smooth in its action, TUV slips quickly through the capillary walls to allow for an easier and more voluminous fluid passage. All of the *dark heavy blood is washed from the capillaries and veins,* preventing any possibility of the flushing of putty gray that so frequently mars embalming results. The widespread effect in the rapid disappearance of surface discolorations and the *greatly stimulated drainage* can be easily seen.

TUV contains efficient, nonhardening preservatives that eliminate all danger of *waterlogging* the tissues but, at the same time, cannot possibly burn, harm, or dehydrate the most tender body. TUV is osmotically balanced to ensure retention of the correct amount of tissue moisture and to maintain naturalness for the maximum period. TUV not only liquifies and removes heavy blood but it *reoxygenates both the blood and tissue cells.* The normal pink cast of the blood and tissues is restored by a natural process homologous to that which exists during life. *For a most satisfactory embalming termination the embalmer must have a proper beginning.* No arterial preparation can accomplish the best results unless the capillary system has been completely cleared of blood and the vessels expanded for maximum capacity.

▶ USE OF COINJECTION FLUIDS

Most coinjection fluids are compatible with the majority of arterial fluids. An arterial fluid and a coinjection fluid should combine to form a homogenous solution that can be distributed and diffused throughout the body. As for the amount to use, remember that the manufacturers' labels are the best guide.

Most coinjection fluids are used in an amount equal to the amount of concentrated arterial fluid. Or, half as much coinjection fluid as concentrated arterial solution is used. Generally, the amount of coinjection fluid should never exceed the amount of concentrated arterial fluid. When too much coinjection fluid is used (plus the use of water softeners), it has a tendency to distribute unevenly and the dyes have a tendency to "blotch." When in doubt, a good rule is to use equal amounts of coinjection fluid and concentrated arterial fluid.

When should a coinjection fluid be used? This chemical, unlike a preinjection chemical, can be employed with every preparation. It assists in distributing and diffusing the arterial solution and helps to control and enhance the arterial fluid. In some special conditions, embalmers use the coinjection fluid as the dilutent vehicle, for example, in the technique of "rapid tissue fixation." Some individuals also practice waterless embalming. In this process, the coinjection fluid takes the place of water in the arterial solution.

Coinjection Fluids

FGH *acts with all arterial fluids.* A few ounces added to the arterial solution will ensure the creation of an unparalleled naturalness and will practically eliminate the possibility of dehydration and feature shrinkage, no matter how long the interval between the embalming and interment. *Distribution and diffusion will be increased to a pronounced degree,* drainage will be more copious, preservation will be more permanent, and the skin will have the same velvety freshness it had in life. FGH is indispensable in every operation in which a standard arterial fluid is used, and especially so in emaciated subjects, infants and the aged—bodies usually susceptible to formaldehyde action—and in all situations where pathologic or climatic conditions necessitate the use of a stronger than normal arterial solution.

FGH diffuses unhindered through the capillary walls and all internal membranes to enter every tissue cell and combine with the cellular protoplasm. It creates a permanent, waxy, moisture-retaining shield, the presence of which can be detected by the velvety texture of the skin.

ABC suppresses reactivation of calcium ion substances and disperses fibrin threads, which are the bonding agents in clots. ABC reduces agglutinated blood and, in addition, washes obstructions from the capillaries, strengthening and lubricating their walls. ABC helps to clear discolorations and amplifies the preserving action of the arterial fluid.

DEF is a *dual-purpose fluid* for addition to each arterial injection. In action, it *softens and lubricates blood clots.* At the same time it conditions and *reduces water hardness to zero,* with an overall improvement in embalming results. It is not a blood solvent, nor is it a preservative. It does, however, contribute importantly to the solution of any drainage problem. It breaks down clots so they may be removed by way of the drain tube.

(To date there is no known chemical that can be used effectively to dissolve a blood clot totally without having, at the same time, an adverse effect on the circulatory system.)

▶ USE OF WATER CORRECTIVE COINJECTION FLUID

Water corrective chemicals can be added (used as a coinjection fluid) to all embalming solutions when water is used as a vehicle. This means that a water conditioner can be added to a preembalming solution as well as to a preservative solution. It is best to follow the manufacturer's guidelines as to the amount to use. Generally, only a few ounces are used for each gallon of solution. Overuse of this chemical can cause blotching of fluid dyes. Details as to the purposes of this chemical can be reviewed in Chapter 6 of this text. Some embalmers use water corrective chemicals for all injections; others rarely or never use this product. In areas of the country where water is exceptionally hard its use can be most valuable.

Water corrective chemical can also be used as a vehicle in formulas for "waterless" embalming solutions. Here one or more bottle of chemical can be used to dilute the arterial fluid.

Water conditioner can also be used for cleaning salts and other solidified chemicals from the embalming machine. Generally 8 ounces or more can be added to warm water to flush and clean the machine.

▶ USE OF ADDED DYES IN ARTERIAL SOLUTIONS

Dye is used in arterial solutions for several reasons. Inactive dye merely colors the arterial fluid. This way, the embalmer knows that the concentrated fluid has been added to the water in the tank. Active dyes serve several functions:

1. They act as a tracer so the location of the arterial fluid can be noted in areas of the body, a sign of arterial fluid distribution.
2. They help restore the natural color of the skin, which changes when blood is drained from the tissues.
3. They help to prevent the body from darkening as a result of reaction with the blood, which remains within the body after the embalming.

There are actually two ways that additional dyes are used with arterial solutions: In the first, dye is added to all of the solution injected. In the second, the embalmer adds the dye to the final gallon that is injected. There are two main objections to the use of additional dye throughout the embalming operation: (1) the tissues will be overstained and create a cosmetic problem, and (2) the embalmer, seeing the dye in the superficial tissue, may tend to underembalm the body.

The amount of dye to add again depends on the fluid manufacturer. Follow the directions on the label; then add or cut back to suit individual preference. For some dyes, only several drops are required per gallon; for other dyes, several ounces are required.

▶ USE OF HUMECTANTS (RESTORATIVES) IN ARTERIAL SOLUTIONS

The separately purchased humectant (antidehydrant) is really a coinjection fluid. The reason for this is quite simple. The humectant is added and injected along with the arterial fluid. Some embalmers use humectants only when the body is dehydrated. Others add extra humectant to all arterial solutions when embalming a body with normal moisture to prevent dehydration. The amount of humectant added to each gallon of solution should follow the manufacturer's directions.

It should be pointed out that most humectants are colloids, and these viscous colloid mixtures, when injected into the arterial system, have a tendency to draw moisture *out of the tissues* and into the capillaries. If additional humectants are used and solutions are injected into the body with continuous drainage, evidence can be seen of dehydration in such areas as the lips, fingers, and backs of the hands. Most embalmers, when adding humectants to the arterial solution, use intermittent drainage. In this manner the humectant is held in the capillaries and tissue spaces and does not draw moisture from the tissues.

For a severely emaciated body, some embalmers add a large amount of humectant to the final gallon injected. In addition, they close off the drainage, causing the facial tissues to distend and restoring them to their natural contour. If this technique is employed, a close watch must be kept on the facial features; gross distention of such areas as the tissues around the eyes can create more problems.

▶ USE OF EDEMA CORRECTIVE COINJECTION FLUIDS

Edema corrective coinjection chemicals have been available for many years; however, in the last few years there has been an increase in the available varieties of this chemical. Manufacturer's instructions should be strictly followed. The amount of chemical to use will depend on the severity of the edema. The corrective chemical is added to the preservative arterial solution as a coinjection fluid. It can be very effective in reducing swollen facial tissues, which often accompany vascular or heart surgery.

The edema corrective chemical changes the osmotic qualities of the embalming solution and draws the edema from the tissue spaces back into the venous drainage. Best results are obtained when a region, such as the head, is separately injected using the corrective treatment. Massage and elevation of the affected area also help to remove the swollen condition. If too much chemical is used, areas such as the facial tissues or hands can become dehydrated. This can produce dark discoloring of the tissues and wrinkles.

▶ CAVITY FLUID

As the name indicates, cavity fluid is injected into the body cavities. Routinely, cavity fluid is injected into the thoracic, abdominal, and pelvic cavities. In some special cases the cranial cavity can also be treated by injecting some fluid via a large needle or infant trocar into the cranial cavity.

For the average body, 32 ounces (or two bottles) of cavity fluid is distributed via the trocar over the viscera of the thoracic, abdominal, and pelvic cavities. The principal ingredient of these fluids is formaldehyde. Obviously, there is little need for dyes, anticoagulants, or humectants in these fluids.

Cavity fluid *preserves, disinfects,* and *deodorizes* organs of the cavities, contents of the hollow viscera, and walls of the cavities. There are, however, other uses for cavity fluids:

- Preservation of viscera removed at an autopsy
- As a surface compress to help treat tissues not reached by arterial profusion
- Injection via hypodermic needle or trocar into tissues that lack sufficient arterial preservation.
- As a surface compress on lesions and pathologic conditions to dry and deodorize
- As an arterial fluid in the preparation of difficult cases such as advanced decomposition, tissue gas, and jaundice. Use only those cavity chemicals recommended by the manufacturer for arterial injection; not all cavity chemicals can be injected arterially.
- As a surface treatment for gangrenous and dropsical limbs to help dry and preserve the tissues
- To bleach blood discolorations
- To dry tissues when excisions have been performed
- For surface preservation of fetal remains

▶ FUMELESS CAVITY AND ARTERIAL FLUIDS

Because formaldehyde is the principal ingredient of most cavity fluids, these chemicals can be very difficult to work with because of the pungent odor produced by formaldehyde. Fumeless fluids, particularly cavity fluids, are produced by many manufacturers. There are three ways in which fumeless fluids can be produced: (1) cover the formaldehyde with a deodorant; (2) substitute other preservatives for formaldehyde (a good example would be the use of phenol); or (3) use formaldehyde donor compounds (these compounds do not release the formaldehyde until it is in contact with the tissues). A problem with the first method, perfuming the formaldehyde, is that the embalmer can breathe these fumes with little irritation at the time, but later notices that large amounts of formaldehyde have been inhaled. The second method is good and is used by many manufacturers, but other preservatives lack the penetrating qualities of formaldehyde. The last method is used mainly in the production of arterial fluids. Its cost is prohibitive in the formulation of most cavity fluids.

▶ ACCESSORY EMBALMING CHEMICALS

Accessory chemicals are chemicals used to treat the dead human body for purposes other than arterial embalming or cavity treatment and include autopsy gels, concentrated cautery chemicals, hardening compounds, concentrated preservative powder, concentrated deodorant powder, concentrated disinfectant powder, mold-preventive agents, powdered seating agents, cream or "putty" sealing agents, and surface sealing agents.

Autopsy (Surface) Gels

Years ago a product called "formal creams" was manufactured for surface or osmotic embalming. Each company had a different name for these emollient creams. Compared with the gels used today, they were very inferior. In the late 1960s, chemical companies began to produce a gel or jellylike surface preservative. These preservative gels are available in two viscosities: a gel that is thin and can be poured, and a more viscous gel that can easily be applied by brush to the skin surface. Not only are these gels easy to work with, but their penetrating abilities and preservative qualities far exceed those of the older formal creams. Autopsy gels are used in several ways. They may be

- Poured over the viscera returned from an autopsy in the plastic bag in which the viscera have been placed.
- Applied to the surface of viscera in partial autopsies.
- Used as a preservative in the orbital area after enucleation.
- Applied to walls of cavities and surfaces, such as the cranial cavity and calvarium in autopsied bodies.
- Applied as a surface preservative to pathologic conditions such as decubitus ulcerations and gangrenous or necrotic areas.
- Applied as disinfectant and as an odor reducer.
- Applied to surface areas of the body that the embalmer feels have received insufficient arterial fluid.
- Helpful in bleaching discolored areas such as ecchymoses and postmortem stains.
- Helpful in preserving, cauterizing, and deodorizing burnt areas.
- Used to pack the anal orifice and colostomy opening.

Autopsy gels are designed as surface or osmotic preservatives. Some manufacturers claim that their product can penetrate several inches beneath the skin. These gels not only preserve tissues but bleach blood and decomposition discolorations. In addition, they help to eliminate odors in such pathologic conditions as gangrene or decubitus ulcerations.

As with most preservative chemicals, care should be taken to use these gels in a well-ventilated embalming room. The embalmer may wish to wear a mask as protection from the fumes. When the gels are applied to an external surface they should be covered with cotton or plastic. This improves the effectiveness of the gel in addition to reducing the fumes.

Each manufacturer recommends the length of time the gels should remain on a surface to be most effective. Several hours would be a good rule. The embalmer can check from time to time on the working action of the gel. When the gels are applied to necrotic areas (as on the legs), plastic stockings should be placed on the body, and the gel should not be removed. The same is true for application over decubitus ulcerations. The compresses should be left in place and plastic garments such as pants or coveralls should be placed on the body.

Cautery Chemicals

Although some may not classify cautery chemicals under the heading of embalming, but rather under the heading of restorative art, they very much belong to the group of chemicals used during or immediately after embalming.

Cautery chemicals are liquids that are basically phenol (carbolic acid). Many of those sold through embalming manufacturers contain about 2 to 5% phenol, whereas those solutions prepared by a pharmacy can be as strong as 70% or more carbolic acid.

It should be emphasized that whenever these chemicals are used, the embalmer must wear eye protection. Unlike most embalming chemicals that irritate the eyes, carbolic acid can actually burn and scar eye tissue. In addition, it is recommended that rubber gloves be worn when handling phenol.

Phenol can be applied to areas where the skin has been removed, for example, abrasions, skin slip, blisters that have been opened, and burned areas. Phenol is a rapid-acting cautery agent and dries these areas in minutes. Phenol can also be used as a surface bleach or be injected subcutaneously and bleach from underneath the skin. It is a good germicide; it can be injected into swollen areas such as black eyes or hematomas and allowed to remain for a time. Then the area is massaged. Some of the phenol is forced from the area along with some of the liquids responsible for the swelling. Thus, phenol is a reducing and constricting agent.

Phenol has many applications during the embalming operation. It can be used as a cautery agent for searing raw tissue, a surface bleach, an internal bleach, a reducing and constricting agent, and a germicidal agent.

Tissue Builder

A tissue builder is a chemical injected by hypodermic syringe and needle **after** arterial embalming. It is injected into sunken areas of the face and hands to help restore their natural contour when the body exhibits a great loss of weight. Individual features such as the lips or fingers can also be treated with this chemical. Once injected beneath the skin it can be spread through the tissues by finger pressure. It is important to not overfill an area; it is almost impossible to remove the tissue builder once it is injected.

Solvents

The embalmer uses three solvents in various embalming treatments. A **general solvent**, such as tri-chloroethylene, is used for cleansing of the skin surface, usually the face and hands. Most of these solvents can also be used for cleansing of the scalp and hair. They are useful in removing cosmetics from the hair, eyelashes, and eyebrows. A **tissue builder solvent** is used to clean hypodermic syringes and needles that have been used for the injection of tissue builder or any other chemicals. Some embalmers like to store syringes with a few ccs of solvent in them. Anytime a syringe is used it should be flushed with this solvent before another chemical is used. A third solvent found in the preparation room is finger nail polish remover, primarily **acetone**.

Hardening Compounds

Hardening compounds are blends of powdered chemicals. They dry moist tissue by dehydrating it. In addition, some hardening compounds contain powdered preservatives, disinfectants, and deodorants. The primary use of this embalming chemical is in treatment of the cavities of the autopsied body. The powdered compound can also be used to treat the visceral organs returned after an autopsy. Hardening compound is often used in the plastic garments placed on bodies with burned tissue, decubitus ulcerations, or edema. Some of the chemicals used in these compounds are plaster of Paris (a hardening agent); paraformaldehyde; aluminum chloride and alum dehydrating, disinfectant, and preservative agents; wood powder (wood flour—very fine sawdust), and whiting and clays (moisture-absorbing chemicals).

Chemical manufacturers have made an effort to develop "dustless" hardening compounds for the safety of the embalmer. When embalming powders are used, the room should be well ventilated and a mask and goggles should be worn. Every effort should be made to reduce the inhalation of any particulate. Consult the Kerfoot studies in Selected Readings for the dangers caused by embalming powders.

The hardening compounds are not as effective preservatives and disinfectants as the autopsy gels. The gels have a much greater penetrating ability.

Embalming Preservative Powder

As the name indicates, embalming powder is designed to preserve tissue. The fumes this powder generates help to preserve and disinfect tissues. Many contain paradichlorobenzene crystals, which arrest mildew and mold. Paraformaldehyde is the chief ingredient of these powdered preservatives. Some embalming powders also serve as deodorants and disinfectants. They do not have the absorbent and drying qualities of a hardening compound. The embalming powder can assist in preservation of the walls and organs of autopsied bodies if placed directly on burned or decomposing tissue. These powders can also be used for preservation of stillborn infants, and can be applied to cancerous tissues, bed sores, and mutilated body parts. They help to preserve the tissues and control odors that may be present.

Embalming powder can also be put into the plastic garments placed on limbs with edema. When bodies are to be shipped to a distant point for interment, embalming powder can be placed in the casket to help control mildews or molds. These powders also help to control maggots and vermin.

Be certain to check the labels of embalming powders; some are preservatives, whereas others are merely disinfectants and deodorants. It would be helpful to purchase an embalming powder that serves all three purposes.

Mold Preventive Agents

Mold retarding chemicals are applied topically. They generally contain phenol or thymol. Mold retardants can be purchased in a prepared form and sprayed or painted on the surface of the body before placing it in storage. Refrigeration can retard mold growth but not stop it; in fact, some molds thrive best at cool temperatures. If mold is present it can be scraped from the skin surface and a phenol mold retardant painted over the area to inhibit further growth. Mold becomes a problem when bodies must be kept for extended time periods. Of course, warm and moist environments encourage their growth.

Sealing Agents

Sealing agents are used to prevent leakage from sutured incisions. The agent is placed in the incised area during suturing. If any moisture develops within the incision these agents absorb that moisture and are converted into a gelatinous material that helps to prevent leakage from the sutures. Two types of powder have been used for many years; more recently, a cream or "puttylike" material has been used.

The "putty" sealing agent can be used in various restorative procedures such as restoration of enucleated eyes, as a base for deep wound restorations, as a substitute for tissue builder, and to fill in sunken temple areas in autopsied bodies. It can be applied with a spatula or a specially designed injector.

Sealing agents are also surface glues. These help to prevent leakage from sutured tissues. Surface glues can be applied with a brush or can be purchased as a spray. Many of these agents can be directly covered with mortuary cosmetics when they are used in restorative work. Surface sealing agents work best on dry tissue **surfaces**.

▶ KEY TERMS AND CONCEPTS FOR STUDY AND DISCUSSION

1. Define the following terms:
   - Arterial fluid
   - Coinjection fluid
   - Hypertonic solution
   - Hypotonic solution
   - Osmosis
   - Preinjection fluid
   - Primary dilution
   - Secondary dilution
2. List and define four special-purpose arterial fluids.
3. List and define four types of coinjection fluid.
4. Give five uses for a preinjection fluid.
5. List eight criteria that help the embalmer to determine the type, strength, and volume of arterial fluid.
6. List several purposes for addition of an active dye to arterial fluid.
7. Give several uses for autopsy gels.
8. List body conditions for which a special-purpose, high-index arterial fluid would be best to use.
9. Give several uses for cavity fluid.
10. How many ounces of a 25-index arterial fluid must be used to prepare a 1-gallon 2.0% strength arterial solution? To prepare a 1.5% strength solution? To prepare a 3.0% strength solution?
11. If 8 ounces of a 20-index arterial fluid is used to prepare a 1-gallon solution of arterial fluid, what will be the strength of this solution? If 12 ounces of arterial fluid was used? If 6 ounces of arterial fluid was used?
12. How much water must be added to make a 2.0% arterial solution if 6 ounces of a 20-index fluid is used? If you desire to make a 1.5% solution? If you desire to make a 3.0% solution?

▶ BIBLIOGRAPHY

Dorn J., Hopkins B. *Thanatocbemistry*, Upper Saddle River, NJ: Prentice Hall; 1998.

General chemical principles of embalming fluids. In: *The Champion Expanding Encyclopedia*, Nos. 365–371; Springfield, OH: Champion CO.; March–October 1966.

Mathews M.C. *Embalming Chemistry Note Outline*. Minneapolis: University of Minnesota; 1998.

Pervier NC. *Textbook of Chemistry for Embalmers*. Minneapolis: University of Minnesota; 1961.

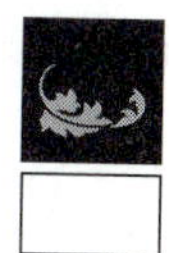

CHAPTER 8
ANATOMICAL CONSIDERATIONS

It is essential that the embalmer possess a sound understanding of and familiarity with the human form to efficiently approach and solve embalming problems. This chapter emphasizes those areas of anatomy most concerned with the embalming process. The orientation is strictly anatomical and space in the text is not consumed with considerations of the functional significance of any structure.

Before one can conceptualize the internal anatomy of the body, he or she must first be familiar with surface features and the manner in which they relate to underlying structures. A thorough knowledge of surface anatomy permits one not only to make appropriate skin incisions but also to anticipate which structures will appear when the incisions are made.

A portion of this chapter is devoted to the fundamentals of surface anatomy as it relates to underlying musculoskeletal and visceral structures. As a complete treatment of these topics is well beyond the scope of this text, this discussion is limited to those aspects of greatest importance to the embalmer.

All descriptions used throughout the text assume that the body is in the *anatomical position:* the subject is standing erect, the arms of the subject are at the sides with the palms of the hands facing the observer, the feet are together, and the subject is facing the observer.

The embalmer should have a detailed understanding of the blood vascular system. For each of the major vessels used in embalming, the anatomical guide, the linear guide, and the anatomical extent (limit) of each artery are given.

An **anatomical guide** is a method of locating a structure, such as an artery or vein, by reference to an adjacent known or prominent structure. A **linear guide** is a line drawn or visualized on the surface of the skin to represent the approximate location of some deeper-lying structure. The **anatomical limit** is the point of origin and point of termination of a structure in relation to adjacent structures.

Because the blood in the veins flows in the *direction opposite* that of blood in the arteries, the anatomical limit and the linear guide for the veins would be the *opposite* of those of the respective artery. The anatomical guides for the arteries and the veins would be the same.

▶ COMMON CAROTID ARTERY AND INTERNAL JUGULAR VEIN

Surface Features and Landmarks

Surface features of the neck that the embalmer should be able to locate and describe are the clavicle, mandible, angle of the jaw, mastoid process of the temporal bone, hyoid bone, sternum, sternoclavicular articulation, suprasternal notch, and thyroid cartilage of the larynx. The embalmer should also be familiar with one muscle, the **sternocleidomastoid muscle (SCM).** In addition, the location of the external jugular vein should be recognized. Underlying the skin in this area is a thin, delicate cutaneous muscle (a muscle of facial expression) called the **platysma,** the presence of which is indicated by the shallow, transverse wrinkles of the neck.

Consider first the anterior triangle of the neck. Draw an imaginary line along the midline of the neck between the tip of the mandible and the sternum. Extend this line superiorly along the anterior border of the SCM and then anteriorly along the lower margin of the body of the mandible. These three lines and their anatomical parallels describe the **anterior triangle.** In the midline, one can palpate (feel), from above downward, the hyoid bone and the thyroid and cricoid cartilages. The external carotid artery and several of its branches are located in the anterior triangle. Here, these vessels are relatively superficial, being covered only by skin and subcutaneous tissue.

Anterior Triangle of the Neck

The skin over the anterior triangle is thin and underlaid by the thin, cutaneous platysma muscle. This muscle acts to alter the contour of the skin of the neck in much the same manner that the muscles of facial expression modify the appearance of the face. The significance of the muscle to the embalmer is that most structures of importance in the embalming process lie beneath the plane of this muscle. With the skin and platysma incised and reflected, the contents of the anterior triangle and the surrounding area are brought into view.

The SCM muscle is a useful guide to the anterior triangle. Attached to the mastoid process of the temporal bone and the manubrium of the sternum, the muscle courses obliquely along the side of the neck. On the muscle surface, one can identify the external jugular vein together with some of its tributaries. The external jugular and the internal jugular veins cannot be confused because of the relationship of the former to the outer surface of the SCM muscle.

Lying posterior and roughly parallel with the SCM muscle are the carotid sheath and its contents. The sheath is an investment of fascia that extends up into the neck and contains within it the common carotid (medial) artery, the internal jugular vein (lateral), and the vagus nerve (between the artery and vein). The lower portion of the sheath is crossed anteriorly by the central tendon of the omohyoid muscle. Identification of this muscle can guide the embalmer to the underlying carotid sheath and provide confidence that the operation has not progressed too deep.

If the sheath is incised, the upper portion of the internal jugular vein and the common carotid artery become visible. The vein lies lateral to and partially overlaps the artery. A few variable tributaries of the internal jugular vein may be seen crossing the carotid artery in this area. The vagus nerve (cranial nerve X) can be identified between and posterior to the two vessels within the sheath.

In the upper portion of the anterior triangle, the common carotid artery divides into internal and external carotid arteries and several branches of the latter may be identified here. The internal carotid, of course, has no branches until it enters the cranium.

Common Carotid Artery

Linear Guide. Draw or visualize a line on the surface of the skin from a point over the respective sternoclavicular articulation to a point over the anterior surface of the base of the respective ear lobes.

Anatomical Guide. The right and the left common carotid arteries are located posterior to the medial border of the sternocleidomastoid muscle, on their respective sides of the neck (Figure 8–1).

Anatomical Limit. The right common carotid begins at the level of the right sternoclavicular articulation and extends to the superior border of the thyroid cartilage. The left common carotid begins at the level of the second costal cartilage and extends to the superior border of the thyroid cartilage.

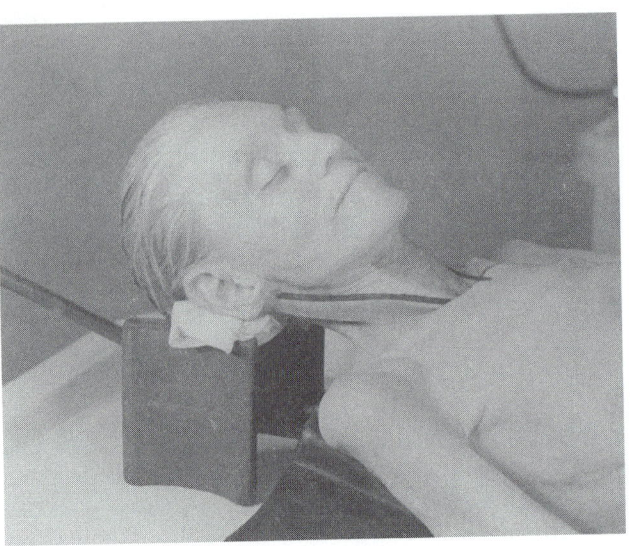

Figure 8–1. Linear and anatomical guides for the common carotid artery.

Origins. The right common carotid is a terminal branch of the brachiocephalic artery. The left common carotid is a branch off the arch of the aorta.

Branches. There are no branches of the right common carotid, except the terminal bifurcation into the right internal and external carotid arteries. The left common carotid also has no branches, except the terminal bifurcation into the left internal and external carotid arteries.

Branches of the Right and Left External Carotid Arteries. Ascending pharyngeal, superior thyroid, lingual, facial,* occipital, posterior auricular, maxillary, superficial temporal (Figure 8–2; also see Figure 9–4).

Branches of the Right and Left Internal Carotid Arteries. Branches arising within the carotid canal, ophthalmic, anterior cerebral, middle cerebral, posterior communicating, choroidal.

Relationship of the Common Carotid to the Internal Jugular Vein. The internal jugular vein lies lateral and superficial to the common carotid artery.

Contents of the Carotid Sheath. Internal jugular vein (lateral to artery), vagus nerve (between and posterior to artery and vein), common carotid artery (medial to vein) (Figure 8–3).

---

* To raise the facial artery for injection, the incision is made along the inferior border of the mandible just anterior to the angle of the jaw.

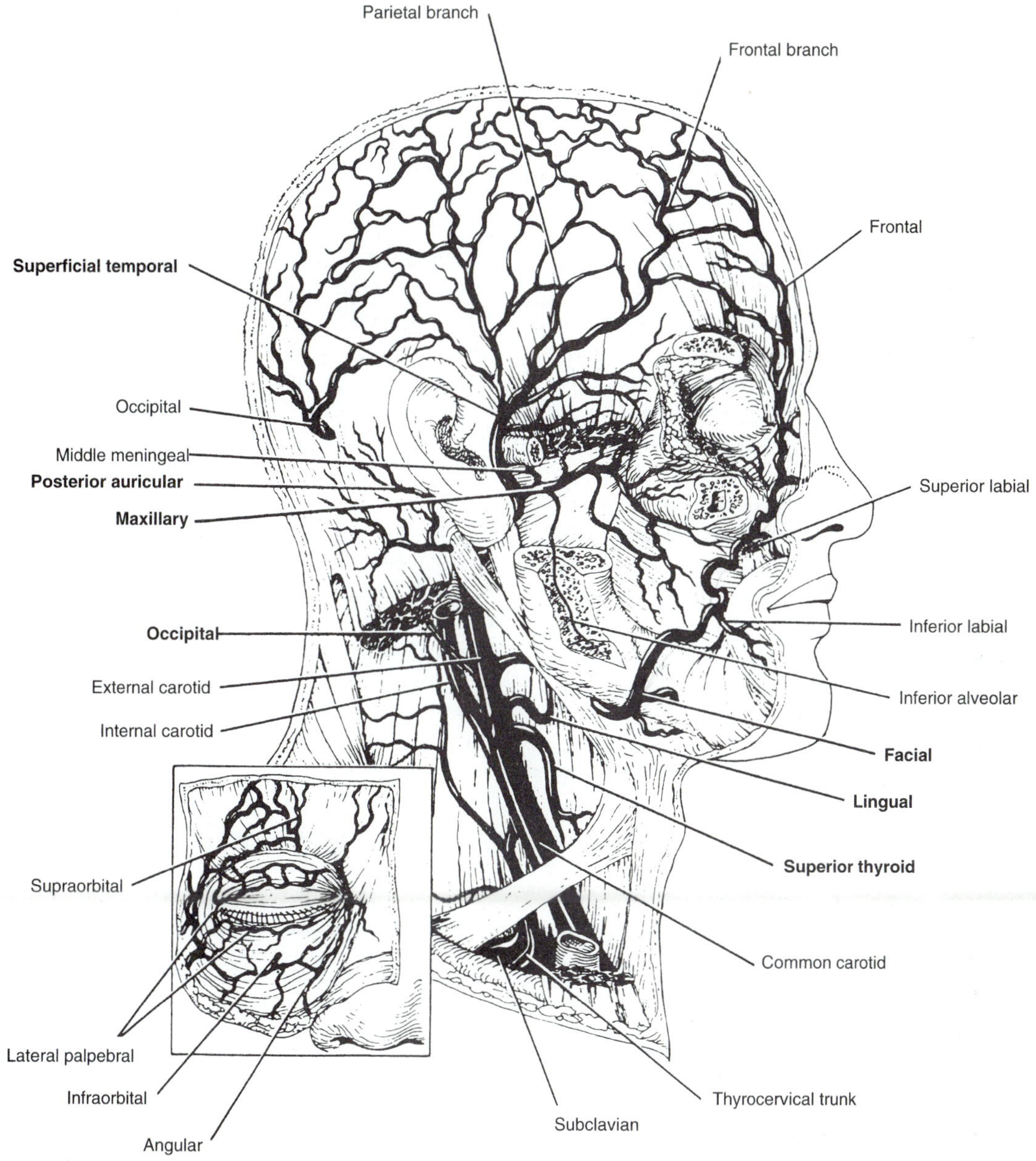

Figure 8–2. Cross section of the head and neck. Branches of the external carotid artery are shown in bold type.

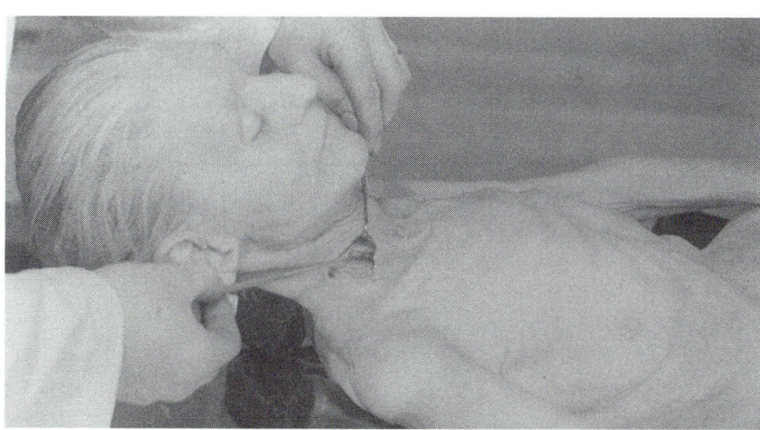

Figure 8–3. Raising the carotid artery. Note the suggested position of the embalmer. This is a posterior parallel incision.

▶ THE AXILLA—SURFACE ANATOMY

When the arm is extended (or abducted) conceptualization of the axilla is easy. Think of a truncated pyramid: four walls, a base, and an apex that has been made flat and parallel with the base. Surface landmarks of the axillary region are the ribs and intercostal muscles and the anterior and posterior axillary folds. The most obvious boundaries of the axilla are its anterior and posterior walls, which comprise the anterior and posterior axillary folds. The anterior fold can be identified by grasping (with one hand) the mass of tissue on the anterior surface of the axilla on the contralateral side of the body. Most of the substance of this fold consists of the pectoralis major muscle with contributions from the pectoralis minor and the subclavius muscles.

The posterior axillary fold can be identified by grasping (with one hand) the tissue mass on the posterior side of the axilla on the contralateral side of the body. This fold consists of the latissimus dorsi, subscapularis, and teres major muscles. The medial axillary wall consists of ribs 2 through 6, which can usually be palpated even if they are not visible on the chest surface.

The serratus anterior muscle also contributes to the medial wall but is visible as a surface feature only in lean, muscular subjects. The shaft of the humerus makes up a portion of the lateral wall, and although it cannot be seen, it is easily palpated.

The biceps brachii and coracobrachialis muscles also contribute to the lateral wall. The former is discernible in virtually all subjects, whereas the latter is clearly defined only in lean, muscular subjects. The apex of the axilla is an opening called the **cervicoaxillary canal,** which transmits structures from the neck into the arm and is bounded by three bony points of interest: the clavicle, the scapula, and the first rib. The cervicoaxillary canal is an important point of interest to the embalmer, particularly in autopsied bodies. Of the three landmarks that demarcate this canal, only the first rib is difficult to palpate. The base of the axilla is closed with dome-shaped fascia and skin on which the axillary hair is found.

Familiarity with the surface features of the axilla guides one to the important axillary contents, including the axillary artery and its six branches, the axillary vein, and the many elements of the brachial plexus. The axillary sheath invests the major structures that leave the neck and pass through the cervicoaxillary canal to enter the axilla. On opening the axillary sheath, the first structure encountered is the axillary vein. If the extremity is abducted, the vein comes to lie over the axillary artery and partially obscures it.

The six typical branches of the axillary artery are fairly consistent and the axillary artery is relatively large. Identification of the artery within the sheath may prove difficult because of the many nerves of the brachial plexus which surround and partially obscure the artery. There are three large nerve cords of the brachial plexus: medial, lateral and posterior. They are grouped around the middle portion of the axillary artery in positions corresponding to their names.

Within the axilla, the nerve cords and some of the terminal branches form specific anatomical relationships with the axillary artery, making access to the artery sometimes awkward. These are large nerves in some cases, and care must be taken to avoid confusing elements of the plexus with the axillary artery. Careful inspection and the knowledge that the nerves surround the artery will remove any confusion. *Approach to the axilla is made through an incision along the midaxillary line.*

Axillary Artery

Linear Guide. Draw or visualize a line on the surface of the skin from a point over or through the center of the base of the axillary space to a point over or through the center of the lateral border of the base of the axillary space. This line is parallel to the long axis of the abducted arm.

Anatomical Guide. The axillary artery is located just behind the medial border of the coracobrachialis muscle.

Anatomical Limit. The axillary artery extends from a point beginning at the lateral border of the first rib and extends to the inferior border of the tendon of the teres major muscle (Figure 8–4).

Origin. The axillary artery is a continuation of the subclavian artery.

Branches. Highest (supreme) thoracic artery, thoracoacromial artery, lateral thoracic artery, subscapular artery, anterior humeral circumflex artery, posterior humeral circumflex artery.

Relationship of the Axillary Artery to the Axillary Vein. The axillary artery is located lateral and deep to the axillary vein.

Incision for Raising the Axillary Vessels. The incision is made along the anterior margin of the hairline of the axilla with the arm abducted.

Brachial Artery

Linear Guide. Draw or visualize a line on the surface of the skin from a point over the center of the lateral border of the base of the axillary space to a point approximately 1 inch below and in front of the elbow joint.

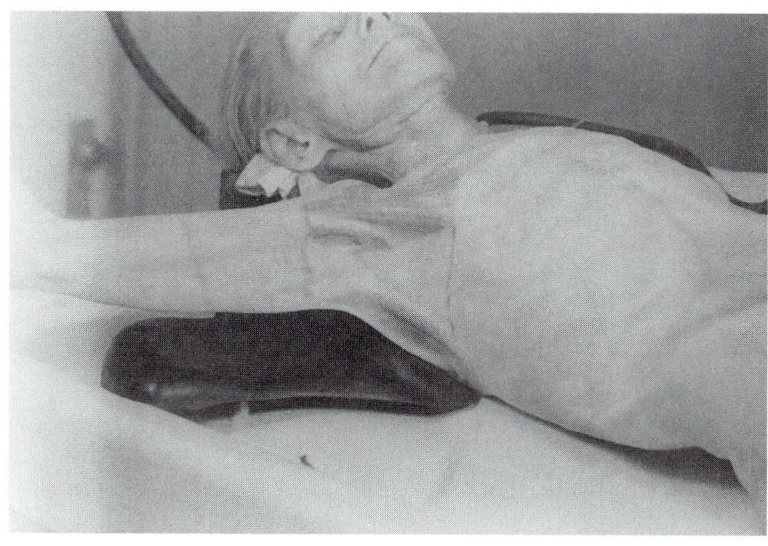

Figure 8–4. The axillary space is outlined and the location of the coracobrachialis muscle illustrated.

Anatomical Guide. The brachial artery lies in the bicipital groove at the posterior margin of the medial border of the belly of the biceps brachii muscle.

Anatomical Limit. The brachial artery extends from a point beginning at the inferior border of the tendon of the teres major muscle and extends to a point inferior to the antecubital fossa (Figure 8–5).

Origin. The brachial artery is a continuation of the axillary artery.

Relationship of the Brachial Artery and the Basilic Vein. The accompanying basilic vein is located medial and superficial to the brachial artery.

Location of the Incision. The brachial artery is usually raised by an incision made along the upper one third of the linear guide.

▶ DISTAL FOREARM

The distal forearm is the area in which the radial and ulnar arteries can be approached should they need to be raised for injection (Figure 8–6). The radial artery lies on the lateral side of the forearm and the ulnar artery on the medial side. The distal forearm permits easy access to the radial artery. Surface features of importance here are the styloid process of the radius and the tendon of the flexor carpi radialis muscle. In the interval between these two structures lies the radial artery on the anterior surface of the styloid.

A pulse may be obtained here easily in the living subject. The styloid is the most distal and lateral bony structure in the forearm, and just medial to this, one can palpate the tendon of flexor carpi radialis. In the distal region, the fleshy bellies of the muscles tend to yield to long, usually well-defined tendons. Here, a lay-

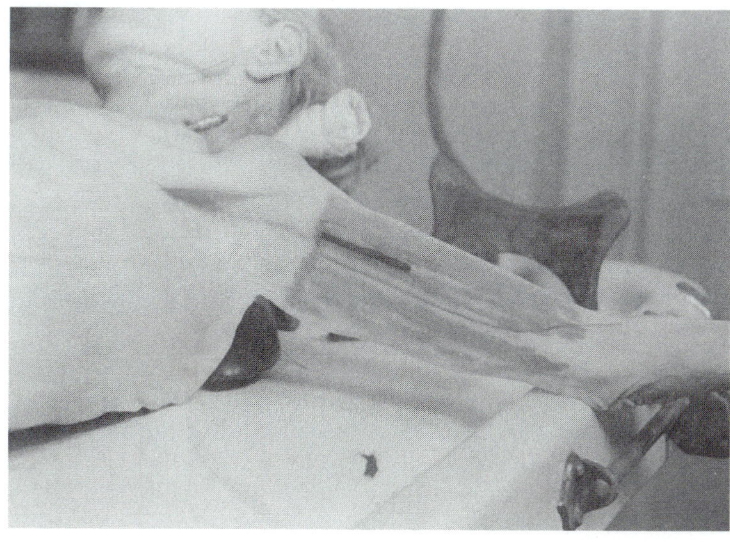

Figure 8–5. Linear guide, anatomical guide, and suggested incision location for the brachial artery.

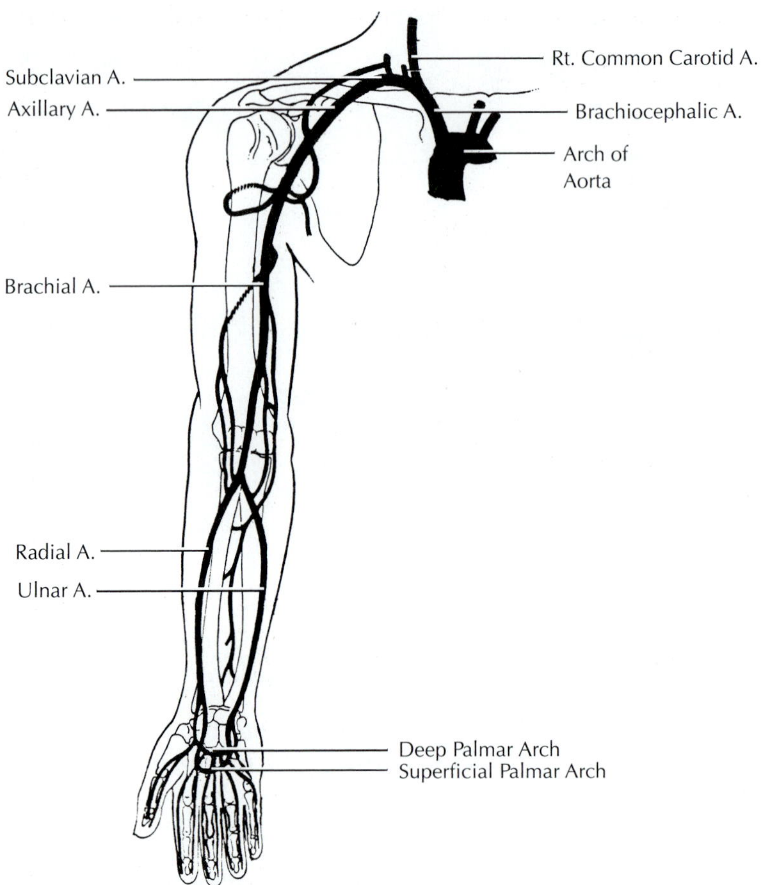

Figure 8–6. Arteries of the distal forearm.

ering of the musculature is evident. In the most superficial layer are four muscles, including the pronator teres, flexor carpi radialis, flexor carpi ulnaris, and palmaris longus. Only the tendon of the pronator teres does not reach the distal forearm.

The second layer consists of one muscle with four tendons, one each leading to digits 2–5. This muscle is the flexor digitorum superficialis. The three muscles in the deep group are the flexor digitorum profoundus, the flexor pollicis longus, and the pronator quadratus. Of these three, only the pronator has no long tendon. Some of these tendons are useful guides to the radial and ulnar arteries.

Consider first the identification of the radial artery. An additional muscle, the brachioradialis, must be introduced here. This muscle is seen partially in the flexor compartment of the forearm. It is, nevertheless, an extensor muscle. In the proximal forearm, the radial artery is overlaid by the brachioradialis muscle but at no point is the artery crossed by this or any other muscle. This situation keeps the radial artery superficial and permits easy access to it at any point along its course in the forearm. In the middle and distal forearms, the radial artery lies medial to the brachioradialis and lateral to the flexor carpi radialis. Its course is described by a line drawn from the middle of the cubital fossa to the medial side of the radial styloid process. It is easiest to approach the artery with an incision in the distal two thirds of the forearm along this line.

The ulnar artery is located on the medial side of the distal forearm. It lies between the tendon of the flexor carpi ulnaris muscle and the tendons of the flexor digitorum superficialis muscle. Here it will always be found traveling with the ulnar nerve, with which it should not be confused. Together with the venae comitantes, the nerve and artery will be found in a connective tissue sheath from which the vessels must be freed before beginning injection.

The course of the ulnar artery is indicated by a line curving medially from the midpoint of the cubital fossa to the pisiform bone in the wrist. An incision along the distal one third of this line permits access to the flexor carpi ulnaris muscle, which is then reflected medially to expose the ulnar artery.

Radial Artery

Linear Guide. Draw or visualize a line on the surface of the skin of the forearm from the center of the antecubital fossa to the center of the base of the index finger.

Anatomical Guide. The radial artery lies just lateral to the tendon of the flexor carpiradialis muscle and just medial to the tendon of the brachioradialis muscle.

Anatomical Limit. The radial artery extends from a point approximately 1 inch below and in front of the bend of the elbow to a point over the base of the thumb (thenar eminence).

Origin. The radial artery originates at the bifurcation of the brachial artery.

Relationship of the Radial Artery and the Vena Comitantes. Two small veins (venae comitantes) lie on either side of the artery. They may be helpful in locating the artery, for they generally contain some blood.

Ulnar Artery

Linear Guide. Draw or visualize a line on the surface of the skin from the center of the antecubital fossa on the forearm to a point between the fourth and fifth fingers.

Anatomical Guide. The ulnar artery lies just lateral to the tendon of the flexor carpi ulnaris muscle. (It lies between the tendons of the flexor carpi ulnaris and flexor digitorum superficialis.)

Anatomical Limit. The ulnar artery extends from a point approximately 1 inch below and in front of the bend of the elbow to a point over the pisiform bone (hypothenar eminence).

Origin. The ulnar artery originates at the bifurcation of the brachial artery.

Relationship of the Ulnar Artery to the Venae Comitantes. Two small veins (venae comitantes) lie on either side of the artery. They can be useful in locating the artery for they generally contain some blood.

▶ ARTERIES OF THE BODY TRUNK

Table 8–1 outlines the arteries of the body trunk and their branches (Figure 8–7).

TABLE 8–1. ARTERIES OF THE BODY TRUNK

Artery	Description	Branches
Ascending aorta	Originates at the left ventricle; at its beginning the aortic semilunar valve should close, thus creating the pathway for arterial solution distribution	Right coronary artery Left coronary artery
Arch of the aorta	Center of arterial solution distribution	Brachiocephalic artery Left common carotid artery Left subclavian artery
Right subclavian	Begins of the right sternoclavicular articulation and extends to the lateral border of the first rib; in the complete autopsy (with neck organs removed), the branches need to be clamped	Vertebral artery Internal thoracic artery Inferior thyroid
Left subclavian	Begins at the level of the left second costal cartilage and extends to the lateral border of the first rib	
Descending thoracic aorta		Its branches include nine pairs of thoracic intercostal arteries
Descending abdominal aorta	Extends from the diaphragm to the lower border of the fourth lumbar vertebra	Parietal Inferior phrenic Superior suprarenals Lumbar Middle sacral Visceral (unpaired) Celiac axis Superior mesenteric Inferior mesenteric Visceral (paired) Middle suprarenals Renals Internal spermatic (male), ovarian (female) Common iliacs (terminal)

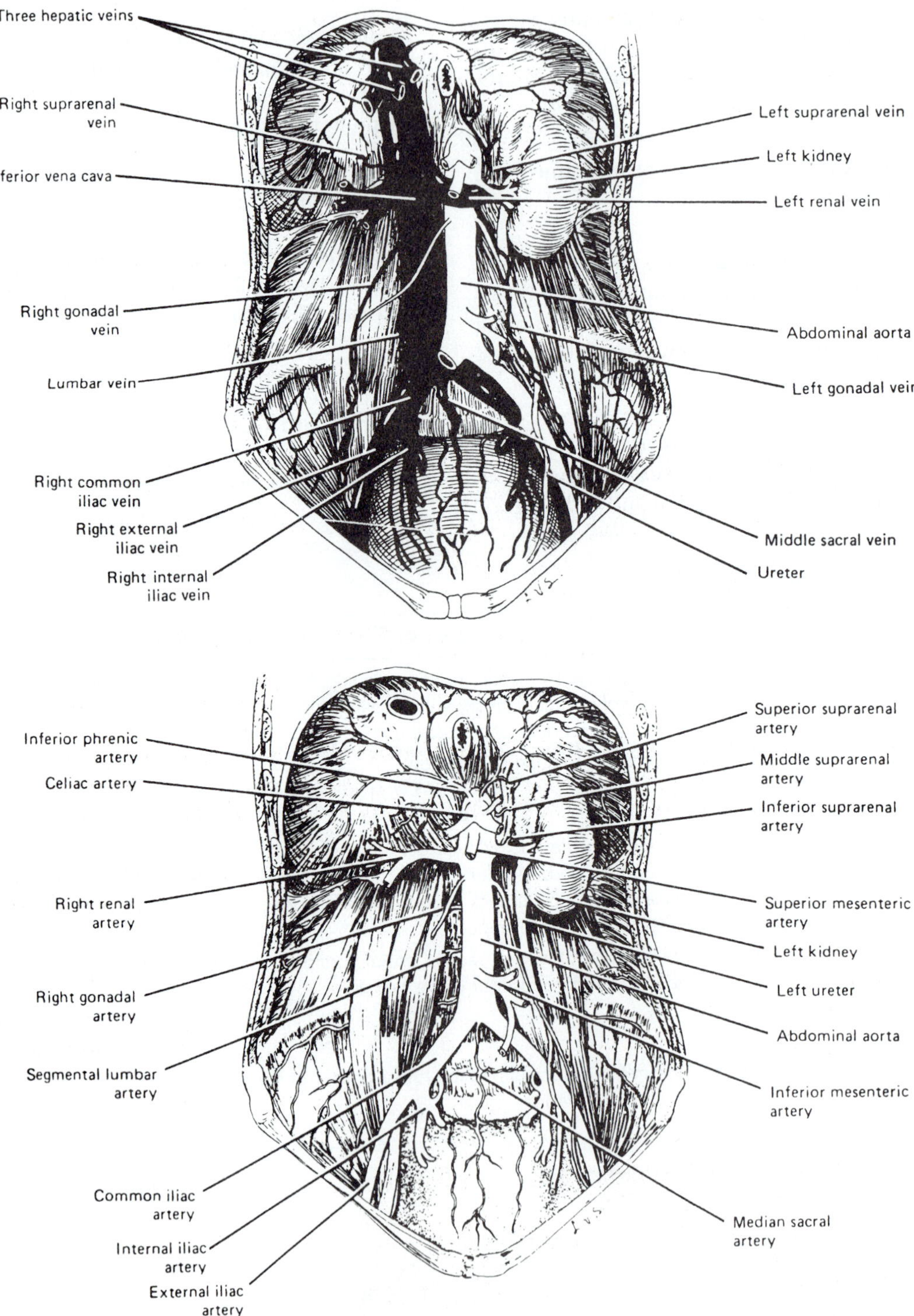

Figure 8–7. Arteries and veins of the body trunk.

In embalming infants the ascending aorta (as it leaves the heart) or abdominal aorta can be used for injection points. A midsternal incision is used for the ascending aorta. An incision from the xiphoid process directed downward and to the left of the midline is used to raise the abdominal aorta.

In the adult, where partial autopsies have been performed or visceral organs are donated without autopsy, the abdominal or thoracic aorta can be used as a point of arterial injection.

External Iliac Artery and Vein

Mention should be made of the use of the external iliac artery and vein as a site for arterial injection and blood drainage (Figure 8–8). The external iliac artery is a continuation of the common iliac artery (the common iliac is one of the terminal branches of the abdominal aorta). The external iliac artery extends to a point under the center of the inguinal ligament. The artery lies exactly at this ligament lateral to the external iliac vein.

In the autopsied body this artery is used for the injection of the lower extremities. Injecting the external iliac artery rather than the common iliac in the autopsied body eliminates the need to clamp off the internal iliac artery (which usually has been cut during the removal of the pelvic organs). In the unautopsied body, when the body is very obese, the femoral vessels are located very deep and are hard to work with; however, the external iliac artery where it passes under the inguinal ligament is quite superficial, and this can be a good location if there is a need to use this vessel in the unautopsied obese body.

Because insertion of an artery tube into the femoral artery (directed toward the upper area of the body) actually places the tip of the tube into the external iliac artery, the term *iliofemoral* is used by many embalmers to indicate use of the vessels at a site near the inguinal ligament.

▶ INGUINAL REGION

The inguinal region is an area below the inguinal ligament in which the femoral vessels may be approached for injection and drainage. As a rule, the subcutaneous tissue in the thigh masks underlying soft tissue structures, so the embalmer must rely on bony landmarks in this area. Fortunately, the anterior superior spine of the ilium and pubic tubercle are easily identified. These two bony processes serve as attachments for the inguinal ligament. The positions of the underlying femoral vessels can be identified if the operator begins by placing the thumb of the left hand on the subject's right anterior superior iliac spine and the left middle finger on the subject's right pubic tubercle. If the operator's left index finger is now allowed to bisect the interval between his thumb and middle finger (i.e., bisect the inguinal ligament), the tip of the index finger will indicate the approximate position of the femoral vessels in the thigh. The procedure can be repeated on the subject's left side using the operator's right hand. The incision to raise the vessel can be made on the linear guide.

▶ FEMORAL TRIANGLE

The inguinal ligament serves as the base for this triangle whose two sides consist of the medial border of the sartorius and the lateral border of the adductor longus muscles (Figure 8–9). In addition to skin and subcutaneous tissue covering the triangle, the roof consists of a dense sheet of fascia, the fascia lata, which attaches firmly to the inguinal ligament and encircles the thigh. This roof must be incised to expose the boundaries and contents of the triangle.

Lying on the surface of the fascia lata is the great saphenous vein which has coursed up the medial aspect of the thigh all the way from the foot. The operator should not mistake the great saphenous for the femoral

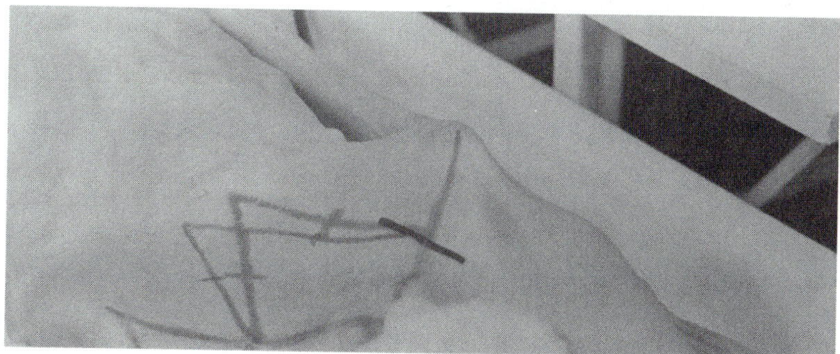

Figure 8–8. Incision location for left external iliac vessels. The linear guides are also shown.

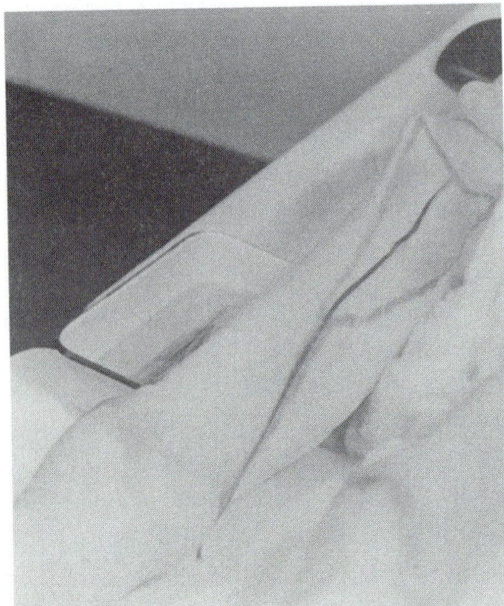

Figure 8–9. Femoral triangle showing the linear guide for the femoral vessels.

vein. This potential mistake can be avoided simply by remembering anatomic relationships. **If the vein in question is lying on the surface of the dense, white fascia lata and if the fascia lata has not yet been incised, then the vein must be the great saphenous or one of its tributaries.**

If the great saphenous is followed, it disappears through an opening in the fascia lata called the fossa ovalis. This opening is not so glamorous as some textbooks would have one believe. Rather, there is a hiatus in the fascia lata and the great saphenous insinuates itself through the fascia and empties directly into the femoral vein. So it is clear that identification of the great saphenous will lead directly to the femoral vein near the base of the femoral triangle. Around the hiatus one is likely to encounter inguinal lymph nodes, which may have to be resected.

When the roof of the triangle is incised and reflected, the contents and borders come into view. The femoral vessels are contained within the femoral sheath, which is a continuation into the thigh of abdominal wall and pelvic fascias. The sheath is subdivided into three compartments which, from lateral to medial, contain the femoral artery, femoral vein, and lymphatic vessels and nodes. The most medial compartment is designated the femoral canal and is the site of femoral hernias. Therefore, a femoral hernia is always situated medial to the femoral vein. This relationship is an important one to remember if preparing a subject whose inguinal region is distorted (such as with a hernia).

To gain access to the femoral vessels, open each of the other two compartments separately. An incision in the sheath over each vessel will cause the artery and vein to be delivered easily. At the base of the triangle, the artery lies slightly anterior and lateral to the femoral vein and its position may be identified at the midpoint of the inguinal ligament. The vessels are best approached 1 to 2 inches from the base of the triangle, where they lie side by side and are easily accessible.

As the vessels approach the apex of the triangle, their relationship shifts to an anteroposterior one so that the femoral artery, femoral vein, deep femoral vein, and deep femoral artery lie one in front of the other, making access to most of them somewhat difficult.

The most lateral structure at the base of the femoral triangle is the femoral nerve, which lies outside the femoral sheath. This very substantial nerve and its many branches should not be confused with the adjacent femoral artery because the nerve lies without the sheath.

The floor of the triangle is entirely muscular and different authors consider that either two or three muscles constitute the floor. Laterally, the iliopsoas muscle emerges beneath the inguinal ligament. Just medial to this lies the pectineus muscle. Certainly these two muscles contribute to the floor of the triangle. The disagreement comes about as a result of whether the medial or lateral border of the adductor longus muscle is considered to be the medial boundary of the triangle. The distinction is academic but in this text the adductor longus is treated as part of the floor for the following reason. The triangle is easily visualized in terms of the number 3. There are three borders: the inguinal ligament, the sartorius muscle, and the adductor longus muscle. Basically, three structures are contained within the triangle: the femoral nerve, the femoral artery, and the femoral vein. Each of these has branches or tributaries, but three major structures are present. Finally, if the adductor longus is considered to be a part of the floor, there are three muscles in the floor: the iliopsoas, the pectineus, and the adductor longus.

At the apex of the femoral triangle the femoral vessels, but not the femoral nerve, enter the subsartorial or adductor canal. Recognizing the relationships of the femoral artery and vein at the triangle apex facilitates the understanding of the anatomical relationships of these vessels after they emerge from the adductor canal and enter the popliteal fossa or space.

Femoral Artery

Linear Guide. Draw or visualize a line on the surface of the skin of the thigh from the center of the inguinal ligament to the center of the medial prominence of the knee (medial condyle of the femur).

Anatomical Guide. The femoral artery passes through the center of the femoral triangle and is bounded laterally by the medial border of the sartorius muscle and medially by the adductor longus muscle.

Anatomical Limit. The femoral artery extends from a point behind the center of the inguinal ligament to the opening in the adductor magnus muscle (Figure 8–10).

Origin. The femoral artery is a continuation of the external iliac artery.

Branches. Superficial epigastric, superficial circumflex iliac, external pudendal, profunda femoris.

Relationship of the Femoral Artery and Vein. The femoral artery lies lateral and superficial to the femoral vein.

Popliteal Fossa

On the posterior aspect of the knee two sets of tendons and two fleshy muscle heads can be identified. This describes the popliteal fossa as a trapezoid and can be subdivided into an upper femoral and lower tibial triangle.

The femoral triangle (not to be confused with the femoral triangle in the inguinal region) is bounded laterally by the long and short heads of the biceps femoris and medially by the tendons of the semimembranosus and semitendinosus muscles. The tibial triangle is limited medially and laterally by the diverging medial and lateral fleshy heads of the gastrocnemius muscle and, to a lesser extent, by the plantaris muscle laterally. The base of each triangle is an imaginary line drawn through the middle of the joint. These surface landmarks serve as guides to the underlying popliteal vessels within the boundaries of the space.

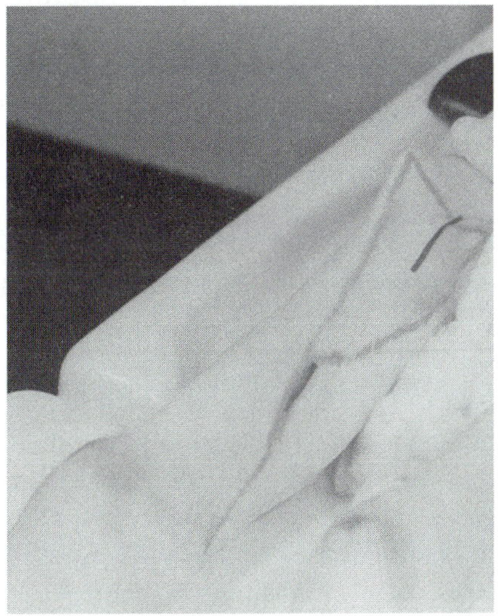

Figure 8–10. Incision for the right femoral vessels.

The muscular boards of this fossa are overlaid by a roof of deep fascia, subcutaneous tissue, and skin. Intrusion into this space provides access to the popliteal vessels for injection and drainage. After recognizing and dispatching minor vascular and nervous branches external to the deep fascia, the fascia is incised to gain access to the vessels. The major contents of the space include the tibial and peroneal nerves (from the sciatic) and their branches, the popliteal vein and its tributaries, the popliteal artery and its branches, and a good deal of fat and lymphatic tissue.

As the space is approached posteriorly, the first structures to be encountered are the tibial and peroneal nerves. The tibial nerve is the larger of the two and is located directly in the midline. The common peroneal nerve, on the other hand, leaves the sciatic nerve at about midthigh and courses down the lateral aspect of the popliteal space.

With the tibial nerve retracted, the popliteal vein comes into view, lying superficial (posterior) to the *popliteal artery, which is the deepest (most anterior) structure in the fossa.* Remember that this relationship was established as these vessels entered the adductor canal. The vessels are bound together by connective tissue, which must be loosened and reflected to gain access to the vessels. Several branches and tributaries of the vessels are also found in the fossa, but these need not be identified by name here.

Deep (anterior) to the popliteal artery, the floor of the fossa is formed by the lower end of the femur and a portion of the capsule surrounding the knee joint.

Linear Guide. Draw or visualize a line on the surface of the skin from the center of the superior border of the popliteal space parallel to the long axis of the lower extremity to the center of the inferior border of the popliteal space.

Anatomical Guide. The popliteal vessels are located between the popliteal surface of the femur and the oblique popliteal ligament.

Anatomical Limit. The popliteal artery extends from a point beginning at the opening of the adductor magnus muscle to the lower border of the popliteus muscle.

Origin. The popliteal artery is a continuation of the femoral artery.

Branches. Five pairs of genicular arteries, muscular branches.

Relationship of the Popliteal Artery and Vein. The vein lies posterior and medial to the artery. Because of the location of these vessels the vein can also be described as lying superficial to the artery.

▶ DISTAL LEG

In the distal leg the superficiality of the anterior tibial artery makes it easily accessible as an injection site. The popliteal artery ends by dividing into two terminal branches: the anterior tibial artery and the posterior tibial artery. The branches begin at the lower border of the popliteus muscle. In the distal portion of the leg the arteries become superficial and can be used as points of injection for the foot. Injection could also be made toward the head to embalm the distal leg and thigh (Figure 8–11).

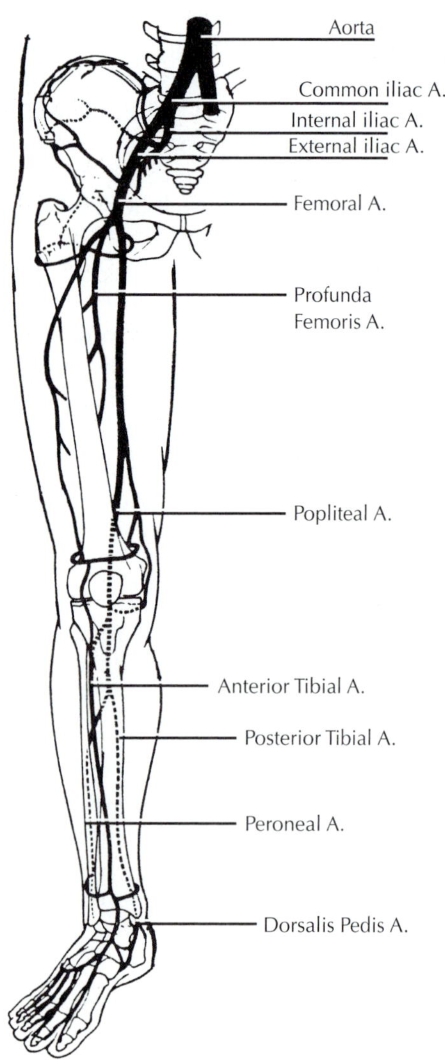

Figure 8–11. Arteries of the distal leg.

The anterior tibial artery is the smaller of the terminal branches of the popliteal artery. As it approaches the distal portion of the leg it becomes very superficial. It can be raised by making an incision just above the ankle, just lateral to the crest of the tibia. In front of the ankle joint the anterior tibial artery now becomes the dorsalis pedis artery.

The posterior tibial artery is also one of the terminal branches of the popliteal artery and passes posteriorly and medially down the leg. In the area between the medial malleolus and the calcaneus bone, the artery can be raised by the embalmer for injection of the foot. The artery terminates by dividing into the medial and lateral plantar arteries.

Anterior and Posterior Tibial Arteries

Linear Guide. *Anterior Tibial Artery:* Draw or visualize a line from the lateral border of the patella to the anterior surface of the ankle joint. *Posterior Tibial Artery:* Draw or visualize a line on the surface of the skin from the center of the popliteal space to a point midway between the medial malleolus and the calcaneus bone.

Anatomical Guide. *Anterior Tibial Artery:* The anterior tibial vessels are located in a groove between the tibialis anterior muscle and the tendon of the extensor hallucis longus muscle. *Posterior Tibial Artery:* The posterior tibial vessels are located between the posterior border of the tibia and the calcaneus tendon.

Anatomical Limit. *Anterior Tibial Artery:* The anterior tibial artery extends from a point beginning at the inferior border of the popliteus muscle to a point in front of the middle of the ankle joint on the respective sides. *Posterior Tibial Artery:* The posterior tibial artery extends from a point beginning at the inferior border of the popliteus muscle to a point over and between the medial malleolus and the calcaneus of the respective foot.

Branches and Tributaries of the Vessels. *Anterior Tibial Vessels, Posterior Tibial Vessels:* right and left peroneal branches, right and left dorsalis pedis arteries.

▶ FOOT

Tendons passing onto the dorsum of the foot from the leg pass posterior to and are restrained by two thickenings of fascia, the superior and inferior extensor retinacula, which lie anterior to the ankle. Additionally, the anterior tibial artery and the deep peroneal nerve also pass deep to these retinacula. Only inconsequential superficial nerves and veins lie superficial to these retinacula.

Skin on the dorsum of the foot is thin and loosely applied. The subcutaneous tissue permits easy visualization of the venous network, which is so prominent here.

Tendons of two extrinsic muscles of the foot, the extensor hallucis longus and the extensor digitorum longus, are easily identified as they pass to the great toe and digits 2–5, respectively. The dorsalis pedis artery is situated in the interosseous spaces between the tendon of extensor hallucis longus and the first tendon of extensor digitorum longus as it passes to the second digit. An incision made from a point midway between the medial and lateral malleoli to the interosseous space will provide access to the dorsalis pedis artery.

Linear Guide (Dorsalis Pedis Artery). Draw or visualize a line from the center of the anterior surface of the ankle joint to a point between the first and second toes.

▶ CONCLUSIONS

The anatomy of several potential injection sites has been considered. More than just vascular anatomy has been presented with the hope that complete familiarity with the anatomy of these regions will facilitate the work of the practitioner. Being aware of the anatomy peripheral to the blood vessels at an injection site and having a solid command of anatomical relationships in these areas should make the embalmer more comfortable with and more confident in his or her operations.

▶ KEY TERMS AND CONCEPTS FOR STUDY AND DISCUSSION

1. Describe the anatomical position.
2. Define anatomical guide, linear guide, and anatomical limit.
3. Give the anatomical limits of the right and the left common carotid arteries.
4. Give the linear guide and the anatomical guide for the common carotid artery.
5. Give the anatomical guide for the facial artery.
6. List the eight branches of the external carotid artery and the areas they supply.
7. Give the bony boundaries of the cervicoaxillary canal.
8. Give the linear and anatomical guides and anatomical limits for the axillary and brachial arteries.
9. Describe the relationship of the internal jugular vein to the common carotid artery; axillary vein to the axillary artery.
10. Give the extent of the axillary artery.
11. Give the linear and anatomical guide for the radial and ulnar arteries.
12. List the branches, from right to left, of the arch of the aorta and the visceral and parietal branches of the abdominal aorta.
13. Give the anatomical and linear guides, and anatomical limits for the femoral artery.
14. Describe the relationship of the femoral artery to the femoral vein.
15. Give the linear guides for the popliteal artery, anterior tibial artery, posterior tibial artery and dorsalis pedis artery.

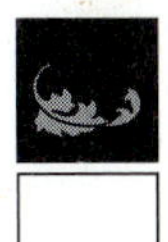

CHAPTER 9
EMBALMING VESSEL SITES AND SELECTIONS

There are several anatomical locations on the dead human body at which arteries and veins may be elevated for the injection of chemical preservatives and subsequent drainage. One of the major objectives of making a preembalming analysis of the body is selection of the most logical and satisfactory vessels to employ for injection and drainage.

The proper selection of vessels should facilitate the most satisfactory results. This selection is based on a variety of intrinsic and extrinsic factors. Embalming analysis is not simply preembalming evaluation. During injection of the body, it may become necessary to select other vessels for injection and drainage. Therefore, an analysis of the progress of the embalming becomes necessary throughout the entire process.

▶ TERMINOLOGY

Vascular Injection Procedures

One-Point Injection. An artery and vein at one location are used for injection and drainage (e.g., injection from the right common carotid artery and drainage from the right internal jugular vein, or injection from the right femoral artery and drainage from the right femoral vein).

Split Injection. The injection is made in an artery at one location and the drainage occurs from a vein at another location (e.g., injection of the right common carotid artery and drainage from the right femoral vein, or injection from the right femoral artery and drainage from the right internal jugular vein).

Restricted Cervical Injection. Both right and left common carotid arteries are raised; tubes are placed into them directed toward the head on both the right and the left side. One tube is directed toward the trunk into the right artery; the inferior portion of the left artery is ligated. Drainage is generally taken from the right internal jugular vein. Some embalmers prefer to open and drain from both the right and left internal jugular veins if the face is badly discolored. During downward injection (toward the trunk), the arterial tubes directed toward the head **remain open.**

Multipoint Injection. Multipoint injection is vascular injection from two or more arteries (e.g., injection is begun from the right femoral artery but the embalming solution does not distribute to the left leg or the left arm; subsequently, the left femoral and the left brachial arteries are raised and injected). Restricted cervical injection, six-point injection and sectional vascular injection are all examples of multipoint injection.

Sectional Vascular Embalming. The embalming of an entire body region is called sectional vascular embalming. Frequently in the unautopsied body the embalming will begin with a one-point injection, and clots freed in the large arteries will move to smaller arteries and block arterial solution from entering an entire body region, such as one of the extremities or side of the head. It then becomes necessary to separately inject this body region; this is sectional injection. The following is a list of the body regions and the artery(s) which can be injected to embalm each area (examples include autopsied and unautopsied selections):

face and head	common carotid artery
upper extremity	subclavian, axillary, brachial artery
hand	radial or ulnar artery
lower extremity	common iliac, external iliac, femoral artery
body trunk	in the unautopsied body, injection of any major artery, injecting toward the trunk region

Sectional embalming is necessary in the preparation of the autopsied body, and is a type of multipoint injection.

Six-Point Injection. Six arteries are raised that will separately inject the head and the limbs: right and left common carotid arteries, right and left axillary (or brachial) arteries, and right and left femoral (or external iliac) arteries. Drainage can be taken from each location or from one location such as the right internal jugular vein. In the autopsied body a six-point injection may include the right and left common carotid artery to embalm the head; right and left subclavian (axillary or brachial) artery to embalm the upper extremity; and right and left common iliac (external iliac or femoral) artery to embalm the lower extremity.

▶ VESSEL SELECTION

Two of the most important objectives in making the embalming analysis of the body is the selection of an artery (or arteries) for injection of arterial solution and the selection of a vein for drainage.

In the unautopsied body the arteries most frequently used for embalming the body are the common carotid, femoral and the axillary arteries. Because of the value of using an accompanying vein for drainage, the femoral and common carotid vessels are preferred over the axillary artery. If a one-point or a restricted cervical injection plan is used by the embalmer after a sufficient quantity of arterial solution has been injected (perhaps one gallon), the embalmer must evaluate what areas of the body **are** receiving arterial solution and what areas **are not** receiving arterial solution. Various embalming techniques can be used in an attempt to stimulate the flow of the solution into the body areas where the solution is lacking. Once the embalmer is satisfied that all body regions have sufficient arterial solution, those areas where there is insufficient solution can be separately injected by sectional embalming. With sectional embalming an evaluation must also be made; if the preservative is not reaching all areas of a body region, perhaps more distant arteries can be raised and injected (e.g. the axillary artery may have been raised to inject the right arm; if solution is not entering the hand the radial or ulnar artery can be raised and injected). After sectional injection an evaluation must again be made. If there is still insufficient solution in an area supplemental methods of embalming (e.g. hypodermic or surface compresses) must be used.

A similar protocol of working from major arteries which supply large regions, to smaller arteries which supply localized body areas, and finally the possible use of supplemental embalming treatments, is utilized in the embalming of the autopsied body.

To summarize a pattern of vessel selection, injection and observation is as follows:

1. Select artery(s) for injection of the body and a vein for drainage.
2. Inject.
3. Observe and evaluate.
4. If needed perform sectional embalming.
5. Inject.
6. Observe and evaluate.
7. If needed perform supplemental embalming treatments, hypodermic and surface compresses or gels.

General Considerations

The right side of the body is used for several reasons. Most embalmers are right-handed and find working on the right side of the body much easier. In addition, if the internal jugular vein is to be used for drainage, the right internal jugular leads directly into the right atrium of the heart and drainage instruments are much easier and more effective when inserted into the right internal jugular vein. It should be pointed out that selecting the left common carotid or left femoral vessels for injection points would afford the same advantages. There are a number of arguments against the use of axillary or brachial vessels as primary points of injection.

Selection of an injection plan involves two criteria: factors concerning the artery or vein itself and general body conditions.

The embalmer should be able to locate and raise all the major vessels of the body without any difficulty. The routes of the vessels can be determined by the surface linear guides, and the embalmer should be thoroughly acquainted with the deeper anatomical relationships so the vessels can be located. ***It is of primary importance that the embalmer be able to locate arteries of the body.*** Drainage can always be taken from a separate vein or directly from the heart, but arterial solution supply into a particular body region must be by way of the arterial system.

Situations in which it may be necessary to isolate severed or cut portions of arteries to inject arterial embalming fluid for preservation include bodies on which extensive autopsies have been performed, bodies on which partial autopsies have been performed or from which only one or more organs and/or tissues for transplantation have been removed, and bodies resulting from traumatic accidents.

Arteries, veins, and nerves tend to be grouped together in their routes through the body. It is essential that the embalmer be able to distinguish between these structures (Table 9–1).

Nerves have a silvery appearance and, when examined with the naked eye, show striations along their surface. When cut, they have no lumen or opening and their cut edges take on a frayed appearance similar to the cut ends of a rope.

Veins are thinner than arteries. They contain valves, which arteries do not, but like arteries, when cut they

TABLE 9–1. COMPARISON OF ARTERIES, VEINS, AND NERVES

Artery	Vein	Nerve
Lumen Creamy white	Lumen Bluish when filled with blood	Solid structure Silvery white
Thick walls are demonstrated when artery is rolled between two fingers; edges of the artery easily felt	When vein is rolled between two fingers, walls collapse and edges are not felt	Solid structure is demonstrated when nerve is rolled between two fingers
Vasa vasorum may be seen on surface	Vasa vasorum not visible	Vasa vasorum not visible
Remain open when cut	Collapse when cut	Solid when cut; ends tend to fray
Generally empty of blood	Generally same blood or clotted material present	No blood present

do have an opening or lumen. When their sides are cut, veins collapse, creating a funnel effect.

Arteries have very thick walls as compared with healthy veins. Arteries are creamy white in appearance, and often, small vessels called the **vasa vasorum** can be seen over the artery surface (especially in arteries exhibiting arteriosclerosis). The most distinguishing feature of an artery is that if it is cut, the lumen remains open and very pronounced. The walls of the artery, unlike those of the vein, do not collapse. In addition, arteries are quite elastic and can easily be stretched after dissection and cleaning. It is most important that the embalmer be familiar with the relationship of arteries to veins where vessels are raised.

▶ SELECTING AN ARTERY AS AN INJECTION POINT

The selection of an artery or arteries for embalming is based on conditions of the individual artery and conditions of the body. Considerations and precautions for each individual artery are first based upon its accessibility with respect to these questions:

1. How superficial or deep is the artery?
2. What structure surround the artery?
3. How close to the aorta is the artery?
4. What is the diametric size of the artery?
5. Can the body be positioned properly if this artery is used?
6. Will incisions for the artery be on an exposed body area?
7. Can drainage be taken from the vein which accompanies the artery?

Second, consideration of what arterial occlusions might be associated with an artery would include: (1) Is arterial clotting present and in what direction will these clots move upon injection?; and (2) What amount of arteriosclerosis is present in the artery?

Other factors governing the selection of an artery or arteries for injection include:

1. Age of the deceased.
2. Sex of the individual with respect to the type of clothing which will be worn.
3. Weight.
4. Fat distribution.
5. Disfigurations present (e.g., arthritic conditions, tumors or scar tissue).
6. Diseases present.
7. Edema, localized or generalized.
8. Location of obstructions or congestion, possibly creating discolorations or a lack of preservative solution flow to a body region.
9. Trauma present from mutilation, accident or surgery.
10. Medico-legal requirements with reguard to autopsies; preparation for medical schools; preparation for international shipping; preparation under military contracts; requirements of a coroner or medical examiner.
11. Cause of the death.
12. Manner of the death.

In addition to these twenty-one variables, two nonvariable guidelines must be considered: (1) Prepare each body with the assumption that the body is dead from an infectious and contagious disease. (2) Prepare each body with the assumption that final disposition and viewing will be delayed.

With respect to size (diameter) of an artery, of the four choices for an injection point, the common carotid artery is the largest, because it is nearest to the heart. The femoral (or external iliac) is the second in size, and the axillary artery is the smallest in diameter. Actually, any artery could be used to inject the entire body, but the use of a vessel such as the radial or ulnar to embalm the entire body allows for a very slow rate of flow of arterial solution. In addition, it is difficult to build sufficient pressure in the arterial system to properly distribute and diffuse the arterial solution. The larger, more elastic arteries such as the common carotid and the femoral allow for use of the higher pressures and faster rates of flow that are often necessary to achieve uniform distribution of the arterial solution.

As for the accessibility of the artery, deep-seated vessels within the thorax or the abdomen are very difficult to use for injection of the adult body. In infants and children these vessels can be considered, for they are easier to reach. In the unautopsied adult body, vessels near the surface of the skin and with few branches can easily be raised to the surface of the incision. The common carotid arteries do not have branches (except their terminals) and, thus, can easily be raised to the skin surface. Likewise, the femoral arteries and the external iliac arteries (at the inguinal ligament) are not held tightly in position by large numbers of branches.

Presence of an accompanying vein is one of the most important factors in selecting an artery for injection of arterial solution. This accompanying vein is also a potential point of drainage. The common carotid artery is accompanied by the large internal jugular vein. On the right side of the neck this vein leads directly into the right atrium of the heart, and the right atrium is the center of drainage.

The size of the artery, its accessibility, and, finally, the possibility of draining from the accompanying vein must be considered in selecting an artery for injection. As previously stated, in the unautopsied adult body, this choice is among four vessels: (1) the common carotid artery, (2) the right and left common carotid arteries, (3) the femoral artery (or external iliac if raised at the inguinal ligament), and (4) the axillary artery (or brachial artery).

The second group of factors that must be considered (and the most important and variable factors in selection of a vessel for injection) is the condition of the body or the external conditions that influence the choice of a vessel.

1. Age of the Body
   A. In the infant, additional vessels may be considered for injection such as the ascending aorta or the abdominal aorta.
   B. With respect to infants, the size of the artery may be the factor that determines which vessel can be used. The common carotid is the largest. A set of small infant arterial tubes should always be available.
   C. In the elderly, many times the femoral vessel is found to be sclerotic; the common carotid artery is rarely found to exhibit arteriosclerosis.
2. Weight of the Body
   A. In obese bodies the femoral artery is found quite deep in the upper thigh. Its depth should not preclude its possible use. If the vessel must be raised it should be raised at the inguinal ligament, or the external iliac artery can be used. At this location the vessel is the most superficial.
   B. Drainage is also a factor to consider with obese bodies. The internal jugular vein affords the best clearing of the body, especially the tissues of the face. Keep in mind that the weight of the viscera in heavy bodies provides resistance to the flow of arterial solution as well as resistance to drainage.
   C. In obese bodies large quantities of arterial solution are needed to adequately preserve the body. To avoid distension of facial tissues, it is best to select the right and the left common carotid arteries, which would be raised at the start of embalming.

      The best approach to embalming obese bodies is to raise both right and left common carotid arteries (restricted cervical injection) and use the right internal jugular vein for drainage. In this manner large volumes (often of a strong solution) can be injected. This allows the use of higher injection pressures and faster rates of flow. It minimizes the necessity of raising other vessels, and in the obese body, especially if edema is also present in the tissues, the raising of secondary vessels can be very difficult.
   D. With very thin bodies care should be taken to minimize any destruction of the sternocleidomastoid muscle of the neck. It generally is very pronounced. All other factors taken into consideration, use of the femoral vessels, if possible, might prove advantageous in the preparation of these bodies.
3. Disease Conditions
   A. A condition such as arthritis may necessitate the avoidance of certain body areas; legs can be in the fetal position in the elderly or in bodies that have suffered from certain brain tumors, making use of the femoral vessel quite difficult (see Figure 11–8).
   B. A goiter condition in the neck may make use of the carotid artery and the jugular vein difficult, because the vessels will be pushed out of their normal location.
   C. Tumors or swollen lymph nodes in the neck, groin, or axillary area should be avoided for injection.
   D. Burned tissues should be avoided if possible; leakage will be a problem and suturing will be difficult.
   E. When edema is present in an area such as the upper thigh, raising a vessel should be avoided in this area; closure (suturing) may be difficult and leakage a problem. When edema is generalized (anasarca), large quantities of arterial solution must be injected. Here it would be

best to use restricted cervical injection, raising both the right and left common carotid arteries. This allows the embalmer to inject large quantities of arterial solution. Many times, these arterial solutions are very strong. The restricted cervical injection allows the use of large amounts of fluid to saturate other body areas without overinjecting the face. A separate, milder solution can then be used for injection of the head.

F. A *ruptured aortic aneurysm* dictates what additional (or secondary) arteries must be injected. Because, many times, arteriosclerosis is responsible for a ruptured aortic aneurysm, the common carotid would be the most logical vessel to use as a starting point for injection. Often, some circulation can be established in these conditions. In the majority, there is direct loss of all arterial fluid to the abdominal cavity, necessitating six-point injection of the body and treatment of the trunk walls, buttocks, and shoulders by hypodermic embalming.

G. When *scar tissue* is seen in a location where a vessel is to be raised (such as the upper inguinal area), no doubt surgery has been performed. Scar tissue beneath the skin can be very difficult to work with in raising vessels, and it may be wise, if possible, to use another vessel. If desiring to inject on the right side of the body it is suggested the left side be used.

H. *Gangrene,* particularly in the lower extremities, indicates the possibility that the deceased suffered from diabetes and that there is poor blood supply into the affected limb(s). Most often that poor blood supply is the result of arteriosclerosis. For example, if the foot or lower leg evidences gangrene, or a recent amputation is evident, the femoral vessel should be avoided as the primary injection point. Use of the carotid arteries is advised, because generally, little arteriosclerosis is associated with these vessels.

4. Interruption of the Vascular System

A. Mutilation or trauma: Automobile fatalities or accidental death can result in severed arteries. These conditions must be individually evaluated by the embalmer; arteries exposed as a result of the trauma may be considered as sites for injection. Likewise, standard points of injection such as the common carotid can be used and the severed arteries clamped during arterial injection. Secondary points of injection will, no doubt, be required.

B. Ulcerations: Ruptured vessels can be the result of ulcerations. If this occurs in the stomach, there will be a great loss of blood during the agonal period. If sufficient arterial solution is lost during injection, the embalmer must select secondary points of injection to treat those areas of the body not reached by arterial solution.

When arterial solution is evidenced in purge from the mouth or nose during arterial injection and there is still blood drainage, continue to inject arterial solution and evaluate the distribution of the solution.

When arterial solution is evidenced in purge from the nose or mouth during arterial injection and there is no blood drainage, it would be wise to discontinue injection, evaluate the distribution of solution, and sectionally treat, by arterial injection, those areas not reached by sufficient arterial solution.

C. Autopsies: Partial autopsies must be evaluated by the embalmer as to the selection of arteries for injection. For example, if the viscera were removed only from the *abdominal cavity,* the portions of the body above the diaphragm could be embalmed by (1) injecting from the thoracic aorta upward and (2) injecting from the right common carotid and ligating the thoracic aorta. Even after a complete autopsy, there can be a choice of vessels depending on the lengths of vessels left by the dissecting pathologist. For example, the subclavian artery or perhaps the axillary artery can be used to inject the arm. If the external iliac arteries have been cut under the inguinal ligament, the femoral vessels may have to be injected. In some autopsies, the entire arch of the aorta may be present and most of the upper areas of the body can be injected from this point. Keep in mind that even in the autopsied body there can be a choice of vessels for injection.

5. Clotting

If an embalmer feels that clots may be present in the arterial system, particularly in the aorta, the femoral artery should *not* be used as the starting point for injection. The best choice in this situation is to begin the injection of the arterial solution from the common carotid, because if any coagula do break loose, it is better that this material be directed toward the legs. If instead the femoral artery is used, the coagula would be pushed up into the common carotid arteries and the axillary vessels. These arteries supply body areas that will be viewed. Clotting may be suspected in bodies that have been dead for long periods, in deaths from systemic infections and febrile disease, and in bodies of persons who were bedfast for long periods.

When the embalmer suspects that the blood vascular system is heavily clotted or that distribution of arterial solution will be difficult, the best vessel to use in beginning the arterial injection is the common carotid artery, and drainage should be taken from the right internal jugular vein. An even better method is to raise both common carotid arteries at the beginning of the embalming (restricted cervical injection). As the head is thus separately embalmed, the embalmer maintains control over solution distribution into the facial tissues.

6. Facial Tissue Distension
The possibility of distension of the facial tissues exists in bodies dead for long periods. Also, the facial tissues can easily distend during arterial injection in bodies that have suffered facial trauma or extended refrigeration or have been frozen. To maintain the most control over arterial solution entering the facial tissues, both common carotid arteries should be raised at the beginning of the embalming (restricted cervical injection).
7. Facial Discolorations
Quite often, after congestive heart failure or pneumonia, bodies show considerable blood congestion of the facial tissues, and the external jugular veins are often distended. If the head has been allowed to remain on a flat surface, it will, many times, exhibit intense livor mortis of the facial and neck tissues, especially if the deceased had been using medication that tended to thin the blood. In the preparation of these bodies, this intense discoloration necessitates the most complete possible drainage of the facial tissues. The right internal jugular vein is the best choice. It may be necessary to open and drain both internal jugular veins. Clearing of these tissues is also assisted by direct injection of arterial solution into the head, which is best achieved by raising and injecting the right and left common carotid arteries.
8. Volume and Strength of Arterial Solution.
If a long delay has occurred between death and embalming, if the body shows evidence of decomposition, if death was due to uremic poisoning or burns, or if skeletal edema is present, the volume of strong arterial solution needed is large. To avoid running excessive amounts of solution through the facial tissues, which can result in dehydration, and to avoid distension and possibly discoloration of the facial tissues, control must be maintained over the amount of arterial solution entering the head and the facial tissues. The best means of controlling solution entering the head and facial tissues is to begin the embalming of the body by raising both right and left common carotid arteries (restricted cervical injection).
9. Medico-Legal Requirements
These two examples illustrate specific requirements in selection of an injection site:
   A. An embalmer preparing a body under orders from the military services must follow minimum standards, which may include the choice of vessels for injection.
   B. Some hospitals allow arterial embalming prior to autopsy; in such situations the hospital may have preference as to the vessels to use for injection of the body.

To summarize, the major factors to consider in selecting an injection site are the age of the body, weight of the body, effects of disease, vascular system interruptions, clotting, facial tissue distension, facial discolorations, volume and strength of arterial solution, and legal considerations.

▶ SELECTION OF SECTIONAL INJECTION SITES

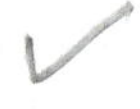

When arterial embalming solution has failed to distribute to a particular area, or if the embalmer feels an insufficient amount of arterial solution is present in a body area, the first consideration should be the direct arterial injection of that area. The artery chosen for injection of the body part needing arterial solution is called a *sectional injection site.* These points of injection all involve treatment of the head or appendages. If there is insufficient arterial solution in any area of the trunk portion of the body, these areas are best treated by hypodermic injection of the area rather than by arterial treatment.

Three methods of embalming can be used to treat body areas that have not received enough arterial solution: (1) sectional arterial embalming, (2) hypodermic embalming, and (3) surface embalming.

Sectional points of injection could include injection of one or more of the following arteries in the *head,* the right and left common carotid and the right and left facial arteries; in the *arms,* the left or right axillary, brachial, radial, or ulnar artery; and in the *legs,* the left or right external iliac, femoral, popliteal, anterior tibial, or posterior tibial artery. As part of the ongoing embalming analysis the embalmer must make at conclusion of the injection of the body, he or she must determine what secondary injections are necessary to properly arterially embalm the areas where solution is needed.

Example 1. Suppose the starting injection site was the right femoral artery. Assume that there is no arterial solution in the entire left arm. It must be assumed that during arterial injection, attempts were made to stimulate the flow of fluid into the left arm, by massaging the arterial pathway, lowering the arm over the side of the table, using intermittent drainage, and increasing rate of flow and injection pressure. Assume there is a blockage before the left axillary artery. A clot or coagulum that was present in the abdominal aorta has been freed and has floated into the left subclavian artery. Now the embalmer must select a secondary injection site. It is almost certain that the left axillary or brachial artery may be used. Injection from this point should establish distribution of solution down the arm and into the hand.

Example 2. Using the same set of circumstances as in Example 1, assume that arterial solution reaches only as far down the left arm as the elbow. Now the embalmer must decide if injection of the left axillary or radial artery will establish distribution of the arterial solution down the remainder of the arm and into the hand *or* if the radial or ulnar artery (or both) should be raised, the hand injected, and then the arterial tube reversed and some solution injected back toward the elbow. Some embalmers would try first to inject the axillary or the brachial artery, hoping that a collateral route may still be open to distribute solution into the hand. If the clotted material is tightly lodged in the area where the brachial artery divides into the radial and ulnar arteries, then one or both of these arteries may have to be raised and injected to properly embalm the hand.

When sectional injection sites are used, drainage can continue to be taken from the primary point of drainage. Some embalmers do, however, prefer to drain from accompanying veins. Exceptions would be the radial and ulnar arteries, where the veins are just too small for practical use.

Example 3. Assume a body has been embalmed using the right common carotid artery. Drainage was taken from the right internal jugular vein. After embalming it is felt that the right leg does not have enough arterial solution. The embalmer raises the right femoral artery for a sectional injection site. She or he may inject the right femoral and drain from (1) the right internal jugular vein, (2) the right femoral vein, or (3) the heart (after beginning aspiration).

▶ ELEVATION AND LIGATION OF VESSELS

After selecting an injection site, the embalmer elevates the vessels to the skin surface, ligates the vessels, and inserts the tubes for arterial solution injection as well as a drainage device into a selected vein for drainage.

After injection of the arterial solution, the embalmer evaluates the body to determine if any further injection is necessary for regions that may have received an inadequate amount of preservative. If such areas are found, sectional injection sites are selected and an artery or arteries raised for direct injection into the areas needing additional solution.

This section of the chapter involves the general protocol for raising and ligating vessels. Later, the specific locations for incisions and the protocol for raising vessels with respect to the individual artery selected are examined.

1. Select instruments and prepare ligatures for the vessels to be used. Be certain arterial tubes, especially very small tubes, are clear and working before inserting them into an artery.
2. Locate vessels and their respective sites for skin incision by the linear guide on the surface of the skin.
3. Generally, make incisions where the vessels are nearest the skin surface.
4. In the dissection for the vessels, remember that muscles do *not* have to be cut to locate vessels, arteries, veins, and nerves. These run in groups *between* the muscles. The only muscle that may have to be divided for locating vessels is the sternocleidomastoid muscle.
5. After making the incision in the skin surface, use blunt dissection to find the vessels based on their anatomical guides and the location of surface vessels. A superficial vessel can be used to locate a deeper vessel by their anatomical relationship.

Example. When the internal jugular vein and the common carotid artery are raised, the vein is the superficial vessel. After a string is placed around the vein, it is pulled laterally, and the artery can easily be located on the medial side of the vein, a little deeper than the vein. The common carotid artery is described as being *medial* and *deep* in its relationship to the internal jugular vein.

6. The order in which vessels are raised varies, depending on the relationship of the artery to the vein. Two general rules should be remembered:

A. **When both the artery and the vein are to be used** (as in a one-point injection), **always raise the superficial vessel first.**

B. **When both the artery and vein are to be used at the same location** (as in a one-point injection), **always insert instruments** (arterial tube or drainage instrument) **into the deepest vessel first.**

Example. When raising the right internal jugular vein and the right common carotid artery, raise the vein *first,* because it is the more superficial. Pull the vein laterally, raise the *deeper* common carotid artery to the surface, open the artery, insert the arterial tubes, return to the vein, open the vein, and insert the drainage instrument.

7. Always use arterial tubes slightly smaller than the lumen of the artery into which they are to be inserted. *Do not* force arterial tubes into arteries.
8. If clotted material is present in an *artery,* especially in the common carotid artery, attempt to gently remove this material.
9. Arteriosclerosis does *not* always preclude use of an artery for injection. Starting from the incision, find the "softest" portion of the exposed artery. Some forms of arteriosclerosis actually form a "wall" around the lumen.
10. If an artery is accidently broken (arteries remain open and do not collapse) merely locate the two open ends and attach a hemostat to each. Carefully apply new ligatures and insert arterial tubes.

▶ INSTRUMENTS AND LIGATURES

To raise an artery for injection and a vein for drainage, the following instruments may be used:

Instrument	Use
Scalpel	Making the incision; opening the artery or vein
Double-point scissors	Making the incision; preparing ligatures; opening the artery or vein
Aneurysm needle	Dissecting fat and fascia; elevating vessels at surface
Bone separator	Elevating vessels at skin surface
Arterial tubes	For insertion into the artery for injection of fluid
Drainage tube	For insertion into the vein for drainage control
Angular spring forceps	For insertion into the vein for drainage control (in lieu of a drainage tube)
Straight spring forceps	Passing ligatures around the vessels
Grooved director	Assisting in expansion of the vein for insertion of the drainage device

This list represents the minimum number of instruments. A variety of other instruments can also be used. These include arterial hemostats (for holding the arterial tubes in place within the artery; this is of great help in autopsy preparation), ligature passers, arterial scissors, and retractors. This list can also be reduced.

Ligatures for securing the arterial and drain tubes are generally linen or cotton thread. The cotton is somewhat thicker and softer, and many embalmers prefer it. Remember to cut these ligatures long enough so that you can get a good grip on the string to make a very secure tie. A length of 8 to 12 inches is comfortable to work with.

▶ VESSELS USED FOR ARTERIAL EMBALMING

The arteries discussed in this chapter from the standpoint of injection site are the common carotid artery, femoral artery, external iliac artery, axillary artery, brachial artery, popliteal artery, radial artery, ulnar artery, facial artery, abdominal aorta, thoracic aorta, anterior tibial artery, and posterior tibial artery. With respect to these arteries, the area supplied, the considerations for their use, precautions, locations for incisions for raising the vessels, and the protocol for raising the vessels and inserting instruments when both the artery and vein are being used for an injection and drainage site are discussed.

Also discussed (along with the accompanying artery) is the use for drainage of the internal jugular vein, femoral vein, external iliac vein, axillary vein, and inferior vena cava. The location and use of the right atrium of the heart as a drainage point are included in the discussion. Because the incisions for the veins are the same as those for the arteries, the student is asked to refer to the artery incisions.

Common Carotid Artery

To be accurate in the discussion of this vessel, consideration is given to the use of a one-point injection, but there follows a discussion of *restricted cervical injection,* which employs both right and left common carotid arteries.

The common carotid artery is the largest vessel the embalmer can raise from a superficial point in a body region outside the trunk area. The incision is made in the inferior portion of the neck. This large artery is closely situated near the *arch of the aorta,* which is the central distribution point for arterial fluid. The common carotid artery can well be described as the "best choice" for injection of the body, especially if there has been any time delay between death and preparation or if vascular difficulties are anticipated.

I. Regions Supplied
   1. If the injection is directed superiorly, the head and face are embalmed.
   2. If the injection is directed inferiorly, the opposite side of the face and head are embalmed as are the trunk and appendages.

II. Considerations
   1. It is very large in diameter.
   2. It has no branches except the terminal branches, so it is easily raised to the skin surface.
   3. It is very elastic.
   4. It is rarely found to be sclerotic.
   5. It supplies fluid directly to the head.
   6. It is situated close to the arch of the aorta.
   7. It is accompanied by a very large vein that can be used for drainage.
   8. Arterial coagula are pushed away from the head.

III. Precautions
   1. The head may be overinjected.
   2. If leakage occurs, it may be seen.
   3. Some types of instruments, if improperly used, may mark the side of the face or jaw line.
   4. The incisions may be visible with some types of clothing.

IV. Incisions for the Common Carotid and the Internal Jugular Vein
   1. **Anterior lateral** (supraclavicular): The incision is made on the clavicle (collar bone) from a point near the sternoclavicular articulation and is directed laterally.
   2. **Anterior vertical** (parallel): The incision is made from a point near the sternoclavicular articulation and is directed upward on the sternocleidomastoid muscle.
   3. **Posterior vertical** (parallel): The incision is made posterior to the sternocleidomastoid muscle, 2 inches below the lobe of the ear, and is directed downward toward the base of the neck.
   4. **Anterior horizontal:** The incision is made at the base of the neck from a point on the sternocleidomastoid muscle and is directed posteriorly.
   5. **Flap incision (semilunar):** This incision is used by the operator when it is necessary to raise the vessels on both the right and left sides for injection or drainage. The incision extends from a point lateral and slightly superior to the sternoclavicular articulation and is directed downward on the upper chest wall, across and upward to a similar location on the opposite side. The pattern may be either a U or an inverted C in shape.
   6. **Strap line:** This incision is adaptable to the embalming of females. The incision is made about 2 inches lateral to the base of the neck on the line where the strap of the undergarments crosses the shoulder (Figure 9–1).

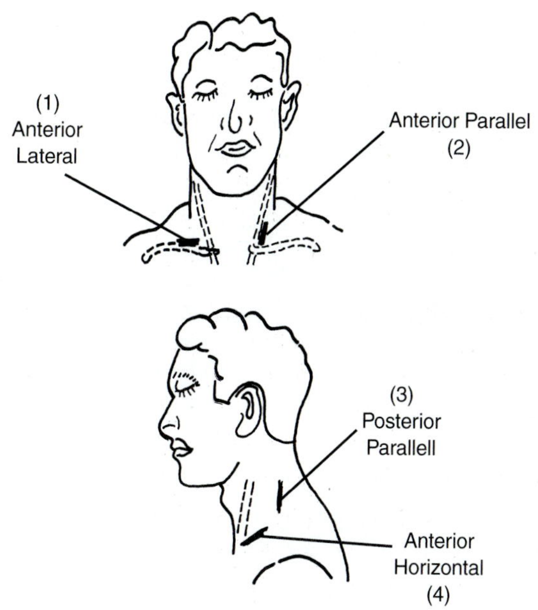

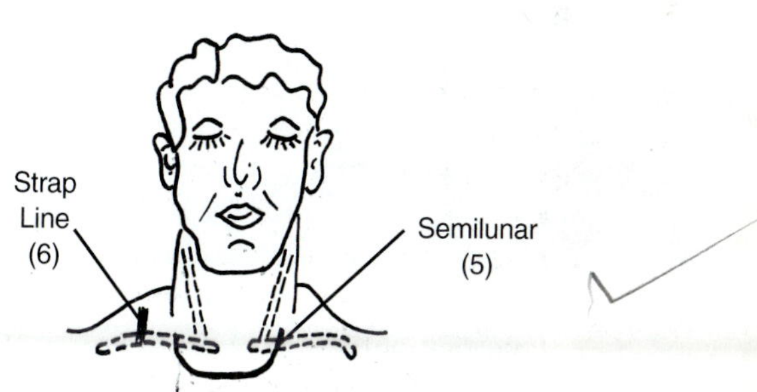

V. Suggested Protocol for Raising the Common Carotid Artery and the Accompanying Internal Jugular Vein
   1. Take a position *at the head of the embalming table.*
   2. Turn the head of the body in the *direction opposite* that of the vessels being raised (i.e., if the right common carotid is being raised, turn the head to the left).
   3. Place a shoulder block under the shoulders

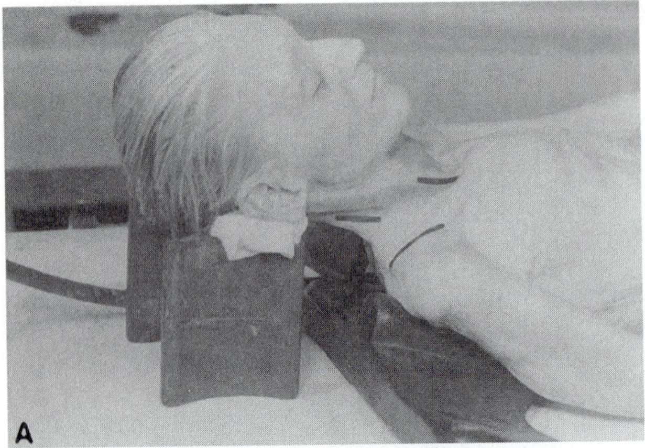

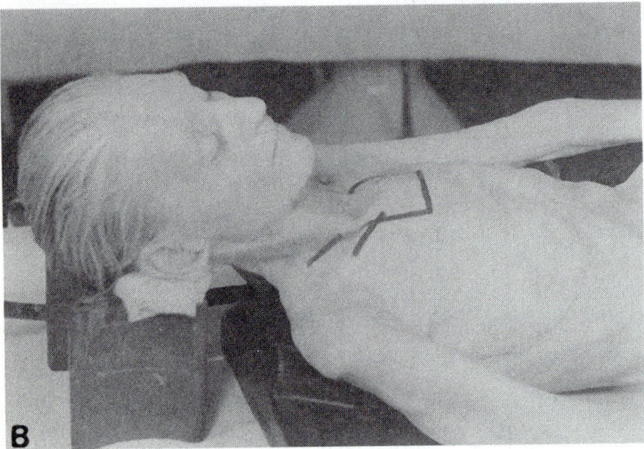

Figure 9–1. A. Anterior vertical, posterior vertical, and strap line incisions. **B.** Supraclavicular, semilunar, and anterior horizontal incisions.

and lower the head of the body on the head block.

4. Make the incision. Dissect through (or cut through) the platysma muscle and the superficial fat and fascia.
5. The sternocleidomastoid muscle will exhibit an area where its fibers part at the clavicle (it looks like a triangle).
6. Raise the *internal jugular vein:* put a ligature around the vein and pull it laterally.
7. Go *medial and deep* and locate the common carotid and bring it to the surface; put two strings around the artery; open the artery; insert arterial tubes superiorly and inferiorly; secure them with a tight ligature.
8. Return to the vein; open the vein and insert a drainage instrument (Figure 9–2).

VI. Protocol if the Internal Jugular Vein Is Collapsed (and Cannot Be Easily Identified)

1. Make the proper incision.
2. Take a position at the *head of the table.*
3. Elevate the shoulders and lower the head.

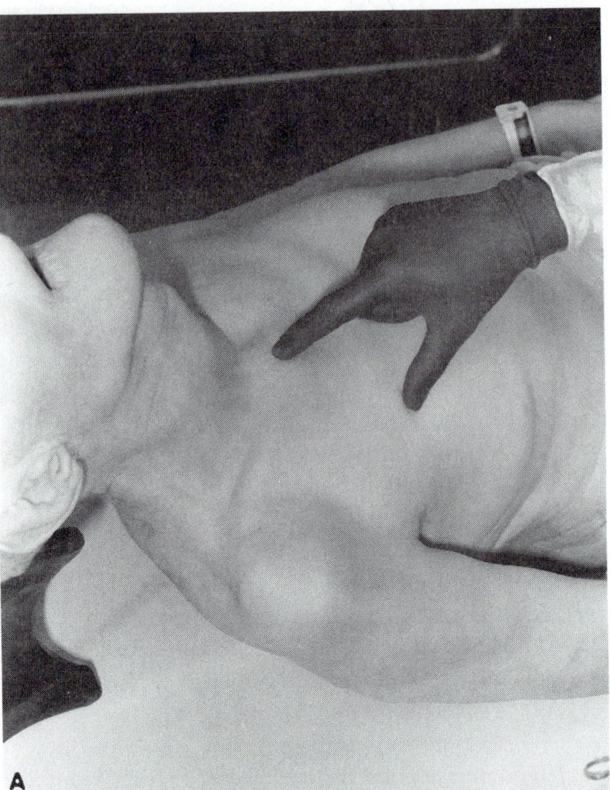

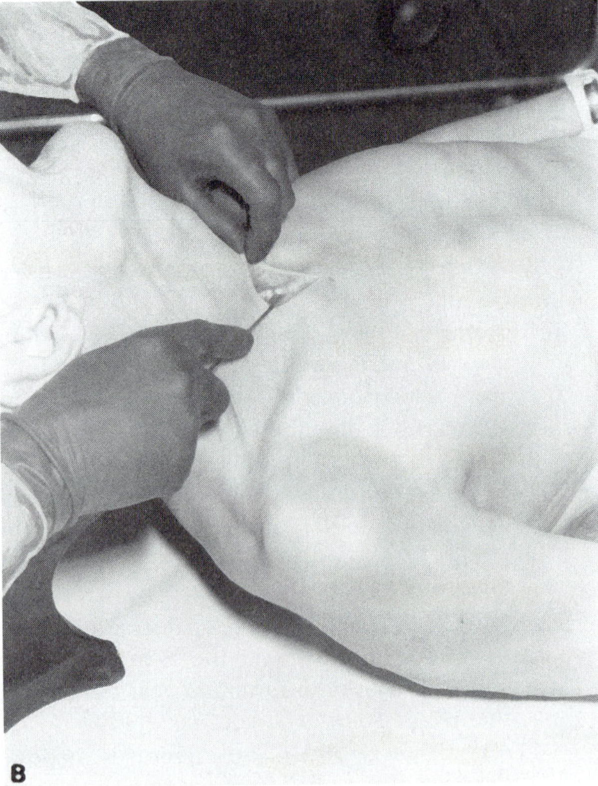

Figure 9–2. A. Point at which an anterior parallel incision is made. **B.** The (superficial) internal jugular vein is raised first.

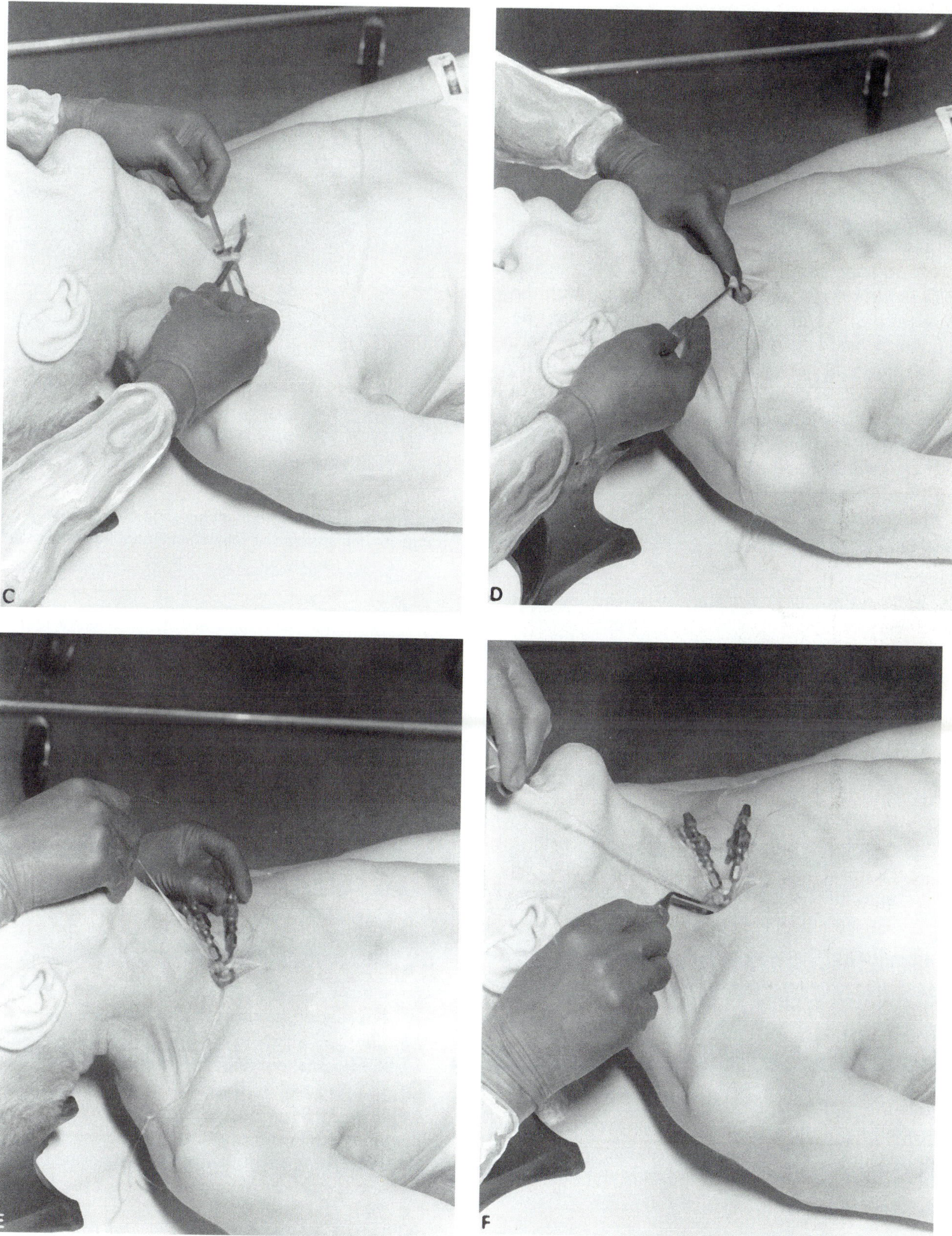

Figure 9–2. *(Continued).* **C.** A ligature is placed around the vein and it is pulled laterally. **D.** With the vein pulled laterally, the artery, which is medial and deep to the vein, is raised. **E.** Arterial tubes are placed into the common carotid and secured with ligatures. **F.** The operator elevates the vein and inserts a drainage instrument toward the heart. Note the suggested position of the operator throughout this procedure.

4. Turn the head in the direction opposite that of the vessels being raised.
5. Palpate the common carotid artery after dissection.
6. Bring the artery to the surface and insert arterial tubes into the artery.
7. Begin arterial injection.
8. When vein becomes dilated, elevate it to the surface and ligate.

Internal Jugular Vein

The right internal jugular vein is in direct line with the right atrium of the heart. The right atrium is the central point of blood drainage in the dead human body. The left internal jugular, although a very large vein, does not lead directly into the right atrium. Instead, it joins with the left subclavian vein to form the left brachiocephalic vein, which crosses to the right side of the chest, joins with the opposite brachiocephalic vein, and forms the superior vena cava. For this reason, the right internal jugular vein is preferred as a drainage site.

I. Considerations
   1. The vein is very large.
   2. There is direct drainage from the face and head.
   3. It is accompanied by the common carotid artery, which can be used for injection.
   4. The right internal jugular vein leads directly through the right brachiocephalic and superior vena cava into the right atrium, allowing easy removal of clotted material that may be present.

II. Precautions
   1. Leakage may be visible.
   2. Drainage instruments, if improperly used, may mark the face.
   3. The incision may be visible with some clothing.

Because of its size, its location with respect to the right atrium of the heart and its ability to directly drain the head, the right internal jugular vein certainly must be considered as one of the best possible sites for drainage during arterial injection.

An excellent method of embalming involves raising *both* the right and left common carotid arteries at the beginning of the embalming process. This method of embalming, ***restricted cervical injection,*** most effectively controls arterial solution entering the head and face (Figure 9–3). The procedure follows:

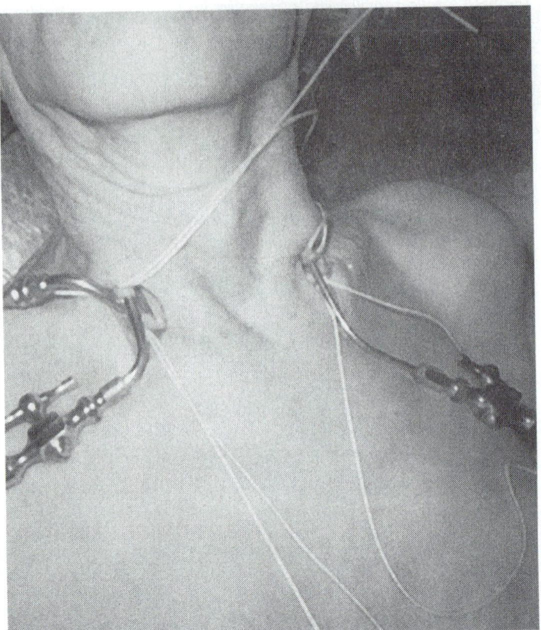

Figure 9–3. Restricted cervical injection affords control over the amount and strength of solution entering the facial tissues.

1. Raise the right common carotid artery and the right internal jugular vein.
2. Insert an arterial tube into the right common carotid artery directed toward the head. Insert a second tube into the artery directed toward the trunk. *Be certain to keep the stopcock open* on the tube directed toward the head.
3. Insert a drainage device into the right internal jugular vein.
4. Raise the left common carotid artery only. Insert a tube into the artery directed toward the head. *Leave the stopcock open.* Tie off the lower portion of the artery.

The following are some advantages to use of the restricted cervical injection:

- The arteries are large.
- Carotids are very elastic and have no branches, so they are easy to elevate.
- The arteries are accompanied by the largest veins.
- The arteries are rarely sclerotic.
- Clots or coagula present in the arterial system will be pushed away from the head area.
- Solution is supplied directly to the head.
- This injection allows the best control over the amount of arterial solution entering the head.
- Two strengths of arterial solution can be used: one for the trunk and another for the head.
- Two rates of flow can be used: one for the trunk and a second for the head.
- Two pressures can be used: one for the head and another for the trunk.
- Large volumes of solution can be run through the trunk without overinjecting the head.

- Features may be set after the trunk is embalmed and aspirated if purging took place during injection.

Facial Artery

The facial artery can be used in two situations: in bodies that have been autopsied and the common carotid and portions of the external carotid removed; and in bodies with clotting or sclerosis of the carotid artery, most frequently found in persons who have suffered from an extracerebral stroke.

The facial artery supplies arterial solution to the soft tissues of the face, the upper and lower lips, the mouth area, the side of the nose, and the medial tissues of the face and some portions of the lower eyelid. The artery is smaller than the carotid or femoral, and requires a very small arterial tube (see Figure 8–2).

In life, the facial artery can be felt pulsating by touching the inferior margin of the mandible just in front of the angle of the jaw. It is in this same location that a small incision is made to raise the artery. Fibers of the platysma muscle have to be opened, and by moving the aneurysm needle along the inferior margin of the mandible, the embalmer can find the artery. This incision is best closed with super glue. If suturing is preferred, the use of dental floss for the stitching will be most beneficial (Figure 9–4).

Axillary Artery

The axillary artery is a continuation of the subclavian artery. It begins at the lateral border of the first rib after passing through the cervicoaxillary canal (this canal is bounded by the first rib, clavicle, and scapula). This vessel can be used to embalm the entire body.

During the early years of embalming, when much work was done at the residence of the deceased, this vessel was preferred. The head received a large amount of solution, and the incision itself was easily hidden from view. It was a very "clean" artery to employ for injection, and drainage was generally taken directly from the right side of the heart by use of a trocar. Keep in mind that early arterial solutions were quite strong, so large volumes were not injected. The small volume would quickly clear the head when injection was from the axillary.

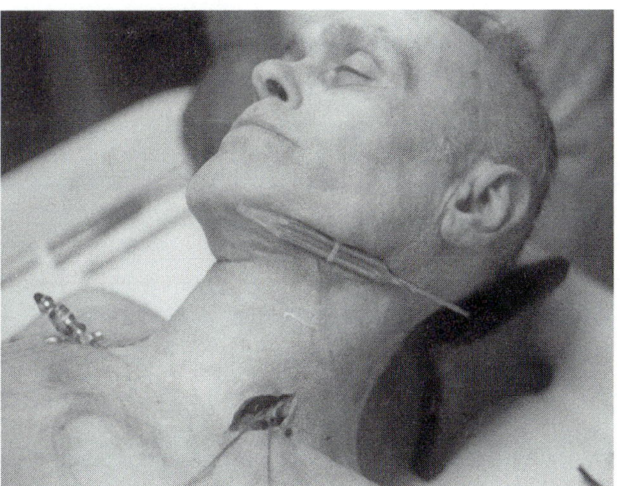

Figure 9–4. Left facial artery.

Today, the axillary is used principally as a secondary point of injection where there is insufficient arterial solution in the arm or hand. Also today, long delays result when hospitals have to request autopsies. Permission must be sought for organ donation, and frequently there are pathological problems such as generalized edema, in which cases the axillary artery is less frequently employed. In addition, the vein that accompanies the artery may not allow easy access for the passage of clotted materials.

I. Regions Supplied
   1. If the arterial tube is directed toward the hand, the axillary supplies fluid directly to the arm and hand.
   2. If the tube is directed toward the body, the entire body can be embalmed from this location.

II. Considerations
   1. Arterial solution flows directly into the arm and hand.
   2. The artery is close to the face.
   3. The vessels are superficial.
   4. The artery is close to the center of arterial solution distribution.

III. Precautions
   1. The arm must be extended, especially if the vein is to be used for drainage.
   2. The artery is small for injection of the whole body.
   3. The artery is accompanied by a vein that is small for drainage.
   4. There exists the danger of overinjecting the facial tissues.
   5. There are numerous branches and, often, anomalies.

IV. Incision for the Axillary Artery and Vein

   The arm should be extended (abducted) a little less than 90° from the body. The incision is made parallel to the linear guide. Many embalmers make this incision along the anterior margin of the hairline of the axilla.

V. Suggested Protocol for Raising the Axillary Artery and Vein

   When the arm is abducted the artery will be found slightly anterior and deep to the axillary vein and the brachial plexus. The vein can be described as being located medial and superficial to the axillary artery (Figure 9–5).

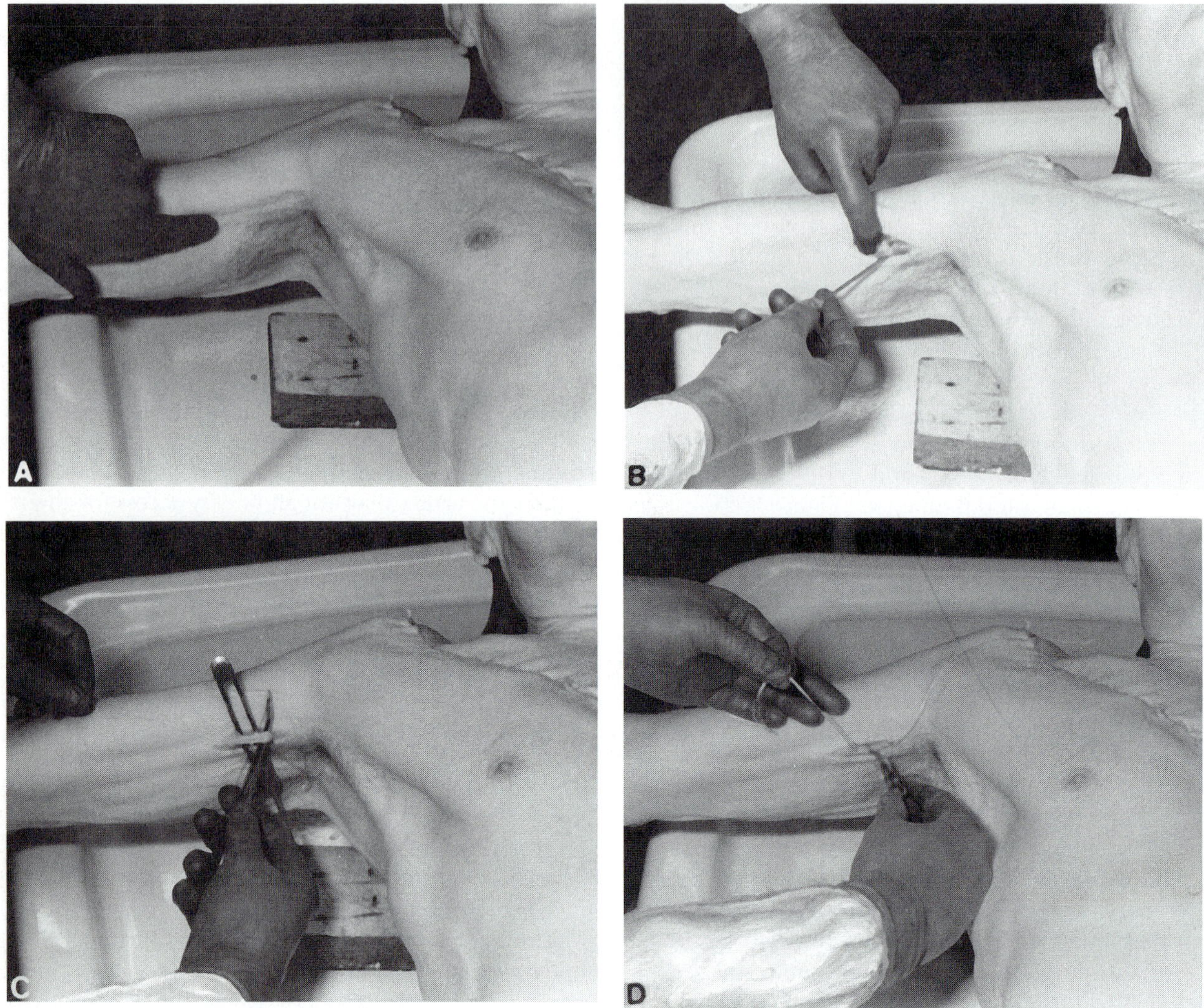

Figure 9–5. A. Location of incision used for raising the axillary artery. This particular incision raises the axillary artery where it becomes the brachial artery. **B.** The artery lies deep (behind) to the vein. **C.** Ligatures are passed around the artery. **D.** An arterial tube is inserted to demonstrate how the arm would be injected.

1. Abduct (extend) the arm and rest the distal portion of the arm on the hip of the embalmer. Try not to abduct the arm beyond 90°, as this tends to compress the structures in the arm.
2. Make the incision along the anterior margin of the hairline.
3. Begin the dissection and first locate the axillary vein. This will be a superficial vessel.
4. Place a ligature around the vein and pull the vein away from the incision and downward.
5. Go "above" and "behind" the vein to locate the artery.
6. Pass two ligatures around the artery.
7. Incise the artery and place arterial tubes into the vessel.
8. Return to the vein; pass a second ligature around the vein; open the vein and insert a drainage tube or forceps toward the heart.

Brachial Artery

The brachial artery supplies fluid directly to the arm and the hand. If the tube is directed toward the body the artery is large enough that the entire body can be embalmed from this point, but because of the small size of the brachial artery, injection would be quite slow and it would be very difficult to build effective arterial pressure. Drainage from the accompanying basilic vein is difficult, as this vein is quite small.

The incision for the brachial artery may be made anywhere along the upper half of the linear guide. The proximal third is preferred. Many embalmers make this incision about 1 inch above and parallel to the linear guide. To raise the artery the arm should be abducted.

Radial Artery

The radial artery supplies solution directly to the thumb side of the hand. It is quite superficial and may easily be palpated through the skin in the area of the wrist. The incision is made parallel to the artery directly on the linear guide, about 1 inch above the base of the thumb (Figure 9–6).

Ulnar Artery

The ulnar artery supplies arterial solution directly to the medial side of the hand. The incision is made parallel to the vessel directly over the linear guide. Generally, the incision should terminate about 1 inch above the pisiform bone (Figure 9–7).

There are times when injection of the axillary or brachial artery alone will establish adequate flow of solution into the arm and the hand. With heavy clotting, however, it is necessary to raise and inject both the radial and the ulnar arteries to adequately embalm the hand. Also, a tube may be directed toward the arm from the radial or ulnar artery in an attempt to inject more solution into the arm area.

If there is difficulty clearing the hand, the embalmer may try injecting only the radial artery. When this is done digital pressure should be placed on the ulnar artery. By application of such pressure, short-circuiting of the solution will not occur and more solution will flow into both sides of the hand.

Some embalmers also raise the brachial artery in the area of the antecubital fossa, where the artery divides into the radial and ulnar arteries. The arterial tube can be directed into each of these arteries from this point, avoiding an incision in the wrist area, which may be a difficult area to tightly suture, especially if edema is present.

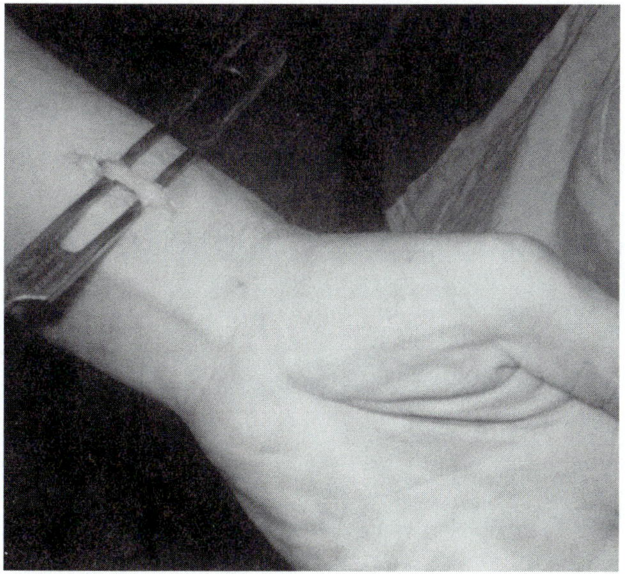

Figure 9–6. Left radial artery.

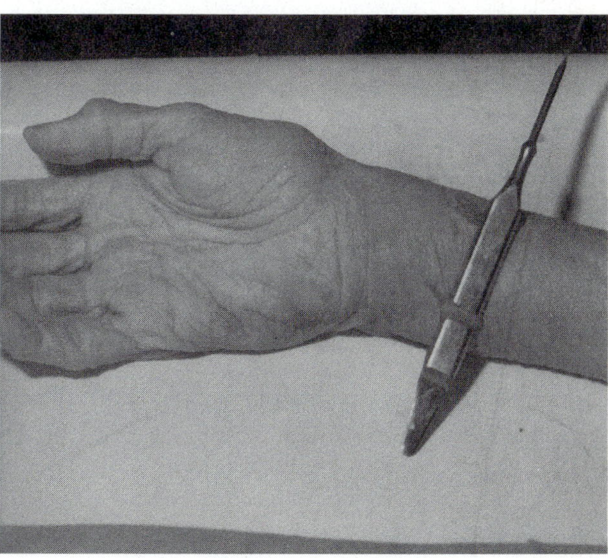

Figure 9–7. Right ulnar artery.

Femoral Artery

The second most frequently used set of vessels for arterial embalming comprises the femoral artery and femoral vein. The artery is located superficial and lateral to the femoral vein. Because it is a continuation of the external iliac artery and vein, this set of vessels is often referred to as the iliofemoral vessels. A tube placed into the femoral artery and directed toward the trunk of the body is actually placed into the external iliac artery. Likewise, a drainage tube inserted into the femoral vein and directed toward the heart is entered into the external iliac vein.

I. Regions Supplied
   1. When the injection is directed toward the foot, the artery directly supplies the leg and the foot.
   2. When a tube is directed toward the head, the artery supplies arterial solution to the opposite leg as well as the remainder of the body.

II. Considerations
   1. The artery is large.
   2. The incision is not visible.
   3. Both sides of the head may receive an even distribution of solution (especially important if dyes are used with the arterial solution).
   4. The artery is accompanied by a large vein, which can be used for drainage.
   5. With the proper instruments, it can be a "clean" method of embalming; no solution or blood will pass under the body.

6. The head and arms can be posed without having to be further manipulated after embalming.

III. Precautions

1. The most frequent reason for inability to use the femoral artery as an injection point is the presence of arteriosclerosis in the artery.
2. In obese bodies, the vessels may be very deep.
3. There is no control over the solution entering the head, especially when large volumes of solution must be injected or when strong solutions are used.
4. Coagula in the arterial system can be pushed into the vessels that supply the arms or the head, areas that will be viewed.
5. Large branches might be mistaken for the femoral artery.

IV. Incision for the Femoral Artery and Vein

This incision is made over the linear guide for the artery beginning at a point slightly medial to the center of a line drawn between the anterior superior iliac spine and the pubic symphysis. Some embalmers prefer to make the incision directly over the inguinal ligament; others prefer to make the incision an inch or more inferior to the inguinal ligament. The external iliac vessels at the inguinal ligament become the femoral vessels. The external iliac artery lies lateral and slightly superficial to the external iliac vein at the inguinal ligament. The code VAN can be used: the Vein is the most medial structure, then comes the Artery, and the most lateral structure is the Nerve.

V. Suggested Protocol for Raising the Femoral Artery and Vein

1. Stand at the right or the left side of the table.
2. Make the incision parallel to the vessels, on the linear guide through the skin and superficial fascia.
3. Dissect superficial fat and fascia bluntly. Observe the great saphenous vein, which is quite superficial.
4. Locate the sartorius muscle. The vessels are found along the medial side of this muscle.
5. Locate the femoral artery and dissect the artery free. Place a ligature around the superior and the inferior portions of the dissected artery.
6. Pull the artery laterally (toward the embalmer) and dissect medially and deeper to free the femoral vein.
7. Clean off the vein, being careful not to rupture it. Also, be careful around the tributaries, which may be full of blood. Bring the vein to the surface and pass one ligature around each end of the dissected portions of the vein.
8. Make an incision into the vein and insert the drainage device, tube, or forceps toward the heart. Tie the tube into the vein. (Keep the vein ligatures on the medial side of the thigh and the artery ligatures on the lateral side of the thigh.)
9. Bring the artery to the surface of the incision. Incise the artery and insert one arterial tube directed toward the head and a second tube directed down the leg. Secure both with the ligatures (Figure 9–8).

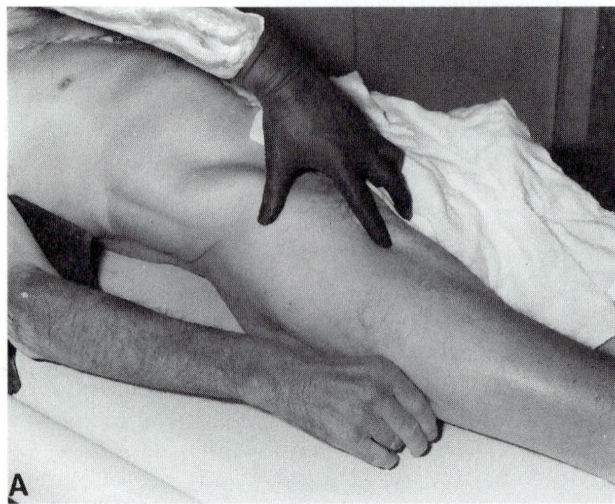

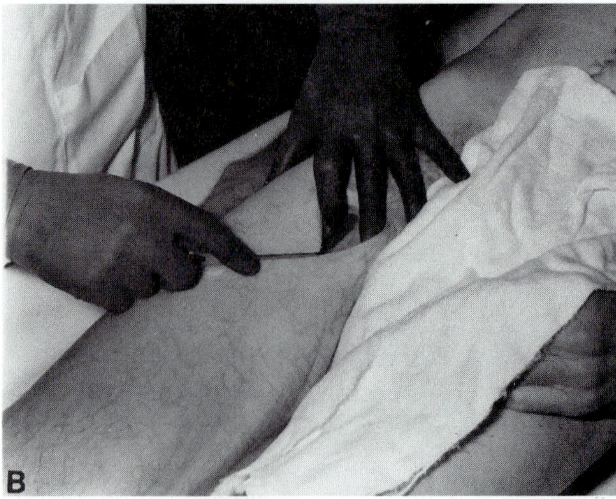

Figure 9–8. A. The femoral artery and veins are raised. **B.** The artery lies just lateral to the sartorius muscle.

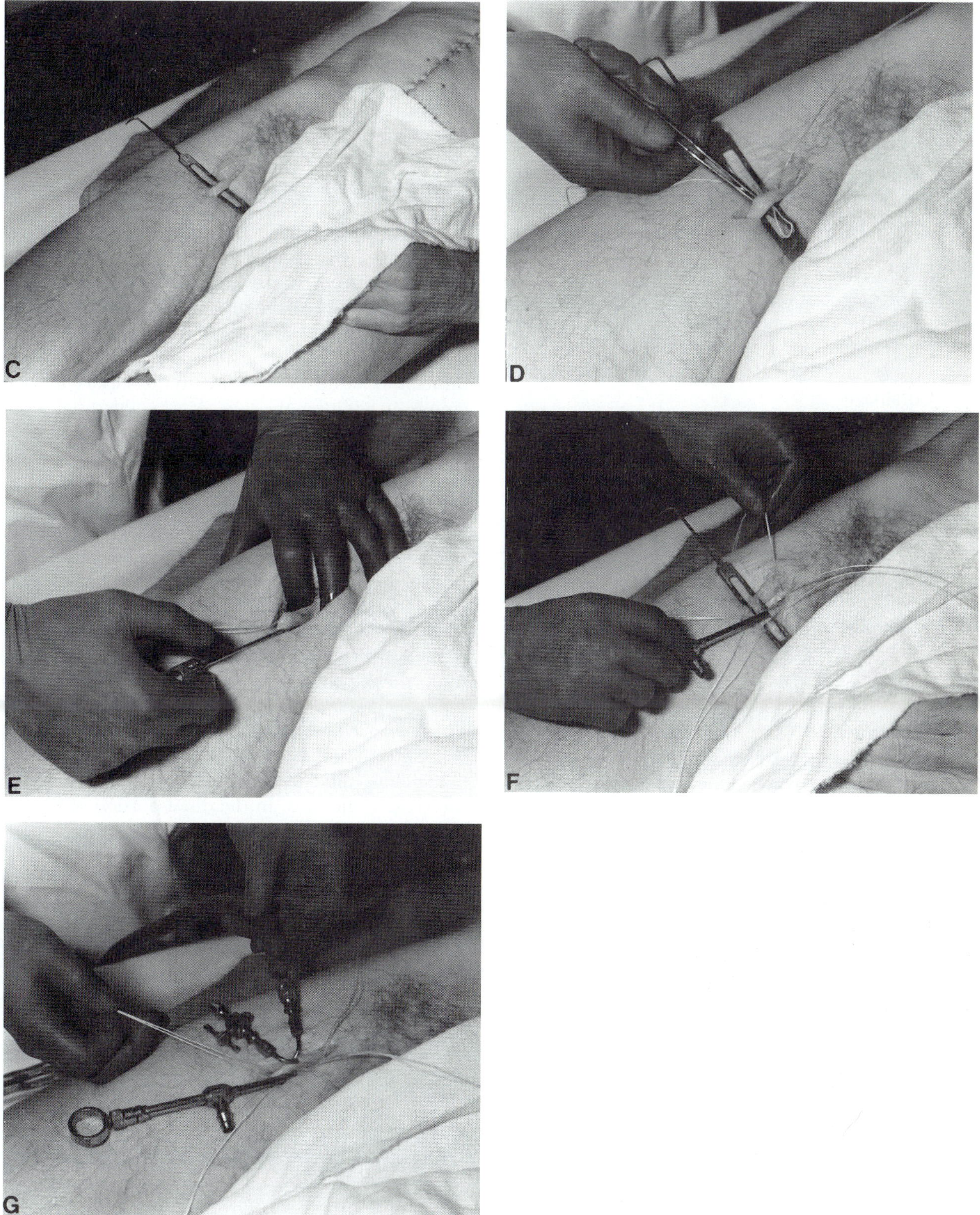

Figure 9–8. *(Continued)* **C.** The femoral artery is superficial and slightly lateral to the vein. **D.** Ligatures are passed beneath the artery and it is pulled laterally, toward the embalmer. **E.** The femoral vein is raised, it is medial and deep to the artery. **F.** Ligatures are passed around the vein and a drain tube is inserted toward the heart. **G.** Arterial tubes are placed in the artery.

Femoral Vein

The femoral vein may be used as a drainage point. The vein is large, and because of its location the incision will not be seen. Because of its location, the femoral vein is assisted by gravity in draining blood from the body.

I. Considerations
   1. The vein is large.
   2. With tubing attached to a drain tube, it can be a very clean method of drainage; water and blood need not come down over the table and under the body.

II. Precautions
   1. The weight of the viscera can restrict drainage from the upper portions of the body.
   2. Abdominal pressure from gases or ascites can exert pressure on the vein and restrict drainage.
   3. In obese bodies, the vein is very deep.
   4. Many tributaries flow into the femoral vein, and care must be taken not to rupture any of them.
   5. Clots in the right atrium and upper areas of the vascular system may be difficult to remove.
   6. Pressure on the heart from hydrothorax (as frequently seen in deaths from pneumonia) may make it difficult to establish good drainage from the right atrium and large veins of the head and arms.

Popliteal Artery

The popliteal artery is used as a secondary injection site when solution has not reached the area of the leg below the knee. Because of the inconvenient location of this artery, it is generally used only in special circumstances. Two examples are bodies resulting from mutilation and accidental deaths and arthritic bodies.

Most tissues of the body are best preserved and more uniformly preserved by arterial injection. As the legs will not be viewed, other methods of embalming can be used, including surface and hypodermic embalming. An attempt should be made, however, to inject the legs. The first choice would be the external iliac or the femoral artery. If these vessels are found to be sclerotic there will, no doubt, also be pathological problems with the other arteries of the leg, especially if gangrene or necrosis is present.

As previously stated, the popliteal is generally used when there has been an interruption of the arterial pathway, as in accidents or mutilations. The limbs of the arthritic body may be in such a position that the femoral vessels cannot be used, and, because of the "swayed" position of the legs, the popliteal artery may be easy to work with.

Two incisions can be used: (1) The body may be turned and the incision made down the center of the popliteal space, parallel to the artery. (2) If the body is not turned the knee can be slightly flexed and a longitudinal incision made along the posterior–medial aspect of the lower third of the thigh, actually just superior to the popliteal space (Figure 9–9). Because of the location of the artery and the size of the vessels, the accompanying vein is not used as a drainage site.

Anterior and Posterior Tibial Arteries

The anterior and tibial arteries supply arterial solution directly to the portion of the leg below the knee and on into the foot. Unlike the superficial radial and ulnar arteries, which supply the distal portion of the arm and the hand, these arteries are deeper, making them more difficult to locate and to bring to the surface of the incisions. In addition, the skin covering the distal portion of the leg is very tight, making suture of the incisions very difficult. When suturing is difficult, leakage can become a problem.

With regard to arteriosclerosis, it would be most impractical to attempt to raise and inject the tibial arteries when the femoral artery is affected by arteriosclerosis, especially if gangrene or necrosis is present in the foot or in the distal portion of the leg. Treatment when the latter conditions are present is best accomplished by hypodermic treatment of the leg with cavity fluid; the leg should be painted with preservative autopsy gel and a plastic stocking containing embalming powder placed on the limb.

The incision for raising the anterior tibial artery is made along the lateral margin of the inferior third of the crest of the tibia. In the distal portion of the leg it

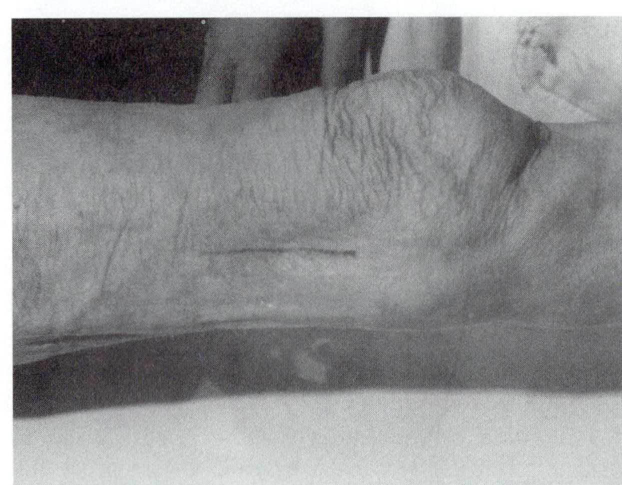

Figure 9–9. Incision location (optional) for the left popliteal artery.

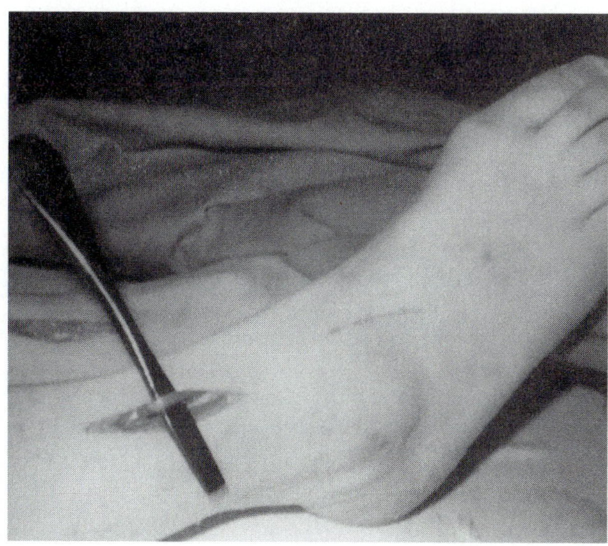

Figure 9–10. Right anterior tibial artery, lateral to the crest of the tibia.

lies at the superficial margin of the tibia. By using the aneurysm needle to dissect down along the tibia, the embalmer can locate the artery (Figure 9–10).

The incision for the posterior tibial artery is made midway between the medial malleolus and the large calcaneous tendon.

Abdominal Aorta and Thoracic Aorta

The abdominal aorta and thoracic aorta are large vessels very deeply seated in the abdominal and thoracic cavities. They lie in the center of the body and can be found on the anterior surface of the spinal column. The thoracic or abdominal aorta may be used for injection after complete or partial autopsy or organ donation and in infants.

The thoracic or abdominal aorta may become a vessel for injection in certain bodies where an incision has been made from which the vessels can be dissected and identified. Such bodies might include those dying following recent surgery; bodies where partial autopsies have been performed or the bodies of organ donors. Drainage may be taken from a vein that the embalmer raises such as the femoral or internal jugular vein. Drainage may also be taken directly from the inferior or superior vena cava. Use of the aorta for injection and the vena cava for drainage is determined by the amount of exposure of these vessels created by the partial autopsy or organ removal.

In the unautopsied infant, the abdominal aorta can be exposed by making an incision to the left of the midline, beginning a few inches below the xiphoid process of the sternum and extending over the abdominal wall about 4 inches in length. The greater omentum is thus exposed. It can be reflected upward, and the small intestines can be pushed aside or lifted out of the abdominal cavity to expose the abdominal aorta and the inferior vena cava resting on the spinal column in the midline of the abdomen.*

The thoracic aorta in the infant can be exposed by making a midline incision down the center of the sternum. Because the sternum is quite soft, a sharp scalpel can be used to divide it. The sternum is retracted and held in this opened position. The pericardium of the heart is now exposed and can be cut open with a pair of surgical scissors. After the pericardium is opened, the right auricle, the little earlike appendage at the top right side of the heart, can be cut open and used as a site for drainage. If the heart is moved to the right the descending thoracic aorta can be exposed as well as the arch of the aorta above it. The aorta can be opened and a tube inserted for injection. (See Chapter 16.)

External Iliac Artery

For considerations on the use of the external iliac artery, see Femoral Artery. The incision is made over the inguinal ligament (Figure 9–11). Because the external iliac artery passes beneath the inguinal ligament it lies on the lateral side of the external iliac vein. If the leg is injected from this point, in the autopsied body, the artery supplies solution to the lower extremity and the anterior abdominal wall.

Internal Iliac Artery

The internal iliac artery is a branch of the common iliac artery that runs medially into the pelvic cavity. In the autopsied body, injection of this artery supplies embalming solution to the gluteal muscles and the peroneal regions.

Inferior Vena Cava

For completeness, at this point the inferior vena cava is discussed as a drainage point. This site can be used for drainage when a partial autopsy has been performed. If the contents of the thorax have been removed, the abdominal viscera and lower extremities can be injected (1) through the abdominal aorta or (2) by clamping off the aorta and injecting the femoral artery. With either point of injection, drainage can be taken directly from the remnants of the inferior vena cava. The inferior vena cava is located to the right of the abdominal aorta at the posterior portion of the diaphragm.

If the contents of the abdominal cavity have been removed in a partial autopsy, the thoracic viscera, head,

*These procedures should only be used when absolutely no other methods would produce satisfactory results; and when used be certain proper permission has been secured.

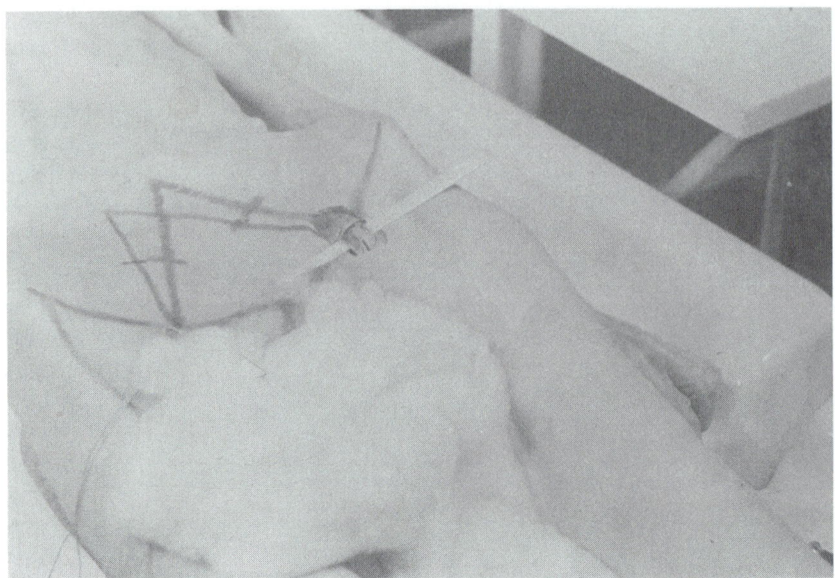

Figure 9–11. Linear guides and incision location for raising the left external iliac artery and vein. The artery is lateral to the vein at the inguinal ligament.

and arms can be injected from the descending thoracic aorta. Or, the aorta can be clamped closed and the upper portions of the body injected from the carotid or axillary vessels. Drainage can easily be taken directly from the remnants of the inferior vena cava.

When drainage is taken from the inferior vena cava it is not necessary to place a drainage device in the vein. To create intermittent drainage the inferior vena cava can be closed shut with a hemostat. A large piece of cotton can also be held over the vena cava with a gloved hand.

Right Atrium of the Heart

When drainage is difficult to establish, the right side of the heart may be pierced with a trocar for drainage. The trocar is inserted into the right side of the heart and should be placed in the right atrium. Piercing of the heart should not begin until one-half to one full gallon of arterial solution has been injected.

To drain from the right side of the heart, the trocar is inserted through the abdominal wall at the standard point of entry (2 inches to the left and 2 inches above the umbilicus). The trocar is directed into the mediastinum area and intersects a line extending from the lobe of the *right* ear to the *left* anterior superior iliac spine. Actually, if the trocar is simply directed toward the right ear lobe, the point should pass into the right side of the heart. The aspirator can be stopped at this point and the drainage established by a gravity system.

It is wise to attach clear plastic tubing to the trocar so further movement of the trocar can be *stopped* immediately after it enters the heart. This very old method for removing blood during arterial injection was used when bodies were embalmed at the residence of the deceased.

▶ MAKING THE INCISION INTO THE ARTERY AND VEIN

To open the artery or vein a scissors or scalpel may be used, depending on the preference of the embalmer. In the method most commonly employed to open the artery or vein, the embalmer simply makes a **transverse** cut into the vessel from the edge of the vessel to the center or just slightly beyond the center. Cutting too far may weaken the vessel enough that it will break into two pieces.

Very elastic arteries such as the carotid and the axillary arteries can easily be stretched to the surface of the incision. With arteries such as the femoral, when some sclerosis is present, raising the vessel to the skin surface can create great tension on the artery. Care should be taken in opening sclerotic vessels to avoid breaking the vessel. As soon as you observe the lumen in this type of vessel, cut no further.

A longitudinal incision may also be used to open vessels. Most embalmers prefer to elevate these vessels on a bone separator. Using a scalpel, cut a longitudinal incision in the center of the vessel running parallel to the vessel. Most embalmers prefer to use a scalpel: however, double-point scissors can also be used. The longitudinal incision is not recommended for opening sclerotic arteries. Many embalmers use this incision for veins, for it provides a large opening for drainage instruments. Two arterial tubes may be placed into position using this incision for the artery.

A combination transverse and longitudinal incision is preferred by many embalmers, especially for opening veins. It is also most helpful when a drainage tube is to be inserted, because it permits drainage from

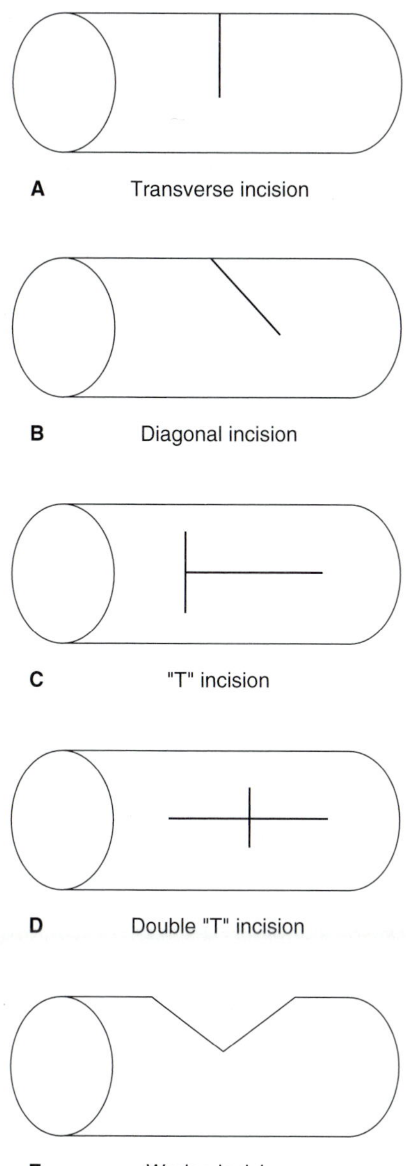

Figure 9–12. A. Transverse incision. **B.** Diagonal incision. **C.** "T" incision. **D.** Double "T" incision. **E.** Wedge incision.

the opposite end of the vein. A wedge can also be cut into an artery or vein with double-point scissors or a scalpel. This method is not recommended for sclerotic arteries (Figure 9–12).

▶ KEY TERMS AND CONCEPTS FOR STUDY AND DISCUSSION

1. Define the following terms:
   multi-point injection
   sectional embalming
   restricted cervical injection
   one-point injection
   six-point injection
   split injection
2. Differentiate between arteries, veins, and nerves.
3. List the twelve major factors to consider in choosing an artery for injection and a vein for drainage.
4. List several advantages to use of the common carotid artery as a vessel for injection.
5. List the steps for raising and inserting instruments into the common carotid artery and the internal jugular vein.
6. List six incisions that can be used to raise the common carotid artery.
7. List the advantages to use of the restricted cervical method of injection.
8. Describe the relationship of the common carotid artery to the internal jugular vein.
9. Describe the relationship of the femoral artery to the femoral vein.
10. Describe the relationship of the axillary artery to the axillary vein.
11. Give the steps for raising and inserting instruments into the femoral artery and vein.
12. Describe where the incisions are made for raising the radial and ulnar arteries.
13. Describe several incisions that can be used to open an artery for insertion of the arterial tube.
14. List the incisions that can be used to raise and inject the popliteal artery.

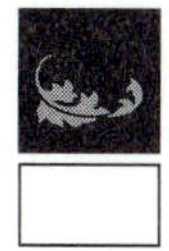

CHAPTER 10
EMBALMING ANALYSIS

No one chapter in any embalming text can really cover embalming analysis. Likewise, one classroom lecture or even a series of lectures cannot possibly cover the entire scope of this subject. Embalming analysis is a summary of the entire embalming process that includes those relevant factors from the disciplines of anatomy, pathology, microbiology, and chemistry. Many think of embalming analysis only as a preembalming "diagnosis" of the body to determine the embalming treatments needed. An embalming analysis is not only a preembalming analysis; it is analysis of the body before, during, and after arterial and cavity embalming. In addition to recognizing the conditions of the body, the embalmer must have a complete knowledge of embalming methodology to make the analysis. **The analysis should be documented in report form.** If the body is being shipped to another funeral home, a copy of this document should also be sent.

EMBALMING ANALYSIS TIME PERIODS

1. Preembalming analysis ⟶ Treatments
2. Analysis during arterial embalming ⟶ Treatments
3. Analysis after arterial embalming ⟶ Treatments

The factors which comprise an analysis can be classified as intrinsic or extrinsic. Intrinsic factors are those conditions present within the body, for example, cause of death; manner of death; pathological conditions; bacterial influence; moisture level; age, weight, and body build; protein level; febrile conditions and effects; presence or absence of discolorations; postmortem changes (decomposition changes, pH of the body, presence or absence of rigor mortis); effects of drugs or medications; trauma; and surgery.

The extrinsic factors of embalming analysis are those conditions outside the body that have had a direct influence on the condition of the body. These include environmental factors (temperature, presence or absence of bacteria, humidity, vermin); length of time between death and preparation; and length of time expected between preparation and disposition.

The aim of this chapter is to approach embalming analysis not as treatment of a specific disease but as treatment of groups of conditions found in the dead human body. A recent death certification listed the following causes of death:

Cause	Duration
Respiratory failure	Hours
Chronic renal failure	1 year
Congestive heart failure	Years

A contributory cause listed *on the same certificate* was arteriosclerosis.

In addition to these disease processes, any one of which could eventually lead to death, this person had received medications for years. It would be impossible for the embalmer to evaluate each disease process and its effects and each drug administered and its effects. The embalmer must consider the effects these diseases and drugs had on the body and the *conditions* they produced.

In the preceding analysis, the embalmer would be most concerned with renal failure, for this disease process can leave nitrogenous wastes in the tissues. These nitrogenous wastes increase the preservative demand. Arteriosclerosis may make use of the femoral artery impossible as an injection site. The best vessels would be the common carotids. The best drainage point to relieve the engorgement of blood in the right side of the heart resulting from congestive heart failure would be the right internal jugular vein. In addition to these factors, the intrinsic general body conditions must be considered—age, weight, and senile changes. Finally, the embalmer must also consider the postmortem changes, the time between death and preparation, degree of rigor mortis, decomposition progress, and refrigeration of the body.

Very few causes of death determine the embalming technique. Three examples are death from a contagious or infectious disease, death from a ruptured aortic aneurysm, and death from renal failure. These causes of death (when known before embalming) can be very important to the embalmer. Some conditions take precedence over others, such as a body dead from renal failure but jaundiced. Preservation of the body must be the first concern of the embalmer. The body dead from renal failure must be treated with strong arterial solutions, and the jaundice condition must be a secondary consideration. The jaundice, no doubt, will worsen from the strong arterial solutions, but the face and hands can be treated later with opaque cosmetics. By using restricted cervical injection, the embalmer is able to inject large quantities of a very strong arterial solution into the edematous areas of the body which will help to overcome edema and the nitrogenous wastes in the tissues, both of which dilute and neutralize formaldehyde. The head could then be injected with a jaundice fluid to modify the effects of the jaundice condition in the facial tissues.

The correct embalming treatment is dictated by the conditions of the body and not solely by the cause of death.

Suppose an apparently healthy man in his mid-fifties is traveling to work and suddenly dies from a massive coronary thrombosis. It is likely in such cases that the coronary arteries are the only vessels occluded by arteriosclerosis. His blood would be of normal viscosity and the tissues in general would not be debilitated. This presents a textbook picture of an "average" or "normal" case. The man would be brought to a medical examiner's office and placed in refrigeration where he would remain until he was identified and a medical examiner had signed a death certificate. This may take as long as 24 hours. The diagnosis on the death certificate might read "coronary thrombosis due to arteriosclerosis."

The embalming treatment required is that for a refrigerated body. Instead of larger volumes of a mild solution as indicated by the facts on the certificate, proper treatment dictates that smaller volumes of stronger solution be used.

To achieve good results the embalmer must learn to observe. When raising the arteries note the condition of the vessels and the blood. When posing the features note the condition of the eyes, the eyelids, and the lips. An eye that is flattened and sunken in its socket can indicate that the interval between death and embalming has been prolonged—the blood possibly has thickened, separated, and settled to the dependent parts. In such cases, regardless of the cause of death, it is wise to raise both common carotid arteries, tie off the superior side, and inject toward the body only. In this manner the body can be injected with large volumes of strong solution under pressure. The head will receive sufficient solution via the vertebrals which are small enough to reduce the volume of solution per minute passing into the head, thereby making it possible to control distension.

While posing the body on the table, the embalmer notes the presence of edema in the lower extremities. This condition can prevail in heart disease or cancer deaths. It is more important for the embalmer to be aware of its presence than its cause. Whether or not edema is noted on the death certificate, it does *dictate* the type of embalming treatment.

Examine the abdomen for masses and the lower quadrant for the telltale green spot of decomposition. At the same time, observe for the presence of ascites. Regardless of the cause of the excess fluid in the abdominal cavity, its presence indicates the need to reduce this abdominal pressure prior to arterial injection. By doing so, pressure on the lower portion of the aorta and the inferior vena cava is eliminated, permitting better distribution of embalming solution and drainage of blood.

Another factor that can influence the embalming treatment is the presence of lesions. For example, decubitus ulcers may be present on the body even though they were not noted on the death certificate. In such cases the subject may have had an old nontraumatic cerebral hemorrhage or a bullet wound in the spine. Either condition would result in long confinement to bed and the resultant ulcerations. Again, regardless of the cause, the ulcers must be treated the same way.

Whatever the cause of death, the condition of the body is affected by the temperature of the environment, environmental moisture, the postmortem interval, the nature and amount of clothing, and airborne bacteria. There have been cases of postmortem contamination of the body with *Clostridium perfringens.* This negates all other pathological considerations for the embalmer. It is, of course, an example of an extreme case, but certainly does not detract from the view that embalming treatment, in general, should be based on the postmortem condition of the body rather than the medical causes of death.

Analysis is not only recognition of the conditions of the body and the effects of disease processes on the body; it is also selection of proper embalming techniques to deal with these conditions.

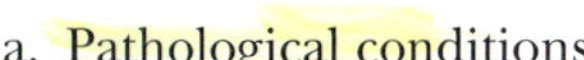

PURPOSE OF THE ANALYSIS

The purpose of an embalming analysis is to select those embalming procedures that provide a thoroughly sanitized and preserved body that closely resembles the lifelike appearance of the deceased.

In making an embalming analysis two important guidelines should always be considered:

1. **Prepare each body as if the deceased were dead from an infectious and highly contagious disease.**
   - This is the premise for using Universal Precautions
   - Sets a standard for embalming solution quality and quantity
   - Sets a standard for disinfection practices with regard to the body and the preparation room environment
2. **Prepare each body as if the disposition (with viewing) of the deceased will be delayed.**
   - Sets a standard for embalming chemical quality and quantity
   - Sets a standard for embalming thoroughness

FACTORS THAT MUST BE DETERMINED BY THE EMBALMING ANALYSIS

1. **VESSELS FOR INJECTION AND DRAINAGE**
2. **STRENGTH OF THE EMBALMING SOLUTION**
3. **VOLUME OF THE EMBALMING SOLUTION**
4. **INJECTION PRESSURE**
5. **INJECTION RATE OF FLOW**

Note: These factors will vary by the individual body and can vary in different areas of the same body.

The 1996 embalming committee of the American Board of Funeral Service Education lists the following factors to be considered in making a preembalming analysis of the body. These factors are given consideration within this chapter and in other chapters of this text. They list the following **variable factors** in making an embalming analysis:

A. Intrinsic factors
   1. Cause and manner of death
   2. Body conditions

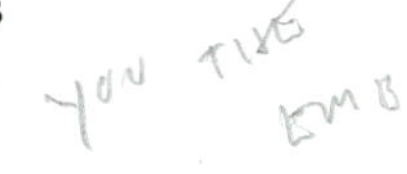

      a. Pathological conditions
      b. Microbial influence
      c. Moisture content
      d. Thermal influences (fever)
      e. Nitrogenous waste products
      f. Weight
      g. Gas in tissues and cavities
   3. Presence or absence of discolorations
   4. Postmortem changes
   5. Pharmaceutical agents
   6. Illegal drugs

B. Extrinsic factors
   1. Environmental
      a. Atmospheric conditions
      b. Thermal influences
      c. Microbial influences
      d. Vermin
   2. Postmortem interval

Older embalming textbooks describe hundreds of diseases, poisons, and traumatic modes of death and the embalming treatment for each. The treatment, however, only concerned the pathological or traumatic problems. No consideration was given to any other factors such as the time between death and preparation, postmortem changes, etc. Later a system of "Typing of bodies" was described. Bodies were classified by conditions of the body rather than by a specific cause of death. Professor Ray E. Slocum of the Dodge Chemical Company published a very complete system of "body types" based primarily on the time between death and preparation, and the degree to which postmortem changes had occurred. Separate categories were established for bodies with jaundice and for infants. In all Professor Slocum established six categories, and with each category he described a specific formulation of chemicals necessary for the preparation of the body. This "recipe" method might be fine for one embalming chemical company, but there are many manufacturers of embalming chemicals, and formulations and fluids vary from company to company.

As can be seen from the Slocum method of body typing, it is not the specific disease that concerns the embalmer but the condition that the disease produces in the body. This method of analysis, or *preembalming observations,* is the approach most embalmers take in determining what embalming techniques to employ. It would be too difficult to approach each body by the specific disease or effects produced by a specific drug.

Professor Slocum published his "typing of bodies" system in the 1950s. This was before the onset of what can be called the "drug era" in medicine. Medicine took a radical change in the early to mid 1960s with the extensive development and use of medications. Now the embalmer had to be concerned with the cause of the death, effects of the medications, and the postmortem body changes. Often the conditions created by the medications became the primary concern in the embalming analysis.

▶ EMBALMING ANALYSIS, PART I: PREEMBALMING ANALYSIS

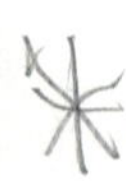

Embalmers consider four major factors in making a preembalming analysis, (factors also used in Slocum's method of analysis): general conditions of the body, effects produced by disease processes, effects produced by drugs or surgical procedures, and effects of the postmortem period between death and embalming.

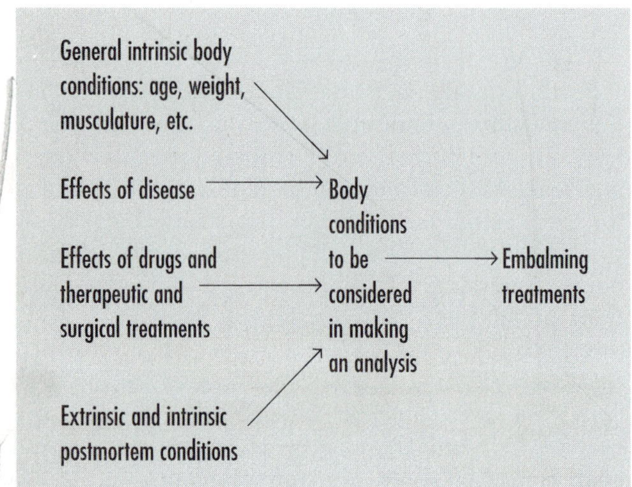

The embalmer must be concerned with the *conditions* of the body he or she can touch or even smell. Most often, the embalmer does not know the cause of death at the time of embalming. The embalmer is also unaware of the medically prescribed drugs that the deceased may have been administered for long-term therapy. If the *conditions* of the body are treated, the exact cause of death or the chemotherapy used need not be known.

General Intrinsic Body Conditions

The general intrinsic conditions of the body include age, body weight and build, musculature, protein level, and general skin condition.

Age. *Child or infant:* Arteries and veins will be much smaller than in the adult; special sized instruments are needed for injection and drainage. Milder solutions may be needed (but preservative demands must determine solution strengths). A needle injector may not be usable for mouth closure. Positioning will vary from that for an adult.

Elderly: Arteriosclerosis may eliminate the use of the femoral artery as an injection point. Absence of teeth and dentures may create problems in setting features. Suturing may be needed for mouth closure if the jaw bone has atrophied.

Weight. *Emaciated:* Solution strengths may need to be reduced. Dehydration may create problems with eye closure and mouth closure.

Obese: Femoral vessels may be too deep to use for injection. Very large quantities of arterial solution will be needed. The internal jugular vein will afford the best drainage site. Restricted cervical injection will best control arterial solution entering facial tissues. There will be positioning problems.

Musculature: In the healthy adult with firm skin and well-developed musculature the embalmer can expect the embalming solution to result in very good firming of the body tissues. If there is a delay between death and preparation, this body can be expected to display intense rigor mortis, making it difficult to establish good distribution of the solution. Where bodies are wasted from disease and the musculature is not well developed and the skin is loose, the embalmer can expect little or no firming of the limbs from the embalming solution; swelling is expected if large volumes of mild solutions are injected. Senile, loose flabby tissue does not assimilate the arterial solution as well as healthy, firm tissues.

Disease Processes and the Cause of Death

The cause of death may not be known at the time of embalming; however, the embalmer can observe the effects that diseases have had on the body. For example, *jaundice* may be caused by the effect of drugs on the liver or red blood cells, obstruction of the bile duct, hepatitis, cancer of the liver, and hemolysis of red blood cells. It is the condition of jaundice that concerns the embalmer, not the disease that caused this condition.

The following excerpts, from an article written by Shor (1972) of the American Academy of Funeral Service, illustrate how the same disease can produce different conditions in different persons. (Remember that it is not the cause of death or the disease but the effects and conditions produced by the disease in the body that should concern the embalmer.)

> Let us begin by examining a very common disease and cause of death today—cancer. This pathological condition may attack and be confined to the stomach. In such an event the patient would not be able to retain foods, either liquid or solid, for weeks just prior to death. He actually might die of starvation although the primary cause of death would be cancer of the stomach.

Primary Condition Unimportant

The embalmer now is presented with a thin, emaciated, dehydrated subject. The primary condition in the stomach is of little significance to him.

Consider next another patient with the same basic disease—cancer. In this subject the malignancy is of the liver or the right suprarenal gland. The attendant enlargement of these structures bears down upon and obstructs the cisterna chyli, the lymph collecting station of the abdomen and lower extremities. This prevents the lymph from returning to the venous system from these areas. All of the parts drained by this system will become edematous and ascites will develop.

The primary cause of death in both examples is cancer. In one case we have a subject with edema, ascites and anasarca; in the other an emaciated, dehydrated subject. We should also note here that many other diseases can cause the above described conditions. (If we learn to treat the conditions, we will treat them successfully—regardless of the cause of death.)

Let me illustrate this further. In incompetence of the right atrioventricular valve of the heart, the valve fails to close efficiently. During the diastole blood will regurgitate from the right ventricle to the right atrium. This, of course, reduces the amount of blood the right atrium can receive from the inferior vena cava. In turn, the amount of blood the vena cava receives from its tributaries is minimized. The resulting venous congestion in the lower venous system increases transudation of plasma and results again in edema and ascites. Whether the excess fluid is a result of cancer of the viscera or damage to the heart valves, the embalming treatment is the same.

Same Basic Treatment

By the same token, emaciation, whether caused by cancer of the stomach, actual starvation or pulmonary tuberculosis, requires the same basic embalming treatment.

Further inquiry into cancer shows that obstruction to the passage of bile into the intestinal tract can lead to the very common embalming problem, jaundice. This condition also can be caused by obstruction of the common bile duct—a disease not usually related to cancer. Here again, it is the symptoms and not the disease that pose an embalming problem.

A disease that is as common as cancer and can produce as varied a group of postmortem conditions is arteriosclerosis. Depending on the vessel or vessels involved, we can get a wide range of different embalming problems.

For example, let us consider renal arteriosclerosis. Here, the blood vessels carrying blood to the kidneys are impaired. As a result, the kidneys diminish in size and efficiency. Nitrogenous wastes and urea instead of passing out of the body via kidney and other excretory organs will remain in the bloodstream and tissue spaces. The result will be uremia, cachexia and possibly edema and ascites, as in some cancers. Arteriosclerosis can affect the vessels of the brain, causing a **stroke** which, in turn, can lead to other abnormalities. One of these is long-term **paralysis** of the extremities with the attendant atrophy and vasoconstriction. Another is long periods of confinement to bed, with the often attendant **decubitus ulcers.** A third is **immediate death** with *no special embalming problems.*

Again, the decubitus ulcers and the atrophied parts can stem from any other disease which confines the patient to bed for extended periods of time. In all these situations the resulting conditions cause much greater embalming problems than the disease that led to them. The embalmer must not overlook the fact that any two or three of the diseases discussed here can and do coexist. So can each disease exist in two or more forms. Therefore, a patient can die with cancer of the stomach and liver. A patient can have cancer of the liver and renal or cerebral arteriosclerosis. In reality, then, **an embalmer should ask, "What conditions exist?" rather than "Of what did the subject die?"**

The reader should not construe this article to mean that the author discourages the study of pathology. It is intended, rather, to encourage the student to correlate his studies of pathology with embalming. It is incumbent upon him to learn the embalming treatments for the basic postmortem conditions that create problems. If the conditions are identified and properly treated, the embalming procedure will succeed regardless of the disease that caused the condition.

Drug Treatments and Surgical Procedures

In the 1960s embalmers became increasingly aware that medications used for the treatment of disease were having a significant impact on embalming results. It was becoming increasingly difficult to establish firmness in the bodies, edema was becoming a frequent problem, and extravascular discolorations in the form of purpura and ecchymosis were more frequently seen along with jaundice and the loss of hair.

During the past 30 years, many articles have been written about the effects of specific drugs on the embalming process (see Chapter 23). Like the hundreds of diseases and their effects on the body, it would be impossible for the embalmer to attempt to embalm a body using chemical formulations designed to combat the effects of a specific drug. Most often a patient is given combinations of drugs, often over a long period. A drug does not always produce the same effects in each person. Here again, it is important that the embalmer have an understanding of the possible effects of drugs and of the fact that embalming problems often stem from the long usage of drug therapy. The embalmer must treat the conditions that can be observed in the dead human body and *not* the effects of a specific medication.

Some of the more common postmortem conditions that concern the embalmer in deciding what embalming treatments to use are those that have been brought about by the long-term usage of drugs. Remember that in addition to the conditions produced by the drugs, the embalmer must observe and consider the conditions produced in the body by disease, general body build, and postmortem changes.

Chemotherapeutic agents are toxic. The one axiom that can be universally applied to ALL chemotherapeutic agents is that they are *toxic*. Cellular changes occur when they are used, no matter which drug is administered. Even the relatively innocuous aspirin pill has its effects. Drugs have an effect on the skin, circulatory system, liver, and kidneys. Such changes may be comparatively minor in nature, limited to slight discolorations that respond readily to cosmetic treatment. But when they assume major proportions such as acute jaundice or saturate the body tissues with uremic poisons, the fixative action of the preservative chemicals contained in the arterial solutions used is seriously impaired (Table 10–1, Figure 10–1).

TABLE 10–1. EMBALMING COMPLICATIONS CREATED BY EXTENSIVE DRUG THERAPIES

Complication	Result
Immediate allergic reaction to the drug	Tissues appear swollen Discolored skin surface Possible skin eruptions
Liver failure	Edema (ascites); edema of lower extremities Increase in ammonia in the tissues (neutralizes formaldehyde) Purges caused by rupture of esophageal veins Gastrointestinal bleeding; fluid loss; possible purge Hair loss Jaundice
Renal failure	Increase in ammonia in the tissues Edema of tissues Gastrointestinal bleeding Pulmonary edema Congestive heart failure Discoloration of the skin (sallow color) Uremic pruritis of the skin
Damage to blood vessels	Skin hemorrhage (ecchymosis, purpural hemorrhage)
Damage to the walls	Breakdown of the skin; skin-slip often present
Clot formation (poor circulation of embalming fluids)	Breakage during arterial injection (causes discolorations)
Loss of cranial hair	
Growth of facial hair and hair on the forehead on women and children	
Creation of resistant strains of microbes	Disinfection treatment more difficult Exposure of embalmer to drug-resistant microbes
Cell membranes become less permeable	Creates "solid" edema that cannot be removed Makes passage of arterial solution into cell very difficult
Killing one type of microbe can stimulate growth of other types	Antibiotics used to kill bacteria give fungal organisms a chance to multiply
Jaundice	Breakdown of the red blood cell Liver failure
Congestive heart failure	Edema Drainage difficulties Facial discolorations
Scaling of skin (seen on facial tissues and between fingers)	Death of the superficial cells
Difficult tissue firming	Protein degeneration Ammonia buildup in the tissues which neutralizes formaldehyde Presence of edema

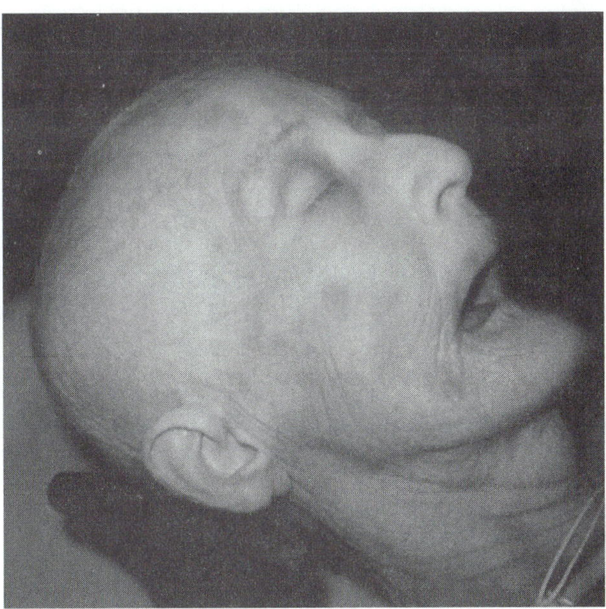

Figure 10–1. Loss of cranial hair but growth of facial hair, and emaciation in this female is the result of extensive chemotherapy.

In making a preembalming analysis, choice of embalming technique may be greatly influenced by whether death occurred during or immediately after surgery. Surgery could be the primary factor in an analysis, as illustrated in the following examples.

Heart Surgery or Aortic Repair. During these procedures the heart may be stopped for a period during which an artificial means of life support is used. Frequently, if death occurs during or shortly after this type of surgery, the face and neck are grossly distended with edema. Repair of an abdominal aneurysm may not always be successful, and the interruption in circulation will necessitate sectional arterial injection.

Abdominal Surgery. Abdominal surgery on the bowel can result in peritonitis. There can be intense distension of the abdomen and bloodstream infection. These conditions require the use of a strong, well coordinated arterial solution.

Whenever death follows surgery, there exists the potential for leakage from arteries and veins involved in the surgical procedure. The embalmer should use dyes to indicate the distribution of arterial solution. It may be necessary to inject a greater volume of arterial solution to compensate for solution that may be lost to the abdominal or thoracic cavities.

All surgical bodies should undergo thorough cavity treatment. Be certain a liberal amount of undiluted cavity fluid is injected into the area where the surgery was performed. It is also a good precaution to inject some undiluted cavity fluid into the tissues surrounding the surgical incision. This decreases the formation of tissue gas in these tissues. Recent surgical incisions should be sutured before cavity aspiration and injection. It is most important in surgical deaths to reaspirate and possibly reinject the cavities.

Postmortem Interval Between Death and Embalming

The fourth component considered in the preembalming analysis comprises those events that can occur during the postmortem interval between death and embalming. Quite often the conditions that evolve during this period take precedence over the conditions created by disease or drugs or the general conditions of the body.

For example, a person dies of cancer and is very emaciated and jaundiced because of the effects of drugs on the liver, and the body is not discovered in its residence for 2 days. If the weather is warm or a furnace is running, the postmortem changes, such as rigor mortis, stain, and decomposition, will determine the treatments that the embalmer must employ to preserve, sanitize, and restore the body. The embalmer is not concerned with the jaundice (a condition that is also treated with mild arterial solutions).

The overriding factor to be considered is the degree of decomposition present. Bodies that have been dead for long periods and have begun to decompose demand the use of very strong arterial solutions injected in such a manner and quantity as to limit the amount of swelling that easily occurs during injection of such bodies.

There are two aspects to the postmortem interval portion of embalming analysis: an **intrinsic consideration** and an **extrinsic consideration.**

The extrinsic consideration is the period between death and preparation. It also includes the environment surrounding the body during this period. It is always best to embalm as soon after death as possible. Embalming generally proceeds with fewer complications in bodies that still retain some heat than when there has been a protracted delay. The distribution and diffusion of embalming solution generally are much easier to establish when there is little time delay between death and embalming.

Two major postmortem factors that interfere most with good distribution of the arterial solution are rigor mortis and decomposition. Embalming the body before these changes are firmly established in the body helps to produce better results.

If there is to be a delay between death and preparation, refrigeration will help to slow the onset of many postmortem changes. Refrigeration, however, can create its own problems depending on how long it is used. Bod-

TABLE 10–2. POSTMORTEM PHYSICAL AND CHEMICAL CHANGES

Change	Embalming Significance
Physical	
Algor mortis	Slows onset of rigor and decomposition Keeps blood in a liquid state; aids drainage
Dehydration	Increases the viscosity of the blood; sludge forms Partly responsible for postmortem edema; increasing preservative demands Darkens surface areas; cannot be bleached Eyelids and lids will separate; lips wrinkle; fingers wrinkle Could retard decomposition if severe enough
Hypostasis	Responsible for livor mortis and eventual postmortem stain Increases tissue moisture in dependent tissue areas
Livor mortis	Varies in intensity from slight redness to black depending on volume and viscosity of the blood Intravascular discoloration; can be cleared Can be set as a stain if too strong an uncoordinated arterial solution is used Keeps capillaries expanded; can work as an aid to distribution If it clears *by itself* it could serve as a sign of arterial solution distribution
Increase in blood viscosity	Sludge is created; intravascular resistance Postmortem edema can accompany problem Blood removal becomes difficult; distribution can be poor
Translocation of microbes	Speeds decomposition in various body regions
Chemical	
Rigor mortis	Extravascular resistance Positioning difficult; features may be hard to pose pH not conducive for good fluid reactions Tissues swell easily False sign of preservation (fixation) After passage, firming is difficult Decomposition is usually minimal when present Increases preservative demand
Decomposition	Color changes; odor present; purges; skin-slip; gases Poor distribution of solutions Increased preservative demand Rapid swelling in affected tissue areas
Postmortem stain	Extravascular; cannot be removed; may be bleached Generally seen after the sixth hour; delayed problems Increased preservative demand False indication of fluid dyes Will turn gray after embalming; cosmetic problem
Postmortem caloricity	Sets off the rigor and decomposition cycles
Shift in the body pH	Interferes with fluid reactions Dyes can splotch

ies in a warm environment rapidly undergo early postmortem changes that can create a number of problems for the embalmer. The embalmer must also keep in mind that many bodies released from a coroner or medical examiner's office were kept first in a warm environment—possibly for a long period—then placed under refrigeration. Frequently, these bodies will also be autopsied. Again, at this point, it is the postmortem conditions that have more influence on the selection of embalming technique than the cause of death or medication.

The intrinsic factors of the postmortem interval include those changes that occur within the body during the delay. Table 10–2 summarizes these changes and lists some of the embalming concerns they can create.

▶ EMBALMING ANALYSIS, PART II: INJECTION OF THE BODY

The analysis is a continuous evaluation of the embalming procedure from the start of the embalming procedure until its conclusion. The second part of the analysis is an evaluation of the treatments begun in the preparation of the body. When a problem is encountered the embalmer must decide what new approach to take to solve the problem. The following are some of the concerns of the embalmer:

1. What areas of the body are receiving arterial solution? This can be noted by the presence of fluid dyes in the tissues and the clearing of discolorations such as livor mortis.
2. What areas are not receiving arterial solution? Dyes will not be present and livor mortis, if present, will not be cleared; no firmness will be present.
3. What can be done to stimulate the flow of arterial solution into areas not receiving solution?
   A. Massage along the arterial route that supplies fluid to the area.
   B. Increase the pressure of the solution being injected.
   C. Increase the rate of flow of the solution being injected.
   D. Lower, raise, or manipulate the body area.
   E. Close off the drainage to increase the intravascular pressure.
4. What areas must receive sectional arterial injection? Areas that did not receive solution even after massage and changes in injection protocol must be injected separately.
5. Has the body as a whole received sufficient arterial solution and has the solution been of sufficient strength?
   A. A high-index arterial fluid can be injected or added to the remaining arterial solution to boost the preservative qualities of the solution.
   B. If there is doubt as to the amount of solution, inject additional amounts as long as there is no distension of the neck or facial tissues; inject until preservation is well established.

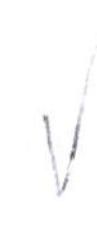

6. Has sufficient arterial solution been retained by the body? The most important portion of the solution being injected is that which **remains** in the body to preserve the tissues after blood and surface discolorations clear; intermittent drainage can be used to help the tissues retain more embalming solution. It has been estimated that more than 50% of the drainage is arterial solution.
7. Is the arterial solution having too much of a dehydrating effect on the tissues? A humectant coinjection fluid can be added.
8. Should additional fluid dye be added for internal coloring of the tissues? Additional dyes may be added throughout the embalming proceure.
9. If purge begins from the mouth or nose, what is its origin and cause? Let the purge continue during the arterial injection **unless** the purge is arterial solution. If the purge is arterial solution and drainage *continues, inject* additional arterial solution to make up for the preservative lost in the purge. If the purge is arterial solution and there is *no* drainage, it can be assumed there is a major rupture in the vascular system. Evaluate the amount of tissues embalmed and consider multipoint injections.
10. Are the tissues firming? This will depend on several factors; in conditions such as *renal failure, emaciation, edema,* and *wasting degenerative diseases,* firming may be very difficult to establish; poor firming can also be a result of the type of arterial fluid being used (some fluids have a slow firming action and others produce less firming of body tissues). If there is doubt as to the preservative needs of the tissues the arterial solution can be increased in strength either by preparing a new solution using a higher-index fluid or by using more concentrated fluid per gallon. A high-index fluid can be added to boost the strength of the solution being injected.

TO INCREASE ARTERIAL SOLUTION STRENGTH

1. Prepare a solution using a higher-index arterial fluid.
2. Add a higher-index arterial fluid to the present solution.
3. Add more concentrated arterial fluid to the present solution.

These are some of the items the embalmer evaluates during arterial injection and drainage of the body in this second phase of an analysis.

▶ EMBALMING ANALYSIS, PART III: EVALUATION OF THE BODY AFTER ARTERIAL EMBALMING

The third phase of the analysis comprises evaluation of the body after the arterial solution and multipoint injections have been completed. Areas that are still lacking solution must now be treated by hypodermic injection or by surface embalming. Some of the following considerations are evaluated during this third phase of the analysis:

1. What body areas have not received arterial solution after primary and multipoint injections are completed?

   A. Look for the absence of fluid dyes, little or no firming of the tissues, and the presence of intravascular discolorations.
   B. Treatment now must be hypodermic injection of the area or surface embalming or a combination of both.
2. Should cavity embalming be done immediately after arterial injection or delayed several hours?
   A. This may depend on the time at which the body must be ready for viewing.
   B. In thin, emaciated bodies, an attempt may have been made to fill out the tissues with a humectant–restorative coinjection; this chemical should be given time to ensure the tissues are firmed before aspiration is done.
   C. If a body is dead from an infectious or contagious disease the embalmer may wish to delay aspiration to help ensure that any blood removed in the aspirated material will have time to mix with the arterial solution injected. With these bodies some embalmers inject a bottle of cavity fluid and wait several hours *before* aspirating; this helps to ensure disinfection of the aspirated materials.
3. Are the features set properly?
   A. Be certain that the mouth is dry. Remove moist cotton and replace it with dry cotton if purge developed during embalming or if moisture leaked from the method of mouth closure where the skin was broken.
   B. Lips and eyelids must not be moist if they are to be glued.
   C. If the eyelids seem soft, cotton can be used for eye closure, and a drop of cavity fluid can be placed on the cotton to make an internal compress before adhesive is applied to the eyelids.
   D. If residual air is present in the mouth after gluing, the lips can be cracked open or limited aspiration of the thorax can be done to remove the air.
4. What if purge developed during embalming?
   A. Be certain the nose is tightly repacked and the mouth has been dried of any purge material.
   B. Purge may be aspirated from the throat and nasal passages using a nasal tube aspirator.
   C. Anal purge can be corrected after cavity embalming; force as much of the fecal material from the orifice; pack the anal orifice with cotton saturated with cavity fluid, phenol cautery fluid, or a chemical solution used for treatment of skin lesions. It may be necessary to use a pursestring suture around the anal orifice to ensure no further purge. Pants and coveralls or a diaper can be used to protect clothing from any further purge.
5. Is the body well groomed? Nails and hands should be cleaned, hands cupped, and fingers together.
6. Are the body and hair clean and dried? The body must be turned on its side to check for clots or debris that were not cleaned away. Turning the body allows it to be dried on all sides.
7. Have decubitus ulcerations been treated? Compresses should be removed from decubitus ulcerations or skin lesions and replaced with clean compresses and fresh chemical or embalming powder. Plastic stockings, pants, or coveralls can be placed on the body to hold the compresses in position.
8. Is there any leakage? Intravenous line punctures leak after arterial injection and even after cavity embalming. They should be properly sealed with a trocar button or super glue.
9. Are tracheotomy and colostomy openings closed? A pursestring suture can be used to close these openings. They should be packed with a cautery chemical and cotton. The tracheotomy can also be filled with some incision seal powder. These openings should be covered with glue and cotton after the suturing is completed.
10. Are incisions sutured? Sutures should be tight and not leaking. If leakage is present the sutures should be removed and the incision resutured.

These 10 items represent the type of evaluation necessary during the third and final stage of embalming analysis.

▶ TREATMENTS

Embalming analysis ⟶ Treatments

The purpose of the analysis is to gather the information necessary to make the correct choices in treating the conditions observed. Through analysis of the body during and after arterial injection, the progress of the treatments is evaluated. If the treatments are not working, then new decisions and plans must be made.

Table 10–3 is by no means complete, but serves to illustrate some of the variables considered by the embalmer in choosing treatments to achieve good sanitation, preservation, and restoration of the body.

TABLE 10–3. EMBALMING TECHNIQUE VARIABLES

Description	Variation
Setting of features	Before embalming, during embalming, after embalming
Method of mouth closure	Needle injector, muscular suture, mandibular suture, dental tie
Method of denture replacement	Cotton, mouth former, kapoc, "pose" material
Method of eye closure	Cotton, eyecaps
Time for raising vessels	Before setting features, after setting features
Artery for primary injection	Right common carotid, right femoral, right axillary
Vein for drainage	Right internal jugular, right femoral, right axillary, heart
Method of injection/drainage	One-point, split injection, restricted cervical, six-point
Method of drainage	Continuous, intermittent, alternate
Drainage instrument	Drainage tube, angular spring forceps, trocar for heart drainage
Body treated with preinjection	Used, not used
Arterial fluid strength	Low index, medium index, high index
Arterial solution injected	Mild fluid solution, moderate fluid solution, strong solution
Coinjection fluid	Used, not used
Fluid dye	Used, not used
Fluid dye color	Pink, tan
Use of fluid dye	Mixed with all solution used, used only in last gallon of solution
Humectant coinjection	Used, not used
Time usage of humectant	Used in all solutions, used in final gallon only
Arterial solution strength	Same used for all solutions injected, mild followed by stronger
Pressure for injection	Low (2–10 pounds), medium (10–20 pounds), high (20 or more pounds)
Rate of flow	Very slow (5–10 ounces), medium (10–15 ounces), fast (more than 15 ounces)
Change of pressure	Not changed during injection, begin low then increase
Change of rate of flow	Not changed during injection, begin slow then increase
Volume of solution injected	Based on weight, edema, time dead, firming of tissues, other
Method of aspiration	Hydroaspirator, electric aspirator, air pressure
Time of aspiration	Immediately after arterial injection, delayed
Reaspiration	Performed, not performed
Method of trocar closure	Trocar button, sutured
Method of cavity fluid injection	Gravity injector, via embalming machine
Cavity fluid reinjected	Done, not done, done only if gases are present
Signs of fluid distribution	Fluid dye, clearing of livor, firming, combinations
Features glued after embalming	Performed, not performed
Type of glue used for features	Rubber-based glue, super glue
Treatment for lack of fluid	Local arterial injection, surface compress, hypodermic injection

▶ COMBINING BODY CONDITIONS AND EMBALMING TREATMENTS

Table 10–4 combines the embalming conditions often observed and of utmost concern to the embalmer. Again, because specific chemicals cannot be listed, a general treatment is described. This list combines the two major parts of an analysis: (1) observation of body conditions and (2) planning of treatment.

▶ SOME GENERALIZATIONS

Whenever it is felt that circulation is going to be a problem because of pathology (arteriosclerosis), time delay since death, and other factors, the first choice should be the common carotid artery and internal jugular vein.

If the preceding conditions exist and it is necessary to run large volumes of solution or very strong solu-

TABLE 10–4. BODY CONDITIONS AND EMBALMING TREATMENTS

Condition	Treatment
Normal body; some livor; dead less than 6 hours; no edema; no chemotherapy	Any vessel for injection and drainage, preinjection; mild to moderate solutions (3–5 gallons, will vary with body size); set tissue to desired firmness
Extensive livor of facial areas; dead less than 6 hours; no extreme pathology	Clear discolorations with a mild to moderate solution; jugular and common carotid recommended; step-up strength to set to desired firmness
Postmortem stain present; body in or out of rigor; dead more than 6 hours	Begin with strong coordinated arterial solutions; continue to increase after circulation is established; restricted cervical injection; slow injection; dye for tracer; section injection where needed; hypodermic and surface treatments where needed
Decomposition evident	Restricted cervical injection; strong coordinated solutions; dye for tracer; sectional/hypodermic and surface treatments where needed
Bodies refrigerated more than 12 hours; some rigor; livor	Solution stronger than average; avoid preinjection; dye tracer; circulation problems expected; restricted cervical injection
Jaundice; no edema; yellow	Jaundice fluid; mild solutions (however, must meet preservative demands); femoral vessels if possible, may respond to preinjection; dye for counterstain
Jaundice green	Cannot be cleared; solution strength based on preservative demands; plenty of dye to counterstain
Generalized edema of body	Start with solution a little above normal strength; continue to increase; if circulation is poor increase to very strong solutions
Localized edema	Treat general embalming based on condition of the tissues; separate sectional embalming of area with edema; hypodermic and surface treatments
Extravascular discolorations from chemotherapy or pathology	Use solutions based on size of body, length of time dead, etc.; treat the discoloration when on hands and face with hypodermic and surface treatments
Autopsied; dead less than 12 hours	Moderate solutions; increase if needed to achieve desired firmness
Autopsied; dead more than 12 hours; refrigerated	Solutions stronger than normal; dyes for tracing; restricted drainage to help achieve circulation; higher pressure may be needed
Death from second-degree burns	Begin with strong solutions; use dye for tracer; death will be related to uremia; may need 100% fluid; do same if autopsied
Localized gangrene/ischemia/possible diabetic	Strong solutions when circulation problems are anticipated; bacterial complications can exist in these bodies; hypodermic/sectional and surface treatments to areas affected; dye for arterial tracing
Frozen bodies	Strong solutions; dye for tracer; restricted cervical injection
Emaciated with edema	Mild to strong solutions depending on circulation (it should be good); again if edema is localized, sectional embalming
Emaciated	Mild solutions in large volume; add humectants to last injection; restricted drainage
Generalized edema with jaundice	Always treat for preservation first; moderate to strong solutions; dye for tracer; inject until edema is treated
Trauma of face/black eyes/lacerations/restorative work needed	Restricted cervical injection if not autopsied; strong solutions; dye for tracer
Infants/children with no pathological complications	Vessels (iliac/carotid/aorta) if not autopsied; standard arterial fluid; inject strength and volume as needed; based on weight and body conditions; dye for tracing
Dehydrated bodies not dead very long	Mild solutions; restricted drainage; humectants in last injection
Bodies with chemotherapy, some edema; skin hemorrhage; expect fixation problems	Use restricted cervical injection; strong solutions into trunk areas; dye for tracing; may help force fluid into tissue spaces
Eye enucleation/no other remarks	To control solution entering head use restricted cervical injection when body not autopsied; use a stronger than normal solution; do not preinject

TABLE 10–4. BODY CONDITIONS AND EMBALMING TREATMENTS (*Continued*)

Condition	Treatment
Contagious disease	Use solutions a little stronger than normal (2–3%); run plenty of volume; avoid personal contact with "first" drainage; run volume and increased strengths depending on other body conditions. (i.e., weight/edema)
Obese	Begin with a slightly stronger than normal solution; after blood discolorations clear, strength may continue to be increased; first vessel choice common carotid/jugular; second choice external iliac
Arteriosclerosis noticed when raising a common carotid	Stronger than normal solutions; high pulsating pressure; dye for tracer; sectional; hypodermic and surface treatments
Arteriosclerosis seen when raising femoral as first vessel	Go to common carotid and jugular; use a solution a little stronger than normal; inject based on other body conditions

tions into the trunk regions, use the restricted cervical injection.

Whenever facial or neck swelling is anticipated or observed, use the restricted cervical injection.

After injecting a strong solution never inject weaker solutions into the same area; always inject *mild solutions* first, after which *stronger solutions* can be injected.

After livor and other intravascular discolorations are cleared, the best response is obtained with average or mild solution. After intravascular discolorations are cleared, solution strengths can be increased. At this time, some form of restricted drainage can be safely used (e.g., intermittent or alternate drainage).

▶ KEY TERMS AND CONCEPTS FOR STUDY AND DISCUSSION

1. Define embalming analysis, intrinsic factors, and extrinsic factors.
2. List the three time periods of embalming analysis.
3. Explain the purpose of embalming analysis.
4. Describe the four categories of information used in embalming analysis.
5. Discuss why the conditions present in the body are more important in an embalming analysis than the actual cause of death.
6. List several effects brought about by long-term drug therapy.
7. List postmortem physical changes and chemical changes.

▶ BIBLIOGRAPHY

Chemotherapy and embalming results. In: *Champion Expanding Encyclopedia.* Springfield, OH: Champion Chemical; 1986:No. 570.

Embalming Course Content Syllabus. American Board of Funeral Service Education; 1996.

Frederick JF. *Effects of Chemotherapeutic Agents.* Boston: Dodge Chemical; 1968.

Shor M. Knowledge of effect of disease simplifies embalming. *Casket and Sunnyside,* September 1960.

Shor M. Conditions of the body dictate the proper embalming treatment. *Casket and Sunnyside,* November 1972.

Slocum RE. *Pre-embalming Considerations.* Boston: MA: Dodge Chemical, 1958.

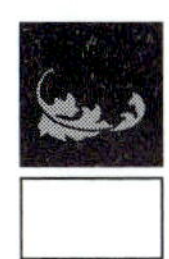

CHAPTER 11
PREPARATION OF THE BODY PRIOR TO ARTERIAL INJECTION

The process of embalming the dead human body can be divided into three time periods, each containing procedures that are best performed within the specified period. The primary reason is that the preservative fluid used for embalming contains formaldehyde, and formaldehyde coagulates the proteins of the body. This coagulation (or preservation) of body protein brings about a firming and drying of the body tissues. Once set in a particular position the tissues are difficult to change.

Three time periods are described:

Preembalming	Period prior to injection of the arterial solution
Embalming	Period during which arterial solution is injected into the body
Postembalming	Period after arterial injection

In each period specific procedures are carried out. They all culminate in the completely embalmed body. In Chapter 1, complete chronologies for embalming autopsied and unautopsied bodies are detailed.

Analysis of the body is performed during each period. The treatments discussed in this chapter are based on the analysis made by the embalmer from his or her first observations of the body (pp. 179–182).

It is important that the student be aware that many procedures carried out in the preembalming period can be performed during the embalming or postembalming period. Because of the fixative and hardening action of the preservative solution, preembalming procedures such as shaving the body, setting the features, and aligning broken skin areas and bones can be done with greater ease prior to injection of the fixative arterial solution.

Body conditions and the skill of the operator may influence the period during which certain procedures are performed. For example, decomposition and the presence of stomach or lung purge may dictate that the mouth be closed after arterial embalming, once the cavity aspiration has been completed. Likewise, the mouth is usually sealed with an adhesive in the postembalming period but, if there is a problem of "buck" teeth, it may be necessary to glue the lips prior to injection of the arterial solution to achieve good mouth closure. The embalmer must learn to be flexible in technique, relying on the conditions of the body to dictate the order of embalming procedures.

An important reason for minimizing the procedures carried out during the period of arterial injection is that the embalmer should devote full attention to observation of solution distribution and drainage during injection of the embalming solution. Attention should be given to drainage problems and techniques to improve arterial solution circulation to all body areas. During the injection phase of embalming it is very important for the embalmer to employ as many techniques as possible to ensure **retention** of the arterial solution (Figure 11–1).

▶ LEGAL REQUIREMENTS

Before the embalming process begins, it is important that the embalmer verifies with the funeral director to make certain that permission has been given for embalming the body. Many states require that permission be given in writing or by verbal order by the person in charge of final disposition. In addition, the Federal Trade Commission requires specific disclosures to the person arranging the funeral as to the price for embalming services and statements as to when embalming is not necessary for final disposition. Before any embalming is begun, it is imperative that the embalmer be certain permission has been given for preparation of the deceased.

▶ PRELIMINARY PREPARATION

The embalming process begins when the deceased is placed on the middle of the embalming table. The body should be temporarily centered on the table with

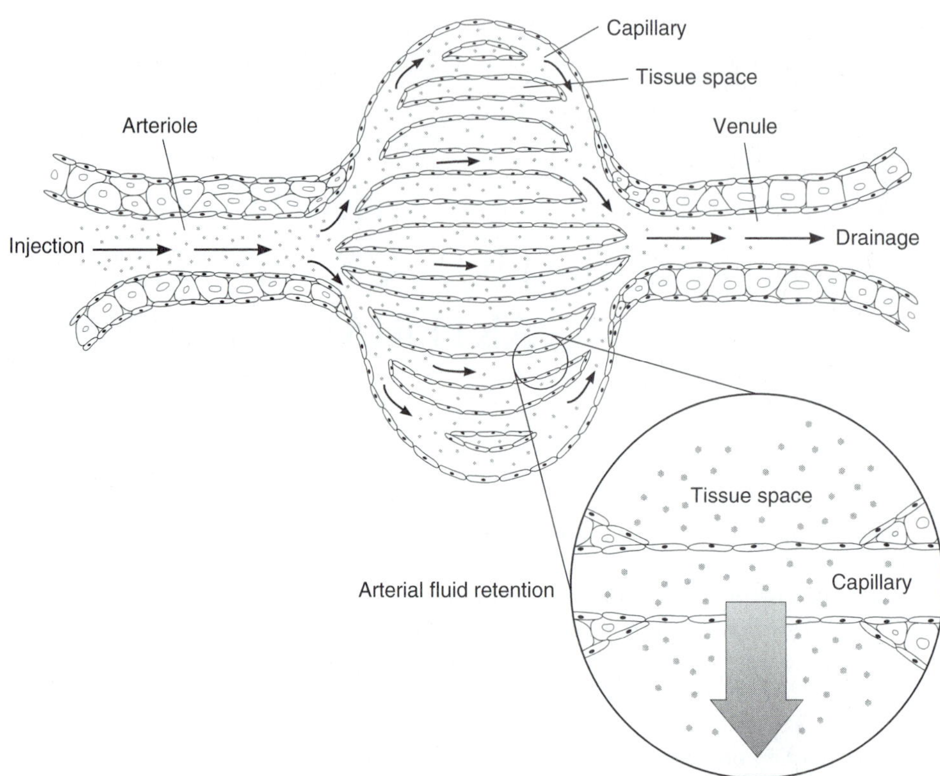

Figure 11–1. Arterial solution retention.

the head as near as possible to the upper end of the table.

Any clothing, sheeting, or body bag should be sprayed with a disinfectant. This helps to control vermin and odors. Standing at the side of the embalming table, the embalmer can gently roll the body toward him* by placing his hands on the shoulder and the hip of the deceased (Figure 11–2A). After the body is slightly turned, the sheets may be pushed beneath the center of the body. (This is also a way to remove clothing.) Next, the embalmer rolls the body back to the supine position. He moves to the opposite side of the body, repeats the rolling process, and, thus, removes the sheeting that enveloped the body (see Chapter 2).

In moving a wrapped body the embalmer should always *pull* the body and not *push* it. For example, transfer of the body from the removal cot to the embalming table can be accomplished in three steps: (1) Place the removal cot next to the embalming table. (2) Stand on the opposite side of the embalming table and reach across the table to the deceased on the removal cot. (3) Pull the legs of the deceased onto the table first; then pull the portions of the sheet that envelop the trunk and shoulders (Fig. 11–2B).

It is easier to position the body on the embalming table while the deceased is wrapped or partially clothed. After clothes have been removed, the deceased can be moved more easily if the embalming table is moistened with water. Clothing should be removed without cutting whenever possible, labeled and properly stored for dry cleaning, and returned to the family. Very soiled clothing and underclothing should be disposed of in a sanitary manner. All clothing should be checked for valuables. Rings, jewelry, and other valuables should be inventoried and securely stored until they can be returned to the family. Some embalmers protect rings on the deceased by placing adhesive tape around the ring finger. Others prefer to place a piece of string or gauze around the ring if it is to be left on the body during embalming. Glasses, jewelry, watches, and religious articles should be removed during embalming.

▶ TOPICAL DISINFECTION OF THE BODY

After the sheeting or clothing has been removed and the body is placed in the center of the table, the surface and orifices of the body are treated with a topical disin-

*As the traditional use of the pronoun *he* has not yet been superseded by a convenient, generally accepted pronoun that means either "he" or "she," the author will continue to use he while acknowledging the inherent inequity of the traditional preference for the masculine pronoun.

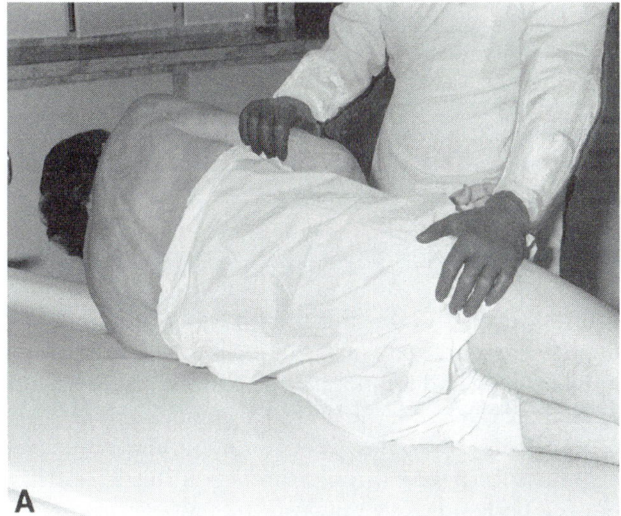

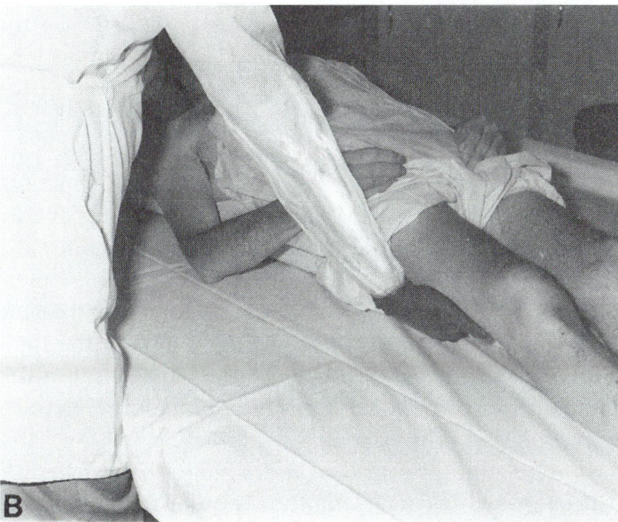

Figure 11-2. A. Turn the body by gripping the shoulder (upper arm) and the hip. **B.** The embalmer can easily move a body by placing one hand under the neck and one under the thigh and pulling the body toward him or her.

fectant.* A good surface disinfectant should be used and should be either washed or sprayed onto the body. A droplet-type spray is preferred over pressurized sprays, which lose too much of the disinfectant to the surrounding air and can then be inhaled by the embalmer. Pressurized sprays also have the tendency to convert surface microbes on the body into airborne microbes. The surface disinfectant should be allowed to remain on the body several minutes. After topical disinfection, the body should be thoroughly washed with lukewarm water and a good germicidal soap. The orifices should be cleaned and packed with cotton and the body dried.

*Disinfectants are discussed in detail in Chapter 3.

QUALITIES OF A GOOD TOPICAL DISINFECTANT

1. It is active, not outdated.
2. It is effective against a wide range of microbes including viruses and fungi.
3. It destroys microbes and their products quickly.
4. It is a good deodorant for the body.
5. It does not bleach or stain the skin.
6. It is not irritating to the embalmer's skin or respiratory tract.

When sodium hypochlorite is used, it is important that the chemical be washed away with water before any contact is made with formaldehyde. Sodium hypochlorite and formaldehyde can combine to produce a carcinogenic product.

Disinfection of the body should also include the destruction of body lice or mites (scabies). If scabies is suspected, a commercial pediculicide should be applied to the skin and hair of the deceased. The embalmer should carefully handle these bodies so that the insects do not infest his skin. The embalmer should also carefully check for fly eggs or maggots, especially in the summer months or in warm climates. Fly eggs appear as yellowish clusters in the corners of the eyes, nostrils, or ears or within the mouth. If present, these eggs can develop into the eating larval stage known as maggots in 24 hours. Great care should be taken to remove all eggs. If the larval stage has begun, a larvicide can be used. Some success is achieved by flushing the affected area with kerosene, concentrated salt water, or a commercial mortuary product.

Maggots eat even embalmed tissue, so it is very important to remove and destroy them. To prevent flies from depositing eggs, keep the body covered. Nostrils can be packed in the summer months and small pieces of cotton can be placed in the nostrils (extending outside the nostril) when the body is left in the preparation room or is shipped. In the summer months, some funeral homes make a habit of covering the face of the body at night. Outside windows and doors of the preparation room should be screened. In addition, insecticides should be used if flies are present in the preparation room. Once fly eggs develop into the larval stage, the problem becomes very difficult, if not impossible, to control.

▶ WASHING THE BODY

The body should be thoroughly washed with warm water and a germicidal soap. Special attention should be given to the areas to be viewed—the face and hands.

These areas must be free of all debris for good cosmetic application after the embalming. If the skin of the hands, particularly between the fingers, is scaly, a solvent such as a dry hair shampoo or trichloroethylene can be used to remove the scaling skin. This condition can also be found on the forehead and parts of the face. This scale must be removed if cosmetics are to be applied. It is also useful to apply massage cream to these areas and wipe the cream away with a cloth after it has been worked into the pores of the skin. After thorough washing and rinsing, the body should be dried with toweling. Use disposable items in these procedures, for they can be destroyed and will not have to be laundered. Manipulation during washing and drying the body also helps to relieve rigor mortis.

The fingernails should be cleaned using soap, water, and a nail brush in the preembalming period. It is much easier to remove debris from under the nails at this time (use great care if an instrument is used to clean the nails). Any stains on the fingers or the nails can be removed with a solvent. Nail polish can be removed with a commercial remover or acetone. Trimming and brushing the nails greatly help to clean the fingers and nails.

▶ CARING FOR THE HAIR

The hair can be washed at the beginning and at the end of embalming. Note the following points:

1. Wash the hair with warm water and a good germicidal soap; a commercial shampoo may also be used.
2. Washing the hair should deodorize the hair.
3. Hair rinses may be used to help untangle long hair. These products usually assist in deodorizing and styling the hair.
4. Blow-drying the hair helps to style the hair, for both men and women.
5. When in doubt as to styling the hair, comb or brush it straight back.
6. When hair is very thin and has a tendency to fall out, dry it before combing or brushing and avoid as much brushing or combing as possible.
7. Use cool water to remove blood from the hair.
8. If lice or mites are suspected, apply a commercial pediculicide before washing. Follow instructions for the use of this chemical.
9. When dandruff or scaling of the skin is present (often seen when therapeutic drugs have been used for longer periods), several washings may be necessary. The hair can also be washed with the "dry wash" solvent shampoos.
10. Do not comb curly hair when wet; knead the hair with a towel while blow-drying. This helps to retain the curl.
11. Plats should be combed out prior to shampooing.

▶ SHAVING THE BODY

After topically disinfecting the body, washing and drying the hair and body surfaces, packing the mouth and nasal orifices, and temporarily positioning the body, the embalmer can shave the body. Facial hair should be removed from all bodies (men, women, and children). The nostrils should also be trimmed at this time. Shaving the body not only improves the appearance of the deceased but greatly assists in the application of cosmetics to facial tissues. If hair were to remain on the face, cosmetics (whether creams, liquids, or powders) would stick to the hair, making the appearance of the deceased quite unnatural.

The embalmer should check with the family with respect to a mustache or beard on a deceased male. It is much easier to remove a mustache or beard before arterial injection. Their removal when the family did not want them removed could create a legal problem for the funeral home. If there is doubt about shaving and the family cannot be consulted, embalm the body and shave later. This process is more difficult, but it is much easier to shave the body after embalming than restore a beard or mustache.

The administration of therapeutic drugs often induces growth of facial hair on women and children. Drug therapy can also induce hair growth on the forehead. In women and children, this facial hair is easily removed by lightly passing a safety razor over the facial tissues. Lather is not always necessary to remove this light growth. Shaving the forehead can be very difficult. Shaving lather should be applied and great care taken not to nick the skin. After shaving the forehead areas apply massage cream.

Note the following points in shaving the face:

1. Use a good, sharp blade; more than one blade may be needed to shave some bodies.
2. Use a double-edged safety razor, single stainless razor or straight edge.
3. Apply warm water to the face with a washcloth first.
4. Use shaving cream to lather the face.
5. When there is doubt about the length of sideburns, mustache, or beard, consult the family. If they cannot be reached, these areas can always be shaved after arterial embalming.
6. When using a new blade, it is wise to begin

shaving on the left side of the face or in the neck area to slightly dull the blade.

7. Shave in the direction of hair growth; bodies vary, and sometimes shaving must be directed against or perpendicular to the growth.
8. Use small, short, repeated strokes over an area to achieve the closest shave; an area can be shaved repeatedly or (as stated in item 7) from one or several different directions (Figure 11–3).
9. Clean the razor frequently with warm water.
10. Try to shave an area without lifting the razor off the face; apply pressure on the razor and "slide" the razor over the area being shaved.
11. Use a small piece of cotton or washcloth (gauze or cheesecloth) to pull the skin taut and make an even area for shaving; this is helpful in shaving the area immediately under the mandible and the upper neck area.
12. After shaving, wash the face with a washcloth and warm water; a thin layer of massage cream may be applied.

Razor abrasions are areas of the face where small pieces of flesh have been removed. Application of massage cream helps to prevent the area from dehydrating and turning brown. During arterial injection, arterial solution may leak through these nicked areas. It is important that a very small piece of wax be placed over these areas after cosmetics have been applied. This prevents the areas from further drying and showing through the cosmetic, especially when alcohol-type transparent cosmetics are used. If the area of the face that has been nicked is discolored and the face is to be treated with opaque cosmetics, use either cream or liquid opaque cover cosmetics. The massage cream can be omitted, for the opaque cosmetic needs dry skin free of any grease products for application.

If a beard or mustache or the face in general must be shaved after arterial injection, lather the face with a very moist, warm lather. Use a sharp, new blade in the razor. To avoid nicking the tissue, shave in small areas and keep applying lather to the area being shaved. When completed, apply a thin film of massage cream.*

In shaving a beard, many embalmers first trim off the longer hair of the beard with shears or hair clippers. This process is not necessary; the beard can be shaved without the preliminary clipping. Shaving should be directed from the cheek areas downward over the face. Heavy growth may necessitate the use of several blades.

*Shaving with an electric razor after vascular embalming and over a dry face is effectively used by some embalmers.

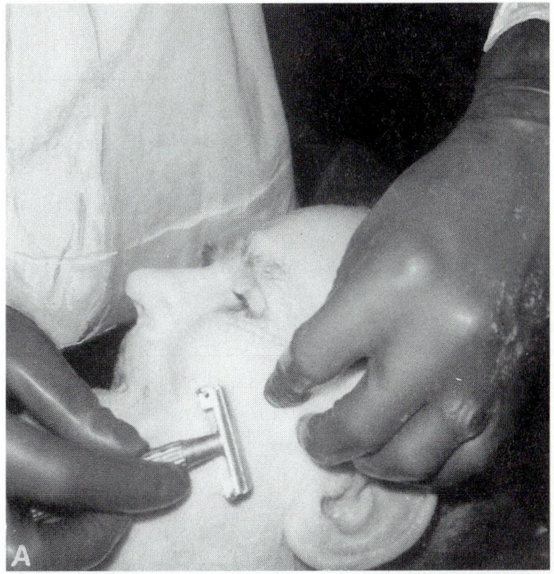

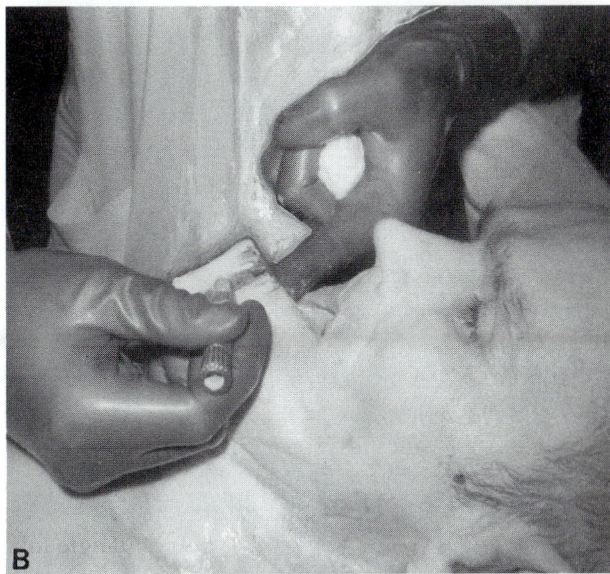

Figure 11–3. A. Slide the razor over the face, shaving in the direction of beard growth. **B.** The best results are achieved by shaving from several directions.

After the body has been shaved, massage cream may be applied. Some embalmers prefer that a light application of this cream be made after the features are set; others prefer to apply massage cream after embalming; some do not apply cream at all because of the type of cosmetic they will use. Massage cream has several uses:

1. It protects the face and hands from surface dehydration.
2. It prevents broken skin areas such as razor abrasions from dehydrating and turning dark brown.

3. It acts as a lubricant when the face is massaged to break up rigor mortis.
4. It is an excellent skin cleanser.
5. It provides a lubricating base that can be used for massaging the facial tissues, neck, and hands during arterial injection.
6. It protects areas of the face from damage if stomach purge from the mouth or nose occurs.
7. It provides a base for cream cosmetics.

There are two types of massage creams. One, the type generally sold by mortuary companies, has a greasy feel. The second is a face or hand cream that has a water base. After application, the cream can hardly be felt. The grease type may be more useful if the embalmer requires massage cream for use with mortuary cosmetics. In addition to creams that can be applied by hand, several spray antidehydrants are available; these are basically silicone or lanolin sprays. Whether a cream or spray, it need not be applied heavily. A very small amount adequately serves to protect the skin areas to which it is applied.

▶ POSITIONING THE BODY

The objective of preembalming positioning is to make the body appear comfortable and restful in later repose in the casket. Preservative arterial solution firms the body proteins of the muscles in the position in which the embalmer places the body prior to arterial embalming. It is very difficult to reposition the body after embalming. The position of the body as it rests on the embalming table should approximate the desired position of the body when casketed. Three position levels are desired: (1) the highest level should be the head, (2) the middle level should be the ventral thoracic wall (chest), and (3) the lowest level should be the ventral abdominal wall (abdomen) (Figure 11–4).

In addition to positioning the trunk of the body, the embalmer needs to properly position the arms, hands, legs, and feet (Figure 11–5). The feet should be placed as close together as possible. During the embalming process, some embalmers prefer not only to place the feet together but also to elevate them. At this time, note should be made of any unusual size problems. If the body is quite obese the straight distance between the elbows should be measured. It is important with overweight bodies to position the arms so that the elbows are as close as possible to the upper area of the abdominal wall. This can save inches in the casket. Using an urn-shaped or oversized casket or turning the body slightly when it is placed into the casket will help to position these heavy bodies in the casket.

If length is a problem, an oversized casket should be ordered. Keeping the feet together and flexing the toes save a little space. Flexing the legs as well as omitting shoes may also help. Oversized caskets may mean that an oversized vault is needed or that the casket cannot be placed in a crypt or a shipping container. In positioning the body, every effort should be made to use a standard-sized casket.

Caskets are available in the following dimensions:

METAL	Standard	6 ft 7 in. × 24 in.
	Oversized	6 ft 9 in. × 26 in.
		× 28 in.
		× 31 in.
WOOD	Standard	6 ft 3 in. × 22 in.
	Oversized	6 ft 6 in. × 24 in.
		× 26 in.
		× 28 in.

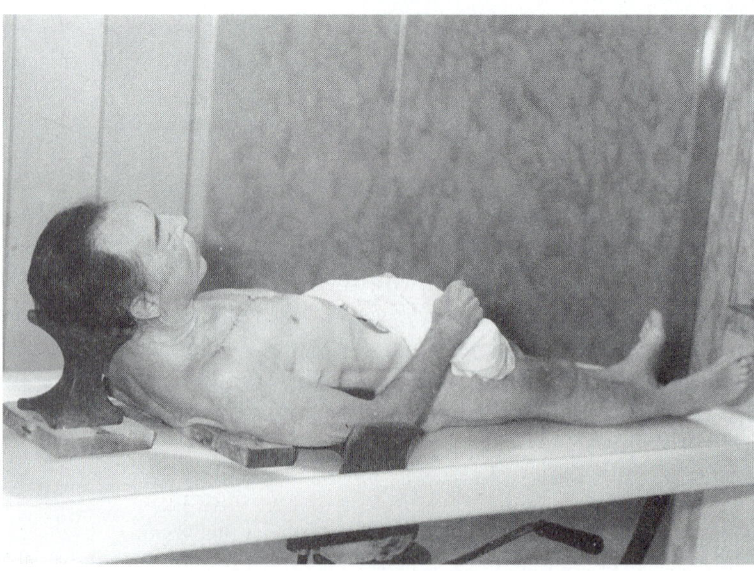

Figure 11–4. The three levels of position: head, chest, and abdomen.

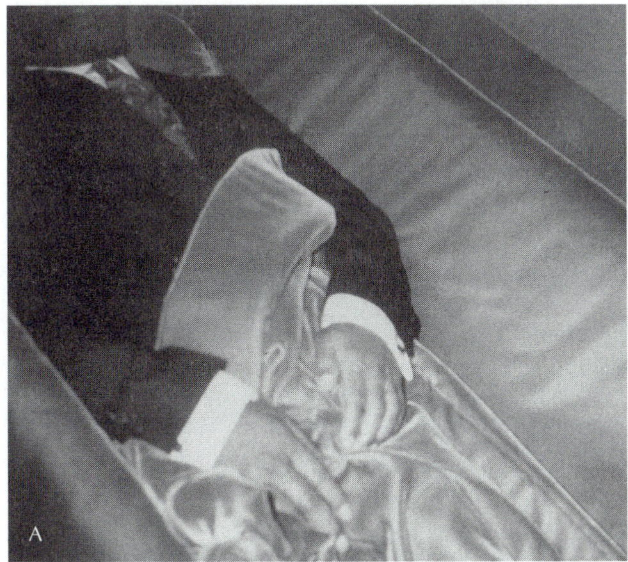

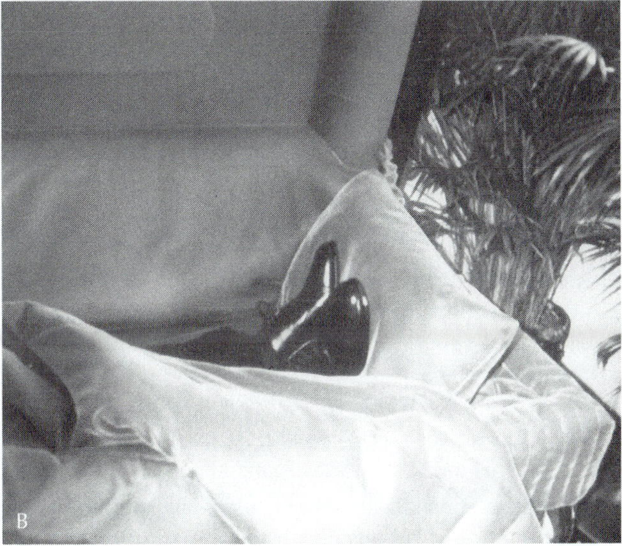

Figure 11–5. A. One pose in which hands, arms, and the blanket may be positioned. **B.** Straight legs and feet allow shoes to be shown, resting on the casket foot pillow.

The body should be undressed, treated with a topical disinfectant, then washed and dried. The embalmer manipulates the limbs while undressing, washing, and drying the body to relieve rigor mortis if present. Rigor mortis may be responsible for the body being in a very undesirable position. It is necessary to remove the rigor by firmly manipulating the muscles.

When limbs are *flexed, rotated, bent,* and *massaged* to relieve rigor, capillaries are torn. This can lead to swelling during arterial injection and is one reason many embalmers do not attempt to relieve rigor. Avoid excessive exercise of the muscles in relieving rigor mortis. Breaking the rigor helps not only in positioning the body but also in removing extravascular resistance in the circulatory system. Relief of the rigor may result in better arterial solution distribution and also better drainage. A routine proposed for relieving rigor mortis follows:

1. Firmly rotate the neck from side to side.
2. Flex the head.
3. Push the lower jaw up to begin to relieve the rigor in the muscles of the jaw. Repeat this several times. If the mouth is firmly closed begin by pushing the mandible upward; then firmly push on the chin to attempt to open the mouth. Massage the temporalis and the masseter muscles on the side of the face. This may help open the mouth.
4. Flex the arm several times, then extend it. Finally, rotate the arm at the shoulder.
5. Grasp the fingers as a group on the palm side of the hand and attempt to extend all the fingers at the same time.
6. Grasp the foot and rotate it inward. Repeat several times. Attempt to flex the legs at the knee. Raise and lower the legs several times.

The body should be placed in a supine position in the center of the embalming table with the head located near the top of the table. This position allows adequate room for positioning devices for the head and arms. The carotid vessels can then be raised by the embalmer standing at the head of the table, the hair can be treated by the embalmer or hairdresser, and, if the table is "ribbed," water run on the table is kept off the body.

Establish the levels of positioning. Rest the buttocks on the table to establish the abdominal level. Next, place supports under the shoulders. Supports promote drainage from the head and neck areas and help relieve pressure on the internal jugular veins should the head be elevated too much. A variety of positioning devices can be used for shoulder supports. Some embalmers prefer that the support elevate the shoulders as much as 4 inches off the table. Additional head support would then be needed for the head rest. The chest and head are so elevated to prevent blood that remains in the heart after embalming from gravitating into the neck and facial tissues and graying these tissues. This discoloration is often referred to as **formaldehyde gray.**

Elevating the shoulders also helps to dry the body, for air can easily pass under a large area of the back. This elevation helps to keep any water on the table from contacting the skin of the back and the neck. It is easier to clean under the body. If the body is obese, a higher shoulder elevation will be needed to establish the three levels of positioning by raising the head and chest above the abdomen. In positioning the obese body, the higher shoulder support allows the embalmer

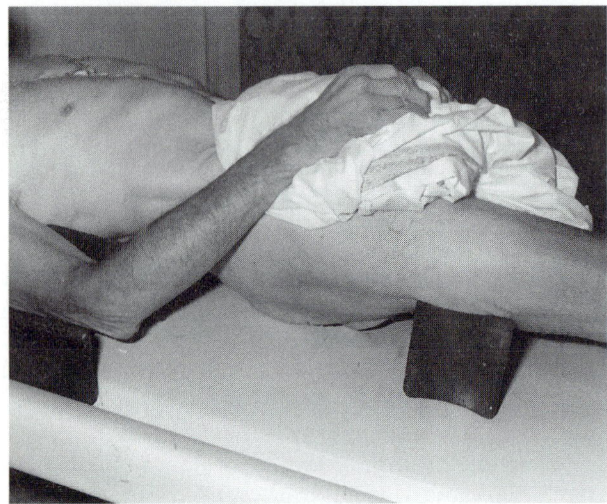

Figure 11–6. Blocking the thigh assists in the positioning of some bodies.

to slightly lower the height of the head. By doing so, the chin can be pushed forward and thus elevated, creating some visible neck area. The neck will appear a little thinner when the chin is pushed upward.

Good elevation of the head and shoulders can also be very important in draining edema from the tissues of the face and neck. At the conclusion of the aspiration phase of cavity embalming as an **operative aid,** a trocar can be passed under the clavicles channeling the neck tissues; this establishes routes for the drainage of edema into the thoracic cavity. As a **manual aid,** a pneumatic cuff or elastic bandage can be applied to the external tissues of the neck to assist in the removal of edema (or swollen tissues).

Shoulders are elevated to (1) assist drainage, (2) keep water off larger areas of the back and shoulders, (3) prevent gravitation of blood into facial tissues after embalming, (4) assist in drying the body by allowing air to pass beneath the body, (5) assist in draining edema from the facial and neck tissues, and (6) position the head and chest higher than the abdomen.

If a problem should arise because of crippling of the limbs (the body cannot lie in an even supine position), a head block can be placed under one of the upper thighs (Figure 11–6). This block prevents the body from turning from side to side. If placed under the left thigh, the block assists in turning the entire body slightly to the right.

▶ POSITIONING THE HEAD

The head is adjusted on the headrest *after* the shoulders have been elevated. If the shoulders had to be elevated greatly, the headrest will need additional elevation. Placing a folded towel between the head and the headrest may be sufficient to elevate the head to the desired position. The head should be slightly tilted to the right about 15°. In some localities, the head is positioned straight without any turn. Custom, of course, dictates such protocol.

With obese persons the chin should be slightly elevated. This makes the neck look a little thinner and somewhat visible. In positioning obese persons it may be helpful to leave the head straight. Turning the head can make the neck and jowl area look swollen and distended. Elevating the left shoulder in the casket turns the entire body slightly to the right. Should there be disfiguration on the left side of the face or if some of the hair has had to be shaved for surgical purposes, leaving the head straight can help to keep these problems from being seen.

If a kneeler is to be used during viewing of the body it should be placed in line with the shoulders. Viewers thus will see the profile of the body and, in particular, only the right side of the face. If the kneeler is placed at the center of the casket, both sides of the face can be seen (bilateral view). Any disfigurement on the left side of the face or any swelling of the face is more easily observed. In some areas of the country a "full-couch" casket is used. Should there be a disfigurement on the right side of the face, the "full-couch" casket allows the body to be turned so the left side of the face is viewed. A reverse-cap or special ordering also makes it possible to reverse the body in the half-couch casket.

▶ POSITIONING THE HANDS AND ARMS

Prior to the start of the injection of arterial solution, the hands should be placed on the embalming table or even lowered over the table. This forces the blood in the veins of the arms to gravitate into the capillaries of the hands and may expand these tiny vessels. Once the embalmer sees that fluid is being distributed into the arms and hands, he can elevate the hands and place them on the abdominal wall. The elbows should be elevated off the embalming table with either a head block or an arm positioning device. Raising the elbows prevents them from interfering with drainage of blood or water that may be passing along the drains on either side of the table. The elbows should be kept close to the sides of the body. This is very important in obese bodies. It may mean that an oversized casket will not have to be used.

Custom again dictates the position in which the hands should be placed. To help hold the hands in a cupped position and in proper place during embalming, a sheet or large towel can be mounded and the hands placed on top (Figure 11–7).

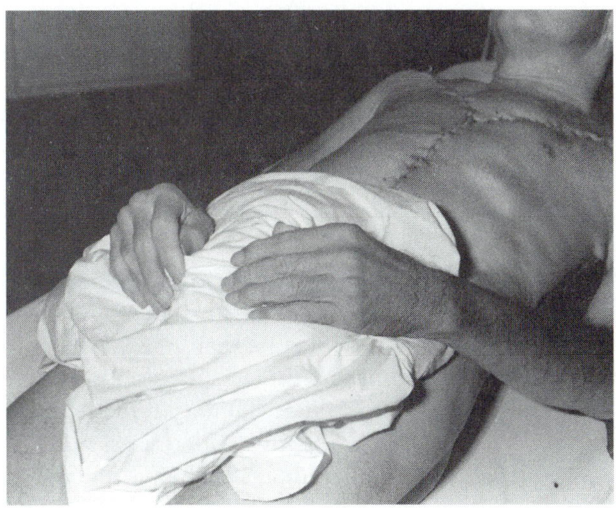

Figure 11-7. A sheet or towel can help in positioning hands and fingers.

Care should be taken to ensure that the fingers remain together (do not separate) and are slightly cupped. A large ball of cotton can be placed in the palm to cup the fingers, and masking tape or gauze can be used to keep fingers together during embalming. A drop of super adhesive between the fingers may be valuable in keeping fingers together.

▶ POSITIONING PROBLEMS

A stroke, paralytic condition, or arthritis may contribute to distorted positions of the extremities (Figure 11–8). Often the arms are drawn up on the chest and the hands are tightly clenched. In addition, there may be severe spinal curvature. When the spine is curved extra elevation of the head is necessary. A head block placed under a thigh helps to keep the body level. It may even be necessary to place straps around the body and table to hold the body in the correct position. Limbs can be gently forced, but if it appears that ligaments or skin will be torn, leave the limbs in their position.

A **manual aid,** such as splinting and wrapping a limb, can be used to position a limb. The **operative aid** of cutting tendons should only be used when absolutely necessary. When the legs are drawn up, as in the fetal position, injection and drainage may be accomplished from the carotid location. Every attempt should be made to obtain good solution distribution, so the iliac or femoral vessels do not have to be raised and injected. After casketing, disfigured arthritic hands can be partly hidden from view by placing the casket blanket around the hands. This procedure and how they will be handled should be explained to the family prior to viewing.

Autopsied bodies present several positioning problems. If the spine is removed, it is very difficult, but very necessary, to place a shoulder block beneath the shoul-

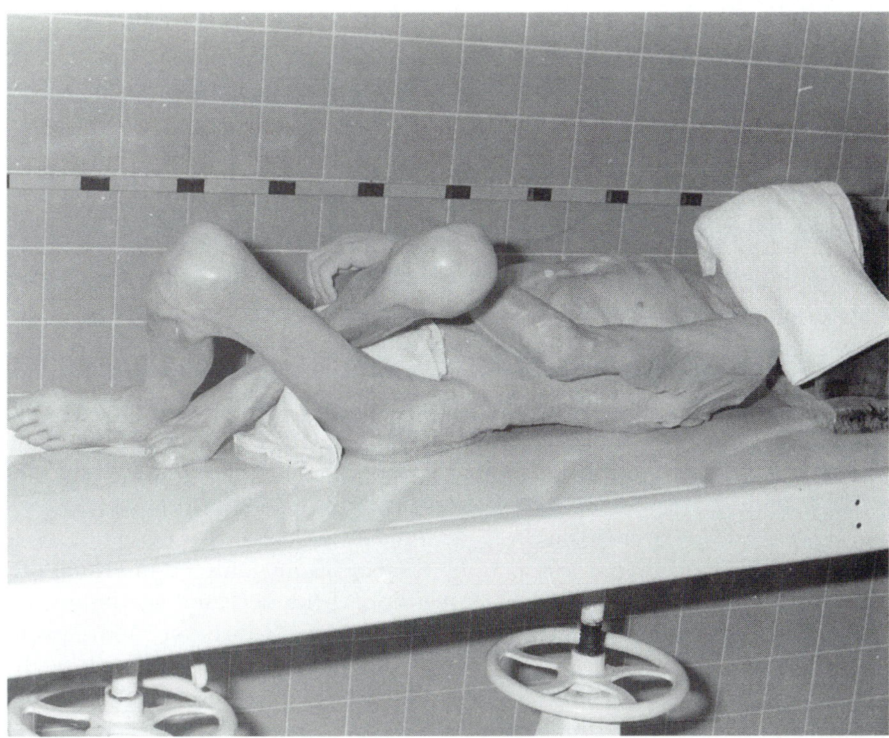

Figure 11-8. Severe arthritis of the lower limbs.

ders. The neck and shoulders have to be lifted to place the support under the shoulders. Some embalmers force a pointed wooden dowel into the foramen magnum at the base of the skull. This dowel extends down into the spinal area of the neck and prevents the head from easily turning from side to side. Once the body is casketed, a wedge of cotton can be placed under the ear to help hold the head in proper position. Rigor mortis may or may not be present in autopsied bodies. If present in the arms, it should be relieved as much as possible. Attempt to keep the arms in the proper position during and immediately after injection.

After autopsy, sutures are completed and the body is washed and dried. It may be necessary to use strips of sheets to tie the arms into proper position. This is very important when the body is to be shipped to another funeral director. Do not let the arms lie at the sides of the body. Be certain they are properly positioned and, if necessary, tie them into position. These ties will later be removed when the body is dressed.

▶ SETTING THE FEATURES

Generally, the features are set in the preembalming period. After the tissues are embalmed it may be difficult to align the tissues to obtain the desired expression. Features can be temporarily set when purge is expected. In this manner the mouth can be dried and the throat packed after the body has been aspirated. Features can be set during embalming, but manipulation of tissues during injection has a tendency to draw arterial solution into the area. This can result in swelling or overembalming of the facial tissues. By doing the steps involved in embalming separately, the embalmer can concentrate fully on each task.

Mouth Closure Sequence

1. Relieve the rigor mortis present.
2. Disinfect the oral cavity and clean it.
3. Remove and clean dentures (if present).
4. Pack the throat area; if natural teeth and dentures are absent, also fill the entire oral cavity.
5. Replace dentures.
6. Close the mouth to observe the natural bite.
7. Secure the mandible by one of the methods of mouth closure.
8. Place the lips in a desired position, attempting to make the line of mouth closure at the level of the inferior margin of the upper teeth.
9. Embalm the body.
10. Check the mouth for moisture or purge material.
11. Seal the mouth.

One of four conditions exists when the mouth is set: (1) natural teeth are present; (2) natural teeth are present but several are missing; (3) dentures are present (complete set—well fitting, lower denture only—no upper denture, upper denture only—no lower denture, old and very loose fitting dentures, new ill-fitting dentures, partial plates); (4) neither dentures or natural teeth are present.

Dentures are personal property and many hospitals and nursing homes return them to the family with the belongings. Funeral directors should make every effort to instruct institutions to keep the dentures with the body. When death occurs at home, the persons removing the body should ask for the dentures. It is possible to open the mouth after embalming and insert dentures, but this task can be very time consuming and often difficult if a hard-firming arterial solution has been used.

The embalmer should relieve the rigor mortis before disinfecting the mouth. The mouth can be cleaned and dried with cotton. If purge is present, a nasal tube aspirator can be used to aspirate purge material. Disinfectant is poured into the mouth. The throat can be packed with cotton to help control purge and odor arising from the stomach or lungs. Some embalmers prefer to cover the cotton with massage cream so that the cotton does not draw purge material from the stomach or lungs, as a wick would do. If the body is to be shipped out of the country or is dead from a contagious disease, it may be mandatory that the throat and nose be packed with cotton saturated with a disinfectant.

The lips should be examined and loose skin removed. Massage cream or a solvent helps to remove any loose skin. A washrag moistened with cool water can be used to remove loose skin off the lips. Fever blisters should be opened and drained, and loose skin removed from the lip. A small cotton pack of a phenol cautery chemical can be placed over the area once the blister is removed to help seal the tissues. If the scab is hard to loosen, massage cream may be helpful. A scab can also be removed by loosening with a sharp scalpel.

Observe the "weather line." This helps to determine the thickness of the lips. A picture of the deceased, if available, is helpful in determining the correct expression. Remember, the upper mucous membrane is generally longer and thinner than the lower mucous membrane. (The mucous membranes are the "red" portions of the lips.)

Many problems may be encountered in setting the mouth. The expression of the deceased can be one of the most criticized areas of the embalming. A rare problem today, but one that is easy to solve, is buck teeth. Protruding upper teeth constitute the most problems. A simple method can be used to correct this condition:

1. Secure the jaw closed using one of the methods of mouth closure.
2. Place a strip of cotton over the lower teeth. This helps to push the lower lip forward.
3. Using rubber-based lip glue, secure the upper and lower lips together (super adhesive may also be used).
4. Embalm the body.
5. Reopen the mouth to be certain there is no purge or air in the mouth; then reglue the lips (Figure 11–9).

Over the years, a variety of methods have been proposed for correcting the problem of protruding upper teeth. The preceding method works very well and is quite simple. The use of a super adhesive greatly facilitates the procedure. If there is a condition that warrants removal of the teeth or showing the teeth, the family should be consulted.

Securing the Mandible for Mouth Closure

Method 1: Needle Injector. A widely used method of mouth closure today involves the needle injector. A pin with an attached wire is driven by a hand-operated device into the center of the maxilla, and a similar pin with a wire attached is driven into the mandible in an opposing position (Figure 11–10). The two wires are

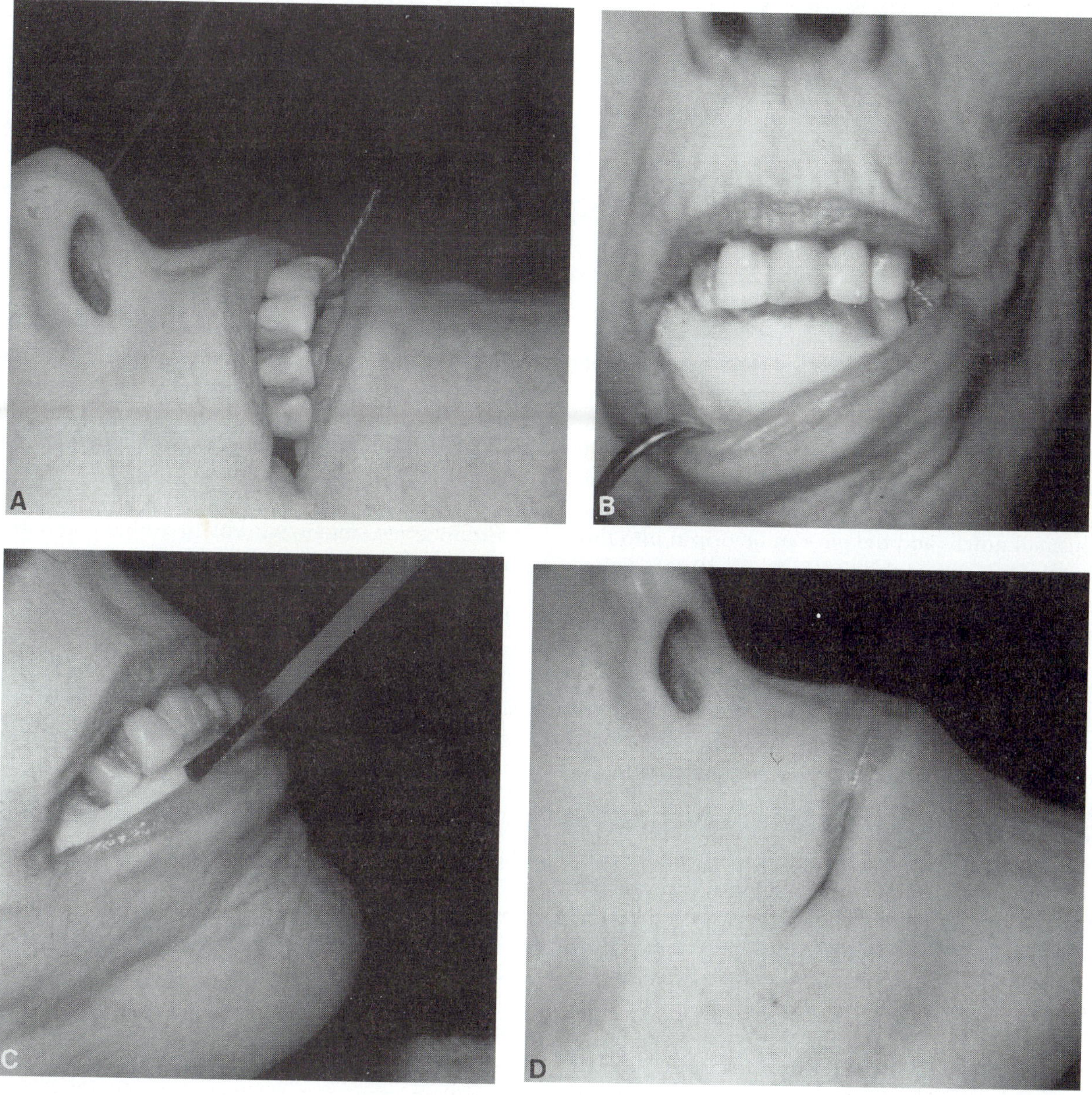

Figure 11–9. A. Preembalming treatment for buck teeth. **B.** Place a strip of cotton over the lower teeth to project the lower lip. **C.** Application of glue. **D.** End result.

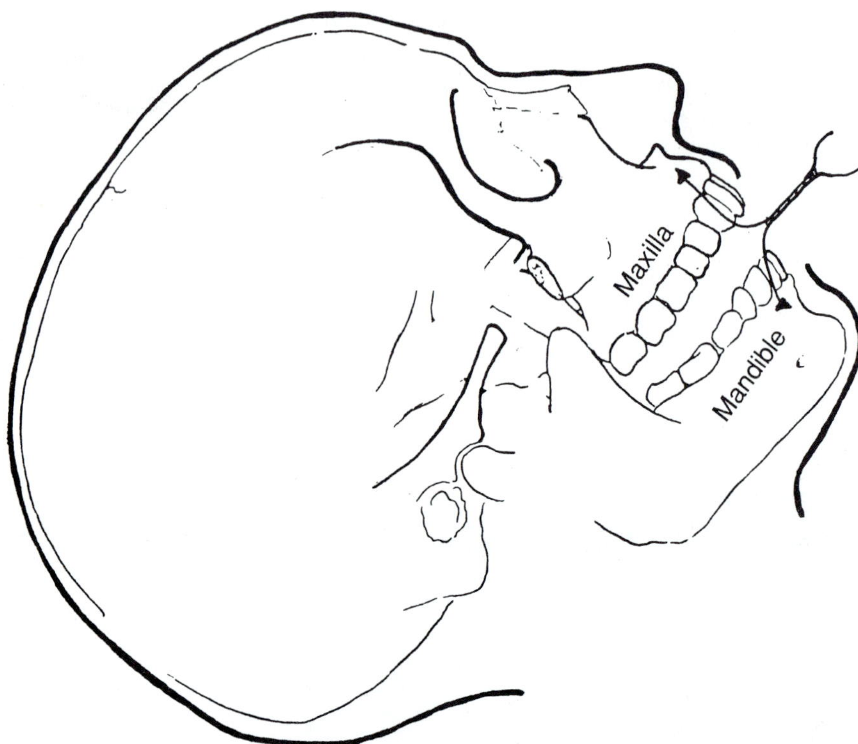

Figure 11–10. Needle barbs are inserted into the mandible and maxilla.

then twisted together to hold the mandible in position. The pin inserted into the maxilla should be placed at the center where the two maxillae fuse. This is called the *nasal spine*. Here, the bone is generally quite strong.

If dentures are to be used it may be wise to insert the teeth before the wire pins are driven into the maxilla and mandible. Most upper dentures at their center have a small notch, and the pin can be driven into the bone at the location of this notch. Some denture wearers exhibit an atrophy of the maxilla and mandible; other bodies exhibit a condition where these bones have become diseased and are very porous. In both instances, it may be difficult, if not impossible, to use the needle injector to close the mouth. Suturing is then necessary. The embalmer can try various points along these bones to locate a solid point for the pins to be placed. The needle injector should be held at a right angle to the bone.

If the bones have been fractured, as often occurs in automobile accidents, four needle injector wires can be used. Place one on either side of the fracture so that two pins are inserted into the mandible. Then, insert two pins into the maxillae. The wires can then be *crossed*, making an ×, and thus the fractured bones can be aligned.

It is important when inserting the pins into the bones that near the point where the skin from the mouth attaches to the gums, the skin be "torn" or pulled over the heads of the pins. This gives the fleshy portion of the lips better contact. Often, when bodies are shipped from another location and the lips are parted, all that needs to be done is to open the mouth and lift the skin over the pin heads to obtain good contact of the mucous membranes.

Method 2: Muscular Suture. In a muscular suture, a variety of needles and suture threads may be used:

*1. Open the mouth and raise the upper lip. Insert the threaded needle at a point where the upper lip joins the maxilla under the left nostril. The needle should slide along the bone and enter the left nostril. Draw the threaded needle out of the left nostril. (By keeping the needle against the maxilla, a "pull" will not be noticed.)
2. Pass the needle through the septum of the nose. Keep the needle as close to the bone as possible. Direct the needle into the right nostril and pull the needle and thread from the right nostril.
3. Insert the needle into the base of the right nostril, keeping the needle against the maxilla. Push the needle into the area where the skin of the upper lip joins the maxilla.

*Order is optional; suturing may begin with the mandible or maxilla.

4. Place the lower denture into the mouth first, then place the upper denture. If the denture is not available, fill the mouth with cotton or use a denture replacement.
5. Pull the lower lip out and insert the needle on the right side of the mandible at a point where the lower lip joins the gum. Be certain to keep the needle against the bone. Make a very wide stitch exiting the needle on the left side of the mandible in the same position where the lower lip joins the gum.
6. Tying the two free ends of the string together pulls the jaw up into position where the two mucous membranes will come into contact (Figure 11–11).

The primary disadvantage of this method of mouth closure is that a pucker might result at the top of the chin that can easily be seen. Keeping all sutures close to the bones helps to relieve this problem.

Method 3: Mandibular Suture. Mandibular suture is identical to muscular suture except that instead of placing the suture in the musculature of the chin, it is passed around the mandible.

1. Open the mouth and insert the needle at the center of the mouth at the base of the tongue behind the lower teeth at a point where the floor of the mouth joins the gum. Push the needle downward, exiting the point where the base of the chin joins the submandibular area.
2. Reinsert the needle into the same small hole at the base of the chin and pass the needle upward just in front of the center of the mandible, where the lip attaches to the gum. Now, the suture has passed completely *around* the mandible. By pulling on both ends of the suture the string will "saw" itself through the soft tissues until it reaches the mandible. The small hole can be covered with a small piece of wax after cosmetics are applied. It should not prove to be a leakage problem. If it does, place a drop of super adhesive on the area.
3. If dentures are used, insert the lower dentures at this point and tie the two ends of the suture together. In this manner, the lower dentures are tied into position. This is an excellent manner for securing loose-fitting dentures.
4. Insert the upper dentures if they are being used.
5. Pass the threaded needle into the left nostril as in the muscular method of mouth closure.
6. Complete the suture by tying both free ends of the suture together (Figure 11–12). A bow may be tied in case an adjustment needs to be made.

This method of mouth closure is excellent to use when the body is to be shipped to another funeral home. It ensures that the mouth will not open during transport.

Method 4: Dental Tie. To use the dental tie of mouth closure the deceased must have natural teeth on both the mandible and the maxilla. A thin thread or dental floss is tied around the base of one tooth in the upper jaw and one tooth in the lower jaw. The two strings are then tied together to hold the jaw in position. Opposing incisor teeth are generally used, but any of the front teeth can be used. It would be too difficult to use the molars. In addition to securing normal mouth closure the dental tie helps to align a fractured jaw. Several dental ties can be used to align a jaw (Figure 11–13).

The following methods of mouth closure are included for completeness. Most are outdated or are specific, but are not used routinely.

Method 5: Drill and Wire. A small hole is drilled through the mandible and a similar hole is drilled through an opposing point on the maxilla. A small wire is passed through the holes and the wire is secured to hold the jaw in position. In lieu of a wire, thread can be passed through the holes with a suture needle. This method has been used over the years to align jaws that have been fractured. Be certain that the drill being used is properly grounded and that care is taken not to cut the fleshy portion of the lips.

Method 6: Chin Rest. The chin rest consists of two small prongs that are inserted into the nostrils. Attached to the two prongs is a sliding support, which can be placed under the chin to hold the chin in the desired position. This method of mouth closure is very old and depended on the harsh, very firm reaction obtained with early embalming fluids. These fluids rapidly and rigidly firmed the tissues. After the tissues of the face and jaw firmed, the device was removed.

Method 7: Gluing the Lips. Gluing the lips has little value as a method of mouth closure. Its use as a method of mouth closure is limited to infants and children. The lips are sealed prior to arterial injection. After the fluid has firmed the body, the lips can be reopened and the mouth dried and checked for air or purge material and then resealed. This method is not recommended for adults.

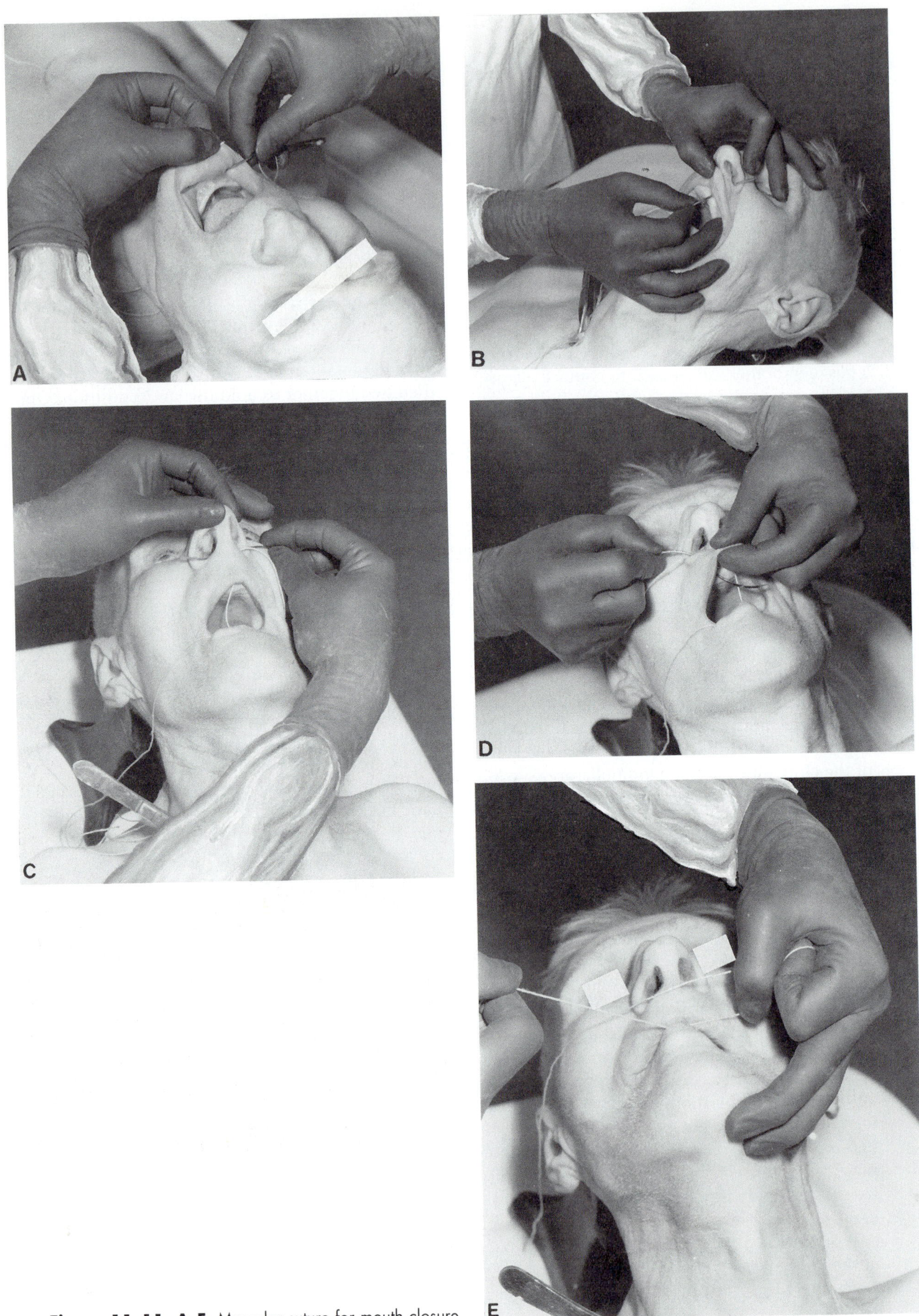

Figure 11–11. A–E. Muscular suture for mouth closure.

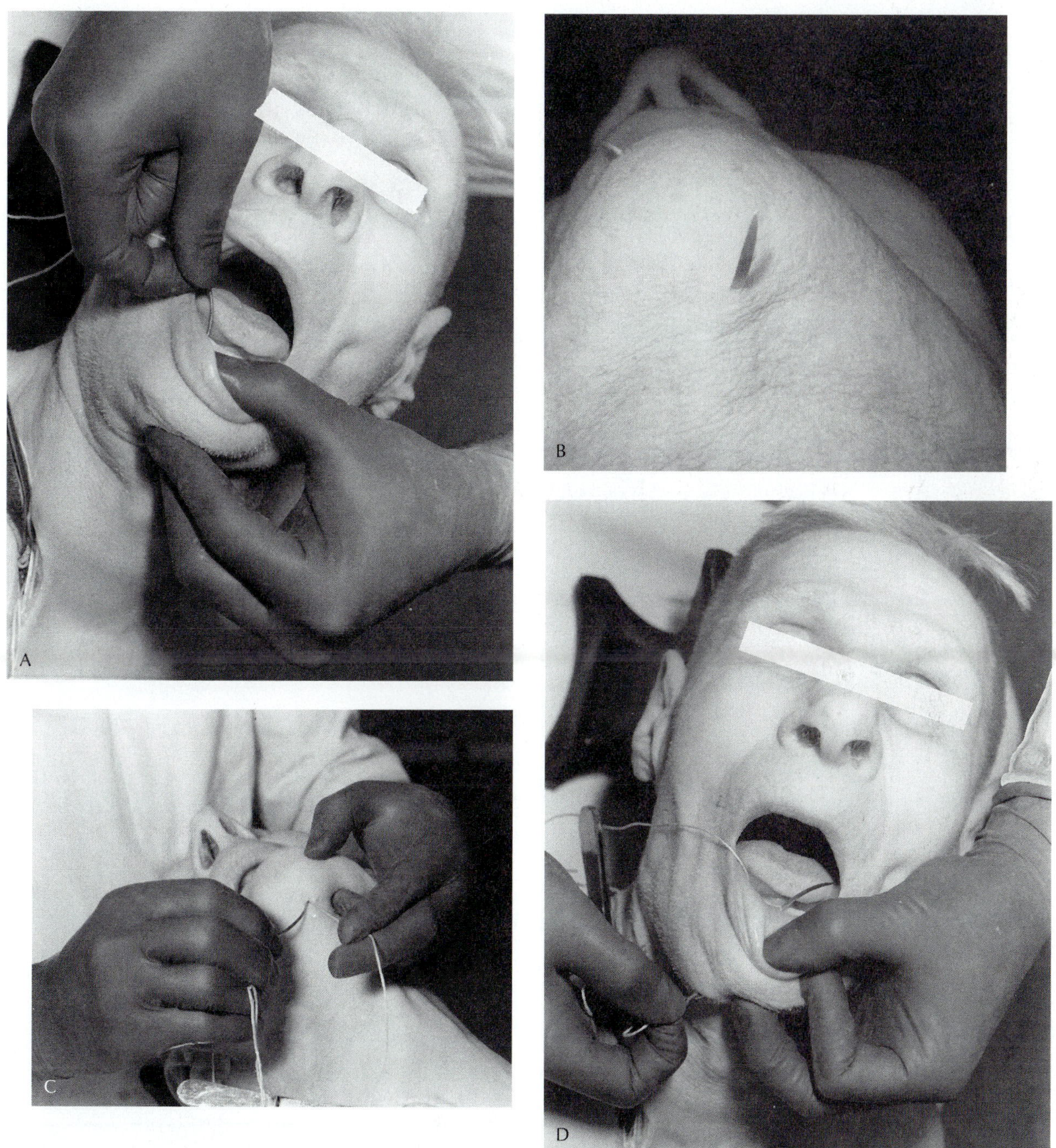

Figure 11–12. A–D. Mandibular suture for mouth closure.

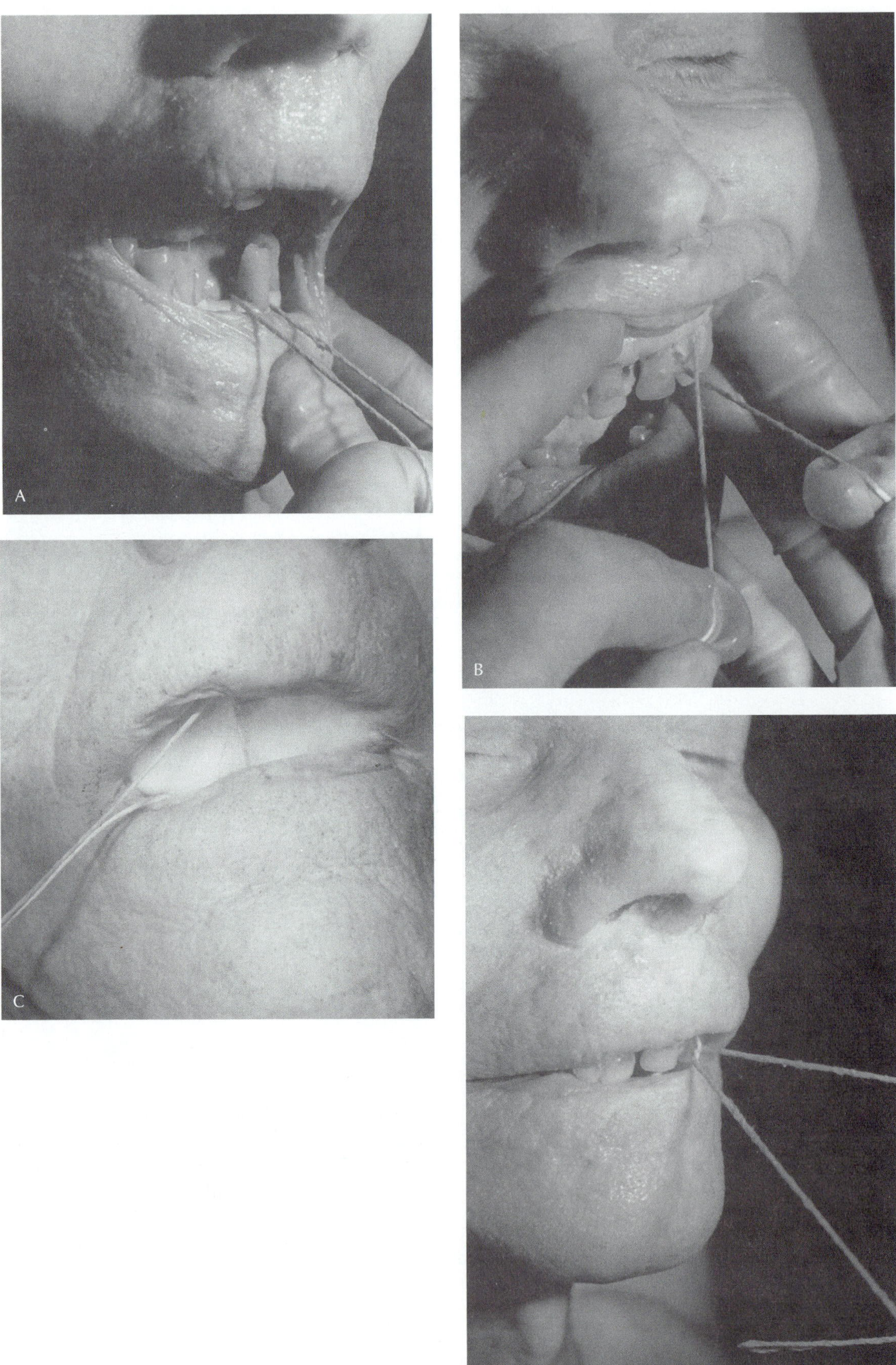

Figure 11–13. A–D. Dental tie.

Modeling the Mouth

Raising the mandible and securing it in position are only parts of the process of mouth closure. Once the lips have been brought into contact the embalmer must create a pleasing and acceptable form.

Natural teeth, when present, create the foundation. It is helpful to place some cotton over the molar teeth to slightly fill out the posterior area of the cheek. This is necessary when the body is emaciated. Keep in mind that with all bodies, gravity tends to result in some sagging of the cheek area. Placing cotton or mortuary putty over the area of the molar teeth helps fill out the area and to slightly lift the tissues into their normal position. After embalming, tissue builder can be injected to elevate these tissues.

When natural teeth are present but several are missing, cotton, mortuary putty, kapoc, or nonabsorbent cotton is used to fill in the missing teeth after the mouth closure is secured. This helps to give an even curvature to the mouth.

When all natural teeth are missing and no dentures are present, the throat can be packed with cotton and the oral cavity with cotton, nonabsorbent cotton, kapoc, or mortuary putty. Secure the jaws into position using one of the methods of mouth closure. A mouth former can be placed over the jaw bones, but if a mouth former is used, it should be placed over the jaws prior to securing mouth closure. The needle injector wires or the suture thread helps to hold the mouth former in position. These formers come in a variety of materials such as plastic, cardboard, or metal, and can be trimmed to fit securely. A substitute can be made with cotton or mortuary putty.

If cotton is used to replace missing dentures, use long strips. **Remember the horseshoe curvature of the mandible and the maxillae.** The cotton should be placed in such a manner that a small portion covers the mandible and the maxillae, the same way a denture does. Always model the upper teeth first. Some embalmers prefer to wet the cotton strips they use to model the mouth. Squeeze out the excess water and place the cotton strips. This prevents the cotton from sinking. If mortuary putty is used as a dental replacement, inject it using a long nozzle injector. The mouth can easily be molded to obtain the horseshoe curvature (Figure 11–14).

When there are dentures but no natural teeth, insert the dentures prior to using the needle injector or suturing the mouth closed. The dentures should be cleaned and disinfected. Cotton placed on the tongue can help to hold the dentures in position. The mandibular suture method of mouth closure can be used to tie the lower denture into position. If dentures do not fit well attempt to use the upper denture. The upper denture gives the best foundation for the curvature of the mouth. It can be held in position by placing cotton or mortuary putty in the area normally occupied by the lower denture. If the denture is new and does not appear to fit, do not use it. When placing dentures in the mouth, **always insert the lower denture first. After it is in position insert the upper denture.** In most people, the line of mouth closure (where the two mucous membranes meet) is located at the inferior margin of the upper teeth. So, establishing the curvature of the upper teeth is the key to a natural appearance.

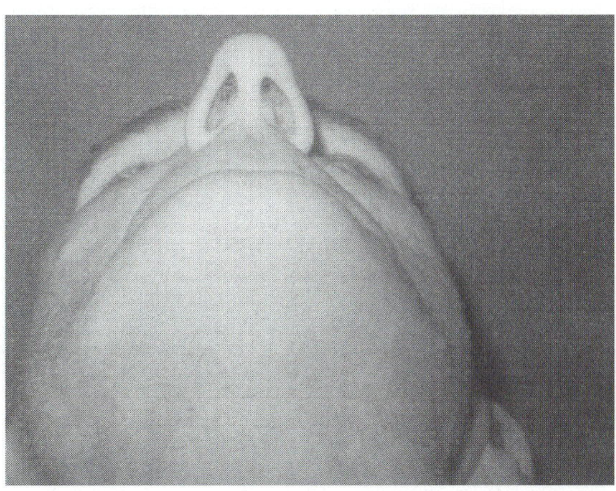

Figure 11–14. Bilateral view of face. Note the curvature of the mouth.

There are occasions when rigor is so intense the jaws cannot be opened. It is still wise to use some form of mouth closure. In these instances, if dentures are in the mouth, it is impossible to remove them for cleaning. Spray a disinfectant into the mouth and dry and clean the buccal cavity with cotton swabs.

Positioning the Lips

After the mouth has been closed and the cheeks padded, the line of closure should be established. Always keep in mind the curvature of the mouth. In the bilateral view of the mouth (looking from the chin upward) the horseshoe curvature of the mouth is easily observed. By keeping this curvature in mind, the embalmer avoids making the mouth look flat and straight. The center of the mouth should give the most projection. Try to obtain some depth at the corners. **The mouth is convex in curvature from corner to corner.** The line of closure is along the inferior margin of the upper teeth. Inserting a small amount of cotton high on the maxillae, on a line from the corner of the mouth to the center of the closed eye, helps to raise the area surrounding the corner (angulus oris eminence) (Figure 11–15).

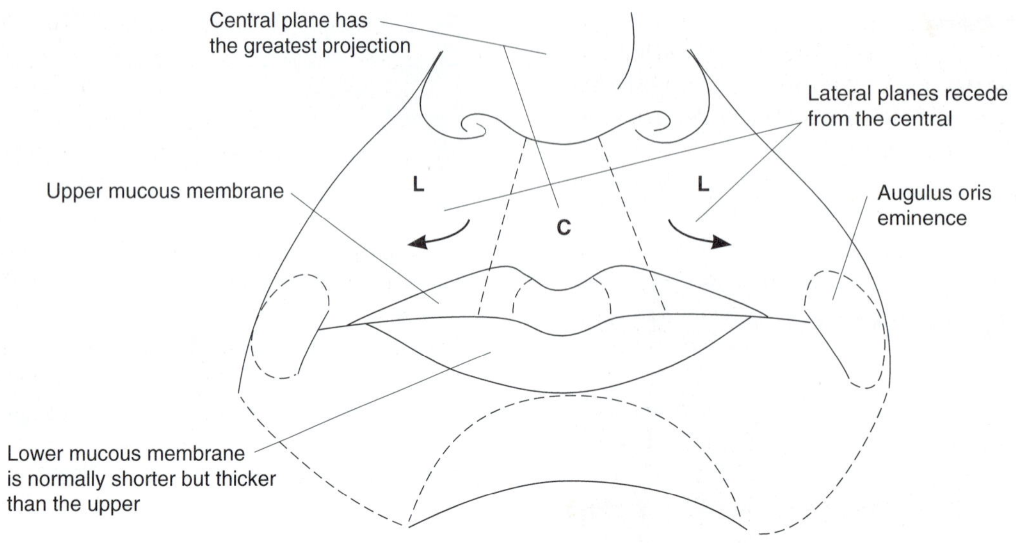

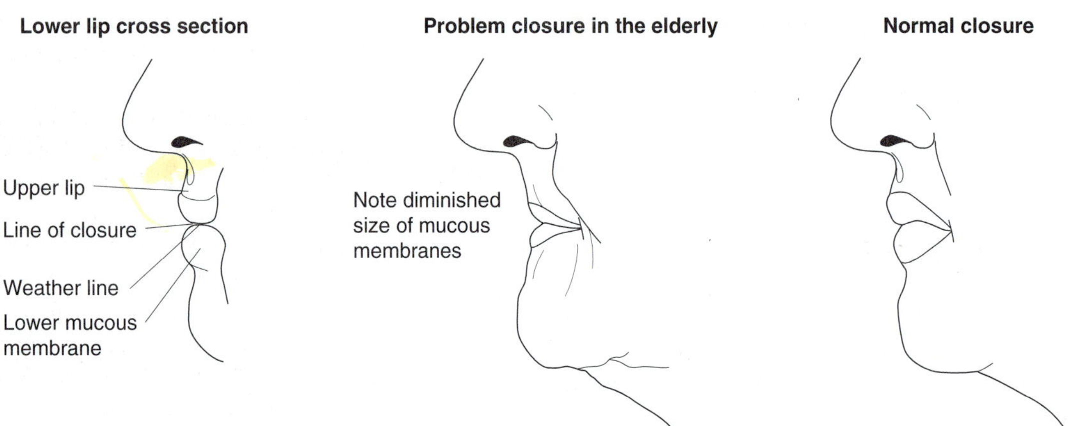

Figure 11–15. Lines of closure for positioning the lips. Various closure profiles are shown.

This angulus oris eminence [the area surrounding the corner of the mouth (angulus oris sulcus)] can be reinstated with tissue builder after arterial embalming. The upper lip (mucous membrane) is usually thinner and longer than the lower lip. This appearance can be reproduced when cosmetics are applied. The weather line (the line between the moist and dry portions of the lips) helps to determine the thickness of the lips. As already mentioned, any scabs or loose skin should be removed from the lips as soon as possible, prior to embalming. To hold the lips in position during embalming the following products can be used (Figure 11–15): lip seal creams (very thick massage creams), petroleum jelly, rubber-based eye and lip glue (for gluing the lips), and super adhesive (for very difficult problems).

Application of a thick cream to the lips during embalming to hold them in position also helps to smooth wrinkles on the lips. Natural wrinkles or lines in the mucous membranes are vertical, but lines from dehydration are horizontal. Place a very thin film of lip cream on each lip, and then bring the lips into contact. They tend to slightly pull away from each other. In doing so, the horizontal wrinkles will be removed. After embalming, wrinkled lips can be corrected by gluing, tissue building, or waxing. These same three methods can be used if the lips are slightly separated after embalming (Figure 11–16). Some embalmers find it helpful to keep the lips *slightly separated* during arterial injection. This allows the mucous membranes to round out and prevents the lip closure from presenting a tight or pursed look.

If the lips are glued *prior* to embalming, they should be opened *after* embalming to be certain there has been no solution leakage into the mouth during in-

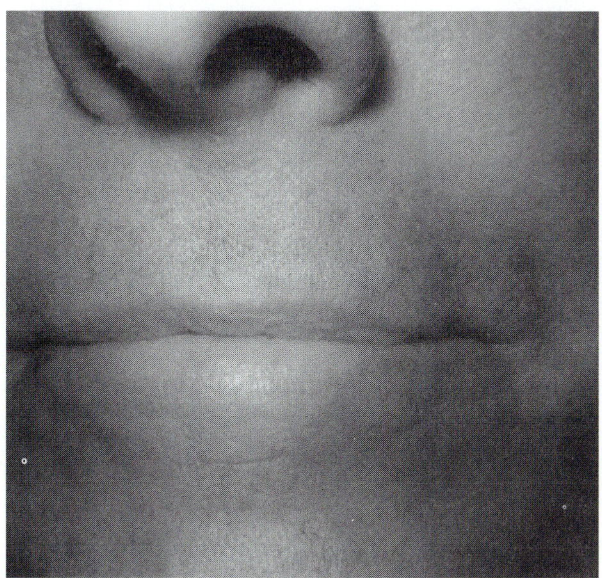

Figure 11–16. Good mouth closure.

jection or that there is no purge material. In addition, air from the lungs can be forced into the mouth and should be released. The lips can then be reglued if desired.

▶ CLOSURE OF THE EYES

In establishing the line of eye closure, keep the following items in mind. The upper eyelid (superior palpebra) forms two thirds of the closed eye; the lower eyelid (inferior palpebra) forms one third of the closed eye. The line of closure is located in the lower one third of the eye orbit. The line of closure is not level and the inner corner of the line of closure (inner canthus) is slightly above the outer corner of the eye (outer canthus).

The general procedure for eye closure can be summarized:

1. Closure of the eyelids is generally done prior to arterial injection. It is easier to close the eye than the mouth after the body has been embalmed, but establishing a good line of closure may be difficult.
2. The eyes can be cleaned with moist cotton. Like all areas of the body, the eyes should be disinfected with a topical disinfectant spray. Conjunctivitis and herpes infections of the eye could be communicable to the embalmer. In addition to cleaning the surface and corners of the eyes, clean the lashes.
3. Cleaning the eyes also helps to relieve rigor mortis in the muscles of the eyelids. If the face is emaciated or dehydrated, the eyelids may have to be stretched slightly to establish closure. This can be done by placing the smooth handle of an instrument such as a pair of forceps or an aneurysm needle, under the eyelid and gently stretching the lids.
4. To help establish the anterior projection of the closed eye and to keep the lids closed, use an eyecap or cotton. These are inserted under the lids.
   A. Eyecap: These plastic or metal disks are approximately the size of the anterior portion of the eyeball. They are generally perforated, and the small perforated projections help to hold the lids closed. The convex shape of the cap helps to maintain the convex curvature of the closed eye. The cap itself prevents the eye and lids from sinking into the orbit should the body begin to dehydrate. Should the eyes be sunken, use several caps or two caps with mortuary putty or a piece of cotton sandwiched between to elevate the closed eyelids.
   B. Cotton: Cotton may be placed under the closed eyelids to keep the lids closed, elevate the lids, and establish the convexity of the closed eye. A piece of cotton about the size of a nickel can be used. Lift the upper lid and insert the cotton under the upper eyelid with an aneurysm handle or forceps. Lift the upper eyelid over the cotton and place it in its proper position. Evert the lower eyelids and insert the cotton into the area covered by the lower eyelid. Lift the lower eyelid into position. If the eyelids do not seem to contain enough arterial solution after embalming, a drop or two of cavity fluid can be placed on the cotton. The lids should then be glued. This will make a preservative pack under the eyelids. If preservation is needed, dehydration from the cavity fluid should not be a concern (Figure 11–17).

In cases of extreme emaciation or dehydration, the eyes can be sunken and the eyeball itself can be dehydrated. The eyelids have to be exercised and stretched to secure closure. Preembalming gluing of the lids may be helpful. The lids should abut but not overlap. In these difficult closures, however, overlapping may be necessary, and if the lids must be overlapped an attempt should be made to show some of the lower eyelid.

Some embalmers place massage cream under the lids. This is easily done by coating the eyecap or the cotton used for closure with a small amount of cream. The

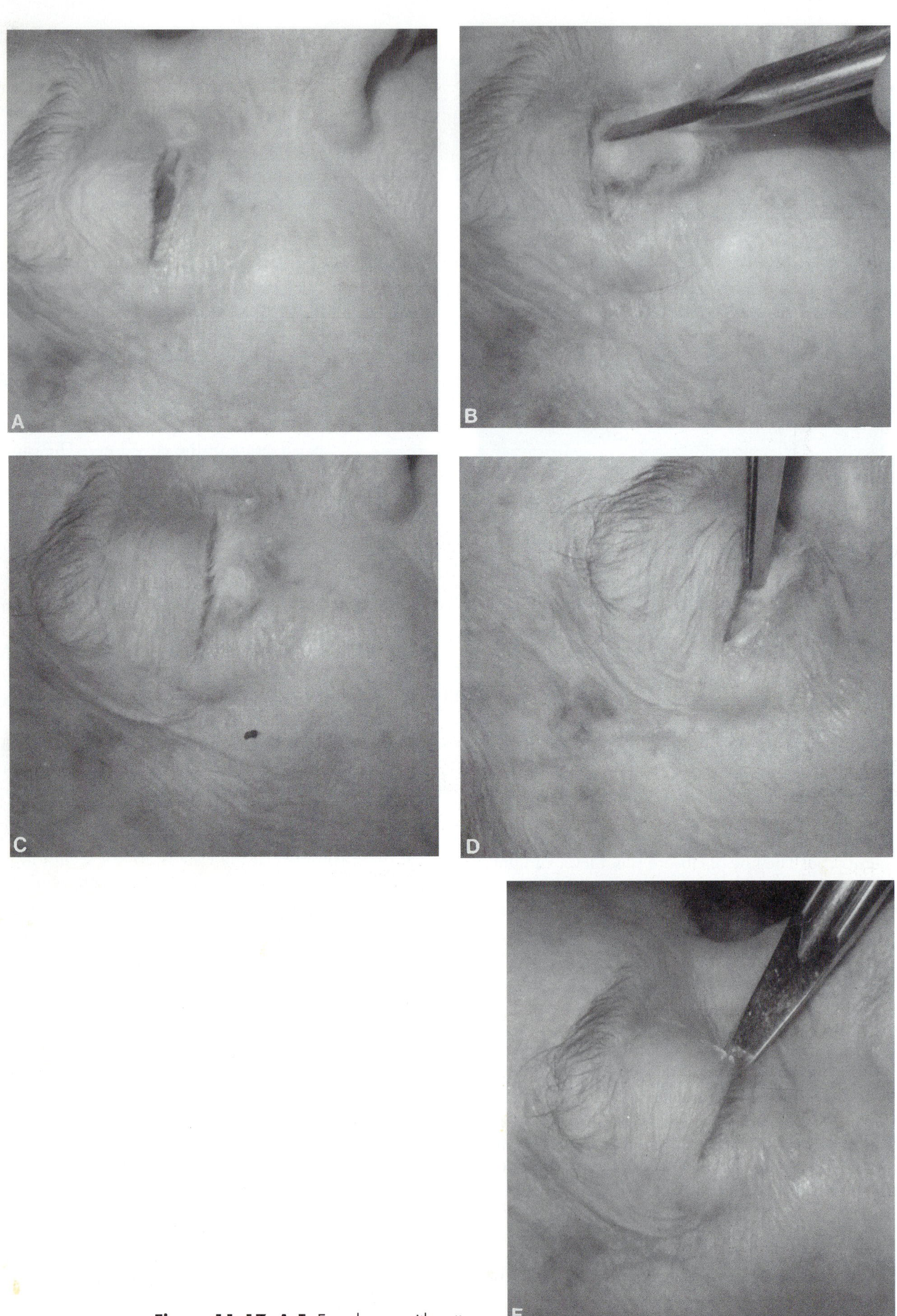

Figure 11–17. A–E. Eye closure with cotton.

difficulty in using massage cream under the eyelids is that a solvent has to be used to clean the cream from the line of closure if the lids have been glued. **Difficult closures can easily be corrected today by using super adhesive to hold the lids together.** Super glue is helpful when during transport from another funeral home, the eyelids have separated. Simply exercise the lids and use super glue to hold them closed. Care should be taken at the start of the embalming to be certain the small inner corner of the eye (the inner canthus) is closed. If this area dehydrates, the brown discoloration can be quite noticeable.

▶ PACKING THE ORIFICES

A topical disinfectant should be sprayed over the outer surfaces of the anal and vaginal orifices. Cotton packing saturated with phenol solution, undiluted cavity fluid, or autopsy gel should be placed into the vaginal and the anal orifices. Some embalmers prefer to do this after embalming, because they prefer that any discharges from these orifices be allowed to exit the body during embalming. After arterial and cavity embalming, the orifices are tightly packed and the body washed.

The nasal cavity as well as the throat and ears should be packed with cotton prior to embalming. The throat must be packed before the features are set. If purge develops, however, all soiled packing should be removed and replaced with dry packing after the body has been thoroughly aspirated.

▶ TREATMENT OF INVASIVE PROCEDURES

The following effects of invasive procedures may be treated by the embalmer before, during, or after embalming. They are listed here because the analysis of the body is made in the preembalming period. Also, several of these conditions should be treated during the preembalming period.

Surgical Incisions. Check the suture to see if the healing process has begun. If the sutures are recent, the area can be disinfected at this time and cauterized with a surface pack or hypodermic injection of a phenol cautery. Temporary metal sutures can be removed with a hemostat after arterial injection, and the surgical incision tightly sutured using a baseball suture. Incision seal powder can be placed within the incision to ensure against leakage. Glue can later be placed over the surface of the suture after the body has been washed and dried. If the incision is in a visible area, super adhesive or a restorative suture may be necessary. The small metal "staples" can be removed by grasping them in their center with a hemostat; then move the hemostat from side to side to allow the small, bent metal edge embedded in the skin surface to be freed.

Feeding Tubes. Tubes that enter the mouth or the nostrils should be removed in the preembalming period. These tubes, if left in place for any time, can mark the corners of the mouth or nose. When the tubes have been in the patient's mouth or nose for several weeks, the surrounding skin may be destroyed. Massage of these areas during arterial injection helps to restore them to their normal contour. After embalming, it may be necessary to use restorative wax, tissue builder, or super adhesive to restore these areas.

Abdominal Feeding Tubes. A feeding tube may also be inserted into the stomach through a small incision in the abdominal wall and a second incision in the stomach wall. These tubes can be removed after arterial embalming. The area of the abdomen should be disinfected. A small piece of cotton saturated with phenol, autopsy gel, or undiluted cavity fluid can be inserted into the abdominal opening after the tube is withdrawn or cut. A small pursestring suture can be used to close the abdominal opening. A trocar button can also be used if the opening is small enough.

Surgical Drains. Surgical drains can be removed after arterial embalming. Drain openings should be packed with cotton saturated with phenol, autopsy gel, or undiluted cavity fluid. A small pursestring suture is used to close the opening. This should be done prior to cavity embalming.

Intravenous Tubes. Any tubing placed into the circulatory system, whether an artery or a vein, should remain in place until the arterial embalming is completed. These invasive devices did not hamper circulation during life, and leaving them in place will not interfere with arterial injection or blood drainage. They can be removed after arterial and cavity embalming is completed. When these tubes are removed from areas that will not be seen after the body is dressed, their openings can be enlarged with a scalpel and a trocar button can be inserted to prevent leakage. Super adhesive can also be applied to these openings, especially in visible areas such as the back of the hands or the neck.*

*Disposal of any invasive device into the blood vascular sys
regulated by OSHA standards if an infectious disease is p

Tracheotomy Tubes. Tracheotomy tubes should be removed in the preembalming period and the area disinfected. Some cotton saturated with a disinfectant or cautery agent can be placed in the opening to disinfect the respiratory passages. It is best not to seal these passages until after arterial embalming. Should any purge develop in the lungs or stomach, this opening in the base of the neck provides an outlet for the purge material. The embalmer may encounter two types of tracheotomies: With the older tracheotomy the skin around the opening contains a great amount of scar tissue. It is not possible to close the opening with a pursestring suture. Pack this type of tracheotomy with cotton and incision seal powder (or mortuary putty) to the surface level of the skin; then place glue over the opening. With the recent tracheotomy there is little or no scar tissue around the opening. After packing with cotton and incision seal powder, a small pursestring suture can be made to close the opening. Dental floss can be used for the suture to hide the opening.

Colostomy. The colostomy bag and the surrounding abdominal wall area should be disinfected. Some embalmers remove the bag, empty its contents, disinfect and deodorize the inside of the bag, then reattach it. Most embalmers prefer to remove the bag after arterial embalming. Insert a piece of cotton saturated with phenol solution, undiluted cavity fluid, or autopsy gel into the abdominal opening. Sometimes a portion of the bowel is exposed. Apply the cotton to this portion of the bowel and use the cotton to gently push the bowel into the abdominal cavity. Close the opening with a pursestring suture. Surface glue and cotton can be applied to prevent any leakage. The bag and its contents (which were removed) should be deodorized and disinfected by pouring some undiluted cavity fluid into the bag. The bag and its contents can then be destroyed.

Urinary Catheter. A catheter can be inserted into the urinary tract through the urethra or the abdominal wall. It can be removed prior to arterial embalming. Cut the small side vent with scissors to allow the dilated balloon located within the bladder to collapse. Then pull the catheter from the body: If the catheter was inserted through the abdominal wall, a small pursestring suture can be used to close the opening. In females, the urethra can be packed with cotton saturated with cavity fluid, autopsy gel, or a phenol cautery chemical after the catheter is removed.

▶ REMOVING CASTS

Sometimes, casts are not removed by the hospital, or death may occur at home where it would be impossible to remove the cast. Most embalmers remove the cast if possible. If the entire leg is in a cast it may be very difficult to remove it and, of course, the cast would not be visible after the body is dressed. The difficulty involved in leaving a cast in place is that the embalmer cannot ensure that embalming solution was distributed to the area covered by the cast. The cast must also be protected from drainage during the embalming; it can, of course, be elevated and covered with plastic.

There are two types of casts: the older plaster type and the new fiberglass type. Both must be sawed open. Sometimes the fiberglass, if thin enough, can be cut open. Some arm casts can be pulled off the body. Some embalmers own a vibrating cast cutting saw or borrow one from a hospital. These devices reduce the time needed to remove the cast. In some locations, the body can be taken to a local hospital, and the hospital personnel will remove the cast. Casts should be removed prior to arterial embalming.

▶ PREEMBALMING TREATMENTS

Skin Lesions and Ulcerations

As the embalmer undresses, disinfects, washes, and dries the body, he should look for rashes, lesions, infected areas, decubitus ulcers, and skin cancers. After cleansing the body the embalmer should begin treatment of these areas immediately (1) to disinfect the affected area, (2) to preserve the tissues surrounding the lesion, (3) to dry the tissues, and (4) to deodorize the tissues. These areas should be of concern to the embalmer for the following reasons:

1. They can be a source of contamination to the embalmer, for example, staph infections and herpes infections.
2. The area is generally necrotic and decomposition of the superficial and deep tissues can already be in progress.
3. Blood supply to the actual necrotic and infected tissues is poor so there will be little or no contact between injected arterial solution and the diseased tissue.
4. Odors may be present that will easily be noticed even after embalming, dressing, and casketing.
5. Necrotic tissue can contain anaerobic gas bacillus microbes that can produce gas gangrene.

A common example of necrotic and infected tissue is the decubitus ulcer. These ulcerations, also known as bedsores, result from limited circulation into areas where there is pressure contact, usually with the bedding. Hospital staph infections result and the necrotic tissue can grow from a small red mark to involve the greater portion of the hip, buttocks, or shoulder. These areas and any area of infection (e.g., pustules) should be sprayed with a topical disinfectant. If one is not available, the area can be swabbed with undiluted chlorine bleach or undiluted cavity fluid. **Do not use the two together.**

If the ulcerated area is covered with a bandage, saturate the bandage with undiluted cavity fluid, undiluted phenol cautery solution, or undiluted autopsy gel. Later, remove the bandage and inject the necrotic tissue with the fluid and solution. If there are no bandages, place a compress of cotton saturated with undiluted cavity chemical, undiluted phenol cautery solution, or autopsy gel over the area during embalming.* This helps to control odors, to preserve the necrotic tissue, and to destroy any microbes and their products that may be present. Hypodermic treatment of the walls of these lesions after embalming is very important, as gas bacillus (*Clostridium perfringens*), a source of tissue gas, may be present.

After embalming and treatment by hypodermic injection and fresh surface preservatives, cotton compresses with embalming powder can be applied to the area. If the hip or buttocks is affected, a large diaper can be made with sheeting. The embalming will do some preserving but, more important, it will control odors. When handling these lesions, the embalmer should always wear gloves (double gloves preferred), gown, and mask. Plastic goods such as coveralls, pants, and plastic stockings can be placed on the treated area.

Lacerations and Fractures

A laceration is defined as a jagged tear in the skin. In the preembalming period, a laceration should be cleaned of any blood or dirt present. This is easily done with germicidal soap and cool water. After the edges of the laceration are cleaned, the torn skin should be aligned. Several small bridge sutures of dental floss can be placed along the laceration to hold the edges in position during embalming. If the laceration is in a body area that will not be viewed after arterial injection, the laceration can be sewn with a baseball suture, using incision seal powder within the laceration to prevent leakage. If the laceration is in an area of the body that will be seen, some massage cream can be placed around the area after the bridge sutures are in place. This protects the good skin.

During embalming, arterial solution escapes from the laceration. After embalming, dry the laceration, treat the edges with a hypodermic injection of phenol cautery solution, and then either suture or glue them closed. Some embalmers prefer to place a compress of undiluted cavity fluid or autopsy gel over the lacerated tissues during embalming to ensure good preservation of the torn tissues.†

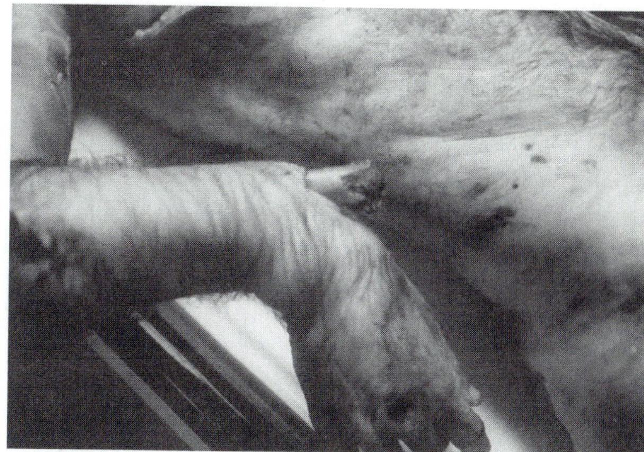

Figure 11–18. Compound fracture of the radius.

When bones are fractured (Figure 11–18), the embalmer is able to observe the distortion by touch or sight. He should make every attempt to align bones, especially facial bones, in the preembalming period. If skull bones or facial bones are fractured, small incisions may have to be made to realign them. Because so many situations can arise regarding fractures, the best advice is simply align all fractures *prior to embalming.*

Abrasions

An abrasion is defined as "skin rubbed off." The embalmer encounters two types of abrasions:

Dry Abrasion. Dry abrasions are abraded areas that have dehydrated. The area resembles a scab. The tissue is dark brown to black, very rough and firm to the touch. It may be the remains of an old abrasion. Or, if it occurred at the time of death, perhaps the body has been dead for a while or the body has been kept in a refrigeration unit, where air passed over the body and dehydrated the abraded tissues.

Moist Abrasions. Moist abrasions are abraded areas that are moist to the touch; some bruising may be present. A fall on a carpeted area can easily bring about an abrasion on that part of the face that came into contact with the carpet.

In the preembalming period, for abrasions located on visible body areas (face, head, neck, arms, or hands), clean the affected area as some blood may be present. Moist abrasions can be covered with a compress of undiluted cavity fluid, phenol cautery solution, or autopsy gel. During embalming, arterial solu-

*Cover with plastic to control odor and fumes and to prevent the chemical from dehydrating.

†Cover with plastic to contain fumes.

tion passes through the abraded tissues. After embalming, the objective should be to dry these abrasions so the tissues *will turn brown.* A hair dryer can be used to dry moist abrasions. *Cosmetics can only be applied to dry tissues.*

Skin-Slip or Torn Skin

Skin-slip should be removed and the underlying tissues treated by immediately packing the denuded tissue with undiluted cavity fluid, phenol solution, or autopsy gel. When the embalmer is satisfied that adequate preservation has occurred and that the area is disinfected and deodorized, he can allow the area to air dry or dry it with a hair dryer. Blisters (Figure 11–19), scabs, torn skin, and other conditions should always be treated in the preembalming period by removing the skin that will not be receiving arterial solution, preserving and cauterizing the denuded skin surface, and, finally, drying the skin. These areas discolor, but they can then be treated with an opaque cosmetic if they are in a visible location. During arterial injection, solution may seep from the affected skin areas. This helps to ensure good preservation.

Gases

During undressing, disinfecting, and cleaning of the body, the embalmer should determine if gas is present in the cavities or body tissues. There are three sources of gas in the dead human body.

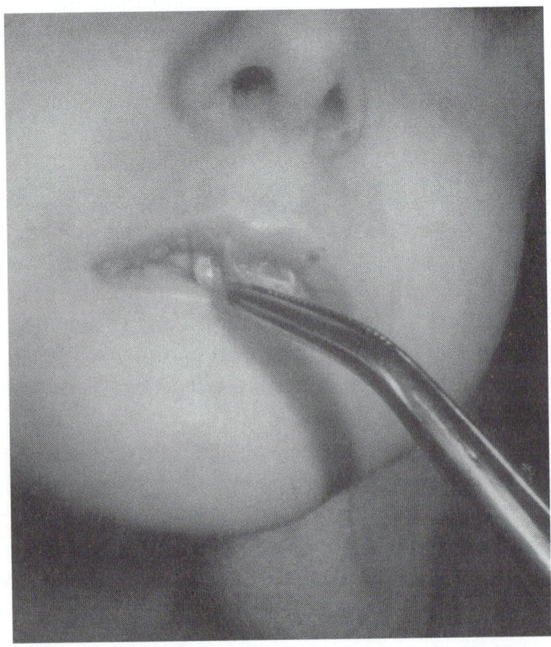

Figure 11–19. Fever blisters.

Subcutaneous Emphysema: Gas or Air in the Tissues. Subcutaneous emphysema originates from invasions into pleural cavities. When gas is detected in the tissues and neither odor nor skin-slip is present, examine the body for punctures that may have been made into the lungs, recent tracheotomy, or fracture of the clavicle, sternum, or ribs. Subcutaneous emphysema can be widespread from the scrotum of the male into the limbs and face.

Gas from Decomposition. If there has been a time delay, signs of decomposition may be present, as may discoloration, odor, purge, skin-slip, and gas. This gas can accumulate in the viscera, body cavities, or skeletal tissues.

True Tissue Gas. The source of this gas is Welch's bacillus (*Clostridium perfringens*). It is an anaerobic spore former and thrives on dead necrotic tissue. The microbe can be passed from body to body through contaminated cutting instruments. A very strong odor of decomposed tissue is present. The condition continues to increase and may begin in the agonal and postmortem periods. Because it spreads so rapidly and is so hard to control, viewing of the body may be impossible. Its presence should immediately be recognized and appropriate steps taken to control it. Use extreme care to disinfect all cutting instruments used in the embalming. Disposable scalpel blades should be removed and placed in an OSHA approved sharps disposal unit and the trocar immersed in concentrated arterial solution using a coinjection chemical specifically designed for bodies with "true tissue gas."

When gases are present in the tissues, distension and swelling may also occur. The gas can be felt by moving the fingers over the tissues. It feels as if it were stuffed with cellophane tissue. This movement may also produce a crackling sound, called *crepitation.* There is only one way to remove gas from tissues. The tissues must be opened and the gas allowed to escape.

In the preembalming period, the greatest concern is distension of the abdomen. Severe distension may restrict the flow of arterial solution and blood drainage. The abdomen should be punctured and the gas allowed to escape.

1. Make a puncture with a scalpel approximately at the standard point of trocar entry—2 inches to the left and 2 inches above the umbilicus. This in itself may allow enough gas to escape that sufficient pressure will be relieved.
2. Insert a trocar at the standard point of entry and, keeping the point high over the viscera, attempt to relieve the gases.

3. Make a small 3- to 4-inch incision over the abdominal wall, possibly opening some of the intestinal viscera, to allow gas to escape.
4. Make an opening with a scalpel on the abdominal wall and insert a "pointless" trocar or large drain tube.

If the facial tissues and the upper chest areas evidence the presence of gas, it would be advantageous to raise both common carotid arteries for injection. The half-moon incision, running from the center of the right clavicle to the center of the left clavicle, is useful. This incision allows gases to escape. Gases already present in the face can be channeled, after embalming, and allowed to exit through these incisions.

It is important that the embalmer determine the type of gas present. True tissue gas is very rare, but most difficult to control. The gas most frequently seen is subcutaneous emphysema. This is generally found when a rib has been fractured during the administration of cardiopulmonary resuscitation (CPR). Table 11–1 outlines the characteristics of these gases.

Ascites

When the abdomen is tightly distended, the embalmer should determine if the distension is caused by gas or edema. Often, simply the insertion of the trocar into the upper areas of the abdomen can determine the difference. If there is generalized edema of the tissues and tortuous veins are visible over the abdominal wall, the presence of edema in the abdomen (ascites) can be expected. If the abdomen is very tense this fluid should be removed prior to arterial injection, for it will create a resistance to the flow of arterial solution and interfere with blood drainage.

Not all the ascitic fluid need be removed, only enough to relieve the intense pressure in the abdomen. An easy method is to insert a trocar, not at the standard point of trocar entry but at a point a little lower on the abdominal wall in the area of the right or left inguinal area or in the hypogastric area (right and left lower quadrants). This lower point allows the ascitic fluid to drain from the cavity by gravity. Insert the trocar, keeping the point directed under the anterior abdominal wall. This instrument can be left in this position during the entire embalming. Drain enough ascitic fluid to relieve the intense pressure. Placing a hand on the abdominal wall and applying slight pressure can assist in drainage. Attaching tubing to the trocar can provide a direct drain of ascitic fluid directly into the sewer system or into a container where it can be disinfected.

TABLE 11–1. GASES CAUSING DISTENSION

Type	Source	Characteristics	Treatments
Subcutaneous emphysema	Puncture of lung or pleural sac; seen in cardiopulmonary resuscitation treatments; puncture wounds to thorax; rib fractures; tracheotomy	No odor; no skin-slip; no blebs; gas can be extreme, present even in toes; can create intense swelling; rises to highest body areas	Gas will escape through incisions; establish good arterial preservation; channel tissues after arterial injection to release gases
True tissue gas	Anaerobic bacteria; *Clostridium perfringens*	Very strong odor of decomposition; skin-slip; skin blebs; the condition and amount of gas increase with time; spore-forming bacterium may be passed by cutting instruments to other bodies.	Use of special "tissue gas" arterial solutions; localized hypodermic injection of cavity fluid; channel tissues to release gases
Gas gangrene	Anaerobic bacteria; *C. perfringens*	Foul odor; infection	Strong arterial solutions; local hypodermic injection of cavity chemical
Decomposition	Bacterial breakdown of body tissues; autolytic breakdown of body tissues	Odor may be present, skin-slip in time; color changes; purging	Proper strong chemical in sufficient amounts by arterial injection; hypodermic and surface treatments; channel to release gases.
Air from embalming apparatus	Air injected by embalming machine (air-pressure machines and hand pumps are in limited use today)	First evidence in eyelids; no odors; no skin-slip; amount would depend on injection time—most would be minimal	If distension is caused, channel after arterial injection to release gases

▶ KEY TERMS AND CONCEPTS FOR STUDY AND DISCUSSION

1. Define the following terms:
   abrasion
   ascites
   colostomy
   dental tie
   embalmer's gray
   eyecap
   laceration
   larvicide
   maggot
   mandibular suture
   mucous membranes
   muscular suture
   needle injector
   subcutaneous emphysema
   tissue gas
   tracheotomy
   weather line
2. List the qualities of a good topical disinfectant.
3. List several rules for shaving.
4. List several uses of massage cream.
5. Name the three levels of position.
6. List several reasons for placing a support beneath the shoulders.
7. List several methods of mouth closure.
8. Describe methods of eye closure.

CHAPTER 12
DISTRIBUTION AND DIFFUSION OF ARTERIAL SOLUTION

Arterial embalming could also be called "capillary embalming." The capillaries, the smallest blood vessels of the body, link the injected embalming solution with the cells of the body. The embalming solution that passes from the capillaries to the tissues effects the embalming. This chapter discusses the movement of arterial solution through the blood vascular (intravascular) and interstitial (extravascular) systems of the body. On reaching the capillaries, the embalming solution, by a series of passive physical transport systems, moves to the cells of the body.* The movement of embalming solution from the intravascular to the extravascular location is called *fluid diffusion.* The remainder of the embalming solution, which passes into the venous system of the body, helps to remove the blood and its discolorations, which exit the body in the form of drainage.

The ability of the embalmer to retain as much preservative within the body as possible without visible distension of the tissues is a key factor in thoroughly preserving and sanitizing the body.

While vascular embalming should be thought of as a **unified process,** this process can be divided into **four** divisions: (1) *Delivery of the arterial solution* from the embalming machine through the connecting tubing and arterial tube into the artery. (2) *Distribution of arterial solution* is the movement of arterial solution from the point of injection throughout the arterial system and into the capillaries (perfusion). (3) *Diffusion of arterial solution* is the movement of arterial solution from inside the vascular system (intravascular) through the walls of the capillaries to the tissue spaces (extravascular). (4) *Drainage,* the discharge or withdrawal of blood and blood clots, embalming solution, interstitial and lymphatic fluids and blood from the body during vascular embalming. The drainage is usually taken from a body vein.

*Passive transport systems require no energy by the cell to operate.

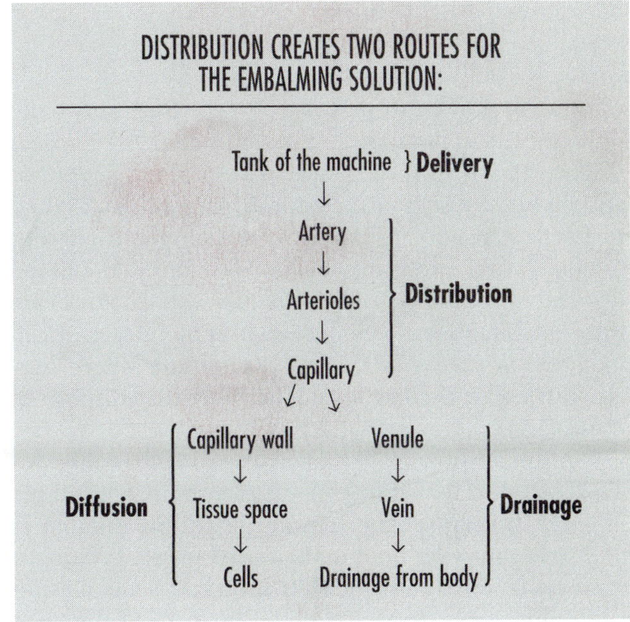

From this simple diagram it is seen that the preservative solution delivery, distribution, diffusion, and drainage occur at the same time once the vascular system has been filled with sufficient embalming solution. These processes work similarly to a lawn sprinkler or soaker hose. Arterial solution fills the vascular system, much like water fills the hose to reach the sprinkler. Some of the arterial solution flows through the walls and pores of the capillaries into the tissue spaces, as water passes through the holes in the sprinkler to reach the grass. The major difference is that all the water is sprayed out of the sprinkler. In embalming, a portion of the arterial solution stays inside the capillaries and flows into the veins to be removed as drainage.

The material drained during embalming of the body is a mixture of blood, arterial solution, and interstitial fluid. It has been demonstrated that as much as 50% of the drainage can be arterial solution. Because the vascular system is **not a closed** system, the arterial

CLINICAL OBSERVATION

In the embalming of a body that has been dead a long time and in which decomposition has begun, injection can result in the immediate swelling of tissues. This swelling occurs because the capillary walls (only one cell in thickness), after being decomposed, can no longer hold arterial solution. Arterial solution thus flows from the large arteries into the small arterioles and then directly into the interstitial spaces. As almost all the arterial solution enters the interstitial spaces, the tissues become distended. In embalming this type of body, it is important to inject a strong arterial solution, so that the maximum amount of preservation is achieved with minimum tissue distension. This is particularly important for the face and hands if the body is to be presentable for viewing.

solution is allowed to pass through the walls and small pores of the capillaries to enter the interstitial spaces (Figure 12–1). In these tissue spaces a fluid surrounds and bathes the cells of the body. In life, this tissue fluid serves to transport the nutrients and oxygen carried by the blood to the cells, as the blood remains in the blood vascular system and does not have direct contact with the cells. The tissue fluid also carries the wastes of cell metabolism to the blood vascular system, where they are carried to the organs of the body that dispose of these wastes.

A similar process occurs in arterial embalming. Arterial solution flows through the arteries into the capillaries. A portion of the solution leaves the capillaries and passes into the fluid in the tissue spaces. Eventually it moves to and enters the cells and makes contact with the cell proteins. In this manner, the cells of the body are preserved or embalmed. The embalming solution that leaves the capillaries and eventually embalms the cells is the **retained arterial solution.** It is the retained arterial solution that embalms.

The arterial solution that remains in the capillaries and is pushed ahead into the venules and veins and is eventually drained from the body serves only to clear the vascular system of blood. This solution can embalm only the walls of the vascular system. The vascular system is extensive and the preservation of arteries, capillaries, and veins would, no doubt, diminish decomposition of the body. Nevertheless, muscle cells and connective tissue cells account for the bulk of the body, and their preservation is essential if decomposition is to be halted and a thorough and extended preservation of the body achieved.

Drainage is a combination of **blood, arterial solution,** and **interstitial fluid.** It is easy to see how blood and embalming solution are elements of the drainage, but interstitial fluid becomes part of the drainage through two routes. In living bodies, excess interstitial fluid is carried away from the spaces between the cells by the lymph system. This system empties into certain large veins of the body. In the embalming process, some embalming solution diffuses into the interstitial fluid and is removed by the lymph system. Even more importantly, embalming solution is present in the capillaries, and as it moves through the capillaries it draws some tissue fluid with it into the drainage. This explains why dehydration often occurs in areas such as the lips and the fingers during injection: more tissue fluid is being removed than is being replaced by embalming solution.

Arterial embalming involves both physical and chemical applications. Filling the arterial system by forced injection with some apparatus that pushes solution into the body under pressure involves physical procedures. Control of the drainage is a physical process. Some of the injected solution is forced through the walls of the capillaries simply by the physical process of filtration.

The arterial fluid is chemical in nature. When properly diluted it makes a homogeneous solution that is described as hypotonic. Through the physical processes of osmosis and dialysis, this hypotonic solution passes from the capillaries into the interstitial spaces. The preservatives in the solution chemically

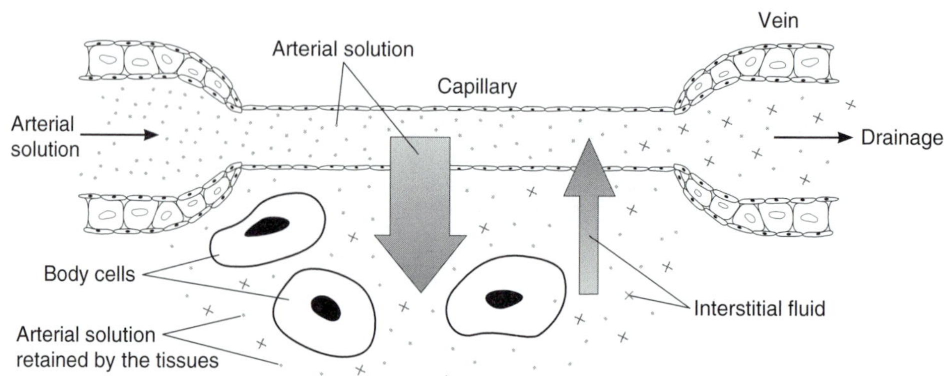

Figure 12–1. Drainage and retention of arterial solution.

combine with the proteins in the body cells and the protein in microorganisms and their products to form new compounds and alter the proteins in such a manner that the tissues are preserved and sanitized.

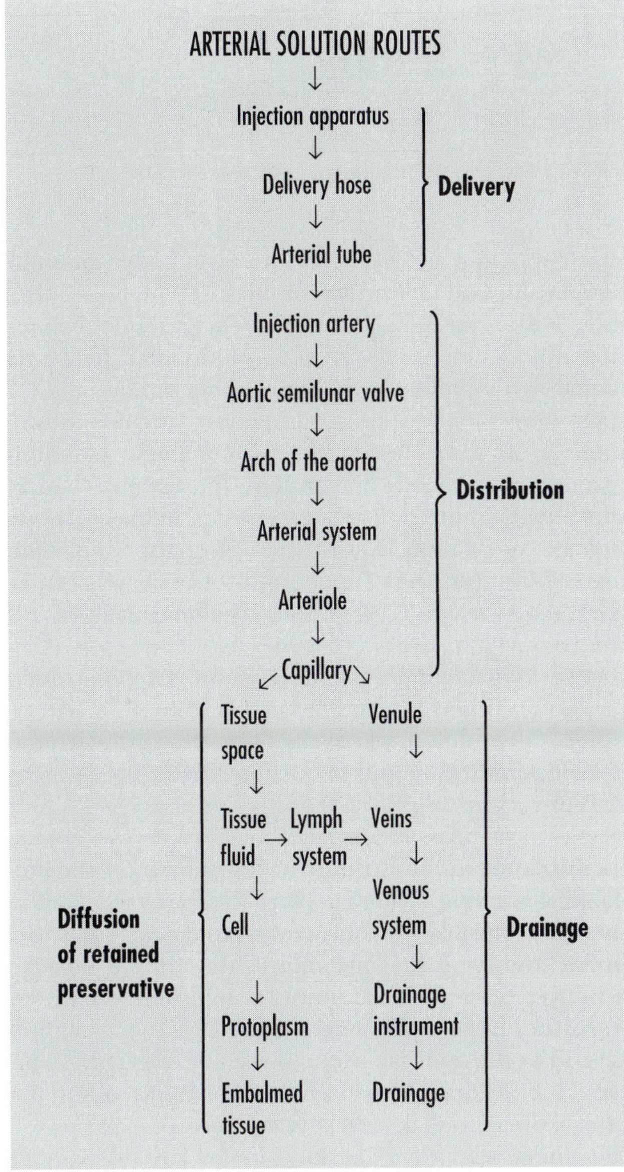

▶ ARTERIAL SOLUTION INJECTION

Arterial embalming begins with the injection of a preservative solution, under pressure, into an artery of the body.* Arterial (vascular) embalming can be defined as the injection of a suitable arterial (embalming) solution, under pressure, into the blood vascular system to accomplish **temporary preservation, sanitation**, and **restoration** of the dead human body. The solution moves from the arteries to the capillaries and then passes through the capillaries to come into contact with the body cells. A portion of the embalming solution remains in the capillaries to remove the blood and its products from the vascular system in the form of drainage. This drainage is taken from a vein of the body.

It is necessary to inject an embalming solution under pressure. Even transfusions of blood into living persons are done under pressure, by elevating the container containing the blood. Some early embalming injection apparatus were just as simple. A solution of embalming chemical was elevated above the body to create the pressure needed to distribute the solution throughout the body. The body offers resistance to the injection of the solution. As the solution is injected into the vascular system by way of an artery, the resistances are described in relationship to the vascular system. Resistances within the blood vessels are called **intravascular resistances;** resistances outside the blood vessels are called **extravascular resistances** (Figure 12–2).

Extravascular and intravascular resistances have their greatest effect on arterial solution distribution. Poor or good distribution of the arterial solution results in poor or good diffusion of the embalming solution, respectively. Pressurized injection is needed primarily to overcome these resistances that interfere with arterial solution distribution. As embalming solution travels from the large central trunk of the arterial system (the aorta) into the arterial branches (arterioles and capillaries), the diameter of the arterial system actually *expands* because of the innumerable branches of the vessels. The injection pressure needed to force the solution through the narrow arteries *decreases* by the time the solution reaches the capillaries.

The arterial solution at the microcirculatory level can take three routes: (1) A portion flows through the capillaries, where some of the embalming solution passes through the walls of the capillaries to embalm the tissues. (2) The portion that remains in the capillaries flows on to the venules. This embalming solution helps to remove the blood from the capillaries and the veins and eventually exits as drainage. (3) The remaining embalming solution flows through direct connections that link arterioles and venules. It eventually exits as drainage.

Intravascular pressure (IVP), which brings about pressure filtration that moves the embalming solution from the capillaries into the interstitial spaces, is no doubt created by the pressure from the machine and the expansion of the elastic arteries. This pressure ef-

*Some embalmers may prefer to begin the arterial embalming (of the unautopsied body) by injecting a preinjection arterial solution.

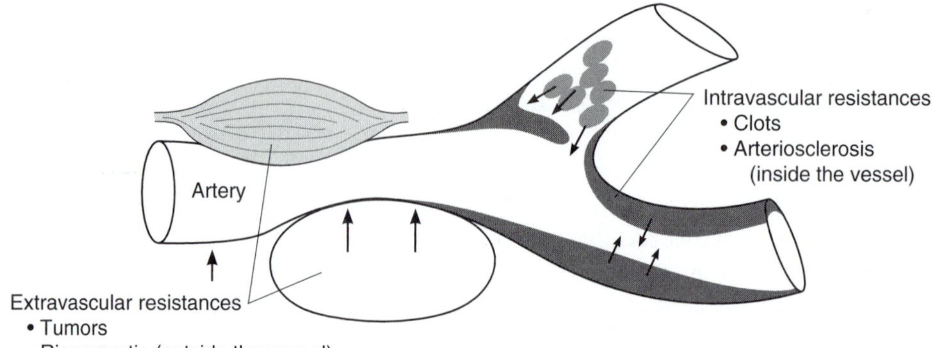

Figure 12–2. Extravascular resistance outside and intravascular resistance within the vessel.

fects embalming solution filtration through the walls of the capillaries. Pressure filtration is one of the major processes by which embalming solution enters the tissue spaces. Intravascular pressure also remains with the embalming solution that flows into the venous system. This is what helps to create the small (approximately $\frac{1}{2}$ pound) pressure that the drainage exhibits. No doubt a lot of the drainage pressure is brought about by arterial solution flowing directly through connecting routes—directly from arterioles to venules and not passing through the capillary routes.

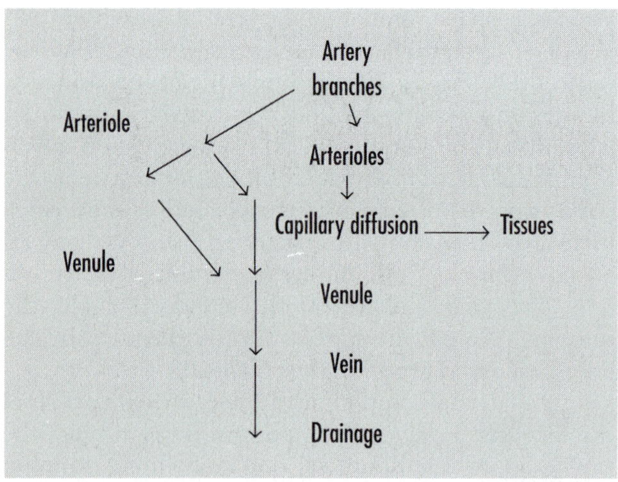

During life, some capillaries remain devoid of blood as a result of vasoconstriction. Also, some areas of the body are engorged with blood because of the activity of the body, which causes vasodilation. For example, in a person who is running, more blood is concentrated in the muscles being used rather than in those muscles not being used. At death, the vascular system relaxes and thus increases its capacity. As a result, the embalmer can inject a large volume of solution without causing immediate distension of the tissues or drainage.

The drainage from the average body generally amounts to one half or less of the total volume of arterial solution injected. It is the intent of the embalmer that 50% or more of the arterial solution injected be retained by the body for the embalming of cells and tissues. The embalmer must make every attempt to promote even distribution of the embalming solution throughout the body and to have the tissues retain as much embalming solution as possible. An old rule was to inject one gallon of a sufficient strength of embalming solution for every fifty pounds of body weight. Today it is necessary to rely on the **embalming analysis** and the **response** of the body tissues as the solution is injected, to determine the amount of solution which needs to be injected and the needed strength of the solution. Observation and evaluation will also determine if multipoint injection is needed to reach all body areas with the preservative solution.

Extravascular and intravascular resistances are responsible for nonuniformity in distribution of the embalming solution. The diameter of the artery, as well as the size of the arterial tube, and the diameter of the delivery hose from the machine to the arterial tube all produce resistance. As a point for injection, the artery with the largest diameter, generally the common carotid or the femoral artery, should be selected. An arterial tube of maximum size should be inserted into the artery. Small radial arterial tubes are of little or no value in vessels as large as the common carotid. Smaller arterial tubes are used for sectional or localized injections. The valve that controls the rate of flow of fluid and the diameters of the delivery hose and arterial tube constitute factors outside the body that determine resistance.

▶ INTRAVASCULAR RESISTANCE

Intravascular resistances can be caused either by narrowing or obstruction of the lumen of a vessel. This narrowing or obstruction is brought about by conditions found either within the lumen of the vessel or within the walls of the vessel. The *lumen* can be *obstructed* by blood, antemortem emboli, antemortem thrombi, and postmortem coagula and thrombi.

As the embalming solution flows from the aorta into the narrowing branches of the arterial tree, the lumen of the arteries also narrows. A coagulum that is loosened and moved along with the solution will eventually clog a small distributing artery. Arterial coagulum could never be reduced to a size where it could pass through arterioles and capillaries. When a coagulum reaches an arterial branch through which it can move no further, distribution of solution beyond this point is stopped. The only way tissues beyond this point can receive embalming solution is through the collateral circulation.

Intravascular resistance resulting from *narrowing of the lumen* can be caused by arteriosclerosis, most frequently seen in the arteries of the lower extremities; vasoconstriction, frequently seen on one side of the body as a result of a stroke; arteritis, brought about by inflammation of the artery; and intravascular rigor mortis, postmortem narrowing caused by rigor mortis of the smooth muscles in the arterial walls. Unlike extravascular resistance, the embalmer can do little to remove intravascular resistance (Figure 12–3).

▶ EMBALMING PROCEDURES FOR INTRAVASCULAR PROBLEMS

The following embalming techniques can be used when intravascular problems are anticipated:

1. Use sufficient pressure and rate of flow to uniformly distribute the arterial solution. A slow rate of flow can help to prevent coagula in the arteries from floating free and clogging smaller branch arteries. Once circulation is established, a faster rate of flow can be used.
2. If arterial coagula are anticipated (i.e., bodies dead for long periods, gangrene evidenced in distal limbs, and death from infections) inject from the right common carotid artery (or restricted cervical injection). This pushes arterial coagula away from the arteries that supply the head and arms (the areas to be viewed). The

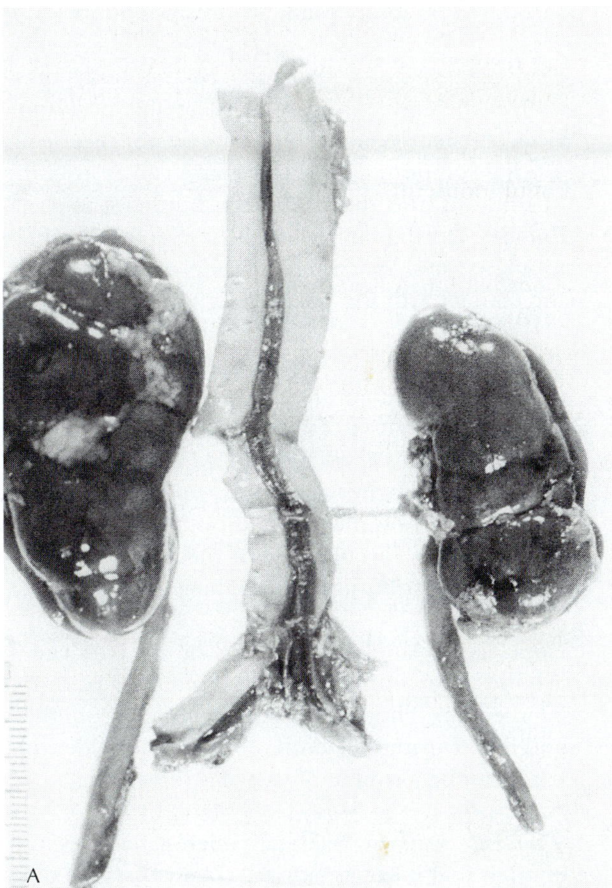

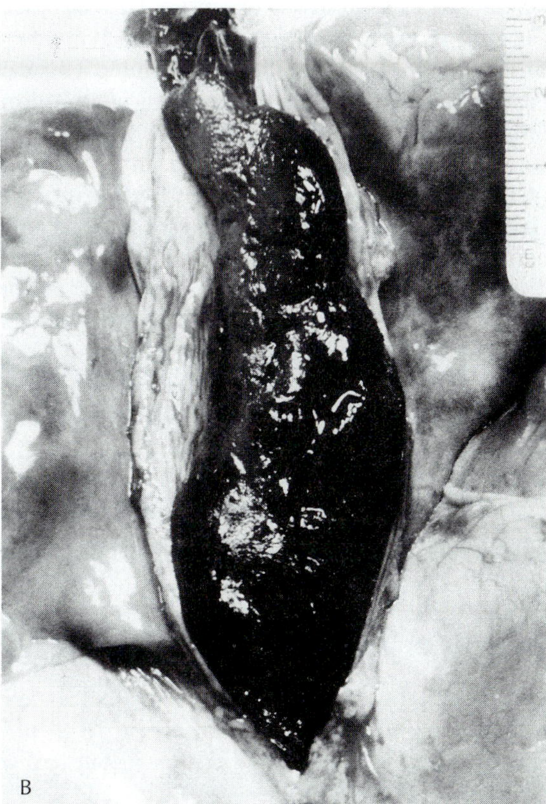

Figure 12–3. A. Example of clots in the aorta. **B.** Example of arterial clotting. *(Courtesy of Debra A. Goethals, Chicago, Illinois.)*

legs can be injected separately, if necessary, or treated by hypodermic and/or surface embalming.

3. Avoid using a sclerotic artery for injection. The common carotid is rarely sclerotic, whereas the femoral and iliac arteries are frequently sclerotic.
4. Use the largest artery possible for the primary injection point. This is usually the common carotid, external iliac, or femoral artery.
5. Use an arterial tube of proper size so that it will not damage the walls of the artery.

▶ EXTRAVASCULAR RESISTANCE

Extravascular resistance is pressure placed on the outside of a blood vessel. This pressure is sufficient to collapse or partially collapse the lumen of the vessel. The embalmer is better able to reduce or remove extravascular resistance than intravascular resistance. Therefore, the following discussion of extravascular resistances includes techniques that can be used to reduce or remove the pressures that these resistances place on blood vessels.

Rigor Mortis. The postmortem stiffening of the voluntary skeletal muscles is a strong extravascular resistance. Rigor mortis is not a uniform condition. It may be present in some muscles and absent in others. This can cause a very uneven distribution of arterial solution. Embalming prior to or during the onset of rigor is generally recommended. When rigor is present, gentle but very firm manipulation and massage of the muscles helps to reduce the degree of stiffness. The massage and manipulation can be done prior to and during arterial injection. During the injection of the first gallon of arterial solution, firm massage and exercise of the extremities can be very important in establishing good distribution. Massage should be done especially along the arterial routes (e.g., axilla, wrist, sides of fingers, groin, popliteal space).

Gas in the Cavities. Decomposition gases in the abdominal cavity can exert enough pressure to push the large abdominal aorta and inferior vena cava against the spinal column, thus causing these vessels to narrow or collapse. Most frequently this pressure can be removed at the beginning of the embalming by puncturing the abdominal wall with a trocar or scalpel. It may also be necessary to puncture some of the large and small intestines. This can easily be done without fear of interrupting the circulation.

Expansion of the Hollow Viscera During Injection. Too rapid an injection of arterial solution, especially in bodies dead for long periods, can result in expansion of the hollow visceral organs. This expansion causes the abdomen to swell and places sufficient pressure on the aorta and vena cava so as to collapse their lumens. Stomach purge often accompanies this abdominal distension. Insert a trocar into the abdominal cavity, keeping the point just beneath the anterior abdominal wall, and puncture some of the distended intestines.

Tumors and Swollen Lymph Nodes. These distended growths and organs can place pressure on the blood vascular system, creating distribution and drainage problems. Sectional injection may be necessary. A higher injection pressure and pulsation may help to obtain good distribution. Massage and manipulation may also help to encourage solution distribution and drainage.

Ascites and Hydrothorax. Enough fluid may accumulate in the thoracic and abdominal cavities to interfere with blood drainage and arterial solution distribution. Drainage from several sites may be necessary. The ascites can be removed or relieved by inserting a trocar into the abdominal cavity or inserting a drainage tube through a puncture made in the abdominal wall.

Contact Pressure. Portions of the body that push against the embalming table or against positioning devices (such as shoulder blocks) may not receive enough arterial solution. Contact pressure can restrict the flow of solution into the shoulders, buttocks, and backs of the legs. During embalming, these areas should be manipulated and massaged to relieve the pressure from the contact with the embalming table.

Visceral Weight. In all bodies, abdominal viscera create some resistance. In obese bodies, however, there can be sufficient visceral weight on the large vessels in the abdomen to restrict drainage and possibly solution distribution. Higher pressures, pulsation, and a more rapid rate of flow may help to overcome this resistance. Manipulation and massage of the abdominal area may also assist distribution and drainage.

Bandages. An elastic bandage or any bandage wound around an extremity should be removed prior to arterial injection. They can disrupt drainage from the hands and feet. During injection, even a patient identification band can be a source of vascular resistance.

Skeletal Edema. Skeletal edema can be intense enough that it exerts extravascular resistance to the distribution of embalming solution as well as a resistance to blood drainage. Numerous conditions, from pathological disorders to drug treatments, can bring this

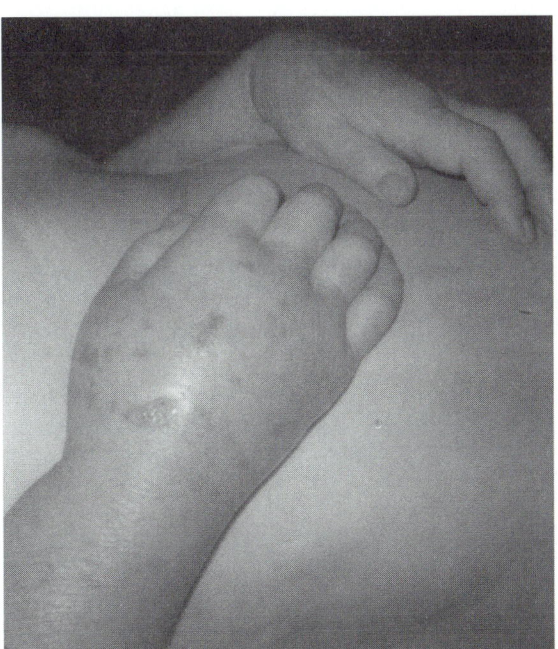

Figure 12–4. A right hand and arm distended with edema.

about (Figure 12–4). These intense edemas are frequently seen postoperatively, particularly after open-heart or vascular surgery. Higher injection pressures, pulsation, manipulation, and massage assist in distribution and drainage. Sectional vascular embalming may be necessary.

Inflammation. Inflamed tissue can swell to the extent that vascular constriction results. Higher injection pressures, pulsation, and massage may assist in distributing arterial solution into these body areas. Sectional vascular and hypodermic embalming may be necessary.

▶ COMBINED RESISTANCE

Extravascular and intravascular resistances rarely exist in and of themselves. In embalming the "average" body, a combination of resistances is found. For example, in embalming a 62-year-old man who died from a myocardial infarction, resistances might originate from rigor mortis (because of delay between death and preparation), arteriosclerosis (some degree of sclerosis can be found), contact pressure (possible in every body), and blood in the dependent portions of the vascular system.

These four sources of resistance demonstrate that even in a sudden death, vascular resistances are present that can restrict good arterial distribution and blood drainage. In the preceding example, the rigor may be intense enough that distribution is reduced to the point where sectional embalming is required. If the person had been taking an anticoagulant the blood may remain in a liquid form and postmortem clotting would be diminished. Thus, arterial distribution and blood drainage would be much better.

At the time of death invasive treatments and drugs administered could cause extensive ecchymoses on the backs of the hands or extreme antemortem subcutaneous emphysema, resulting in gross distension of the tissues of the neck and face. Delays between death and preparation greatly increase the amount of postmortem coagula in the vessels.

All these hypothetical factors demonstrate that the embalmer must prepare each body on the basis of the conditions exhibited by the individual body. The embalming analysis must be based upon the individual body conditions. As the embalming progresses, further analysis must be made as to the extent of arterial distribution, volume of drainage, clearing of discolorations, amount of tissue distension, degree of firming, and any new conditions that arise.

▶ NEED FOR RESISTANCE

Resistance is not a totally negative factor in arterial embalming. If there were total resistance on the arteries no distribution could take place. If there was total resistance on the veins, drainage would not be possible and distension of the tissues would result. In embalming any body a certain amount of resistance is found throughout the vascular system. The injection pressure is greatest on the arterial side of the capillaries. This pressure overcomes arterial resistances and helps to distribute the embalming solution. The resistance in the capillaries and on the venous side of the capillaries slows the embalming solution and helps to hold it within the capillaries, giving the solution an opportunity to diffuse; brings about a more even distribution of the embalming solution, because it reduces short-circuiting of the embalming solution; and helps the tissues to retain more embalming solution, for it allows for better filtration of the embalming solution into the tissues.

If there were no resistance, the embalming solution would pass directly through the capillaries and into the drainage. To illustrate the problems that arise when there is little or no resistance, take the case of a person who dies from a ruptured aneurysm of the abdominal aorta. Some solution may be distributed, but most of the embalming solution will follow the path of least resistance through the torn artery and fill the abdominal cavity.

During injection and drainage of the body, most embalmers create resistance to effect better penetration of the embalming solution and reduction of the loss of solution. Intermittent or alternate methods of drainage are used. The solution is injected against a closed drainage system, which creates the resistance. In addition, some embalmers inject the last $\frac{1}{4}$ to $\frac{1}{2}$ gallon of embalming solution with the vein used for drainage tied off. Aspiration can be delayed several hours. This technique helps the capillaries to hold the embalming solution and gives the solution time to diffuse.

Figure 12–5 illustrates the need for some degree of resistance. Figure 12–5A shows little or no resistance. The solution rushes through the tissues, resulting in tissue dehydration. Filtration is reduced, solution can easily short circuit, and the evenness of distribution is reduced.

Figure 12–5B demonstrates total resistance, perhaps a situation in which there is very extensive blood clotting. Once the system is filled, tissue distension becomes a major problem and uniformity of distribution is reduced.

Figure 12–5C represents a movable resistance, such as liquid blood in the venules and veins or the use of intermittent drainage. Blood removal is more complete, distribution is more uniform, and, most important, more embalming solution is retained by the body with a minimum of tissue distension.

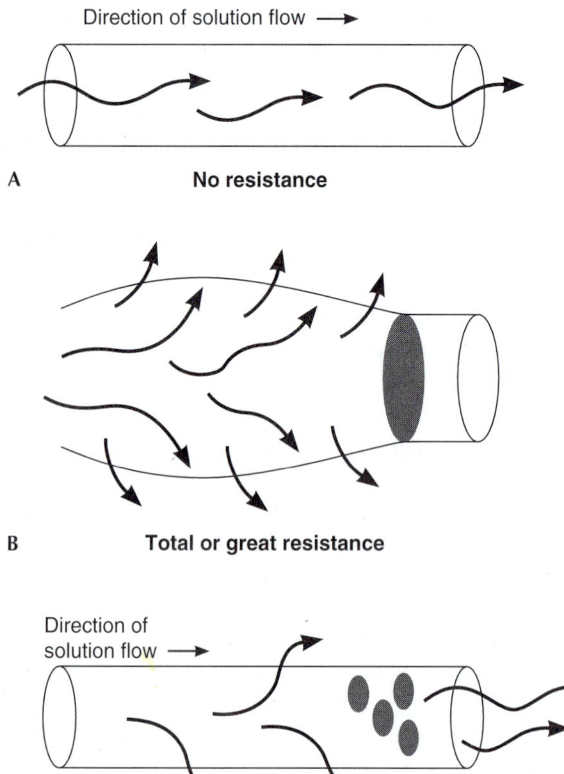

Figure 12–5. A. No resistance. **B.** Total or great resistance. **C.** Movable resistance.

▶ PATHS OF LEAST RESISTANCE

When vascular resistances are present in a body, the arterial embalming solution always distributes to those areas where little or no resistance exists. As a result, certain body areas receive too much solution and others do not receive enough. Three questions must be asked: (1) Is the embalming solution flowing into the blood vascular system? (2) What body areas *are* and what areas *are not* receiving embalming solution? (3) Has a body area received *sufficient* arterial solution?

Three indicators can be used to tell if arterial solution is being distributed throughout the vascular system:

1. A drop in the solution volume in the tank of the embalming machine.
2. When the rate-of-flow valve is opened on the centrifugal injection machine, there should be a drop on the pressure gauge. This drop is the **differential pressure.** The greater the drop, the greater the rate of flow. The differential reading of "10" in Figure 12–6B indicates that the embalming solution is being injected twice as fast as it would if the differential reading were "5" (Figure 12–6A). The fact that the dial dropped to 5 or 10 from the reading of 15 when the rate-of-flow valve was closed indicates that solution is entering the body. As the solution fills the vascular system, the dial reading may rise. This shows that more resistance is being encountered. To keep the rate of flow at the original speed, the pressure has to increase. Increasing the pressure increases the differential reading.

Example. The machine is turned on with the rate-of-flow valve (or the stopcock) turned off. (*No* solution is entering the body.) The pressure is set at 20 pounds. The rate-of-flow valve is now opened and the dial drops to 15 pounds. The differential reading is 5. After a gallon and a half is injected, the needle on the dial rises to 18. This indicates the system has been filled and more resistance is being encountered. To establish the original rate of flow, try to open the rate-of-flow valve so the needle drops to 15. If this does not happen, increase the pressure to 23 pounds. If the dial remains at 18 the differential is again 5, and this was the original rate of flow. Differential "pressure" is a good indicator of the resistance in the body. It may also indicate that an arterial tube is clogged. (The tube should always be checked prior to use to be certain it is clean.)

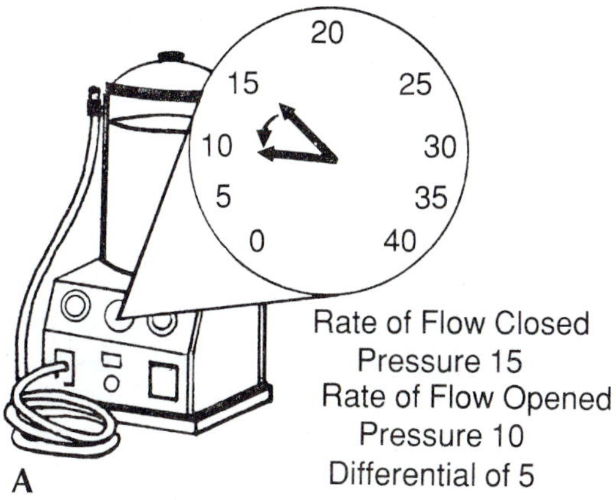

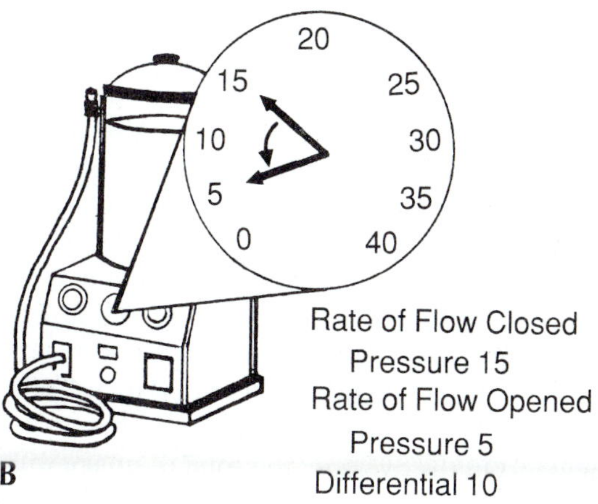

Figure 12–6. Pressure–flow differentials. **A.** Slower rate of flow. **B.** Faster rate of flow.

3. There should be drainage if the solution is entering the body and making the proper circuit through the arteries, capillaries, and veins.

Once it has been determined that the arterial solution is entering the body at a rate of flow and pressure that do not cause distension, the embalmer must determine which body regions are receiving arterial solution and which areas are not. A group of indicators known as the ***signs of arterial solution distribution and diffusion*** help to make this determination. Most of these indicators, such as the presence of fluid dye in the tissues, demonstrate only the presence of embalming solution in skin regions.

The dermis, the deep layer of the skin, is very vascular and offers little resistance to the flow of embalming solution, as the solution flows rapidly and easily into the surface areas of the body. The embalmer can easily detect the presence of embalming solution in the skin. Concern must be given to the deep tissues such as the muscles. It is very important that solution distribute to these body tissues, which offer more resistance. To achieve this deeper penetration of solution, the drainage can be restricted and massage must be very firm. Penetrating agents in the arterial solution also promote the passage of solution into the deeper tissues.

The skin areas offer little resistance to the flow of solution; also, some localized areas can receive large amounts of arterial solution. These areas are generally in the vicinity of the artery injected. Solutions will establish pathways where they quickly pass through a group of capillaries near the artery being injected. The solution then passes rapidly into the drainage. This frequently happens when injection and drainage occur at the same location. This short-circuiting reduces the total volume of solution available for saturation of other body areas.

Many direct connections exist between arterioles and venules in the microcirculation of the blood. Here, again, is a route that offers little resistance to the flow of fluid. Embalming solution can rapidly pass from the arterial system to the veins without distributing to the tissues. Restricting the drainage can reduce the amount of arterial solution lost in these direct routes.

Once the embalmer determines that solution is entering the body and where it is within the body, it must be determined which body areas have received sufficient solution. There is no positive test for determining if a body area has sufficient solution. If there is any doubt, the embalmer should raise an artery that supplies the area and make a separate injection. If the area is very localized, hypodermic or surface embalming can be used. With local injections, it may be wise to increase the strength of the injected chemical to help ensure good preservation. It is better to slightly overembalm an area than to risk the chance that an inadequate amount of preservative has reached the area.

▶ INJECTION PRESSURE AND RATE OF FLOW

Injection pressure is needed to overcome intravascular and extravascular resistances. The pressure needed is created by the injection apparatus (embalming machine); it can be as simple as a gravity percolator or as complex as some of the centrifugal pumps (Figure 12–7).

Injection pressure is the amount of pressure produced by an injection device to overcome initial resistance within the vascular system.

Rate of flow is the amount of embalming solution injected in a given period, or the speed at which the embalming solution enters the body. The rate of flow is generally measured in ounces per minute.

Injection pressure and rate of flow are related, but not identical. Of the two, the rate of flow is the factor of

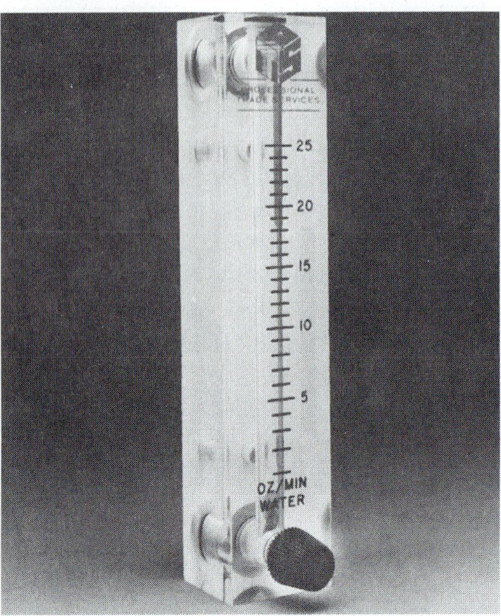

Figure 12–7. Rate-of-flow meter.

most concern to the embalmer. The ideal rate of flow can be as much arterial solution as the body can accept as long as (1) the solution is evenly distributed throughout as much of the body as possible, and (2) there is little or no distension of the tissues. The ideal pressure is the amount needed to establish this rate of flow.

By use of a centrifugal pump it is possible to have a set pressure with the rate-of-flow valve closed. It is then possible to open the rate-of-flow valve to a certain point and establish the desired rate of flow. ***In use of a centrifugal pump injector, it is recommended that the pressure be set with the rate-of-flow valve closed.*** The pressure set with the rate-of-flow valve closed is called the ***potential pressure.*** When the rate-of-flow valve is opened the resultant pressure reading is called the ***actual pressure.*** The difference between actual pressure and potential pressure is the rate of flow or the ***differential pressure.***

There are many theories as to the amount of pressure and rate of flow that should be used. Keep in mind that these factors vary in different ways:

1. From body to body: Bodies injected shortly after death when rigor is not present. These bodies can be injected much faster than bodies that have been dead for a long period of time with rigor fully established. A low pressure can be used to establish a high rate of flow in a recently decreased body.
2. In different body areas: Fluids always follow the path of least resistance. Areas such as the skin and vascular visceral organs and glandular tissues easily accept fluid. Resistance is greater in tissues where arteriosclerosis is present in the arteries or in body areas where blood has clotted or coagulated in the vessels.
3. As embalming proceeds: As embalming proceeds, resistance increases (a) when vessels are empty and the solution rapidly enters (after the vessels fill, more resistance is created), (b) when the preservative in the solution acts on the capillaries, allowing less solution to flow into the tissue spaces (more solution will then be directed into the drainage), (c) when the tissue spaces become filled to capacity with arterial solution, and (d) when arterial clots move and block small arteries and venous coagula are hardened by the preservative solution, making them more difficult to remove.

It can easily be seen that the needed pressure and rate of flow can vary from body to body and at different times in the embalming process.

It may be necessary to increase, possibly for short intervals, the pressure normally used. After death, and depending on the cause of death, some blood vessels may collapse because the volume of circulating blood has decreased. Increase in the pressure or rate of flow may well promote filling of the vessels and start good distribution. When this has been accomplished, the amount of pressure can be reduced. The pressure used at that time should be sufficient to maintain a rate of injection that is slightly greater than the amount of drainage. (On the average, the total drainage will equal approximately one half of the total volume of solution injected.)

FACTORS WHICH MUST BE DETERMINED BY THE EMBALMING ANALYSIS

1. VESSELS FOR INJECTION AND DRAINAGE
2. STRENGTH OF THE EMBALMING SOLUTION
3. VOLUME OF THE EMBALMING SOLUTION
4. INJECTION PRESSURE
5. INJECTION RATE OF FLOW

Note: These factors will vary by the individual body and can vary in different areas of the same body.

Ideal pressure is then defined as the pressure needed to overcome the vascular resistances of the body to distribute the embalming solution to all body areas. It can easily be seen that a one-point injection may require very little pressure; however, if the left leg does not receive arterial solution, a high pressure may be needed to inject solution down this leg using the left femoral artery if the vessels of the leg are sclerotic because of diabetes.

The *ideal rate of flow* is defined as the rate of flow needed to achieve uniform distribution of the embalming solution without distension of the tissues. In embalming a body dead from a sudden myocardial infarction, a faster rate of injection can be used if death occurred within 2 or 3 hours of embalming rather than if death occurred several days previously and there was some evidence of decomposition. In the latter situation, a rapid rate of flow could easily bring about distension of the tissues.

There are two strong schools of thought on injection rate. Some embalmers prefer a low pressure and a rapid rate of flow. (Note: Injection machines have been developed on this idea of low pressure but high rates of flow.) Other embalmers feel a high pressure but a very slow rate of flow is ideal. One study has suggested a moderate rate of injection for the *average unautopsied* body as a rate of 1 gallon of solution over a 10 to 15 minute time period. They have recommended a pressure of 2 to 10 pounds to achieve this rate of flow.* Postmortem coagula are found in the arteries as well as the veins. Using slower rates of injection may help to keep these coagula from moving to smaller distal arteries where the vessel would become blocked and diminish or completely stop the distribution of arterial solution from that point.

Not all bodies can be injected within the same set time at the same rate of flow and injection pressures. As soon as distension is evident, injection should be stopped. The injection pressure can be reduced, the rate of flow can be reduced, or sectional embalming can be done. Likewise, if arterial solution is not entering some areas of the body, the rate of flow can be increased, the pressure can be increased, or sectional embalming may be necessary.

The use of ideal pressure and rate of flow with intermittent or restricted drainage after surface discolorations have been cleared, the following effects are possible: removal of blood from the main as well as the collateral circulation; saturation of soft tissues by the injected solution; and buildup of intravascular pressure, restoring moisture and retaining a sufficient amount of solution to produce thorough preservation without tissue distention.

For the injected embalming solution to accomplish its function of preservation, it must reach and penetrate *all* tissue areas. Merely flushing the solution through the blood vascular system and out the drain tube does not achieve the intended purpose. It requires time for the preservative solution to diffuse out of the capillaries and penetrate, and saturate tissues.

Clinical studies have demonstrated that 50 to 55 percent of the embalming solution is lost through the drainage, regardless if a high or a low pressure is used for embalming. Techniques such as restricted drainage may help to retain more embalming solution within the body.†

The foregoing would be true under "ideal" conditions. The *ideal rate of flow* and the *ideal pressure* will vary from body to body. The "ideal" values of these two factors is the pressure necessary and the rate of flow necessary to overcome the resistances and evenly distribute the preservative solution throughout the entire body, while at the same time the body retains as much of the preservative solution as possible without distension or dehydration of the body tissues.

From a historical point of view **pressure** was the single most important factor controlling the entry of the preservative solution into the body. When gravity devices and air-pressure machines were used for injection simply increasing the pressure also increased the rate of flow of the solution. With the centrifugal pump, rate of flow could also be controlled. Some embalmers prefer to set the pressure of the centrifugal pump (with the rate of flow valve closed **or** the stopcock of the arterial tube closed); then **fully open** the rate-of-flow valve or the stopcock valve. The rate of flow is now determined by the size of the delivery hose, size of the arterial tube and the resistance within the body. If the rate of flow seems too slow (indicating resistance) the pressure is increased.

▶ CLINICAL DISCUSSION

To many embalmers the gauge on a pressurized fluid injection machine indicates the pressure that is being exerted within the body's blood vessels. Such a belief, however, is fallacious. The pressure gauge actually relates the resistance to the flow of the arterial solution. The pressure or force of the stream of embalming solution depends on a number of significant influences within the body and on the mechanical arrangement of the injector itself.

For example, if a centrifugal embalming machine is filled with fluid and the end of the rubber tubing is allowed to discharge the fluid back into the tank unin-

* See selected readings: Rose GW, Rendon L. Coping with the present and the future: Minimum standards for performance of embalming. In: *The National Reporter.* Evanston, Il: National Research and Information Center; 1979; vol. 2. No. 9.

† Kroshus J, McConnell J. The measurement of formaldehyde retention in the tissues of embalmed bodies. *Director* 1983; March/April 10–12.

hibited, the volume of fluid pumped out would increase as the pressure is increased if the rate of flow remains unchanged. If the pressure is set at a constant rate, the volume pumped out would decrease as the rate of flow is reduced, and the pressure would tend to increase as the resistance to the flow increases. A simple illustration of the effect of end resistance on rate of flow and pressure is obtained by filling the tank of a centrifugal machine and setting the controls to deliver a moderate amount of pressure and rate of flow. After the machine is running, pinch off the rubber tubing so as not to totally occlude the fluid from flowing, and note the gauge readings. The restriction (resistance) causes the pressure to *increase* markedly and the rate of flow to *decrease* substantially.

The relationship between machine gauge pressure, rate of flow, and events within the blood vascular system is difficult to equate. There is a steady decline in pressure from the high point recorded on the embalming injector pressure gauge to the smallest arteries. Pressure is dissipated against the channel walls while moving through the rubber tubing (the size of arterial tube), through blood vessels, and against the blood (thick or thin) and clots within the blood vascular system.

In a living person, blood pressure falls from its exit at the left ventricle through the blood vascular system to its entrance into the right atrium. It is commonly acknowledged that within a normal healthy aorta, blood flows at about 15 inches per second. By the time the blood reaches the capillary bed, which has 700 to 800 times the volume capacity of the aorta, flow diminishes to about one-fiftieth of an inch per second. As the blood flow passes into the venous side, the vessels increase in size and diminish in volume capacity. Thus, blood pressure and flow slowly increase.

Many factors influence blood pressure and the blood vascular system in life. In younger people, free from vascular diseases, the arteries expand on systole and, thus, exert pressure to move the blood as their elastic walls contract and return to normal size in response to the pressure. In persons with arteriosclerosis the walls are no longer fully elastic; the arteries do not expand and, therefore, offer more resistance, which is reflected as an increase in blood pressure. Additional factors influence blood flow when arteriosclerosis is present. There is usually a reduction in the diameter of the lumen of the artery almost to the point of occlusion. The roughening of the intimal coat resulting from the calcium deposits interrupts the flow of blood.

Temperature plays a part in increasing or decreasing blood flow in the living. Cold tends to cause vasoconstriction, whereas heat tends to cause vasodilation. When considering possible postmortem influences on the rate of flow of embalming solution and pressure, remember that rigor mortis may restrict the flow of the solution if not relieved; warm fluid (at or near 100°F) may be more efficient than cold fluid; and various tumors, accumulations of ascites, and body position may exert profound alterations in rate of flow and/or embalming solution pressure by compressing blood vessels and increasing resistance to the flow of embalming solutions. Ruptured blood vessels further alter the "normal" postmortem pressure/resistance relationship by permitting the escape of embalming solution from blood vessels into surrounding tissues at low pressures. Increasing the injector pressure output rarely improves the situation.

▶ CENTER OF ARTERIAL SOLUTION DISTRIBUTION

The ascending aorta and the **arch of the aorta** are the center of arterial distribution. The arch is a continuation of the ascending aorta and gives off three large branches from its superior surface. From right to left, these are the **brachiocephalic artery,** which supplies the right side of the head and right arm; the **left common carotid artery,** which supplies the left side of the head and face; and the **left subclavian artery,** which supplies the left arm. The *arch* continues as the *descending thoracic aorta* through which the embalming solution is distributed to all other parts of the body.

The arch of the aorta is a continuation of the *ascending aorta,* which begins at the left ventricle. The embalming solution is injected into the arteries of the body and not into the veins because of the valve at the beginning of the ascending aorta called the *aortic semilunar valve.* This valve is situated between the left ventricle of the heart and the ascending aorta. As embalming solution is injected, the ascending aorta fills and causes the aortic semilunar valve to close (Figure 12–8). Once it is closed, the arteries of the body can begin to fill with the embalming solution. If the valve fails to close, or leaks, the left ventricle fills with embalming solution. If this happens, the cusps of the left atrioventricular (bicuspid) valve close, allowing the arteries of the body to fill.

If, for some reason, both the aortic semilunar valve and the bicuspid valve fail to close (solution injected under too much pressure), arterial solution will flow to the lungs through the pulmonary veins, which could

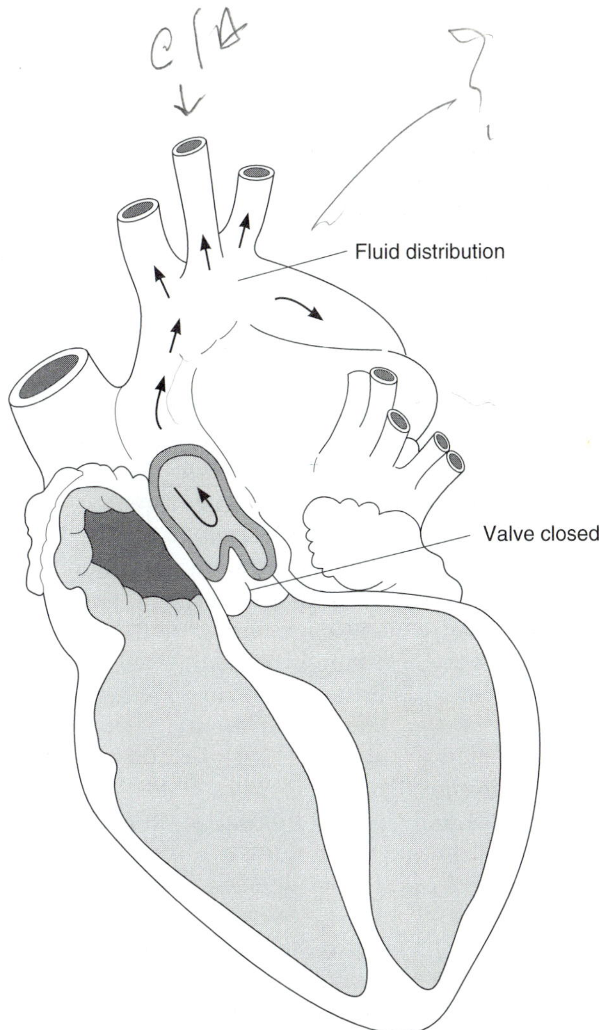

Figure 12–8. Arch of the aorta, ascending aorta, and the closed semilunar valve.

create a purge. The solution might flow into the right ventricle through the pulmonary artery, and from the right ventricle to the right atrium, from which it would exit through the drainage.

▶ SIGNS OF ARTERIAL SOLUTION DISTRIBUTION AND DIFFUSION

Each embalmer has a set of criteria that he or she uses to tell if arterial solution has reached an area of the body. It is best that more than one indicator be used. Remember that even if embalming solution is present in an area, sufficient solution of the proper strength must be present. Most of the signs of distribution and diffusion are surface indicators. Concern must always be given to the deeper tissues and organs that cannot be seen. These indicators of distribution and diffusion can occur at the same time.

SIGNS OF ARTERIAL SOLUTION DISTRIBUTION

- Fluid dye
- Distension of superficial blood vessels
- Blood drainage
- Leakage from intravenous punctures
- Clearing of intravascular blood discolorations

SIGNS OF ARTERIAL SOLUTION DIFFUSION

- Dye in the tissues
- Firming of the tissues
- Loss of skin elasticity (beginning firming)
- Drying of the tissues
- Rounding of fingertips, lips and toes
- Mottling of the tissues (bleaching)
- Fluorescent dye observed using "black light"

Dyes. The most reliable sign of arterial distribution and diffusion is the presence of an active fluid dye in the tissues of the skin. As active fluid dyes stain the tissues, they act not only as a sign of solution distribution, but clearly demonstrate solution diffusion. The dyes help to prevent formaldehyde gray and provide an excellent internal cosmetic. They are available in pink and suntan. Many arterial fluids contain active dye, but additional dyes may be added separately to the arterial solution.

Fluorescent Dye. A coinjection arterial chemical that contains a fluorescent dye that cannot be seen without the use of a "black light" is available for injection with the preservative arterial solution. When the lights of the embalming room are extinguished and a "black light" is held over the body, areas of the body in which the coinjection fluorescent dye is present glow a bluish white. This coinjection fluid is similar to active fluid dye, except that the coinjection dye cannot be seen on the body surface. It is important to remember that fluid dyes indicate only surface profusion of the embalming solution.

Clearing of Intravascular Blood Discoloration. It is most important that the livor mortis be observed prior to the injection of arterial solution (Figure 12–9). Livor is found in the dependent body areas. The fingertips and nail beds should be carefully inspected. Depending on the cause of death and the position of the body, livor may be present even in the face. If this blood discol-

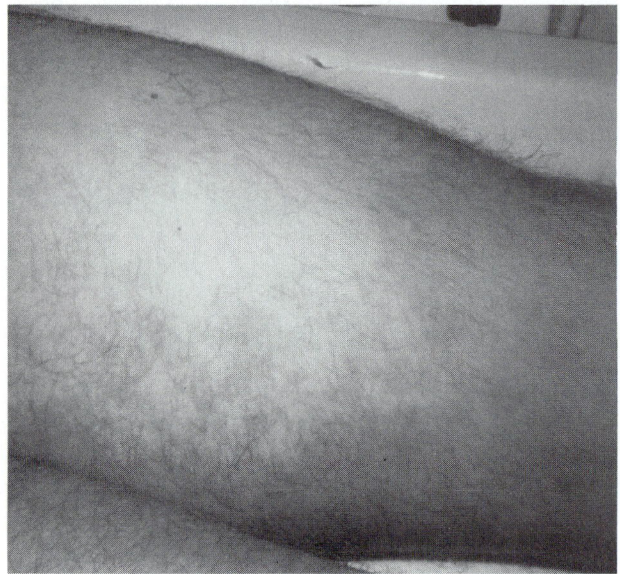

Figure 12–9. Livor mortis starting to clear in the legs.

oration is pushed on, it should lighten, indicating that the blood present is still in the vascular system. During injection, the livor mortis should be removed. Many times the "breaking up" of large areas of livor mortis can easily be observed. Once this breakup begins, the area can be massaged.

Distension of Small Surface Vessels. When fluid reaches certain body areas such as the hands, feet, or temple of the face, small vessels can often be observed by their distension. It should be pointed out that gravitated blood can also cause the veins to rise when hands are placed on the embalming table. Gas in the cavities can cause small vessels to distend. Observe vessel areas (e.g., temples, backs of hands) prior to and during arterial injection to be certain any distension of the vessel(s) is brought about by arterial injection.

Loss of Skin Elasticity. As the solution begins to firm the tissues, skin areas exhibit a loss of elasticity. When the skin is gathered and gently pulled upward, it slowly settles back into proper position.

Firming (Fixation) of the Tissues. Rigor mortis can easily be mistaken for firming of the tissues by the arterial solution. It is most important that in making the preembalming analysis of the body, the **presence of rigor** be noted. Some bodies exhibit little or no firming after good embalming. These are usually bodies that have been treated with large doses of drugs, that have small amounts of muscular protein, or that have been dead for long periods. Most bodies exhibit some degree of firming depending on the amount and strength of embalming chemical injected. Firming, although not a foolproof sign of embalmed tissue, is nevertheless an indicator that most embalmers rely on as a sign of arterial distribution. Some embalming chemicals are designed to produce tissues that are only slightly firm or that exhibit no firming. Different embalming chemicals affect the degree and speed of tissue firming.

Drying of the Tissues. As arterial solution reacts with the tissues to the skin, the surface of the body dries slightly. Areas not reached by the embalming solution often appear shiny and somewhat moist to the touch. This is not a very reliable sign of distribution and should *not* be relied on as an accurate indicator. Bodies that are dehydrated prior to embalming exhibit dry skin tissues *before* arterial solution is injected.

Bleaching of the Tissues. Some arterial fluids produce a mottled effect of the skin when the solution is present. This mottled coloring is caused by the bleaching quality of some arterial fluids. Dyes in the embalming solution, however, can mask this bleaching effect. Bleaching is not a reliable sign of arterial fluid distribution.

Blood Drainage. The presence of blood drainage indicates that embalming solution is being distributed to the tissues and organs of the body. It does not, however, indicate what specific areas of the body are receiving arterial solution. As a sign of distribution, it does not account for short-circuiting of arterial solution. Some body areas might be receiving too much and other body areas might not be receiving any solution. Excellent preservation can be accomplished with little or no drainage. In embalming bodies for dissection, many medical schools take no drainage. The blood is used as a vehicle for the concentrated embalming solutions; however, distension is generally very evident. In "waterless embalming," very concentrated solutions but in much smaller volumes are used than in standard embalming (i.e., 1 to $1\frac{1}{2}$ gallons would be injected in waterless embalming; 2 to 4 gallons would be injected in standard embalming). Limiting drainage again helps to make the blood the vehicle for dilution and distribution of the concentrated chemical solution.

Leakage From Punctures. When intravenous needles are removed by the hospital after death, during the embalming process, fluid or blood drainage can be seen exiting from these intravenous sites. This is a good indication that arterial solution is reaching these body areas. Some embalmers puncture the skin with a large-gauge needle or the tip of a scalpel (in an area not to be viewed) to see if embalming solution seeps from the skin.

Rounding of Fingers, Lips, and Toes. With some embalming formulations the tips of the fingers, lips, and toes slightly plump when reached by the arterial solution. Depending on the method of drainage and the strength of the embalming solution, the reverse can happen; these areas can wrinkle when fluid reaches them as a result of dehydration. It is an unreliable test of distribution but may be very evident in some bodies.

Most embalmers use several signs of distribution to ensure that a sufficient amount of arterial solution has reached a body area. The most reliable in the preceding list are dyes, clearing of intravascular blood discolorations, and firming of tissues.

▶ OBSERVATIONS PRIOR TO INJECTION

Several signs of arterial solution distribution and diffusion can be confused with several postmortem changes. It is important that the embalmer note these changes prior to injection so they are not mistaken as a sign of arterial distribution.

Observe for the presence or absence of livor mortis in all body areas prior to the start of the arterial injection. Examine the nail beds. Some degree of livor is generally present. In some bodies, however, depending on the position of the hands, the livor may gravitate from the fingers and hands. If this were not noted at the start of the embalming, the *absence* of the livor could be mistaken for clearing of the livor by the arterial injection.

Note the degree of rigor mortis present in the tissues. An attempt should always be made to relieve the rigor prior to injection. This is not always possible in areas such as the legs or jaw. Rigor can easily be mistaken for firming of the tissues by the arterial solution.

Observe the distension of veins or small arteries. Veins on the backs of the hands can be distended before arterial solution is injected as a result of gravitation of the blood. Gases in the cavities or conditions such as ascites or hydrothorax can put pressure on the diaphragm and heart and cause small vessels to fill with blood. This distension or its absence should be noted prior to arterial injection.

Note any discoloration of the skin. Skin of refrigerated or frozen bodies or bodies dead from carbon monoxide poisoning may have a pinkish hue. If fluid dyes are used, this color gives the appearance of embalmed tissue. It is important to note this discoloration (resulting from hemolysis) prior to arterial injection.

Check for firmness of the tissues. Tissues of bodies placed in refrigeration, as many are done today, not only appear to be embalmed (hemolysis) but also feel slightly firm, as embalmed tissue. This firming is due to the slight firming of subcutaneous fatty tissues as a result of the refrigeration. This condition should be noted with refrigerated bodies so it is not mistaken for distribution and firming by the arterial solution.

These factors should all be noted in making a preembalming analysis. Active dyes in the arterial fluid serve as the best indicator for the presence of arterial solution in a body region.

▶ IMPROVING ARTERIAL SOLUTION DISTRIBUTION

Several mechanical (or physical) procedures improve the distribution of the arterial solution. The embalmer may also use a combination of these procedures. **During the injection of the first gallon of arterial solution, firm massage and exercise of the extremities can be very important in establishing good distribution.**

1. Increase the rate of flow of the arterial solution being injected.
2. Increase the pressure of the arterial solution being injected.
3. Inject the arterial solution using pulsation.
4. Restrict the drainage; use intermittent drainage and the alternate method of drainage.
5. Massage the body. Massage should be firm, not merely rubbing the surface of the body. Massage should be directed along the arterial routes (e.g., if solution is not entering the legs, massage should first be concentrated on the inguinal areas; once solution enters the leg the remainder of the arterial route can be massaged and flexed).
6. Inject an adequate volume of embalming solution. Often, when large volumes of embalming solution are injected, body areas that received little or no arterial solution during the early part of the embalming receive solution after 2 or 3 gallons have been injected.
7. Relieve extreme abdominal extravascular pressures caused by gas or abdominal edema (ascites). A trocar can be entered from the left inguinal area keeping the point under the anterior abdominal wall; the transverse colon can be pierced to relieve gas; if edema is present, some of the fluid can be drained.
8. If distribution of the solution appears to be happening but there is little drainage, selection of

another drainage site may improve not only the drainage but the distribution of the solution. Some embalmers may even use direct heart drainage to establish a better drainage flow.

Treatments for specific areas may also be applied. For *facial tissues,* massage the neck where the common carotid arteries are located. For the *arms,* lower them to the sides or over the embalming table; massage should first be concentrated in the axilla (Figure 12–10). For the *fingers,* massage the radial and ulnar artery areas of the forearm and then massage the sides of the fingers (where the vessels are located); pressure can also be applied to the nail beds. For the *legs,* massage the inguinal areas over the femoral arteries, flex the legs, and turn the foot inward; this helps to "squeeze" the muscles of the legs.

Massage can attract arterial solution to an area. Areas such as the lips and eyelids often respond well to massage (when it is needed). Squeezing the lips can attract solution into the labial tissues. Care should be taken that swelling or dehydration (wrinkles) do not result.

Body areas that receive no solution or inadequate amounts of arterial solution should be injected separately. If distribution is still a problem, restricting drainage from the limb, massaging, increasing the pressure or rate of flow of injection, or using pulsation with higher pressures may all help to distribute solution into a particular body area.

CLINICAL EXAMPLE: ONE-POINT INJECTION USING THE COMMON CAROTID ARTERY

The right arm does not appear to be receiving arterial solution. The axillary area is massaged and the arm lowered over the side of the table. There is still no solution in the arm. Raise and inject the axillary or brachial artery. Use a higher pressure if desired. Thoroughly massage along the arterial route. Assume that the hand does not receive solution. Raise the radial or ulnar artery and inject.

A preservative solution must enter a body region before it can reach a specific location. Arterial solution cannot enter the fingers if it is not entering the arm.

When doubt exists as to whether a body area has received any or an adequate amount of arterial solution, make every attempt to raise the artery that supplies the area and separately inject the area.

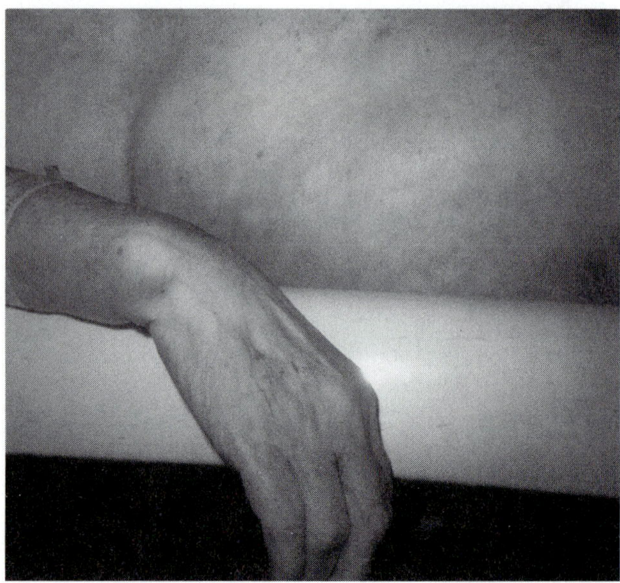

Figure 12–10. The hands are lowered to facilitate circulation.

Stimulation of arterial solution distribution is a three-step procedure:

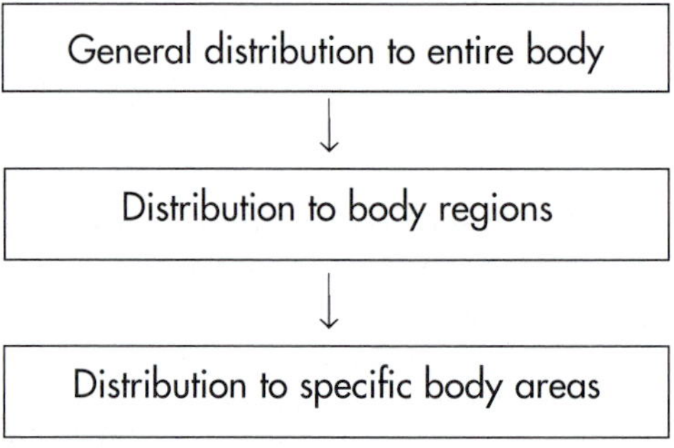

▶ DIFFUSION OF THE EMBALMING SOLUTION

The key to arterial embalming is arterial fluid *diffusion.* Fluid diffusion can be defined as the passage of some elements of the injected embalming solutions from within the capillary (intravascular) to the tissue spaces (extravascular). The capillary network of the blood vascular system is so vast that a pin can hardly be inserted into the living skin without rupturing a sufficient number of these smallest of blood vessels to cause bleeding (Figure 12–11).

Capillaries are the smallest blood vessels. They link the smallest arteries (arterioles) to the smallest veins (venules). They are actually the extensions of the inner linings of these larger vessels. Their walls are composed of endothelium, which lines the entire vascular system

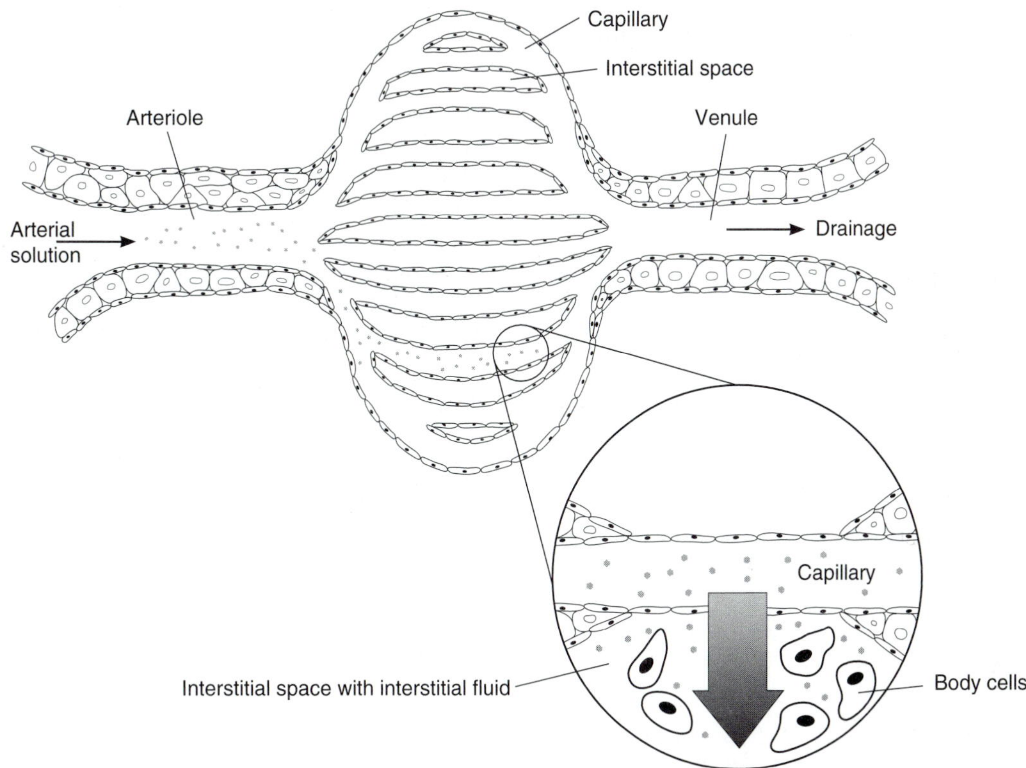

Figure 12–11. Diffusion of the embalming solution.

and is made up of flat, single-layered cells called *squamous epithelium.* These very thin-walled cells form the semipermeable membranes through which substances in the blood must pass to reach the body cells.

Blood does not have direct contact with body cells. All of the cells (e.g., muscle cells, nerve cells) are surrounded by a liquid called interstitial (tissue) fluid. Blood nutrients and oxygen must pass through the walls of the capillaries and into the interstitial fluid. These products diffuse through the tissue fluid to reach the body cells. This same movement occurs in embalming. The arterial solution must pass from the capillary, through the walls of the capillary, into the interstitial fluid, and finally to the body cells. It must then enter the cells of the body and react with the protoplasm protein.

▶ METHODS OF ARTERIAL SOLUTION DIFFUSION

The start of this chapter stated that "arterial embalming could actually be called capillary embalming." It is at the capillary level that most embalming begins. (Additionally, the contents of the blood vascular system, including any microbes or their agents in the blood, and the lining of the blood vascular system are disinfected and preserved as the embalming solution passes through the vessels.) From the capillaries, embalming solution moves to the interstitial fluid that surrounds each cell. The solution makes contact with proteins in the interstitial fluid, proteins in the cell membranes, and proteins in the cytoplasm of the cell.

Physical (or passive) transport mechanisms are responsible for the movement of embalming solution from within the capillaries to the tissue spaces. The energy needed to move the solution through the walls of the capillary originates from a nonliving mechanism. Passive mechanisms can move materials through dead cell membranes (capillaries). The major passive (or physical) transport processes for the movement of embalming solutions are pressure filtration, osmosis, and dialysis.

Pressure Filtration

Pressure filtration caused by intravascular pressure (IVP) is one of the most important passive transport systems for the passage of embalming solution from the capillary to tissue fluid. In this process both the solute and solvent portions of the embalming solution pass into the interstitial fluid. Penetrating agents (wetting agents, surface tension reducers, or surfactants) in the concentrated embalming fluid lower its surface tension. The reduction of surface tension makes the embalming solution "wetter," and it can more easily pass through the minute pores and the cell membranes of the capillaries.

Intravascular pressure places enough pressure on the embalming solution to force it through the pores and cells of the capillary walls. This is similar to the effect of a lawn soaker hose. Some of the solution enters the tissue spaces to mix with the interstitial fluid. The embalming solution that remains in the capillary pushes on to remove the blood and exits as part of the drainage.

In the agonal period, respiration can become difficult and shallow. Sufficient oxygen is not delivered to the blood. As a defense mechanism, the pores between the cells of the capillaries expand in an attempt to get more oxygen. It is theorized that at death the capillaries are permeable, for their pores are still expanded. As a result, embalming solution can easily be filtered (or pushed) through these pores (caused by intravascular pressure). In some bodies, the capillaries may have begun to decompose. The injected solution can now easily flow through the broken capillaries into the tissue spaces. When this happens the body tissues easily distend. This is seen in bodies that have been dead for long periods. These bodies easily swell and there is little or no drainage.

Likewise, when the limbs are exercised to break up rigor mortis, many capillaries may be torn. The muscle tissues can rapidly swell on injection and, again, drainage is minimal. In bodies in which decomposition is evident or rigor is present, stronger solutions should be used so preservation can be achieved with a minimal amount of solution. This keeps swelling at a minimum. Pressure filtration is, no doubt, one of the primary mechanisms by which embalming solution comes into contact with the interstitial spaces and fluids (Figure 12–12).

Osmosis

Osmosis is a passive transport mechanism involved with liquid (or solvent) movement. It is the passage of a solvent (such as water) through a semipermeable membrane from a dilute to a concentrated solution. Embalming solutions are more dilute (or less dense) than the interstitial fluids that surround the body cells. The interstitial fluids and the embalming solution are separated by the walls of the capillaries, which are semipermeable. Some of the chemical compounds found in the interstitial fluid cannot move through the capillary walls into the blood vascular system. The more dilute solution, in this case the embalming solution, is described as hypotonic, meaning it is more dilute or less dense than the interstitial fluid. For example, in mixing a 1-gallon solution of embalming solution, assume that 8 ounces of concentrated fluid is added to 120 ounces of water; for every ounce of embalming fluid, 15 ounces of water is used as a dilutant.

Some of the hypotonic embalming solution will easily pass through the walls and minute pores of the capillary to enter the interstitial spaces and mix with the interstitial fluid. It will then travel through the interstitial fluid and come into contact with the cells. Again, the process of osmosis will occur. This time the mixture of interstitial fluid and embalming solution will pass through the cell membrane and the preservatives will enter the cytoplasm of the cell. All along this route, contact of the preservative solution is made with proteins whether they are in the walls of the capillaries, in the interstitial fluid, in the membranes of the cells, or in the cytoplasm of the cell. New substances are being produced from the reaction between the protein and the preservative. In this manner, the process of preservation occurs.

When the directions are not followed and embalming solutions are made too weak (too dilute), these solutions will rapidly pass through the capillaries into the tissue fluids. Not only can swelling occur, but inadequate preservation results. These tissues become "waterlogged" with the weak solution, and the process of decomposition can actually be accelerated. A reverse condition can be created by mixing solutions that are too concentrated. These concentrated solutions can cause the moisture in the interstitial fluid to move into the capillaries, bringing about dehydration. In conditions such as edema, a more concentrated (or dense) embalming solution can be used.

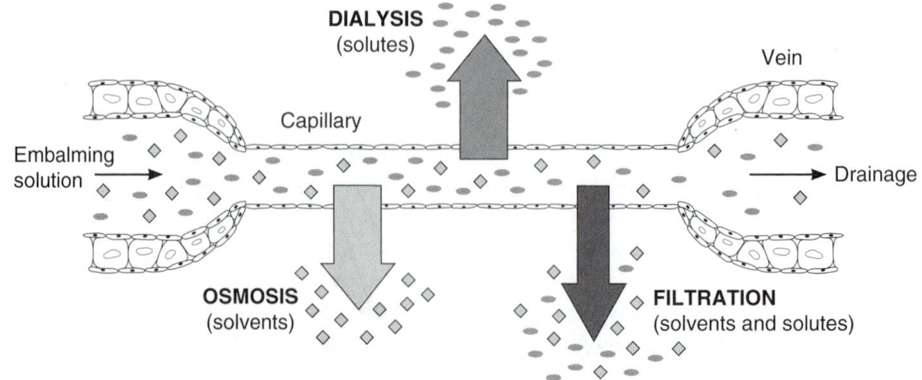

Figure 12–12. Summary of solution diffusion: pressure filtration, osmosis, and dialysis.

When the embalmer dilutes the concentrated arterial fluid with water, this dilution is called **primary dilution.** In addition to water, coinjection fluid may also be used as a diluent in addition to such chemicals as humectant and water softener. These solutions are described as being hypotonic for embalming the average body under normal moisture conditions. They allow some moisture to be added to the tissues and assist in retaining tissue moisture.

Within the tissue spaces, where the interstitial fluid is present, dilution of the arterial fluid continues. This dilution of the embalming solution that occurs in the tissues of the body is called the **secondary dilution.** The moisture found in the tissues dilutes the fluid. In addition, the fluid that remains in the capillaries and exits with the drainage is also diluted by the liquid portion of the blood. The secondary dilution of the fluid can be very great in bodies with skeletal edema.

In making an embalming analysis the embalmer must evaluate the moisture conditions of the body. Are the tissues dehydrated? Are the tissues moist as a result of edema? Or are the tissues normal? On the basis of these observations the primary dilution is prepared. On the labels of embalming fluid most chemical manufacturers indicate the number of ounces of concentrated fluid to use per gallon based on the moisture content of the body.

Dialysis

The third method of passive transport by which the embalming solution passes from the capillaries to the cells is dialysis. Dialysis is the diffusion of the dissolved crystalloid solutes of a solution through a semipermeable membrane. Interstitial fluid, cytoplasm of the body cells, and embalming solutions are composed primarily of the solvent water. Dissolved in these solutions are very small solutes called **crystalloids** and very large solutes called **colloids.**

The embalming solution in the capillary is separated from the interstitial fluid by the semipermeable membrane of the capillary wall. The cytoplasm within the cell is separated from the interstitial fluid by the semipermeable **cell membrane.** In dialysis, small crystalloids can diffuse through the semipermeable membranes, but large colloids in the solutions cannot. Water is the primary solvent in embalming solutions; alcohols and glycerine are other examples. The solutes in embalming fluids are various crystalloids such as salts, preservatives, and germicides and colloids (humectants). Interstitial fluid comprises the solvent water and various crystalloid salts and colloids (proteins, enzymes, etc.). Crystalloids in the embalming solution can diffuse through the capillary semipermeable membrane into the interstitial fluid. These preservatives, germicides, dyes, and so on then spread through the interstitial fluid and again pass through the cell membrane to enter the cytoplasm of the cell.

To repeat, dialysis is the diffusion of crystalloids across a semipermeable membrane that is impermeable to colloids. It is the process of separating crystalloids (smaller particles) from colloids (larger particles) by the difference in their rates of diffusion through a semipermeable membrane.

▶ MOVEMENT OF EMBALMING SOLUTIONS FROM OUTSIDE THE CAPILLARIES TO INSIDE THE CELLS

Fluid diffusion was defined as the movement of embalming solution from within the capillary (intravascular) to the interstitial fluid (extravascular). Embalming solution does not stop moving once it leaves the capillary and enters the interstitial space to mix with the interstitial fluid. The interstitial fluid (intercellular or tissue fluid) is a viscous solution similar to the cytoplasm found inside the cells of the body. It contains inorganic chemicals, proteins, carbohydrates, and lipids dissolved in water. This fluid surrounds the cells of the body and is the connection between the blood vascular system (capillaries) and the body cells. Embalming solution must pass from the capillaries into the interstitial fluid, spread through the interstitial fluid, and finally enter the cells of the body (Figure 12–13). Once inside the body cells, the embalming solution again diffuses to come into contact with all portions of the cell.

The concentrated embalming elements are spread through the interstitial fluid by the passive transport systems called *diffusion* and *filtration gravitation.* Passage of embalming solution into the body cells is brought about by the passive transport systems of **adsorption, osmosis,** and **dialysis.**

Diffusion

Diffusion means scattering or spreading. Small particles such as molecules are always moving in all directions. For example, place a drop of fluid dye into a gallon of water and let the solution of dye and water set without stirring. In a short period, the entire gallon of water is slightly and evenly colored by the dye. The concentrated drop of dye has spread through the water. Diffusion occurs from a region of high concentration to a region of lower concentration. In a similar manner, once the embalming solution passes into the interstitial fluid it spreads (or diffuses) through the interstitial fluid to come into contact with the cells of the body. By the processes of dialysis, adsorption, and osmosis it passes into the cell and, once in the cell, spreads through the cytoplasm by diffusion.

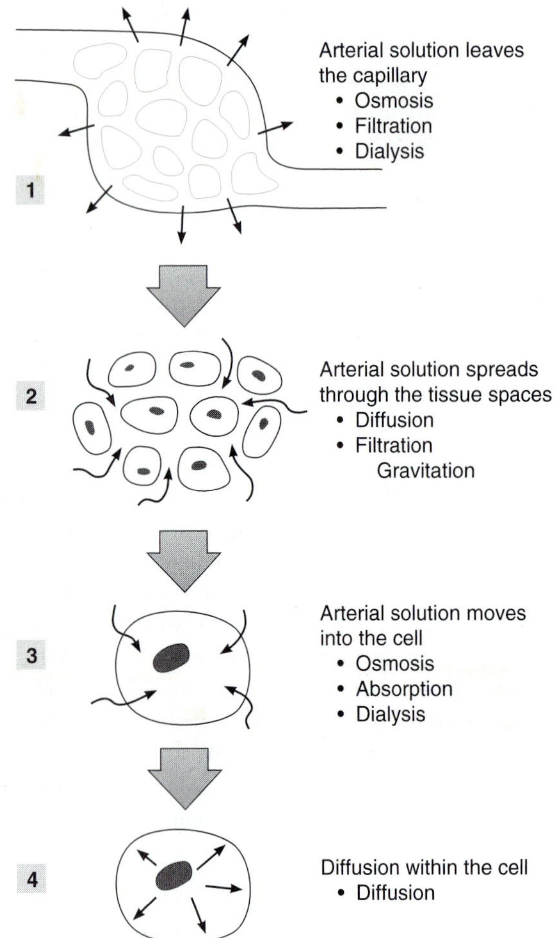

Figure 12–13. Movement of embalming solution from outside the capillaries to inside the cells.

Adsorption

The cytoplasm of the body cells is composed of a continuous aqueous solution (cytosol) with all the organelles (except nucleus) suspended in it. The fluid inside the cells of the body is called a **colloidal dispersion.** The large colloid molecules, because of their large surface area, tend to *adsorb* molecules. Colloidal dispersions in cells adsorb molecules from the surrounding interstitial tissue fluids. In this manner, some of the embalming solution present in the interstitial fluid is adsorbed into the body cells.

Gravity Filtration

Gravity filtration is the extravascular settling of embalming solution by gravitational force into the dependent areas of the body. This passive transport system helps to move embalming solution throughout the interstitial fluid. In the embalmed body gravity filtration is responsible for the movement of embalming solution into the dependent tissues—lower back, buttocks, and backs of arms, legs, and shoulders. It may be of some value in moving embalming solution into those areas that are in contact with the embalming table. This slow movement continues for some time after the injection of solution. This is *not* a gravitation of fluids through the vascular system. It is extravascular movement of the solution through the interstitial fluid.

Summary

Passive transport systems require some amount of time to work. Pressurized injection, the penetrating agents found in the arterial fluids, and pressure filtration constitute the primary transport system for the movement of arterial solution from the capillaries to the tissue spaces. Osmosis, dialysis, gravitation filtration, and diffusion all take longer. Many embalmers prefer a delay between injection and cavity aspiration. In addition to a delay, many embalmers prefer to inject the last half-gallon of arterial solution with the drainage closed. This method allows a maximum filtration pressure to be established. The delay after injection can be 1 or 2 hours. Some embalmers feel several hours is needed. There should be some interval between injection and aspiration, even if it is only the time in which incisions are sewn and the body washed and dried. This interval gives the solutions an opportunity to fully penetrate the capillaries.

▶ KEYS TERMS AND CONCEPTS FOR STUDY AND DISCUSSION

1. Define the following terms:
   Actual pressure
   Adsorption
   Arterial fluid
   Arterial solution
   Arterial solution diffusion
   Arterial solution distribution
   Arterial solution perfusion
   Arteriole
   Capillary
   Center of arterial solution distribution
   Contact pressure
   Crystalloid
   Dialysis
   Differential pressure
   Diffusion
   Drainage
   Extravascular resistance
   Gravity filtration
   Hypertonic solution
   Hypotonic solution
   Ideal pressure
   Ideal rate of flow
   Injection pressure

Interstitial
Interstitial fluid
Intravascular resistance
Lumen
Osmosis
Passive transport system
Potential pressure
Pressure filtration
Primary dilution
Rate of flow
Retained embalming solution
Secondary dilution
Semipermeable membrane
Signs of diffusion
Signs of distribution
Solute
Solvent
Venule

2. Discuss the movement of arterial solution from the machine to an individual body cell.
3. Why would the ascending aorta and the arch of the aorta be considered the "center of arterial solution distribution"?
4. Why is some resistance valuable to drainage?
5. Discuss fluid dilutions for the normal (moisture content) body; emaciated and dehydrated body; body with skeletal edema; and body with ascites and/or hydrothorax but no skeletal edema.

▶ BIBLIOGRAPHY

Anthony CP. *Textbook of Anatomy and Physiology*. St. Louis, MO: CV Mosby; 1979:40–53.

Arnow LE. *Introduction to Physiological and Pathological Chemistry*. St. Louis, MO: CV Mosby; 1976:66–73.

Dhonau CO. *The ABCs of Pressure and Distribution*, File 86. Cincinnati, OH: Cincinnati College of Embalming.

Dhonau CO. *Manual of Case Analysis*. 2nd ed. Cincinnati, OH: The Embalming Book Co.; 1928.

Frederick JF. The mathematics of embalming chemistry, Parts I and II. *Dodge Mag*, October–November 1968.

Johnson EC. A study of arterial pressure during embalming. In: *Champion Expanding Encyclopedia*. Springfield, OH: Champion Chemical; 1981:2081–2084.

Kroshus J, McConnell J, Bardole J. The measurement of formaldehyde retention in the tissues of embalmed bodies. *Director* 1983; March/April 10–12.

Zweifach BW. The microcirculation of the blood. *Sci Am*, January 1959.

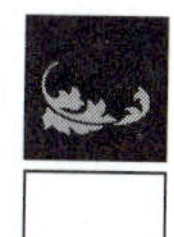

CHAPTER 13
INJECTION AND DRAINAGE TECHNIQUES

During arterial embalming of the body, four processes take place *at the same time:* (1) *injection* of the arterial solution at a set rate of flow and pressure from the machine, (2) *distribution* of the embalming solution through the blood vascular system, (3) *diffusion* of the embalming solution from the blood vascular system (capillaries) to the cells and tissues, and (4) *drainage* of the contents of the blood vascular system, some of these tissue fluids, and a portion of the embalming solution.

When all four of these processes are successful, a sufficient amount of embalming solution is delivered to the tissues to achieve a uniform preservation and sanitation of the body tissues without distension. These processes remove intravascular discolorations, color the tissues, and establish the proper moisture balance in the tissues so that dehydration or overly moist tissue is not a problem.

In Chapter 12, discussion centered on the distribution of arterial solution and the mechanisms by which arterial solution is retained by the body. Injection involves not only pressurized injecting apparatus but the equally important artery (or arteries) used for injection and the vein (or veins) used for drainage. In the unautopsied body, the ideal artery for injection is the largest artery, the aorta. Its location, however, makes the aorta an impractical choice. The best location for drainage is the right atrium of the heart, but again, its location within the thoracic cavity makes it an impractical choice. Therefore, the vessels used for injection and drainage should be as close as possible to both the aorta and the right atrium.

▶ WORK CONTROLS

Work practice controls are those work procedures taken to reduce the exposure levels to formaldehyde and other chemical vapors during the embalming of the body. Some examples include the following items:

1. Adequate and properly operating air exchange system
   a. The exhaust ventilation should draw fumes *away* from the embalmer
   b. There needs to be a good supply of incoming clean, fresh air
2. Prevent spillage of chemicals
   a. Gently mix embalming solutions and avoid splashing
   b. Keep the rate of flow valve on the embalming machine closed or stopcocks on arterial tubes closed to prevent leakage, before and after injection, or when the delivery hose is being moved between injection sites
3. Keep embalming machines in good repair
   a. No leakage from within the machine apparatus
   b. No leakage where hose attachments are made to machine or arterial tube
4. Rinse fluid bottles and empty into the arterial solution
5. Cap all chemical bottles
6. Keep a lid on the embalming machine reservoir
7. Use continuous aspiration of body cavities during injection of the autopsied body
8. Clamp all accessible leaking arteries during the injection of the autopsied body
9. Restrict drainage as much as possible after blood discolorations have cleared
   a. Helps to retain embalming solution within the body
   b. Lowers the volume of chemicals placed into the waste system
10. Use closed drainage
    a. Attach tubing to the drain tube
    b. Direct heart drainage with trocar
11. Cover the waste sink to avoid splashing and aerosolization
12. Use moving water to immediately remove drainage from the embalming table
13. Avoid high water pressure to avoid splashing

These work controls combined with personal protective attire will greatly reduce exposure to chemicals or their vapors. Consult Chapter 3 of this text for a discussion of personal protective equipment.

▶ ARTERIES FOR INJECTION/VEINS FOR DRAINAGE

FACTORS DETERMINED DURING THE EMBALMING ANALYSIS

1. **VESSELS FOR INJECTION AND DRAINAGE**
2. **STRENGTH OF THE EMBALMING SOLUTION**
3. **VOLUME OF THE EMBALMING SOLUTION**
4. **INJECTION PRESSURE**
5. **INJECTION RATE OF FLOW**

Note: These factors will vary by the individual body and they can vary in different areas of the same body.

Arteries are used for injection of arterial solution, because, unlike some of the long veins of the body, they *do not* have valves. When arterial solution is injected "down" the leg, the drainage is returned "up" the leg through the veins. In life, blood flows back to the heart. In embalming, drainage flows in a similar direction, toward the heart.

▶ INJECTION TECHNIQUES

Embalming of the unautopsied body begins when the embalmer selects a suitable artery or combination of arteries (as in restricted cervical injection) from which the arterial solution can be distributed throughout the *entire body*. Should injection of the embalming solution from this injection site fail to distribute the fluid to all body areas, other arteries must be raised and injected.

Embalming analysis continues throughout the embalming process. In the preembalming period, an artery and vein are selected for the primary injection and drainage sites on the basis of the following criteria:

One-point injection	Injection and drainage from one location
Split injection	Injection and drainage from separate locations
Multipoint injection	Injection at two or more sites
Restricted cervical injection	Raising of both common carotid arteries at the start of injection
Sectional injection	Multipoint injection where direct injection of a body region is made

One-Point Injection

In single-point injection, one location is used for both injection and drainage, requiring only one incision to be made. The most frequently used one-point injection sites are the right common carotid artery and the right internal jugular vein, the right femoral artery and the right femoral vein, the right external iliac artery and the right external iliac vein, and the right axillary artery and the right axillary vein.* The common carotid and the femoral arteries are the most frequently used one-point injection sites today. The axillary artery is least used. Years ago, when most embalming was performed at the residence of the deceased and a minimum amount of very concentrated fluid was injected, the axillary, no doubt, was the most frequently used artery because the head could easily be cleared of discoloration, and drainage could easily be collected from this site or by drainage from the right atrium of the heart. Also, the incision would not be seen by the family after the preparation.

CRITERIA FOR SELECTION OF AN ARTERY AS AN INJECTION SITE

1. Size (diameter) of the artery
2. Practicality of drainage from the accompanying vein
3. Depth of the location of the artery
4. Flexibility of the artery because of its branches
5. Effect on posing the body
6. Incision location if leakage is a possibility (if edema is in the area of the artery)
7. Proximity of the vessel to the arch of the aorta

CRITERIA FOR SELECTION OF A VEIN FOR DRAINAGE

1. Size (diameter) of the vein
2. Proximity to the right atrium of the heart
3. Discolorations of the face and neck (blood)
4. Ease with which vein can be brought to the surface because of tributaries
5. Depth of vein

* Reference is made to Chapters 8 and 9 concerning the advantages and disadvantages of each artery and vein as a point for injection or drainage. The left vessels could also be used.

Often embalming necessitates the use of large volumes of embalming solution. The internal jugular or femoral vein allows for better drainage than the small axillary or basilic veins. Good drainage is essential when a large amount of solution is being injected. Some embalmers prefer to drain from each injection site when sectional embalming is performed in the unautopsied body; others prefer a central site such as those just mentioned. There are three major injection sites: the common carotid, femoral, and axillary arteries. These arteries are large in size (especially the femoral and common carotid) and they are located as close to the aorta as is possible in the unautopsied body. An arterial tube comparable to the size of the artery is recommended (when arteriosclerosis is not a concern) for maximum rate of flow of the embalming solution. The diameter of the arterial tube determines to a great degree the volume and velocity of embalming solution injected in any given time period and under any given pressure. Procedures for such an injection from the three major sites are as follows:

RIGHT COMMON CAROTID INTERNAL JUGULAR VEIN

1. Insert an arterial tube into the right common carotid artery directed downward toward the trunk of the body.
2. Insert an arterial tube into the right common carotid artery directed upward toward the right side of the face, leaving the stop cock *open.*
3. Insert a drainage instrument into the right internal jugular vein *directed toward the heart.*
4. *Inject* the trunk of the body; several gallons of solution are required for the adult body.
5. Inject sufficient solution up the right side of the head.

RIGHT FEMORAL ARTERY AND VEIN

1. Insert a drainage tube *directed toward the heart* into the femoral vein.
2. Insert an arterial tube directed toward the right foot into the femoral artery.
3. Insert an arterial tube directed toward the trunk (head) of the body.
4. Inject the right leg first.
5. Inject the trunk, arms, and head.

See Figure 13–1.

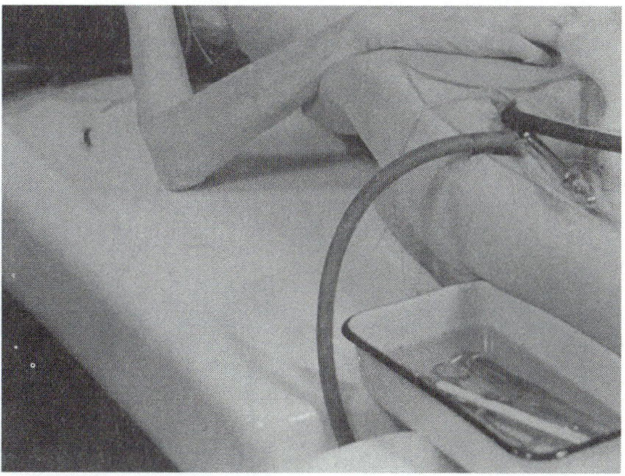

Figure 13–1. Single-point injection and drainage from the right femoral artery and vein. Note the concurrent disinfection of the instruments. A hose is attached to collect drainage from the drain tube, closed drainage.

RIGHT AXILLARY ARTERY AND VEIN

1. Insert an arterial tube into the axillary artery directed toward the right hand.
2. Insert an arterial tube into the right axillary artery directed toward the trunk and head of the body.
3. Insert a drainage instrument in the axillary vein directed toward the heart.
4. Inject the head and trunk first.
5. Inject the right arm.

See Figure 13–2A.

A disadvantage of the one-point method of injection and drainage is the short-circuiting of arterial fluid. Fluid has a tendency to find direct routes from the arterioles to the venules or through only portions of the capillaries in the region around the injection site. This can account for overembalming of the area near the injection site and loss of a great amount of arterial solution through the drainage.

Short-Circuiting of Arterial Solution

Fluids follow the path of least resistance. Quite often the skin area is the path of least resistance, for the skin has a greater amount of capillaries than most deeper body tissues. The skin areas surrounding the injection and drainage points frequently receive a greater volume of solution (Fig. 13–2B). Embalming in which only the skin and superficial portions of the body and not the deeper tissues receive solution has been referred to as **shell embalming.** Massage, manipulation, and restric-

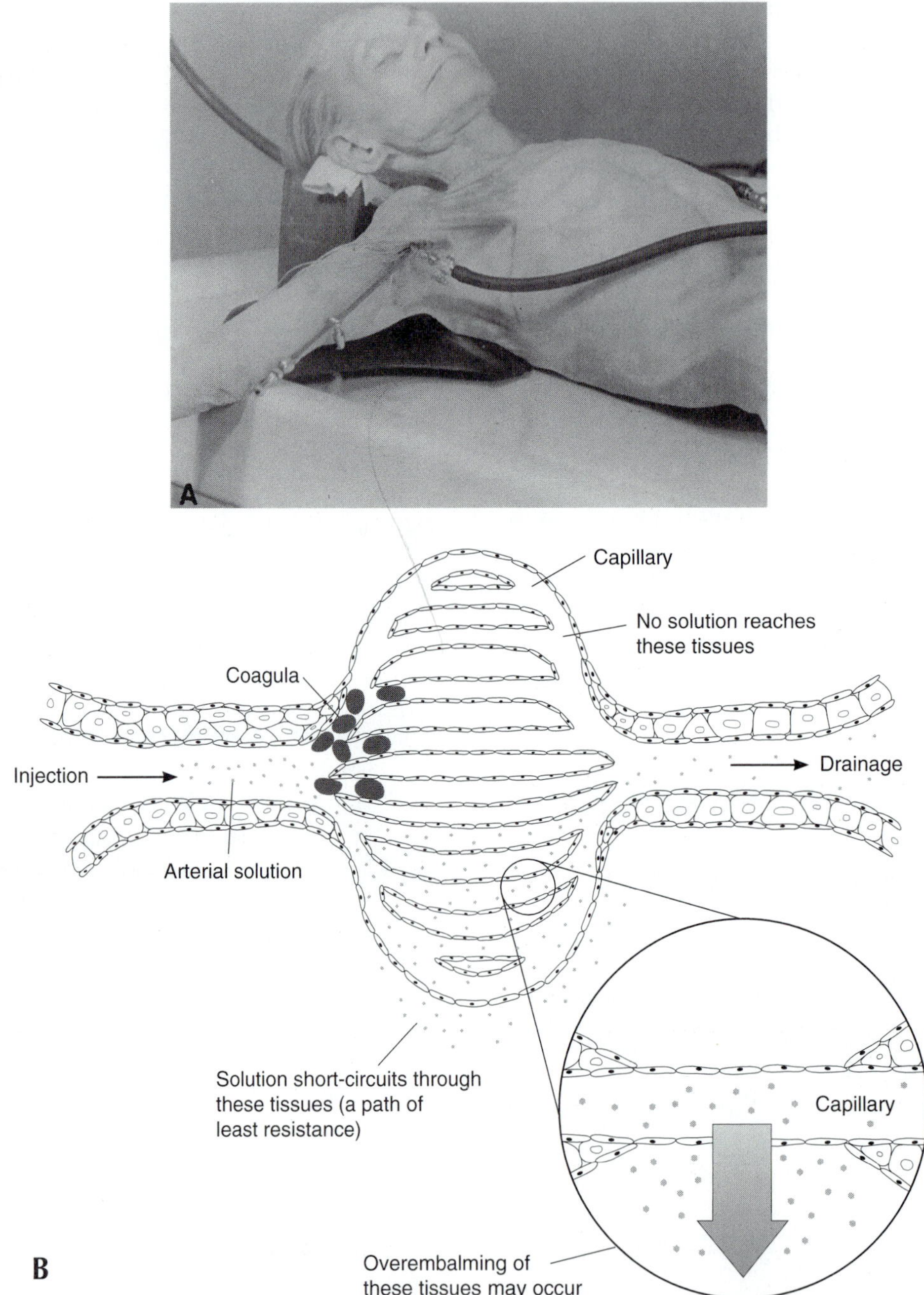

Figure 13–2. A. Injection and drainage from the axillary artery and vein. Because of the small size of these veins, this method is not used often today. **B.** The greatest disadvantage of the one-point method of injection and drainage is the short-circuiting of arterial solution. Solution has a tendency to find direct routes from the arterioles to the venules in the region around the injection site. This can account for overembalming of the area near the injection site and loss of a large amount of arterial solution through the drainage.

tion of drainage all help to reduce shell embalming and to encourage movement of arterial solution into the muscles and deep tissues.

There are direct connections between arterioles and venules. In life, direct connections between arterioles and venules help to divert blood into tissues that need the most nourishment. After one-point injection, such short-circuiting pathways are quite frequently established. As a result, the solution does not enter some capillaries, but, instead, rapidly passes from the arterial side to the venous side of the blood vascular system, where it is drained from the body. This is often seen in regions that surround a one-point injection and drainage site.

Coagula in the arterial system can easily be pushed into minute arterial tributaries. Solution then seeks out paths of least resistance and quickly finds its way into the venous system. Once there, it can easily be removed at the drainage site. The short-circuiting of this problem is caused not so much by the use of one-point injection as by the unrestricted drainage (Fig. 13–2B).

Split Injection

Split injection is the injection of solution from one site and the drainage from another location. This method reduces short-circuiting of the solution and attempts to establish a more even distribution of the arterial solution. The most frequently used combination of vessels in the split injection method is the right internal jugular vein (drainage) and the right femoral artery (injection). Often, the embalmer begins with a one-point injection using the femoral vessels, but soon finds difficulties with the drainage. Raising the internal jugular vein generally solves the drainage problem. Some embalmers prefer to use this type of injection and drainage process. Examples of split injection include the following:

RIGHT FEMORAL ARTERY, RIGHT INTERNAL JUGULAR VEIN

1. Insert a drainage instrument into the right internal jugular vein directed toward the heart.
2. Insert an arterial tube into the right femoral artery directed toward the right foot.
3. Insert an arterial tube into the right femoral artery directed toward the trunk and head of the body.
4. Inject the right leg and foot first; drainage is taken from the jugular.
5. Inject the trunk and head of the body, drainage is taken from the jugular.

RIGHT COMMON CAROTID ARTERY, RIGHT FEMORAL VEIN

1. Insert a drainage instrument into the right femoral vein directed toward the heart.
2. Insert an arterial tube into the right common carotid artery directed toward the right side of the head.
3. Insert an arterial tube into the right common carotid artery directed toward the trunk of the body.
4. Inject down the right common carotid first to embalm the trunk of the body and left side of the face; drainage is taken from the femoral vein.
5. Inject the right side of the head; drainage is taken from the femoral vein.

A similar process is used to inject from the axillary artery and to drain from either the internal jugular vein or the right femoral vein. If pathological or physical problems exist in the body, the veins and arteries on the left side can be used. Most operators, being right-handed, find working on the right side of the body more convenient. Split injection does require two incisions and, therefore, requires more time for suturing and for the preparation of vessels.

Multipoint Injection

Multipoint injection is vascular injection from two or more arteries. Multipoint injection can be used as the primary injection technique. If the embalmer is preparing a body dead for a long period and anticipates poor solution distribution and possibly tissue distension, he or she can *begin* the embalming using a multipoint injection. The embalmer would raise several arteries for injection; drainage is taken from each injection location or from one drainage point. More often, multipoint injection is used after a onepoint injection has resulted in poor distribution. In this case several secondary arteries must be raised to embalm the various body areas receiving inadequate amounts of solution.

Restricted cervical, sectional, and six-point injection are all forms of multipoint injection. A *six-point injection* is a multipoint injection. It involves the injection of six paired arteries, usually the right and left common carotids; right and left subclavian (axillary or brachial) arteries; and the right and left femoral (common, external iliac) arteries. The six-point injection is used in the preparation of most autopsied bodies. It can also be used in the preparation of the unautopsied body. Preparation of bodies of members of the armed services and bodies being shipped to some foreign countries may require a six-point injection.

The multipoint procedure ensures thorough distribution throughout a body region. This type of injection allows different solution strengths to be used in different body regions. Each area is directly injected, and the volume and strength of solution injected into an area can be varied.

The procedure for the **six-point injection** follows:

1. Raise the right internal jugular vein and insert a drainage instrument directed toward the heart.
2. Raise the right common carotid artery and insert an arterial tube directed toward the trunk of the body. Also insert a tube directed toward the right side of the head.
3. Raise the left common carotid and insert a tube directed toward the left side of the head. Tie off the lower portion of the artery.

4. Raise the right axillary (or brachial) artery and insert an arterial tube directed toward the right hand. Tie off the upper part of the artery.
5. Raise the left axillary (or brachial) artery and insert a tube directed toward the left hand. Tie off the upper part of the artery.
6. Raise the right femoral artery and insert an arterial tube directed toward the right foot. Tie off the upper portion of the artery.
7. Raise the left femoral artery and insert an arterial tube directed toward the left foot. Tie off the upper portion of the artery.
8. Inject in the following order: right leg, left leg, right arm, left arm, trunk of the body (inject down the right common carotid), left side of the head, right side of the head.
9. Drainage can be taken from the right internal jugular vein for all body areas injected, or drainage may be taken from each accompanying vein.
10. The body may be aspirated before injecting the head, if purge has been a problem.

SITUATIONS THAT MAY REQUIRE A MULTIPOINT INJECTION

1. When a body area does not receive arterial solution
2. Bodies dead for long time periods
3. Bodies that show evidence of decomposition
4. Death caused by a ruptured aortic aneurysm
5. Bodies dead of highly contagious diseases involving the blood vascular system (this method of injection maximizes tissue saturation with embalming chemicals)
6. When disposition of the body is delayed for some period
7. In following military regulations
8. When a one-point injection has been used but embalming solution purge develops and drainage stops (distribution cannot be observed)
9. Bodies with generalized edema
10. Bodies that are difficult to firm
11. Bodies that exhibit poor peripheral circulation
12. Bodies that exhibit poor distribution after a one-point injection is completed
13. Bodies with true tissue gas
14. Bodies that must be reinjected because of poor preservation *after* cavity embalming
15. Autopsied bodies

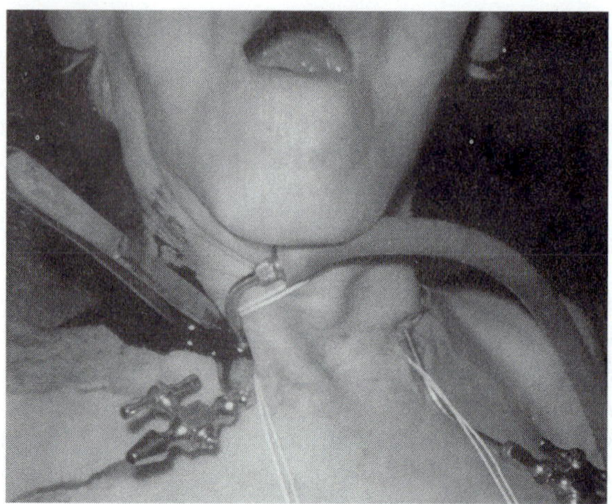

Figure 13–3. Restricted cervical injection.

Restricted Cervical Injection*

In restricted cervical injection, both common carotid arteries are raised so that the head can be separately injected (Figure 13–3). With many of the distribution and drainage problems encountered in embalming today, this method has become a standard practice in many funeral establishments.

1. Raise the right common carotid artery and insert an arterial tube directed toward the trunk of the body. Insert an arterial tube directed toward the right side of the head and leave the stopcock *open.*
2. Insert a drainage instrument into the right internal jugular vein directed toward the heart.
3. Raise the left common carotid artery and insert an arterial tube directed toward the left side of the head; *tie off the lower portion of the left common carotid artery and leave the stopcock open.*
4. Inject the trunk of the body *first;* drainage is taken from the right internal jugular vein. (Solution entering the head by collateral circulation exits through the two open stopcocks. Only the trunk of the body is embalmed.)
5. Inject the left side of the head.
6. Inject the right side of the head.

The restricted cervical injection is recommended in several situations.

Bodies with Facial Trauma. With restricted cervical injection a minimum volume of a very strong solution is injected to preserve and firm tissues with a minimum amount of tissue distension.

* Much of this information was supplied by David G. Williams, Pittsburgh, Pennsylvania.

Bodies in Which Facial Distension Is Anticipated. When there has been a long delay between death and preparation, when bodies have been refrigerated, or when frozen bodies exhibit decomposition changes, restricted cervical injection allows the trunk to be saturated with large amounts of strong solution while the head and facial tissues are injected separately to control distension.

Bodies in Which Eye Enucleation Has Been Performed. Restricted cervical injection allows complete control over the strength and amount of solution entering the facial tissues and thus helps to control distension of the eyelids.

Bodies with Generalized Edema. A large volume of solution can be injected into the trunk areas. Frequently, if facial tissues are not edematous, a milder solution can be used for injection of the head to prevent distension and/or dehydration of the tissues.

Difficult-to-Firm Bodies. With many of the drugs used today protein levels in the body can be low. Restricted cervical injection allows the embalmer to inject large quantities of preservative solutions without overembalming the facial tissues.

Bodies with Distribution Problems. Restricted cervical injection allows the use of high pressures and high rates of flow without distending the facial tissues.

Bodies with a High Formaldehyde Demand. Burned bodies and bodies dead from renal failure require large amounts of preservative. Restricted cervical injection allows the embalmer to inject strong solutions of special-purpose high-index fluids without overembalming the facial tissues.

Bodies in Which Purge is Expected. In a body that purges prior to arterial injection, the purge often continues during the embalming process. Examples include bodies with esophageal varices (as in alcoholism); bodies that suffered pneumonia, tuberculosis of the lungs, and ulcerations of the upper digestive organs; and bodies that show decomposition changes. Restricted cervical injection allows the embalmer to embalm the limbs and trunk areas, then *aspirate the body,* set the features, and embalm the head. This eliminates the necessity to reset the features if purge occurs.

Jaundiced Bodies. The head can be embalmed with a jaundice fluid preparation or other jaundice treatment. Restricted cervical injection allows thorough distribution of the solution to the facial tissues. The remainder of the body can be injected using arterial solutions suitable to the body conditions. First inject the body, then inject the head and face.

It can easily be seen that restricted cervical injection can be a routine embalming technique, similar to the one-point injection. With the difficulties encountered in embalming today (time delays, poor distribution as a result of vascular clotting, edema, and difficulty in firming as a result of drug therapy), more embalmers are using restricted cervical injection as their primary injection method.

The restricted cervical method of injection affords the *greatest control* over entry of arterial solution into the head. Because the tubes that are directed upward are left open while the trunk is injected, any solution that does reach the face and head via the collateral circulation *exits* the carotid arteries through the open arterial tubes.

ADVANTAGES TO THE USE OF RESTRICTED CERVICAL INJECTION

1. Amount of arterial solution entering the facial tissues can be controlled.
2. Large volumes of arterial solution can be injected into the trunk without overinjecting the head and face.
3. Two solution strengths can be used: one for the trunk and limbs and another for the head and face.
4. Arterial coagula, if present in the aorta, are pushed toward the lower extremities.
5. Different pressures can be used to inject the head and the trunk.
6. Different rates of flow can be used to inject the trunk and the head.
7. The trunk can be injected first and the body aspirated to stop purging; the features can be set *after aspirating,* and then the head injected last.
8. The *instant tissue fixation* technique can be employed for trauma and decomposition cases.
9. For jaundiced bodies, only the head is treated with jaundice fluids.

ADVANTAGES TO USE OF THESE VESSELS FOR RESTRICTED CERVICAL INJECTION

1. Arteriosclerosis is rarely seen in the carotid arteries; they are very large vessels and very elastic.
2. The common carotid arteries have no branches (except their terminal branches) and, thus, are easily raised to the surface.
3. Clots present in the right or left carotid artery can be identified and removed.
4. The carotid arteries allow direct injection of the head and facial tissues.
5. The carotid arteries are accompanied by the large internal jugular veins, which directly drain the head and face.

▶ INSTANT TISSUE FIXATION

A variation of the restricted cervical injection in which a very strong arterial solution is used is **instant tissue fixation.** This embalming technique is used for injection of the head (although other body areas can be similarly treated) when swelling of the face is anticipated (as in bodies that show evidence of decomposition) or when trauma has damaged facial tissues. This technique is used when the tissues must be dry and firm for restorative treatments, when pathological conditions such as tumors exist, or when cancerous tissue must be dry and very firm for its excision and facial reconstruction. In this method of injection very little drainage is taken as only a minimal amount of arterial solution is injected. The restricted cervical injection is used with both common carotid arteries and the right internal jugular vein.

Solution Strength. A very strong arterial solution is prepared, and in some cases, 100% arterial fluid is used. One solution suggested contains 16 ounces of a high-index arterial fluid (25-index or above), 16 ounces of a coinjection chemical, 16 ounces of water, and 1 to $1\frac{1}{2}$ ounces of arterial fluid dye. This solution is designed to immediately preserve, dry, and firm the tissues.

Pressure. The solution is mixed in the machine. When a centrifugal injection machine is used, the pressure with the rate of flow valve *off* should be set at 20 pounds or above.

Method of Injection. Connect the injection hose to the arterial tube in the left common carotid artery. Be certain that the arterial tubes used are as large as the arteries allow. Turn the machine *on* with the rate-of-flow valve closed. Set the pressure at 20 pounds. Once the hoses are connected, open the rate-of-flow valve a full turn and immediately turn it *off.* This creates a "pulse" type of fluid flow. The solution is injected in a strong spurt, under high pressure, for only a moment. Repeatedly turn the rate-of-flow valve on and off until sufficient solution has been injected. Only a minimum amount of solution is needed because of its strength. The excess dye indicates the presence of the solution in the tissues. In addition, the dye helps to prevent graying of the tissues. Next, the right side of the head is injected in the same manner. High pressure is used, but the rate-of-flow valve is turned on and off for only a moment each time. The purpose of this method of embalming is to inject a very strong solution throughout all the facial tissues but to use the minimum amount of solution. In this manner, maximum preservation is achieved with a minimum of tissue distension (Figure 13–4).

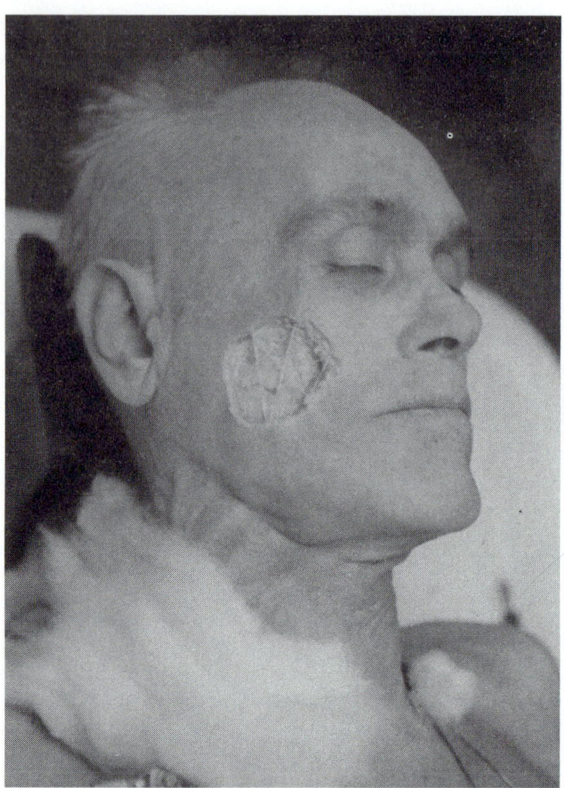

Figure 13–4. Facial tissues embalmed using the instant tissue fixation technique prior to the removal of a cancerous tumor of the right cheek.

▶ VARIATIONS OF INJECTION TECHNIQUES

The autopsied body presents its own injection problems. When the body has undergone a complete autopsy, generally a six-point injection is used; each body extremity is embalmed separately. After partial autopsies, or when organs have been removed for donation, the routine varies with the access to the abdominal or thoracic aorta.

After the partial autopsy and in bodies from which abdominal or thoracic organs have been removed, the aorta may be an injection point. Infants may also be embalmed from the ascending or abdominal aorta, for this vessel is much easier to raise in the unautopsied infant than it is in the adult body. Secondary injection sites may also be needed in autopsy preparations and would most likely involve the more distal arteries such as the radial, ulnar, popliteal, and facial.

▶ DRAINAGE

As stated at the beginning of this chapter, four processes occur at the same time in the embalming of the average body: (1) injection of the solution, (2) distri-

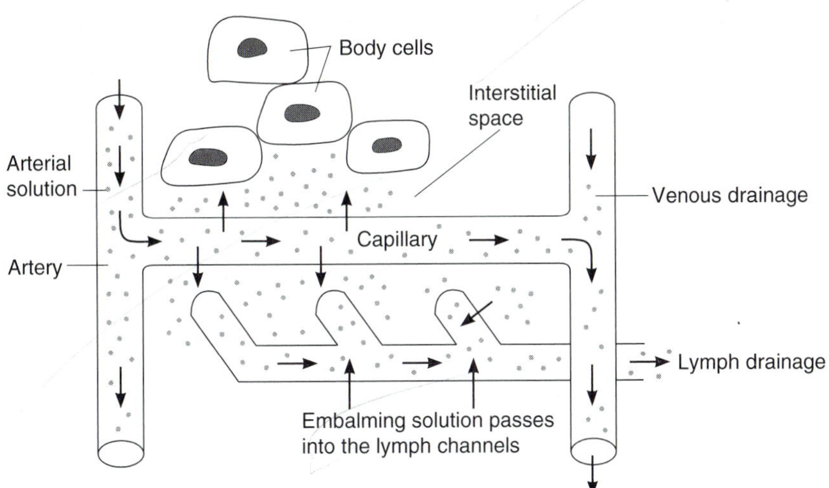

Figure 13–5. Drainage consists of blood, interstitial fluid, embalming solution, and lymphatic fluid.

LYMPHATIC CIRCULATION

The lymphatic vessels originate as blind-end tubes called lymph capillaries (Figure 13–5). These tubes are located in the spaces between the cells. The lymph capillaries are larger and more permeable than the blood capillaries. They converge to form lymph channels called the lymphatics. These lymphatics have valves similar to those of veins and contain lymph nodes along their routes. Their fluid eventually enters the blood vascular system by flowing into the thoracic and the right lymphatic ducts. The thoracic duct empties lymph into the junction of the left subclavian vein and the left internal jugular vein. The lymph from the right lymphatic channel empties into the junction of the right subclavian vein and the right internal jugular vein.

In life, the lymph is composed of the fluids that pass from the blood through the walls of the capillaries. Here it is called tissue or interstitial fluid. More fluid enters the interstitial spaces from the blood than is directly reabsorbed back into the bloodstream by the capillaries. This excess fluid is drained by the lymph system. Once the interstitial fluid enters the lymph capillaries it is called lymph. At the time of death these lymph channels can be the site of large numbers of microbes. The lymph system is part of the defense system for protecting the body from pathological microbes. Embalming solution will diffuse from the interstitial spaces into the lymph channels. Massage and manipulation of the body during injection combined with the use of restricted drainage help to move embalming fluid throughout the lymph system.

Embalming solution can be diffused through the lymphatics in the following order: lymphatic capillary → lymphatic vessel → lymph nodes → lymph vessels → lymphatic trunk → subclavian veins.

bution of the solution, (3) diffusion of the solution, and (4) drainage. Distribution and diffusion of arterial solution are discussed in Chapter 12.

Drainage is brought about by displacement. As the arterial solution fills the vascular system the contents of the vascular system are displaced. There are 5 to 6 quarts of blood in the vascular system of the average body. This accounts for approximately 8% of the body weight. At death, there is generally a wave contraction of the arterial system. This contraction forces the greatest volume of blood into the capillary and venous portions of the blood vascular system after death.

It has been estimated that after death, 85% of the blood is found in the capillaries, 10% in the veins, and 5% in the arteries. Amounts of blood in the vascular system vary depending on the cause and manner of death. In addition, the blood will gravitate into the dependent body regions over time. This engorges the dependent capillaries with blood (livor mortis) and leaves the less dependent tissues free of most blood.

Contents of Drainage

Drainage is composed of blood and blood clots, interstitial fluid, lymphatic fluid, and embalming solution. As arterial solution flows into the capillary, a portion of the solution passes through the walls of the capillary and is retained by the body. This retained preservative is the portion of the embalming solution that preserves, sanitizes, moisturizes, and colors the body tissues. Some of the embalming solution moves through the capillaries, into the venules and veins, and exits as part of the drainage. It has been estimated that 50% or more of the drainage taken during embalming is actually embalming solution.

The color and consistency of the drainage change during injection of the body. During injection of the first gallon of embalming solution, drainage contains more blood than in subsequent injections. As the blood in the vascular system is gradually displaced and replaced with embalming solution, the drainage lightens in color and becomes thinner. The initial drainage is the most dangerous; however, all drainage should be carefully controlled and splashing should be avoided. Collection and sanitation of drainage may be warranted with diseases such as hepatitis and AIDS.

As the embalming solution passes through the capillaries some of the interstitial fluid in the tissue spaces enters the capillaries by osmosis because of the high concentration of the embalming solution, especially when strong arterial solutions are used. Some interstitial fluid may enter the drainage through the lymphatic system. Dehydration can result when too much interstitial fluid is removed. In bodies with edema, the edema is removed in much the same way that interstitial fluid is taken from the tissue spaces.

Drainage can then be said to consist of blood, interstitial fluid, and arterial solution (Figure 13–6). Bacteria and microbial agents and their products that have entered the blood vascular system before or after death are also removed in the drainage. In bodies with skeletal edema, the edematous fluid may be part of the drainage. Coagula should also be included in the contents of drainage. Several types of clotted materials are present in drainage; however, all clotted material comes from the *veins* or from a heart chamber. It is impossible for any arterial coagula to pass through the capillary beds and enter the venous side of the circulatory system. The following coagula can be identified:

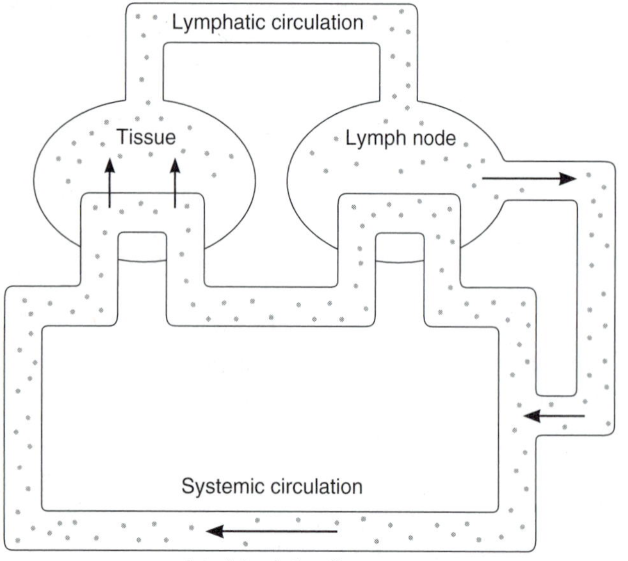

Figure 13–6. Lymphatic and systemic circulation.

- Postmortem coagula: These coagula are not actual clots, but simply blood inclusions that have congealed and stuck together; they can be large and dark.
- Postmortem clots: These clots are multicolored. The bottom portion of the clot is dark, for it was formed by red blood cells that gravitated to the dependent part of a vessel. The clear layer on the top of the clot is a jellylike layer of fibrin.
- Antemortem clots: Clots such as thrombosis form in layers—a layer of platelets, followed by a layer of fibrin, followed by another layer of platelets, and so on.

The viscosity of the blood can vary depending on the cause of death and the time between death and embalming. As the body gradually dehydrates after death, the viscosity of the blood increases. Bodies that have been refrigerated for very short periods after death, have been administered drugs such as heparin or dicumarol, or have died from carbon monoxide poisoning exhibit low blood viscosity.

The volume of drainage is not equal to the volume of embalming solution injected. A large portion of the blood vascular system, particularly the arteries, is empty at death. This entire area must be filled, which accounts for the delay often noted between injection and the start of the drainage. At the conclusion of the embalming, the arterial system is filled; some of the injected solution is found in the capillaries and the veins, and some has passed through the capillaries to be retained by the tissues and cells.

In some bodies, there will be little or no drainage.

As long as the solution is distributing and there is no swelling or discolorations in the tissues, drainage need not be a concern.

Sometimes, there is little to drain, as illustrated in these examples.

1. In cases of esophageal varices and ruptured ulcerations of the digestive tract (blood has been lost to the lumen of the esophagus, stomach, or intestines), drainage actually occurs within the intestinal tract.
2. Accidental death could cause the spleen or other internal organ to rupture; blood is lost from these sites and drainage also occurs at these ruptures.
3. Traumatic death may result in a large loss of blood outside the body. This hemorrhage decreases the volume of blood available for drainage.
4. Insertion of the drainage tube into the femoral

or external iliac vein may tear the vein, allowing drainage to flow into the abdominal cavity.

5. When a preinjection embalming solution is used, a portion of the blood is removed. At the time of arterial solution injection, there is less blood to drain.
6. Pathological or tubercular lesions may account for a blood loss in life and an internal site of drainage at the time of solution injection.
7. Bloodstream infections frequently cause extensive clotting, and anemic diseases reduce blood volume; these factors contribute to poor distribution and low drainage volume.

Often in bodies in which hemorrhage into the digestive tract or abdominal cavity occurred prior to death, there may be a gradual swelling of the abdomen as the solution is injected and some of the drainage (and arterial solution) fills the digestive tract or abdominal cavity. This drainage can be removed with a trocar. Likewise, hemorrhage into the stomach, esophagus, or lung tissues can result in a purge during injection. The purge will take the form of drainage. It is possible to drain from the mouth if a stomach ulcer has ruptured large veins. Aspiration can later remove these fluids. Some medications cause gastrointestinal bleeding. If this bleeding was intense, a major portion of the drainage may flow into the intestinal tract during arterial injection.

The bodies just described may demonstrate two forms of drainage: internal, into a cavity or hollow organ, and external, through the drainage tube or exit as purge.

Good drainage may be expected under the following conditions:

1. The interval between death and preparation is short; the body retains some heat.
2. The body shows early evidence of livor mortis, indicating that the blood has a low viscosity and can easily be moved.
3. Death was not the result of a febrile disease or a bloodstream infection.
4. Skeletal edema is present.
5. The body is jaundiced.
6. The person had been treated with blood thinners (e.g., heparin and dicumarol), resulting in low blood viscosity.
7. The body was refrigerated shortly after death but not for a long period.
8. Death was due to carbon monoxide poisoning.

Purpose of Drainage

Bodies to be used for dissection are often embalmed but not drained. Bodies dead for long periods can be slowly embalmed without draining, and are suitable for viewing. Years ago, small volumes (1 to $1\frac{1}{2}$ gallons) of arterial solutions were injected, drainage was limited, and the blood that remained in the vessels was expected to act as a vehicle to gradually spread the fluid through the body. Machine injection not only improved arterial solution distribution and diffusion but increased the volume of blood drainage. Fluid is drained for many reasons:

1. To make room for the arterial solution. Distension would result without removal of some of the blood (especially today, when 3 to 5 gallons of preservative solution is injected into the average body).
2. To reduce a secondary dilution of the arterial fluid. The blood in the capillaries can dilute the embalming solution. This dilution would be very small if a major portion of the blood is drained as the result of injecting large volumes of arterial solution.
3. To remove intravascular blood discolorations. Livor mortis is a postmortem intravascular blood discoloration. Discolorations such as carbon monoxide and capillary congestion are antemortem blood discolorations. Injection of arterial solution accompanied by blood drainage should greatly reduce or remove these discolorations.
4. To remove a tissue that rapidly decomposes. Blood is a liquid tissue that rapidly decomposes after death, and decomposition of the blood can result in discolorations, odors, and formation of gas.
5. To remove an element that speeds decomposition. Blood, a portion of which is liquid, can hasten hydrolysis and the decomposition of the body tissues. Moisture is needed for decomposition and blood can provide that medium.
6. To remove bacteria present in the blood. With some diseases, microbes normally found in the intestine can translocate to the bloodstream. After death, this translocation greatly increases. Removal of blood as drainage helps to reduce microbial agents in the body.
7. To prevent discolorations. When the blood in the body (hemoglobin) mixes with the formaldehyde of the arterial solution methyl-hemoglobin can form, which produces a gray color in the tissues (formaldehyde gray).
8. To reduce swollen tissues. When pitting edema is present in the skeletal tissues, it is possible to remove some of the edematous fluid via the blood drainage from the body.

In some bodies drainage is most important in clearing very pronounced discolorations, especially when the face, neck, and hands are affected. In some very thin bodies, with little or no livor mortis, drainage is not as copious, nor as necessary. The importance of drainage varies from body to body. If a primary purpose for drainage must be stated, it would be that the drainage makes room for the arterial solution so it can be evenly distributed to all tissues of the body with a minimum of distension.

Center of Drainage

The center of drainage in the dead human body is the right atrium of the heart (Figure 13–7). The superior vena cava returns blood to this chamber from the head and the upper extremities. The inferior vena cava returns blood from the visceral organs, trunk, and legs. If the internal jugular vein is used as a drainage point, all blood from the lower extremities and visceral organs must pass through the right atrium to be drained. Likewise, if drainage is to be taken from the right femoral vein, blood from the arms and head must pass through the right atrium. After death, blood in the right atrium frequently congeals. This condition warrants drainage from the right internal jugular vein where an instrument, such as angular spring forceps, can be placed directly into the right atrium to fragment this coagulum.

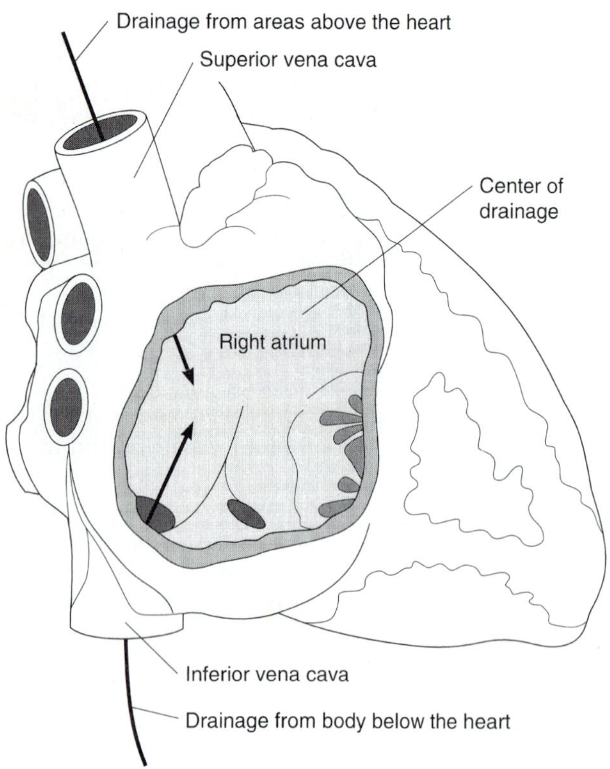

Figure 13–7. The center of drainage in the dead human body is the right atrium of the heart. The superior vena cava returns blood to this chamber from the head and the upper extremities. The inferior vena cava returns blood from the visceral organs, trunk, and legs.

Some embalmers also use two locations for drainage. An example of the two-point (above and below the heart) drainage technique would be when the primary drainage site is the femoral vein. When the face and upper extremities begin to flush and discolor, the internal jugular vein is opened as the "above heart" drainage site.

Drainage instruments are inserted into the vein and directed toward the heart.

Drainage Sites

The primary drainage site is the location from which drainage is first taken. In the unautopsied body, the veins most commonly used for drainage are the right internal jugular vein, the right femoral vein, and the right external iliac vein.

Axillary and basilic veins can be used, but their small size and the need to extend the arm make these veins an impractical choice. *Any vein can be used for drainage whether it is large or small or on the right or left side of the body.* In unusual circumstances, even the external jugular vein can be used if the internal jugular vein is obstructed by a cancerous growth or a large attached thrombosis.

A broken vein can still be used as a drainage site; if an instrument such as angular forceps cannot be inserted, a groove director may be used. Following injection the area can be dried and the ends of the broken vein ligated.

Should a vein tear while it is being raised, the following steps can be taken to attempt to place an instrument in the portion of the vein leading to the heart:

1. Force as much blood from the vein as possible.
2. Clean the area using a very large piece of absorbent cotton.
3. Observe where blood is seeping from the broken portion of the vein.
4. Clamp an edge of the wall of the broken vein with a small serrated or rat-toothed hemostat, or place the hemostat across the entire broken portion of the vein.

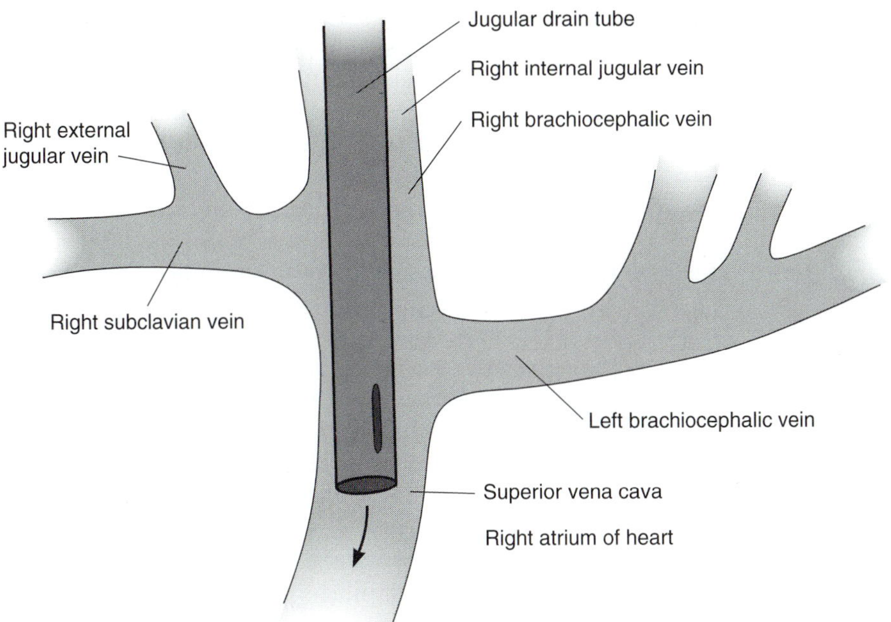

Figure 13–8. Drainage tube placed in the right internal jugular vein.

5. Gently insert a drainage device toward the heart; if the vein has been torn into two pieces do not remove the hemostat.
6. After embalming, pass a ligature around the distal portions of the vein (holding the torn vein with the hemostat).

In Chapter 9, the advantages and disadvantages of the various veins for drainage are discussed, as are the incision locations and the relationships of veins to arteries. The internal jugular vein is the most valuable drainage point. It is the largest systemic vein that can be raised in the unautopsied body. The right internal jugular vein leads directly into the right atrium of the heart. Figure 13–8 illustrates why the *right* and not the left internal jugular vein is most frequently used for drainage. Should there be a complication with the right internal jugular vein, the left can be used, but note that the vein turns to the right, often making insertion of a drainage instrument difficult.

A second drainage point is often used when the femoral vein is used as the primary injection and drainage point. If there is a blockage in the right atrium or the right internal jugular vein, the neck and face can begin to flush. The neck veins distend and the neck tissues may begin to distend. The right internal jugular vein should be raised and opened as a second drainage site. If it is impossible to use the jugular veins as drainage sites attempt to use the axillary or direct heart drainage.

Direct Heart Drainage*

The right atrium of the heart can be directly drained using a trocar (Figure 13–9). This very old method of drainage was often used when embalming was performed at the residence of the deceased. The drainage could be conveniently collected in bottles, which could be taken back to the funeral parlor to be emptied.

To drain directly from the right atrium of the heart, start by injecting approximately $\frac{1}{2}$ to 1 gallon of embalming solution to fill the vascular system. To drain the heart, insert the trocar at approximately the standard point of entry, 2 inches to the left and 2 inches above the umbilicus. Draw an imaginary line across the body connecting the *left* anterior superior iliac spine and the lobe of the *right* ear. Direct the trocar toward a point where this line crosses the right side of the sternum. This point is approximately at the level of the sternum where the fourth rib joins the sternum. Be certain to keep the trocar slightly to the right of the sternum. The trocar point should be kept in the anterior portion of the mediastinum. If there is sufficient pressure in the right atrium, simply placing the trocar in the heart chamber should be sufficient to start drainage. The trocar can be attached to the hydroaspirator.

Do not turn the hydroaspirator on to full suction; half is quite sufficient. Insert the trocar with the hydroaspirator running. As soon as the heart is pierced

* This method is not intended for use as a primary drainage technique but only in special situations where a vein cannot be used for drainage.

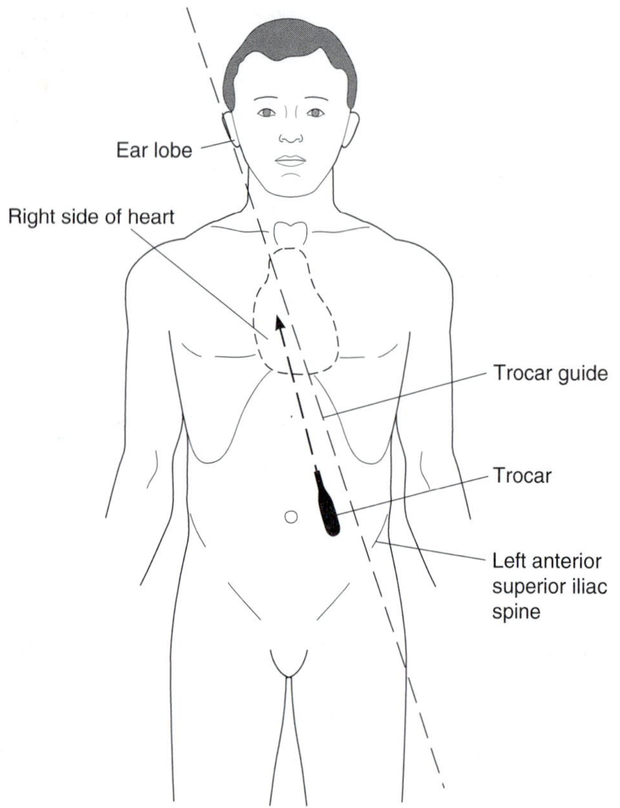

Figure 13–9. Direct heart drainage.

the hydroaspirator can be turned off. Most hydroaspirators are lower than the height of the embalming table, so a natural gravity system is established. It is important that a plastic hose be used on the trocar, for the embalmer can then see immediately when the right side of the heart has been punctured.

If the embalmer is unfamiliar with this technique of drainage it can easily be practiced. Begin cavity aspiration by aspirating the right side of the heart first. The embalmer need not pierce only the right atrium with the trocar; the right ventricle can also be pierced. There should be sufficient pressure in the right side of the heart that the suction of the aspirator on the trocar can open the right atrioventricular valve and, in this manner, drain the right atrium. Should the trocar puncture the ascending aorta or the arch, sufficient embalming solution may be lost to necessitate a six-point injection. This method of drainage is efficient to use on the body of an infant, child, or adult.

Drainage Instrumentation

A large variety of drainage devices are available. The most standard drainage instruments are the drainage or drain tube and the angular spring forceps. Drainage tubes are made especially for use in the internal jugular vein (Figure 13–10). These tubes are very large in diameter and short in length. Axillary drain tubes are long and slightly curved for insertion into the axillary vein.

Axillary drain tubes are not very large in diameter. A variety of drainage tubes are made for the femoral vein; they come in a wide range of diameters and lengths. One type of iliac drain tube is designed to be inserted into the external iliac vein, and the tip of the tube reaches into the right atrium of the heart; they are approximately 2 to $2\frac{1}{2}$ feet long and can be made of

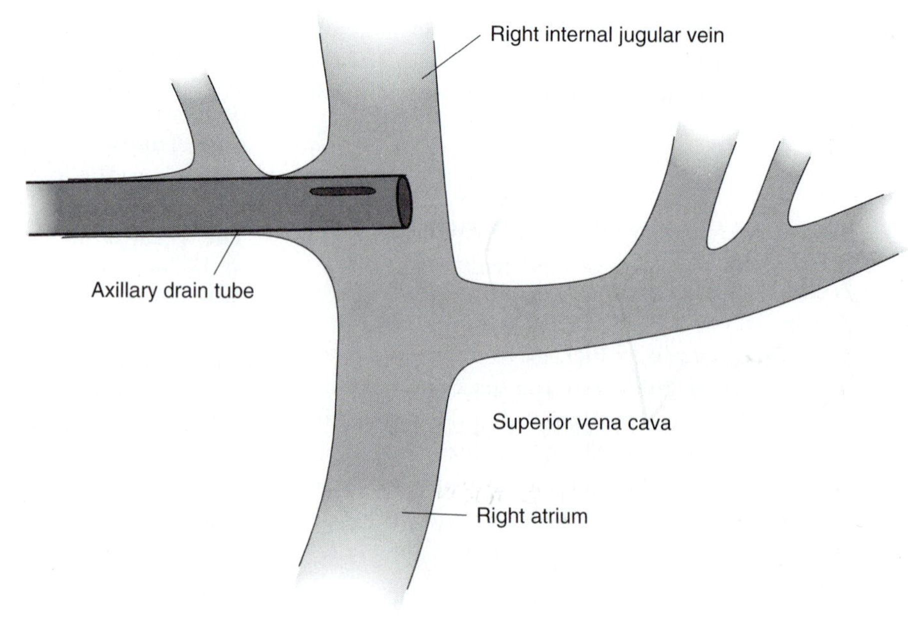

Figure 13–10. Drainage tube insert.

plastic, metal, or rubber. **Drain tubes are inserted into veins and directed toward the heart.** Some embalmers prefer to lubricate these devices with massage cream to facilitate their entry into the vein. Drain tubes contain a plunger rod, which also can be lubricated with massage cream. After each use drain tubes should be disassembled and flushed with cool, soapy water.

Many times, a drainage tube cannot be fully inserted into the vein; it should not be forced. As long as a portion of the tube can be inserted, it will keep the vein expanded. Changing the position of the tube in the vein often assists with the drainage. Tubes should be tied into a vein, but loosely enough so that their position can be changed.

Advantages of the Drain Tube	Disadvantages of the Drain Tube
The tube keeps the vein expanded.	The size of the opening is limited to the diameter of the tube.
The "stirring" rod helps to fragment coagula.	The tube can block the opposite portion of the vein. The tube can block other veins.
Drainage can be shut off to build intravascular pressure.	Coagula cannot be grasped.
Closed drainage technique can be used.	The tube may mark the face or interfere with positioning of the head.
	The tube can easily be pushed through the vein into a body cavity.

Angular spring forceps can be used to assist drainage from any vein; however, this drainage device is generally used with the right internal jugular vein. The 8-inch angular spring forceps fits conveniently into the superior vena cava and the upper portions of the right atrium.

Advantages of the Angular Spring Forceps for Jugular Drainage	Disadvantages of the Angular Spring Forceps
It provides a very large opening for the drainage.	It may have to be removed to close the vein for intermittent drainage.
The head can be positioned to the right.	Drainage may splatter onto the table.
The forceps does not mark the face.	Embalmer's contact with the drainage is increased.
Coagula can be grasped.	
It does not block other venous tributaries.	

The angular spring forceps is convenient to use for drainage from the right internal jugular vein. It *does not block* drainage from the left innominate vein, right subclavian vein, or upper portion of the right internal jugular vein. These tributaries can be blocked if the jugular drain tube is used. It provides a wide opening for the passage of coagula and it allows the right side of the head to drain. Large masses of coagula can be broken and easily removed from the superior vena cava and the right atrium. The head can easily be positioned without the forceps marking the side of the face.

The **groove director** is used to assist in the insertion of a drainage tube or forceps into the vein. The groove director is inserted into the vein first. Once it is in place, the drainage instrument is slid along the grooved portion of the instrument. The grooved portion should face the lumen of the vein.

Methods of Drainage

Most embalmers use a compromise of embalming techniques. For example, it is recommended that 1 gallon of arterial solution be injected over 10 to 15 minutes. Embalmers can, however, inject this amount of solution in a shorter period if necessary. A 2% arterial solution is recommended as the standard solution. Many embalmers would be hesitant to begin injections with a solution of this strength so they begin with a milder solution and increase to the 2% level once circulation is established.

The same is true of the relationship between injection and drainage. Many embalmers use a combination of drainage methods. They begin the injection using continuous drainage and then restrict the drainage (using intermittent drainage) after the blood discolorations clear.

METHODS OF DRAINAGE IN RELATION TO INJECTION

Alternate
Concurrent
Intermittent

Alternate Drainage. In alternate drainage, the arterial solution is never injected while drainage is being taken. A quart or two of arterial solution is injected; then the arterial injection is stopped and venous drainage commences. This is allowed to continue until drainage subsides; then the drainage instrument is closed. The process is then repeated. Injection and drainage are alternated until the embalming is completed. Because 1 or 2 quarts of fluid is constantly injected into a confined system, it is believed that a more uniform pressure is developed in all parts of the body. More complete distribution of arterial solution is achieved and more complete drainage results. Fluid diffusion is enhanced, for pressure filtration is increased. This method increases preparation time and care must be taken to avoid distension.

Concurrent (Continuous) Drainage. In concurrent drainage, injection and drainage are allowed to proceed at the same time throughout the embalming. This method is less time consuming than the alternate method, and there is less chance of distension.

Distension is possible with any method of drainage or injection. As soon as distension is evident, stop injection.

Because of the open drainage, it may be difficult to attain a pressure sufficient to saturate tissues throughout the body. Clots (in the venous system) may not be dislodged when the concurrent method is used. Fluid will follow the path of least resistance and "short-circuit," and more embalming solution may be lost to the drainage. This method of drainage may dehydrate and wrinkle body tissues. It has value in the preparation of bodies with skeletal edema, for which dehydration is encouraged.

Intermittent Drainage. Another method of drainage involves continuous injection and intermittent drainage (Figure 13–11). When drainage is difficult the vein is closed to build up pressure and encourage drainage. The intermittent method is considered a compromise between the alternate and the concurrent methods. In this process the injection continues throughout the embalming and the drainage is shut off for selected periods. Some embalmers stop drainage until a particular amount of solution is injected (1 or 2 quarts); others stop drainage until surface veins are raised. It is important that surface intravascular blood discolorations clear before intermittent drainage is begun. This method is less time consuming than the alternate method, encourages fluid distribution and pressure filtration, helps to prevent short-circuiting of the embalming solution and its loss to the drainage, and promotes retention of the embalming solution by the tissues. Intermittent drainage helps the body to retain tissue fluid (which provides a proper moisture balance) and is recommended when colloidal fluids such as humectants or restorative fluids are used to slightly distend emaciated tissues.

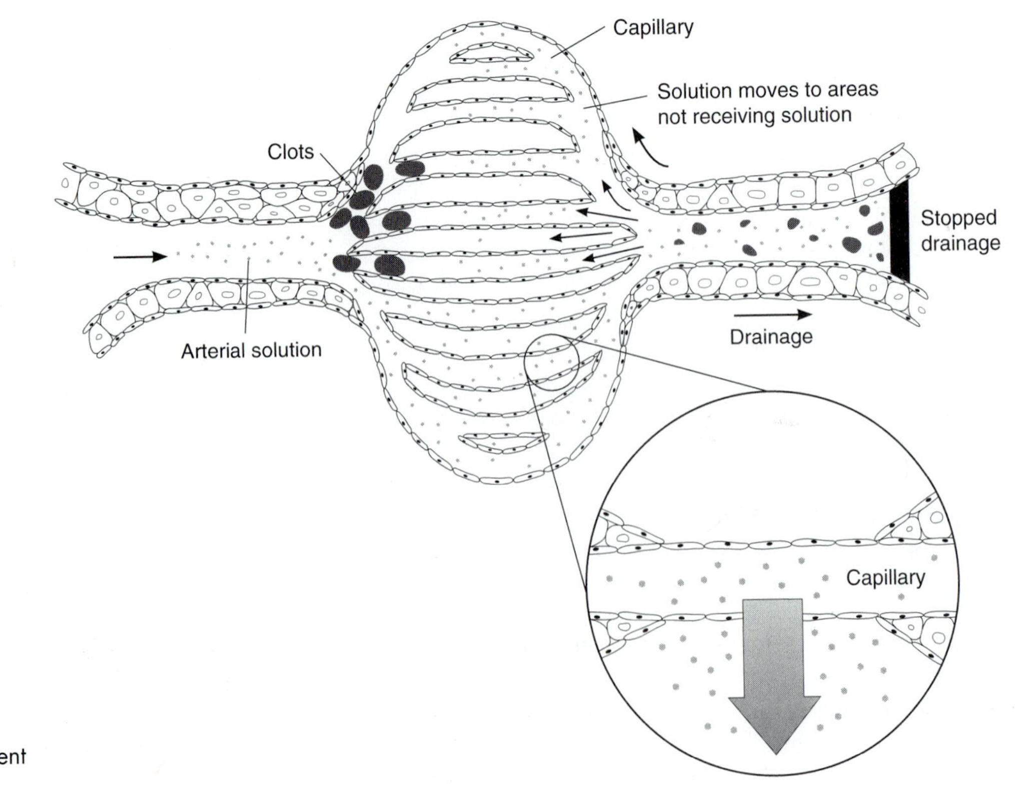

Figure 13–11. Intermittent drainage.

Techniques for Improving Drainage

The necessity for drainage has already been discussed. In summary, drainage (1) allows for a thorough distribution of the embalming solution, (2) prevents distension of the body tissues, and (3) prevents adverse discolorations. Creation of good drainage can be done in two periods, prior to injection of the preservative solution and during injection of the preservative solution.

Preembalming techniques include the following:

- Selection of a large vein: Preference is generally the internal jugular or the femoral, or external iliac vein.
- Selection of a large drainage instrument: An angular spring forceps or drainage tube is used.
- Injection of a preinjection fluid: Follow the manufacturer's dilution of the chemical and volume of the chemical injected. If a preinjection chemical is not used, a mild arterial solution can be injected to clear blood discolorations and establish circulation.
- Removal of extravascular pressure such as gas and fluids in the abdomen.

During injection, techniques include the following:

- Use of drainage devices to fragment clots
- Use of massage and pressure applied over the heart and/or liver to move venous clots
- Increase in the rate of solution injection or increase in the pressure of the solution being injected
- Intermittent and alternate forms of drainage techniques
- Selection of another drainage site if necessary

Closed Drainage Technique. Exposure to the contents of the drainage, which can contain viable pathogens, can be reduced by using a closed drainage technique. A clear plastic hose is connected to the drain tube and the free end is placed directly into the sanitary receptacle. Drainage may also be collected in a holding tank and sanitized before being emptied into a sanitary system. For direct heart drainage a clear plastic tube can be attached to the trocar and from the aspirator directly into the drain.

Disinfection of the Drainage

The initial drainage presents the greatest risk to the embalmer when the cause of death was bloodborne infection (AIDS, hepatitis, or bloodstream sepsis). At present, the Occupational Safety and Health Administration permits bulk blood, suction, and aspirated fluids to be carefully drained into a sanitary sewer system. To minimize contact as blood is being drained, tubing may be attached to the drain tube. If a drainage forceps is used running water should direct blood drainage immediately into the sewer system.

As drainage and injection proceed, formaldehyde from the fluid becomes part of the drainage and disinfects the blood and its microbial contents. Some embalmers recommend injecting as much arterial solution as possible prior to draining into bodies dead from contagious disease and, several minutes later, beginning the drainage. This interval allows the blood and the embalming solution to mix.

▶ KEY TERMS AND CONCEPTS FOR STUDY AND DISCUSSION

1. Define the following terms:
   alternate drainage
   closed drainage
   concurrent drainage
   instant tissue fixation
   intermittent drainage
   multipoint injection
   one-point injection
   path of least resistance
   restricted cervical injection
   six-point injection
   split injection
2. List the advantages of using restricted cervical injection.
3. List the contents of drainage.
4. List the purposes for drainage.
5. List several techniques for stimulating drainage.
6. Complete the following distribution problems:

Embalming Solution Tracing Problems

One-Point Injection and Drainage

Skeletal tissues — Trace arterial solution from the femoral artery (tube directed downward) to the right great toe; drain from the right femoral vein

Skeletal tissues — Trace arterial solution from the right femoral artery to the left side of the upper lip; drain from the right femoral vein

Visceral tissues — Trace arterial solution from the right femoral artery to the fundus of the stomach; drain from the right femoral vein

Split Injection and Drainage

Skeletal tissues — Trace arterial solution from the right femoral artery to the right great toe; drain from the right internal jugular

Skeletal tissues	Trace arterial solution from the right common carotid to the left upper lip; drain from the right femoral vein
Visceral tissues	Trace arterial solution from the right common carotid to the appendix; drain from the right femoral vein

Restricted Cervical Injection

Skeletal tissues	Inject the right common carotid down to reach the left lower lip; drain from the right internal jugular
Skeletal tissues	Inject the right common carotid down to reach the right upper lip (with the stopcock directed upward closed); drain from the right internal jugular
Visceral tissues	Inject down the right common carotid to the tissues of the left lung; drain from the right internal jugular

▶ BIBLIOGRAPHY

Investigating factors relating to fluid retention during embalming, Parts I and II. In: *Champion Expanding Encyclopedia.* Springfield, OH: Champion Chemical; August–September 1979: Nos. 499 and 500, 2013–2020.

Johnson EC. A study of arterial pressure during embalming. In: *The Champion Expanding Encyclopedia.* Springfield, OH: Champion Chemical; 1981:2081–2084.

Kroshus J, McConnell J, Bardole J. The measurement of formaldehyde retention in the tissues of embalmed bodies. *Director* 1983; March/April:10–12.

Mechanics of proper drainage. In: *Champion Expanding Encyclopedia.* Springfield, OH: Champion Chemical; November–December 1973: No. 442, 1785–1788.

Removal of blood via the heart. In: *Champion Expanding Encyclopedia.* Springfield, OH: Champion Chemical; May 1976: 1885–1888.

Shor M. An examination into methods old and new of achieving greatest possible venous drainage. *Casket and Sunnyside* 1964; July:20.

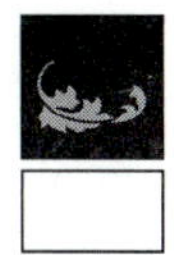

CHAPTER 14
CAVITY EMBALMING

Cavity embalming, or cavity treatment, is the second major procedure in the preservation and sanitation of the dead human body.

The oldest methods of embalming, dating back to the Egyptians, included treatment of the viscera. Until the "modern era" of embalming, most embalming techniques involved not only removal of the viscera (evisceration) from the thoracic and abdominal cavities, but removal of the brain from the cranial cavity. Embalmers using these early embalming processes recognized the difficulty in preserving the body if some method of visceral treatment was not practiced. With the invention of the "trocar" toward the end of the 19th century, embalmers began to move away from a direct incision approach to preserve and sanitize the contents of the body cavities.

There is a need to continue the preservation and sanitation process after arterial embalming. Purulent materials, blood, and edematous fluids within the body cavities, along with possibly unembalmed tissues, continue to decompose and remain an excellent medium for bacterial growth. Untreated microbes can become a source of gases and possibly contagion.

Even preserved tissues are subject to reversal and breakdown as long as there are untreated or partially embalmed body areas. The aspiration procedure and subsequent perfusion with cavity fluid are designed to reach the substances and microbes found in the spaces within the thoracic, abdominopelvic, and sometimes cranial cavities. In addition to these substances, those materials found within the hollow viscera and portions of the visceral organs themselves that are not reached by arterial injection are treated in the process of cavity embalming.

Cavity treatment is normally a two-step process: aspiration of the cavities and their contents and injection of a strong preservative/disinfectant chemical. This process takes place after the arterial embalming. Often, depending on the condition of the body, the process involves subsequent steps of reaspiration and reinjection of the cavities.

There may be occasions when cavity treatment is *not* employed in preparation of the body, for example, when the body is bequeathed to a medical school (where the school permits vascular preparation of the body for viewing by the family and public), and when a hospital allows the body to be arterially embalmed prior to a postmortem examination (autopsy).

There are also situations in which arterial embalming is not possible. Cavity embalming along with surface and hypodermic embalming woud be the principal means of preserving and sanitizing the remains. These cases include badly decomposed and badly burned bodies.

This is *not* a visible process. The work should proceed in an orderly fashion so that all areas of the cavities are treated. Large numbers of microbes may be found within these spaces, which are perfect media for postmortem microbial growth. Thorough cavity treatment prevents gas formation and subsequent purging of the body.

▶ CHRONOLOGY OF CAVITY TREATMENT

1. Arterial embalming
   - A. Limited treatment of the abdominal cavity prior to or during arterial injection if the abdominal wall is very tense.
     - a. Drainage of edema from the abdominal cavity if ascites exists
     - b. Removal of gases if the abdomen is tightly distended with gas
   - B. Limited treatment of the thoracic cavity
     - a. Limited aspiration of the thorax if subcutaneous emphysema is present
2. Aspiration of the cavities
   - A. Time of treatment
     - a. Immediately after arterial injection
     - b. Several hours after arterial injection
3. Order of aspiration
   - A. Thoracic cavity and its contents

B. Abdominal cavity and its contents
C. Pelvic cavity and its contents
4. Injection of the body cavities
5. Closure of the trocar point of entry
6. Washing and drying of the body
7. Possible reaspiration
8. Possible reinjection

Direct treatment in cavity embalming other than arterial injection of the contents of the body cavities and the lumina of the hollow viscera is usually accomplished by aspiration and injection.

Cavity treatment after vascular injection accomplishes as complete a preservation and sanitation of the dead human body for funeralization as possible. Vascular injection alone does not reach all spaces of the body and may not treat all tissues of the body whether visceral organs or skeletal tissue.

Not all microorganisms die with the host. Many survive some time after somatic and cellular death. During the agonal period and then the postmortem period following somatic death, microbes from the hollow intestinal organs enter the bloodstream and lymph channels where they translocate to the skeletal tissues and interstitial fluids. In tissues not reached by arterial treatments, the decomposition cycle can occur and produce undesired effects. Cavity treatment attempts to treat visceral tissues that may not have been reached by arterial solution. It creates an unfavorable environment in the internal organs and destroys the media on which these microbes can grow and multiply.

Cavity embalming treats the **contents** of the hollow viscera (Table 14–1), the **walls** of the visceral organs not embalmed by arterial injection, and the **contents** of the spaces between the visceral organs and the walls of the cavities.

The contents of the hollow portions of the viscera are not perfused during arterial injection. Materials within these spaces continue to decompose if untreated, and the resulting products of decomposition may cause **odors, gas formation, and purge.** The gases may move into the skeletal tissues and cause distension of viewable areas such as the face and hands.

It is impossible to determine which visceral organs did or did not receive arterial solution. The embalmer cannot look at these organs for signs of arterial distribution, so cavity embalming serves to *ensure* that the walls and parenchyma of the hollow viscera and the stroma and parenchyma of the solid organs are embalmed.

The solid organs treated by cavity embalming are the pancreas, spleen, kidney, brain, liver and lungs.

TABLE 14–1. CONTENTS OF THE HOLLOW VISCERA THAT MUST BE TREATED

Organ	Contents to be Aspirated or Treated
Lungs, trachea, bronchi	Blood, edema, purulent material, gases
Stomach	Hydrochloric acid, undigested food, blood, gases
Small intestine	Gases, undigested foods, partially digested foods, blood
Large intestine	Gases, fecal material, blood
Urinary bladder	Urine, pustular material, blood
Gallbladder	Bile
Pelvis of the kidney	Urine, pustular material, blood
Heart	Blood
Inferior vena cava, portal veins	Blood

Undigested or partially digested foodstuffs within the stomach and small intestines, as well as the gases and liquids resulting from the breakdown of these materials, are removed by the aspiration process. Those not removed are treated by the injection of cavity fluid (Table 14–2). If these materials are not removed or treated, gases could form, placing sufficient pressure on the stomach and diaphragm to create purge from the oral or nasal cavities.

Purge from the *mouth* originates from either the contents of the *lungs*, the contents of the *stomach*, or the throat area (esophageal veins that hemorrhage) (Table 14–3). Purge from the *nose* can also originate from the lungs, stomach, or throat. If fecal material is not removed or treated by cavity chemicals, it can cause sufficient gases to form within the abdomen to cause a lung purge (by pressure on the diaphragm) or stomach purge. In addition, purge from the *anal orifice* is quite possible. Rectal hemorrhage can be a source of bloody purge from the anal orifice.

Cranial purge is very rare. Gases within the cranial cavity can spread into the facial tissues through the var-

TABLE 14–2. CAVITY CONTENTS THAT MUST BE TREATED

Cavity	Material to be Treated
Thoracic	Blood, edema, purulent material, gases
Pericardial	Blood, edema
Abdominal	Blood, edema, purulent material, gases
Pelvic	Blood, edema, purulent material, gases
Cranial	Blood, edema, gases

Note. The liquids in these cavities not only *decompose;* they serve as *media for bacteria* and as a *diluent* for cavity chemicals.

TABLE 14–3. DESCRIPTION OF PURGE

Source	Orifice	Description
Stomach	Nose/mouth	Liquids, semisolids, dark brown "coffee ground" appearance; odor; acid pH
Lungs	Nose/mouth	Frothy; any blood present is red in color, little odor
Brain	Nose/ear/ eyelids	Gases can move into tissues of the eye, fractures can cause blood to purge from the ears, creamy white semisolid brain matter may exit through a fracture or the nasal passage

ious foramina that lead from the cranial cavity to the soft facial tissues. Generally, a liquid or semisolid purge from the cranial cavity is the result of a fracture of the temporal bone. The point of exit of the purge is the ear. If gas is of sufficient pressure to exit the cranial cavity, the eyes and eyelids will be distended.

In some diseases, infections of the brain or meninges may lead to formation of gases or edema in the cranial cavity. Hemorrhages from a stroke can also cause blood and edema to accumulate in the cranial cavity. **It is rare for disease to cause cranial purge.** In bodies in which decomposition is advanced, sufficient pressure may be present to cause a purge from the cranial cavity.

Foramina in the area of the *eye* that serve as pathways for gas that affects the eye and surrounding tissues include the optic foramen, superior orbital fissure, inferior orbital fissure, infraorbital foramen, supraorbital foramen, anterior ethmoidal foramen, and posterior ethmoidal foramen.

In certain preparations such as after recent cranial surgery (gunshot or trauma to the head) or advanced decomposition, aspiration and injection of a few ounces of cavity fluid into the cranial cavity may prevent the buildup of gas in the cranial cavity. The point at which the aspirating device is introduced into the cranium is discussed later in this chapter.

It should be mentioned here that it is not necessary to aspirate the brain of an adult who suffered from hydrocephalus. The bones at this time in life are ossified and the condition should present little problem in embalming.

Some embalmers routinely aspirate and inject the cranial cavity on every body. There is a very heavy arterial supply to the brain through both the internal carotid arteries and the vertebral arteries. In the majority of embalmings these routes should supply sufficient arterial solution to the brain and even to the cerebrospinal fluid.

In preparation of the unautopsied stillborn child or infant, the embalmer should consider the need for cranial treatment. The stillborn or infant brain can decompose very rapidly. Carefully evaluate for the presence of gases in the tissues around the eyes and give consideration to the time between death and preparation. It may be most advantageous in these preparations to at least inject some cavity fluid into the cranial cavity with a large hypodermic needle.

▶ INSTRUMENTATION AND EQUIPMENT REQUIRED

A scalpel, pointed trocar, several feet of rubber or plastic hose, a device to create a suction or vacuum, and a receptacle (usually a sewer service, jar, or pail) are the items needed to accomplish the process of aspiration. After aspiration, a gravity cavity injector or other injection device is connected with tubing to the trocar to apply the disinfectant/preservative chemicals. To close the opening in the body wall, a needle and ligature or trocar button and inserter are used. A disinfection tray or basin is needed for cleaning and disinfecting the scalpel, needle, trocar, and tubing (see Chapter 4).

Instruments Used to Create a Vacuum

Hydroaspirator. The hydroaspirator is installed on a cold water line, preferably over a flush sink; when the water is turned on, a vacuum is created. Proper operation of the equipment depends on the water pressure of the water line. A vacuum breaker is normally a part of the hydroaspirator and protects against a backflow into the water line. Local ordinance directives for proper installation of the aspirator may require other vacuum breakers at different heights above the water level of the receptacle into which the aspirant flows.

The student unfamiliar with the hydroaspirator should experiment with this device. A few ounces of material such as blood passing through the water of the hydroaspirator can give the appearance of a very large quantity of material. Although it is helpful to observe the material passing through the hydroaspirator, it is more important to observe the material being withdrawn from the body at a position near the trocar. A piece of plastic or glass tubing can be inserted into a portion of the tubing used for aspiration. Clear tubing can be used so the aspirated material can be observed. Some trocars have a glass portion in the handle that allows the material flowing through the trocar to be observed.

Hydroaspirators can become clogged with small pieces of solid or semisolid material, for example, fatty tissue from the abdominal wall. There is a distinct sound change when this happens. Water then *reverses* and flows into the tubing, trocar, and body cavity. The hydroaspirator should be shut off immediately and the hose removed from the trocar. An attempt should be made to "flush" the material from the hydroaspirator. If this is unsuccessful, the hydroaspirator may be disassembled and the material removed from the inside of the device.

Electric Aspirator. An electric aspirator contains an electric motor with an encased impeller on the shaft. The impeller creates the suction. A small-diameter water line may be attached to the encasement for lubrication of the impeller. The electric aspirator is perhaps more expensive and requires more maintenance than the hydroaspirator. The electric aspirator may be the preferred device in funeral homes where there is low water pressure. An attachment to the electric aspirator allows the embalmer to add a disinfectant solution to the materials being aspirated.

Hand Pump. A dual-purpose piece of equipment, the hand pump, permits removal of air or forces air into an enclosed airtight container. Drawing the air out of the container creates suction and is used for aspiration. Forcing the air into the container of embalming solution forces the solution out and is used to generate flow for injection. In the past, a glass jar with a "gooseneck" and the hand pump were commonly used. The "gooseneck" is the rubber stopper that makes the jar airtight. The stopper has two openings for two hose attachments. One hose allows air movement out of the jar, and the second hose leads to a trocar. This method is little used today.

Air Pressure Machine. The air pressure machine operates on the same principle as the hand pump. The machine has two outlets. One creates a vacuum; the other can be used to force air into a jar. Again, a "gooseneck" is employed. The concentrated aspirated material is collected in the jar. Care should be taken to use jars specially made for aspiration, as there is a danger of glass implosion. The contents of the jar can be poured into the sewer line, or, if the embalmer desires to disinfect the contents, they can be treated in the jar prior to being released into the sewer system.

Instruments Used in Aspiration

Trocar. A trocar is a long hollow needle (metal tube) with a removable sharp point that is available in varying lengths and bores. Whetstones or other sharpening devices can be used to keep the points honed, or the point can be replaced. The trocar is used to pierce the wall of the abdomen and the walls of the internal organs in the thoracic and abdominal cavities. The trocar, attached to the suction device, is used to withdraw the contents of the organs and residual fluid that has pooled in the cavities. The trocar is also used to introduce the disinfectant/preservative solution over and into the internal organs.

An 18-inch long, $\frac{5}{16}$ inch-bore trocar is used in aspiration of the abdominal and thoracic cavities of the adult body. Opening the cavities after the trocar has been used would reveal all of the organs in their *proper positions.* The embalmer would have to examine the viscera for the *pierce marks* made by the trocar, as these punctures close.

The *infant trocar* is approximately 12 inches in length and about $\frac{1}{4}$ inch in diameter. It is used in cavity treatment of infants and children. Many embalmers also use it for hypodermic injection of preservative chemicals into areas of the limbs or trunk not reached by arterial embalming.

Complete disinfection/sterilization of the trocar is important. Microorganisms have been carelessly transferred from one body to another via the trocar. Trays of sufficient size and length for the trocar are needed whether the chemical or autoclave method of sterilization is used. For example, after its use in a body with true tissue gas, an improperly cleaned trocar can harbor the spore-forming *Clostridium perfringens.*

Tubing. Clear plastic or rubber tubing 6 to 8 feet in length and $\frac{3}{8}$ to $\frac{1}{2}$ inch in diameter is needed to connect the trocar toaspiration devices. The wall of the tubing must be thick enough to preclude collapse as the suction is generated. Clear or semiclear tubing permits visual examination of the material being removed and aids in determining which organ or space is being aspirated.

Nasal Tube Aspirator. A 10-inch, 90° curved metal tube with a $\frac{3}{16}$-inch bore, the nasal tube aspirator is designed for aspiration of the nasal/oral cavity. It is placed through the nasal opening or between the lips. The primary problem in the use of this instrument is the diameter of its opening. Even a small semisolid particle can easily clog this instrument.

Autopsy Aspirator. The autopsy aspirator is an 8- to 10-inch long, $\frac{3}{8}$-inch-bore metal tube. A collector is attached to one end and a hose to the other. This equipment is used for aspiration of the cavities of the autopsied body, and has a number of openings to prevent clogging of the instrument. The aspirator can be set to operate while the body is being embalmed. The non-clogging feature is designed to free the embalmer's hands so constant attention is not needed.

▶ VISCERAL ANATOMY

The embalmer should constantly be aware of the internal structures he or she is attempting to preserve. Although comprehensive treatment of the internal anatomy is beyond the scope of this textbook, it is appropriate to include here limited descriptions of internal soft tissue structures to provide the embalmer with a quick reference source should he or she encounter a simple anatomical question or problem. Resolution of more complex problems is, of course, deferred to complete textbooks of anatomy.

Head

The interior of the cranial vault comprises anterior, middle, and posterior cranial fossae in which portions of the brain and brain stem are located. The frontal lobes of the cerebrum rest on that portion of the skull floor created by the anterior cranial fossa. The temporal lobes, hypothalamus, and midbrain cover the floor of the middle fossa. The large, posterior fossa houses the medulla, pons, and entire cerebellum.

Neck

The thyroid gland is a bilobed endocrine gland that partially covers the thyroid cartilage of the larynx and extends inferiorly as the sixth tracheal ring. The two lobes are usually, but not always, connected by an isthmus, which crosses the midline at about the level of the second, third, and fourth tracheal rings. The common carotid and inferior thyroid arteries are found posterior to the two lobes. Lateral to the lobes are the internal jugular veins. Posteriorly, the trachea is related to the straight muscular tube of the esophagus.

Thorax

Although the lungs are properly described as contents of the thorax, remember that their apices extend above the level of the first rib into the neck under the cupola. The right lung comprises three lobes and the left lung two lobes, although this is subject to some variation. The left lung is further characterized by the presence of a cardiac notch or impression to accommodate the ventricles of the heart. Medially, both lung surfaces relate to the contents of the mediastinum and contain the hilar structures, that is, the pulmonary vessels and the main-stem bronchi. Inferiorly, the lungs are related to the diaphragmatic pleura and the diaphragm.

The heart is positioned retrosternally in the middle mediastinum and extends from the second intercostal space inferiorly to the fifth. The lateral cardiac margins extend beyond the lateral margins of the body of the sternum. The great vessels arise from the base of the heart at the level of the second intercostal space, behind the upper portion of the body and the manubrium of the sternum.

Abdomen

The majority of abdominal viscera consist of some part of the digestive apparatus, which is mainly tubular with some modifications and specializations of this basic structure in various locations. As the straight-tubed esophagus passes through the diaphragm and enters the abdomen, it quickly gives rise to the stomach. The remainder of the alimentary or digestive tube, in order, consists of the duodenum, jejunum, ileum (small intestine), cecum, ascending colon, transverse colon, descending colon, sigmoid colon, rectum (large intestine), and anus. Organs that facilitate digestion include the gallbladder, liver, and pancreas.

A rather peripatetic organ, the stomach is one whose location varies with changes in the position and orientation of the body. It is, therefore, difficult to describe specific relationships of the stomach. Similarly, the shape of this organ is dependent on the amount and type of food-stuffs contained therein as well as the extent to which the digestive process has progressed. A "typical" stomach possesses greater and lesser curvatures, a fundic region that extends above the level at which the esophagus enters, and a pyloric region at the junction of the stomach and the duodenum.

The C-shaped duodenum is the first part of the small intestine and consists of four parts, which are either numbered one, two, three, and four or named superior, descending, transverse, and ascending. The superior portion is only partially covered by peritoneum and is, therefore, the most mobile of the four parts, as the others are entirely retroperitoneal. The descending portion typically receives the common bile duct and the main pancreatic duct, the contents of which facilitate digestion. The transverse portion crosses the body from right to left at the level of fourth lumbar vertebra and continues as the ascending portion, which emerges from the peritoneum and gives rise to the jejunum.

The first 40% of the remainder of the small intestine is the jejunum, which cannot be grossly distinguished from the other 60%, which is the ileum. Internal and microscopic structures, together with vascular patterns associated with each organ, allow discrimination between the two. The distinctions are most obvious at the extreme ends. These organs occupy much of the abdomen and both are suspended by a fan-shaped mesentery from the posterior body wall.

The large intestine can be distinguished grossly from the small bowel by the presence of three longitudinal strips of muscle, the taeniae coli, sacculations, and fatty appendages called epiploic appendices, none of which is found on the small intestine.

A diverticulum, the cecum, marks the beginning of the large intestine and extends inferiorly beyond the level at which the ileum joins the ascending colon. The cecum is situated in the right iliac and hypogastric regions. Opening from it is the vermiform appendix. Extending superiorly from the cecum is the retroperitoneal ascending colon, which continues to the right colic or hepatic flexure, inferior to the liver in the right lumbar region. Here, the colon turns sharply to the left in the umbilical region, as the transverse colon. This is a freely movable portion of the large bowel, suspended by the transverse mesocolon from the posterior body wall and extending to the left colic or splenic flexure in the left hypochondriac and lumbar regions. Here, the colon again becomes retroperitoneal and descends to the level of the iliac crest as the descending colon. In the left iliac region, the descending colon forms the sigmoid colon which is once again freely movable, being suspended by the sigmoid mesocolon. Anterior to the third sacral vertebra, the sigmoid colon gives way to the rectum which in humans is not really straight as its name implies but is curved, following the curvature of the sacrum and coccyx.

The largest gland in the body is the liver, which develops as an outgrowth of the digestive tract and retains a functional and anatomical relationship with it. It rests in the right hypochondriac and epigastric regions. The upper surface of the liver is higher on the right than on the left and lies in relationship with the inferior surface of the diaphragm from which it is suspended by the coronary ligaments. On the inferior surface of the liver is the gallbladder, whose cystic duct is joined by the common hepatic duct from the liver to form the common bile duct which empties into the second (descending) portion of the duodenum. The gallbladder and the lower portion of the right lobe of the liver lie anterior to the right hepatic flexure in the right lumbar region.

The pancreas lies cradled in the arms of the C-shaped duodenum and extends across the midline from the right to the left at about the level of the second lumbar vertebra. The major subdivisions of the pancreas include the head, neck, body, and tail. The main duct of the pancreas typically joins the common bile duct immediately as they both enter the second part of the duodenum, but the patterns of the ducts from the liver, gallbladder, and pancreas are subject to considerable variation.

The remaining unpaired organ in the abdomen is the spleen, which is located in the left hypochondriac region. Lying in the umbilical left and right lumbar regions are the usually paired kidneys. These lie along the posterior body wall, with the right slightly lower than the left because of encroachment by the large right lobe of the liver. Both kidneys lie at the level of the umbilicus and both are retroperitoneal. In its own separate capsule at the superior pole of each kidney is a suprarenal gland.

Pelvis

Internal pelvic viscera in the male include the prostate gland, seminal vesicles, urinary bladder, and rectum. The last structure was already discussed; the first three are considered here. The prostate gland is situated at the base of the urinary bladder, surrounding the prostatic or initial portion of the male urethra. The gland is difficult to visualize in the pelvis but can be palpated as a firm structure if fingers are introduced into the pelvis around the neck of the bladder immediately anterior to the rectum. In addition to its continuity with the urinary bladder, the prostate also receives secretions from the paired seminal vesicles, which lie posterior to the prostate and communicate with it by means of ejaculatory ducts. The latter structures form as a result of the union of the ducts of the seminal vesicles and the distal ends of the vasa deferentia.

The urinary bladder is situated behind the pubic symphysis in the midline and its shape and size are dependent on the volume of urine contained within it. This muscular, distensible structure receives urine from the kidneys via the paired ureters, which open posterolaterally into the bladder.

In the female, the urinary bladder occupies a position similar to that in the male but is separated from the rectum by the intervening uterus and its adnexa. In addition to the uterus and bladder, other visceral structures in the female pelvis include the ovaries, uterine tubes, and vagina. The muscular unpaired uterus is positioned in the midline and is supported by a double layer of peritoneum called broad ligament. The uterus is divided into several parts including the fundus, body, and cervix.

The fundus projects above the level at which the uterine tubes communicate with the uterine cavity. At the distal end of the body is a thick, muscular constriction known as the cervix. Through the cervix, the cavity of the uterus communicates with the vagina, which is a distensible tube, flattened anteroposteriorly. The uterine tubes communicate with the opening directly into the abdominal cavity and the uterine cavity. The abdominal cavity, therefore, opens to the external environment via the uterine tubes, the cavity of the uterus, the cavity of the cervix, and the vagina. The paired ovaries are located on the posterior aspect of the broad ligament on either side of the uterus. The uterus, tubes, and ovaries are supported by an elaborate system of "ligaments" derived from reflections of the peritoneum.

▶ CONTENTS OF THE ABDOMEN: THE NINE-REGION METHOD

To establish the nine abdominal regions (Table 14–4), extend two *vertical* lines upward from a point midway between the anterior superior iliac spine and the symphysis pubis. Draw two *horizontal* lines. Join the upper line to the lowest point of the costal margin on each side, at the level of the inferior margin of the tenth costal cartilage. Join the lower horizontal line to the tubercles on the respective iliac crests (Figure 14–1).

Quadrant Method

There is a second method of dividing the abdomen into regions and that is the **four region plan**. A *horizontal* line is drawn from left to right through the *umbilicus*, A *vertical* line is drawn down the midline of the body. This establishes upper right and left quadrants and lower right and left quadrants (Figure 14–2).

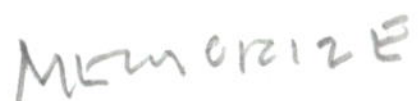

TABLE 14–4. THE NINE ABDOMINAL REGIONS

Right Hypochondriac	Epigastric	Left Hypochondriac
Part of the liver Part of right kidney Greater omentum Coils of small intestine Gallbladder	Stomach including cardiac and pyloric openings Portion of liver Duodenum, pancreas Suprarenal glands and parts of kidneys Greater omentum	Part of liver Stomach, fundus and cardiac regions Spleen Tail of pancreas Left colic splenic flexure Part of left kidney Greater omentum
Right Lumbar	**Umbilical**	**Left Lumbar**
Lower portion of liver Ascending colon Part of right kidney Coils of small intestine Greater omentum Right colic (hepatic) flexure	Transverse colon Part of body kidneys Part of duodenum Coils of small intestine Greater omentum Bifurcation of the abdominal aorta and inferior vena cava	Part of left kidney Descending colon Coils of small intestine Greater omentum
Right Inguinal (iliac)	**Hypogastric**	**Left Inguinal (iliac)**
Cecum, appendix Part of ascending colon Coils of small intestine Greater omentum	Bladder in adults if distended Uterus during pregnancy Coils of small intestine Greater omentum	Part of descending colon Sigmoid colon Coils of small intestine Greater omentum

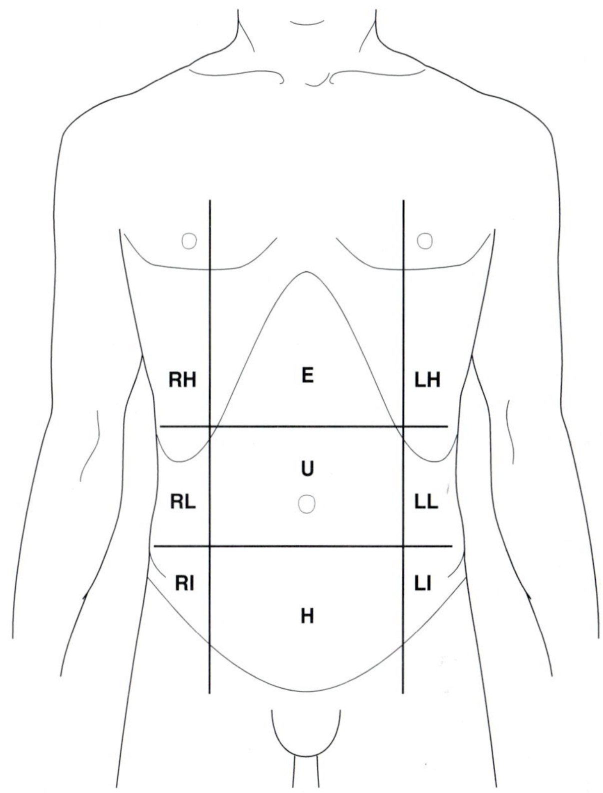

Figure 14–1. The nine regions of the abdomen. RH, right hypochondriac; E, epigastric; LH, left hypochondriac; RL, right lumbar; U, umbilical; LL, left lumbar; RI, right inguinal; H, hypogastric; LI, left inguinal.

These topographical systems of dividing the abdomen serve to give the practitioner an approximate location of the various abdominal organs. The embalmer should have a thorough knowledge of the location of the visceral organs. This understanding is important in the process of cavity embalming. It is also valuable when one or more organs have been donated to an organ bank or when partial autopsies have been performed. In addition, the embalmer should have a complete understanding of the relationship of the vascular system to the visceral organs.

Trocar Guides

The efficiency of using the trocar to pierce the internal organs and aspirate their contents is enhanced by the use of trocar guides. **The main guides are to reach the stomach, cecum, urinary bladder, and the heart.** The guides all originate at the common insertion point—2 inches to the left and 2 inches superior to the navel. The point of the trocar is inserted into the abdomen and kept close to the anterior abdominal wall until the specific organ is reached.

Guide for the Right Side of the Heart. Move the trocar along a line from the left anterior–superior iliac spine and the right earlobe. After the trocar has passed through the diaphragm, depress the point and enter the heart (Figure 14–3).

Guide for the Stomach. Direct the trocar point toward the intersection of the fifth intercostal space and the left mid-axillary line (established by extending a line from the center of the medial base of the axillary space inferiorly along the rib cage); continue until the trocar enters the stomach (Figure 14–3).

Guide for the Cecum. The trocar is directed to a point three fourths of the distance on a line from the pubic symphysis to the right anterior superior iliac spine. When the point of the trocar is approximately 2 inches from the line, the point is depressed 2 inches and then thrust forward to pierce the cecum as it is trapped against the pelvis (Figure 14–3).

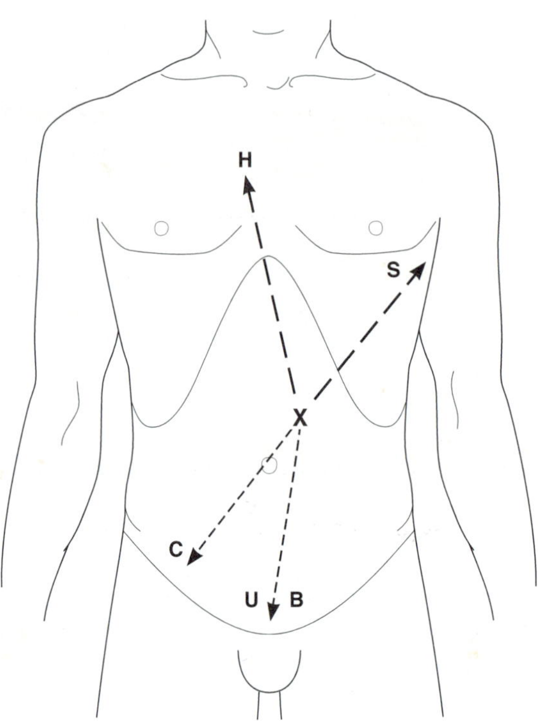

Figure 14–3. Trocar guides. S, stomach; C, cecum; UB, urinary bladder; H, heart; X, insertion point.

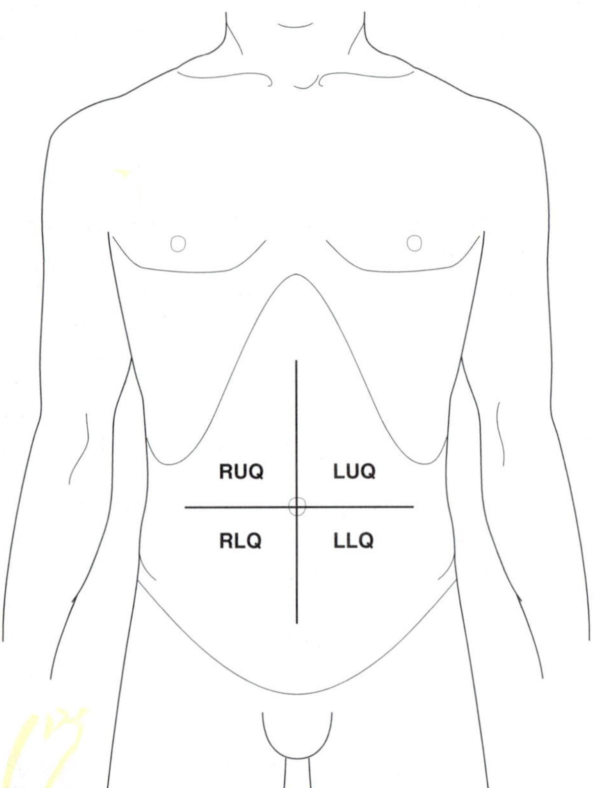

Figure 14–2. Division of the abdomen into quadrants. RUQ (LUQ), right (left) upper quadrant; RLQ (LLQ), right (left) lower quadrant.

Trocar Guide for the Urinary Bladder. Keep the point up near the abdominal wall directing the trocar to the median line of the pubic bone (symphysis pubis) until the point touches the bone. Retract the trocar slightly, depress the point slightly, and insert into the urinary bladder.

▶ PARTIAL ASPIRATION PRIOR TO OR DURING ARTERIAL TREATMENT

Cavity embalming, complete aspiration and injection of cavity fluids, *follows* arterial injection and drainage. There is one exception to this rule: When the abdomen is tightly distended with gas or edema this pressure should be relieved *prior to or during* arterial injection. The presence of fluid (as in ascites) or gas in the abdomen can be great enough to act as an *extravascular resistance.* This resistance may also interfere with drainage. Drainage may be difficult to establish until this extravascular pressure is relieved.

Two methods can be employed:

First, using a scalpel, puncture the abdomen at the standard point of trocar entry 2 inches left and 2 inches superior to the umbilicus. (Later, this point can be used for aspiration and injection.) Then insert a trocar or blunt instrument such as a large drain tube into the cavity and aspirate the gases or edema. It may be more use-

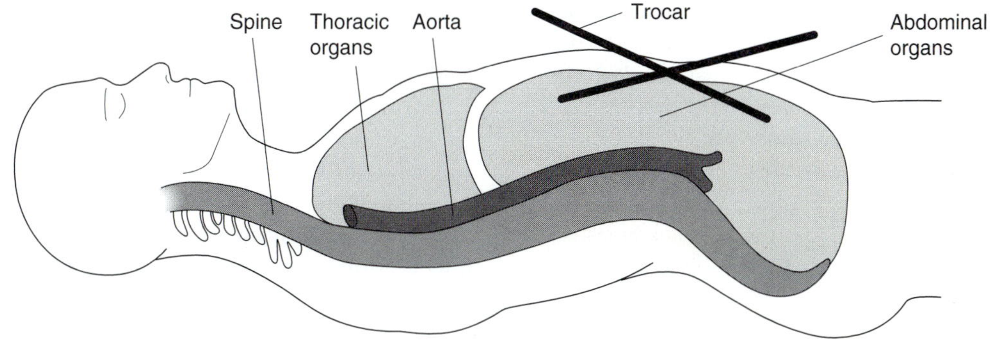

Figure 14–4. Trocar levels to relieve abdominal distension from edema (ascites) or gases.

ful to make this puncture in the lower area of the abdomen in the right or left inguinal area or the hypogastric region of the abdomen. From this point edema will be able to gravitate easier from the abdomen, and if gases are the trouble, it may be easier to pierce the *transverse colon* with a trocar from this more distant point (Figure 14–4).

Second, using a scalpel, make a small incision in the abdominal wall. Dissect into the abdominal cavity. A portion of the large intestine can be incised if gas is the problem; edema drainage can be taken from the opening. Cover this opening with cotton or gauze saturated with a disinfectant so microbial agents are not released into the air.

The first method using the trocar is much cleaner and will be found to be generally more effective in relieving abdominal pressure (gas or edema) prior to or during arterial injection.

If the neck is distended and discolored prior to injection, using the standard trocar point of entry, direct the trocar along the lateral abdominal wall through the diaphragm and into the thoracic cavity. The problem could be hydrothorax, and this can be removed to relieve pressure on the heart and neck veins. Care must be taken not to interrupt circulation.

▶ ANTEMORTEM SUBCUTANEOUS EMPHYSEMA

A condition where there is an exceptional and noticeable amount of gas in the tissues *prior to embalming* is antemortem subcutaneous emphysema. Many times the facial tissues will be quite distended, the tongue will protrude, gases may be felt all along the thoracic walls, and, in the male, the scrotum may be distended with gas.

If there is no odor and if there are no signs of decomposition, palpate for a broken rib or examine the body for a puncture wound to the thorax or a very recent tracheotomy opening. Look for large needle punctures over the skin of the rib cage. This condition is brought about by a rupture or by the puncturing or tearing of the pleural sac of the lung. Air was forced into the tissues as the person struggled to breathe air. If the condition is severe enough, try and remove some of this gas *prior to arterial embalming.*

Insert the trocar into the abdomen at the standard point of entry, then direct the point through the diaphragm, keeping the point just under the rib cage so as not to damage any of the large vessels. This should help to relieve some of the gases. Likewise, using a carotid incision will help to relieve gases from the neck tissues. Removal of these gases can be better accomplished by channeling and/or lancing the tissues after the arterial injection is completed.

▶ TIME PERIOD FOR CAVITY TREATMENT

There are two periods during which cavity aspiration and injection can take place: immediately following arterial injection and several hours following arterial injection. Most embalmers will certainly delay aspiration for a short period following arterial injection if it is only for a matter of a few minutes while the arteries and veins used for injection are being ligated and the embalming machine rinsed and cleaned. This time delay will allow the intravascular pressure to assist the diffusion of the arterial solution from the capillaries into the interstitial spaces. It is best to inject the last quarter to one-half gallon of arterial solution with the drainage closed, being careful to remove the arterial tubes and drainage devices quickly and to tie off the vessels so as much pressure as possible remains within the vascular system. A short delay of several minutes can then follow.

Now the aspirating begins. It is wise to do the aspirating *prior to suturing.* Aspiration takes the pressure off the vascular system and, thus, decreases the chances of leakage from the incision should some small vessels leak.

It should be stated that some funeral homes do not do the cavity embalming until the time of dressing and casketing. Many embalmers do the cavity embalming immediately at the conclusion of the arterial embalming. The theory of aspiration shortly after arterial injection has the following advantages:

1. Large numbers of microbes that can easily multiply and accelerate decomposition are removed as soon as possible.
2. Removal of the microbes prevents the possibility of translocation of the microbes to the skeletal tissues.
3. Removal of these microbes prevents or minimizes the production of gases that could cause purge.
4. Immediate aspiration removes materials that could purge if sufficient gases were generated during the delay.
5. Removal of the contents of the hollow viscera and cavities eliminates a bacterial medium.
6. **Most important,** removal of blood from the heart, liver, and large veins helps to prevent blood discolorations.
7. If there has been some distension of the neck or facial tissues during arterial injection, immediate aspiration decreases the swelling. This is often seen in bodies dead from pneumonia when hydrothorax is present.

The second theory is to have a long delay prior to aspirating the body. Some embalmers delay aspirating for 8 to 12 hours. The theory is to allow a maximum time for the arterial solution to penetrate into the tissue spaces. Some embalmers feel the delay helps to preserve the walls of the visceral organs. This will then make the walls easier to pierce with the trocar when the aspirating is done. If a humectant coinjection or a humectant restorative "to fill out" emaciated tissue has been used, some chemical manufacturers suggest that the last half-gallon be injected with the vein ligated and a delay made between arterial injection and aspiration. This delay gives the tissues time to firm.

▶ ASPIRATION TECHNIQUE

The standard point of trocar entry is located 2 inches to the left of and 2 inches superior to the umbilicus. This point is used for the standard trocar; from it the embalmer is able to reach all areas of the thoracic, abdominal, and pelvic cavities. The trocar should also be able to reach above the clavicle into the base of the neck. A second reason for using this point, especially with infants and children, is that the liver is on the right side of the body. At the location where the trocar is inserted, it is easier to move the instrument from point to point. If it were inserted on the right side, the trocar would be entangled in the solid tissues of the liver.

During the aspiration of the cavities, the trocar can be withdrawn enough to let some air pass through the instrument. This helps to "clean out" materials in the tubing and the instrument. Some embalmers withdraw the trocar several times during aspiration and plunge it into a container of water to flush out the tubing and trocar.

A moistened cloth saturated with a disinfectant solution can be used to clean the barrel of the trocar as well as any matter that may exist around the abdominal opening during the aspiration process.

An orderly method of aspiration should be employed. Remember that gases are usually found in the anterior portions of the abdominal and thoracic cavities. Liquids gravitate to the posterior portions of the cavities. If each cavity is "fanned" from right to left, most of the viscera are pierced. This "fanning" can be done in about three levels of depth.

Begin by inserting the trocar and aspirating the most anterior portions of the cavity. Then progress from right to left within the middle portion of the cavity, and finally from right to left through the deepest portions of the cavity. Treat both abdominal and thoracic cavities in this manner. The trocar guides can be used to aspirate the hollow viscera such as the stomach, heart, urinary bladder, and cecum.

Let the trocar "sit" for a while until an area filled with liquid is thoroughly drained. This is necessary when treating bodies with ascites, hydrothorax, or ruptured vessels such as the aorta.

▶ RECENT SURGERY OR ORGAN REMOVAL

If the deceased was an organ donor or died during the course of an operation and no autopsy was performed, the surgical incision or the incision used to remove the organ(s) may or may not have been loosely closed by the hospital. For such bodies, the following protocol simplifies treatment of the cavities:

1. Disinfect the surgical incision with a *phenol solution.*
2. Arterially embalm the body.
3. Remove loose sutures, surgical staples, and so on, and open the incision.
4. Swab the edges of the incision with a phenol solution.
5. Suture closed the incision using a tight baseball suture. If possible, use sufficient quantities of incision seal powder.
6. *Aspirate the cavities and inject cavity fluid.*

Any surgical drainage openings should be closed by suture or trocar button *prior* to aspiration of the cavities.

▶ PARTIAL AUTOPSIES AND ORGAN DONATIONS

After a partial autopsy on an adult, the unautopsied cavity can be difficult to treat from the cavity that has been opened. It is much simpler to treat the walls of the autopsied cavity by hypodermic treatment and painting with autopsy gel. Fill the cavity with an absorbent material and saturate the material with a cavity fluid. Suture the cavity closed. *Now treat the unautopsied cavity* by aspirating the cavity and its visceral contents. Inject a sufficient quantity of cavity fluid.

▶ DIRECT INCISION METHOD

In the treatment of bodies that have recent surgical incisions or from which organs were removed after death, resuturing followed by aspiration and injection with the trocar is recommended.

An alternate method can be used, a method that was employed as an alternative to cavity treatment via trocar many years ago. In this *direct incision method* of cavity treatment, the *embalmer* makes a midline incision over the abdominal wall and, from this point, treats the visceral organs and the cavities by lancing and draining the organs and sponging or aspirating their contents within the cavity. Either cavity fluid is poured over the various organs or the organs are directly injected with a parietal needle or large hypodermic needle.

This method of direct cavity treatment can be used when the cavity has been opened by recent surgery, an organ(s) has been removed for donation, or partial autopsy has been performed. The method is not only time consuming and unsanitary, but access to both thorax and abdomen is difficult.

▶ ORDER OF TREATMENT

There is no specific order of treatment, but the embalmer should proceed in an orderly fashion in treating the cavities to ensure that no areas are missed. Years ago some instructors taught that each organ should be separately treated. That is, the stomach was aspirated (with one puncture) and then, without removing the trocar, the stomach was filled with cavity fluid. The embalmer then moved on to treat another organ until all hollow viscera and cavities had been embalmed.

A suggested order might be *thoracic* cavity, abdominal cavity, and pelvic cavity. Likewise, when injecting cavity fluid, inject the thoracic cavity first, then the abdominal and pelvic cavities.

▶ ASPIRATION OF THE THORACIC CAVITY

At the standard point of entry, direct the trocar into the thoracic cavity. A good point at which to begin aspiration is the right side of the heart, using the trocar guide as an imaginary line running from the left anterior superior iliac spine to the lobe of the right ear. Intersect this line with the trocar in the mediastinal area. This technique also provides practice for those occasions on which the trocar may have to be used as a drainage instrument (which will have to be inserted into the right atrium of the heart). Next, aspirate the anterior chambers of the right and left pleural cavities. Direct the trocar a little lower and pierce the central portions of the lungs and the heart.

Observe what is being aspirated. Clear tubing is a help. Remember, the hydroaspirator may be 10 feet away from the body. Look through clear tubing at what is being immediately removed from the body.

Finally, aspirate the deep areas of the pleural cavities. If hydrothorax is present, edematous liquids will be found, often in great quantities. Be certain that the trocar is directed to either side of the vertebral column where the great vessels enter and leave the lungs. This also aspirates the bronchial tubes leading to the trachea.

▶ ASPIRATION OF THE ABDOMINAL CAVITY

After aspiration of the thorax, the trocar can be withdrawn and the stomach aspirated. Use the trocar guide. Move the trocar toward a point established along the *left* midaxillary line, at about the level of the fifth intercostal space. As the trocar moves toward this point it should pierce the stomach.

Several passages can be made through the stomach wall. Aspiration not only *removes* gases, liquids, and semisolids from the organs, but also *pierces* the viscera so that cavity fluid can better penetrate the visceral organs. Next, the cecum and bladder can be aspirated again using the trocar guides.

In similar "fanning" movements, aspirate the entire abdominal cavity again. Try to establish three levels.

Remember, gases, when they can move, will be in the anterior portions and liquids in the posterior portions of the cavities.

In aspiration of the abdomen, the small intestines and the greater omentum have a tendency to cling tightly to the small holes located in the point and shaft of the trocar. For this reason, it is best to keep the instrument in constant motion, except when a large amount of liquid such as edema in bodies with ascites is being drained. Removing the trocar from time to time helps to prevent clogging of these small holes.

Pay special attention to the posterior of the liver. It is here that the great vessels enter and leave this organ. The liver is very difficult to preserve. Therefore, numerous passes with the trocar should be made through the solid portions of this organ. Also give special attention to the large intestine, especially the *transverse colon.* Check the previous charts to observe the location of this intestinal organ. The large intestine, especialy the transverse portion, should be thoroughly pierced to allow the escape of gases and to assist later in penetration of the cavity fluid.

To assist the trocar in piercing the abdominal organs, place external pressure on the abdominal wall. Do this with a gloved hand. Hold the trocar with one hand and apply the pressure with the other. Apply pressure gently on the abdominal wall. To facilitate passage of the trocar through the coils of the small intestine, in addition to applying pressure on the abdomen, pass the trocar to a bony part such as the ilium or pubic bone. In this way, the point of the trocar will pass through the intestine rather than push it aside or slip around it.

Another method that can be used in aspirating the *abdomen* and inferior portion of the thorax is to insert the trocar in the center of the right or left inguinal region of the abdomen. Long passes can be made with the trocar, which will pass through the lumen of the intestines as the point forges ahead through the diaphragm. Many embalmers feel they can better pierce the large and small intestine from this point of trocar entry.

▶ TREATMENT OF THE MALE GENITALIA

After aspiration of the pelvic and abdominal cavities of the male, the trocar need *not* be inserted into the scrotum to aspirate this organ. Cavity fluid should, however, be injected into the shaft of the penis and the scrotum if these organs appear not to have received arterial solution.

To enter the scrotum direct the point of the trocar to the most anterior portion of the symphysis pubis. Draw back slightly on the trocar and direct the point over the top of the symphysis pubis into the scrotum. In cases of hydrocoele, edema of the scrotum, make several such passages into the scrotum. Be careful not to puncture the organ. Then, with a cloth placed around the scrotum, much of the water can be forced into the pelvic cavity. Later, undiluted cavity fluid can be injected into the scrotum.

Another condition less frequently encountered is a hernia involving the scrotum. A portion of the intestines moves into the scrotum. This condition can be severe enough to make dressing the body difficult. The trocar should be directed into the scrotum to pierce the loops of the intestine and remove as much of the content as possible. Later, this area should be injected with cavity fluid. The embalmer can also use the trocar to pull the intestine back into the abdominal cavity. This is slowly accomplished by pulling on the intestine with the point of the trocar. Gradually, the intestine can be manipulated into the abdominal cavity. This will make dressing of the body much easier.

▶ CRANIAL ASPIRATION

The point of entry in cranial aspiration is the right or left nostril. A small trocar is introduced into the nostril and pushed through the *cribriform plate of the ethmoid bone.* At this point the instrument enters the anterior portion of the cranial cavity (Figure 14–5). It is not possible to move the trocar into the posterior portion of the cavity; therefore, any gases present must be removed from this anterior position.

Inject only a few ounces of concentrated cavity fluid. This is done by using a hypodermic syringe with a long needle. After injection, tightly pack the nostril with cotton to prevent leakage.

▶ INJECTION OF CAVITY CHEMICALS

After the complete aspiration of the thoracic and abdominal cavities, preservative/disinfectant cavity chemicals are placed within the cavities over the viscera. *Concentrated cavity fluid* is always used. In cases of hydrothorax or ascites or where blood has escaped during arterial injection or during aspiration of the organs, the fluids—blood and edema—dilute the cavity fluid.

The volume of chemical is determined by the mass of tissues to be treated, which is estimated on the basis of body size and weight. On the average, for a body weighing 150 pounds, 16 ounces of undiluted cavity chemical is used for each (thoracic, abdominal and pelvic) cavity. Larger bodies may require considerably more chemical. Smaller bodies, such as infants, require less.

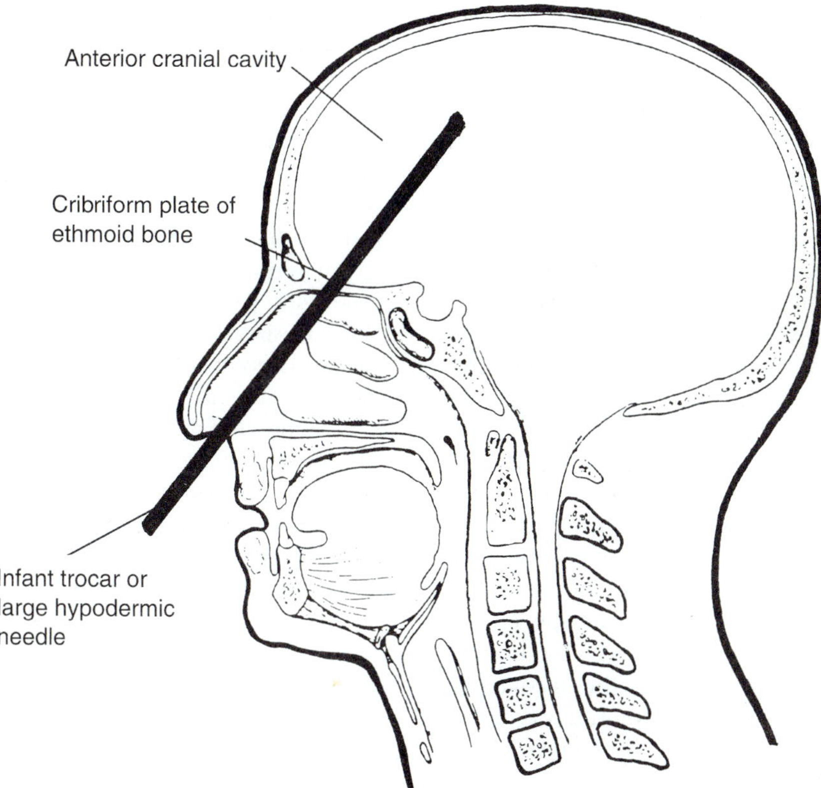

Figure 14–5. Anterior cranial cavity and cribriform plate of the ethmoid bone.

Prior to cavity chemical injection, it is necessary to wash and flush the trocar thoroughly. All organic materials must be flushed from the trocar if concentrated cavity fluid is to pass through the instrument. The undiluted cavity chemical may be injected by two methods: gravity injector and machine injection. The gravity injector is attached directly to the 16-ounce bottle of cavity fluid. A hose connects the injector to the trocar. The higher the bottle is raised, the faster the fluid flows into the body. A small opening on the side of the gravity injector allows air to flow into the cavity fluid bottle. By placing a finger over this opening, the embalmer stops the flow of cavity fluid. This can be done when the trocar must be withdrawn to change its position within a body cavity. After use, the gravity injector, tubing, and trocar should be rinsed with cold water to disperse all the cavity fluid. The trocar can then be immersed in a cold liquid sterilant.

In machine injection, three bottles of cavity fluid are placed in the tank of the embalming machine. The delivery hose is then connected directly to the trocar. Pressure and rate of flow should both be set very low. The tubing alone can hold several ounces of cavity fluid. Following injection, make certain that the cavity chemical is thoroughly rinsed from the machine. Wash the machine with warm water and ammonia and then run fresh cold water through it.

The chemicals are sprayed or made to flow over the *anterior surface* of the viscera close to the anterior wall of the thoracic and abdominal cavities. The cavity chemicals gravitate through the openings in the viscera made by the trocar and are absorbed by or rest on the posterior surface of the cavity walls.

After the cavity fluid is injected, some embalmers make several passes with the trocar through the abdomen and thorax to release gases that may have been displaced to the surface of the cavities. This movement of the trocar helps to distribute the cavity fluid. Cover the open end of the trocar with a cloth saturated with disinfectant so formaldehyde fumes and/or body gases are not released into the air.

After the trocar puncture has been closed and during the postembalming washing and drying of the body, *turn the body on its sides* not only to wash and dry the back and sides of the body, but also to distribute the cavity fluid and bring any trapped gases to the surface of the cavities.

The cavity chemicals should be kept in the body and not be allowed to spill or run onto the surface of the abdominal wall. Use a wet cloth to wrap the trocar and cover the opening in the body as the fluids are injected. If cavity chemicals accidentally flow onto the surface of the body, immediately flush with cold running water.

It is possible to inject cavity fluid into the trachea or esophagus. If the nasal passages or throat have not been tightly packed with cotton when the features were set, this fluid can exit when the body is turned to be dried after it is washed. Limited aspiration can be done with the nasal tube aspirator after the body is placed into a supine position. The nasal passages can be tightly packed with cotton. Open the lips and, using dry cotton, make certain all the liquid is dried from the mouth. Likewise, clean and pack the nose again. If the embalmer feels that cavity fluid purge may be a problem during dressing and casketing, he should reaspirate the thoracic cavity at this time, giving special emphasis to the posterior of the neck, where the trachea and esophagus are located. Packing the throat and nasal passages with an abundant amount of cotton prior to embalming can help reduce the chance of cavity fluid purge.

▶ CLOSURE OF THE ABDOMINAL OPENING

To complete the aspiration procedure, the opening in the body wall is closed. Several methods can be used. Each embalmer uses his or her own preferred method. The plastic, threaded trocar button provides complete closure and is easily removed if further aspiration and reinjection are necessary later.

Two sutures are commonly used to close the trocar opening: the **purse-string** (Figure 14–6) and the **"N" or reverse stitch.** Sutures offer the advantage of a complete closure. A bow can be used to secure the suture. It can easily be opened if reaspiration is necessary. To minimize exposure to any fluid that may leak from the abdominal opening, if the embalmer plans to suture the opening closed, place the stitch after aspiration, just before the cavity fluid is injected. After injection, pull the suture tight to close the opening.

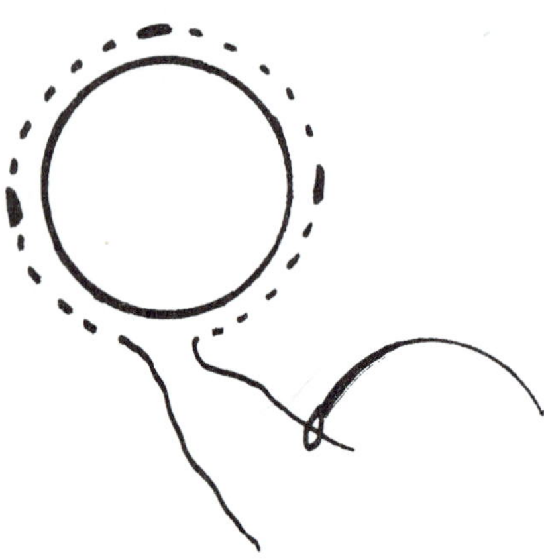

Figure 14–6. Purse-string suture.

The barrel of the trocar can enlarge the abdominal opening if there is poor integrity to the abdominal skin to a size where a trocar button would be impossible to use. This condition necessitates the use of sutures for closure.

Some embalmers do not close the trocar openings but allow them to remain open for the escape of any gases. If this is done the opening should be covered with cotton and the cotton covered with plastic to prevent any soilage of the clothing. This technique is not recommended when the body is being shipped.

▶ REASPIRATION/REINJECTION

A body must be reaspirated and reinjected with cavity embalming chemicals whenever the possibility exists that tissues or cavity contents (liquids, gases, semisolids) have not been thoroughly saturated with disinfectant preservative chemicals. The procedures are the same as those used in the initial cavity embalming. The entire cavity is aspirated and cavity chemicals applied.

In some funeral homes, policy mandates that *every body* be reaspirated prior to dressing and casketing, whereas others reaspirate only when it is felt absolutely necessary. Some embalmers not only reaspirate but reinject at least one full bottle of cavity fluid after reaspiration.

The following situations require reaspiration and reinjection:

1. A noticeable amount of gas escapes when the trocar button is removed.
2. The body is to be transported to another funeral home.
3. Final disposition of the body is to be delayed.
4. Decomposition is evident prior to embalming.
5. Abdominal surgery has been performed recently.
6. The body is obese.
7. The body shows evidence of gas (distension of the veins of the neck or backs of the hands) or purge or distension of the abdomen is present.
8. Death was due to blood infections or infectious diseases of the abdomen, thorax, or visceral organs (e.g., bacteremia, peritonitis, pneumonia).

9. Death was due to drowning, or purge was evident prior to, during, or after arterial embalming.
10. Ascites is present.

▶ KEY TERMS AND CONCEPTS FOR STUDY AND DISCUSSION

1. Define the following terms:
   aspiration
   cavity embalming
   electric aspirator
   hydroaspirator
   infant trocar
   purge
   reaspiration
   trocar
2. Give several reasons for aspiration.
3. Distinguish between stomach purge and lung purge.
4. Describe how the abdomen is divided into nine regions; name each region.
5. Describe how the abdomen is divided into quadrants.
6. List the major visceral contents of the nine abdominal regions.
7. Give the trocar guides for the following organs: (a) right side of the heart, (b) stomach, (c) cecum, and (d) urinary bladder.
8. Describe four means of creating a vacuum for aspiration.
9. Discuss the various means of closing the trocar opening in the abdominal wall.
10. Give the standard point of trocar entry into the abdomen and explain why this location is used.
11. List conditions that necessitate reaspiration of the body.
12. Explain why partial aspiration may be necessary prior to or during arterial injection.
13. Explain why cavity embalming is performed.
14. List the advantages and disadvantages of immediate cavity treatment and delayed cavity treatment.

▶ BIBLIOGRAPHY

Burke PA, Sheffner AL. The antimicrobial activity of embalming chemicals and topical disinfectants on the microbial flora of human remains. *Health Lab Sci* 1976;13(4):267–270.

Cavity fluids. In: *Champion Encyclopedia.* Springfield, OH: Champion Chemical; 1975:No. 454, 1833–1836.

Dorn JM, Hopkins BM. *Thanatochemistry.* Reston, VA: Reston; 1985.

Grant ME. Cavity embalming. In: *Champion Encyclopedia.* Springfield, OH: Champion Chemical; 1987:2338–2341.

Proper cavity treatment. In: *Champion Encyclopedia.* Springfield, OH: Champion Chemical; 1974:No. 449, 1813–1816.

Rose GW, Hockett RN. The microbiological evaluation and enumeration of postmortem specimens from human remains. *Health Lab Sci* 1971;8(2): 75–78.

Tortora GJ. *Principles of Human Anatomy.* 3rd ed. New York: Harper & Row; 1983.

Weed LA, Baggenstoss AH. The isolation of pathogens from tissues of embalmed human bodies. *Am J Clin Pathol* 1951;21:1114.

Weed LA, Baggenstoss AH. The isolation of pathogens from embalmed tissues. *Proc Soc Mayo Clin* 1952; 27:124.

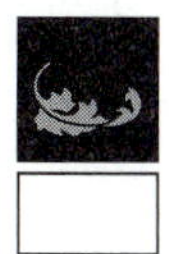

CHAPTER 15
PREPARATION OF THE BODY AFTER ARTERIAL INJECTION

▶ POSTEMBALMING TREATMENTS

The process of embalming is divided into three periods: preembalming, embalming, and postembalming. Preembalming procedures are carried out before arterial injection of the body and include setting of the features, positioning of the body, selection and elevation of vessels for injection and drainage, and selection and preparation of the embalming fluid.

During embalming the arterial solution is injected. In this period, activities include the selection of proper pressures and rates of flow to distribute the arterial solution, massage and manipulation of the body to promote fluid distribution, control of drainage to help distribute the fluid, removal of surface blood discolorations and promotion of the retention of arterial fluid for preservation, use of humectants and dilute arterial solutions to moisturize dehydrated bodies, use of high-specific-gravity, concentrated arterial solutions to dry bodies with skeletal edema, and maintenance of a good moisture balance in the "normal body."

In the embalming period an embalming analysis is made to determine what body areas have not received arterial solution. Procedures to promote fluid solution distribution to these areas are instituted, and, if necessary, a secondary artery is raised to inject the area devoid of fluid. Most embalmers pause a short time between injection and cavity embalming to flush and clean the embalming machine, remove drainage instruments and ligate veins, remove arterial tubes and ligate arteries, and clean blood and drainage materials from the embalming table. Cavity embalming is usually carried out during the embalming period; however, some embalmers prefer to wait several hours between injection and cavity embalming. When this is done, cavity embalming is considered to be carried out during the *postembalming* period.

The following treatments are generally carried out after the arterial and cavity embalming. **The order of treatment is optional.** Each is discussed in detail in this chapter.

1. Preservative treatments for areas that did not receive arterial solution or did not receive *sufficient* arterial solution
2. Closure of embalming incisions
3. Removal (and closure of the opening) of invasive devices, for example, pacemaker, intravenous needles, surgical drains, colostomy apparatus
4. Washing of the body, turning of the body to dry and inspect for posterior lesions
5. Final treatments for ulcerations and discolorations
6. Corrective treatments for purge and packing of all orifices
7. Removal of gases or edema from viewable facial areas
8. Inspection of mouth for purge or moisture; resetting of features if necessary, and insertion of false teeth if these were not available before embalming
9. Application of adhesives to eyes and mouth
10. Dressing with plastic garments
11. Repositioning, if necessary
12. Terminal disinfection of instruments and preparation room and personal hygiene
13. Preparation of documentation, shipping instructions, and so on

▶ TREATMENT OF AREAS NEEDING ARTERIAL SOLUTION

The primary embalming point is the artery (or arteries) that the embalmer chose as a site from which to embalm the entire unautopsied body. If areas of the body have not received fluid or have not received sufficient arterial solution, the embalmer should inject the area through a secondary injection point.

Example. If the embalmer began by injecting and draining from the right femoral artery and vein, and solution did not reach the left forearm and hand, he or she should first inject the axillary, brachial, radial, or ulnar artery to secure preservation of the forearm and hand by arterial injection. If fluid is not distributed to these areas through the secondary injection sites, the embalmer must now use one or more other methods of embalming to preserve these tissues.

Appearance of Areas Not Receiving Arterial Solution. Areas that have not received arterial solution do not show evidence of fluid dye. Intravascular blood discolorations may still be present. The tissues exhibit no preservative fixation.

When doubt exists as to whether an area has received any or sufficient solution, the simplest corrective treatment is to inject the area arterially with a slightly stronger arterial solution.

Appearance of Areas Receiving Insufficient Arterial Solution. Determining if a body region contains arterial solution is not as easy as determining if a body area has received NO FLUID. Fixation is not as intense as normally would be expected. Dyes may be blotchy and not as intense. If there is doubt, follow the preceding rule and inject the area. Later, these areas can darken, gases may form, and skin-slip is a possibility.

▶ SUPPLEMENTAL EMBALMING TREATMENTS

There are two supplemental methods of embalming: *surface embalming* and *hypodermic embalming.* These supplemental embalming methods are used to treat small areas, such as the eyelids, mouth, and fingers, or to treat large body areas that could not be injected because of arteriosclerosis, trunk walls that did not receive arterial fluid, or the side of the face when the common carotid is occluded.

Surface Embalming*

Surface embalming can be used to treat intact skin that has not received sufficient arterial fluid. It can also be used in "raw" skin areas, for example, broken skin, skin-slip, burned tissues, and surface lesions. Surface embalming may be applied to both *external* and *internal* body surfaces, for example, the buccal cavity of the mouth, underneath the eyelids, within the nasal cavity, underneath the scalp in autopsied bodies, and the inner trunk walls in autopsied bodies.

The chemicals used for surface embalming may be liquids, gels, or powders. The liquids most frequently used include accessory surface embalming chemicals and cavity fluid. Cotton compresses saturated with an accessory chemical specifically formulated for the treatment of intact skin are most frequently used both for viewable and for nonviewable body areas. Surface chemicals also include strong formulations of phenol. These chemicals are designed to bleach, dry, and cauterize tissue. Cavity fluid compresses may be used to treat intact and broken skin.

Cavity fluid and the accessory surface chemicals may be milder than phenol solutions and are designed to preserve, bleach, dry, and deodorize the tissues. The stronger phenol solutions bleach, preserve, dry, and cauterize tissues. Cotton should be soaked with the chemical and applied to the skin area needing fluid. The cotton should then be covered with plastic. The plastic reduces the fumes and keeps the compress from drying. The compress may need to be left on several hours.

Gels constitute a second surface embalming chemical. Years ago, formalin creams were used for surface embalming. In the early 1960s, surface preservative gels were introduced. These can be applied directly to the skin with a large brush or they can be poured onto cotton and applied as a pack. The gels are available in an almost-liquid form of very low viscosity or in a very heavy "jelly" of very high viscosity. When used on external surfaces, gels should also be covered with plastic to reduce fumes and to prevent evaporation. These chemicals are designed to penetrate the tissues. They should remain affixed to nonviewed body areas. Cotton compresses with the liquid surface preservatives should also remain on body areas that will not be viewed. In areas that will be cosmetically treated and viewed, the chemicals should be left on the skin several hours.

Arterial fluid is not recommended as a surface embalming chemical, for the dyes present in the fluid stain the skin surface. Their penetrating strength and preservative strength may be less than those of cavity fluid, accessory surface chemicals, or gels. When a surface compress (gel or liquid) is removed from an area to which cosmetics will be applied, the area should be cleaned with a solvent before cosmetic treatment begins.

Specific Treatments

Specific areas are discussed to show how surface embalming can establish good preservation.

Mouth, Lips, and Cheeks. Cotton can be placed over the dentures and saturated with cavity fluid, using a hypodermic needle and syringe to moisten the cotton. The lips can then be glued; the preservative works from

* When any surface chemicals are used, the compress or gel should be covered with plastic so as to reduce fumes and to prevent the surface chemical from evaporating.

the inside of the mouth to preserve the tissues. Cosmetic treatment can be immediately implemented using this method of preservation.

Eyelids. Cotton can be used for eye closure or a small piece of cotton can be inserted over the top of an eyecap. The cotton can be moistened with a few drops of cavity fluid and the eyelids sealed with an adhesive. Cosmetic treatment can begin immediately (Figure 15–1).

Dehydration. If tissues need the preservative they will not dehydrate. Underembalmed tissue can dehydrate faster than well-embalmed tissue. Gluing the eyes and mouth further reduces any dehydration problems. Visible areas treated by internal surface compresses or hypodermic preservative treatments can be cosmetized using a cream-based cosmetic to retard dehydration.

Nose. Cotton saturated with preservative fluid can be inserted into the nostrils. It can later be pushed back far enough that it will not be noticeable.

The preceding areas can also be treated with external surface packs; however, the application of cosmetics must be delayed.

For areas that will not be seen, such as the leg or foot, the gel can be applied to the skin surface or poured into a plastic stocking. The latter reduces fumes and makes application easier.

Surface embalming powders have been used for many years.* Diapers can be used to apply the powder or the powder can be placed in plastic garments such as stockings, coveralls, or pants after the garments are in position. Powders can also be used to treat the interior walls of the abdomen and thorax in the autopsied body. Powders are not as effective as gels or liquids. Read the label to be certain the powder is a preservative and not just a deodorant. (Note: *An excellent way to treat a gangrenous limb is to pour preservative gel into a plastic stocking along with some preservative powder. Place the stocking on the leg. The powder sticks to the sides of the stocking along with the gel. This combination helps to establish preservation and control odors.)*

Hypodermic Embalming

The second and most effective supplemental method of embalming is hypodermic embalming. This method is used to treat small localized body areas or large areas, such as the trunk walls of the autopsied body or a limb that did not receive sufficient arterial fluid and cannot be injected arterially.

Hypodermic injection involves the use of a hypodermic syringe and needles ranging from 6 to 19 gauge and of varying lengths. The larger needles (6 gauge) are useful for large areas. An infant trocar or specially designed hypovalve trocar can be connected to the centrifugal embalming machine for the injection of large body areas.

* When embalming powders are being used, the embalmer must wear a protective particulate mask and the room should be properly ventilated to remove powder particulate and fumes.

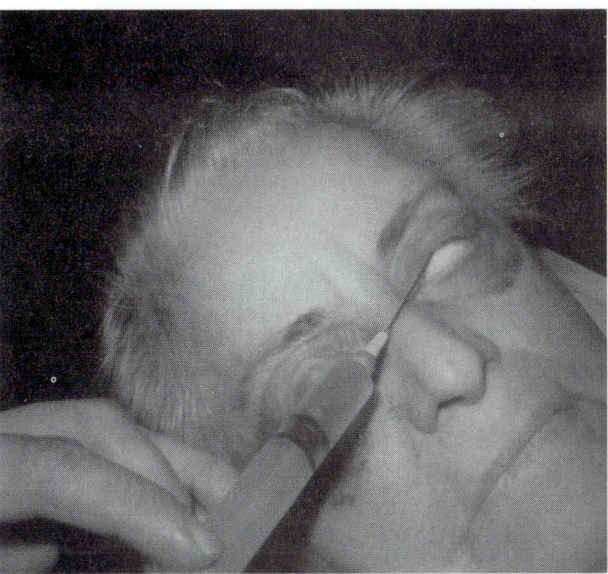

Figure 15–1. Placing cotton moistened with several drops of concentrated cavity fluid under the eyelids ensures good preservation of the lids. Seal eyelids with superglue. Cosmetic treatment can then begin.

The arterial solution used for arterial injection can be used for hypodermic injection. It is recommended that it be strengthened with cavity fluid or a high-index arterial fluid. This type of solution should be used only on body areas that will not be viewed, as the dye in the fluid can blotch the skin. Cavity fluid as well as specially designed accessory embalming chemicals may be used for hypodermic embalming. Phenol solutions should be reserved for localized treatments of discolored areas or tissues when bleaching of tissues is necessary. The phenol solutions would not be used for routine supplemental hypodermic embalming.

In nonviewable areas where the infant trocar or hypovalve trocar has been used, the punctures can be sealed with a trocar button. In facial areas, where hypodermic needles would be used, most of the injections can be made from inside the mouth. In this manner, leakage will not exit onto the face. Unlike tissue builder, these chemicals have a tendency to seep from the point of puncture. If the inside of the nose is to be used as an entry point for hypodermic embalming, use the nostril **opposite** the side of the face being treated. For example, if the right cheek needs arterial fluid, inject the right cheek from the left nostril. Pass the needle under the septum and enter the right cheek or upper right mouth. This reduces fluid leakage. In the autopsied body large portions of the face can be reached through scalp incisions.

The hands and fingers can be injected from the palmar surface of the hand or from between the fingers. Super adhesive can be applied to prevent leakage.

The nose can be treated hypodermically by inserting the needle inside the mouth. The ear can be reached by hypodermic injection from behind the ear. Application of super adhesive to the punctures prevents leakage.

For larger areas such as the arm and leg, the infant trocar can be inserted into the area of the cubital fossa of the arm to reach the arm and forearm. The leg can be treated by inserting the infant trocar on the medial side of the leg just inferior or superior to the knee. From this point, both the thigh and lower leg can be reached.

Combination Treatments for Large Areas

Certain conditions such as arteriosclerosis, gangrene, and edema require additional injection of the legs. If arterial treatment is unsuccessful the legs can be injected hypodermically. In addition, surface embalming can also be used. The legs can be painted with autopsy gels and embalming powder can be placed into the plastic stockings. A combination of supplemental embalming methods (hypodermic and surface) is used.

In the trunk area, hypodermic injection is used when edema is present. Coveralls can be applied and embalming powder or autopsy gel painted over the areas being treated. When edema is a problem in the elbow area, hypodermic treatment can be used and the area painted with autopsy gel and wrapped with gauze. A plastic sleeve can then be placed over the treated area.

▶ CLOSURE OF INCISIONS

Today, two methods are used to close incisions: sutures and super adhesive. Regardless of the method of closure, the embalmer must follow several steps to prepare all incisions for closure:

1. Be certain all vessels are securely tied. This prevents any further leakage.
2. Dry the incision with cotton.
3. If there is edema in the surrounding tissues, force as much liquid out of the incision as possible.
4. Do not suture until after cavity aspiration; aspiration relieves pressure on the vascular system and helps to prevent leakage.
5. Tightly close all sutures.
6. During suturing or prior to gluing, place an absorbent powder (or absorbent clay, "mortuary putty") in the incision to absorb any moisture that may accumulate.
7. Make several sutures before applying the incision seal powder to the incision. In this manner, a "pocket" is created and the powder is retained within the incision and not spread on the surface of the body (Figure 15–2D).
8. After suturing, apply a surface glue over the area to prevent leakage.

Suturing

Cotton or Linen Thread. Linen thread is stronger than cotton thread and is recommended for autopsy and vessel incision sutures. For restorative sutures, which are located on visible areas, dental floss is an excellent material to use.

A $\frac{3}{8}$-inch Circle Needle. The $\frac{3}{8}$-inch circle needle is used for restorative sutures and to suture incisions made to raise vessels.

Double-Curved Autopsy Needle. The double-curved autopsy needle is easy to grip with the gloved hand. It is used to close autopsy incisions, surgical incisions, and incisions made to raise vessels.

Needles come in a variety of sizes and shapes, for example, single-curved autopsy needles, loopyt needles, and circle needles. Some have a "patented eye." These eyes are threaded by merely pushing the thread against the eye portion of the needle, which eliminates the need to pass thread through the eye of the needle. Regardless of the size or the shape of the needle, it is most important to keep it sharp. Suturing can be very dangerous if the needles are dull, as extra pressure must be applied. In doing so, the embalmer increases the chance of the needle breaking or piercing her or his skin. A sharp needle makes suturing much easier, safer, and faster.

Keep in mind that when suturing, one should pull on the thread and not on the needle to tighten the suture. Pulling on the needle weakens the suture cord where it passes through the needle's eye. In closing long sutures, as in autopsies, this may cause the cord to break.

The embalmer can suture using single- or double-stranded thread. This depends on the strength of the suture cord or on the type of suture. It is wise to double the cord when cotton thread or three- or four-twist linen thread is used. Single-stranded suture cord works best with five- and six-twist linen thread, dental floss, and single and double intradermal and worm sutures.

Direction of Suturing

To make suturing more efficient, follow these directions for the various sutures.

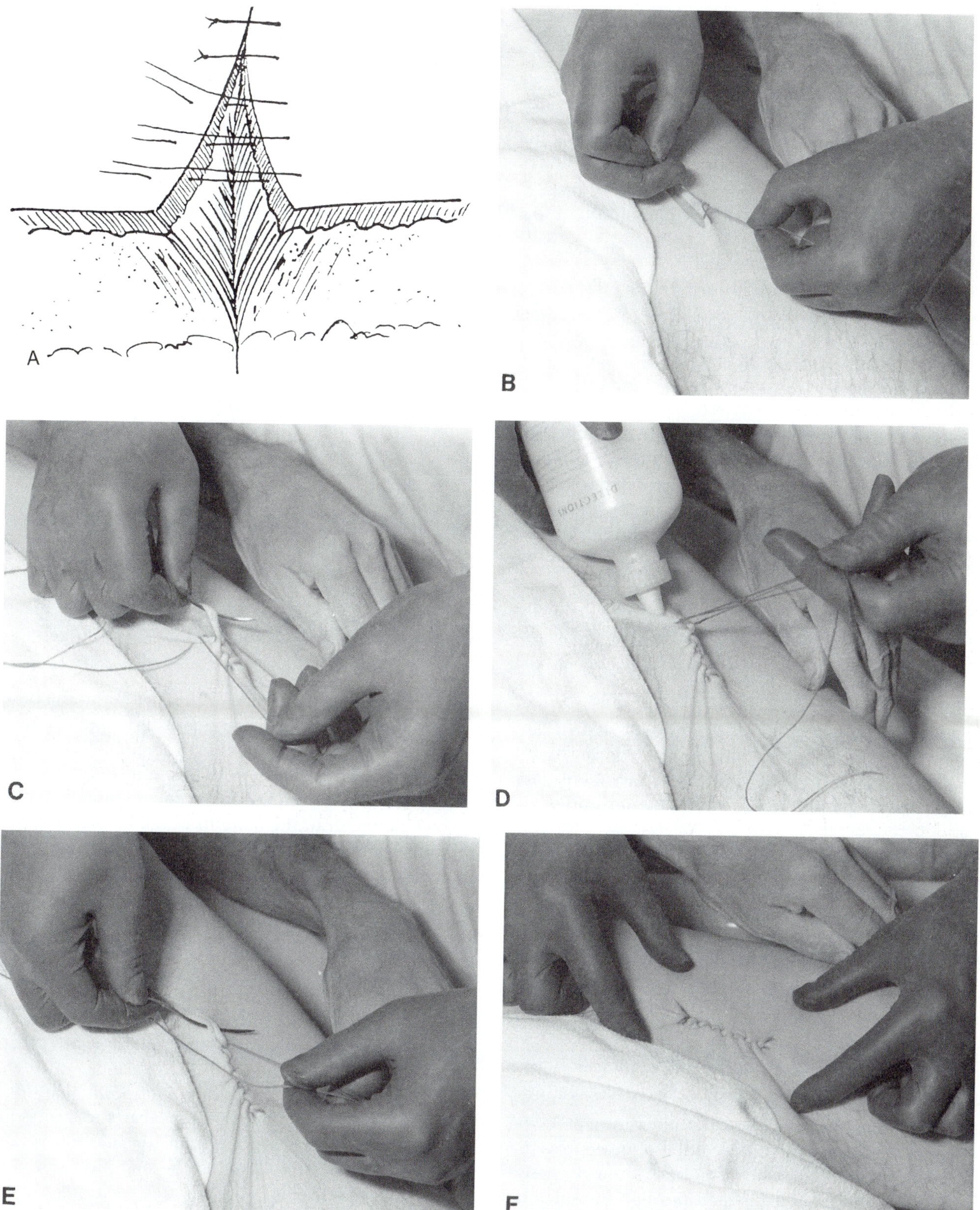

Figure 15–2. A. Individual (bridge) sutures. **B.** Baseball stitch. The ligature is tied in place. Knots should be avoided. **C.** Sutures are made from inside the incision. **D.** A pocket is made before the suture ends and incision seal powder is inserted. **E.** When properly sewn, no string should be visible. **F.** The completed suture. The ligature cord should not be visible. These sutures are airtight.

Common Carotid Artery. If using the parallel incision, suture from the inferior portion of the incision superiorly. Suture from the medial portion of the incision laterally if using a supraclavicular incision.

Axillary Artery. Suture from the medial area of the incision laterally (with the arm abducted).

Brachial Artery. Suture from the medial portion of the incision laterally.

Radial and Ulnar Arteries. Suture from the distal portion of the incision medially.

Femoral Artery. Suture from the inferior portion of the incision superiorly.

Autopsies (Trunk Standard "Y" Incision). Use bridge sutures to align the skin into position. Begin the trunk suturing at the pubic symphysis and suture superiorly.

Popliteal Artery. Begin the suture at the inferior (or distal) portion of the incision and suture superiorly.

Anterior and Posterior Tibial Arteries. Begin the sutures distally and suture superiorly.

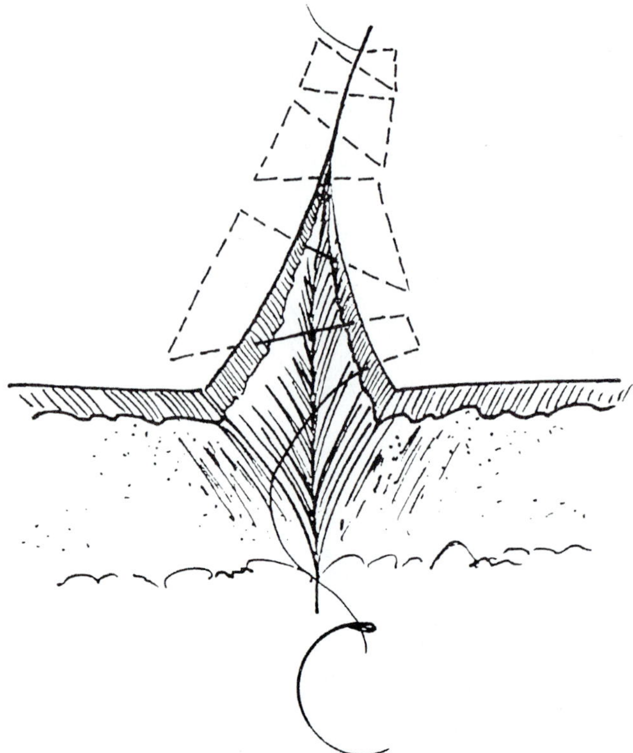

Figure 15–3. Single intradermal (hidden) suture.

Common Sutures

Individual (Bridge) Sutures. Individual sutures are used to align tissues into position prior to, during, or after embalming (Figure 15–2A). They are temporary and are later replaced by more permanent sutures.

Baseball Sutures. Considered the most secure and commonly used, the baseball suture can be airtight. In addition to the injection site incisions, it is used for autopsy stitching. To make this stitch, pass a suture needle and thread from beneath the incision up through the integument, and cross the needle from side to side with each stitch (Figure 15–2B). This creates a strong tight closure. In the process, however, the tissues adjacent to the incision are pulled up into a ridge.

Single Intradermal (Hidden) Suture. The single subcutaneous or intradermal suture is made with one needle and a single thread (Figure 15–3). It is referred to as the "hidden stitch," because it is used on exposed areas of the body and is directed through the subcutaneous tissue only. To begin the closure, insert the needle deep into the tissues at one end of the incision. Make a knot in the thread a short distance from the end and pull the knot to the position of the needle puncture in the integument. Keeping the needle directed through the dermal tissues only, develop a back-and-forth pattern from one side of the incision to the other. Take care to line up the margins as the thread is drawn so that there are no gaps between stitches. To complete the closure, direct the needle through the integument as far as possible from the end of the incision. Once this is completed, draw the margins of the incision together by pulling the free end of the thread. Puckering may result if the thread is pulled too tight. The excess thread is cut off close to the incision as slight pressure is applied, concealing the ends of the thread.

Double Intradermal Suture. The double intradermal suture is made with two needles threaded with opposite ends of the same thread (Figure 15–4A). Because this suture is permanently fixed at each end, it has greater holding ability than the single intradermal suture. Pass each needle through the dermis at opposite margins so that both stitches are parallel, similar to the lacing on a shoe. Continue the process until the incision is completely sutured. After drawing the margins tight, knot the two ends together within the incision. Correct puckering by light massage or smoothing with the finger. To end the suture, insert both threads onto one needle and insert it under the skin from the end of the incision to a point $\frac{1}{2}$ inch away. The excess threads are then cut as pressure is applied, resulting in the ends of the threads being hidden.

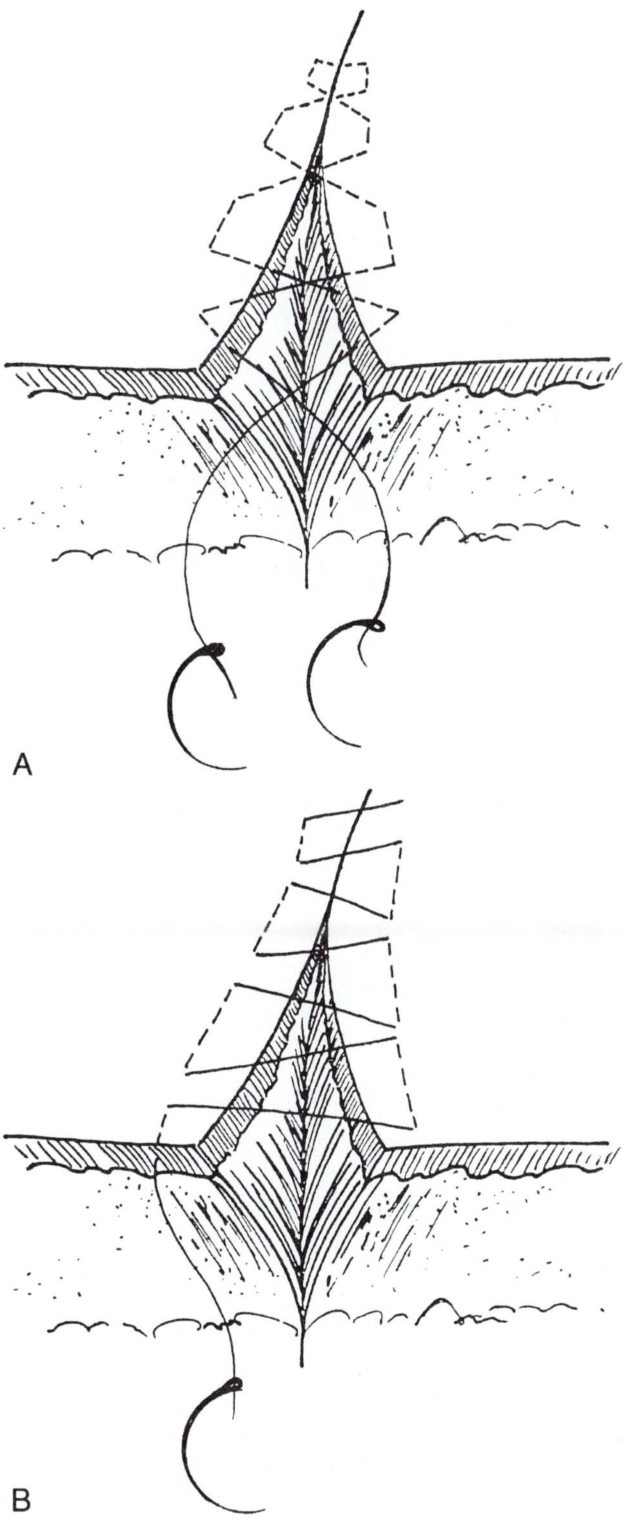

Figure 15-4. A. Double intradermal suture. **B.** Inversion (worm) suture.

Inversion (Worm) Suture. The inversion suture is used to gather in and turn under excess tissues (Figure 15–4B). The pattern of this suture is the same as that of the single intradermal suture, except that the stitches are made parallel to the incision edges and do not pierce the margins of the incision. The stitches are generally made as close to the margins as possible. The best results are obtained by making the stitches uniform in length. The stitches do not enter the incision except to start the suture. Each stitch should be drawn taut as sewn. The worm suture is not visible and may be waxed as needed. It is an excellent suture for closing a carotid incision or closing the scalp on the cranial autopsy (Figure 15–5).

Interlocking (Lock) Suture. The interlocking suture creates a tight, leakproof closure. It has a disadvantage in that an unsightly ridge appears on the surface of the incision. Begin the suture at one end of the incision and direct the needle through the tissue so that it passes through both sides of the incision from the outside. Keep the thread tight with the hand not holding the suture needle. Then, lock the stitch by looping the needle through the thread. When completing the loop, pull the thread tight. Repeat this process until the incision is closed. The needle insertion should be made consistently from the same side of the incision.

Continuous (Whip) Suture. The continuous suture is generally used to close long incisions (Figure 15–6). Frequently, it is used by the autopsy technician to close the long incisions from the autopsy. This suture prevents leakage of fluids from the body cavities during transfer from the hospital to the funeral home. The suture is also seen in people who have died during surgery; the incision has been drawn closed to prevent leakage of fluids. Organ transplant retrieval teams use the stitch to close long incisions after the removal of visceral organs. To make this stitch, anchor the suture thread. Pass the needle through both sides of the incision, starting on the outside of the tissue on one side of the incision and passing directly through and out the tissues of the opposite side of the incision. Pass the thread over the top of the incision and begin the next stitch $\frac{1}{2}$ to 1 inch beyond the previous stitch. The process is completed when the incision is closed.

Adhesives

The other method of closing incisions involves the use of a super adhesive. Many brands are available today in local stores. Most super glues can work in the presence of moist tissues. These adhesives are excellent for closing jagged tears in the skin.

Many embalmers use the glues to close the incisions made to raise vessels. Some use the glues to close

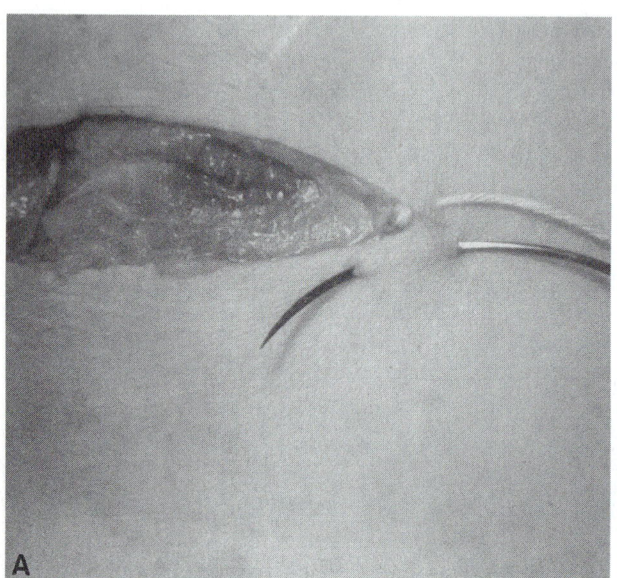

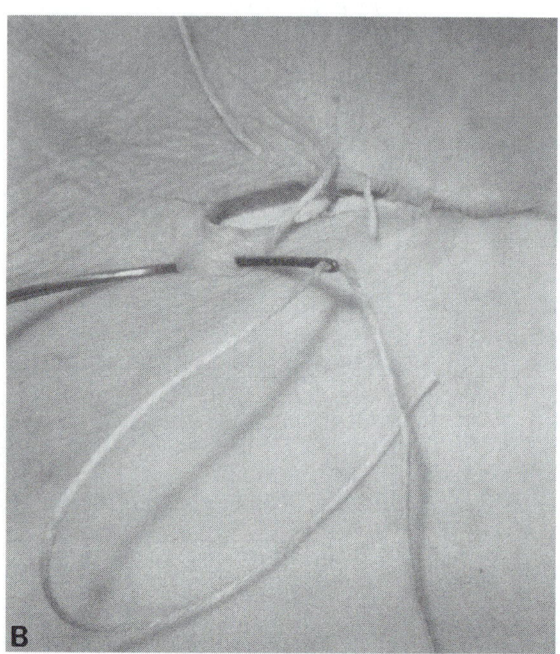

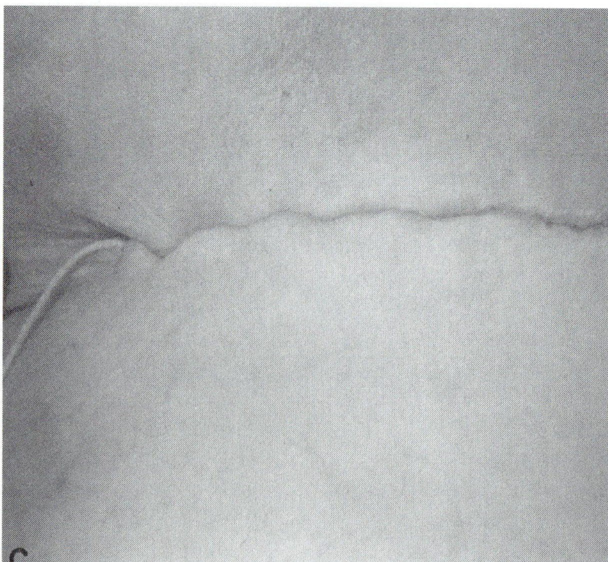

Figure 15–5. Worm suture. All stitches are made on the surface of the skin. **A.** Worm suture begun. **B.** Worm suture concluded. **C.** A flat (easily waxed) surface is created with the worm suture.

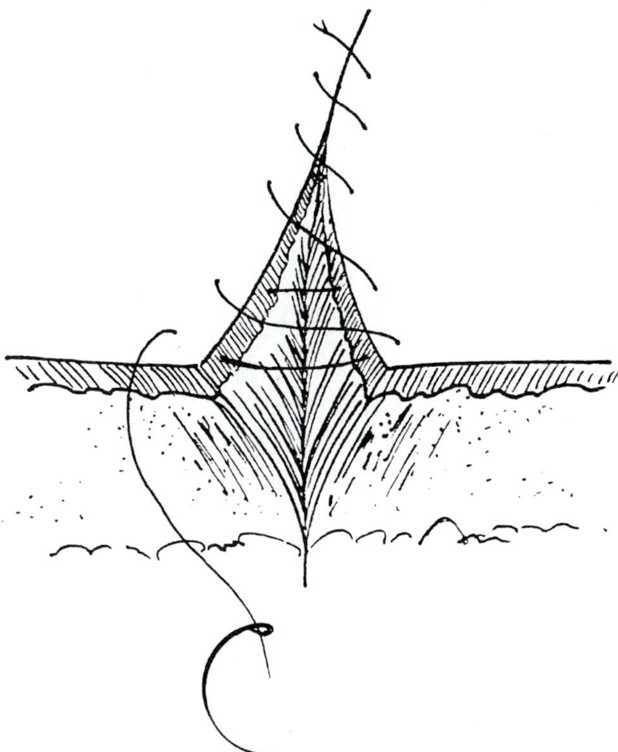

Figure 15–6. Continuous (whip) stitch.

the scalp in cranial autopsies. Long autopsy incisions, however, are closed with sutures. As there are many uses for these glues in the embalming room, super glues should be kept in stock.

▶ REMOVAL OF BODY-INVASIVE DEVICES

Many hospitals do not remove the intravenous needles or tubes from bodies after death. It is best to leave these needles and tubes in place until *after* arterial injection. If the needle is in an artery, considerable swelling will result if the needle is removed prior to arterial injection. A similar problem arises when needles or tubes inserted into veins are removed prior to embalming. A large ecchymosis or swelling and discoloration can develop. These punctures can be sealed with a drop of super glue. Tissue builder or a phenol solution injected beneath the skin also helps to seal these punctures on visible skin areas. When the needle or tube has been placed into the subclavian or jugular vein a small incision can be made, and the area filled with incision seal powder, then sutured with a small tight baseball suture. If the area will not be seen, a trocar button may be used to seal the puncture.

Pacemakers. A pacemaker should be removed if the body is to be cremated. Certain radioactive powered

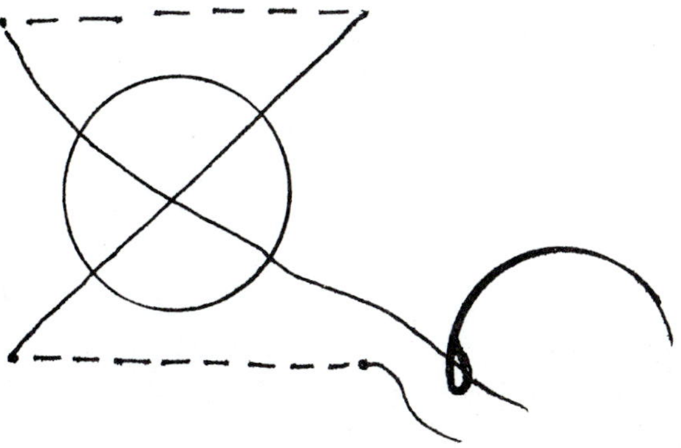

Figure 15–7. "N" suture.

units must be returned to the manufacturer. A small incision can be made over the device, which is usually located in the upper right pectoral region. The wire leading to the heart is cut. Incision seal powder is placed in the pocket and the incision sutured.

Colostomy Closures. Remove the colostomy collecting bag. Pour some cavity fluid into the bag for disinfection before destroying it. Disinfect the body area and colostomy stump with cavity fluid or a phenol solution on cotton. By placing pressure on the stump and slightly twisting, force the piece of bowel back into the abdominal cavity. A purse-string or "N" suture can be used to close the colostomy (Figure 15–7). Surface glue may be applied to the closure after the body is washed and dried. The colostomy opening may be closed before or after arterial injection.

Surgical Drains. Remove surgical drains and close the openings using a purse-string suture. Surface glue may be applied after the body is washed and dried to prevent leakage.

▶ FINAL WASHING AND DRYING OF THE BODY*

After all sutures are completed and points of leakage sealed, the body should be washed and thoroughly dried. Particular attention should be given to the removal of blood from the surface of the body. A washcloth or rough-surfaced material will help to loosen the blood. Lukewarm water and plenty of antiseptic soap should be used. Care should be given to the washing of the hair, especially if the jugular vein has been used for

* Proper preparation room attire—gown, gloves, and, if necessary, mask and eye protection—should be worn during these postembalming procedures.

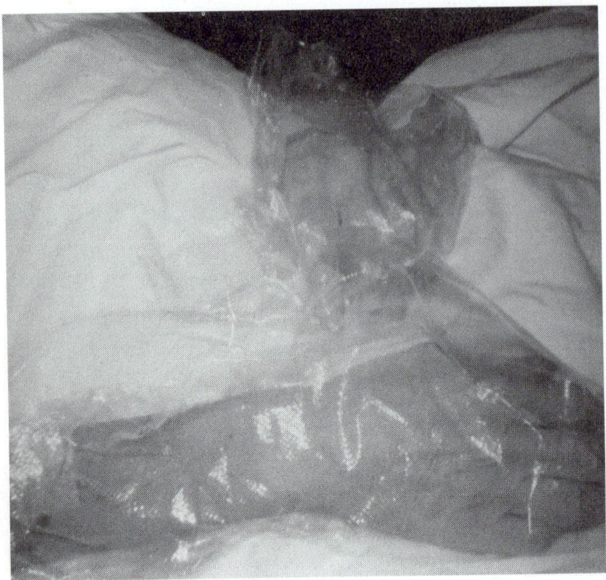

Figure 15–8. Cosmetized hands protected by plastic during dressing and casketing.

drainage. A conditioner rinse can be massaged into the hair during washing to help eliminate tangles and deodorize the hair. If the scalp exhibits a lot of dander of flaking, wash the hair several times and thoroughly dry with a hair dryer. (This pertains to men as well as women.) Attached hairpieces, natural curly hair and permed hair should be dried with cool air so the hair does not straighten. If plats are present, especially in an African-American, it may be wise to consult with the family prior to combing them out when the hair is washed.

The body should be carefully dried. Good drying eliminates mold growth on the skin surface, especially in warm climates. Turning the body on its side gives the embalmer an opportunity to examine the posterior area. After the body has been dried, any intravenous punctures or punctures used to draw postmortem blood samples can be sealed with a super adhesive (Figure 15–8).

▶ TREATMENT OF ULCERATIONS, LESIONS, AND DISCOLORATIONS

After the body has been washed and dried, the sutures have been closed, and invasive devices have been removed and their punctures sealed, the embalmer should treat those lesions (e.g., decubitus ulcers) and discolorations (e.g., an ecchymosis on the back of the hand) on visible areas. Of course, decubitus ulcers should have been treated (preservative surface compresses) at the beginning of the embalming. After embalming, these ulcerations are redressed with compresses of phenol solution, accessory surface embalming chemicals, cavity fluid, or autopsy gels. This redressing helps to ensure preservation and sanitization.

Dry the tissues and deodorize the ulceration. Plastic clothing (overalls, pants, and stockings) can be placed on the body to help control odors. The buttocks may be diapered. The embalmer can inject the area around the decubitus ulcer with cavity fluid or accessory chemicals designed to combat the gas bacillus that forms tissue gas. The solution may be injected with a large-diameter hypodermic needle (6 gauge) or an infant trocar. Gloves should be worn in dressing these ulcerations. A mask is also advisable. Decubitus ulcers will be located at pressure points—the buttocks, shoulders, and heels.

Surface compresses containing phenol solution, an accessory bleaching solution, or cavity fluid can be applied to discolorations (e.g., an ecchymosis on the back of a hand). These discolorations can also be treated internally by hypodermic injection of the same chemical into the discolored areas. With this method, cosmetics may be applied without the delay needed for surface chemicals to work.

If any "raw skin areas" are present in viewable areas, the tissues should be dried at this time. Chemical compresses of a surface preservative chemical (or cavity chemical) can be applied over the areas. These compresses should remain in place for several hours. When the compresses are removed, the tissues should be cleaned with a solvent and thoroughly dried with a hair dryer. If arterial fluid seeps through these broken skin areas during injection, some embalmers simply remove all loose skin, clean with a solvent, and dry with a hair dryer.

▶ TREATMENT OF PURGE

After arterial and cavity embalming, there always exists the possibility of purge from the anus, mouth, or nose, generally because cavity fluid is present in a position or an amount that allows its exit from one of these orifices. The injected cavity fluid may have built up enough pressure to purge materials from the upper respiratory tract, upper esophageal area, or rectum. Tightly packing the nasal passages, throat, and rectum prior to arterial injection should eliminate this problem. This will help to contain odors, prevent purging, and prevent any soiling of the clothing or casket interior.

When anal purge is present after embalming, force as much purge as possible from the rectum by firmly pressing on the lower abdominal area. Pack the rectum using cotton saturated with cavity fluid, autopsy gel, or a phenol solution. Dry packing should be inserted into the anal orifice after the moistened cotton. Leave a portion of the dry cotton so it can be seen. This will help to fully block the anal orifice.

When purge is present from the mouth or nose immediately following arterial injection and cavity treatment, it may be necessary to immediately reaspirate the body and reinject cavity fluid. Clean out the orifices and be certain they are tightly packed with plenty of dry cotton or cotton webbing.

The purge observed at the conclusion of embalming is not the same purge observed several hours after embalming (caused by the buildup of pressure from gases that form in the body cavities). This immediate postembalming purge is generally the result of cavity embalming. Prior to dressing and casketing, reaspirate the body cavities and, if gas is present, reinject the cavities.

▶ TREATMENT OF DISTENSION

Visible areas—face, neck, and hands—that are distended often need to be reduced for viewing of the body. These treatments can be carried out during the postembalming period. Some swellings, such as edema, can be treated by specific arterial solutions during arterial injection. It is necessary to know the cause of the distension to perform a corrective treatment. Swellings present prior to arterial injection should be noted on the *embalming report*. Examples of such conditions include edema, tumors, swellings caused by trauma, distension from gases of decomposition in the tissues or cavities, tissue gas produced by *Clostridium perfringens*, distension caused by allergic reactions, distension brought about by use of steroid drugs, and gases in the tissues from subcutaneous emphysema.

Distension of facial tissues, the neck, or glandular tissues of the face or the tissues surrounding the eye orbit during embalming of the body can be caused by an excessive amount of arterial solution in these tissues. Some of the causes of this swelling are very rapid injection of solution, use of too much injection pressure, poor drainage from these tissues, breakdown of the capillaries (possibly decomposition) in these tissues, excessive massage, and use of arterial solutions that are too weak. It is essential during embalming of the body that the embalmer is alert to any tissue distension. Injection should be immediately stopped and the situation evaluated. If correction of distended tissue involves excision of tissue (e.g., goiter, tumor), permisson must be obtained from the persons in charge of disposition of the body.

Areas of the body that contain skeletal edema should be treated during the embalming period with fluids of sufficient strength to meet the preservative demands of the tissues and, at the same time, reduce the edema. Edema of the face and hands can be somewhat corrected in the postembalming period, if adequate preservation has been achieved.

In pitting edema, excess moisture is present in the tissue spaces. In solid edema, the excess moisture is within the cells. Pitting edema can be moved by mechanical aids such as gravitation, massage, channeling of the area, and application of pressure (e.g., pneumatic collar, weights, elastic bandage, water collar, digital pressure) to move the moisture to another area. Elevation of the head and firm digital pressure slowly drain pitting edema from the facial tissues. During cavity aspiration, the trocar can be used to channel the neck, which allows the edema to drain from the facial tissues into the thorax. Edema of the eyes can be treated in several ways: (1) surface compresses using cavity fluid, phenol compound, or autopsy gel, during and after injection; (2) cavity fluid on cotton under the eyelids, during and after injection; (3) hypodermic injection of phenol compound or cavity fluid after embalming.

After preservation of the lids is accomplished channels can be made under the skin (e.g., from within the mouth, temple area): carefully applying external pressure to the distended tissues, "massage" as much of the edema from the tissues of the eyelids as possible. Drainage areas, such as in the temple area, can be sealed later with a drop of super adhesive. The primary problem that arises in removing edema from the facial tissues or hands is that the skin may become very wrinkled. Tissue preservation must always be the first concern.

Subcutaneous emphysema is frequently seen when the lung has been punctured. It may be the result of a surgical procedure (e.g., tracheotomy), a bullet wound in the thorax, or a broken rib that tears into the lung. Cardiopulmonary resuscitation can fracture a rib and tear the lung. Gas escapes into the subcutaneous tissues. As the individual struggles to breathe, more air is forced into the body tissues. Gases can easily be detected after death by palpating the tissues. The term **crepitation** is used to describe the spongy feel of the gas as it moves through the tissues when they are pushed on. Arterial injection and blood drainage remove a small portion of the gas, but gas that is trapped in the facial tissues must be removed by channeling. This channeling can be done after the body is embalmed. The lips can be opened and a scalpel, bistoury knife, or large hypodermic needle used to channel the tissues of the face from inside the mouth (Figure 15–9). Once the channels are made the gas can be pushed out of the tissues. If the eyes are affected the lids can be everted and the underside of the lids incised with a suture or hypodermic needle. Cotton can be used to close the eyes; it will also absorb any leakage.

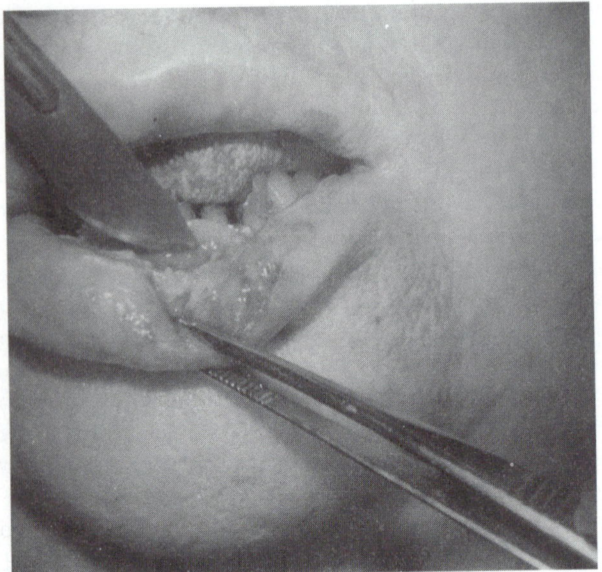

Figure 15–9. After embalming, the lips are lanced to release gases in the tissues.

Subcutaneous emphysema can be differentiated from true tissue gas. True tissue gas has a very distinct foul odor that worsens progressively and is caused by an anaerobic bacterium. Blebbing and skin-slip develop with true tissue gas. (See Chapter 24 for treatments of true tissue gas.)

▶ RESETTING AND GLUING THE FEATURES

The features can be corrected after embalming. Additional cotton or feature posing compound can be inserted to fill out sunken and emaciated cheeks. If the cotton that was originally used to set the features becomes moist during the embalming, as a result of contact with purge or blood and fluid from the suture or needle injector used for mouth closure, it should be replaced with dry cotton.

The dentures are not always available at the beginning of the embalming. The mouth can be reopened and the dentures inserted afterward. These procedures are, of course, more difficult when the tissues are firm. Eyes, too, can be closed or reset after arterial injection. (Refer to Chapter 18 for a discussion of the postembalming procedures employed when eye enucleation has been performed.)

After the features have been properly aligned and the cavity embalming has been completed, the features can be glued. Adhesive applied to the lips and eyelids helps to avoid the separation caused by dehydration. The area where the adhesive is to be applied should first be cleaned with a solvent. Rubber-based adhesive, which is often used for the mouth and eyes, does not work well on a moist or oily surface. The skin of the lips and margins of the eyelids should be clean, dry, and free of moisture or oils. Super adhesive works very well for securing the eyelids. It ensures good closure of the inner canthus.

When glue is applied to the mucous membranes it is advised that it be kept behind the "weather line." This is not always possible. In some elderly persons or in individuals in whom blisters are removed from the mucous membranes after the gluing, the mucous membranes are not even visible. New mucous membranes

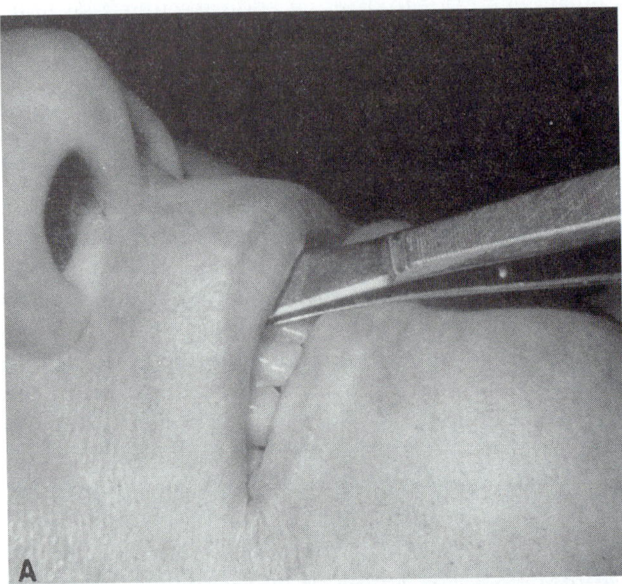

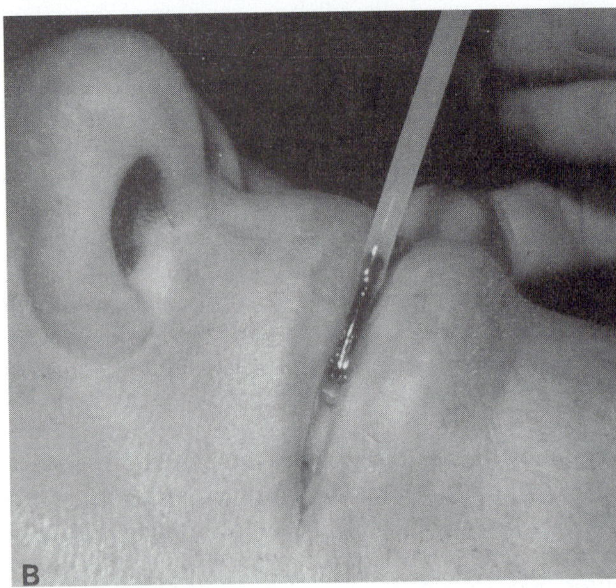

Figure 15–10. A. The lips are exercised with the blunt handle of a pair of forceps. **B.** A rubber-base adhesive or a super adhesive is used to seal the lips.

can be drawn with cosmetics. Gluing helps to place tension on the mucous membranes, and this tension often "pulls" wrinkles from the membranes. Wrinkled lips can be corrected by gluing, waxing, or injecting the mucous membrane with tissue builder.

If the body was shipped, the lips may separate as a result of flight vibrations. Because of the delay, the tissues have time to become very firm. In such cases, the lips can be stretched or exercised with the blunt handle of an aneurysm needle or a pair of forceps (Figure 15–10A). If the eyelids separate, they may also have to be "exercised" or stretched to obtain closure. Super adhesive is more effective in securing the mouth and eyes when the tissues are very firm (Figure 15–10B).

▶ PLASTIC GARMENTS

Prior to dressing, protective plastic garments can be placed on the body. Pants or coveralls can be placed on the trunk and plastic stockings on the legs. Embalming powder should be sprinkled into these plastic goods. The powder deodorizes the body and helps to control mold growth. Plastic sleeves may be applied to broken skin at the elbows or on the arms. Coveralls do not cover the shoulders, however. So, if edema is present in the shoulder area, place the body in a unionall. The unionall covers the arms, trunk (including the shoulders), and legs. Unionalls are very helpful in bodies that show advanced decomposition or extensive burns.

▶ TERMINAL DISINFECTION

Terminal disinfection comprises the disinfection practices carried out after the embalming process to protect the environment and includes personal hygiene for the embalmer as well as disinfection of the instruments, equipment, and preparation room.

Care of the Embalming Machine

After use, the embalming machine should be flushed with warm water. Fluids that contain a humectant such as lanolin or silicon often leave a thick residue in the tank. Ammonia and lukewarm water should be flushed through the machine to remove the residue. Many embalmers prefer to flush the machines with a water softener or the powder used in electric dishwashers. Additives for machine cleaning can be purchased through fluid manufacturers. A final flush with warm water is necessary. It is recommended that the machine be filled with water at this time for the next preparation. This keeps the gaskets moist. Give the water time to release any dissolved gases such as chlorine. Adding embalming fluid (later) to an already filled machine decreases the release of formaldehyde fumes. A lid must be placed on the water tank of the machine.

Surfaces

All surfaces should first be cleaned with cool water and a small amount of antiseptic soap to remove organic debris. Torn-up sheets make good washcloths and can be disposed of after use. A preliminary wash removes organic debris and also any formaldehyde present. Remember that a number of good disinfectants contain chlorine, and this chemical should not come into contact with formaldehyde. Bleach and warm water make a very good cleaning solution. The table, countertops, and drains can be wiped clean and disinfected with this solution. Lysol products are good disinfectants and are easily available. Be certain to clean the area *under* the table surrounding the drainage outlet. Tops of overhead lighting should also be given attention. Tubing used for aspiration should be soaked in a disinfectant solution. Pay attention to handles on cabinets and drawers. Commercial products used for cleaning the preparation room contain dilution instructions. (Refer to Chapter 3 for a review of disinfection practices.)

Instruments

Clean instruments prior to disinfection. Removing organic material from the instrument makes disinfection more effective. Immerse all instruments including trocars in a solution of Bard–Parker disinfectant (8% by volume formaldehyde in 70% ethanol or isopropanol) or in 200 to 300 ppm of an iodophor for 45 minutes or longer. If possible, destroy cutting blades in a biohazards sharps container. Take special care with cutting instruments when gas gangrene or "tissue gas" has been encountered. The causative agent of this condition, *Clostridium perfringens*, is a spore-forming bacillus and can easily be passed via contaminated cutting instruments. They should remain in this solution several hours. After disinfection, instruments should be rinsed, dried, and properly stored (Figure 15–11).

Disinfectant Checklist

In selecting a disinfectant for instruments and other preparation room paraphernalia, keep in mind the characteristics of a good disinfectant:

- Has a wide range of activity (works against viruses, bacteria, and fungi)
- Is of sufficient strength (active against spore-forming organisms of bacilli and fungi)
- Acts in the presence of water
- Is stable and has a reasonably long shelf-life
- Is noncorrosive to metal instruments
- Acts fast
- Is not highly toxic to living tissues or injurious to the respiratory system

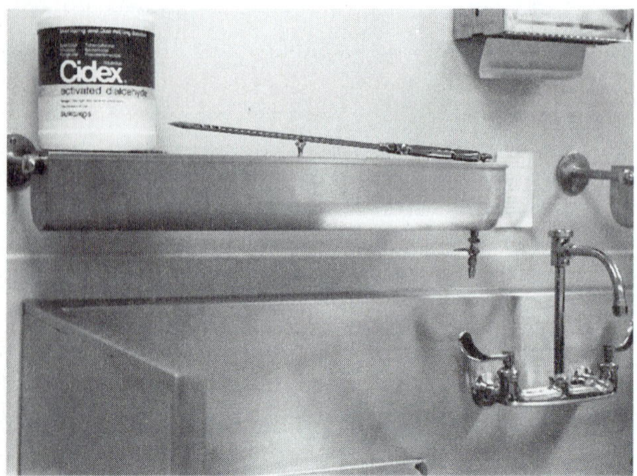

Figure 15–11. Containers of sufficient size must be provided so all instruments can be completely immersed for disinfection.

▶ PERSONAL HYGIENE

Terminal disinfection also concerns the embalmer. *Destroy* gloves after use; gloves are made to be used *once*. Thoroughly wash hands after removing gloves. Keep fingernails short and trimmed to prevent tears in the gloves. Numerous antiseptic preparations are available for washing or applying to the skin after the hands are dried. Consult a hospital supply catalog. Treat all cuts and punctures immediately: disinfect the area, induce bleeding, and consult a physician. Review Chapter 3 for preembalming and postembalming sanitation techniques.

▶ DOCUMENTATION AND SHIPPING PREPARATION

After embalming, the work should be documented. The report should contain information pertaining to the embalming and to all personal property received with the body. Particular attention should be made to the list of jewelry and clothing. A report should accompany all bodies being shipped. When the body has been autopsied and is being shipped, the report should contain information indicating if viscera were returned from the hospital or morgue. Organs and tissues removed at autopsy or for donation must be noted, especially if the eyes have been removed. If the viscera were returned from the hospital and replaced in the body cavities, note how the organs were preserved and note that they have been placed in the cavities.

Later, when the death certificate is available, the cause of death and contributing causes should be added to the report. This may be valuable information for health records of the funeral home employees. If the person died of a contagious or infectious disease, properly label the body if it is being shipped to another funeral home. Bodies should never be shipped without some partial dressing. Place plastic coveralls or pants and undergarments on the body. If undergarments are not provided, clothe the body in pajamas or a hospital gown.

Place the body deep enough in the shipping container that the lid does not press against the face. Remember, in moving bodies on and off planes, the shipping container may be slightly tilted. The body should be firmly secure in the shipping container. Position casket pillows or cardboard packing at the sides, head, and foot of the body to keep it from shifting. Place a large piece of plastic under the body to protect the container from leakage or purge. Arrange cotton around the head and neck and in the nares to absorb any purge that may be released. Let the cotton stick out from the nostrils, so that flies are less likely to be attracted to the body. This practice should always be followed in the summer months when the body is in the preparation room. Careful packing of the nasal, throat, and oral passages prior to embalming is an important factor in preventing any postembalming purge.

When positioning instructions have *not* been given by the receiving funeral home, make certain one of the hands is *not* placed over the other. Hands should be placed on the abdomen. Resting one on top of another (which is a custom in many communities) can mark the covered hand.

A very light coating of massage cream can be placed on the face and hands when the body is to be shipped. Large amounts are not necessary and may be difficult to remove even with a solvent.

If they have not been given instructions by the receiving funeral home, many embalmers do NOT seal the mouth when the body is being shipped. The lips are coated with massage cream. This allows the receiving funeral home an opportunity to be certain the mouth is dry, allows any gases created by the movement of the shipping of the body to escape from the mouth, and permits tissue building to be done from inside the mouth. The body will be reaspirated by the receiving funeral home; any reconstruction work will be performed by them.

▶ MONITORING: SURVEILLANCE OF THE CASKETED REMAINS UNTIL DISPOSITION

It is the duty of the funeral establishment having custody of the remains (either casketed or waiting to be casketed or to be shipped uncasketed) during the postembalming period to observe the appearance of the body and to correct any problems that might arise.

Detailed examinations should be made before and after each visitation period. Likewise uncasketed remains should be daily inspected for any changes.

Postembalming problems include, but are not limited to, dehydration of tissues, purge, leakage from incisions (embalming or antemortem surgical), leakage from any antemortem invasive treatments, softening and discoloring of tissues, gas formation, separation of lips or eyelids, leakage from areas where edema is present, odors, maggots, and needed cosmetic changes. If any of these conditions are noted, immediate steps should be taken to make a correction.

Cosmetic Corrections

Areas of the face, neck, hands, or arms may reveal color changes in the skin. The causes include greening of tissues affected by jaundice, darkening of the skin due to dehydration, darkening of the skin due to insufficient preservation of the area, and darkening from minor trauma. Where softening of the skin or darkening from trauma or ecchymosis has occurred, the area should first be treated by hypodermic injection of undiluted cavity fluid or application of a surface compress (it needs to remain in contact with the skin for several hours). These areas and dehydrated areas can be covered with a variety of opaque cosmetic "undercoats"; an adjustment can easily be made with cream cosmetics.

Separated Tissues

Tissues such as the lips and eyelids may separate due to dehydration, improper gluing, or motion and handling if the body has been shipped. These tissues should be "exercised" to establish good contact. The contact surfaces should be cleaned with a good solvent and a super adhesive applied. Lips may also be "filled out" with tissue builder to establish contact of the surfaces or they may be waxed.

Leakage

Potential areas of leakage could include some of the following:

- Any area of trauma to the face or hands where the skin was broken or torn
- Cranial autopsy incisions
- Autopsy sutures
- Surgical sutures
- Sutures at sites where vessels were raised for arterial injection
- Areas where edema is present
- Intravenous punctures
- Punctures used for drawing postmortem blood samples
- Any point where the skin has been broken

Minor seepage (e.g., intravenous puncture) may be corrected by wiping away the accumulated liquid, injecting a phenol compound to cauterize the area, and sealing the puncture with a super adhesive. Where the skin has been torn, a phenol compound surface compress (or a cavity fluid compress) can be applied; later the area can be cleaned with a solvent, dried with a hair dryer, and sealed with a super adhesive or surface glue.

Clothing can be protected by sheets of plastic. The casket interior, pillow, and clothing should be inspected for any signs of leakage. If leakage is judged severe, the body should be removed from the casket and carefully undressed. Incisions can be opened, dried, checked to be certain vessels are ligated, and resutured using large amounts of incision seal powder within the incisions. Plastic garments can be placed on the body and, if necessary, edges sealed with duct tape. Interior damage may be severe enough to require replacement. Casket pillows can be reversed for minor leakage. Blankets and clothing may need to be replaced.

Purge

If purge has occurred it will be necessary to reaspirate the body. No doubt the body will have to be taken back to the preparation room for this procedure. Not only should the body be thoroughly reaspirated, but the cavities should also be reinjected with undiluted cavity fluid. If gases were noted when the trocar button was removed leave the body in the preparation room, if possible, for several hours and repeat the treatments again before redressing the body. The mouth and nasal cavities should be checked for dryness and tightly repacked with cotton or cotton webbing. The lips can then be resealed and recosmetized. Distended eyelids may indicate the presence of gases in the tissues. It may be necessary with this condition to aspirate the cranial cavity and inject some cavity fluid into the anterior cranial cavity. The presence of true tissue gas may necessitate reembalming of the body.

Maggots

Infestation of body with maggots is a nightmare experienced by few embalmers today. In the summer months, bodies should be carefully examined for fly eggs, in particular the corners of the eyes, within the mouth, and the nostrils. If maggots are present, they can be picked from the surface of the body with cotton saturated with a dry hair wash. To stimulate maggots to emerge to the surface from areas beneath the skin or from the mouth or nostrils, the areas can be swabbed with a petroleum product (kerosene has been used by many embalmers). As the maggots emerge on the skin surface they can be removed with cotton saturated with dry hair wash. They should be placed in plastic bags before being discarded. The problem with maggots is not knowing if all have been found. If they persist it may become necessary to close the casket. Maggots in the clothing and hair can be vacuumed with a suction vacuum. The dust bag then can be destroyed.

Mold

In warm climates, mold can be a problem when bodies are being held for long periods. Bodies should be thoroughly dried to discourage mold growth. Mold needs to be carefully removed with a scalpel or spatula. The area is then swabbed with a phenol compound chemical and later thoroughly dried before cosmetics are applied. Placing embalming powder inside plastic coveralls, pants, and/or stockings helps to control mold growth.

▶ KEY TERMS AND CONCEPTS FOR STUDY AND DISCUSSION

1. Define the following terms:
   autopsy gel
   baseball suture
   bridge suture
   coverall
   crepitation
   hypodermic embalming
   postembalming analysis
   purge
   single intradermal suture
   surface embalming
   terminal disinfection
   unionall
   worm suture
2. Describe a body area that is well embalmed.
3. Describe a body area that has not received any arterial solution.
4. Describe a postembalming treatment for a large decubitus ulcer of the buttocks.

▶ BIBLIOGRAPHY

Grant ME. Chronological order of events in embalming. In: *Champion Expanding Encyclopedia.* Springfield, OH: Champion Chemical Co.; October 1986: No. 571.

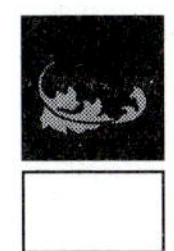

CHAPTER 16
GENERAL BODY CONSIDERATIONS

A factor that must always be considered in the preembalming analysis of a body is **age.** Embalmers often think only of the extremes—the techniques that will be used in the preparation of children as compared with those used for adults. If age is taken into careful consideration as a factor influencing embalming technique, four categories become evident:

Infant to child	Birth to about age 4
Child to young adult	About age 4 to approximately age 12
Young adult to adult	Approximately age 12 to about midseventies
Old age	Midseventies to late nineties

Not only does age influence the techniques used in the embalming process; age also leads the embalmer to expect certain difficulties and conditions with respect to positioning, setting of features, sites for injection and drainage, strength and volume of embalming solution, and injection pressure and rate of flow.

FACTORS THAT MUST BE DETERMINED IN THE EMBALMING ANALYSIS

1. Vessels for injection and drainage
2. Strength of the embalming solution
3. Volume of the embalming solution
4. Injection pressure
5. Injection rate of flow

Note: These factors will vary by the individual body; these factors can also vary in different areas of the same body.

The hands and head of an infant are positioned differently than those of the adult. Elderly persons may present positioning problems if arthritic conditions are present. Methods of mouth closure in adults and infants differ because the bones of the infant have not yet ossified. In old age the mandible and maxillae may have undergone degenerative changes to the point where a needle injector cannot be used and the mouth must be sutured closed.

This chapter deals with some of the problems encountered in the preparation of bodies of different age groups and the techniques required. The embalmer should remember that many factors other than *age* influence technique. Size and weight of the body, cause of death, moisture conditions in the body, postmortem changes, and discolorations are a few of these other factors considered in the preembalming analysis.

The embalmer should not stereotype bodies by age. For example, not all elderly persons are thin-skinned, emaciated, and toothless. Many very elderly persons are in excellent health. Their vessels are free of sclerosis and they may have a normal or above-normal weight, good musculature, and excellent teeth. Likewise, not every middle-aged adult will have vessels free of sclerosis, good teeth, good muscular build, and normal weight.

Even in children, it is not always the rule that small quantities of a mild-strength arterial fluid should be used. Many children die from diseases that produced edema or show evidence of advanced postmortem changes. In these cases, seemingly large volumes of strong arterial solutions are needed.

Every body must be individually judged in making a preembalming analysis.

▶ INFANTS AND CHILDREN—GENERAL CONSIDERATIONS

Infants and children require the use of several definite techniques that vary from those used in an adult or very elderly person. As defined in pediatric medicine, the infant period ranges from birth to 18 months and the toddler period from 18 to 48 months. Obviously there are considerable variations in both total weight and development between individuals in these classifications.

In embalming infants, it is important to realize the relationship of body water to body fat. Both contribute to total body weight. At birth, body water is approximately 75% of total body weight. At 1 year of age the body water declines to about the normal adult level of 60% of total body weight. It is therefore easy to understand the need for special embalming care for infants.

Similarly, body fat in the newborn is about 12% of total body weight and normally doubles to 25% at 6 months of age and then increases to about 30% at age 1.

Infant skin is much more delicate than adult skin and can easily distend and wrinkle on injection of the arterial solution. The vessels in the infant are extremely small but should be free of sclerosis. Most infants are autopsied, but infants dead from birth defects and systemic disease may not be autopsied. **It is important that the embalmer be familiar with the preparation of both autopsied and unautopsied infants.**

Several important facts should be stated at this point. The embalmer must have arterial tubes available for embalming infants. These tubes should be cleaned thoroughly after each use because they clog easily. They should always be tested prior to use to be certain they are in working order.

With regard to embalming solutions, it must be remembered that the infant body normally contains a large amount of moisture. In addition to this moisture, disease processes and medications can further increase moisture in the body. Renal and liver failure can bring about the accumulation of toxic wastes in the blood and tissues. This moisture and the toxic wastes can greatly increase the preservative demand of the body. It is suggested that the embalmer *not* use preinjection as the preservative solution for embalming infants. Many of these small bodies do not demand as much preservative as an adolescent or adult, but require a similar strength of arterial solution. **Use regular arterial and supplemental fluids.**

Certain factors characterize the different cases encountered in the embalming of infants and children:

1. Autopsied bodies
   A. Complete autopsy: cranial, thoracic, and abdominal cavities, spinal autopsy, limbs examined
   B. Partial autopsy: examination of only cranial, thoracic, or abdominal cavity, spine, or limbs
   C. Organ examination only: removal of only one organ
2. Unautopsied bodies
3. Organ donors: removal of eyes and/or any of the visceral organs or skin that may be used for transplantation
4. Infants whose embalming has been delayed but who have been neither refrigerated nor frozen
5. Infants that require restorative treatments (these bodies may or may not be autopsied)
6. Fetuses
   A. Premature infants: referred to as "preterm" in pediatric medicine today, any infant weighing less than $5\frac{1}{2}$ pounds at birth or born prior to the end of the 37th week of gestation
   B. Stillborn: fetus that dies prior to delivery from the uterus (In many states the definition of a stillborn includes a specified number of weeks of gestation, and if that specified time has passed, a death certificate and burial permit are required.)

▶ EMBALMING THE INFANT

All treatment should begin with topical disinfection followed by a good soap and water washing of the body, cleaning of the nasal, oral, and orbital areas, and gentle extension and manipulation of the head and extremities to relieve any rigor mortis. Intravenous tubes or any other invasive connections to the arterial or venous systems should be left in place and removed *after* arterial injection. Tracheotomy tubes or any tubing placed into the mouth or nose should be removed *prior to* arterial injection.

Eye Closure

Eyecaps may be "cut down" and inserted under the lids, or cotton pads can be placed under the lids to effect closure. After embalming, the lids may be glued with rubber-based glue or affixed with super glue. Most embalmers close the eyes prior to arterial embalming, but it should be pointed out that closure can also be done after arterial preparation. In addition, some embalmers prefer to cover eyecaps or the cotton with a thin film of massage cream. Care should be taken when using massage cream that the free margins of the eyelids are cleaned with a solvent if the lids are to be glued.

Mouth Closure

In the infant, the needle injector method of closure is not possible; however, in an older child this method can easily be used. In the infant, a muscular suture can be used (passing the needle for the suture just in front of the mandible). The suture is completed by passing the needle through the septum of the nose. As the mandible and maxillae are very soft in the infant, closure can also be made by passing a sharp $\frac{3}{8}$-inch circle needle directly through the mandible. The needle can then be passed either through the septum of the nose or directly through the maxillae.

In some small infants the embalmer may wish to use a rubber-based adhesive prior to embalming as a method of closure rather than suturing. After embalming, the mouth can again be cleaned and reglued with a rubber-based glue or super adhesive. Depending on the customs of the community, some embalmers leave the mouth of an infant open. When this is done, massage cream should be placed on the tongue and walls of the mouth. The corners of the mouth can be glued.

It may be difficult to create a good line of mouth closure in an infant. If a suture has been used for mouth closure the embalmer may also want to use a rubber-based glue or super glue to obtain a good line of closure. The mouth is generally glued *after* arterial and cavity embalming because air from the lungs can be trapped in the mouth. If gluing is necessary before embalming, use of a rubber-based glue is advised, as the mouth can easily be reopened by the use of a solvent or by reapplication of glue. (The glue acts as its own solvent.) After the features are set, a light cover of massage cream is applied over the face, hands, and arms. Massage cream should *not* be placed over discolored areas where opaque cosmetics will later be applied.

Positioning

After washing and drying of the infant, the body is placed on a towel. The towel can be gathered to hold the head in a proper position. It later is discarded and replaced with a clean, dry one. The position of the arms and head can vary considerably. Generally, the funeral home will have a policy. In some cases the arms are arranged along the sides of the trunk, and forearms and hands are placed on the body, barely touching, so as to encircle or clasp a toy, doll, or stuffed animal. In other cases, the arms are positioned bent at the elbows, forearms flexed, and hands placed near the shoulders. One arm may be placed across the body to hold some object while the other arm is positioned upward near the head and shoulder area.

The head may be so placed that it rests on its side (the right cheek area) or, like an adult, is slightly turned to the right. As it may be impossible to use a head block, pads of cotton or towels can be used. The infant body can firm as strongly as that of the adult. Changes in position can be difficult in the casket. Attention should also be given to the positioning of the legs. Often, the legs are visible during viewing of the infant. If the legs are flexed, they may be straightened by wrapping them with strips of sheeting during the injection of arterial solution.

Blood Vessel Selection: Unautopsied Infants

Common Carotid Artery. All arteries should be usable; size is the varying factor. The common carotid is the largest of the nonaortic arteries. It is easily accessible and very shallow. The infant has little neck musculature so the incision area can easily be concealed by the chin. This artery is accompanied by a relatively large adjoining vein (the internal jugular vein) and affords excellent drainage. A special incision is available in addition to the conventional carotid/jugular skin surface incisions. Placing support under the shoulders helps to elevate this neck area. Dropping the head backward brings the vessels closer to the surface. Keep in mind that the thymus gland can be quite large in the infant. Turn the head in the direction opposite that of the vessel being raised (i.e., to raise the right common carotid turn the head to the left). In using this variant incision, place a horizontal incision in one of the horizontal neck wrinkles present in all infants. Later, a super adhesive, a subcutaneous suture, or an inversion (worm) suture can be employed to close the incision. If, because of damage, it is not possible to drain from the right jugular vein, raise and attempt to take drainage from the left internal jugular vein. If this is not successful, use a small trocar to drain directly from the right atrium of the heart. Insert the trocar at the standard entry point over the abdomen and direct the point toward the lobe of the right ear.

Femoral (External Iliac) Artery. The second largest nonaortic vessel that can be used is either the external iliac artery or the femoral artery. The external iliac is slightly larger than the femoral. The same incisions can be used to raise these vessels as are used to raise the vessels of an adult. The accompanying veins are relatively large and may be used as points of drainage. If a small drain tube is not available, these veins can be expanded by inserting a small pair of forceps into the vessels. **Always inject the distal leg first.** This gives the embalmer a chance to observe the effects of the fluid solution on the skin of the leg and to determine if too much or too little fluid dye has been used. If drainage is difficult to establish from the femoral location, the right internal jugular vein can be raised and used as a drainage point.

Use of the axillary vessels is *not* advised in preparation of the unautopsied infant. The vessel is too small for efficient use, and establishing drainage may be very difficult. In the autopsied infant, however, it may be necessary to inject this vessel. If possible, the embalmer should try to use the larger subclavian artery for arterial injection of the arm.

Abdominal Aorta

The abdominal aorta is a large artery and is accompanied by the largest vein that could be used for drainage. The artery and vein are deep-seated, resting on the anterior surface of the spine. A 2- to 3-inch incision can be made just to the left of the midline in the middle of the abdomen, and inferior enough to avoid the liver, which is very large in the infant. The greater omentum must be opened and some of the small and large intestines either held away from the spine or removed from the cavity during arterial injection. The aorta is held in position by its parietal branches (the four pairs of lumbar arteries in particular). Once located, the aorta can be opened and a tube placed in the direction of the legs and another tube in the direction of the upper portions of the body. The vein can be opened and the blood allowed to drain into the cavity. It is not necessary to place a drainage instrument into the vein. The lower portion of the body should be injected first, then the upper portion. During injection the viscera can greatly expand. The viscera can be clipped and drained prior to return to the cavity (Figure 16–1).

Ascending Aorta

In a variant technique involving the aorta as a primary injection point, the ascending aorta is used. Several incisions are used to reach the ascending aorta as it leaves the heart. In one incision for drainage, the right auricle of the heart (the small earlike appendage of the right atrium of the heart) is clipped open. An incision can be made directly down the midline of the sternum. Because this bone is not ossified but is actually cartilage, a sharp scalpel or strong surgical shears can be used to make this incision. The difficulty is that the incision must be held open with some form of retraction. A 2-inch block can be placed in the spread incision to hold it open and to allow the embalmer to work. A second incision, a U-shaped one, is made straight down from

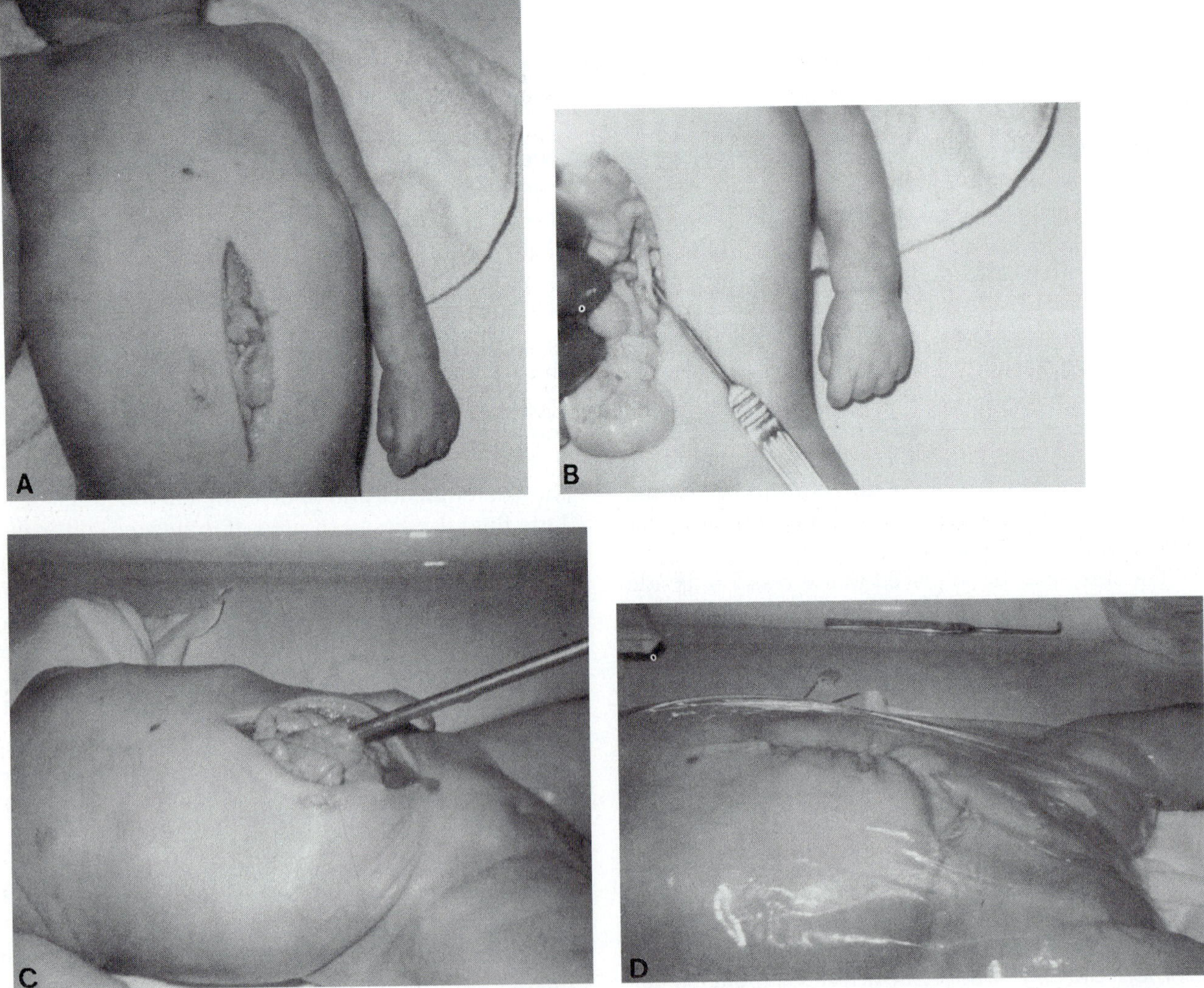

Figure 16–1. Preparation of an infant using the abdominal aorta. **A.** The incision is made to the left of the midline to raise the abdominal aorta. **B.** The abdominal aorta is exposed. Note that the small intestine has been carefully pulled out and set to the right. The small intestines are lifted out during the injection. These should not be severed. **C.** Viscera are treated after injection. **D.** Plastic is placed over the incision after preparation.

the midclavicle to the bottom of the rib cage, where it makes a right angle across the inferior margin of the sternum to a point identical to the original midclavicle incision. From this point, the cut is directed upward to the midclavicle position. The skin is then dissected upward, thus disclosing the sternum, which is then opened by severing the sternal cartilage at its junction with the ribs.

When the sternum is severed free of its lateral attachments it can be bent upward toward the head. With this incision, the internal thoracic arteries may need to be clamped during arterial injection. Once the incision has been made and the pericardium exposed, the embalmer must cut open the pericardium and expose the heart and the great vessels (Figure 16–2). The ascending aorta is observed as it rises from the left ventricle of the heart. It can be opened, or an opening can be made in the arch of the aorta and an arterial tube inserted. The entire body can be embalmed from this one point.

With respect to use of the abdominal aorta or the ascending aorta (or the heart) method of embalming, it is necessary to point out the possibility of legal ramifications. In many areas of the United States, all hospital deaths require hospital personnel to solicit autopsies. Obviously, in the cases just described, an autopsy has not been performed, the legal next of kin having denied consent for the autopsy. The family may suspect that an autopsy was performed without their consent and thus want to examine the body of the embalmed infant at their first opportunity. The incisions for raising the abdominal aorta or the arch of the aorta closely resemble autopsy incisions. Laypersons can arrive at a false conclusion in these circumstances and blame both the funeral home and the hospital using the mistakenly identified incisions as evidence of a surreptitious autopsy.

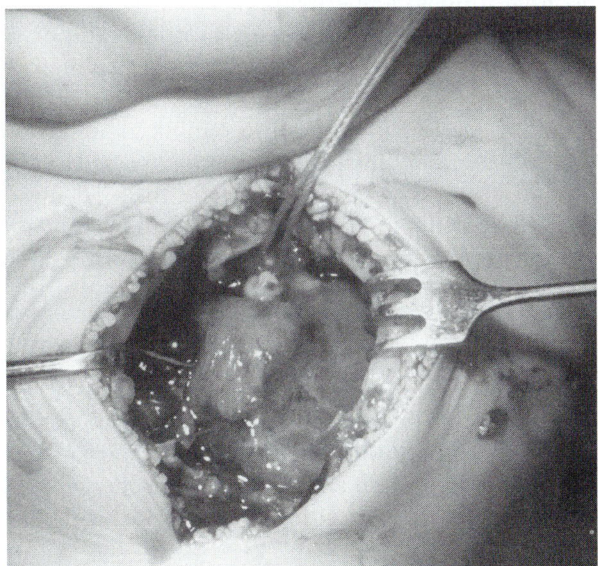

Figure 16–2. The pericardium is opened. Note the string around the ascending aorta. The right auricle is in the center; it will be incised and used for drainage.

Infant Cavity Treatment

For aspirating and injecting the unautopsied infant, use an infant trocar. These trocars are generally about 12 inches in length with an inside diameter of at least $\frac{1}{4}$ inch. The standard trocar point of entry or a lower point, such as the right or left inguinal abdominal area, may be used.

Cavity embalming may either immediately follow arterial injection or be delayed several hours. Injection of an undiluted cavity chemical follows aspiration. The amount of cavity chemical depends on the size of the infant. The trocar point of entry can be closed by suture or the trocar button. Reaspiration several hours later is recommended.

Preparation of the Autopsied Infant

The embalmer should try to prepare autopsied infants by arterial injection, which produces very satisfactory results. Although this process may be very time consuming, every attempt should be made to effect complete arterial distribution of embalming fluid. Those areas not reached by arterial injection or that cannot be embalmed by arterial injection can be treated in several ways. Regardless of the techniques employed, preservation is accomplished by hypodermic or surface embalming.

The proportion of infants autopsied in some large hospitals in major cities approaches 70% or more. In these communities, autopsies of infants by coroners or medical examiners may approach 100%. (It should be noted that in some areas of the country, the hospital or coroner may permit arterial embalming of the body prior to autopsy. The same is true of autopsies on adult bodies; however, the majority of hospital and medical examiner autopsies are performed prior to arterial embalming.)

Four types of autopsies are performed on infants:

- *Complete autopsy:* Cranial and trunk cavities are opened and enclosed viscera removed.
- *Partial autopsy:* Only one cavity is opened (cranial, thoracic, abdominal, or spine).
- *Special or local autopsy:* Only one organ is removed or a special examination is made of the route of blood vessels or nerves.
- *Organ donor autopsy:* Eyes may be removed, for the eye is quite large in the infant and the cornea of great value. The heart, heart/lungs, liver, kidneys, or skin may be removed as in the adult, and these donations can be treated as partial autopsies.

When viscera are removed in the autopsy, they may or may not be returned with the body. Generally, any viscera removed by a coroner or medical examiner are returned with the body. With hospital autopsies, the viscera are not always returned.*

Blood Vessel Selection: Autopsied Infants

Neither the common carotid, common iliac, or external iliac arteries and their accompanying veins, the iliac and internal jugular, of the adult and infant vary greatly except in *size*. If the autopsy pathologist has left vessels of reasonable length, the difficulty encountered is no greater than when working with an adult. If the vessels are severed excessively short (iliacs at the inguinal ligament, carotids at thyroid cartilage), considerable extensive dissection will be required to locate the vessels and to ligate arterial tubes within them. In lieu of string for ligation, an arterial tube hemostat may be helpful. Do not attempt to locate veins. Drainage can be taken without the use of any instruments. Remember that arteries remain open when cut. This can often help in locating the tiny arteries. It is also most important that the embalmer be certain of the anatomical locations and relationships of the vessels.

If the iliac arteries cannot be located or if they are too small for the arterial tubes, supplemental methods of embalming can be used to preserve the legs. Hypodermic treatment with long large-gauge needles can be employed. Painting the surface of the legs with an autopsy gel and wrapping the painted limbs in plastic could serve to embalm the limbs. When the carotid arteries are missing the embalmer can place cotton saturated with cavity fluid in the mouth and under the eyelids. With a diluted cavity fluid, deep hypodermic treatment can be made from inside the mouth, from the scalp incisions of the autopsy, and from the opened neck areas of the autopsy. If arterial fluid is going to be injected hypodermically, one with little dye should be used. The dye can create blotches of color as the fluid spreads through the facial tissues. Likewise, the face can be painted with autopsy gel and covered with plastic for several hours. This treatment often bleaches the skin, and corrective cosmetics will be needed. The inside of the scalp and the base of the cranial cavity can also be painted with autopsy gel.

Subclavian arteries can be located at the usual adult site. If they have been cut short, the axillary artery can be raised at its largest point, as the artery passes into the axilla just at the lateral border of the first rib. To reach the axillary at this point it may be necessary to dissect the pectoralis major and minor muscles. Some embalmers prefer to raise the subclavian artery by elevating the clavicle bones. This exposes the subclavian arteries where they have been severed. An arterial hemostat may again be more useful than string ties in securing the arterial tube.

Instruments and Chemicals

Very small arterial tubes are a necessity. These can be made by filing off the tip of a hypodermic needle.

There are many suggested chemical combinations, strengths, and dilutions for infant arterial embalming. A false theory is that infants must always be embalmed with very dilute low-index arterial fluids. Infant body tissue contains a higher percentage of water than adult body tissue. In addition, disease processes and drugs may have increased tissue moisture and toxic wastes. It may be necessary to use solution strengths similar to those used for adult bodies. Harsh tissue reactions may be reduced by the addition of supplemental fluids such as humectants and coinjection chemicals or the use of arterial fluids, which contain large amounts of humectants. Some fluid companies even have arterial fluids designed for infants and children. Guidelines for fluid use are provided by the manufacturers. A small amount of fluid dye to add color to the tissues is recommended.

In the autopsied body, the legs are embalmed before the head or arms. This allows the embalmer to adjust the fluid strengths and dyes.

The volume to be injected is best determined by guidelines similar to those for the adult. Intravascular blood discolorations should be cleared and the fluid dyes must appear uniform throughout the tissues. Generally, the tissues may plump slightly. Massage may be necessary to assist distribution of the fluid. Pinching the fingertips and lips helps to clear these areas of blood discolorations. If the eyelids wrinkle after discolorations have cleared, it is recommended that injection be stopped. If any swelling occurs, the arterial solution can be strengthened and only a minimum amount injected. In addition, all injection can be stopped and the untreated areas preserved by hypodermic and surface embalming. Keep in mind that *weak* solutions can easily distend tissues, another reason to use arterial solution at a strength close to that used in the adult.

Treatment of Areas Not Reached by Arterial Injection

Hypodermic Injection. The head may be injected hypodermically from within an incised neck area or natural openings (mouth and nostrils) or an incised scalp area; arms and legs may be injected from within the open trunk cavity.

In larger children this may entail injection of the arm from the point of insertion of the hypodermic needle or trocar from the antecubital fossa upward toward the shoulder, and then, utilizing the same point of in-

---

* Refer to Chapter 17 for treatment of viscera.

sertion, down toward the fingers. The puncture incision is closed with a trocar button and later covered by glue, cotton, plastic sheeting, and adhesive tape.

The legs may similarly be injected by inserting the hypodermic needle or trocar from a point within the abdominal cavity or on the inner aspect of the knee area. The instrument may be directed upward first and then, when injection is completed, downward using the same point of insertion. The point of insertion may be closed in the same manner as previously described. Diluted cavity fluid can be used for injection. Cosmetic arterial fluid should not be used.

Internal Compresses. Internal compresses, sometimes referred to as inlays, are cotton or sheeting (well dampened with cavity fluid) inserted into such areas as the interior of the neck, the cranium, and the trunk cavity, when devoid of viscera. Internal packs can also be inserted under the pectoral chest flaps (over the sternum) before trunk incision closure. Autopsy gel can be used in lieu of cavity fluid.

Preservative Gels. Preservative gels are semisolid chemicals that are inserted over the calvarium as well as under the anterior chest and abdominal skin flaps before skin suturing.

External Compresses. Cotton saturated with undiluted cavity fluid or other special chemical preparations may be needed to preserve areas as small as the ears or, in other cases, the entire body. An attempt should be made to secure a smooth cotton surface, for irregular application to the skin surface impresses the unevenness onto the skin. Compresses should be left in place long enough to accomplish complete preservation.

Treatment of the Trunk Walls of the Autopsied Infant

The back, shoulders, trunk walls, and buttocks, and the scrotum and penis of the male may require additional chemical treatments for preservation. An infant trocar, a large-diameter hypodermic needle, or a straight long arterial tube can be used to inject these areas with a strong chemical solution. This solution is injected either through the embalming machine or with a large hypodermic syringe. In addition, the inside walls may be treated with autopsy gel or embalming powder. If the viscera are not returned, cavities can be filled with sheeting saturated with cavity fluid.

Autopsy Viscera Treatments

The viscera of the autopsied body may be immersed in undiluted cavity fluid. Some prefer to place the viscera and cavity fluid together within a plastic bag and then, later, place the plastic-encased viscera in the abdominal and thoracic cavities. The organs should be clipped and freed of gases after the addition of cavity fluid. It is also recommended that the cavity fluid not be added until the bag of viscera has been positioned within the body cavity. Some embalmers also prefer to make a cut in the thick solid organs (e.g., lungs and liver) to ensure contact with the cavity fluid.

Closure of Cavities in Autopsied Infants

In small infants the scalp has been opened by the usual transverse incision from ear to ear. Access to the floor of the cranial cavity would have been necessary to control leakage from the internal carotids and, possibly, the vertebral or basilar arteries during arterial injection. The scalp should be reflected and the floor of the cavity dried. The walls of the cranial vault can be liberally coated with autopsy gel, and the inside surface of the reflected scalp can likewise be coated with a preservative gel. To repair the area, a quantity of cotton may be used to fill the cranial cavity and to reproduce the normal contours as well as act as an absorbent for seepage. The scalp is drawn back to its normal position, and then carefully sutured.

When the fontanelles are still present, it may be helpful to fill the cranial cavity with cotton. With dental floss and a $\frac{3}{8}$-inch circle needle, the soft cranial bones are sutured together. The fontanelle areas can be filled with "mortuary putty." If this is not available, the cranial cavity must be tightly filled with cotton. If the cavity is not tightly filled, sunken areas may be noticed at the locations of the fontanelles. Many embalmers do not want the scalp to rest on the cotton at the fontanelles, so they coat the cotton with massage cream. This prevents dehydration of the scalp around the fontanelles.

For the scalp, suturing begins on the right side of the cranium and ends on the left side. The inversion (worm) suture is excellent for infants. It helps to tighten the scalp. When the autopsy incision has been made high on the head and the hair is very thin, it is recommended that the funeral director request that a bonnet be used. It is not necessary to discuss the reason unless questioned by the family. Most hospitals make these incisions low enough that the sutured incisions can be hidden by the pillow. Super adhesive can provide a closure that is not easily detected. If the embalmer prefers, a small baseball or interdermal suture using dental floss may be used for closure instead of the worm suture.

In infants in whom the bones of the cranium are well calcified and the calvaruim has been removed as in an adult case, the same procedure used for such repair in the adult is recommended.

If the temporalis muscles have been cut from the cranium or calvarium, the area can easily be filled in with "mortuary putty" to prevent a sunken appearance.

Tissue building of the temple is not possible if the muscular tissue has been removed. When the calvarium has not been "notched" it may be very difficult to maintain the calvarium in correct position during and after suturing. Calvarium clamps might possibly be used to hold the calvarium in place. As the bones are not completely ossified, small holes can easily be made on either side of the calvarium and the calvarium wired into proper position.

The abdominal, thoracic, and pelvic cavities should be coated with autopsy gel or a preservative-drying powder, following aspiration and drying of the cavities. If neck organs have been removed the neck area should be filled with cotton and saturated with a preservative such as cavity fluid. The trunk cavities should be filled with an absorbent material and also saturated with a preservative chemical. The breast plate should be laid into proper position (and if necessary anchored with sutures); paper toweling can be laid over the plate and saturated with preservative chemical. The skin flaps are tacked together to ensure proper alignment. Suturing is begun at the pubic symphysis and directed upward; a small baseball suture provides a good closure. The body is bathed and the skin surfaces thoroughly dried. The sutures may be coated with a surface sealer glue. The trunk area can be covered with a thin sheet of plastic to ensure protection of the clothing.

To reemphasize, although many premature infants are autopsied and may be extremely small (less than 1 pound), there may exist a need to preserve them temporarily for funeral, burial, or cremation services.

Optional Treatments. If the premature infant has not been autopsied, arterial injection may be attempted. Some success is achieved by injection of the internal carotid artery followed by cavity aspiration and injection of a small amount of cavity fluid. Injection of the arterial umbilical vessel has occasionally been advocated, but difficulty in identifying the artery from the other two veins as well as the poor results obtained when the proper vessel is injected make this procedure unattractive. Other large vessels that could be injection sites are the abdominal aorta, the ascending aorta, and the arch of the aorta.

External compresses constitute the easiest treatment. The premature infant is wrapped in cotton saturated with cavity fluid or painted with autopsy gel.

The limbs, trunk cavity and walls, and head are injected hypodermically with a strong concentration of preservative chemicals. Cavity treatment and external compresses are additionally applied as necessary.

General Treatments. In other treatments for autopsied infants, the entire body and hair should be rewashed, the nails cleaned and trimmed, and all incisions sealed. Cosmetics should be applied in accordance with the requirements of the individual case. Trunk autopsy incisions as well as other incised or lacerated areas should be covered with plastic. Also recommended are long-sleeved dresses, shirts, and jackets, long trousers (boys), and tights (girls). This, obviously, minimizes the skin area to be cosmetized.

▶ EMBALMING THE 4- to 12-YEAR OLD

The second age group relative to embalming ranges from approximately 4 years to approximately 12 years. Although the special techniques used for the infant or the aged are not required, some difficulties are encountered because of the body size.

Vessel Selection

The vessels in this age group should be healthy and much larger than those of the infant, but still smaller than those of the adult. The two major injection sites used in embalming the adult are also used for preparation of the child: (1) the common carotid artery and the internal jugular vein and (2) the femoral artery and femoral vein. There is no need to consider use of the abdominal aorta or the arch of the aorta in this age group. Likewise, the many disadvantages of the axillary artery and vein do not make this a good primary injection site. Many members of this age group are autopsied, so most of the embalming is done from the primary autopsy sites—right and left common carotid, right and left external and internal iliac, and right and left subclavian arteries.

In the unautopsied body, the right internal jugular vein is the largest vein that can be used for drainage. It also affords direct access to the right atrium of the heart. Whenever facial blood discolorations are present, this vein affords the best possible clearing of the facial tissues.

Some embalmers prefer the femoral vessels for this age group strictly because their location permits the use of clothing that can be opened at the neck. The possibility of leakage or visibility of the carotid incision should be of little concern if properly prepared, sutured, and sealed.

Remember that in this age group (4–12 years), if there has been any trauma to the face or head or if there has been a long delay between death and preparation, the facial tissues may swell during injection. The best control over fluid flow into the head and face is obtained by use of restricted cervical injection.

The arteries of children in this age group should all be in excellent condition with no evidence of arteriosclerosis.

FACTORS THAT MUST BE DETERMINED IN THE EMBALMING ANALYSIS

1. Strength of the embalming solution
2. Volume of the embalming solution
3. Injection pressure
4. Injection rate of flow

Note: These factors will vary from body to body; these factors can vary within different areas of the same body.

Fluid Strengths and Volume

Fluid strength is determined by the condition of the body. As 4- to 12-year-olds have more delicate skin than adults, for routine embalming, a medium-index fluid in the range 18 to 25 is most satisfactory. Dilutions should follow those recommended by the manufacturer. Two schools of thought exist as to embalming solution strengths: the first is to use one mixture strength throughout the entire operation; the second is to begin the injection with a mild solution but following the clearing of intravascular blood discolorations the solution is gradually strengthened. Supplemental chemicals may be used to control harsh reactions of the embalming chemicals. Dye can always be used for its cosmetic effect and to indicate the distribution of arterial solution. In these bodies, however, dyes should be kept to a minimum for, no doubt, cosmetic application will be minimized to produce the most natural appearance.

In cases of trauma and the effects of diseases, such as edema and renal failure, appropriate fluid strengths should be used and, if necessary, special-purpose high-index fluids.

Four- to twelve-year-olds require a smaller volume of fluid than adults, but a greater volume than used for infants. Intravascular blood discolorations should have cleared, some firming of the tissues should be present, and there should be evidence of good distribution as indicated by the presence of dye. All of these indicators help to establish the volume of fluid to be injected.

In this age group, the causes of death include infectious and contagious diseases (e.g., meningitis and pneumonia), childhood viral diseases, and systemic diseases (e.g., leukemia and cystic fibrosis). When contagious or infectious disease is the cause of death, the arterial solution strength should be of sufficient strength to sanitize the body tissues without any noticible effect on the appearance of the body. A thorough aspiration of the cavities is necessary, followed by injection of sufficient concentrated cavity fluid to reach all areas of the cavities. Reaspiration and reinjection of the cavities may be necessary.

Pressure and Rate of Flow of Injection

The rate of flow should be a greater concern than pressure to the embalmer, especially in embalming a child. If arterial solution is moved too quickly into the body, the tissues may distend. Injection must be slow enough that the drainage can be restricted at times during the injection. This helps to prevent a loss of the solution through low-resistance paths, especially those vessel connections located near the injection site.

The embalmer must remember that sufficient force is necessary to establish good distribution, especially in distal body areas such as the hands and feet. By the use of intermittent drainage, short-circuiting of solution is reduced and retention of solution increased. Rapid injection with continuous drainage often has the tendency to remove moisture from a child's tissues. This could lead to wrinkling of the skin. A sufficient pressure and rate of flow should be used to achieve a uniform distribution of the solution.

Setting of Features and Positioning

Positioning of the child is similar to that of the adult. The arms can be a little more "relaxed" than those of the adult and, generally, are placed straighter (Figure 16–3). The head should be slightly tilted to the right.

Facial hair must be removed for good cosmetic treatment. Some drugs stimulate growth of facial hair, and this hair can easily be removed with shaving lather and a sharp razor. It is best not to attempt to shave the forehead.

Mouth closure may pose some difficulty if the child has buck teeth or is wearing braces. For buck teeth, place a small layer of cotton over the *lower* teeth and gum. This helps to push the lower lip forward. The lips can now be glued together with a rubber-based glue prior to arterial injection (Figure 16–4). Some embalmers prefer to inject the body with the lips slightly

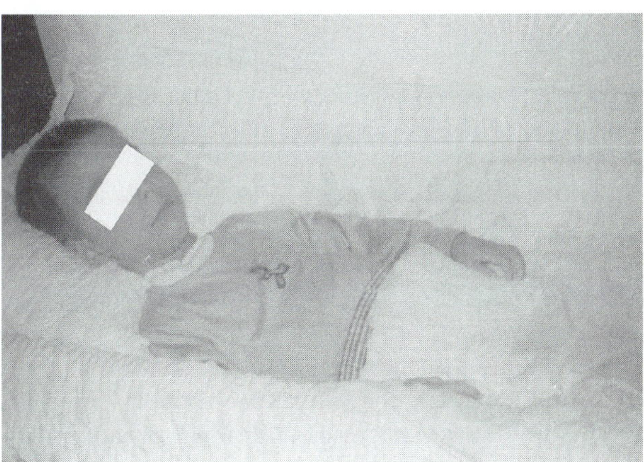

Figure 16–3. Positioning of the child. Note that the arms are placed at the sides.

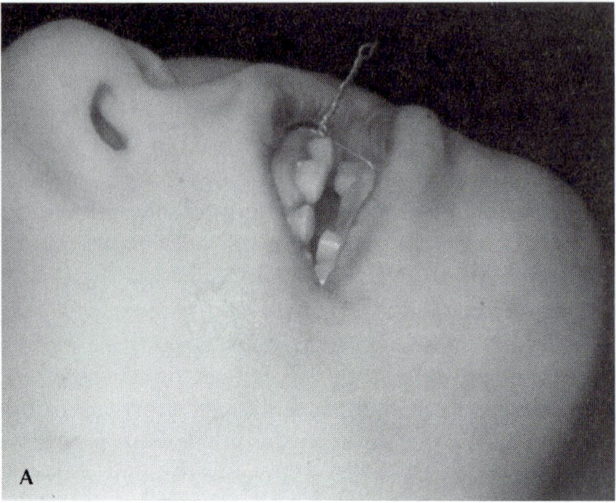

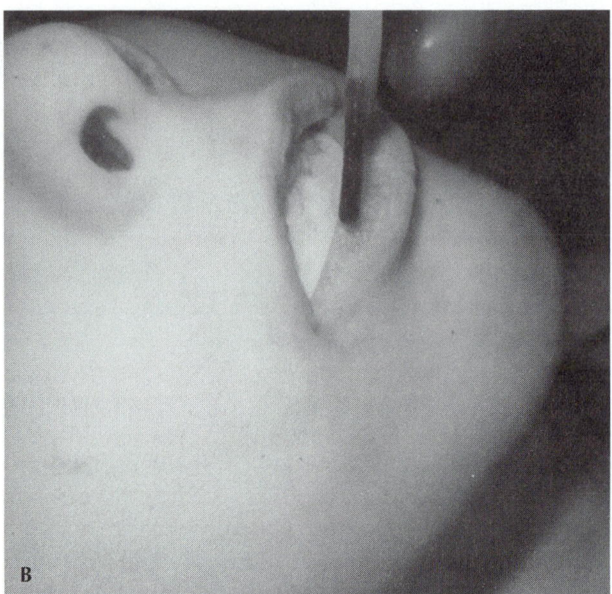

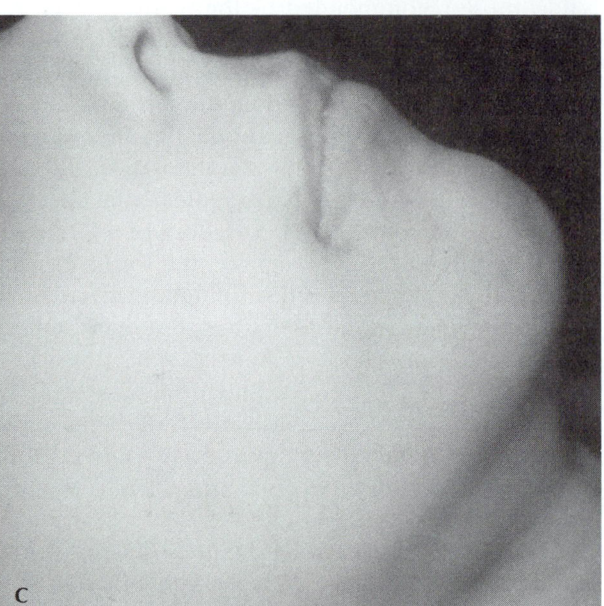

Figure 16–4. A. Note the large separation of the lips with this child. **B.** The lips are glued prior to arterial injection with a rubber-base glue. **C.** A glued closure is made prior to arterial injection.

parted. This allows the tissues of the lips to "round out." The super adhesives can assist, after injection, with difficult closures.

▶ EMBALMING THE ADOLESCENT AND ADULT

For embalming purposes, the adolescent/adult group comprises persons from 13 to approximately 75 years of age. As in all age categories, individual variations and exceptions exist. Because this age group is characterized by average body conditions for which average embalming treatments are practiced, embalming of the "routine" or "normal" body is outlined. For the beginning practitioner, this overview is suggested in an outline of the step-by-step preparation of the unautopsied or autopsied body (see Chapter 1).

Causes of death in this group include heart disease, malignancies, and accidents. It is important that the embalmer remember that age is only one factor in the embalming analysis. Other factors are time between death and preparation, progress of decomposition, moisture content, discolorations, condition of the blood vascular system, protein and nutritional condition, traumatic or surgical considerations, time between preparation and disposition, weight, autopsy and organ donation considerations, and pathologic changes.

Chapter 1 provides a recommended sequence for complete embalming of the body. Here, certain points of the chronology are discussed in greater detail.

Vessel Selection

In the embalming of the "normal" adult body, the order of injection sites would be to first employ *restricted cervical* injection, using both right and left common carotid arteries and the right internal jugular vein for drainage; second would be the use of the right common carotid artery and right internal jugular vein; third would be the use of the right femoral artery and vein. This order is based on the fact that should there be any arterial coagula in the aorta, it would be best that this material be pushed toward the legs rather than toward the head. The internal jugular vein is the largest vein that can be used for drainage, and any coagula present in the right atrium of the heart can easily be removed with angular spring forceps. Rarely does the common carotid artery show arteriosclerosis, whereas the femoral is the first vessel used for embalming to exhibit this condition. Use of both common carotids gives the embalmer control of the strength and volume of arterial solutions entering the head and trunk areas of the body.

Supplemental Fluids

Supplemental chemicals can be used in the embalming of all bodies. These chemicals are designed to enhance the preservative and disinfecting qualities of the preservative fluids, control moisture, add color to the tissues, and adjust pH of the tissues as well as the arterial solution. Supplemental chemicals include preinjection and coinjection fluids, humectants, dyes, and water conditions. In addition, there are specialized supplemental fluids to control tissue gas, bleach internal discolorations, and remove excessive moisture from the tissues. The conditions present with the body to be embalmed will determine the need for the use of specific supplemental fluids.

Preinjection is a supplemental embalming fluid as well as an embalming procedure. As a fluid it is a chemical containing very little or no preservative. As a process it is the injection of this chemical—diluted as recommended by the manufacturer—into the vascular system (via an artery) for the purposes of preparing the vascular system and the body tissues for the injection of the preservative solution. This solution is injected **before** the preservative solution is injected. It is also used to clear intravascular blood discolorations, remove blood in the vascular system, and adjust the pH of the tissues. Preinjection is done with the unautopsied body; it is rarely done with the autopsied case. There seem to be two schools of thought—those embalmers who frequently practice preinjection and those who never use this process.

Coinjection is a supplemental embalming fluid used to enhance the action of the preservative solution. It is added to the embalming solution to build up almost all of the embalming chemicals with the exception of the preservatives. A purpose of coinjection fluid is to better control the harsh reactions of the preservatives without simply adding more water to the solution. Some embalmers will use coinjection chemicals as a substitute for water, thus producing a **waterless solution** for injection. Coinjection fluids can be used with almost all arterial solutions.

Both preinjection and coinjection fluids can be used in the preparation of the same unautopsied body. Likewise, some embalmers do not preinject or coinject any bodies. Many embalmers feel that preinjection should be used only when good distribution is anticipated. When circulatory problems are expected (e.g., bodies dead for long periods of time, bodies that evidence early signs of decomposition, arteriosclerotic vessels), the filling of the vascular system and the tissues with a very weak preinjection solution will only bring about tissue distension when the preservative solution is injected. Bodies that have the greatest need for preservative chemicals, such as the previous examples, generally have the least capacity to accept the preservative solution without tissue distension. Preinjection treatment is used by some embalmers as a clearing method for jaundiced bodies. In these cases only the head needs to be preinjected; use of restricted cervical injection makes this technique possible.

Both adolescent and adult bodies can be treated with preinjection and coinjection chemicals. The use of these supplemental chemicals along with the preservative chemical will be determined by the condition of the body.

FACTORS THAT MUST BE DETERMINED IN THE EMBALMING ANALYSIS

1. Strength of the embalming solution
2. Volume of the embalming solution
3. Injection pressure
4. Injection rate of flow

Note: These factors will vary from body to body; these factors can vary within different areas of the same body.

Solution Strength and Volume

Age alone cannot be the **single factor** in determining the strength and volume of the preservative solution to be injected. Conditions within the body such as weight, body build; moisture in the tissues; effects of disease, surgery, or trauma; blood discolorations; and effects of long use of medications all assist in determining arterial solution strength and volume. Several time elements are equally important—the time lapse between the death and the embalming and the time that will lapse between the embalming and the disposition of the body. Sufficient strength and volume of the embalming chemical must be used to assure thorough sanitizing and preservation of all body areas. With respect to the factor of age, in general, it can be stated that infants, children, and the very elderly may display a delicate skin texture, easily subject to the dehydrating and possible wrinking effects of preservative chemicals.

Several simple rules can be established in determining strength and volume of the embalming solution:

1. *Selection of a particular fluid.* Most fluid companies make a variety of arterial fluids; consider the recommendations of the manufacturer. In producing fluids, some are formulated for infants and children or older individuals where dehydration and wrinkling of the skin might be a concern. Other formulations are produced for bodies with problems such as edema, refrigerated, frozen, or decomposition conditions. If formaldehyde is used as a primary preservative, various indexes and buffers in the fluids will produce varing degrees of firmness.
2. *Follow the recommendations of the manufacturer* for the dilution of the concentrated chemical. This is usually measured in ounces per gallon or ounces per half-gallon. These dilutions are often based on the moisture content of the body (e.g., dehydrated, normal, or edema).
3. *For the "average body,"* a milder solution can be used at the start of the embalming. After good distribution of the solution has been established and the intravascular blood discolorations have been cleared, if necessary, the solution can be strengthened. This can be accomplished by (1) adding more of the same concentrated arterial fluid, or (2) adding a stronger arterial fluid to the original dilution. Here are two examples of this process. It may even be necessary to make a gallon or more using not only more of the original fluid but adding to that mixture a number of ounces of a concentrated stronger arterial fluid. It is possible to find body conditions that will call for the use of the injecting of pure concentrated fluid without the use of a water dilutant.

Pressure and Rate of Flow of Injection

With most embalming machines the pressure and the rate of flow are related. The important factor is the rate of flow—how fast or in what volume the fluid enters the body.

In Chapters 2 and 3 the ideal speed of 10 to 15 minutes per gallon was recommended for the first gallon of solution. Discussion of the ideal rate of flow indicated that sufficient pressure and rate of flow should be used to overcome the resistances of the body and to distribute the arterial solution without causing tissue distension. The greater the resistance in a body, the greater the pressure required. A pressure setting of 5 to 20 pounds, using the centrifugal machine, should be sufficient to overcome most body resistances. This range is very wide; many embalmers prefer a low pressure, whereas others prefer a higher setting. The rate of flow can be varied with either setting (Figure 16–5).

The first injection, while the vascular system is filling, should be slow, to prevent any arterial coagula from loosening and moving. The arterial solution can then "ride over top" of the coagula. After the first gallon, the speed of injection is increased. Many embalmers inject a gallon of solution at a rate of 10 to 15 minutes per gallon. Healthy body tissues can accept fluid at this rate of speed without distension.

The skin of adolescents should be much firmer and dryer than that of adults, indicating a good protein level. Adolescent tissues are able to assimilate injected

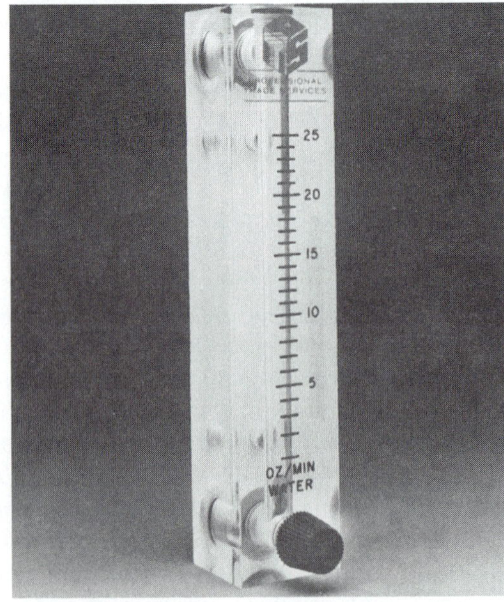

Figure 16–5. Rate-of-flow meter can be installed on any centrifugal embalming machine.

arterial solution much better than those of the elderly, in whom skin support is often weak and swelling occurs easily. For this reason, a wide range of pressures and rates of flow can be used to embalm bodies in this category.

Some embalmers prefer to inject at a rapid rate of flow from the very beginning (5–10 minutes per gallon). The theory is that this places greater pressure on the arterial side of the capillaries and increases filtration of the embalming solution through the capillaries. With this method, continuous drainage is used throughout the preparation. The body must be observed carefully to detect any facial or neck distension. This method can also loosen coagula in the arteries. Multipoint injection and hypodermic embalming may then be required to overcome the problems thus produced. Pressure and rate of flow must be sufficient to evenly distribute the preservative solution to all body areas without distension of any tissues. Injection speed should be such that restricted drainage can be employed to assist with the solution distribution, penetration, and retention.

▶ EMBALMING THE ELDERLY PERSON

Modern medicine has provided health care and control of disease with the result that the average life expectancy has increased to 72.6 years for men and 77.6 years for women. The number of persons living into their eighties and nineties is expected to double within several years. Embalmers are, as a consequence, required to prepare greater numbers of those dying in these upper age groups. Of course, certain afflictions and pathologic conditions are more frequently encountered in the elderly than among the other previously described three age groups. It is useful to identify some of the more common conditions associated with advanced age and to give some general comments on them. As in all age groups, drug therapy can greatly alter the classic conditions of certain diseases, so the medications in and of themselves will play an important role in determining what postmortem conditions exist in the body.

Arthritic Conditions

Many elderly are afflicted with arthritis. This condition, which may be long-standing, may be accompanied by atrophy of many muscles. These conditions are manifest many times in a patient restricted to bedrest. Legs are drawn up and curvature of the spine is evident. Frequently the arms are drawn up onto the chest and the fingers clenched (Figure 16–6).

These conditions create a number of positioning problems for the embalmer. Placing head blocks under

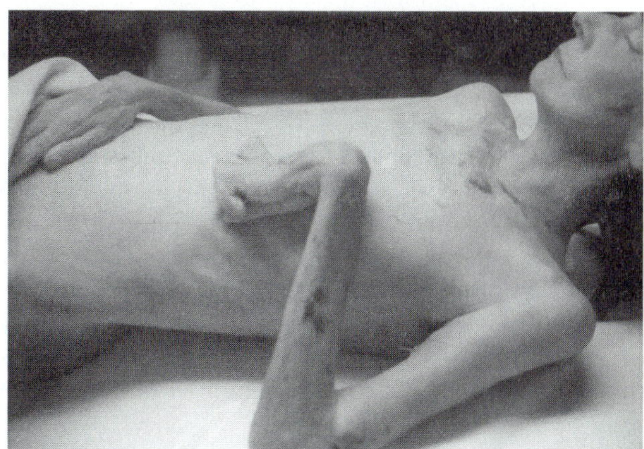

Figure 16–6. Arthritic arm and hand.

the things helps to position the body on the embalming table. It may also be necessary to tie the body in position. Generally, blocks under the thighs and head blocks under a shoulder provide adequate support. Turkish towels placed under the shoulders also help to achieve temporary position. After casketing, the bedding of the casket along with pillow supports places the body into a comfortable-looking position. The neck may be difficult to position. Application of firm pressure to arthritic limbs and arms may change their position. It is possible to tear tendons and atrophied muscles. It must be remembered that the person has had this arthritic condition for many months or years, so leaving the arms and legs in these positions may be acceptable to the family. It is not recommended that tendons or skin be cut to achieve good positioning. It is almost impossible to open and expand arthritic fingers. These can be left in their clenched position and partially hidden by the blanket in the casket. When the legs are drawn to one side or into the fetal position, use of the femoral vessels is limited.

The common carotid would be the best site for a primary injection. If it becomes necessary to inject the legs, an attempt can be made to raise the femoral or external iliac artery. The popliteal artery may also be a choice. If these vessels are found to be sclerotic, an attempt should be made to inject using a small arterial tube; if this is not possible the legs should then be hypodermically injected using a small trocar and a dilute solution of cavity fluid injected through the embalming machine. In addition, plastic stockings can be placed on the legs. Autopsy gel can be poured into the stockings so that the viscous preservative coats the legs.

Mouth Closure Problems

Frequently a loss of weight is manifested in the facial tissues of the elderly. After mouth closure, it is necessary to place either cotton or "mortuary putty" over the teeth or dentures. This helps to fill out the sunken cheek areas. These areas should not be overfilled, especially if it is known that the deceased did not wear dentures. In this age group there are natural depressions of the facial tissues. The biggest problem with mouth closure is atrophy of the maxillae and mandible. The mandible in particular has a tendency to atrophy, and for this reason, it is more difficult many times to use the needle injector method of mouth closure. It is necessary to suture using either a muscular or a mandibular suture. The mandibular suture holds the dentures forward and in a tight position in the mouth.

Arteriosclerosis

Although not a problem exclusively of the elderly, arteriosclerotic arteries are frequently encountered in this age group. (Persons who live into their late nineties frequently exhibit very little sclerosis. This is a factor in achieving their longevity.) The vessel that most frequently exhibits sclerosis and that would be used for embalming is the femoral artery. Many times in a very thin individual, the sclerotic condition of the femoral can be palpated. The common carotid artery is thus the best choice in embalming the elderly. Rarely is the carotid found to be sclerotic, and if there is sclerosis, it is generally not sufficient to occlude the carotid (refer to Chapter 22). Restricted cervical injection, which uses both common carotid arteries, would be the first choice.

In addition to bringing about occlusion of the arteries, arteriosclerosis can also bring about poor peripheral circulation. As a result of poor circulation, bedfast individuals tend to form bedsores (decubitus ulcers). These sores develop where there is pressure contact with the bedclothing. Bacteria invade these areas. Of first concern to the embalmer is control of the odor from these ulcerations. It is important to properly disinfect these areas. Undiluted cavity fluid can be applied on cotton compresses to the ulcerated areas. If bandages cover these areas it may be useful to saturate the bandages with undiluted cavity fluid or a phenol cautery–disinfectant during the embalming procedure. It is also wise to hypodermically treat the areas around these ulcerations using a small trocar and undiluted cavity fluid. This prevents continued bacterial activity and decreases the possibility of tissue gas (Figure 16–7A).

At the time of dressing, fresh cotton saturated with undiluted cavity chemical, a phenol solution, or autopsy gel is applied to the ulcerations; then the area is wrapped or, if possible, plastic garments should be used to cover these areas. Embalming powder should be placed in the garments to control odors. Some of these ulcerations are quite small, as frequently seen on the shoulders. Others are very large, often involving the entire buttocks or hip area.

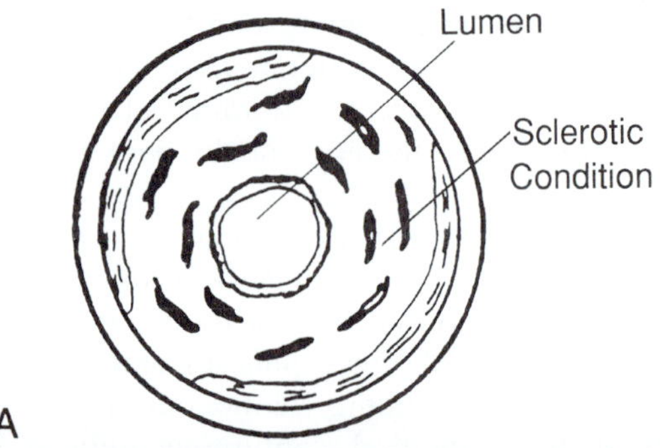

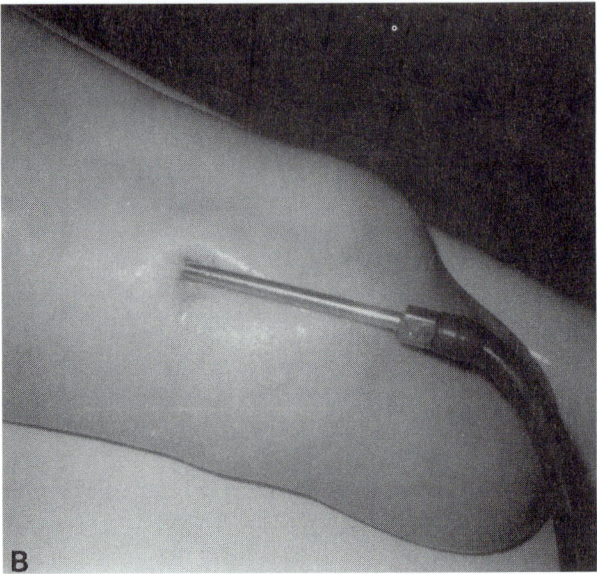

Figure 16–7. A. Diagram of medial sclerosis. **B.** The lower leg had been removed because of arteriosclerosis. This illustrates treatment of upper leg. Arterial fluid did not enter this area of the body.

Arteriosclerosis can also result in loss of a limb. If the limb was amputated recently, the stump should be treated by hypodermic injection with undiluted cavity chemical (Figure 16–7B). If stitching is still present, a plastic stocking is placed over the stitches in case there is leakage. Many times the embalmer is faced with gangrene of the leg. It is very important that these limbs be hypodermically injected with undiluted cavity chemical. They can also be wrapped in cotton saturated with undiluted cavity chemical, phenol solution, or autopsy gel. A plastic garment containing embalming powder can be placed over the leg. It is important to thoroughly hypodermically inject the tissues immediately superior to the gangrene area.

Arteriosclerosis can also lead to a ruptured aneurysm. When an aneurysm ruptures in the aorta, death results within minutes. This rupture is a site for leakage of embalming fluid during arterial injection. Many times the embalmer is unaware that a ruptured aortic aneurysm is the cause of death. On injection there is little or no drainage. The abdomen distends during injection and there are no signs of arterial fluid distribution such as the presence of dye in the tissues. A six-point injection becomes necessary. The trunk walls will have to be hypodermically injected with a small trocar as in an autopsied body for preservation.

Senile Purpura

Senile purpura (or ecchymosis) is an extravascular irregularly shaped blood discoloration that often appears on the arms and backs of the hands. The condition is brought about by fragility of the capillaries. In the elderly, drug usage, blood thinning, vitamin deficiencies, uremia, hypertension, thin skin, and slight bruising can easily bring about senile purpura. These discolorations vary greatly in size. The embalmer's concern in senile purpura lies in the fact that these discolorations do *not* clear during arterial injection. Often, these areas become engorged with fluid and swell during arterial injection. Purpural areas often darken after embalming and are prone to separate from underlying tissue, causing the tissues to tear open. Care should be taken in handling these areas. (Quite often the persons removing the body place a tight strap across the hands, and when the embalmer receives the body, skin areas on the backs of the hands are torn.)

If senile purpura is evidenced over the hands and arms (and often the base of the neck) the arterial solution should be strengthened. A fast rate of flow is *not* recommended. A slower rate of flow helps to limit further rupture of capillaries. It may be necessary to use multiple injection points. If the arms are separately injected, a special-purpose high-index fluid can be used in an attempt to dry these areas. Surface compresses of cavity fluid, phenol, or autopsy gel can be used. **If the skin over the purpural areas has been torn or broken open, all loose skin should be removed. This should be done at the beginning of embalming.** After surface compresses have had time to cauterize or bleach these discolored areas, the surface of the skin can be dried with a hair dryer and restorative and cosmetic treatment performed. Unseen hemorrhaged areas can be packed with cotton saturated with a proper preservative solution (a phenol solution is preferred) and then covered with plastic. Leakage is always possible with this condition. Care should be taken to protect the clothing of the deceased.

Care should be taken when massage is used to assist in fluid distribution and senile purpura is present. This condition is often the result of the use of blood thinners. Rough handling of the tissues can bring about postmortem bruising. This bruising is frequently seen when the eyes of the elderly or of individuals on blood thinners have been enucleated.

Malignancy

Improved medical procedures have done much to lengthen the life expectancy. With the extension of life, there is also an increased probability of a malignant tumor. Cancers or neoplasms that begin as localized tumors can easily invade healthy tissues, spread via the blood vascular system, and invade organs. This can interrupt vital functions to the point where death ensues. The embalmer is concerned with the following systemic effects of a malignancy:

- Disseminated intravascular coagulation
- Disruption of metabolism by uncontrolled secretion of hormones (This can greatly affect weight control, cell membrane activity, and metabolism of sugars, fats, and proteins.)
- Secretion of both peptide and steroid hormones by many tumors (Some of these hormones can bring about sustained hypercalcemia.)
- Anemia
- Cachexia (caused by the tumor's competition with the body for metabolites and resulting in a wasting away of tissues)

The local effects of a malignant tumor include invasion and destruction of normal tissues; obstruction of intestines, airways, urinary tract, and biliary tract; pathologic fractures; perforation of the hollow viscera; erosion of blood vessel walls, creating acute and chronic hemorrhage; and establishment of portals of entry for infections.

Both local and systemic effects of a malignancy have an effect on the embalming. There can be a loss of weight and emaciation; often, the skin is loose and flabby and has no support. The skin can be dry because of the body's inability to take in proper amounts of water. Localized edema can result when local tumors exert pressure on veins and lymphatics. If the hormone balance has been interrupted and a condition such as sustained hypercalcemia exists, the calcium can easily create a barrier, making it very difficult for embalming solutions to enter the cell and preserve the protoplasm. Because the fluid cannot penetrate the cells, tissue firmness is difficult to establish. When there is loose, flabby tissue, what appears to be firming is only a plumping of the tissues with embalming solution (actually, distension of the tissues). After the solution gravitates away, the tissues become soft along with being underembalmed.

The malignancy in and of itself may not be the cause of death. Most often the actual cause of death is pneumonia leading to respiratory arrest. In embalming these bodies fluid solutions should be of moderate strength (at least 2% or above) and should be well coordinated. Use of a coinjection fluid is advised. The coinjection helps to increase the distribution and diffusion of the arterial solution. It is especially helpful in the passage of the arterial solution through the cell membranes.

Metabolic disturbances and renal and respiratory failure, which often accompany a malignancy, result in the buildup of metabolic wastes in the tissues. These wastes increase the demand for preservative. Use of a strong arterial solution helps to ensure satisfactory preservation. The rate of flow should be adequate to distribute the fluid throughout the entire body, but if the skin appears flabby and loose, a slower rate of injection may be helpful. Senile, flabby tissue does not assimilate fluid as well as healthy tissue and swelling can result.

If the facial tissues are emaciated, restricted cervical injection is recommended. This allows for separate embalming of the head, at which time a slightly milder solution can be used or a solution containing humectant can be used to moisturize and restore the facial tissues.

If local edema is present as in the arms or legs, it may be necessary to use multiple sites for injection. In the elderly, the femoral arteries are often sclerotic. If it is not possible to inject the femoral, the legs can receive supplemental preservation by hypodermic treatment with undiluted cavity chemical. In addition, autopsy gel can be painted on the legs and plastic stockings placed over the gel.

A colostomy may be present if there has been a malignancy in the intestinal tract. The collecting bag can remain in place during arterial injection and cavity treatment. After cavity treatment the bag should be removed and its contents disinfected with cavity fluid. Cotton saturated with cavity fluid or a phenol solution can be inserted into the colostomy opening in the abdominal wall. Closure of the opening is easily achieved with a purse-string suture.

Cardiac Disease

In some diseases of the heart the medical treatment may include surgical procedures. If the patient died shortly after surgery and if no autopsy was performed, the embalmer may be confronted with extensive incisions of one or both legs and of the anterior chest wall and possibly the abdominal wall. In addition, very pronounced amounts of edema may be present in the facial tissues, especially if death occurred within a day or so of the operation. Generally, the surgery involves bypass repair or valve repair.

The common carotid artery and the internal jugular vein would be the best primary points for injection and drainage on these cardiac patients. A moderate to strong arterial solution should be used. Addition of dye to the solution from the start helps to indicate the distribution of arterial fluid.

If local obstructions exist, sectional embalming is necessary. If there is extensive edema of the facial tissues, restricted cervical injection should be used and strong solutions for treatment of the edematous face employed. If the sutures are recent and leak during injection, the metal staples used to hold them closed should be removed with a hemostat. Dry the incisions and inject a phenol cautery agent by hypodermic needle within the open incisions. Tightly suture them closed with a baseball stitch using incision seal powder to prevent leakage. After washing and drying the body, paint the incisions with a surface glue.

Some surgical procedures, such as the installation of a pacemaker, require only a small incision. This device is generally placed in the upper lateral portion on the right side of the chest. The contacts for the pacemaker run from the device into the right internal jugular vein and then into the heart. Drainage may be difficult to secure from the internal jugular vein. The angular spring forceps is the easiest drainage device to use. A drainage tube may be very difficult to insert. The left internal jugular vein or the femoral vein may be a necessary second choice for a point of drainage. If the body is to be cremated, the pacemaker should be removed. Some hospitals also require removal and return of the pacemaker.

Diabetes Mellitus

Diabetes mellitus may be defined as both an acute and a chronic metabolic disorder characterized principally by hyperglycemia (an excess of sugar in the blood) resulting from a deficiency of insulin.

Medical authorities estimate that up to 5% of the population are afflicted with diabetes mellitus, and that over the age of 40, women outnumber men so afflicted by about 3 to 2. Individuals who are obese are more frequently diabetic than those who are not. The disease usually manifests itself during adult life at the age of 50 to 60. The exception is an acute juvenile type that has a far younger age of onset. Remember that even though the onset of the disease can be in middle age, its effects continue into old age and may contribute to a middle-age death. The affliction affords some merit to the congenital theory of the origin of the disease as researchers have observed that when both parents are diabetic, offspring have a 90% (estimated) chance of acquiring diabetes mellitus.

The principal manifestations of diabetes mellitus include *hyperglycemia*, excess sugar in the blood; *glycosuria*, sugar in the urine; and *ketosis*, acidosis characterized by the presence of ketones in the blood and body tissues.

Pathologic changes resulting from the disease include poor peripheral circulation brought about by accelerated arteriosclerosis and degenerative changes in small blood vessels that result in poor circulation, particularly in the lower extremities. This often results in gangrene (Figure 16–8). Kidney failure and enlargement of the liver (very often resulting in infestation of the liver because of the high sugar content of the tissues) and fungal infestations of the lung can also be prevalent. The skin often exhibits scratch marks and infections brought about by pruritus and itching. A strong odor of acetone may be noted, as it is present in the urine and the perspiration.

In embalming these bodies a strong arterial solution is needed. Peripheral circulation is often poor; therefore, dyes should be added so the embalmer can detect where fluid is present. Areas of the face such as the ears, tip of the nose, and cheeks often do not receive an adequate amount of fluid. Likewise, the hands and the legs should be carefully evaluated. The common carotid artery (restricted cervical) would be the best injection point. This artery is the least likely to exhibit arteriosclerosis.

The **restricted cervical injection** is recommended so that higher pressures and two arterial solutions can be employed. Restricted cervical injection also allows the embalmer to inject both sides of the head. This helps to ensure good circulation to all facial tissues. If the lower extremities or the stump of an amputated leg do not receive sufficient fluid by arterial injection then hypodermic and surface treatment may be needed. Plastic garments, containing surface preservatives or gels, may also be placed on the lower extremities.

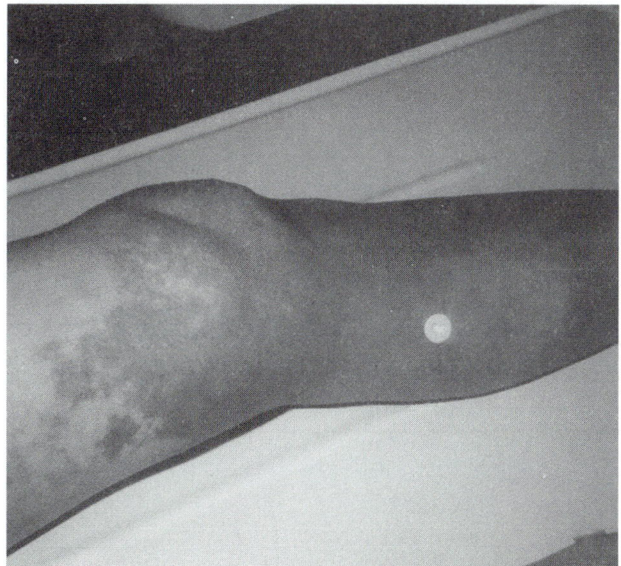

Figure 16–8. Gangrene of the left leg in a diabetic. Treatments included hypodermic injection of cavity fluid and application of surface preservative gel with a plastic stocking.

If the hands or fingers do not receive sufficient fluid, a small-gauge hypodermic needle can be inserted between the fingers and arterial or cavity fluid injected to secure preservation. The hands can also be wrapped with cotton saturated with a surface preservative such as a cavity fluid compress or autopsy gel. Manufacturer's directions may inform how long compresses should be left in place. One must be certain that the preservative is applied to the palm side of the hand in addition to the back of the hand.

The following list summarizes the recommended treatment for diabetics:

1. Use the carotid vessels for primary injection.
2. Use strong arterial solutions.
3. Use fluid dyes for tracers.
4. Carefully disinfect the respiratory tract, as fungal infections may be present.
5. Institute hypodermic treatment and surface treatment for areas receiving insufficient arterial fluid.

Cavity embalming should immediately follow arterial injection. The embalmer should be certain that a liberal amount of cavity fluid is injected into the liver and lungs.

▶ KEY TERMS AND CONCEPTS FOR STUDY AND DISCUSSION

1. Define the following terms.
   ideal fluid strength for embalming the "normal" adult body
   ideal pressure for embalming the "normal" adult body
   ideal rate of flow for embalming the "normal" adult body
   infant
   senile purpura
   stillborn
2. Describe in detail several arterial methods of injection for embalming an infant.
3. Explain why it may be necessary to use the same strength arterial solution for embalming an infant or child and an adult.
4. Discuss the following complications in embalming of the elderly:
   arteriosclerosis
   arthritis
   atrophy of the mandible and maxillae
   senile diabetes

▶ BIBLIOGRAPHY

Bickley HC. *Practical Concepts in Human Disease.* Baltimore, MD: Williams & Wilkins; 1974:92–95.

Slocum RE. Type six classification. In. *Pre-embalming Considerations.* Boston: Dodge Chemical Co; 1969:79.

Smith AL. *Microbiology and Pathology.* 12th ed. St. Louis, MO: CV Mosby; 1980:513–514.

Spriggs AO. Preparation of children's bodies. In: *The Art and Science of Embalming.* Springfield, OH: Champion Chemical Co.; 1963:Chap. 29, pp. 127–128.

The elderly cases. In: *Champion Expanding Encyclopedia.* Springfield, OH: Champion Chemical Co.; January–March 1971: Nos. 413–415.

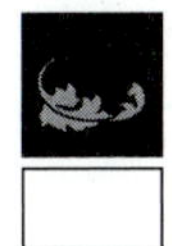

CHAPTER 17
PREPARATION OF AUTOPSIED BODIES

An autopsy (necropsy or postmortem) is a postmortem examination of the dead human body. There are two types of autopsy: the medical (hospital) autopsy and the medicolegal (forensic) autopsy. In some communities the pathologist prefers that the arterial embalming of the body be done prior to the autopsy. In contrast, most coroners and medical examiner offices **do not** want the body embalmed prior to the autopsy.

Before an autopsy can be performed proper permission *must be given* by the family member who has the right of disposition of the remains.

In certain autopsies, particularly hospital autopsies, the family not only must give permission for the autopsy, they also have the right to limit the extent of the autopsy. Where special instructions have been given, it is important that the pathologist follow the limitations established by the family. A family often gives permission only for what is called a partial autopsy, which consists of external examination and removal of one or two organs.

With respect to liability, the embalmer should also note in the funeral home records the type of autopsy performed. In addition, a memorandum should be made as to the disposition of the visceral organs: Were they returned with the body? *This is very important. In a number of instances a second autopsy has been ordered to support insurance claims or to confirm a cause of death. This is especially true in communities where black-lung and industrial deaths have insurance relationships.*

▶ TYPES OF AUTOPSIES

Medical or Hospital Autopsy

Permission for the medical or hospital autopsy is obtained from a family member who has the proper authority to take charge of the body after death. Several reasons are given by the College of American Pathologists for the performance of the hospital autopsy*:

- When doctors have not made a firm diagnosis
- When death follows unexpected medical complications
- When death follows the use of an experimental drug or device, a new procedure, or unusual therapy
- When death follows a dental or surgical procedure done for diagnostic purposes and the case does not come under the jurisdiction of medical examiner or coroner
- When death occurs suddenly, unexpectedly, or in mysterious circumstances from apparently natural causes and the case does not come under the jurisdiction of medical examiner or coroner
- When environmental or workplace hazards are suspected
- When death occurs during or after childbirth
- When there are concerns about a hereditary disease that might affect other members of the family
- When there are concerns about the possible spread of a contagious disease
- When the cause of death could affect insurance settlements (e.g., policies that cover cancer or that grant double indemnity for accidental death)
- When death occurs in a hospital and the patient comes from a nursing home and the quality of care is questioned

In addition to the preceding reasons, hospital autopsies are requested to confirm or to verify a diagnosis. Also, many of these institutions are teaching hospitals, and the autopsy serves as a tool in explaining a diagnostic technique or disease process.

Coroner or Medical Examiner Autopsy

In the coroner or medical examiner autopsy, discovering the cause of death and the manner of death are the goals. The cases that come under the jurisdiction of a coroner or medical examiner vary from state to state

* Adapted from recommendations of the College of American Pathologists headed by Dr. Hans J. Peters, *N. Y. Times*, July 21, 1988.

and from county to county *within* a state. The following list represents typical cases that would be reported to a coroner or medical examiner. This will vary from state to state and even county to county.

- All sudden deaths not caused by readily recognizable disease or wherein the cause of death cannot be properly certified by a physician on the basis of prior (recent) medical attendance
- All deaths occurring in suspicious circumstances, including those where alcohol, drugs, or other toxic substances may have had a direct bearing on the outcome
- All deaths occurring as a result of violence or trauma, whether apparently homicidal, suicidal, or accidental (including those caused by mechanical, thermal, chemical, electrical, or radiation injury, drowning, cave-ins, and subsidences), regardless of the time elapsed between injury and death
- Any fetal death, stillbirth, or death of a baby within 24 hours of birth, where the mother has not been under the care of a physician
- All therapeutic and criminal abortions, regardless of the length of pregnancy, and spontaneous abortions beyond 16 weeks gestation
- All operative and perioperative deaths in which the death is not readily explainable on the basis of prior disease
- Any death wherein the body is unidentified or unclaimed
- Any death where there is uncertainty as to whether or not it should be reported to the coroner's office

Death within 24 hours of admission to a hospital is not considered a reportable death unless it falls into one of the specific categories defined.

▶ GUIDELINES TO DETERMINE WHEN AUTOPSIES ARE TO BE PERFORMED

The following list includes not only the cases that fall under the jurisdiction of a coroner or medical examiner, but **specific cases on which an autopsy must be performed.** (This list is only representative.) Autopsies must be performed on all of the following cases, which fall under the jurisdiction of the coroner; this varies from state to state and even county to county.

- Victims of homicide
- Victims of deaths in the workplace
- Motor vehicle drivers who have been involved in accidents
- Pedestrians who have been involved in accidents
- Passengers who have been involved in accidents but who lack clear evidence of trauma
- Victims of intra- and perioperative accidental deaths
- Epileptics
- Possible victims of sudden infant death syndrome
- Infants or children with evidence of bodily injury
- Inmate fatalities in correctional facilities, nursing homes, or medical institutions
- Victims of trauma
- Victims of nontraumatic, sudden, unexpected deaths
- Victims of anorexia nervosa
- Multiple victims of coincidental, unexplained death at one location
- Victims of possible poisoning or overdose deaths
- Any other case in which the pathologist holds a bona fide belief that the death is unexplained and/or an autopsy is in the best interest of the public or that it is necessary for the proper administration of the statutory duties of the office of the coroner.

▶ GENERAL CONSIDERATIONS IN AUTOPSY TREATMENT

WORK PRACTICE CONTROLS

1. Be aware where cutting and sharp instruments are laid during preparation.
2. Cover broken or cut bones (e.g., ribs) prior to placement of embalmers hands into a body cavity.
3. Wash gloved hands or change gloves often during the embalming procedure.
4. Avoid use of high water pressure when water is used to flush blood and fluids from the embalming table.
5. Practice continuous aspiration of the cavities during arterial injection.
6. Clamp leaking arteries and small veins to avoid excessive embalming solution loss during arterial injection.
7. Run table water continuously to dilute and carry away any blood or chemicals on the table surface.

Order in Working

Do one item at a time in preparation of the autopsied body. In injection of the legs, that must be the only concern—

that is, check for distribution, use intermittent drainage by clamping off the external iliac vein, massage the leg to assist distribution, and so on. Do not try to set features or raise other vessels while injecting the legs. Do one procedure at a time. In the long run, this makes the work more thorough. Time is not saved by doing several things at the same time.

FACTORS THAT MUST BE DETERMINED IN THE EMBALMING ANALYSIS

1. Vessels for injection and drainage
2. Strength of the embalming solution
3. Volume of the embalming solution
4. Injection pressure
5. Injection rate of flow

Note: These factors will vary by the individual body; these factors can vary in different areas of the same body.

Fluid Strength

Preparation of the autopsied body is usually *delayed.* The delay may occur between death and autopsy or between autopsy and release of the body. Most institutions *refrigerate* bodies during these time delays. These factors combined with the pathologic conditions of the body generally require that somewhat **stronger-than-average arterial solutions** be used; however, improper and delayed refrigeration could also produce dehydrated tissues, which will demand a different type of arterial solution. Delays increase the possibility of **distension** during arterial injection and also increase the preservative demand of the tissues.

Use of Fluid Dyes

Delay also brings about rigor mortis and, if long enough, the passing of rigor. Rigor can cause poor arterial solution distribution and may also be a false sign of fluid firming. Fluid reactions with body proteins do not proceed normally when a body is in rigor mortis. Refrigeration can bring about hemolysis of blood trapped in the superficial tissues. This hemolysis can create an appearance similar to that of the dye present in arterial solutions. The tissue thus appears "embalmed." In addition, refrigerated tissues feel "embalmed" because the artifacts in the subcutaneous region have hardened. Use dye in the arterial solution; it serves as the best sign of arterial solution distribution. Keep in mind that dyes show only *surface* distribution of arterial solutions. Massage deep tissues, such as the muscles of the legs (especially in rigor). Employ intermittent drainage to "force" fluids into the deep tissues.

▶ PRESSURES AND RATES OF FLOW

Tissues can assimilate only a certain amount of fluid in a given time period. Often, arterial solution is injected too fast into the body and swelling results. In preparation of the autopsied body, inject each section separately. During injection into a specific body region, such as an arm or leg, higher pressures and faster rates of flow can be safely used to help establish good circulation. The embalmer can vary the rate of flow for each area and, if necessary, vary the pressure to overcome the resistances of a particular body part. In addition, intermittent drainage and pulsation can be used for each area to establish good distribution and diffusion.

▶ DRAINAGE

With the autopsied body it is **not** necessary to insert drainage devices (drain tubes or angular spring forceps) into the veins. Drainage can be taken directly from the cut vein and the drainage material can flow directly into the body cavities. Once in the cavities, an autopsy aspirator is used to keep accumulated drainage at a minimum. These instruments are useful because they are designed not to clog. These accumulated fluids can be aspirated into a sanitary sewer system. Intermittent or alternate drainage can also be used for each area injected in the autopsied body. Clamping the vein with a hemostat or applying digital pressure with a piece of cotton temporarily stops the drainage. Intermittent and alternate drainage greatly assists in fluid distribution, diffusion, and retention.

▶ COMPLETE AUTOPSY/PARTIAL AUTOPSY

In this chapter, autopsies are divided into two categories (based on the extent of the autopsy): the *complete autopsy* and the *partial autopsy.* The hospital or forensic autopsy can be either type. The coroner or medical examiner autopsy is generally a complete autopsy. Complete examination of the body is necessary when the findings will be challenged in a court of law (Figure 17–1).

The **complete autopsy** involves opening of the following body cavities and removal of the following organs:

1. Cranial cavity and its contents
   A. Possibly removal of the inner ear
   B. Brain
   C. Removal of the pituitary gland

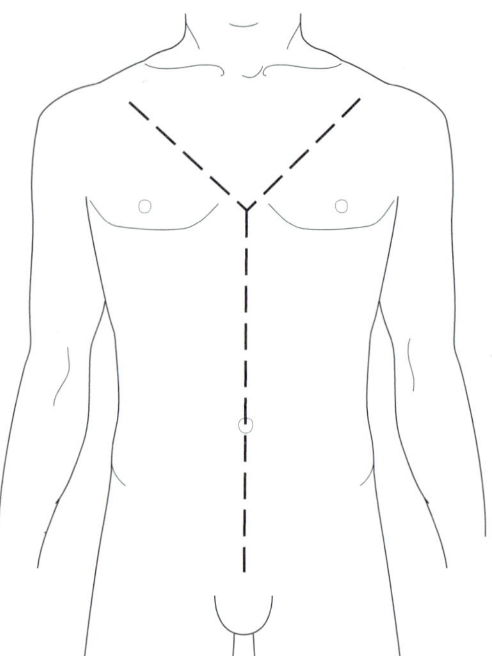

Figure 17–1. Standard Y autopsy incision.

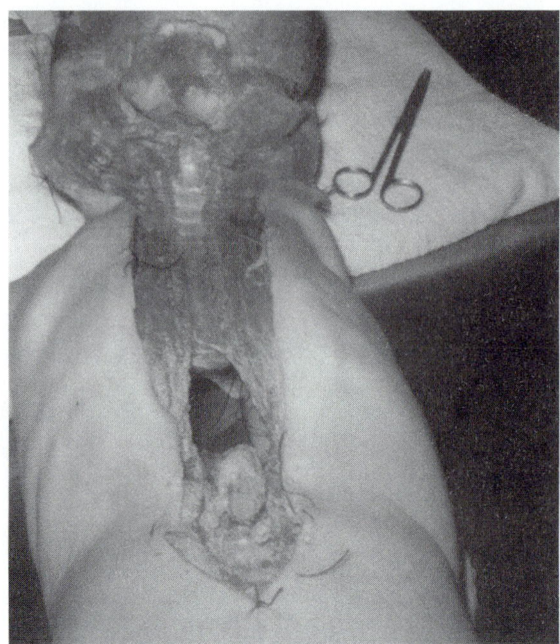

Figure 17–2. Spinal cord removed for examination by the dorsal approach.

2. Eye enucleation
3. Removal of the neck organs
   A. Thyroid gland
   B. Larynx
   C. Cervical portion of the esophagus and trachea
   D. Possibly removal of the common carotid arteries
   E. Possibly removal of the tongue (especially if a "cafe coronary" is suspected)
4. Thoracic cavity and its contents
5. Abdominal cavity and its contents
6. Pelvic cavity contents
7. Removal of spinal cord
   A. *Dorsal* approach: body is turned over and vertebral column opened (Figure 17–2).
   B. *Ventral* approach: vertebral column is opened from within the body cavities and cervical area
   C. Removal from the foramen magnum

OR

8. Sample removal of the spinal cord, usually through the ventral approach (a "wedge" cut from the vertebral column)

In the **partial autopsy**, generally only one body cavity (cranial, thoracic, or abdominopelvic cavity) is opened to examine one specific item. This type of autopsy is most frequently performed as the medical (or hospital) autopsy.

Some institutions remove and examine only one organ, usually because they are limited by the person granting permission for the autopsy. If only one organ is removed and all vessels ligated, the embalmer should have little difficulty. Many pathologists, however, remove the one organ but do not ligate the vessels. This often leads to extensive prosection of the cavity and contributes to interrupted circulation in the embalming process.

▶ SUGGESTED ORDER FOR PREPARATION OF THE AUTOPSIED BODY

1. Unwrap the body. To disinfect, apply a topical droplet spray to the surface of the body and the orifices. Wash the body with germicidal soap and dry it. Relieve (as much as possible) any rigor mortis present. Position the head and shoulders.
2. Shave the body and set the features.
3. Open the cavities. Remove the viscera if they have been returned. Disinfect the internal surfaces of the body cavities with droplet spray.
4. Locate and place ligatures around the six vessels needed for sectional arterial injection:
   A. Right and left external-iliac arteries*
   B. Right and left axillary or subclavian arteries
   C. Right and left common carotid arteries
5. Prepare the arterial solution. Consider a variety of factors in determining the strength of the solution:

---

* Common iliacs can be injected when present. Internal iliacs may be injected if they are present.

A. Cause of death
B. Size and weight of body
C. Time between death and preparation
D. Presence of decomposition changes
E. Moisture content of tissues
F. Protein content of body
G. Refrigeration
(Different solutions may have to be prepared for different sections of the body, e.g., if edema is present in the legs but not in the arms or head.)

6. Inject at rates of flow and pressures that meet the demands of the various body areas. Drainage may be concurrent or intermittent.
   A. Inject the legs first, one at a time.
   B. Inject the arms second, one at a time.
   C. Inject the head.
      a. Inject the left side *first.*
      b. Inject the right side.
7. Institute supplemental treatments: hypodermic injection of the *trunk walls, shoulders, neck,* and *buttocks.*
8. Drain all liquids from body cavities and treat internal surfaces with hardening compound or autopsy gel.
9. Prepare abdominal and thoracic cavities and neck area.
   A. Return the bag of viscera and add preservative chemical.
   B. Fill cavities with absorbent material such as sheeting or cotton and saturate material with preservative chemical.
   C. Fill out neck area with cotton saturated with preservative chemical or autopsy gel.
10. Suture thoracic and abdominal cavities.
11. Dry cranial cavity. Treat walls with preservative powder or gel and attach calvarium.
12. Suture scalp.
13. Wash and dry body.
14. Apply glue to incisions of the thoracic and abdominal cavity.
15. Dress body in coveralls, adding embalming powder to surface of abdominal and back areas.
16. Prepare the embalming report.

▶ PREPARATION OF THE AUTOPSIED BODY

Carefully open the zippered pouch or plastic or cotton sheeting enveloping the autopsied remains. Liberally, using a droplet spray, disinfect the exposed surfaces and inner wrappings. Several minutes later, roll up the covering material, and gently roll the body from side to side to remove all of the wrappings. Place these immediately in a biohazard container. Next, wash the body with a disinfectant solution. Let this topical solution remain on the body for at least 10 minutes. The body can then be rinsed and dried. Relieve any rigor mortis present and proceed to position the body.

1. Remove the pathologist's stitches and lay back the flaps of skin, exposing the thoracic and abdominal and cranial cavities. Spray these cavities with a broad-spectrum disinfectant droplet spray. Remove the stitches from the scalp and remove the calvarium. Disinfect the cranial cavity or better yet, swab it with autopsy gel, especially in cases of systemic infection (meningitis, hepatitis, AIDS). Support the scalp in the forehead area, especially during arterial injection, to avoid a "creased" area across the forehead and to assist distribution of fluid through the scalp.
2. Inspect the arteries needed for injection.
3. *Option:* Some embalmers prefer to shave and set the features at this time; others prefer to inject the legs and arms prior to setting the features.
4. Mix arterial solution. Remember that if there has been a delay between death and preparation or if the body has been refrigerated, or both, a slightly stronger arterial solution is needed: *either a higher-index fluid or a standard arterial solution to which 4 to 6 ounces of a high-index fluid has been added.* Add some tracer dye to indicate the distribution of arterial solution in the body.
5. Inject the lower extremities.
   A. The ideal vessels to use for injection of the legs are the right and left common iliac. Any leakage from the internal iliac branch can be clamped (vessels were severed when the pelvic organs were removed). Arterial solution will reach the legs by the external iliac and the internal iliac artery will supply solution to the buttocks, anal area, and perineal tissues. Injection of the common iliac would also supply solution to the trunk walls through branches off the external iliac artery. In some autopsies the common iliac and internal iliac arteries have been excised. In this situation the embalmer will use the external iliac artery to inject each leg. Injecting each common iliac artery or external iliac artery separately permits more control over the flow of the solution into the extremity being injected. The embalmer can control massage, pressure, rate of flow, and strength of the solution being used for each leg. Separate direct injection of the internal iliac artery accompanied by massage to the buttocks and upper thighs can bring about a noticeable amount of arterial solution distribution to these areas. It should always be at-

tempted; leakage may need to be controlled with hemostats.

B. Some autopsy technicians and/or pathologists sever the external iliac artery directly beneath the inguinal ligament. It is important to remember that arteries remain open when severed. In the nose of a hemostat, grasp the cut end of the artery and gently expose it sufficiently to insert an arterial tube. If possible place a tight ligature around the artery to secure the tube; if this is not possible use an arterial hemostat to secure the tube in the artery. Always attempt to place strings around arteries to hold arterial tubes in place rather than holding them in position using hemostats.

C. If necessary, raise the femoral artery to inject the lower extremities.

D. Allow drainage to enter the abdominopelvic cavity. If intermittent drainage is desired, use a hemostat to stop drainage for intervals.

E. If fluid does not reach the foot, institute the following procedures:
   a. Very firmly massage the leg, pushing strongly along the arterial route (femoral, popliteal, and anterior and posterior tibial arteries). Rotate the foot medially. This squeezes all the muscles of the lower leg.
   b. Use a higher injection pressure and pulsation.
   c. Limit drainage by using intermittent drainage.

Many times, the vessels of the leg are sclerotic. If injection of the lower arteries is impossible, inject the legs hypodermically (using an infant trocar) with a preservative. Then paint the legs with autopsy gel and clothe them in plastic stockings.

The volume and strength of solution depend on pathologic conditions, leakage, and postmortem conditions. Sometimes, $\frac{1}{2}$ gallon is sufficient. With edema, 2 or more gallons might be needed per leg. *There is no set volume or strength.*

Some embalmers prefer to aspirate drainage material continuously while injecting the legs and arms. Others prefer to let the excess fluids that accumulate sit in the cavities during arterial injection, the theory being that these fluids preserve the tissues of the inner surface of the back area. The problem with the latter method is that the working environment may become quite uncomfortable for the embalmer because of the excess fumes. It is easier to aspirate the excess fluids from the cavities and thus reduce exposure to formaldehyde fumes.

6. Inject the upper extremities.

A. If the arch of the aorta or its branches are present, use the subclavian arteries for injection. In this way fluid is distributed to the shoulders, to the back of the neck, and to the upper back regions. In the complete autopsy, however, the following vessels must be clamped if the subclavian artery is injected:
   a. Vertebral artery (if a cranial autopsy has been done)
   b. Internal thoracic artery
   c. Inferior thyroid artery (when neck organs have been removed)

   The right subclavian is a branch of the brachiocephalic artery. It can be distinguished from the right common carotid artery, because the subclavian is usually larger in diameter. Follow the direction of the insertion of an arterial tube to determine if the right subclavian artery has been entered; it heads laterally toward the arm. The left subclavian branches off the arch of the aorta. If, after clamping off the leakage from the severed branches of the subclavian, leakage still continues, it may be necessary to raise and inject the axillary artery. The problem with using the axillary is that the shoulder, upper portions of the back, and deep muscles of the neck do not receive arterial solution distribution.

B. The axillary artery can be raised by cutting the pectoralis major and minor muscles (Figure 17–3). It is easy to raise this artery just as it leaves the cervicoaxillary canal. This canal is bounded by the scapula, the first rib, and the clavicle. If the axillary artery is raised at this point, all its branches can be used to distribute fluid to the trunk walls and shoulder areas. In addition, the arm can be placed in a natural position. Use of the axillary artery avoids many of the leakage problems seen with the subclavian artery, and the axillary can be raised from the incision the pathologist has already made (if that incision rises to the shoulder area). *If fluid does not flow easily down the arm, pull the arterial tube out a little. This usually frees the tube of any blockage.*

C. Drainage can be taken from the subclavian vein. If intermittent drainage is desired, place a hemostat on either the subclavian or the axillary vein.

D. Fluid strength and volume vary from body to body or even from right side to left side. Continue injection until the hand has cleared and distribution is evident. Manipulate the arm, flexing at the elbow and wrist, to assist distribution along with intermittent drainage. It may also be necessary to place digital pressure

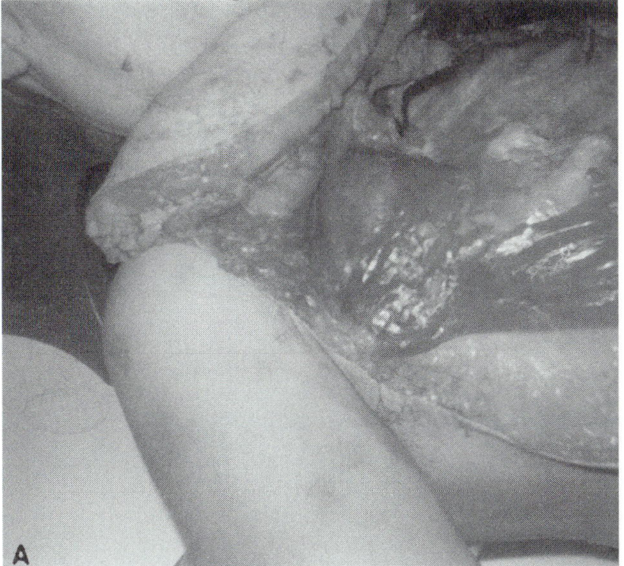

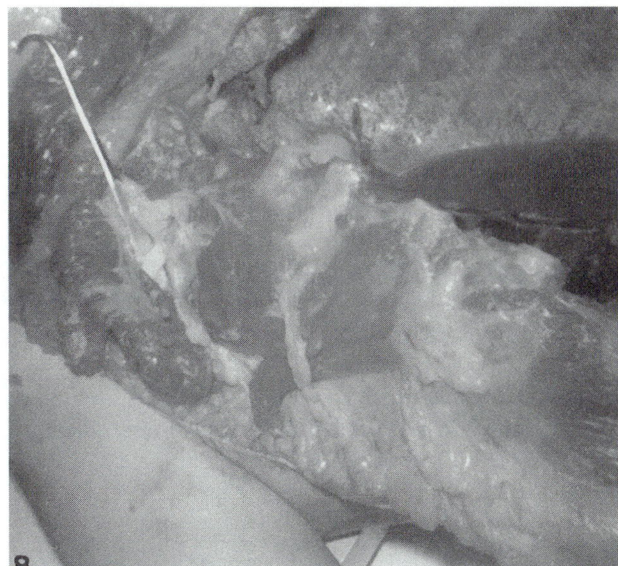

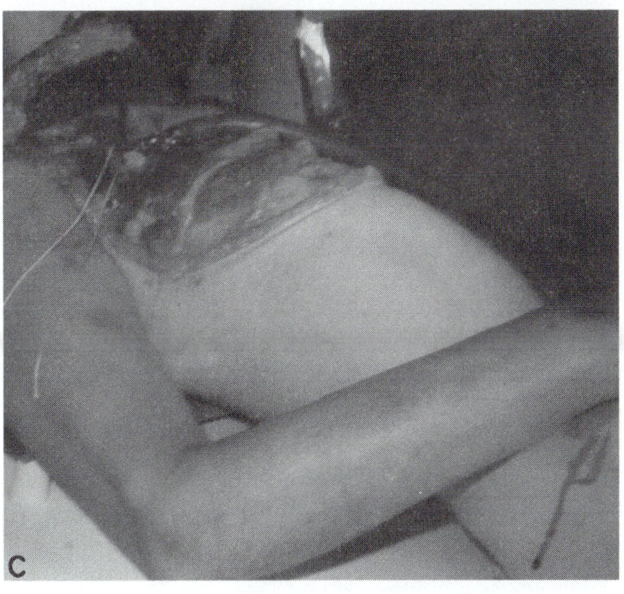

Figure 17-3. Autopsy injection of arms using the axillary artery. **A.** Note the pectoralis muscle. **B.** The axillary artery is shown; inject from this location. **C.** The arm may be positioned during injection.

on the cephalic vein to increase distribution by blocking the loss of fluid from the superficial drainage route.

If fluid is not flowing into the hand, try the following: lower the hand while injecting, massage by pushing very firmly along the arterial route (axillary, brachial, radial, and ulnar arteries), increase injection pressure (using pulsation if available), and use intermittent drainage. Finally, the radial and ulnar arteries can be raised and injected. If fluid still does not enter the fingers, treat by hypodermic injection of a preservative fluid.

7. Inject the head.
   A. Place arterial tubes in the right and left common carotid arteries. If the common carotid has been cut by the pathologist, try to find the external carotid. Remember that the common carotid bifurcates at the level of the superior border of the thyroid cartilage. This point is quite high in the neck. If the artery can be located, insert a small arterial tube. Clamp it in place with an arterial hemostat.
   B. If the eyes have been enucleated, loosely pack the eye orbits with cotton saturated with autopsy gel.
   C. If the inner ear has been removed, tightly pack the area of the temporal bone from which the tissues were removed with cotton saturated with autopsy gel. If this area leaks profusely during injection, apply a hemostat to the leaking vessels.

D. *Option 1:* Inject the left side of the head first. Certain arteries must be clamped for leakage if the left common carotid artery is injected. The *left internal carotid* is located inside the cranial cavity just lateral to the sella turcica of the sphenoid bone. Clamp this vessel after arterial injection has begun. In this way, filling of the vascular system supplied by the common carotid artery can be observed. The *superior thyroid artery* is located in the neck; this branch of external carotid artery leaks if the neck organs have been removed.

   Inject the right side of the head. The left is injected first so that a certain amount of fluid flows to the right side via anastomosis. It also gives the embalmer a chance to observe the effects of the fluid and the dyes on the left side. If there is any problem, the arterial solution can be changed before the right side is injected. This method also prevents overinjection of the right side of the face. Arteries to be clamped are the *right internal carotid,* found lateral to the sella turcica in the cranial cavity, and the *right superior thyroid,* found in the neck if the neck organs have been removed.

E. *Option 2:* Once tubes are in place in the right and left common carotid arteries, attach them to a Y tube. Inject both right and left sides at the same time. Clamp all arteries, such as internal carotids and superior thyroids or any other major leaking arteries, with hemostats.

F. Observe the parotid, sublingual, and submaxillary glands for swelling. Use of a stronger solution and pulsation, a slower rate flow, and a reduced pressure during the injection helps to limit swelling of these glands. If swelling occurs, apply digital pressure against the glands. These glands can also be pierced from under the skin with a scalpel, which, together with digital pressure, helps to reduce swelling. If the swelling is too pronounced, the glands may have to be excised from under the skin by going up through the neck.

▶ SUPPLEMENTAL HYPODERMIC INJECTION

Depending on the incisions made by the pathologist and the extent of vessel removal, only a small portion of the trunk may receive arterial fluid. It now becomes necessary for the embalmer to preserve those areas lacking fluid, as best as possible, by hypodermic embalming (Figure 17–4). Preservative solution is injected via a trocar attached to the embalming machine. Some embalmers prefer arterial solution for this work; others use a mixture of cavity fluid and water.

It is important that all tissues be channeled: the trunk walls (anterior, lateral, and posterior), with special emphasis on injection of the buttocks, breasts in the female, and shoulder and neck regions. Channel these regions first; then turn on the machine or allow the fluid to pass through the trocar into the channels. Avoid accidents that expose the embalmer to excessive amounts of embalming solution. Universal Precautions require eye protection during all embalming proce-

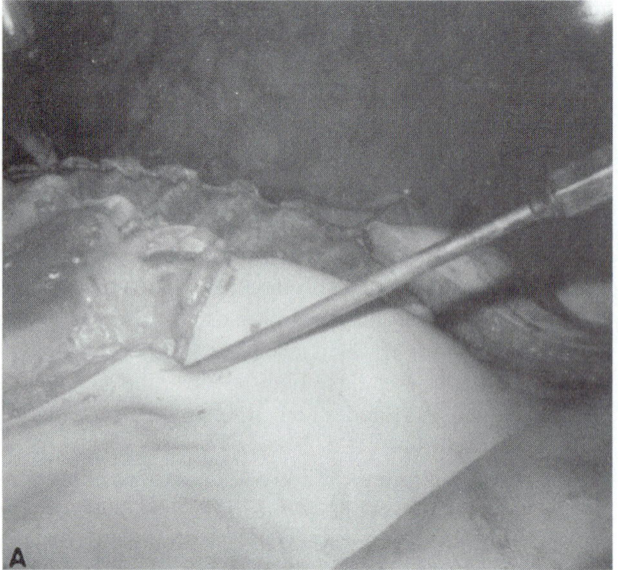

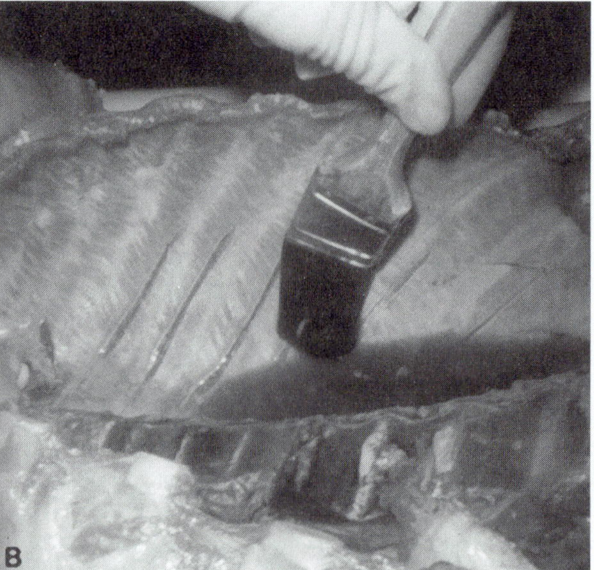

Figure 17–4. A. Hypodermic treatment of the walls after autopsy. **B.** After the intercostal muscles are incised, the cavity walls are painted with autopsy gel.

dures; hypodermic treatments certainly demand this protection. In addition to the hypodermic treatment of the trunk walls, surface embalming can be used in the following ways.

1. A scalpel can be used to cut the intercostal muscles in the thoracic area. Later, this area can be painted with autopsy gel, which, over time, penetrates the tissues of the back (Figure 17–4B).
2. The trunk walls on the outside of the rib case can be cut further back (some embalmers do this as far back as the vertebral column) and then painted with autopsy gel. In lieu of autopsy gel, cotton, paper towels, or strips of sheeting can be placed between the trunk wall and the rib cage and saturated with cavity fluid.
3. All inside surfaces of the cavities can be painted with autopsy gel.
4. If viscera are not returned, sheeting can be placed in the cavities and saturated with cavity fluid. This provides an "inside compress" for surface embalming.
5. Even if viscera are returned, the cavity can be lined with cotton, paper towels, or sheeting and saturated with cavity fluid before the plastic bag of viscera is placed back in the cavity. This material can be saturated with preservative or cavity fluid, in lieu of autopsy gel.

Autopsy gels are made to cling to the lateral walls. In addition, they are formulated to penetrate the tissues, so their use may be preferred to that of inlays of cavity fluid. The autopsy gels are a little easier to work with from the standpoint of formaldehyde irritation.

Care should be taken to pack the pelvic cavity so there is no leakage from the rectum. If the pathologist has removed the entire rectum, it may be necessary to turn the body over and suture the area closed. The rectum, esophagus, and trachea can be tightly ligated from within the cavities.

Attention should also be given to the neck area if the neck organs have been removed. Cotton is used to replace the missing organs, and once it is in place, the cotton is saturated with preservative fluid. This is necessary, because circulation to the skin of the neck is interrupted when the neck organs are removed. Again, all inside areas of the neck can be painted with autopsy gel before cotton is inserted.

▶ TREATMENT OF THE VISCERA

The embalming report should indicate if the viscera were or were not returned with the remains. If the viscera were returned the report should state whether they were (1) placed within the body, or (2) prepared and placed in a separate container with the body in the casket or shipping case. If returned, the viscera are usually enclosed in a plastic bag. Several methods can be used to treat the viscera.

If the viscera are to be returned to the abdominal and thoracic cavities, a new plastic bag should be used. A minimum of two bottles of cavity fluid should be mixed and poured over the viscera before the bag is returned to the cavities. It is much easier to position and "find room" for the viscera in the cavities if the preservative fluids are not poured over the viscera until the bag is in position. After being covered with cavity chemical, the hollow organs can be incised using shears to release any gases.

Some embalmers return the viscera to the cavities but *not* in plastic bags. The viscera should be soaked in cavity fluid several hours, returned to the abdominal and thoracic cavities, and covered well with absorbent autopsy hardening compound, absorbent cotton, and a piece of sheet. Then, the cavities are sutured closed.

▶ CLOSURE OF THE CAVITIES

After *walls of the cavities* have been treated *hypodermically* and by *surface embalming* and the viscera returned (preferably in a plastic bag) to the abdominal and thoracic cavities, the next step is closure of the cavities.

If the viscera are not returned to the abdominal and thoracic cavities, the cavities should be filled with absorbent material such as sheeting, kapoc, or cotton. This material should be saturated with cavity fluid or autopsy gel to prevent it from molding or developing odor. The sheeting or cotton also serves as an internal preservative compress.

Position the breastplate, being certain it is coated on both sides with autopsy gel or preservative powder.

Begin to suture using a double-curved needle and linen suture cord. Linen suture cord is much stronger than cotton suture cord. A minimum of a five-twist (strand) linen suture cord should be used. When pulling the cord to tighten the stitches, **pull on the thread, not on the needle.** Otherwise, the thread may break as it rubs against the eye of the needle.

If cotton is used as filler for the cavities, be certain that paper toweling or sheeting is placed over the cotton. Cotton has a tendency to get caught in the suturing and can be quite troublesome to work with.

Bring all three flaps of the incision together and tie them together with one suture. From this point, if desired, sew to the shoulder area along one of the branches of the incision extending from the xiphoid process of the sternum to the shoulder (Figure 17–5).

Start the suture for the abdominal cavity at the level of the pubic symphysis. Begin the suture by *tying*

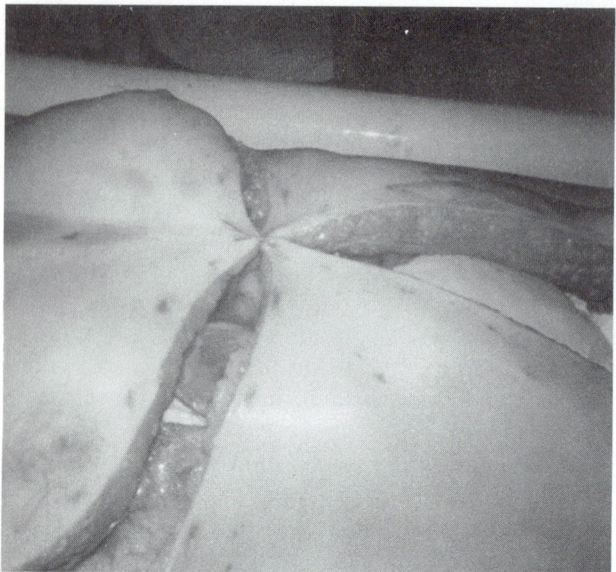

Figure 17–5. Align autopsy incisions before suturing the abdominal incisions.

the suture in place rather than just tying a knot on the end of the suture. Knots have a tendency to pull through the skin. Use a baseball suture for closure. This suture is very tight. In fact, if properly done, it is airtight. String from the suture pattern should not be seen. If the suture looks like the lacing pattern of a baseball, it is *too loose.* Pull the sutures *very tight.* Single- or double-cord suture thread may be used. If linen is used, single-strand thread should be sufficient and not cause any breakage. [If the hole made by the suture needle appears large, double-stranded thread may be preferred to close (fill) the hole.]

If the suture thread should break, assess the situation. Rather than tearing out all the suturing and starting over, it may be more convenient to begin sewing from another direction and tie the two sutures together.

When the tie at the location of the xiphoid process is reached, continue the suture up the branch of the Y incision that was not previously closed to the shoulder. It is important, especially in the shoulder areas, to use *incision seal powder* to prevent any leakage. This is the one area of the Y incision that is most likely to leak.

The skin of bodies with certain wasting diseases may be difficult to suture because it tears easily. Try using a large inversion suture to close these incisions. In extreme cases, it may be necessary simply to wrap the trunk closed by wrapping strips of sheeting around the body.

In the female, suturing is easier if the pathologist made a Y incision over rather than under the breasts. This might be suggested to the pathologist.

During the embalming of the body, a phenol cautery chemical can be placed on cotton compresses and laid along the autopsy incision where the scalp has been opened. This will assist in drying the marginal tissues and reduce the possibility of leakage from this incision when the scalp is closed by suturing.

Arterial solution or blood that has accumulated in the posterior portion of the cranial cavity should be removed by aspirating or sponging. The walls of the cavity can be painted with autopsy gel or dusted with a preservative powder. An absorbent material should be placed in the cavity to absorb liquids that may accumulate. In addition, some embalmers place incision seal powder in the foramen magnum and the posterior areas of the cranium to absorb liquids that might leak.

Some embalmers force (by hammering) a long wedge of wood into the foramen magnum. This holds the head steady if the vertebral column has been cut open.

Next, the calvarium should be replaced. If the autopsy has been properly performed, there should be one *notch* in the area of the *frontal bone* and other *notches* laterally in the *area of the temporal bone.* If notches are present, the calvarium will not be able to move forward, backward, or laterally (from side to side). If notches are not present, several methods of attachment can be used to prevent the calvarium from moving:

1. Suture through the temporalis muscles and up across the calvarium. Suture through the cut portion of the temporalis muscle still attached to the temporal bone and through that portion of the muscle still attached to the calvarium.
2. Separately suture the cut temporalis muscles on either side of the head.
3. Use calvarium "clamps." Several varieties are available.
4. Drill opposing holes in the calvarium and the temporal bone and wire the calvarium into position.
5. Use super glue to help hold the calvarium in position.
6. Use plaster of Paris. This older method of attachment may have advantages if the skull was fractured. The base of the skull would be aligned and plastered into position (prior to arterial injection). Later, the cranial cavity can be filled with cotton and this covered with plaster, and the calvarium (or its pieces) can be placed into position.
7. Use needle injector wires. Use four wires on each side: two attached to the calvarium and two attached to the temporal bone. Then crisscross the wires.

After the calvarium is attached, place a small amount of "mortuary putty" along the cut line of the calvarium in the region of the *forehead*. Mortuary putty can also be used to fill in the area of the temple where some of the muscle may have been cut away.

Mortuary putty is a useful substitute for incision seal powder along the scalp incision. The putty helps to prevent leakage, especially if some of the material is pulled through the punctures made by the suture needle. If "mortuary putty" is not available and the temple muscles have been cut away, use mortuary wax as well as cotton and glue as a filler. "Tissue builder" cannot be used if the muscles are missing.

Next, coat the calvarium with autopsy gel or preservative powder (Figure 17–6). Reflect the scalp over the calvarium. While attaching the calvarium, pull the scalp down over the face. Doing so prevents wrinkles in the area of the forehead. After reflecting the scalp, spread some incision seal powder or mortuary putty along the posterior portion of the area where the scalp meets the occipital and temporal bones, to help prevent leakage through the sutures.

Begin sutures on the right side of the head and end them on the left side.

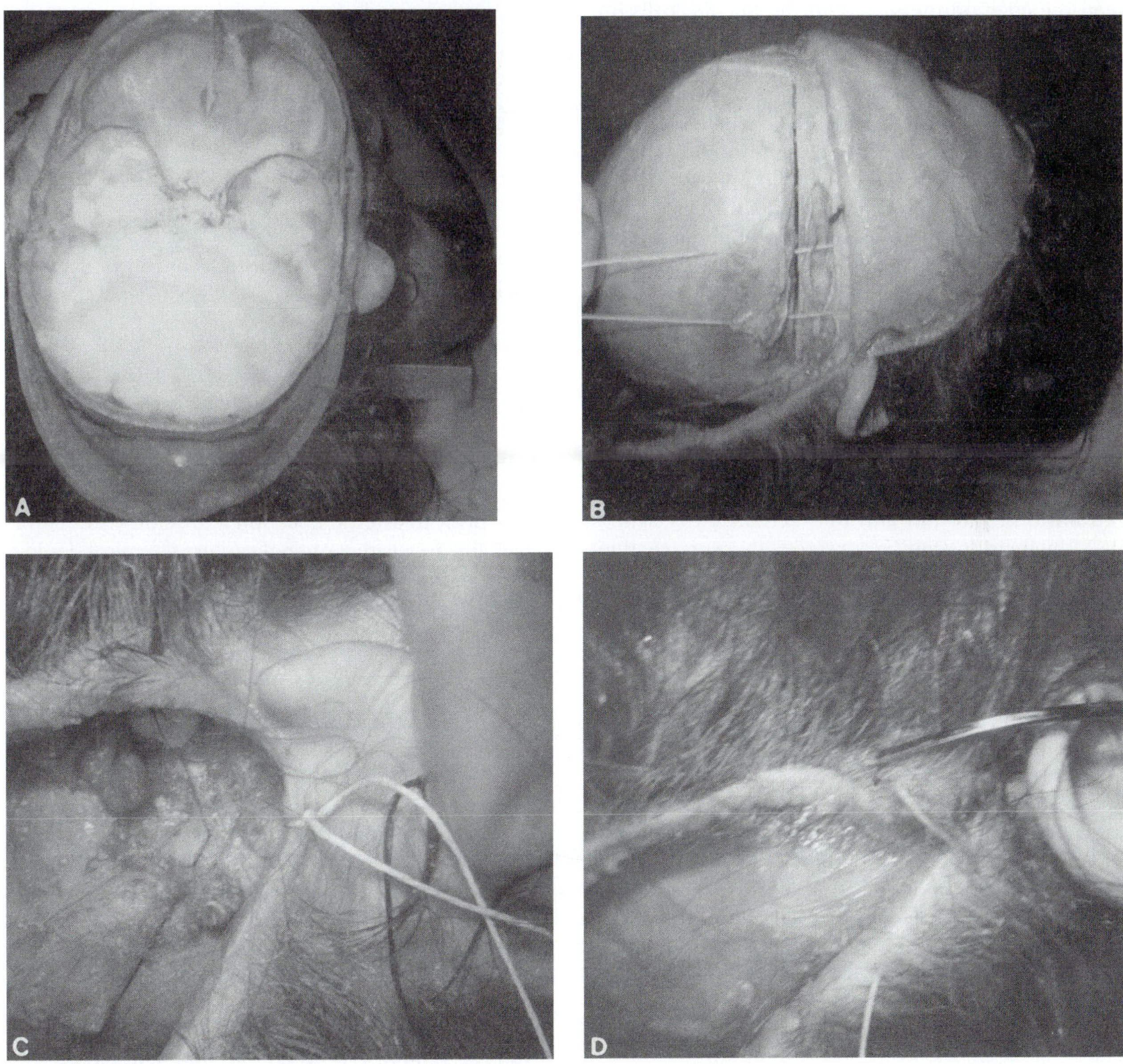

Figure 17–6. Treatment of the autopsied skull. **A.** The base of the skull is prepared using absorbent powders and cotton. Cavity walls are painted with gel preservatives. **B.** The temporalis muscle is sutured to the calvarium. The scalp is painted with a preservative gel. **C.** Begin on the right side when suturing the scalp. **D.** Use a "worm" suture for scalp closure. Spread incision seal powder along the incision.

There are many ways in which the hair can be kept out of the suture line. Comb the hair with water as the suturing proceeds. Use hair clamps to "clamp" the hair away from the sutures. Moisten the hair with liquid soap and comb the hair away from the incision line.

Using a double-curved needle, tie the first suture into place behind the right ear. *Do not use knots;* they have a tendency to pull through the scalp. Single- or double-linen suture cord can be used. Single is preferred and the cord should be a minimum of five-twist (strand) linen suture cord. Two sutures can be used to close the scalp incision. The *inversion (worm) suture* is made entirely on the surface of the scalp. The area between the edge on the scalp and the needle "rolls under" if each stitch is tightly pulled when the sutures are completed. Only a straight line should be seen. On a bald body the line can easily be waxed or covered with glue, and cosmetics placed over the dried glue. If a *baseball suture* is used, be sure each suture is tightly placed. No thread should be seen.

Some embalmers use *super adhesive* in place of sutures on the scalp. In the preparation of infants and in difficult circumstances (such as when surgery has been performed on the cranium), super adhesive may be advantageous.

▶ FINAL PROCEDURES

After closure of the cranial incisions, the body and the hair should be again washed and dried. A hair dryer dries not only hair but also the incision. After skin is dried, the incisions can be covered with a surface glue. Some embalmers then cover the incisions with cotton or a cotton webbing while the glue is still wet. Others prefer to wait until the glue has dried and place the body in coveralls.

In yet another method, the incisions can be covered with glue, then cotton, and the body clothed in coveralls. An embalming powder should be sprinkled inside the coveralls to control odors, prevent mold, and assist in preservation.

If air appears to be trapped in the thoracic area, insert a trocar through the abdominal wall just under the skin surface to draw out the air. Also, use forceps to separate one of the thoracic sutures. This allows the air to be expressed through the gap in the forceps. Keep in mind that a properly sewn "baseball suture" should be airtight.

▶ ADDITIONAL EXAMINATIONS

In some autopsies the posterior of the cervical vertebrae is opened externally and examined (Figure 17–7).

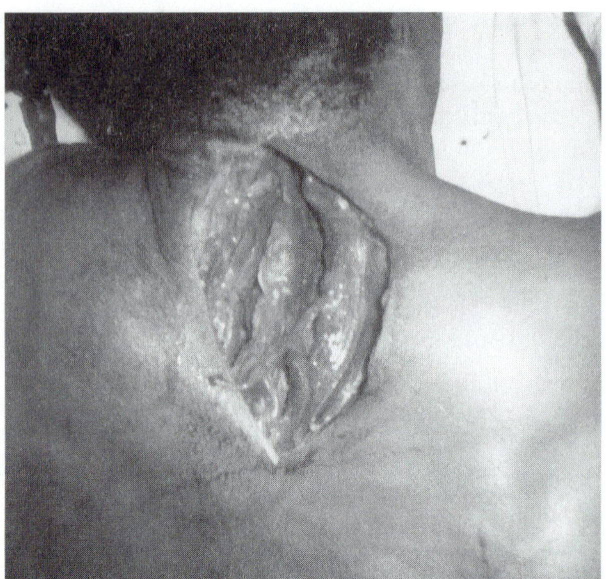

Figure 17–7. Examination of cervical vertebrae.

Cervical vertebrae are usually examined when a broken neck is suspected or when bleeding may have occurred along the vertebrae (as might occur in falls or automobile accidents).

For the pathologist to examine the vertebrae, an incision is made along the back of the neck, above the line where the shirt collar would pass to as high as the hair-line.

Roll the body on its side or, if necessary, completely over prior to arterial injection and remove any sutures. Pack the area with a phenol cautery chemical. Hold the edges together with bridge sutures or several strips of duct tape. After the body is embalmed again roll the body on its side or completely over. Remove the cautery packing, dry the deep tissues, fill the incision with incision seal powder or "mortuary putty," and tightly suture closed using a baseball stitch. The sutures can be coated with a thick layer of surface glue.

Tissues are sometimes taken from the knee areas. These incisions can be opened prior to arterial embalming. They should be dried with cotton and packed with a cautery agent on cotton swabs. After injection, dry out the area, fill with incision seal powder, and suture tightly closed with a baseball stitch. The incisions can then be glued. If leakage might be a problem, place plastic stockings on the body.

Death from Pulmonary Embolism

After a pulmonary embolism, the pathologist often makes incisions along the medial portions of the legs. The pathologist is looking for the source of the clot that moved into the lungs. These incisions can be filled with cotton packs dipped in a phenol cautery solution or cavity fluid while the rest of the body is embalmed. After the other incisions have been closed, the cotton packs can be removed and the incisions packed with dry, absorbent cotton. Use sufficient amounts of incision seal powder or mortuary putty when suturing these long incisions (some of these incisions may be 2 feet or longer). A baseball suture is the tightest stitch and the easiest to use. The stitching can be coated with a surface glue. Plastic stockings may be used if any leakage is anticipated.

Death from Drug Overdoses

In the autopsy of persons dead from suspected drug overdoses, the pathologist is likely to excise tissue where old keloid scars (fibrous tissue) have formed from the use of needles. Generally, a square of tissue is cut out, quite often in the bend of the elbow. **The excision cannot be closed by suturing.** It is best to cover these open areas with cotton saturated with phenol chemical prior to embalming. After arterial injection, remove the cotton, dry with a hair dryer, and paint the area with glue. Apply fresh cotton and wrap the area. If the possibility of leakage exists, place a plastic "sleeve" on the arm or self-clinging food wrap around the arm. Some embalmers cut out a portion of plastic stocking to make a sleeve, slip it onto the arm, and tape it in place with duct tape.

▶ PARTIAL AUTOPSIES

Cranial Autopsy Only

In this partial autopsy the cranial cavity is opened and the brain is removed. The body can be embalmed by one of three procedures.

Method 1. Raise the right and left common carotid arteries. Insert tubes in both, directed upward toward the head. Insert one tube directed downward toward the trunk in the right common carotid. Tie off (ligate) the lower portion of the left common carotid.

Use the right internal jugular vein for drainage.

Inject downward *first* to embalm the extremities and trunk. Clamp off leakage in the cranium from the right and left vertebral arteries (which are branches of the subclavian arteries). Inject the left and right sides of the head, clamping off the left and right internal carotid arteries.

Method 2. Raise the right common carotid artery and the right internal jugular vein. Insert two tubes directed upward toward the head and one tube directed downward toward the trunk.

Inject downward, clamping off the right and left vertebral arteries and the left internal carotid artery. These are found in the base of the cranial cavity.

Inject up the right side of the head. Clamp off the right internal carotid artery in the base of the skull.

Method 3. Raise the right femoral artery and vein. Insert into the artery one tube directed upward and one tube directed to the foot.

Inject the right leg.

Inject upward toward the trunk and head. Clamp off the right and left internal carotid arteries and the right and left vertebral arteries. After arterial injection, dry the cranial cavity, paint it with autopsy gel, and fill it with cotton.

Attach the calvarium and suture the scalp back into position using the inversion or baseball suture. Spread plenty of incision seal powder or mortuary putty within the incision as the suturing progresses. Begin suturing on the right side of the head and end on the left side.

▶ THORACIC AUTOPSY ONLY

In a thoracic partial autopsy, one or more organs of the cavity have been removed (assuming that the neck organs have not been removed). Drainage taken for the lower extremities and the abdomen are drained through the inferior vena cava, which is located at the lower right area of the diaphragm (Figure 17–8).

There is only one way to prepare the head and the arms. It is similar to the technique used after a complete autopsy, when the head and the arms are separately injected. Inject the left arm using the left subclavian or left axially artery. Inject the right arm using the right subclavian or right axillary artery. Inject the left side of the head using the left common carotid artery. Inject the right side of the head using the right common carotid artery. Two methods can be used to inject the abdomen and the lower extremities.

Method 1. Locate the terminal portion of the thoracic aorta on the vertebral column at the central posterior portion of the diaphragm. Insert a large arterial tube into the aorta. Either clamp the tube in place with an arterial hemostat or, if possible, tie the tube in place. Inject downward through the arterial tube. This embalms the abdominal walls, abdominal contents, and lower extremities. Leakage may occur from the right and left inferior or superior epigastric arteries, depending on how the pathologist made incisions.

Method 2. Raise the right femoral artery and insert a tube directed upward toward the abdomen. Also, insert a tube downward to inject the right leg. Inject the right leg first. Next, inject upward. This embalms the left leg, abdominal contents, and trunk. Ligate by

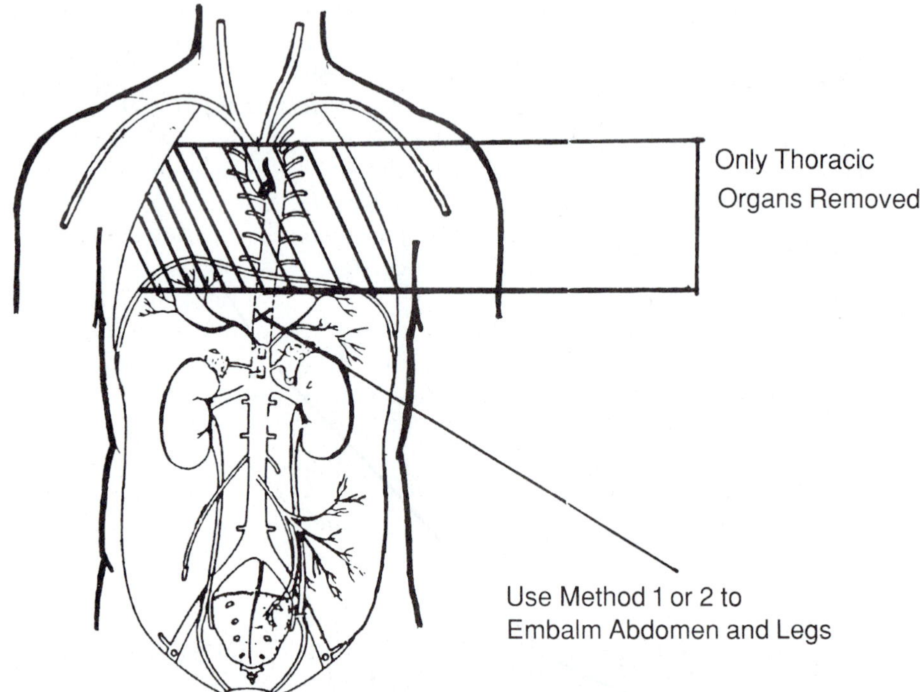

Figure 17–8. Thoracic autopsy only.

tying or clamping the thoracic aorta when fluid is observed flowing from this artery into the thoracic cavity.

After arterial injection, check for preservation of the thoracic walls and the back and shoulders. If the preservation is inadequate, the walls should be treated by hypodermic injection. The thoracic cavity can be painted with autopsy gel and filled with sheeting or an appropriate absorbent material. This material, in turn, can be saturated with cavity fluid or some other preservative, the breastplate put into position, and the incisions closed with a baseball suture. Aspirate the abdominal cavity and inject cavity fluid over the abdominal viscera (Figure 17–9).

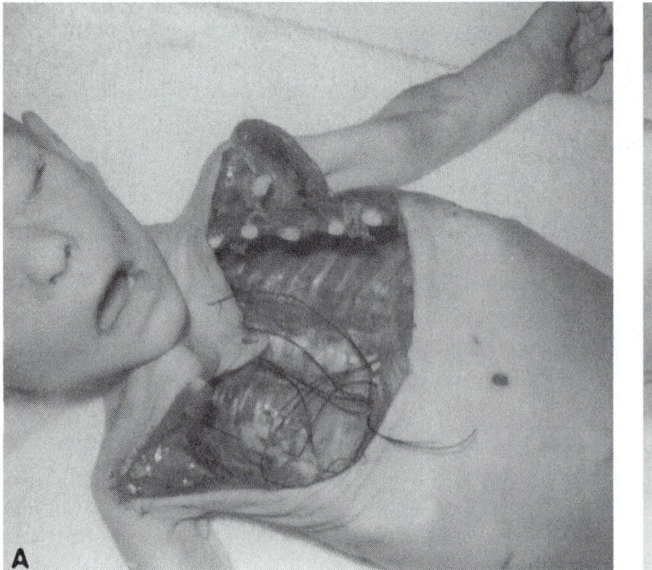

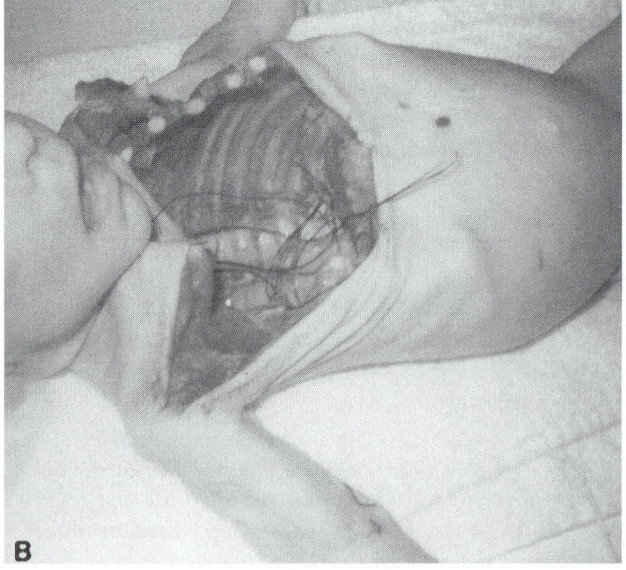

Figure 17–9. Partial autopsy of an infant (the abdominal aorta was used). **A, B.** Only the thoracic organs have been removed.

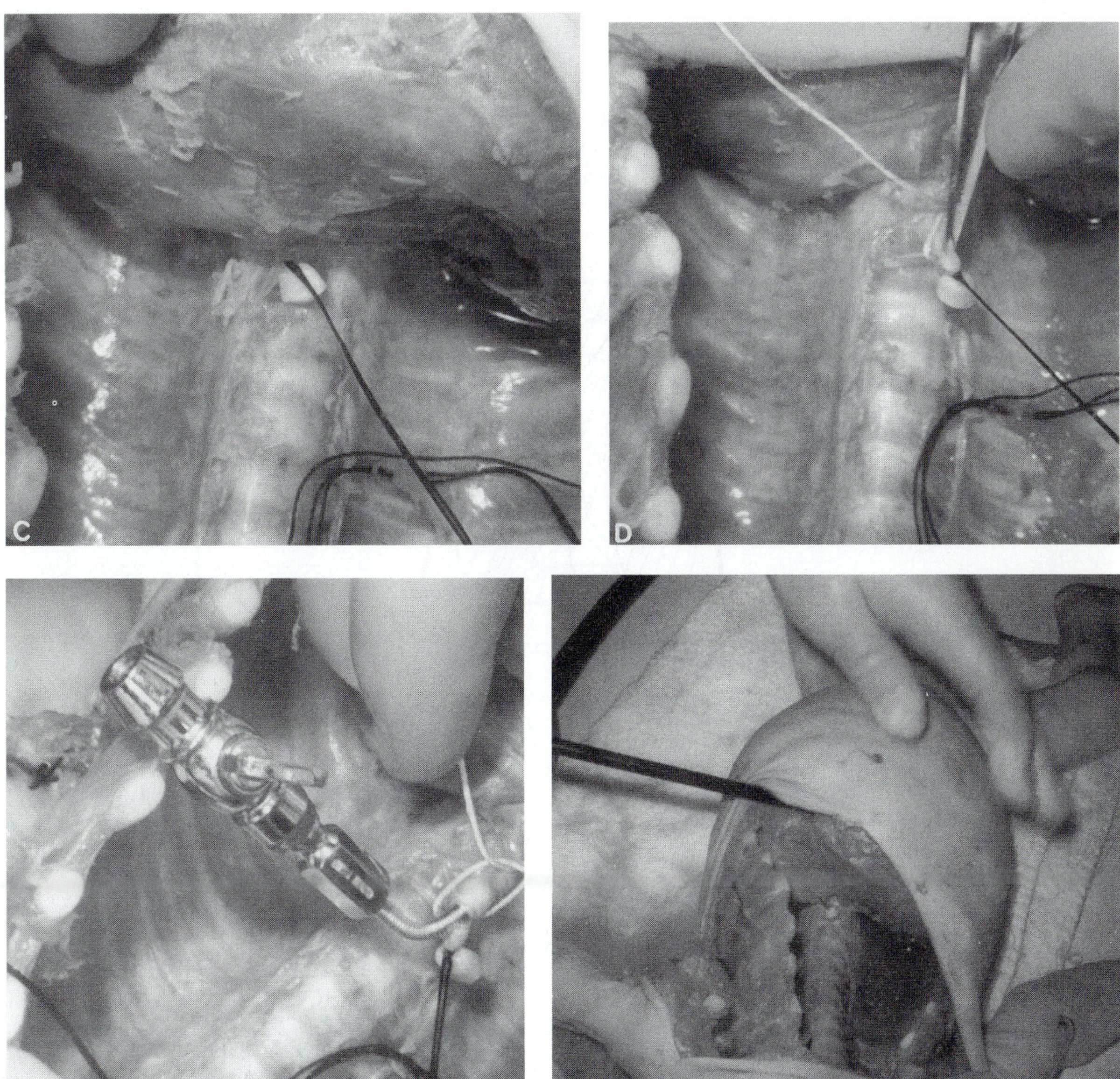

Figure 17–9. *(Continued)* **C.** The thoracic aorta is located on the spinal column. The diaphragm is at the top of the picture. **D.** The aorta being opened. Drainage is taken from the inferior vena cava located at the diaphragm. No drainage instruments are needed. **E.** The arterial tube is inserted into the aorta. **F.** Treatment of the abdominal viscera.

▶ ABDOMINAL AUTOPSY ONLY

In an abdominal partial autopsy, the contents of the abdominal cavity are removed (Figure 17–10). If only the abdominal cavity is opened and the organs are removed, two methods can be employed for arterial embalming of the thorax, upper extremities, and head. The legs can be injected from the external iliac arteries. Drainage from the arterial injection of the upper trunk, arms, and head can be taken from the *inferior vena cava,* found in the lower right area of the diaphragm, where it would be attached to the liver.

Method 1. To inject the thorax, upper extremities, and head, locate the abdominal aorta as it passes through the diaphragm. The aorta can be located at the level of the vertebral column in the central posterior position of the diaphragm. Tie or clamp an arterial tube into the aorta. Upward injection should embalm the thorax and its contents, the arms, and the head.

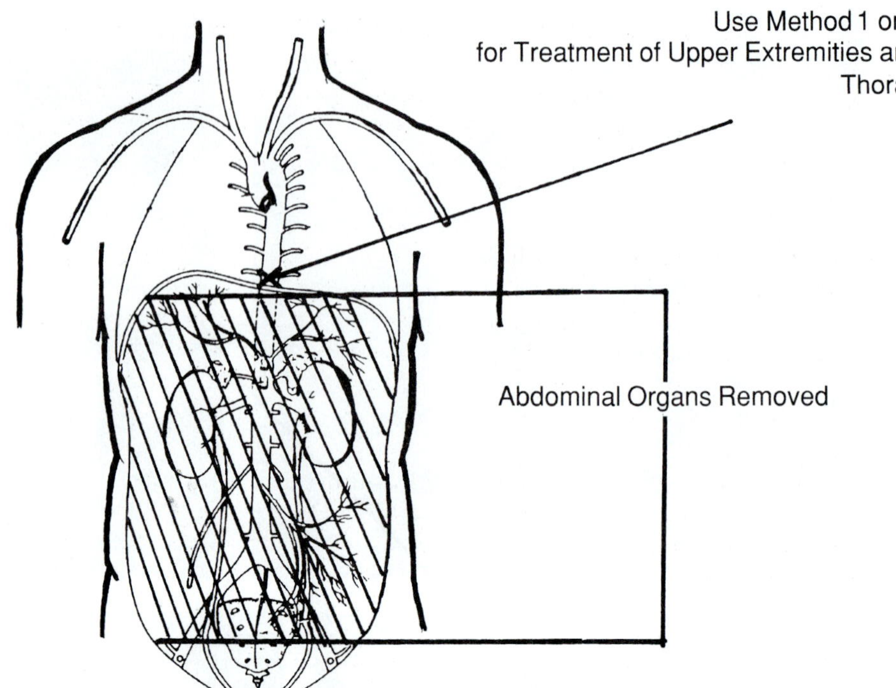

Figure 17–10. Abdominal autopsy only.

Method 2. Raise the right common carotid artery. Insert a tube upward for the right side of the head. Insert a tube downward. Inject downward toward the trunk; the arms, thorax, and left side of the head should receive arterial solution. When leakage is noted from the aorta, clamp or tie the aorta in the abdominal cavity. After the downward injection, inject the right side of the head. (The restricted cervical method of injection could also be used.)

Check the abdominal walls, the buttocks, and the back for fluid distribution. Depending on the pathologist's incision there may be leakage from the superior epigastric arteries during injection. (*Hypodermic injection can be used to preserve the abdominal walls and buttocks.*) Injection of the male genitalia may also be necessary. Direct injection of both internal iliac arteries will provide good distribution of arterial solution to the buttocks, genitalia, and upper thighs. The walls of the cavity can be painted with autopsy gel and the abdominal cavity filled with sheeting or other absorbent material. This filler can then be saturated with cavity chemical or other preservative.

Suture the abdominal incisions using a baseball suture. After washing and drying the body, cover the incisions with surface glue.

In both partial autopsies, thoracic and abdominal, the cavity *not* opened and examined should be treated by trocar. Aspiration can be done either through the diaphragm or by inserting the trocar through the rib cage for the thorax or through the abdominal wall for the abdomen. This treatment can be done *before or after* the autopsied cavity has been closed by suturing. The cavity not autopsied should also be injected with a minimum of one bottle of concentrated cavity fluid.

▶ PROTOCOL FOR THE TREATMENT OF AUTOPSIED BODIES WHEN RESTORATIVE TREATMENTS ARE NECESSARY

Restoration of the deceased to natural **form** and **color** is directly related to *embalming*. Many restorative treatments begin in the preembalming period and some are carried out during embalming. The majority of restorative work, however, is accomplished in the postembalming period. Accidental deaths may involve *trauma*, which involves visible regions of the body such as the face and hands. Because these deaths are accidental, the certification of death is under the jurisdiction of the coroner or medical examiner. In most instances the official will have the body autopsied to determine the exact cause of death.

The outline that follows suggests the order of preparation of bodies that have sustained traumatic injuries to the face and have also been autopsied. Restorative art is a subject unto itself, and this protocol involves only some of those restorative treatments that should be carried out before and during arterial embalming. Two important criteria must be achieved for good restorative work. Tissues of the body must be *firm* and completely *dry*. It is the goal of the embalmer to adequately preserve and, thus, firm the tissue. By the use of embalming chemicals, solvents, and manual aids, the embalmer can dry the tissue.

In addition to trauma—be it lacerations, abrasions, bruising, or fractures—pathologic conditions may exist in the body prior to accidental death. Consideration must also be given to postmortem changes. Preparation of the body with facial trauma and a complete autopsy allows the embalmer to use a different strength of arterial solution for each area of the body injected. If trauma is in the facial tissues, a stronger solution can be injected to control swelling, and dry and firm these tissues; a milder solution may be desired for the arms and/or legs. These factors, taken together, constitute the basis for the embalming analysis.

1. Disinfect and position the body.
   A. Be cautious of shards of glass that may be embedded in the skin if glass was involved in the accident. Sometimes these shards can be flushed out with water or picked out with forceps.
   B. Use cool water and plenty of liquid soap to remove blood, grease, and oils.
2. Assess the damage to all body areas.
3. Begin with injection of the legs; then, inject the arms.
4. Prepare the head and face.
   A. Open the cranial cavity and check for fractured bones. Inspect for scalp lacerations or abrasions.
   B. Shave the body. Observe punctures, lacerations, abrasions, and hematomas. Remove all loose skin and dehydrated edges of lacerated tissues using a sharp razor or scalpel.
   C. By application of digital pressure to face, inspect for fractures of the mandible, maxillae, and nasal bones and for the presence of air (subcutaneous emphysema).
   D. Close the mouth using a method that keeps the lips in contact and align the jaw bones if they are fractured. Suturing may be required. Use several needle injector barbs. Temporarily gluing lips may help.
   E. Close the eyes using cotton support or eyecaps. Depending on the damage to the eyelids, it may be necessary to glue the lids prior to injection.
   F. Attempt to realign fractured bones and support depressed fractures.
   G. Align lacerated tissues. Temporary individual sutures of dental floss or super glue can be used. After embalming, remove the temporary sutures or glue anchors and place permanent sutures or glue.
   H. Prepare a very strong arterial solution using a high index fluid (25-index above), for example, (1) 16 ounces of fluid and 32 ounces of water or (2) 16 ounces of fluid, one bottle of co-injection, and one bottle of water. Then add the fluid dye.
   I. Inject the left side of the face first. Pulse the fluid into the head and observe the dye to check fluid distribution.

In many of these bodies there will be a great amount of fluid leakage. This leakage helps to control some of the swelling. What is important is that the tissues receive fluid, as indicated by the presence of dye.

▶ KEY TERMS AND CONCEPTS FOR STUDY AND DISCUSSION

1. Define the following terms:
   autopsy gel
   baseball suture
   calvarium
   cranial autopsy
   forensic autopsy
   hardening compound
   hypodermic embalming
   necropsy
   partial autopsy
   surface embalming
   worm suture
   Y tube
2. Describe the general order for embalming the autopsied body.
3. Describe several methods for securing the calvarium.
4. List the branches of the external carotid artery.
5. Give the location where the common carotid artery divides.
6. In the complete autopsy (neck organs removed), name the major arteries that must be clamped if the *left subclavian artery* is injected.
7. In the complete autopsy (neck organs removed), name the major arteries that must be clamped.

8. List the branches of the internal iliac artery and the area each supplies.
9. Describe several methods for preserving autopsy viscera.
10. Discuss several treatments for embalming the trunk walls in the autopsied body.
11. Describe two methods of injection to embalm the abdomen and legs when a partial autopsy has been performed and the contents of the thoracic cavity have been removed.

▶ BIBLIOGRAPHY

Altman LK. Sharp drop in autopsies stirs fears that quality of care may also fall. *N.Y. Times,* July 21, 1988.

Altman LK. Diagnosis and the autopsies are found to differ greatly. *N.Y. Times,* October 14, 1998.

Ninker R. Ethics goes beyond self interest. *The Director* 1997;7:18.

Slocum RE. *Pre-embalming Considerations.* Boston: Dodge Chemical Co.

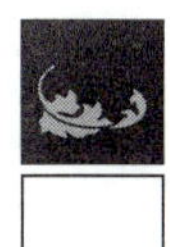

CHAPTER 18
PREPARATION OF ORGAN AND TISSUE DONORS

Although **tissue donation** and **organ donation** share many similar goals and objectives, they are not exclusively the same. The differences are better understood by comparing the definition of *tissue* with the definition of *organ*. **Tissue** is defined as a collection of similar cells and the intercellular substances surrounding them. There are four basic tissues in the body: (1) epithelium; (2) connective tissues, including blood, bone, and cartilage; (3) muscle tissue; and (4) nerve tissue.* Tissue donation refers to the procurement and transplantation of tissues that fall into one of the four categories. An **organ** is defined as any part of the body exercising a specific function, such as respiration, secretion, digestion.† Organ donation refers to the procurement and transplantation of a body part that fulfills such a specific function. Organ transplantation would include procedures to transplant a kidney, heart, liver, and so on. Thus, a cornea transplant is not an organ transplant, it is a tissue transplant; a heart transplant is not a tissue transplant, it is an organ transplant.

There are common issues and objectives that arise from the procurement and transplantation of organs and tissues. The nature of transplanting organs versus transplanting tissues also gives rise to different conditions and circumstances, which must be carefully controlled. For example, it can generally be said that the window of opportunity for recovering and transplanting an organ is much more restrictive than for tissues. Organ recovery and transplantation is very time sensitive. Tissue recovery and transplantation is not nearly as time sensitive.

The involvement of embalmers in procedures utilized to solicit, document, and perform organ and tissue donations varies. In some instances, in some states, the embalmer may have extensive involvement in the process. In other instances, the embalmer would have no participation in the solicitation or procurement, and would not become involved until such time that the body was transported to the funeral home for embalming.

▶ CONSENT FOR ORGAN AND TISSUE DONATION

The *Uniform Anatomical Gift Act* has been enacted in all states and the District of Columbia to provide statutory regulations regarding postmortem organ and tissue donation. The Act allows any person 18 years or older to donate all organs and tissues of his or her body for transplantation, research, or educational purposes after his or her death. Many people make known their desire to be an organ donor by completing and carrying a Uniform Organ Donor Card; although such cards are legal documents, in practice, however, consent must be obtained from the legally responsible next-of-kin. The Uniform Anatomical Gift Act provides the order of priority for consenting persons and specifically protects physicians who act in good faith from civil liabilities and criminal prosecution. The Act provides for consent for organ donation from a next-of-kin in the following order of priority: (1) spouse, (2) adult son or daughter, (3) either parent, (4) adult sibling, (5) guardian, and (6) any other person authorized or under obligation to dispose of the body. In situations where objections are raised, or where there are competing interests within a family, the donation will likely be declined.

▶ ORGAN DONORS

Every effort is made to recover as many organs from a donor as possible. Currently, the following organs are being recovered for transplantation: heart, lung(s), heart and lungs en bloc, liver, kidney(s), pancreas, and small bowel. The number of organs that are actually recovered may depend on consent or on the viability of each individual organ. For example, the next-of-kin may only give consent for the procurement of a certain

* *Stedman's Medical Dictionary*, 26th ed. Baltimore: Williams & Wilkins, 1995, p. 1816.

† *Stedman's Medical Dictionary*, p. 1257.

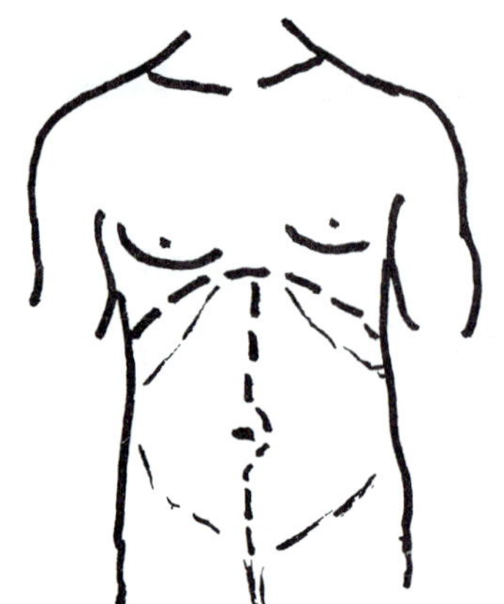
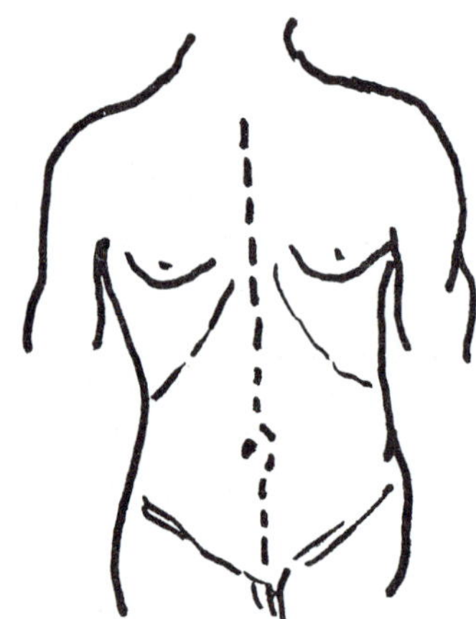

Figure 18–1. Incisions frequently used for organ transplantation.

organ, or the cause and circumstances of death may affect the viability and transplantability of organs. Because of the variations that can occur in organ recovery, the embalmer must be prepared to deal with a variety of embalming issues that arise from organ donation. Dealing with embalming complications of organ donation will require the embalmer to: (1) assess the situation, (2) analyze the embalming complications, (3) develop a plan for the application of embalming treatments, (4) implement the embalming plan, and then (5) engage in concurrent evaluation of the effectiveness of the embalming treatments, making any changes in procedure that might be indicated.

The embalming consequences of the organ procurement will be determined by the nature and location of the vascular disruptions, and how the embalmer deals with the problems associated with the disruptions.

The embalmer has two options for the arterial injection of an organ donor. First, there is the option of **external access,** where embalming is accomplished by raising vessels at one of the commonly used injection and drainage sites. Second, there is the option of **internal access,** where the embalmer opens the procurement incision(s) and attempts to inject the body utilizing the arterial structures that remain intact in the area(s) where organ recovery has taken place.

Embalming of an organ donor using the external access option requires the embalmer to raise arteries and veins at one of the commonly used injection and drainage sites. Realistically, the embalmer can anticipate having to use two or more injection sites, depending on the extent of vascular disruption. In addition to the considerations for the organ procurement, the procedure would involve many of the same case analysis considerations that embalmers routinely apply. As the embalming proceeds, the embalmer needs to carefully monitor the body for signs that arterial solution is being adequately distributed in the body, and for indicators that the ligatures on vessels affected by the procurement are preventing leakage. If procurement ligatures are absent, or if they fail, the embalmer can anticipate excess leakage from the procurement incision or distention caused by an accumulation of liquids in body cavities. If the leakage and/or distention are too severe, the procurement incision will likely have to be opened to deal with the complication.

If the internal access option is selected for embalming an organ donor, the embalmer can anticipate finding one of four procurement incisions* (Figure 18–1).

1. A midline incision that runs from the base of the neck to the base of the sternum for a heart, lung, or heart and lung procurement
2. A midline incision that runs from the base of the sternum to the pubic bone for liver, kidney, pancreas, and/or small bowel recovery
3. A 'T' incision that transverses the abdomen along the inferior margin of the rib cage, and a midline incision from the base of the sternum to the pubic bone for liver, kidney, pancreas, and/or small bowel recovery
4. A midline incision that runs from the base of the neck to the pubic bone if a full recovery was done

Modern embalmers have become very adept at embalming autopsy cases. The knowledge, skill, and experience of autopsy embalming can be applied when the embalmer is called upon to embalm an organ donor. In cases where the procurement has been limited, embalming can be approached in a manner similar to embalming a partial autopsy. In cases where a full organ procurement has taken place (heart, lungs, liver, kidney, pancreas, and small bowel) the embalming can be

* From Toledo-Pereya LH. *Organ Procurement and Preservation for Transplantation*, 2nd ed. Austin: Landes Bioscience, 1997.

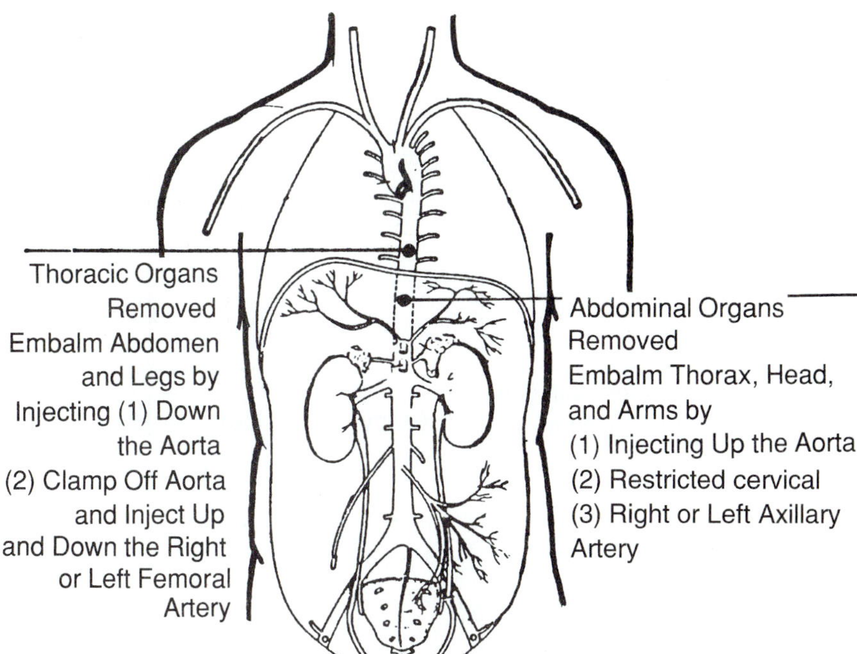

Figure 18–2. Embalming sites in bodies from which organs have been removed.

approached in a manner very similar to a full autopsy (Figure 18–2). Keys to successful autopsy and organ donor embalming include: (1) knowing anatomical structures and relationships, (2) anticipating which vessels have been cut, and (3) an ability to locate the ends of the vessels which have been cut.

Other Issues

The embalmer can expect that an organ donor has been given **heparin** prior to the removal of the donated organ as a means to keep blood from clotting. The embalming implications of heparin are positive and negative, depending on circumstance. The fact that blood clotting has been decreased can lead to more effective drainage from the body. A time lapse between death and embalming, however, would predispose livor mortis and postmortem stain because the thinned blood would more readily gravitate to dependent parts of the body.

Embalmers can also anticipate that the organs will have been perfused with a liquid solution prior to recovery. The perfusion may increase the amount of moisture in the body, but generally not to an extent that would cause the embalmer to make any substantive changes in the composition of arterial solution or in injection procedures. For example, in the recovery of a heart, the organ itself is infused with 1000 cc of cardioplegic solution, which causes a rapid cardiac arrest. Because the solution is infused into the heart, however, most of it also leaves the body when the heart is removed.

▶ TISSUE DONORS

Eye Enucleation

One of the tissues most commonly transplanted today is the human cornea. Every year, thousands of individuals undergo corneal transplantation. Although the cornea itself can be removed from the organ donor, most frequently the entire eyeball is removed, or **enucleated.**

The most common problem in the aftermath of an enucleation is swelling or distention in and around the orbital cavity. In addition, ecchymosis may be present, and there is always the possibility of small lacerations.

To help control swelling of the eyelids during embalming, the following procedures are recommended: (1) use restricted cervical injection to control arterial solution entering the head; (2) avoid preinjection procedures; (3) **do not** use weak arterial solutions—it is recommended that the solution be slightly stronger than average; (4) avoid excessive manipulation of the eyelids prior to and during embalming; (5) let embalming solution drain from the eye during arterial injection; (6) avoid rapid rates of flow and high injection pressure during arterial injection.

The following treatments have produced very satisfactory results:

1. Remove packing from the eye.
2. Saturate pieces of cotton with autopsy gel and loosely fill the orbital cavity. Autopsy gel on the outside of the eyelids will not create additional problems.

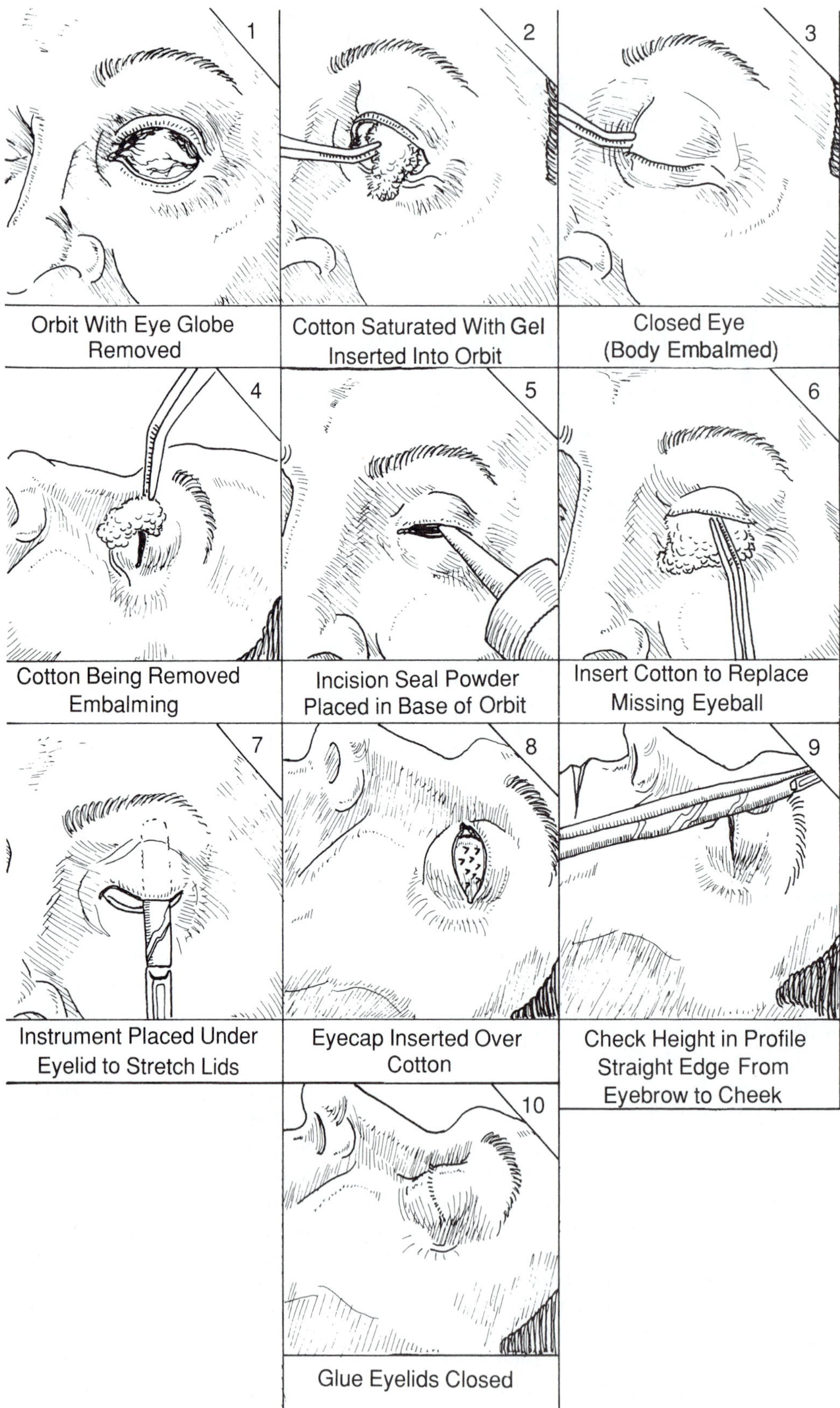

Figure 18–3. Procedure for eye enucleation restoration.

3. Fill the eye with sufficient cotton to recreate the normal appearance of the closed eye.
4. Embalm the body; use the procedures previously suggested to avoid swelling. If swelling does begin, strengthen the arterial solution so only a minimum amount can be injected. Stop injection if swelling becomes excessive and, if necessary, use surface embalming.
5. After arterial injection, remove the autopsy gel saturated cotton and dry out the orbit.
6. Carefully place a small amount of incision seal powder or mortuary putty in the base of the orbit.
7. Pack the orbital cavity with cotton, kapok, or mortuary putty.
8. Exercise the eyelids and insert an eyecap over the filler.
9. Glue the eyelids closed.

With this method, major treatment of the eye occurs after the arterial injection (Figure 18–3).

Cornea Removal

When only the cornea has been removed, the preparation work is greatly reduced. The body can be embalmed using whatever injection technique and arterial solution strength the embalmer feels necessary. The eyes can be set after the arterial injection.

As the front of the eye is opened when the cornea is removed, the embalmer may find it necessary to aspirate the fluids from the eye to prevent leakage. A large-diameter hypodermic needle can be used to aspirate these fluids. The needle is inserted through the opening created by the removal of the cornea. During embalming the hollow eye globe can be filled with cotton saturated with autopsy gel or undiluted cavity fluid. The eye is then filled with mortuary putty or incision sealer. An eyecap can then be placed over the eyeball to support the eyelids, and create a natural contour and form. The eyelids can be secured with super glue (Figure 18–4).

Vertebral Body Donor

Recovery of vertebral bodies involves removing sections of the spinal column. Once removed the tissue is processed into biomedical products that are used in a number of orthopedic surgical procedures. As a rule, tissue procurement specialists will attempt to recover as large a section of the spinal column as possible, but the size of the section removed may vary depending on the use to which the tissue will be put, the accessibility of the spine, and other factors. The embalmer can anticipate that varying lengths of spine may be removed from the donor depending on circumstances.

Access to the vertebral bodies can be gained in a number of ways. Vertebral bodies may be harvested following organ recovery or autopsy where an incision already exists, and the spine is partially or completely exposed. Vertebral bodies may be harvested from an anterior incision where no organ recovery or autopsy has been performed. Vertebral bodies may be harvested through a posterior incision. This usually occurs when no previous postmortem invasive procedures have occurred, but can also be used in cases where autopsy or organ recovery has taken place.

Recovery Following Autopsy or Organ Recovery. As embalmers well know, an autopsy will include the removal of thoracic, abdominal, and pelvic organs, exposing the spinal column. In this instance, removal of vertebral bodies will not significantly alter injection and drainage techniques for the embalmer, because recovery of the vertebral bodies requires no additional disruption to the cardiovascular system beyond what has already taken place at autopsy. One major concern will be the possibility that the tissue specialist has punctured skin on the donor's back during vertebral body recovery. The embalmer must carefully inspect the donor's back for leakage. Another major concern will be the loss of rigidity that results from having a section of the spinal column removed. Many tissue banks are reconstructing vertebral body donors with prosthetic devices intended to recreate the support previously provided by the tissues that have been removed, thus making the spine and back area rigid. One of the most effective of these devices is a Limbz product, which is made of adjustable lengths of PVC piping and end caps containing surgical screws. The device's adjustability allows it to be fitted to the size of the opening in the spinal column. Turning the surgical screws into the remaining bony structures allows the device to be securely attached at the top and the bottom of the opening. The secure, custom-fitted device assures stability during dressing and casketing.

In those cases where vertebral bodies have been removed following organ donation, the embalmer will encounter circumstances quite different from autopsy. In such cases, a majority of viscera will be left in the body, with the notable exception of the organ or organs that have been harvested.

The embalming procedures required for this type of case would include locating the transected vascular structures, watching for leakage from skin punctures that may have been made in the back during vertebral body recovery, and the loss of rigidity in the spinal column.

For example, in a case where the heart has been removed for transplant, the embalmer deals with the vascular disruptions of the organ donation during the arterial injection and the structural disruptions of the vertebral body recovery during reconstruction. The

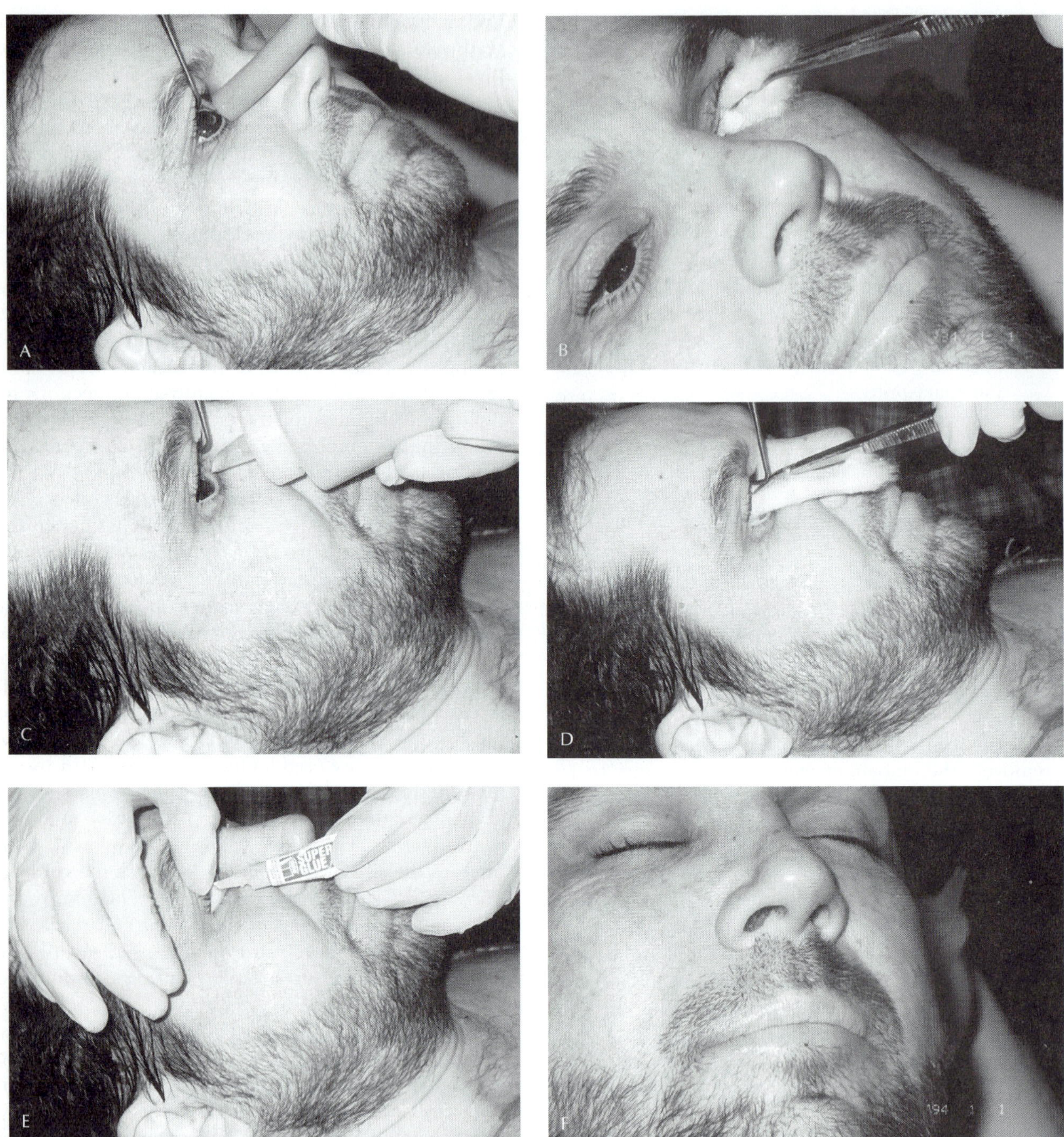

Figure 18–4. A. Aspiration of the eye globe after the cornea is removed. **B.** Packing inserted into aspirated eye globe. The packing is saturated with autopsy gel or cavity fluid. **C.** After embalming, the eye globe is dried and incision seal powder is placed in the globe to prevent any leakage. **D.** Cotton is placed over the incision seal powder to fill the eye globe. An eye cap is placed over the filled globe. **E.** The lids are sealed with glue. **F.** Completed restoration. Only the cornea was removed from each eye.

transected ends of the subclavian arteries and common carotid arteries are located and injected to embalm the head, neck and arms, in much the same manner as an autopsied case. The lower portion of the body can be embalmed by injecting interiorly from the thoracic or abdominal aorta.

Recovery Via an Anterior Incision. Some tissue banks recover vertebral bodies using an anterior midline incision that runs from the xiphoid process to the pubic bone. The primary consideration in this method is to avoid making an incision on the back of the donor, which creates obvious complications for the embalmer.

When the anterior incision is utilized, however, the embalmer can anticipate that the aorta will be cut in both the thoracic and abdominal cavities, and that a renal vein(s) will be cut. Once the incision has been made, the tissue specialist mobilizes and retracts the necessary organs to allow the spinal column to be visualized. It is at this time that the aorta will be cut. Once the vertebral tissue has been recovered, a prosthesis may be put in position. The tissue procurement specialist will then place the viscera back into position. Although it is necessary for some vascular structures to be sacrificed, procurement procedures caution the tissue specialist to avoid cutting or damaging vascular structures needlessly. Procurement procedures also instruct tissue procurement specialists to ligate any vessel that is damaged or cut. The embalmer would be wise to anticipate the possibility that accidental damage or disruptions will occur from time to time. As such, it is prudent for the embalmer to open the incision to determine whether vascular disruptions exist, and take the appropriate steps to deal with them. The embalmer may be able to arterially inject such a case using the ends of the transected vessels, carefully watching for signs that solution is being lost in the abdominal or thoracic cavities.

Recovery Via a Posterior Incision. Tissue banks in the American Red Cross National Tissue Services system use a posterior incision as the recommended method of vertebral body recovery. This method requires that a posterior midline incision be made beginning at the level of the scapula, ending at about the level of the sacrum. Once the incision is made, the surrounding tissues are dissected to expose the spine. The section of spine to be removed is transected, and rotated in such a manner that leaves the spinal cord in the body. If proper skill and care are utilized, this procedure should not cut or damage the vascular structures that are necessary for embalming. Once the section of spine is taken from the body, the tissue procurement specialist will install a prosthetic device as described previously, and suture the incision closed.

Because the vascular system should not be disrupted by this procedure, the embalmer can approach arterial injection and venous drainage in a manner that is determined by evaluating factors common to case analysis. The embalmer must consider leakage from the procurement incision as a major postembalming problem, and take appropriate steps to stop leakage and seal the incision.

The embalmer must be aware of several factors that will effect embalming results in the aftermath of vertebral body recovery. First and foremost, vertebral body recovery seldom takes place without other tissues also being taken. If the patient is a full tissue donor, the embalmer will be dealing with a multitude of conditions that will require special attention. Second, depending on the procedure utilized by the tissue bank, the embalmer will most certainly have to deal with the possibility of leakage from the body following vertebral body recovery. Third, again depending on the procedure utilized by the tissue bank and the length of spine taken, the embalmer will need to take steps to reconstruct the body in such a way as to provide rigidity previously provided by the tissue that has been removed.

Long Bone Donor (Femur, Tibia, Fibula, Hemi-pelvis)

The recovery of long bone tissue from a donor involves making an incision along the anterior surface of each leg from the hip to the ankle. Long bone procurement is the most dramatic of all tissue recovery. It involves a great amount of time, not only for the removal of the tissue, but also for the treatments that will be applied by the embalmer. Because of the delays that are involved in this process, and the large-scale disruptions of the circulatory system, it is recommended that arterial injection be accomplished with a stronger arterial solution than normal. These bodies should not be preinjected. The increased strength of the arterial solution accomplishes two things: (1) if a smaller volume of solution is distributed to the tissues and muscles, the higher concentration of preservative will, to an extent, offset the lack of volume; (2) there is some possibility that arterial solution which pools in the tissue spaces will penetrate the tissues and provide some preservation (Figure 18–5).

Two methods of preparation for the legs are discussed. In the first technique the incisions are opened; in the second, if the sutures are tight, they are not opened.

Method 1. Supports, such as head blocks, can be placed along the medial and lateral sides of the legs in preparation of removing the sutures. This work practice helps to create a "channel" to drain blood and embalming chemicals flow to the foot of the table, thus allowing the embalmer to maintain a cleaner work area.

In those cases where the donor's legs have been sutured, *all* suture lines are removed from the extremities, followed by removal of the prosthesis. This provides unobstructed access to the tissue beds. The embalmer then locates and identifies any ligatures that have been put in place by the tissue procurement team. The practice of ligating vessels during procurement varies widely, and it will not be uncommon for the embalmer to find no ligatures.

The embalmer will then dissect and ligate the left and right femoral arteries to isolate each extremity for injection separately from the rest of the body.

The trunk, hips, head, neck, and upper extremities of the body can be injected by using cervical and/or femoral vessels as injection and drainage sites. If neces-

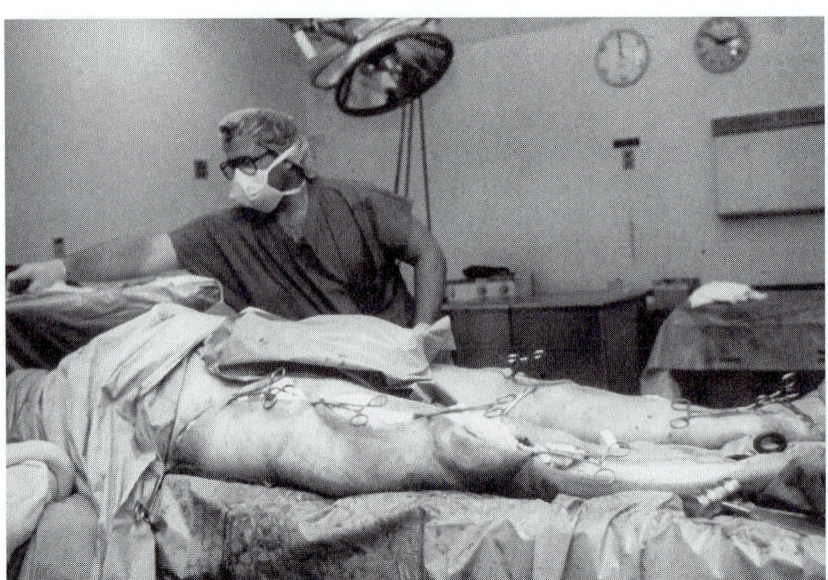

Figure 18–5. Removal of long bones from the legs. Performed under sterile conditions.

sary, the embalmer can choose other injection sites as needed to complete this portion of the preparation. Care is taken to ensure that embalming solution does not freely flow into either the lower extremities during injection of the trunk, hips, head, neck, and upper extremities.

The thigh and leg areas are injected by using the left and right femoral arteries. Care is taken to clamp off other vessels as loss of embalming solution becomes apparent. Particular attention is paid to the multiple branches of the genicular arteries found just above the knee, because they will likely have been cut during sharp dissection. A large number of hemostats may be required.

The leg and foot are injected by using the left and right popliteal arteries. In some instances, the popliteal may not be accessible and the embalmer may use the superior aspects of either the anterior or posterior tibial artery for injection. Care is again taken to clamp off other vessels as loss of embalming solution becomes apparent. Here, also, the multiple branches of the genicular arteries found just below the knee will likely have been cut during sharp dissection. A large number of hemostats may be required.

Hypodermic injection may be required to supplement arterial injection. The embalmer must carefully assess the success of arterial injection to determine where hypodermic supplement might be required.

At the conclusion of the arterial and hypodermic injections, the embalmer dries the tissue bed with absorbent cotton. The prosthetic device is then placed back into position.

A light coating of preservative/drying compound is applied to the tissue beds. It is to the embalmer's advantage to use a substance that has both preservative and absorptive qualities.

The incisions are then sutured closed. Care is taken to make the sutures tight. Additional preservative/drying compound may be added during the suturing process. Following suturing, the body is thoroughly bathed. Cotton and liquid sealer are then applied to the incision to provide an additional barrier to leakage. Finally, plastic stockings are placed on the legs as a further barrier to leakage. The body is now ready for dressing and casketing.

Method 2. There is a second method of preparing the lower extremities when the long bones (femur, tibia, and fibula) have been removed. This method leaves the procurement sutures in place. If tight baseball stitches have been used to close the incisions, leakage from these sutures should be minimal. Raise the right and left external iliac arteries (or right and left femoral arteries) and insert arterial tubes directed down the legs in each vessel. Prepare an arterial solution of very strong concentration: a high-index arterial fluid with equal parts of water or 100% arterial fluid. Inject each leg using at least a half-gallon of solution. The tissues of the leg will distend slightly, (Figure 18–6). Be certain the solution has reached portions of the leg below the knee. Stop the injection and let the arterial solution saturate the tissues while the arms and head and trunk areas of the body are embalmed. After the solution has had time to thoroughly saturate the tissues of the leg; with a scalpel, place a puncture in the area of the lower leg. Insert a drain tube or trocar and force as much of the solution as possible from the leg. The tissue procurement specialists will have placed prosthetic devices into the legs and heavily padded them with gauze

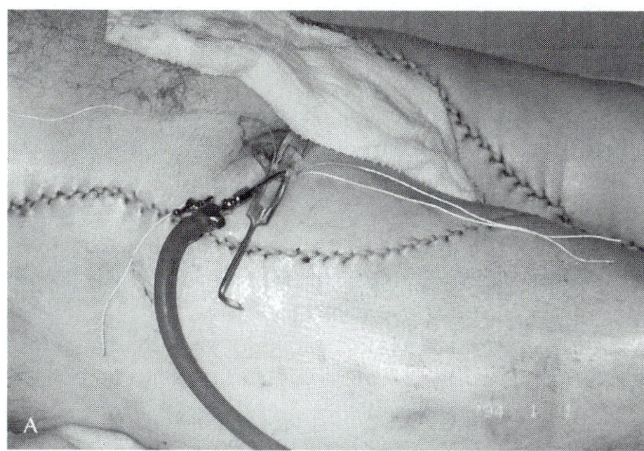

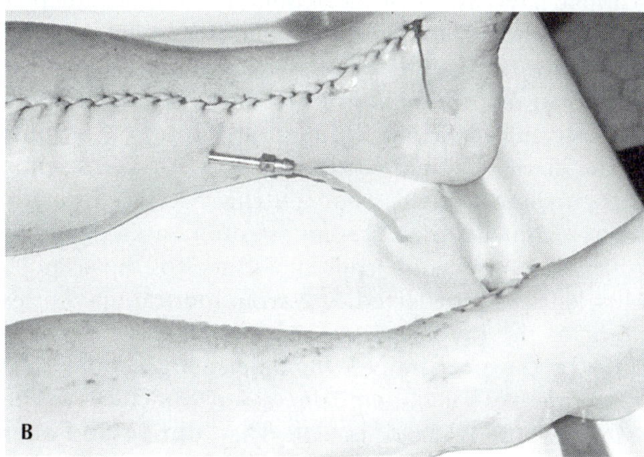

Figure 18–6. A. Injection of the leg using the femoral artery. The recovery team has sutured the leg using a tight baseball suture. **B.** Drainage of excess fluids, 1 hour after injection, from the lower leg.

sponges. These will now act as internal compresses. The procurement team's suturing can then be coated with a surface glue and the leg placed in a plastic stocking containing preservative powder or autopsy gel.

Proximal Humerus and Scapula Donors

In spite of the steady increase in the number of bone donors encountered by embalmers, tissue banks still operate in an environment where demand for tissue products far exceeds the supply. As a result of this shortage, tissue banks are constantly evaluating the possibility of harvesting bones in addition to the pelvis and long bones from which suitable tissue products can be processed.

The proximal humerus and scapula have been identified as additional sources of bone, and embalmers can anticipate seeing cases where these structures have been harvested. The term *proximal humerus* is used by tissue banks to indicate that only the humeral head and upper portion of the humerus are recovered. The scapula is commonly known as the shoulder blade. In those cases where both the proximal humerus and the scapula are taken, procurement technicians will usually take them en bloc. In those cases where the scapula will not be recovered, only the proximal humerus will be taken from the donor.

Recovering the Proximal Humerus. The procedures for recovering a proximal humerus are relatively straightforward. The procurement technician first prepares the work area and the donor to assure that the procurement is done under aseptic conditions. Then, with the donor in a supine position on the table, an incision is made laterally along the anterior/superior surface of the shoulder starting just below the acromion and continuing for about 4 inches down the anterior surface of the upper arm (Figure 18–7). The acromion is a process on the dorsal side of the scapula that articulates with the clavicle at a point on the superior surface of the shoulder. After the initial incision is complete, the technician deepens the opening so the shaft of the humerus is visible. Once the humeral shaft has been visually identified, all muscle attachments are cut so that the bone is mobile and more fully exposed. At this time in the procurement procedure, the technician needs to exercise great care to avoid cutting the axillary

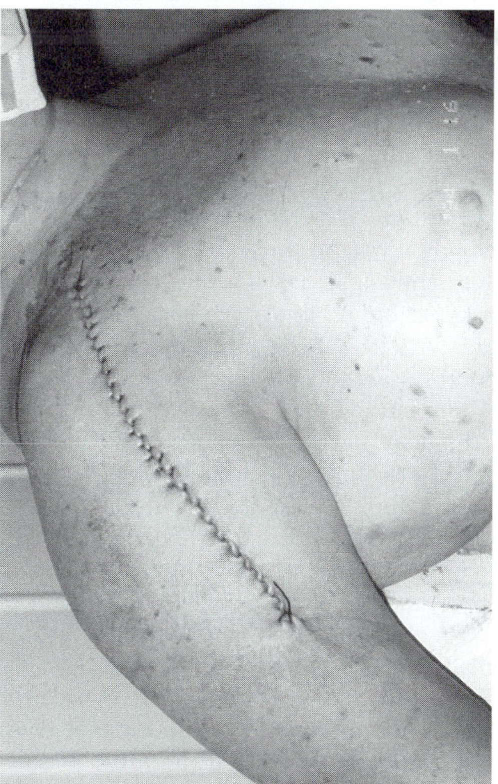

Figure 18–7. Anterior incision for removal of the proximal humerus.

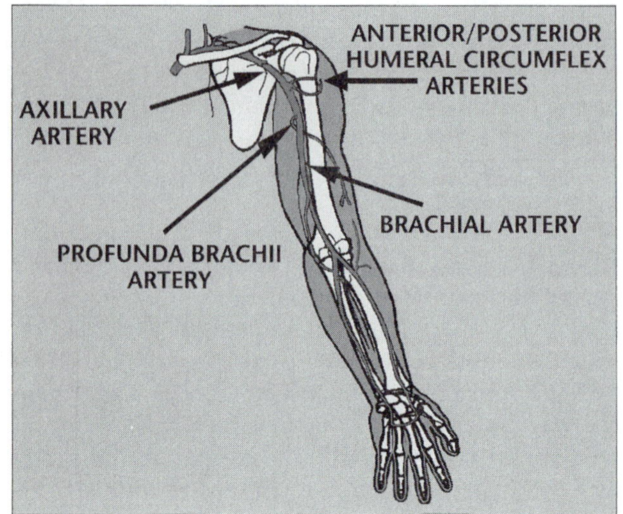

Figure 18–8. Arteries of the upper arm. *(Courtesy of National Funeral Directors Association [NFDA].)*

artery, axillary vein, anterior humeral circumflex artery, posterior humeral circumflex artery, brachial artery, profunda brachii artery, or basilic vein (Figure 18–8). Detaching muscles on the anterior surface of the humerus includes cutting attachments for the supraspinatus muscle, the subscapularis muscle, the latissimus dorsi muscle, the pectoralis major muscle, and the teres major muscles. On the posterior side of the humerus, attachments for the infraspinatus muscle, the teres minor muscle, and the triceps muscles are cut. Next, the technician uses a Gigli's (jel'yez) saw or other type of surgical saw, and cuts through the humerus at a point about 4 inches down the shaft. This is another point in the procedure where the technician needs to exercise great care to avoid cutting the blood vessel in the area. The Gigli's saw is a wire saw ideally suited to this task because it allows the procurement technician to maneuver the cutting wire into the space between the blood vessels and the bone. Thus the bone can be cut without putting the blood vessels in the area at risk. Once the bone has been cut, the technician will carefully cut the ligaments that attach the humeral head within the glenoid cavity. After the ligaments have been cut, the humeral head is disarticulated from the glenoid cavity, and the proximal humerus can be lifted from the arm.

Recovering the Proximal Humerus and Scapula En Bloc. This procedure requires an incision on the back side of the donor's shoulder, and for that reason the donor must be placed face down on the procurement table. The procurement technician must exercise great care in handling the body so that no postmortem damage or injuries occur. The embalming implications arising from having a body face down on the table are many, but the main concerns for embalmers center on disfigurement, the development of discolorations, and the engorging of facial tissues with blood and other body fluids. For these reasons, in addition to handling the body with extreme care, procurement technicians need to support the head and face with soft padding, keep the face elevated off the table surface, and work quickly so that the body is not face down for any longer than is absolutely necessary.

The procurement technician begins the procedure by prepping the work area and the body to assure the procurement is done under aseptic conditions. An incision is made along the superior margin of the scapula, laterally across the shoulder, and down the posterior portion of the upper arm, ending about 4 inches down the arm (Figure 18–9). Skin and soft tissue are reflected so that the bones of the shoulder are exposed. The acromioclavicular ligament attaching the scapula to the clavicle is then cut (Figure 18–10). The scapula is then disarticulated from the clavicle. The procurement technician then uses an osteotome to separate or cut muscle insertions from all surfaces of the scapula. Muscle tissue is dissected away from the scapula. At this point in the procurement, there is potential for mistakes by the procurement technician that could have consequences for the embalmer. Any punctures in the skin are potential points of leakage during and after embalming. Also, if the technician punctures a lung or the heart, embalming complications could result. Obviously, the procurement technician needs to exercise great care to avoid creating problems for the embalmer.

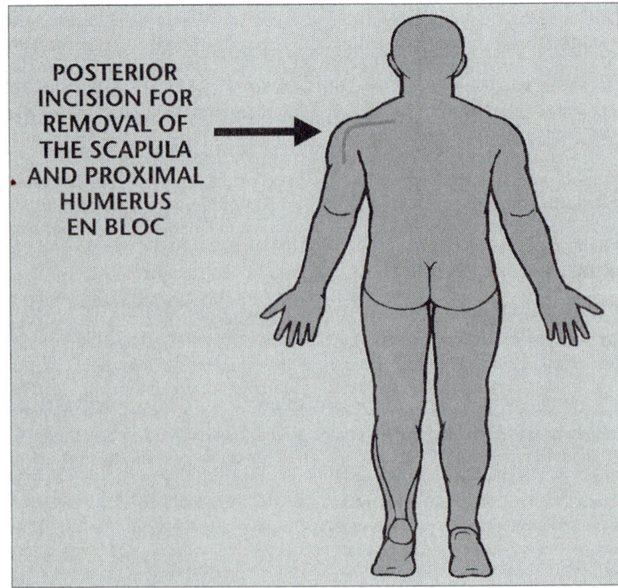

Figure 18–9. Incision for scapula harvesting. *(Drawing used with permission from NFDA.)*

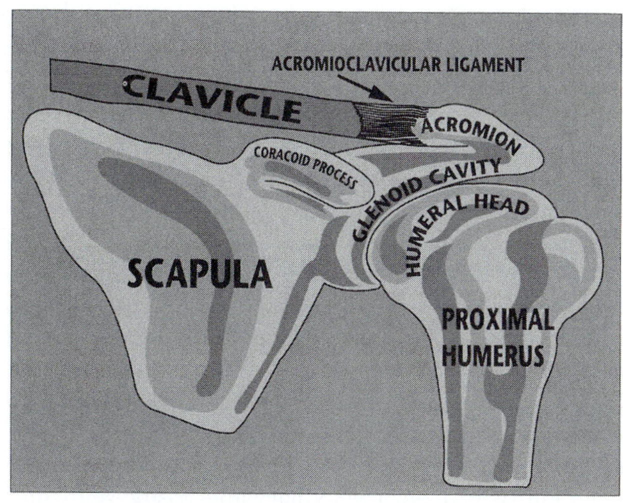

Figure 18–10. The acromioclavicular ligament attaches the scapula to the clavicle. *(Used with permission from NFDA.)*

The procurement technician then cuts the muscle attachments on the anterior and posterior surfaces of the humerus. The technician needs to be very careful to avoid cutting blood vessels in the area. A Gigli's saw or other surgical saw can be used to cut the humerus at a point about 4 inches down the humeral shaft. The scapula and proximal humerus can then be lifted from the body en bloc.

Restoration by the Procurement Technician. It is the responsibility of the procurement technician to restore the body to a condition and appearance as similar to the pre-procurement condition and appearance as possible.

In those cases where the tissue has been harvested in a funeral home preparation room, the funeral home staff may request that the procurement technician *not* do the restoration at the conclusion of the procurement. It makes little sense for the procurement technician to do restorative work on a donor, only to have the embalmer come in and remove the sutures and prosthesis in order to prepare the body. The funeral home can request that the prosthesis and any other materials needed for the restoration be left for use at the time of postembalming restoration. Communication between the tissue bank and the funeral home is important in these cases, so that both know the other's capabilities, needs, and preferences.

In those cases where the restoration is completed by the procurement technician, it will be necessary to utilize a prosthetic device to recreate the shape and support that was once provided by the harvested bone. Some tissue banks employ devices made of plastic tubing that can be secured by means of surgical screws to the glenoid cavity and to the distal end of the humerus. Once the prosthesis is in place, the incision is closed with a tight suture.

Any leakage that might occur after a proximal humerus recovery would generally be easier to manage because the procurement incision occurs on the anterior surface of the shoulder. The anterior location of the incision causes blood and other fluids to gravitate away from the opening of the incision. Greater difficulty could be anticipated for a proximal humerus and scapula en bloc procurement where the incision is made on the posterior surface of the shoulder. The posterior location of the incision would cause blood and other fluids to gravitate toward the opening of the incision.

Embalming. Unlike many other types of tissue procurement, proximal humerus and scapula removal can be done with little disruption to the blood vascular system. If the procurement technician exercises the necessary skill and care, major blood vessels in the arm and shoulder will be intact for arterial embalming. This circumstance has obvious implications for the embalmer.

EMBALMING WITHOUT OPENING THE PROCUREMENT INCISION. If proper technique has been employed in procurement and restoration, it may be possible to embalm the body without opening the procurement incisions. Selecting this option requires that the embalmer know, or trust, that the technician has done the procurement without disrupting major blood vessels. In this situation the embalmer employs standard procedures, using either a cervical or a femoral injection and drainage site. As the arterial injection proceeds, the embalmer must carefully monitor the procurement site for distention and/or leakage. If neither occurs, the embalming can be completed with a normal application of embalming procedures. If distention occurs, it is likely that either blood or embalming solution is causing the problem. The embalmer must assess the problem, and make a determination as to whether the procurement incision should be opened, and alternative embalming procedures be applied.

OPENING THE PROCUREMENT INCISION. In cases where the procurement incision is opened before or during arterial injection, the embalmer first examines the procurement site for cut or broken blood vessels. If no disruption is found in either the axillary or brachial arteries, the embalmer looks for cuts or breaks in the anterior and/or posterior humeral circumflex arteries, or in the profunda brachii artery (Figure 18–11). Cuts or breaks in smaller branch arteries may not represent a significant enough disruption to prevent the perfusion of arterial solution into the arm and hand. If either the axillary or brachial artery is cut or broken, the em-

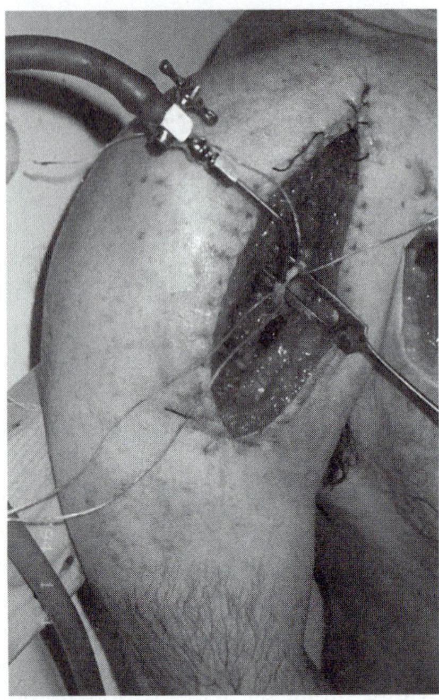

Figure 18–11. Injection of the arm using the brachial artery.

balmer ligates the proximal (close to the midline) and distal (away from the midline) end of the vessel. Ligation of the proximal end helps to control leakage as the rest of the body was embalmed. Ligation of the distal end would serve as an anatomical marker for locating the vessel as an injection site when the arm and hand are embalmed. If either the axillary or basilic vein has been cut or broken, the embalmer will clamp the proximal and distal ends of the vessel so that they are marked. The embalmer may choose to allow drainage to flow from cut or broken veins as arterial injection takes place. If controlled drainage is desired, the open ends of the axillary or basilic vein can be clamped.

Other Embalming Considerations. Opening the incision and examining the procurement site may not always reveal cut or broken vessels. As the arterial injection is proceeding, the embalmer will monitor the site for signs of leakage. Blood leaking into the procurement site during arterial injection should prompt the embalmer to look for a cut or break in the axillary vein, basilic vein, or one of their tributaries. In this case, it is possible to continue embalming from the primary injection site. Leakage from the veins is not a significant problem during arterial injection, but it is necessary for the embalmer to make certain that any cut or broken veins are properly ligated at the conclusion of the arterial injection to prevent postembalming leakage.

Arterial solution leaking into the procurement site indicates that vessels providing circulation to the arm and hand have been disrupted. The embalmer can thus conclude that the arm and hand are likely to have to be injected separately from the rest of the body. The embalmer examines the procurement site for a cut or break in the axillary artery or the brachial artery. If either has been cut or broken, the embalmer must locate the distal and proximal ends of the vessel. The proximal end is clamped, and the distal end used as a secondary injection site to embalm the arm and hand separately from the rest of the body. If examination reveals the artery has only been punctured, the embalmer may attempt to clamp the puncture and continue with the injection. It may also be possible for the embalmer to utilize the puncture as a secondary injection site. For those cases where the axillary or brachial arteries have been cut or broken, the axillary and basilic veins may also have been cut. Leakage or drainage from these vessels can be controlled with hemostats.

At the conclusion of arterial injection, the embalmer should assess embalming results to determine if supplemental embalming techniques are necessary. The embalmer must securely ligate all vessels that have been cut or broken. Once the embalmer has determined that leakage has been stopped, the procurement site should then be thoroughly dried with absorbent material, and treated with powdered incision sealer. A tight suture will then be used to hold the incision closed. The sutures should be treated with a coating of liquid sealer, and a layer of absorbent material. The embalmer should take effective steps to stop or contain any postembalming leakage that might occur.

Embalming proximal humerus and scapula donors does not present great difficulty, providing the procurement has been done with reasonable skill and care. Many of the procedures are not significantly different from procedures frequently applied in autopsied cases or in sectional embalming.

Skin Donors

Donor skin is taken in a thin layer, usually from areas of the body such as the back, chest, and thighs, where there is a flatter surface that has a larger area. An instrument called a **dermatome** is used to peel or shave very thin layers of the skin (Figure 18–12).

The recovery of skin from the dead human body presents two major problems for the embalmer: drying of the effected areas from which skin has been taken, and control of the seepage or leakage from the area where skin has been taken. To deal with these problems the embalmer should:

1. Spray the effected areas with disinfectant.
2. Wash the body with liquid soap and warm water. This step removes the sterilant, which is often betadine, from the surface of the body. The

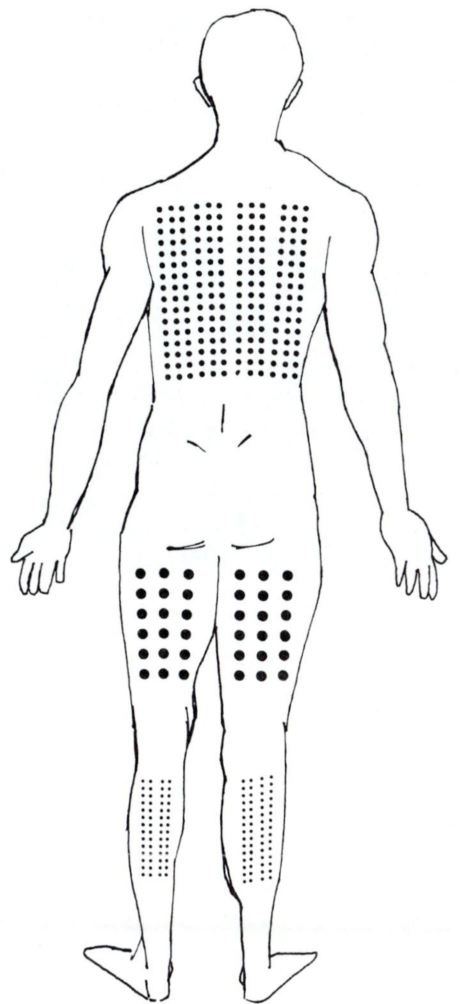

Figure 18–12. Areas from which skin is most often removed.

sterilant can cause a discoloration of the skin. Bathing the body should also remove blood and body fluids that may have leaked or seeped from the affected area.

3. Once the bathing is completed, the embalmer should properly position the body on the table. Because the affected areas may be on both the anterior and posterior surface of the body, a fair amount of moving and rolling might be necessary to bathe the body. These movements can easily cause the body to slip out of proper position.
4. Procedure as determined by embalming analysis for shaving, feature posing, raising of vessels, and so on.
5. Consider condition of the body, in concert with other factors identified during case analysis that determine decisions regarding the volume and concentration of arterial solution injected into the body. The embalmer will certainly want to be aware of the need to dry the tissues where skin has been removed, but this need will also have to be balanced with the desire to embalm the body in such a way as to produce the best chance for satisfactory viewing.
6. Paint the affected areas with a cauterant, or apply surface compress(es) saturated with cauterant, or both, once arterial injection is completed. Commercially produced products which have a phenol base (cauterants and/or autopsy gel) can be used for this procedure. Or, the embalmer can utilize a compress saturated with undiluted cavity fluid. The embalmer must allow sufficient time for the products to work and for body surfaces to dry. In those cases where time becomes a critical factor, the drying process can be aided by the use of a hair dryer.
7. The embalmer should consider measures that can be employed to create barriers to leakage. For example, once the affected surface is dry, some embalmers prefer to coat the raw skin with a glue or surface sealer, over which a layer or layers of cotton is placed. Or, the embalmer can place plastic garments, inside which preservative/drying compound or embalming powder has been sprinkled, on the body. Some embalmers prefer to use sealer, cotton and plastic garments to aid and supplement each other.

Mandible Donors

Mandible recovery does not occur as frequently as other types of tissue donation. In most cases, mandibles are recovered from bodies that will not be viewed. There are two methods by which mandibles are removed from the body. Both methods have significant embalming and restorative consequences.

Method 1. An incision is made on the undersurface of the jaw starting at the angle of the jaw on one side, following the jawline under and around the chin to the angle of the jaw on the other side. The skin, muscle, and fascia are then dissected away, exposing the bone. Once the bone has been freed from soft tissue, it is manually disarticulated from the temporomandibular joint, and removed.

Method 2. An incision is made between the lip and gum on the inside of the mouth, following the jawline from approximately the angle of the jaw on one side of the face, passing over the chin to the angle of the jaw on the other side of the face. The soft tissues are then dissected away so that the mandible can be freed, disarticulated, and removed.

In both cases the arterial system supplying the facial surface will be disrupted. In particular, the facial artery will be cut and/or broken in the process. The external incision method will leave obvious restorative problems, although the internal incision method, if not done carefully, can result in tears or cuts in the surface tissue along the jawline as well.

Rib Donors

Ribs are usually recovered through the same incision used for vascular organ recovery. After organ recovery, a scalpel is used to peel back the skin, and every other rib is removed. The embalmer will have to contend with disruptions to the intercostal arteries as a result of this procedure. This may not present a problem that would cause the embalmer to make any significant changes in procedure, but will definitely contribute to leakage during embalming. The embalmer must ensure that the leakage is stopped so that it does not create problems after embalming.

Temporal Bone Donors

Two techniques are employed to recover the temporal bone: (1) exterior approach, and (2) interior approach.

Method 1. The internal approach is most commonly used to recover the bone during autopsy. The advantage of the internal approach from an embalming standpoint is that it ensures that there is no disfigurement to the body's facial area. The recovery process in both procedures is very similar. Soft tissues and periosteum are scraped from the mastoid with a sharp instrument. All tissue forward of the external auditory canal is elevated. After the external auditory canal is identified, it is transected. Soft tissue is further elevated from the bone around the open ear canal.

A plug cutter is placed on the mastoid bone so that it is centered over the external auditory canal. It is moved posteriorly so the front of the blade is at the anterior edge of the external auditory canal. The plug cutter is angled 20 degrees backward so that it points toward the opposite temple. Pressure is applied to a drill attached to the plug cutter, and the drilling is continued until the plug cutter is completely embedded in the incision. After drilling is complete, chisel cuts must be made around the temporal bone specimen to sever the deep bony attachments. At this point, any soft tissue attachments can be cut by sharp dissection. As the temporal bone becomes more mobile, a twisting motion frees it from its last attachment. If an internal approach is used, there should be no problems with embalming (Figure 18–13).

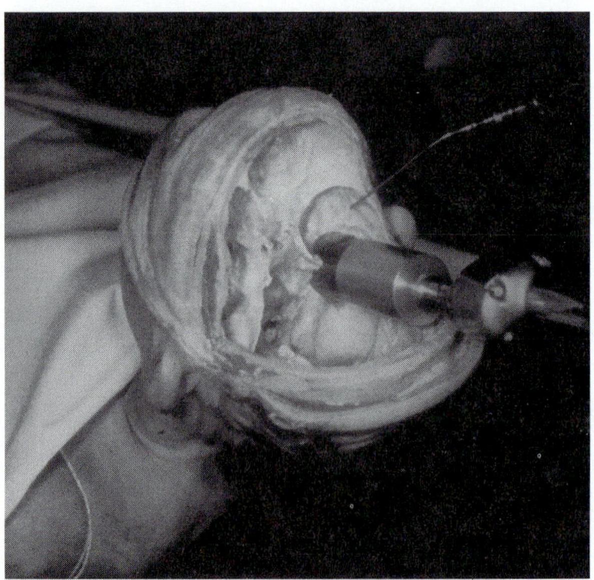

Figure 18–13. Temporal bone recovery—internal approach.

Method 2. The external approach begins with a curved incision 1 inch behind the ear crease that extends from above the ear to the mastoid tip. This poses some additional challenges for the embalmer. The major problem encountered after removal of the inner ear bone by the internal approach is that the upper portions of the face and eyes do not receive sufficient amounts of arterial solution. The embalmer can use tracer dye to check circulation to the various facial regions. Care should also be taken to check for arterial fluid leakage from the base of the skull, where the temporal bone was removed.

Generally, leakage can be controlled with hemostats or by tightly packing cotton into the area where the temporal bone has been removed and applying hand pressure. After embalming, mortuary putty or incision seal powder can be placed in the area from which the bone was removed. Some embalmers prefer plaster of Paris as a filler for this cavity. These measures ensure against further leakage from the external ear as well as from the scalp. Plenty of absorbent cotton filler can be placed in the cranial cavity prior to suturing the scalp. It is wise to pack the external auditory meatus with cotton and some incision seal powder to prevent leakage from the external ear.

If the bone was removed by the external approach and the ear has been partially excised after embalming, the temporal area should be packed with a phenol cautery agent. This material should be left in place for a time, then replaced with dry cotton and incision seal powder. Mortuary putty can also be used as a filler. The ear can be reattached with intradermal sutures or super glue.

▶ CONCLUSIONS

In an environment where the demand for tissue exceeds supply, tissue banks will continue to work very hard to perpetuate the growth in donations that has already been realized. Embalmers can anticipate an ever-increasing number of cases where the deceased has been a tissue donor. Knowing what steps to take in the preparation of tissue donors is a professional requirement for the embalmer.

There is a great need for embalmers and tissue bankers to become professional colleagues because the work done by each group is vital to fulfilling the wishes of the deceased and/or the deceased's next of kin. Unfortunately, the lack of regard which sometimes exists between the two groups has created a number of adversarial situations. It is important to remember that both the funeral home and the tissue bank are involved in postdeath activities at the invitation of, and with the permission of, the donor and/or the donor family.

The funeral service community, however, has every right to insist that tissue procurement be done in a manner that preserves options for open-casket viewing. Tissue banks go to great lengths to assure donor families that consent to harvest tissues will not significantly disrupt funeral plans. Donor families, therefore, have a right to expect that tissue banks are true to that claim. Funeral directors are in a unique position, because they know when procurement agencies have failed to keep their word. Funeral directors, therefore, can serve families by communicating with tissue banks regarding any issues and problems that arise from tissue procurement. That *does not* mean the funeral director becomes a watchdog; rather, the funeral director and the tissue banker are colleagues who must deal in a professional manner with each other, and the families they serve.

▶ KEY TERMS AND CONCEPTS FOR STUDY

1. Define the following terms:
   dermatome
   enucleation
   Gigli's saw
   heparin
   organ
   organ donation
   prosthesis
   proximal humerus
   temporal bone
   tissue
   tissue donation
   vertebral bodies
2. Describe an embalming technique for:
   eye enucleation
   heart removal
   heart and lung removal
   kidney(s) removal
   liver removal
   long bone removal (hip/legs)
   lung(s) removal
   mandible removal
   multiple organ removal
   pancreas removal
   proximal humerus and scapula removal
   rib removal
   skin donors
   small bowel removal
   temporal bone removal
   vertebral body removal

▶ REFERENCES

Koosmann S. Bone transplantation. *Champion Expanding Encyclopedia.* Springfield, OH: Champion Chemical Co., 1984: 2210–2217.

Kroshus J, et al. Embalming techniques in long bone donor cases. *American Funeral Director* 1995;118: 26–27, 30.

Kroshus J. Embalming the vertebral body donor. *The Director* 1997; 69:30, 32–34.

Kroshus TJ, et al. Heart transplantation. In Hakim NS, ed. *Introduction to Organ Transplantation.* London: Imperial College Press, 1997:121–132.

Kroshus J. Embalming proximal humerus and scapula donors. *The Director* 1998;70: 44–48.

Mayer RG. Enucleation restoration. *Champion Expanding Encyclopedia,* Springfield, OH: Champion Chemical Co., 1987:2322–2325.

Toledo-Pereya, LH. *Organ Procurement and Preservation for Transplantation,* 2nd edition. Austin, TX: Landes Bioscience, 1997.

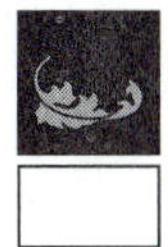

CHAPTER 19
DELAYED EMBALMING

The postmortem period between death and preparation of the body plays an important role in determining the proper embalming technique. It is during this period that postmortem changes occur within the body. These changes include algor mortis, hypostasis of the blood, livor mortis, dehydration, increase in blood viscosity, decomposition, change in body pH, rigor mortis, postmortem stain and postmortem caloricity.

These changes do not always occur in a uniform manner in the tissues of the body. For example, rigor may be present in some muscles but will have passed in others. Also, tissue pH varies and heat is retained by some tissues (e.g., viscera) but rapidly lost from others (e.g., extremities). Decomposition may be present in a gangrenous limb but not in other body areas. These changes are greatly influenced by the length of time between death and preparation as well as the temperature of the environment during that period.

As a general rule, most postmortem changes are speeded by a warm environment or by the presence of heat. An exception is algor mortis. The longer the period between death and embalming the more changes can be expected to occur. From an embalming standpoint, the longer the delay the more problems the embalmer may expect to encounter. As time passes, the preservative demands of the various tissues increase.

Figure 19–1 illustrates the gradual increase in the demand for preservative. Increased temperature increases the preservative demand, because the higher temperature speeds decomposition of the proteins. A shift to a more alkaline pH increases preservative demand. Autolysis and putrefaction produce an increased number of sites for the union of preservative and the products of protein decomposition. Bodies from which rigor has passed and those showing early signs of decomposition have a very high preservative demand. Bodies in a state of rigor mortis have very little preservative demand, for the proteins are engaged in such a manner that they are not free to make contact with the preservative. After the rigor passes, however, the demand increases. Thus, in preparing a body in which most of the muscles are in a state of rigor, the embalmer must saturate the tissues with a strong arterial solution so that the preservative is available to make contact with the protein as the muscle fibers begin to pass from this contracted state of rigor.

Bodies in three postmortem states are discussed in this chapter: (1) bodies in a state of intense rigor mortis, (2) bodies from which rigor has passed and in which early signs of decomposition are observed, and (3) bodies refrigerated for long periods. The techniques used to prepare all of these bodies are almost the same. The embalmer must understand the specific problems presented by each body type as well as the reasons for using the prescribed technique. These techniques vary with other body factors, such as age, weight, general body nutrition, and the effects of diseases or medications.

The three body types listed all show some degree of delay. Generally, the longer the period between death and preparation, the more problems can be anticipated. Temperature also affects all three categories. Elevation of environmental temperature speeds both rigor mortis and decomposition cycles. Low temperatures can also slow these cycles, but during refrigeration, *autolysis* and bacterial enzymes continue tissue breakdown. Low temperatures can slow arterial solution diffusion but increase capillary permeability. Increased capillary permeability can result in tissue distension during arterial solution injection. Lowered temperature affects all chemical reactions, so bodies can be expected to firm more slowly after refrigeration.

Preservative absorption by tissue proteins is usually greatest immediately after injection. Most bodies exhibit some degree of firming during the injection process. One reason for this early fixation is that the concentration of preservative (fixative) is greatest when the arterial solution is first introduced into the tissues. If a sufficient amount of preservative has been injected, complete firming of the body will occur several hours to a day later. Degree of decomposition, tissue pH, and temperature and concentration of arterial solution all play a role in determining the speed and degree of fixation. Cool temperature slows these reactions; alkaline

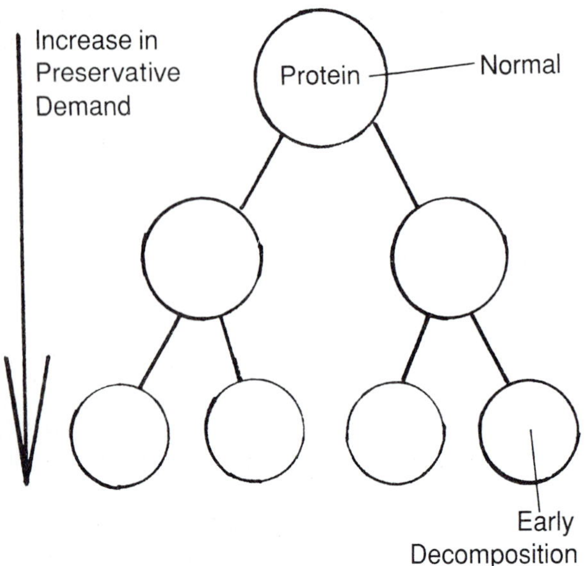

Figure 19–1. Demand for preservative is increased in bodies as protein breaks down.

pH above 7.4 slows fixation; and decomposed protein demands more concentrated preservative.

Arterial fluids vary. Some are buffered to act slowly (slow-firming fluids) and others are buffered to fix tissues rapidly (buffered-acid fast-firming fluids). It is imperative that the embalmer provide sufficient preservative to the tissues to meet the total preservative demands of the tissues. **It is better to overembalm than to underembalm body tissues.**

All these bodies have a high preservative demand. This increased fluid need is brought about by the breakdown of tissues. As circulation is impaired in most of these bodies, distribution problems can be anticipated. As these bodies are all subject to distension, use *of a minimum amount* of *a stronger* arterial solution best establishes good preservation and minimizes tissue distension. Strong (hypertonic) arterial solution helps to minimize swelling to the tissues.

▶ MECHANICAL AND MANUAL AIDS

Achieving adequate distribution of the preservative solution with a minimum amount of tissue swelling is of great concern in the preparation of bodies where there has been an extended time delay between the death and embalming. Manual aids such as lowering the arms; firm but limited massage; squeezing the sides of the fingers and the nailbeds; bending, rotating and, flexing of limbs; and massaging the areas of the buttocks and shoulders where there is contact with the embalming table surface will help to distribute the arterial solution. Manual aids such as elevation devices, weights, compresses, and pneumatic collars can be used to correct minor swellings. Mechanical aids in the form of drainage tubes, controlled pressure and rate of flow, use of pulsation, and size of the arterial tube will all help to control the speed and amount of embalming solution entering the body or a body area.

Operative Corrections

When localized swelling of unsupported tissues such as the eyelids or neck occurs, invasive treatments such as channeling, incising, and if necessary excising can be used to correct the swollen condition.

▶ INJECTION PROTOCOL

The suggested order of arterial treatment for the bodies discussed in this chapter follows.

Injection and Drainage Sites

For injection and drainage, *restricted cervical injection* is the first choice in the embalming of the unautopsied body. *Both* the right and the left common carotid arteries are raised. A tube is placed in each artery directed toward the head, and the tubes are left open. Another tube placed in the right common carotid is directed toward the trunk. The trunk is injected first. The head is injected through the left common carotid and then the right common carotid. Drainage may be taken from the right internal jugular vein.

The second choice would be to begin the preparation using a six-point injection.

The third choice is use of the right common carotid artery for injection and the right internal jugular vein for drainage.

Use of the one-point injection is not recommended. It affords no control over the amount of arterial solution entering the head or over swelling of neck or facial tissues.

FACTORS THAT MUST BE DETERMINED IN THE EMBALMING ANALYSIS

1. Vessels for injection and drainage
2. Strength of the embalming solution
3. Volume of the embalming solution
4. Injection pressure
5. Injection rate of flow

Note: These factors will vary by the individual body; these factors can vary in different areas of the same body.

Arterial Solution Strength

As previously stated, a stronger-than-average arterial solution is needed for the bodies discussed in this chapter, especially when signs of decomposition are evident. A *high-index special-purpose fluid* is best for the preparation of these bodies. If this fluid is not available, an arterial fluid of 25 index or higher should be selected.

In preparing the arterial solution the first recommendation is to follow the suggestions of the manufacturer. Many labels carry dilution instructions for delayed, refrigerated, or decomposed bodies. Preinjection fluids should be avoided. Use of a coinjection would be a better choice.

The first half-gallon may be made milder in an attempt to clear blood discolorations in the unautopsied body, but should be followed by stronger fluid solutions, 2.0% strength or higher. In the treatment of bodies that show evidence of decomposition, 100% arterial fluid with a coinjection fluid (waterless) may be required. Fluid dye should be added to the embalming solution because it will serve as an indicator of arterial solution distribution. The dye will also help to prevent graying of the embalmed tissues. If a body is exhibiting advanced signs of decomposition and restricted cervical injection or a six-point injection is used, the head can be injected using a waterless embalming technique. For extreme situations, the instant tissue fixation method may be helpful. This helps to minimize swelling of the face and establishes maximum fluid distribution throughout the facial tissues.

Volume of Arterial Solution

The amount of solution injected depends on the size of the body and the success in distributing the arterial solution. The tissues of these bodies can easily distend, necessitating the use of a concentrated, well-coordinated embalming solution. Such a solution should require less amount (volume) to establish preservation, thus resulting in a minimum amount of tissue swelling.

Order of Injection

The following order of injection is recommended when there has been a delay between death and preparation, when intense rigor is present, when the body has been refrigerated a long time, or when decomposition is evident:

1. Raise the right and the left common carotid arteries.
2. Use the right internal jugular vein for drainage.
3. Place tubes directed toward the head into the right and left common carotid arteries; leave these tubes open. Place one tube directed toward the trunk.
4. Slowly inject about 1 gallon of arterial solution toward the trunk using extra fluid dye.
5. Evaluate the distribution of fluid. If the extremities of the body are not receiving arterial solution, separately arterially inject those areas needing arterial solution.
6. Inject strong arterial solutions by using sufficient pressure and rate of flow to distribute the solution and minimize swelling. Increased pressures and rates of flow can be used for sectional embalming. Pulsation injection is usually helpful. Use firm massage and manipulation to encourage fluid distribution.
7. Embalm the head last, first the left side and then the right side, using a strong arterial solution. Use dye to trace the fluid. For extreme conditions, consider using waterless solutions and instant tissue fixation injection techniques.
8. Evaluate the body and use hypodermic and surface embalming for areas not receiving arterial solution.

Pressure and Rate of Flow

When there has been a long delay between death and embalming, the unautopsied body should be very slowly injected. Slower injection helps to prevent clots in the arterial system from moving (solution flows over the coagula) into the smaller distal arteries. Rapid injection can easily cause abdominal distension, which can create purge. Even in embalming the "normal" body, the first gallon of arterial fluid is slowly injected; then, the process may be speeded to facilitate distribution of the arterial solution.

In the injection of arms or legs of the autopsied body, higher pressures and faster rates of flow may be needed to establish distribution. Pulsation may be helpful in distributing fluid to the extremities, and higher pressures can be used with pulsation.

A pulsed flow can be created in several ways: use an embalming machine with a pulse setting; manually turn the rate of flow valve on and off; turn the stopcock valve on and off; bend the delivery hose, starting and stopping the flow of fluid.

▶ PREPARATION OF BODIES IN RIGOR MORTIS

One of the most difficult preparations is that of the body in the intense state of *rigor mortis*, in particular, the body that is well nourished and has a well-developed musculature. The death may have been accidental or sudden as in a heart attack or fatal stroke. These bodies with well-developed musculature develop a very intense rigor mortis. It may be impossible for the embalmer to remove this rigor by manipulating the body prior to injection of the arterial solution. Thin bodies, bodies that demonstrate the effects of wasting disease, and bodies in which the musculature is not well developed undergo as complete and intense rigor as the body with good musculature, except that the muscles are not as large and the rigor can be relieved prior to injection.

Rigor is first observed in the average body approximately 2 hours after death. Depending on cause of death, environmental temperature, and activity prior to death, the rigor can occur sooner or be delayed beyond the 2 hours. (See Chapter 5 for further details concerning the rigor mortis cycle in the dead human body.) Rigor comprises three general stages: (1) primary flaccidity, the period in which the rigor develops and is hardly noticeable; (2) the period of rigor; (3) secondary flaccidity, in which the rigor passes from the body. The most problems are encountered when the body is to be embalmed while in intense rigor.

Table 19–1 summarizes the preservative demand of the muscle tissues during the stages of rigor.

As noted in Table 19–1, a body in rigor requires or absorbs a very small amount of preservative. The problem, however, arises in that once the rigor passes, the demand for preservative increases greatly. **It is imperative that the embalmer saturate the tissues with a well-coordinated solution of sufficient strength to meet the preservative demands of the body when the rigor has passed.** Otherwise, the body will soften not only from the passage of rigor, but from the decomposition processes that break down body proteins. Therefore, bodies embalmed prior to the onset of rigor should be injected with a sufficient strength of arterial solution to meet the preservation needs as determined from body weight and effects of disease or drugs; bodies embalmed during and after rigor mortis need a strong arterial solution.

Problems Associated with Embalming Bodies in Rigor

Rigor may be relieved by physical manipulation of the muscle tissues. Firmly massaging, rotating, flexing, and bending the joints helps to relieve the rigor condition. Once broken, the condition does not recur. As previously stated, rigor may be broken when the musculature is not well developed. In well-developed individuals, it may be very difficult to attempt to relieve rigor in areas such as the thighs or upper arms. The following problems may be encountered in the preparation of the body in intense rigor:

1. Positioning may be difficult.
2. The features may be difficult to set if the jaw is firmly fixed.
3. Distribution of fluid may be poor because of the pressure on arteries and the narrowed arterial lumens resulting from contraction of muscle cells in the arterial walls.
4. Drainage may be poor because of the pressure exerted by contracted muscles on the small veins.
5. Tissues tend to swell, because fluid does not penetrate muscles during rigor but flows to surface areas where there is little resistance.
6. The pH of the tissues is not ideal for fluid reactions.
7. Tissues may not firm well after the passage of rigor, because it may not have been possible to inject sufficient quantities of the arterial solution.
8. Firmness of rigor can be a false sign of tissue fixation.

Features. In setting the features of a body in intense rigor, use a towel to firmly manipulate the jaw. Begin by raising the jaw, even if the lips are firmly pressed together. Massaging the temporalis muscles may also be helpful. Firmly push the chin, covering the chin with a towel and pressing firmly with the palm of the hand. Cotton may also be forced into the mouth to help open it. As soon as the lips can be properly aligned, suture or use a needle injector to ensure that the lower jaw remains in the proper position.

TABLE 19–1. PRESERVATIVE DEMAND OF THE MUSCLE TISSUES DURING RIGOR

Prerigor	Great absorption of preservative	The protein centers to which preservative attaches and crosslinks the proteins are readily available. Tissue pH is slightly alkaline and fluids work best in this pH range.
Rigor	Little absorption of preservative	The protein centers to which preservative attaches are engaged in maintaining the state of rigor mortis; vessel lumens are reduced so distribution is decreased. Muscle protein is contracted so fluid does not penetrate the muscle fibers well. The acid pH retards the absorption of preservative.
After rigor	Great preservative demand	Proteins have disorganized (or broken) and many centers are available for preservative attachment. The alkaline pH increases preservative absorption; nitrogenous wastes increase the need for preservative.

Positioning. Firmly rotate, bend, flex, and massage the joints and muscles of the neck, arms, and, if possible, legs. This may be necessary to position the body properly. Relieve the rigor in the arms by first rotating the shoulder joint. Next, flex the elbow and wrist areas. Grasp all the fingers and gently pull them into a straightened position if the hand is firmly closed. To relieve rigor in the legs, exercise the hip joint first. Next, flex the knee joint. Finally, rotate the foot inward very firmly. These manipulations help to relieve some of the rigor present.

Injection. Both common carotid arteries should be raised for the injection of bodies in intense rigor mortis. The right internal jugular vein can be used for drainage. A medium to strong arterial solution should be used. Follow the manufacturer's recommendations for dilutions. Dye and coinjection fluid can be added to the solution. The extra dye not only serves as a fluid tracer, but helps to prevent the tissues from graying. In the embalming of these bodies, blood drainage is often minimal and formaldehyde gray can easily develop hours after the embalming. The coinjection fluid assists in fluid penetration and adjustment of tissue pH. Keep in mind that the dye merely indicates that surface tissues have received fluid; there is no indicator for the deeper tissues.

Some embalmers prefer to begin the injection of most bodies with a mild arterial solution (1.25–1.50%) until surface blood discolorations are cleared. Subsequent injections are then made using stronger arterial solutions. Avoid the use of preinjection fluids with the body in intense rigor condition. Whenever distribution difficulties are expected, preinjection should not be used.

Inject slowly. During arterial injection, massage and manipulate the limbs to encourage distribution. When drainage is established, the injection speed can be slightly increased to encourage better distribution. Inject the trunk first. Both arterial tubes directed toward the head should be left open and no fluid should enter the head or facial tissues while the trunk is being injected in the unautopsied body.

Frequently, the autopsied body exhibits intense rigor, because the delay for the autopsy allows the rigor mortis to become firmly established in the body muscles. As each area of the body is separately injected, a faster rate of flow may be used. This is an excellent opportunity for the embalmer to use pulsation injection.

Using a mild to strong arterial solution, inject the head separately in the unautopsied body, first the left side then the right. Remember that swelling may be a problem, so a minimum amount of arterial solution should be injected. Injection should be stopped as soon as fluid dye is evident or if there is any distension in the eyelids, neck or glandular areas of the face, or neck. If parts of the face require additional treatment, hypodermic or surface embalming can be employed. **Use of a minimum amount of a strong solution helps to control swelling and achieve good preservation and tissue fixation.**

Injection of Limbs in Rigor. Physical manipulation of the limbs removes some of the intense rigor. The muscles should be manipulated before arterial injection is begun. As an example, take the healthy, well-developed, well-nourished man who dies as the result of trauma or sudden heart attack. Delay has resulted in intense rigor. If the arms and legs are to be separately injected, try first to relieve some of the rigor. This will be very difficult; more success will be possible with the arms than with the legs. Attempt to manipulate the arms so they can be positioned as they will appear in the casket. Inject from the brachial, axillary, or subclavian artery in the autopsied body. The brachial artery is most frequently used in the unautopsied body and the axillary in the autopsied body. The femoral artery can be used to inject the legs in the unautopsied body, and the external iliac artery can be used to inject the legs in the autopsied body.

The arterial solution used for injection should be stronger than the "average" arterial solution. A high-index arterial fluid can be used or several ounces of a high-index fluid can be added to the standard arterial solution. When injecting the arms or the legs, begin at a slow rate of flow (i.e., set the pressure with the rate-of-flow valve closed at 20 psi; open the valve until the pressure drops to 18 psi). By lowering the arms and using gentle but firm massage, attempt to distribute the fluid into the hands and fingers. Once distribution is established, a higher rate of flow can be used. If slow injection is not very successful in establishing distribution, use pulsation. Try pulsing the fluid into the limb (inject, pause, inject, pause, etc.) until distribution is established. Pulsation allows the use of higher pressures but also greater rates of flow.

Keep in mind that some swelling of the arms can be expected. Again, the stronger fluid helps to limit the swelling because less fluid is needed. Inject until blood discolorations clear and dye is present in the tissues. Intermittent drainage helps to achieve penetration of the fluid. The same procedure can be used to inject the legs. If distribution to the legs is unsuccessful, use hypodermic treatment to ensure thorough preservation of the leg tissues. If the hands do not receive adequate fluid, raise and inject the radial or ulnar artery. Individual fingers can be treated by hypodermic injection of a preservative solution.

Other Considerations for Bodies in Rigor Mortis. During the period in which rigor occurs, the pH of the tissues is slightly acid. It has been found that the preservative–protein reaction occurs most readily at slightly basic pH, about the same as that of normal, healthy tissues (7.38–7.4). **Rigor mortis does not occur in all muscles simultaneously.** Rigor may pass from those muscles where it first occurs (the face and upper extremities) while it is still very intense in the lower areas of the body, such as the leg muscles. Also, pH will not be the same in the various muscles. Where rigor has passed from the muscles, autolysis and hydrolysis have proceeded to a point where protein has decomposed and the pH has become increasingly alkaline (basic).

Increase of tissue pH into the alkaline pH range after rigor mortis indicates that the muscle proteins have begun to break down or decompose. There are now additional sites for reaction with preservative. During rigor there are few sites for the reaction of preservative and proteins. A body being embalmed while in rigor should be saturated with sufficient preservative, so that it will be available later as the state of rigor passes.

Rigor and varying pH combine to make it very difficult for the embalmer to obtain uniform preservation of the body. Some of the factors that contribute to this lack of uniform embalming are outlined in the following chart:

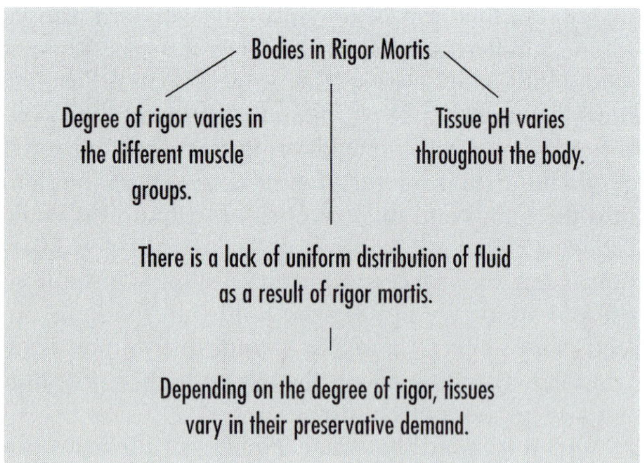

As the absorption of preservative results in firming, there is a relationship between the rate of preservative absorption by tissues and the rate of firming. This is why bodies embalmed prior to the onset of rigor rapidly firm; preservative is rapidly absorbed and rapidly attaches to the proteins. During rigor the proteins are "locked" together, and it is difficult for the preservative to attach to the proteins. As a result, there is little absorption of preservative by muscles in the state of rigor mortis. Most of the firming that occurs during the injection of a body in rigor is caused by the swelling of the tissues. If a mild or weak arterial solution is used, these tissues soften later. After the passage of rigor, demand for preservative increases greatly.

As well as a need to use strong solutions in the preparation of bodies in rigor, there is a need for a coinjection chemical. This chemical helps to adjust tissue pH as the various areas of the body are at different pH. The buffers in arterial fluids help to achieve the uniform pH necessary for the action of the preservative. It is easily seen that distribution is not uniform in these bodies, dyes are not evenly distributed, firming is not uniform, and the preservative needs of the tissues vary throughout the body.

PRESERVATIVE ABSORPTION AND FIRMING

Prerigor	Good absorption	Firming is good
Rigor	Little absorption	Firming is due to the rigor present and swelling
Postrigor	Great need for preservative	Firming is difficult to achieve

Firmness cannot be relied on as a test of preservation, for the firmness may be a result of the rigor present in the muscles. Firmness can also result from the distension of tissues during injection of arterial solution. In addition, if the embalmer attempted to relieve the rigor by manipulating the muscles, many capillary beds may have been torn, which would also account for the swelling of muscles and tissues during arterial injection. Tissues also swell because fluid follows the path(s) of least resistance. These paths lead to surface areas, as the deep muscle tissues, because of the rigor, resist the flow of fluid.

Causes of Swelling in Bodies in Rigor

1. Capillary beds are torn when muscles are flexed, bent, rotated, and massaged.
2. Fluid flows to surface areas because the deep muscles and tissue in rigor offer resistance to flow.
3. Drainage is limited because muscles in rigor exert pressure on veins.

▶ PREPARATION OF REFRIGERATED BODIES

Today, almost all bodies removed from hospitals and other institutions have been refrigerated for some period. It is difficult to set an exact length of time after which refrigeration would pose special problems for the embalmer. Up to approximately 6 hours after death, few problems should be encountered. The cool environment slows the progress of rigor mortis and decomposition. In addition, the cold environment helps to maintain blood in a liquid state. Because the blood remains liquid, livor mortis can be expected to be more intense.

There are three advantages of short-term refrigeration: (1) the rigor cycle is slowed, (2) the decomposition cycle is slowed, and (3) the low viscosity of the blood is maintained. Long-term refrigeration, however, can cause a number of problems for the embalmer.

For years, one effect of refrigeration has been a major subject of discussion—*dehydration;* however, this situation is gradually changing. When bodies were wrapped in cotton sheets and refrigerated, surface dehydration occurred easily. Lips and eyes soon showed the brown discolorations associated with drying of the tissues. The blood gradually thickened as the moisture was removed from the surface tissues. Movement of water out of the surface tissues forced the liquid portion of the blood into the dry tissues, causing a postmortem edema. Gradually, this moisture also worked itself to the skin surface. If the body were exposed to the cool, dry air for a sufficient period, the tissues mummified as a result of dehydration. Today, however, most bodies are wrapped in plastic, and many are also placed into large zippered plastic pouches. Dehydration is no longer a problem. The plastic wrapping does cause other problems for the embalmer. Plastic traps heat and moisture, and refrigerated bodies show signs of decomposition and skin-slip because of the moisture trapped on the skin.

There is usually a slight elevation of body temperature after death (postmortem caloricity) because metabolism continues until the oxygen trapped in the body is exhausted. As the blood no longer circulates, the heat produced by the catabolic phase of metabolism is trapped in the body. Therefore, the body temperature increases slightly. Heat speeds rigor mortis and decomposition as these are both chemical reactions. Because of this trapped heat, it is not unusual to find green discolorations on abdominal areas when the bodies are removed from refrigeration. Autolysis and bacterial activity continue while the body is in refrigeration, faster at first while the body is still warm and then slower as the tissues gradually cool.

Figure 19–2 illustrates some of the problems associated with refrigeration.

When bodies have been refrigerated for long periods and wrapped in plastic or placed in a plastic pouch, the embalmer can expect some of the following problems:

- Increased capillary permeability
- Easy rupture of the capillaries during arterial injection
- Tissue structure breakdown as a result of the slow, continuous processes of autolysis and bacterial enzymes
- Increased coagula in the vascular system
- Gravitation of blood and body liquids into the dependent body tissues, resulting in an increase in moisture in these tissues
- Intense livor mortis
- Rapid hemolysis resulting in postmortem extravascular stain
- Moist clammy tissues caused by the plastic wrapping of the surface tissues; possibly skin-slip
- Decomposition signs (e.g., abdominal discoloration, purge, and skin-slip)
- Rapid distension of abdominal organs during

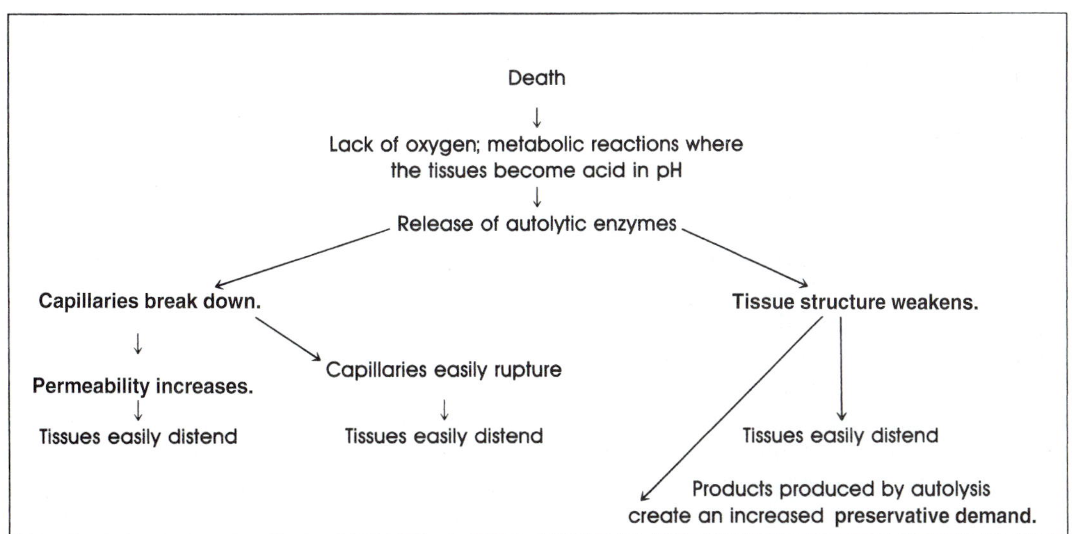

Figure 19–2. Problems associated with refrigeration: time–temperature effects.

injection, resulting in stomach and/or lung purge

Blood gravitates to dependent areas. As the body cools, hemolysis easily occurs, causing the blood cells to rupture and release **heme** into the tissues. This results in *postmortem staining*. This type of blood discoloration cannot be removed by arterial injection and blood drainage. If the head has not been raised, these discolorations may be present in the facial tissues. Some bleaching is possible with the use of a strong arterial solution, a bleaching coinjection fluid, and surface bleaches. This stain can, however, be lightened but *not* removed. Opaque cosmetics are needed to hide the discoloration.

If the body has been refrigerated for a long period and wrapped in cloth sheeting, dehydration will be a problem. The amount of moisture in the dependent tissues increases because of hypostasis of the blood and settling of the liquids in these areas. The upper areas of the body may be browned from dehydration. Of particular interest to the embalmer are the drying and browning of the lips, eyelids, fingers, and base of the nose. The cheeks and forehead may also exhibit the brown discoloration of dehydration. This discoloration cannot be removed by arterial injection. Opaque cosmetics are used to hide the discolorations. Loss of water also results in a loss of moisture from the blood vascular system. There will be increased numbers of coagula in the vascular system, making distribution of the arterial solution very difficult.

During refrigeration, the progress of rigor mortis slows, but still occurs. Rigor usually passes 36 to 72 hours after death. Because it is slowed by cooling, it may still be present in some muscles at the time of embalming. Decomposition is what breaks rigor, and it too is slowed in a body that is cooled.

Arterial Preparation

Swelling is not the only concern. The viscera can easily distend, which can lead to *purge*. There is an increased demand for preservative, as the processes of autolysis and decomposition slowly continue. If rigor is present there is additional need for stronger arterial solutions. Blood discolorations can be bleached with strong arterial solutions. Distribution may be difficult to achieve, so strong solutions would again be the best type. There is an increase in moisture in the dependent tissues and, thus, an increased demand for preservative.

As strong arterial solutions are necessary, the best vessels to use as a primary site of injection are both common carotid arteries (restricted cervical injection). Drainage may be difficult to establish because of large numbers of coagula; therefore, the right internal jugular vein would be the best choice for the primary drainage site. Multipoint injection should be used for arms and legs not receiving sufficient arterial solution. Injection should be slow to prevent abdominal distension and to keep arterial coagula from moving and blocking smaller arteries.

Because of tissue distension, it is not possible to use large volumes of a mild arterial solution. Use of limited quantities of a strong solution produces the best results. The volume of fluid, of course, is determined by the size of the body and the embalmer's satisfaction that the tissues have received sufficient preservative solution. Because such a variety of arterial chemicals are available, the best advice that can be given with respect to fluid dilution is to follow the instructions of the manufacturer. Some manufacturers recommend the use of a coinjection fluid. Others advise that when their arterial chemicals are used to make strong arterial solutions, no coinjection fluid be used (Figure 19–3).

Extra amounts of fluid dye should be used to trace the distribution of arterial fluid. When postmortem stain is present, the tissues can easily gray several hours after embalming. The dye helps to cover the gray discoloration produced when formaldehyde and hemoglobin combine. Most refrigerated bodies appear pink prior to embalming. This is caused by the hemolysis of red blood cells trapped in surface tissue capillaries. The tissues appear to be embalmed. In addition, the cold has a tendency to solidify the fatty tissues of the body, so the tissues may also feel embalmed.

Dependent areas of the trunk, buttocks, and shoulders that do not receive sufficient fluid can be treated by hypodermic injection. Cavity fluid can be injected (by infant trocar) into these areas through use of the embalming machine. These dependent areas are very moist and, thus, may be sites of bacterial activity. Thoroughly hypodermically inject these areas. Surface treatment is of little or no value in these high-moisture areas.

Cavity Embalming

If restricted cervical injection is used the cavities can be aspirated before the features are set and the head and facial tissues are embalmed. If purge develops during embalming of trunk areas, aspirating *before* setting of the features eliminates the need to reopen the mouth and remove *purge*. Cavity embalming should be thorough. A minimum of one bottle of concentrated cavity fluid should be injected into each major body cavity. Reaspiration is always advised. If any gases escape when the trocar button is removed for reaspiration, if the abdomen appears distended, or if the large surface veins of the neck appear distended, the cavities should also be reinjected with concentrated cavity fluid after reaspiration.

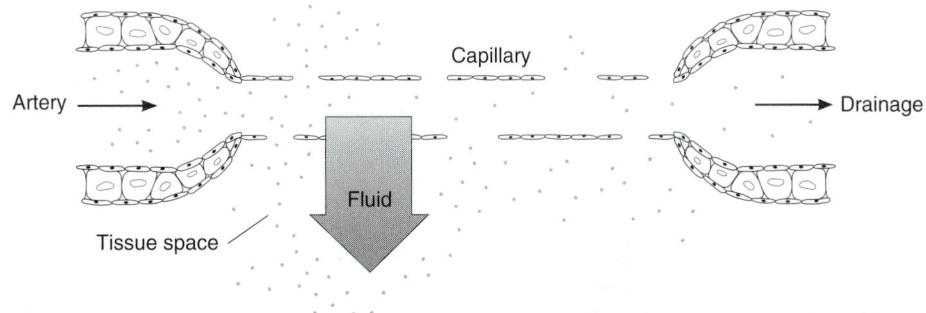

Figure 19–3. Refrigerated bodies and bodies in which decomposition has begun easily swell because of capillary breakdown and increased capillary permeability.

Cosmetic Treatment

Application of cosmetics may pose some problems if the tissues are still cold after arterial treatment. Condensation from the air is possible and the skin surface will feel moist to the touch. Cosmetic application may be delayed until the tissues have had time to warm and condensation has stopped.

Desquamation

Desquamation (skin-slip) has been mentioned several times as a problem in bodies that have undergone long refrigeration. Such bodies should be massaged carefully, for desquamation can easily be caused by the embalmer. Run as little water as possible over the skin of these bodies. Pat rather than rub the surface dry with toweling. Keep water from running over the skin surfaces during injection. Water should run along the sides of the table, not onto the skin surfaces.

Loose skin should be removed prior to embalming. Apply surface compresses of autopsy gel, cavity fluid, or surface embalming agents over these areas to help ensure preservation. After embalming remove the surface compresses and force the tissues to dehydrate with a hair dryer. If there is a sufficient delay between embalming and cosmetic application, enough air may pass over the body to dry the areas of nude skin. When skin-slip occurs on areas that will not be viewed, apply surface compresses and later plastic garments.

Frozen Tissues

Some refrigeration units may freeze body tissues. It is very important to remember that ice crystals form in these tissues. These crystals tear tissues. The body should not be warmed by pouring warm water over it. Allow the body to warm gradually by letting it sit in the preparation room for several hours. Manipulation of the tissues while ice crystals are still present will cause more tearing. Try to manipulate the body as little as possible.

Restricted cervical injection is vital. Some embalmers prefer to inject these bodies as soon as it is possible to raise an artery and a vein. There will be little or no blood drainage. A strong arterial solution should be used and injected very slowly. The blood acts as a vehicle for the arterial solution as it does in bodies from which blood is not drained. Some embalmers prefer to use a strong arterial solution prepared with warm to hot water.

The facial tissues will, no doubt, be thawed so a stronger-than-average solution can be used to inject the head. If the embalmer feels that distension of the face will be a problem, he should use the instant tissue fixation method of injection to achieve preservation of the face.

Additional fluid dyes should be used in embalming these bodies.

▶ PREPARATION OF BODIES THAT SHOW SIGNS OF DECOMPOSITION

Heat speeds chemical reactions. In the period between death and embalming, the cycles of rigor mortis and decomposition are speeded if the body is not cooled, but left in a warm environment. If the environment is warm and moist (conditions present during summer months), decomposition can be very rapid. After passage of rigor, tissues begin to break down, and many changes are noted (Figure 19–4).

Color Changes

Trunk Areas. The right quadrant of the abdomen turns green; in a short time, the outline of the large intestine can be identified by the green discoloration over the abdominal wall. Hydrogen sulfide produced in the colon after death reacts with hemoglobin breakdown products to produce the greenish discoloration seen in the bowel and the structures that contact the bowel. The color change proceeds up the anterior abdominal and thoracic walls to the neck and chin.

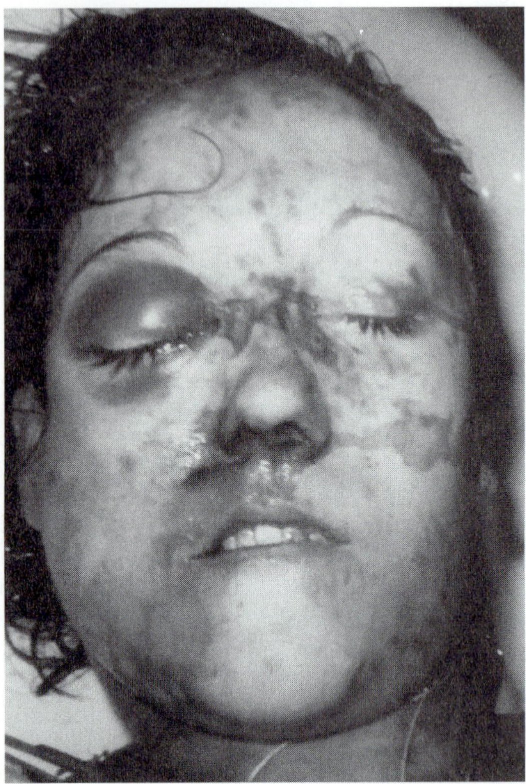

Figure 19–4. Early signs of decomposition (color changes, purge). Note ecchymosis of the right eyelid.

Vascular Changes. Early decomposition color changes can affect the small veins in almost any area of the body. The blood in these superficial vessels breaks down and the coloring matter of the hemoglobin makes the veins appear as brown lines over the surface of the skin.

Livor Mortis and Stain. Livor mortis is completely established in the dependent tissues of these bodies. Some of these purple discolorations clear during injection of the arterial solution. The majority, however, become postmortem stains. Stain develops as the hemoglobin breaks down (hemolysis) and allows the heme portion of the molecule to pass from the capillaries into the tissue spaces. This light red discoloration cannot be removed by arterial injection. At best it may be bleached, which will aid in the cosmetic treatment if the stain occurs in facial tissues or tissues of the back of the hand.

Odors

As autolysis and putrefaction occur, some products of protein breakdown emit very foul odors. Foul amines and mercaptans combine with ammonia and hydrogen sulfide to produce the odors of decomposition. Embalming converts the amines, mercaptans, and hydrogen sulfide to odorless methylol compounds. Formaldehyde converts ammonia to odorless hexamethylene. Nutrition, body weight, and presence of bacterial disease prior to death all contribute to the extent of these odors.

Purges

If gases have developed in the abdominal cavity and products of partial digestion were present in the stomach at the time of death, purge can be expected (Figure 19–5). Ruptured capillaries and congested lung passageways may also create a "lung" purge (i.e., pneumonia, tuberculosis, influenza). Abdominal pressures may also cause purging from the rectum through the anal orifice.

Gases

In some bodies, especially those in which bacterial activity increased after death, the tissues and cavities may contain gases. Conditions favoring gas formation are heat and humidity; those hindering formation are cold and dry environments. Gas can cause bloating and swelling of the body, protrusion of the tongue and eyes, and distension of the male genitalia. The pressure resulting from distension of the abdominal cavity creates lung, stomach, and anal purges.

Desquamation

The autolytic changes that begin immediately after death weaken the superficial layer of the skin. Gas can easily move into the weakened superficial tissues, resulting in blisters and separation of the skin layers. Fre-

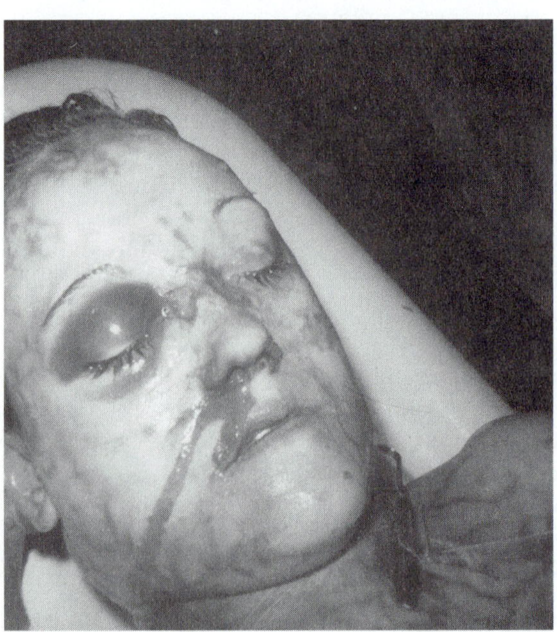

Figure 19–5. Early decomposition. Purge, discolorations, and distension from gases are evident.

quently, the embalmer encounters skin-slip when there are no gases in the tissues. Then, mere handling of the body causes the epidermis to loosen and separate.

Dehydration

Some of these bodies exhibit local dehydration in the fingers, lips, nose, eyelids, and ears.

Chemical Changes

Although not visible postmortem changes, important chemical changes occur in the tissues that the embalmer must be concerned about. Autolytic and proteolytic decomposition of the body proteins result in numerous nitrogenous products. These products greatly increase the preservative demand of the body. Their presence also shifts the body pH to alkaline (basic). Embalming solutions react best with proteins under slightly (not strong) alkaline pH conditions.

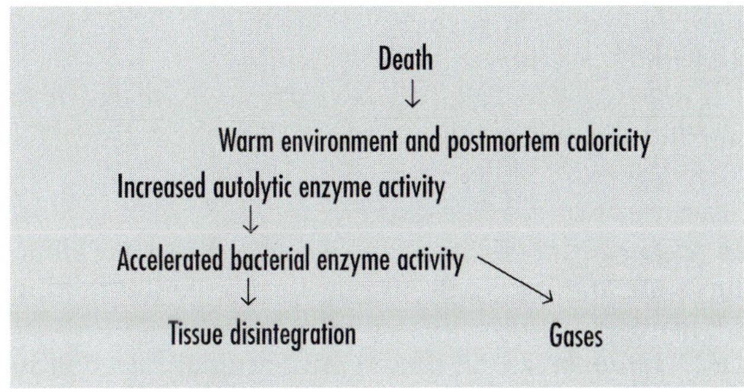

These classic signs of decomposition may also be accompanied by rigor mortis in some muscles. Rigor can be found in bodies that show early signs of decomposition in the hands, legs, and jaw muscles.

Embalming Protocol

The following factors concerning the body enter into a **preembalming analysis:** (1) general conditions of the body, (2) effects of disease on body tissues, (3) effects of drugs on body tissues, and (4) postmortem changes. The postmortem changes may be the most important factor in determining the embalming techniques to be used.

The protocols for embalming the bodies discussed in this chapter are similar, because all of these bodies have undergone a delay between death and preparation and all have a high preservative demand. Some of the complications encountered during embalming of the body with early signs of decomposition follow:

1. Fluid distribution is poor, because coagula are present in the arterial system.
2. Drainage is poor because blood elements have decomposed.
3. Tissues easily swell, because capillaries have broken down or are easily torn by the pressure of the fluid; tissue structure has been weakened by autolytic and putrefactive changes.
4. Ammonia and nitrogenous products in the tissues greatly increase the preservative demand.
5. Little or no firming is exhibited because of protein breakdown.

Maximum-strength fluid can be used to prepare these bodies—25 to 30 index or higher. For this type of body, maximum-strength arterial solutions are necessary. Supplemental chemicals can be used to increase the working ability of these arterial solutions. Again, follow the instructions of the manufacturer. The goal here is to use a minimum amount of a very strong arterial solution. **Do not preinject these bodies.** Only a strong arterial solution should be injected into the vascular system. Use additional fluid dye, because firming cannot be used to judge distribution or preservation. Remember, the dye only indicates the presence of fluid in the surface tissues.

Two protocols can be used for injection. Drainage can be taken from each injection site or from the right internal jugular vein. Little or no drainage can be expected from these bodies.

The purpose in using *injection protocol 1* is to minimize the number of arterial coagula that may move into the smaller arteries. Keep in mind that the aorta may contain a number of large coagula. If these coagula move, they will block small arteries.

1. Raise the right and left common carotid, right and left axillary (brachial), and right and left femoral (external iliac) arteries.
2. Inject the right femoral artery.
3. Inject the left femoral artery.
4. Inject the right axillary artery.
5. Inject the left axillary artery.
6. Inject the right common carotid artery through the tube directed toward the trunk. Be certain the left common carotid is tied off and a tube has been inserted and directed upward to the left side of the head; leave this tube open.
7. Aspirate the body after the trunk is injected.
8. Set the features.
9. Inject the left side of the head.
10. Inject the right side of the head.
11. Aspirate the cavities again and inject them with a suitable undiluted cavity chemical.
12. Evaluate the distribution of fluid and use hypodermic and surface embalming treatments where fluid has not been distributed.

Injection protocol 2 makes use of restricted cervical injection.

1. Raise the right and left common carotid arteries; drain from the right internal jugular vein.
2. Inject down the right common carotid to embalm the arms, legs, and trunk. The left common carotid should be tied off and a tube directed toward the head inserted; this tube should remain open.
3. Evaluate the distribution of arterial solution. Inject the arms and legs separately if these areas lack fluid.
4. Aspirate the body cavities.
5. Set the features.
6. Inject the left side of the head.
7. Inject the right side of the head.
8. Reaspirate the cavities and inject a suitable undiluted cavity chemical.
9. Evaluate the distribution of arterial solution and treat area needing fluid with hypodermic and surface embalming.

If the abdomen is distended tightly with gas prior to arterial injection, introduce a trocar into the abdominal cavity to relieve this pressure. The trocar should be kept just beneath the anterior wall. An attempt can be made to puncture the transverse colon and the distended stomach.

The trunk should be injected at a very slow rate of flow to prevent swelling of the abdominal viscera and purge. Limbs can be injected slowly at first, and then at a higher pressure and faster rate of flow to secure distribution. Pulsation is recommended. If desired, each extremity can also be injected by the instant tissue fixation method (100% arterial fluid injected in pulses under high pressure) or by using waterless embalming.

If sectional arterial embalming has produced unsatisfactory results, sectional hypodermic injection will be necessary. Undiluted arterial or cavity fluid may be injected by machine through an infant trocar. To inject the arms, insert the trocar into the area of the bend of the elbow; from this point the upper as well as the distal portion of the arm can be reached, possibly as far as the palm of the hand. To inject the legs, insert the trocar on the medial side of the leg either above or below the knee; from this point fluid can be injected as far as the buttocks and as far as the foot. An alternative point of entry is the base of the foot. From this point of entry, fluid could be injected as far as the knee. The trunk walls can be injected from points of entry on the lateral walls of the trunk at approximately the level of the midaxillary line. It may be necessary to insert the infant trocar into the upper shoulder area to inject the posterior portions of the back, shoulder, and neck. All of these points of entry can be closed with trocar buttons or, if necessary, sutured closed with a purse-string suture. Glue can be applied over the trocar button or suture to ensure against leakage. Fingers and the foot can be separately injected with a hypodermic syringe and a small gauge needle. The use of super adhesive helps to ensure against leakage from each point where the needle is inserted.

It is most important that these bodies be reaspirated several hours after embalming. Reinjection is strongly advised, especially if any gases are evident during the reaspiration. If desquamation is present, the loose skin should be removed at the beginning of the embalming. Surface compresses can be applied to help dry these areas. Air drying also helps to dry the raw skin after the compresses have been removed.

Plastic garments can be used, but embalming powder or moisture-absorbent kitty litter should be placed inside these garments. This powder produces some surface preservation but, more importantly, helps to control odors. Odors can be reduced by bathing the surface of the body with a solution prepared by mixing 2 pints of hydrogen peroxide with $\frac{1}{2}$ cup of baking soda and adding a tablespoon of liquid soap. This solution is left on the skin surface for several minutes before rinsing and drying.

Treatment of the Features

In preparing a body in which decomposition is evident, the embalmer may wish to vary the technique used to set features.

The man can be shaved after arterial injection to limit skin removal on the facial areas. Facial skin that appears easily removable can be painted with autopsy gel during embalming of the body, or the face can be covered with surface compresses of cavity fluid. Use shaving cream to lather the face. Avoid the use of warm water to soften the beard. A new, sharp razor blade makes the shaving much easier and puts less tension on the skin. Several blades may be needed to shave dense facial hair growth.

The mouth can be closed after arterial injection. As the lips and areas around the mouth may swell, it may be easier to obtain a proper closure after injection. Firming is not a problem in these bodies, because it is delayed. Also, if purge develops during arterial injection, the mouth can be properly dried and packed after cavity treatment.

The embalmer should evaluate the preservation of tissues surrounding the mouth. It may be necessary to place cotton in the mouth and saturate it with concentrated cavity fluid to help ensure preservation. Dehydration should not be a concern. The lips can be secured with a super adhesive.

Eyes can also be closed after arterial injection. In this way, the embalmer has an opportunity to observe if the eyelids have received sufficient fluid. Cotton can be used for closure, and this cotton can be saturated with some concentrated cavity fluid to help ensure preservation of the lids. Be very careful in handling the eyelids, because this skin is very easily removed. A super adhesive can be used to secure eye closure. Let the cavity fluid remain under the eyelids. It helps to secure preservation and to bleach the tissues. Dehydration is not a concern in the preparation of these bodies.

Areas of the face that appear not to have received sufficient arterial solution can be reached by hypodermic injection from inside the mouth. Cavity fluid should be used to treat these areas. Do not dilute the cavity fluid; use the concentrated fluid. Make all injections from inside the mouth, because cavity fluid, unlike tissue builder, has a tendency to leak from the tissues. This leakage occurs on the inside of the closed mouth. The sides of the nose can be reached as well as the cheeks and the lower eyelids from inside the mouth. A 19-gauge needle is excellent for this work.

In bodies dead for a long period, the submaxillary, sublingual, and parotid glands tend to swell during injection. If this happens, apply very firm digital pressure to these areas immediately after arterial injection. If the swelling is not reduced, make a flap incision at the base of the neck. Using an infant trocar as an operative aid, lance the glandular tissue several times and apply digital pressure again. If this treatment is unsuccessful, another operative correction—excision of the swollen tissues—may be necessary.

In bodies exhibiting decomposition, the tongue often protrudes and is swollen. Attempt to force the tongue back into the mouth by using firm digital pressure prior to arterial injection. The protruding tongue can be covered with a piece of cloth and firm pressure applied to the cloth. When teeth or dentures are present, try to force the tongue behind them and then secure the jaw shut. This helps to contain the tongue. Excision of the tongue should be a last resort.

Advanced Decomposition

There should be some preparation of the body in advanced stages of decomposition. If removing the body from a residence, use rubber gloves, masks, a plastic or rubber pouch, and disinfectant and deodorant sprays. In an emergency, wrap the body in a wool blanket to help absorb liquids and odors. These bodies should not be removed until they are placed in a zippered pouch. As much soiled clothing and bedding as possible should be removed from the residence and the family should be informed that these soiled articles will be destroyed.

If the embalmer thinks it is possible, raise and inject the right common carotid artery with about 1 gallon of undiluted high-index fluid. Coinjection fluids are made for such cases (decomposition, burns, etc.). One or two bottles of the coinjection fluid can be added to undiluted arterial fluid (at least 30 index). Some cavity fluids (undiluted) can be injected arterially in special situations. Do not attempt to drain.

The abdominal and thoracic cavities should be aspirated and filled with three or more bottles of undiluted cavity fluid. The extremities and trunk walls can be treated by hypodermic injection of undiluted cavity fluid by use of an infant trocar and the embalming machine. The primary purpose here is to diminish some of the odor and slow the progress of decomposition.

The body can be wrapped in one or more sheets and placed in a clean, zippered pouch. Before wrapping the blankets around the body, sprinkle embalming powder over the surface of the body. The entire body surface may also be painted with autopsy gel. Place the wrapped body in the pouch. If desired, saturate the sheets surrounding the body with cavity fluid or an external preservative solution. Any chemical used to saturate the sheeting should be concentrated and not diluted.

Before zippering the pouch, sprinkle additional embalming powder over the sheeting and the inside of the pouch. Placing moisture-absorbent kitty litter inside the pouch will assist in the control of odors. Some embalmers prefer to place a surface glue along the zipper of the pouch to help control the escape of any odors. A double pouch may be necessary to ensure that the odors are contained and the pouch does not rip when it is lifted. To prevent the pouch from tearing, place a sheet under it; the pouch can be lifted and moved with the sheet.

▶ KEY TERMS AND CONCEPTS FOR STUDY AND DISCUSSION

1. Define the following terms:
   autolysis
   decomposition
   dehydration
   desquamation
   postmortem stain
   purge
   restricted cervical injection
   rigor mortis
   special-purpose high-index fluid
   waterless embalming
2. List the postmortem chemical and physical changes.
3. Explain why restricted cervical injection should be used when strong arterial solutions are to be injected?

4. Describe the effects of rigor mortis on the embalming process.
5. Describe the postmortem pH changes in the unembalmed body.
6. Describe the effects of cooling on the body.

▶ BIBLIOGRAPHY

Boehringer PR. *Controlled Embalming of the Head.* Westport, CT: ESCO Tech Notes; Feb–March, 1969, No. 57.

Jones, H. A chemist looks at embalming problems. *Casket and Sunnyside,* May 1968.

Pervier NC. *A Textbook of Chemistry for Embalming.* Minneapolis: University of Minnesota; 1961.

Sanders CR. Refrigeration (Parts 1-2-3). *Dodge Magazine,* March/April/May 1987.

Slocum RE. *Pre-embalming Considerations.* Boston: Dodge Chemical Co.

Strub CG. Why bodies decay. *Casket and Sunnyside,* February/March 1959.

Weber DL. *Autopsy Pathology Procedure and Protocol.* Springfield, IL: Charles C Thomas; 1973:69–70

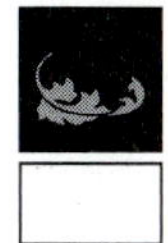

CHAPTER 20
DISCOLORATIONS

The embalmer soon learns that nearly every body embalmed today has some discolorations. They might be localized, such as an ecchymosis on the back of a hand, or generalized, such as a simple condition of livor mortis or as complex a condition as jaundice. Even intravenous lines begun when a body is received "DOA" (dead on arrival) at the emergency room in an attempt to resuscitate can create a postmortem bruise.

Discolorations are of utmost concern to the embalmer. These deviations from normal skin coloration may require a change in the embalming technique, the chemicals employed, and the cosmetic and restorative techniques. The embalmer should be able to identify any and all discolorations present on the body. Quite often, a family member asks questions concerning the antemortem discolorations and if they will be visible after the preparation. The embalmer should also recognize those discolorations that necessitate notification of the proper authorities if a doctor was not in attendance at the time of death or did not examine the body after death. The embalmer should be able to recognize the *cause* of a discoloration, know which *can* and *cannot* be cleared by arterial injection, know which can be altered or bleached by proper chemicals, and know which will have to be treated by opaque cosmetics to hide the discoloration.

FACTORS THAT MUST BE DETERMINED IN THE EMBALMING ANALYSIS

1. Vessels for injection and drainage
2. Strength of the embalming solution
3. Volume of the embalming solution
4. Injection pressure
5. Injection rate of flow

Note: These factors will vary by the individual body and can vary in different areas of the same body.

A discoloration is defined as any abnormal color in or on the skin of the human body. In embalming, discolorations are classified according to the time at which they appeared and the cause.

There are two classifications of discolorations by time of occurence: **antemortem** (before death) and **postmortem** (after death). A discoloration that was present during life and remains after death is classified as antemortem.

There are six classifications of discolorations by cause that the embalmer can identify:

1. Blood discolorations are discolorations resulting from changes in blood composition, content, and location. (Blood discolorations, in addition to being classified as antemortem or postmortem, are also classified as **intravascular** or **extravascular.**)
2. Drug or therapeutic discolorations are antemortem discolorations resulting from the administration of drugs or chemotherapeutic agents.
3. Pathological discolorations are antemortem discolorations that occur during the course of certain diseases.
4. Surface coloring agent discolorations are antemortem or postmortem discolorations that occur prior to (or during) embalming as the result of the deposit of matter on the body surface.
5. Reactions to embalming chemicals are postmortem discolorations present before embalming that become more intense, change in hue, or evolve as a result of the embalming.
6. Decomposition changes are postmortem discolorations brought about by the action of bacterial and/or autolytic enzymes on the body tissues.

The following charts summarize the classifications of the various discolorations. Examples are given for each category. Some brief explanation should be made regarding discolorations labeled as blood, pathological, and drug discolorations. Keep in mind the classification is by cause of the discoloration. Thus, "ecchymosis" is a blood discoloration if caused by trauma, is a pathological discoloration if it occurs during a disease, and is a drug discoloration when brought about by a drug. Jaundice can be classified as a drug or a pathological discoloration depending on its *cause.*

Classification of Discolorations According to Cause

1. Blood discolorations
   A. Intravascular
   B. Extravascular
2. Drug and therapeutic discolorations
3. Pathological discolorations
4. Surface coloring agent discolorations
5. Reactions to embalming chemicals on the body
6. Decomposition changes

Classification of Discolorations According to Time of Occurrence

1. Antemortem
   A. Blood discolorations
   B. Drug and therapeutic discolorations
   C. Pathological discolorations
   D. Surface coloring agent discolorations
2. Postmortem
   A. Blood discolorations
   B. Surface coloring agent discolorations
   C. Reactions to embalming chemicals on the body
   D. Decomposition discolorations

Examples of the various classifications follow.

I. Blood discolorations
   1. Antemortem blood discolorations
      A. Intravascular
         a. Hypostasis of blood (blue-black discoloration)
         b. Carbon monoxide poisoning (cherry red coloring)
         c. Capillary congestion (hypostatic, active or passive)
      B. Extravascular
         a. Ecchymosis: a large bruise caused by escape of blood into the tissues
         b. Purpura: flat medium-sized hemorrhage beneath the skin surface
         c. Petechia: small pinpoint skin hemorrhage
         d. Hematoma: swollen blood-filled area within the skin
   2. Postmortem blood discolorations
      A. Intravascular: livor mortis
      B. Extravascular: postmortem stain

II. Drug and therapeutic discolorations: There are many discolorations under this classification. Some are specific to a particular drug. Large amounts of drugs, in time, affect the vascular, renal and hepatic systems. Frequently, drug discolorations such as ecchymosis and purpura result from the breakdown of capillaries by the drugs. Often, the capillaries are fragile and bruising occurs easily. A second frequently encountered drug discoloration is jaundice, a result of the toxic effect of drugs on the liver. All drug discolorations are antemortem and are caused by specific drugs or combinations of drugs. These discolorations are very common. Usually, the arms are affected by hemorrhagic discolorations, and the entire body is affected by jaundice.

III. Pathological discolorations: These discolorations, all antemortem, are brought about by specific diseases.
   1. Gangrene
      A. Wet: infected tissues red to black in color
      B. Dry: caused by arterial insufficiency; a dark red-brown to black color

      When gangrene occurs in a facial area or affects the fingers, it becomes of cosmetic concern to the embalmer. Frostbite and diabetes can be responsible for this condition in the facial areas and hands. Arterial preservation is difficult to establish, and surface and hypodermic preservation are necessary.
   2. Jaundice: caused by many disease processes, for example, diseases of the liver, a bile problem, or a blood problem
   3. Specific diseases
      A. Addison's disease: a bronze discoloration produced in the skin
      B. Leukemia: petechiae
      C. Meningitis: rashes on the skin surface
      D. Tumors: discolorations in and around the tumor itself may be caused by pathological changes

   These are only some of the discolorations resulting from pathological disorders. Discolorations may also be brought about by a reaction to drugs or radiation therapy.

IV. Surface coloring agent discolorations: These may be antemortem or postmortem depending on when the agent was applied to the skin surface. Examples include blood, adhesive tape marks, gentian violet, paint, Mercurochrome, mold, and tobacco tars. This list could be more extensive as the embalmer encounters many surface discolorations. Most can easily be removed with soap and water or with a solvent such as the dry hair washes and trichloroethylene.

V. Reactions to embalming chemicals: These are postmortem discolorations that occur before, during, or after embalming of the body. Examples are razor burns, dehydration of tissues, formaldehyde gray, and conversion of yellow to green jaundice.

VI. Decomposition discolorations: These postmortem color changes occur during decomposition and may be yellow, green, or blue-black to black. Examples are progressive skin color changes and mottling of the veins on the skin surface.

▶ GENERAL TREATMENT OF BLOOD DISCOLORATIONS

Intravascular Blood Discolorations

Intravascular blood discolorations respond best to arterial injection and blood drainage. These discolorations include antemortem hypostais, cyanosis, carbon monoxide poisoning, capillary congestion, and livor mortis. A preinjection fluid can be used to flush the vascular system if the body has been dead a short period and the embalmer feels distribution and drainage will be good. A mild arterial solution could also be used as a beginning injection in an attempt to flush the vascular system of the discoloration.

Very strong solutions should be avoided, as they may convert an intravascular discoloration into an extravascular stain. Many of the high-index arterial fluids today promote distribution and drainage without creating postmortem stains. Concurrent drainage also promotes clearing of the intravascular discolorations. Intravascular blood discolorations can be gravitated from visible areas by elevation of the face, neck, and hands. Massage may also be helpful in removal of intravascular discolorations. Once surface discolorations have cleared, intermittent drainage may be the preferred method for effecting the best diffusion of the embalming chemical.

If these intravascular discolorations are localized, such as in the legs, arms, or side of the face, and do not respond to injection and drainage, then local injection may be necessary to clear the discoloration. In essence, failure of the discoloration to clear is a very good sign that fluid has not entered the area. Therefore, selection and injection of an artery closest to the discoloration may be necessary. If a condition such as arteriosclerosis exists in the femoral arteries and the discoloration in the legs does not clear, use of the femoral or external iliac arteries may be impractical for arterial injection. Hypodermic and surface embalming of the legs is then necessary (Table 20–1).

Livor mortis is a postmortem intravascular blood discoloration. It is also a postmortem physical change, a discoloration brought about by the gravitation of blood into the dependent capillaries (Fig. 20–1). It is first observed approximately 20 to 30 minutes after death and is well established by the sixth hour after death. Refrigeration and drugs such as blood thinners speed the onset and increase in intensity of livor mortis. If the darkened area is pushed on and the area clears, this is an indication that the discoloration is intravascular. Livor mortis can be gravitated. If a body is laid on a flat surface, the heart is slightly higher than the head. Blood, thus, has a tendency to gravitate into the facial and neck tissues.

The head and shoulders should always be elevated to help drain blood from these upper tissues. While the body is shaved, the face and hair washed, and the features set, most of the blood gravitates from facial and neck tissues if the shoulders and head have been elevated. If the discoloration does not clear, this may be an indication that there is blockage (e.g., a coagulum) in the right atrium of the heart or in the right or left internal jugular veins. The best vessels for injection and drainage of this body would be the right and left common carotid arteries and the right internal jugular vein. The internal jugular allows access to the right atrium of the heart. Any coagula present can be removed with an angular spring forceps.

Preinjection fluids were developed to help clear blood discolorations such as livor mortis. If the body has not been dead very long, the embalmer may wish to inject a preinjection fluid solution. A large enough volume of solution should be injected to clear the livor mortis. If a preinjection fluid is not used, a mild arterial solution may be used to clear the blood discolorations. Subsequent injections can be stronger. This method helps to prevent setting of the livor mortis as a stain. Most of the fluids manufactured today are of such a nature that strong solutions can be injected and the fluid will clear the blood discolorations without setting the livor mortis as a stain. Many of these fluids are labeled "reaction controlled fluids," meaning that they are able to be distributed throughout the body and diffuse into the tissue spaces before the chemical reaction with the proteins of the body. *Note:* In attempting to clear livor mortis, the drainage used should be concurrent (or continuous) until the livor has cleared. Then, intermittent or alternate methods of drainage can be employed.

Livor mortis can also be an advantage for the embalmer. The breaking and clearing of the livor mortis indicates that fluid has been distributed into those tissues. Most bodies exhibit some degree of livor mortis. Some, however, are quite dramatic and the face may be almost blue-black. Elevation, continuous drainage, use of the internal jugular veins for drainage, and a mild arterial solution all help to clear the discoloration of livor mortis.

In making an embalming analysis, the nail beds should be observed for livor. This is especially important in the embalming of African-Americans in whom the livor in the skin tissues is not always evident.

TABLE 20–1. EMBALMING CONSIDERATIONS AND BLOOD DISCOLORATIONS

Antemortem Hypostasis	Postmortem Hypostasis	Time →	Livor Mortis	Time →	Postmortem Stain	Time →	Formaldehyde Gray
Occurs prior to death or during the agonal period	Begins at death		Seen as soon as blood fills superficial vessels; begins approx 20 minutes after death; depends on postmortem/antemortem hypostasis		Normally occurs about 6 hours after death; rate varies with cause of death and blood chemistry		Occurs after embalming
Intravascular	Intravascular		Intravascular		Extravascular		Intravascular or extravascular
Movement of blood to dependent tissues	Movement of blood to dependent tissues		Postmortem blood discoloration as a result of postmortem/antemortem hypostasis		Postmortem blood discoloration as a result of hemolysis		Embalming discoloration
Antemortem physical change	Postmortem physical change		Postmortem physical change		Postmortem chemical change		—
	Speed depends on blood viscosity		Color varies with blood volume and viscosity and amount of O_2 in blood		May occur prior to, during or after arterial injection		Seen after arterial injection
Antemortem	Postmortem		Postmortem		Postmortem		Postmortem
—	—		Clears when pressed on		Does *not* clear when pressed on		Seen as a gray stain
—	—		Removed by blood drainage		Not removed by blood drainage		Methemoglobin (HCHO & blood)
—	Arterial injection stops progress		Arterial injection (mild) clears with drainage		Strong solutions bleach and "set" livor as stain		—
—	Speeded by cooling of body, low blood viscosity		Speeded by cooling, blood "thinners," low blood viscosity, CO deaths		Speeded by cooling, rapid red blood cell hemolysis, CO deaths		Speeded by poor drainage, small amount of arterial fluid Vascular system not well cleared of blood.

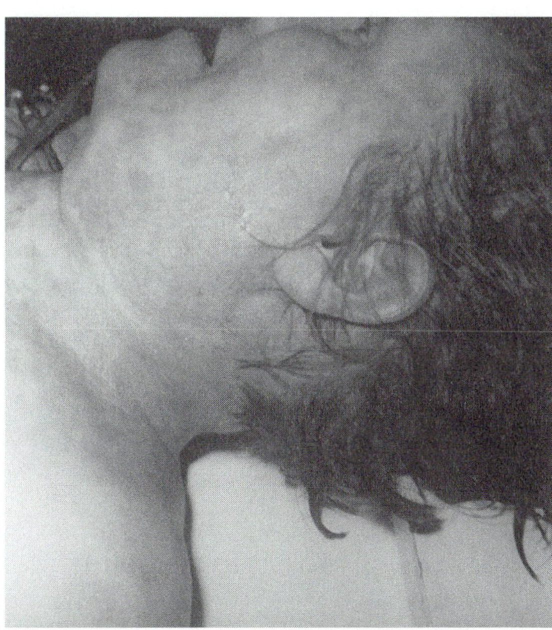

Figure 20–1. Livor mortis of the facial tissues, ear, and neck.

Clearing of the nail beds indicates distribution of the fluid.

Areas such as the trunk and buttocks where livor does not clear should be treated hypodermically to ensure preservation. When livor does not clear from the limbs or head, arteries should be raised and sectional embalming performed.

Antemortem as well as postmortem intravascular discoloration should respond to arterial injection and subsequent blood drainage.

Carbon monoxide discolorations are antemortem blood discolorations classified as intravascular and, thus, should be cleared by arterial injection. Remember, however, that many times there is a delay between death and preparation. The body might not be found for a while or the death must be investigated by the coroner or medical examiner. Quite frequently the *intra*vascular condition becomes an *extra*vascular condition because of the delay. The blood in these bodies rapidly breaks down allowing for hemolysis and staining of the tissues. The embalming is routine, but the bright discoloration may not clear. Care should be taken to use a dye with the arterial solution to be certain of the distribution of the arterial fluid.

To summarize, the embalmer must consider several factors in embalming the body with livor mortis:

1. It is a postmortem physical change.
2. It appears in dependent tissues.
3. It is speeded by refrigeration and blood thinners, carbon monoxide deaths, low blood viscosity, and large blood volume.
4. Sometimes it begins even before death and is seen rapidly after death.
5. It is an intravascular condition.
6. It may be cleared by arterial injection and blood drainage.
7. It may be gravitated and massaged from a body region.
8. Color varies from light pink to almost black depending on blood volume and viscosity.
9. When pushed on (or palpated), tissues clear.
10. It is cleared best by the use of mild arterial solutions or preinjection solutions.

Extravascular Blood Discolorations

Extravascular blood discolorations do not respond well to arterial treatment. Examples of these discolorations are ecchymosis, purpura, petechia, hematoma, and postmortem stain. Specific treatments for ecchymosis, hematoma, and postmortem stain are discussed later. Injection of a stronger arterial solution assists in bleaching some of these discolorations. Keep in mind that livor mortis and postmortem stain can both be present in a dependent area. The livor might be "washed out" but the stain remains. The stronger solution helps to bleach and to preserve these affected areas. Local treatment such as surface compresses and hypodermic treatment are frequently needed. No preinjection, coinjection, or "special arterial" fluids can completely remove these extravascular discolorations. Some may be lightened by the bleaching action of these fluids.

Ecchymosis, purpura, and petechia are all extravascular. They are classified as blood discolorations but can also be classified as pathological and drug discolorations, for they can be *caused* by diseases as well as by extended use of many drugs. A good example of both is the ecchymosis caused by use of the drug thinner coumadin. The disease leukemia produces hemorrhagic petechiae on the body surface. The treatment of these extravascular conditions can involve all three types of embalming: arterial, hypodermic, and surface.

Compared with ecchymoses, purpura and petechiae are smaller discolorations, and very frequently, simple arterial embalming satisfactorily bleaches and preserves these discolorations. Ecchymoses are of concern when they occur in a visible area such as on the face or the back of the hands, the most frequently seen areas. If the ecchymosis was caused by a needle puncture, the area may distend during arterial injection (Figure 20–2A).

Let us assume that a large ecchymosis on the back of the hand was caused by a hypodermic puncture (Fig. 20–2B). Three things can happen during arterial injection of this body: (1) Arterial solution will perfuse the area, there will be little distension, and the area will be well preserved and may even bleach a little.

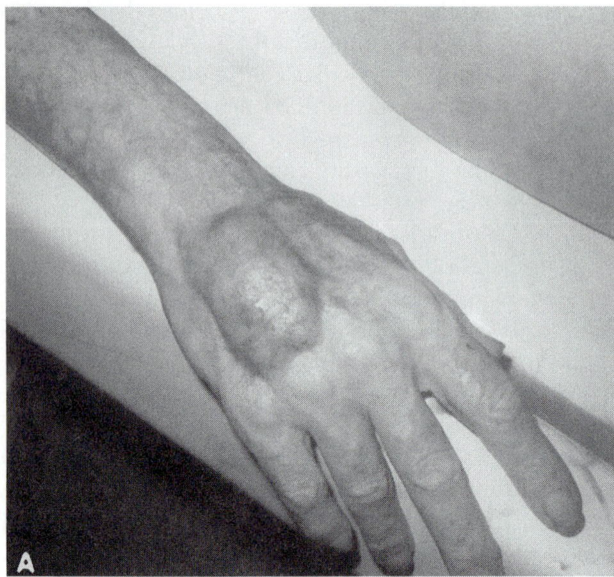

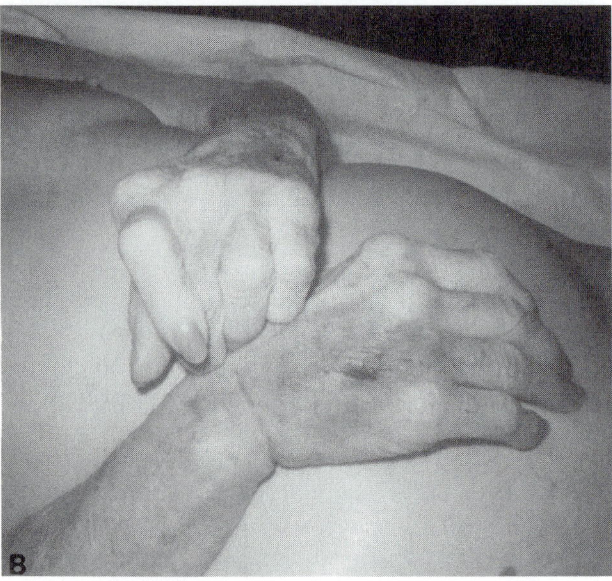

Figure 20–2. A. Swelling of an ecchymotic area during arterial injection. **B.** Large ecchymosis caused by intravenous needles. Application of super glue after embalming can easily prevent leakage.

(2) The area will distend, oftentimes very dramatically. (3) Nothing will happen. The area will not receive arterial solution. It will be neither preserved nor bleached. The ecchymosis must now be treated by hypodermic or surface embalming, or both.

Hypodermic Treatment (After Arterial Injection). Two chemicals can be used: a phenol cautery solution or formaldehyde (a cavity fluid). The phenol solution is a better bleaching agent. It also works much faster and cauterizes as well as preserves and disinfects the area.

1. Insert a hypodermic needle between the fingers.
2. Repeatedly push the needle through the discolored tissues prior to injecting any of the solution.
3. Inject the solution and massage the area to uniformly distribute the chemical beneath the skin.
4. Some of the chemical will leak out of the points of entry between fingers; some may also exit from the needle puncture on the back of the hand.
5. Let the chemical remain for 15 to 20 minutes. Then, massage as much of the chemical as possible through the punctures in item 4.
6. Seal the needle punctures with a drop of super adhesive.

Surface Embalming. In addition to formaldehyde and phenol solution, a variety of surface preservatives are available. The autopsy gels are quite popular for surface embalming. Surface treatments can be done before, during, or after arterial injection.

1. Coat the surface of the ecchymosis with autopsy gel. Or, saturate cotton compresses with the preservative chemical and apply the cotton packs to the ecchymosis.
2. Cover the cotton compresses with plastic. This helps to decrease odors and prevent dehydration of the chemical.
3. Allow sufficient time for these chemicals to penetrate and preserve the ecchymotic tissues. Several hours will, no doubt, be required. Keep in mind that phenol solutions work very fast. Autopsy gels have a good penetrating ability.
4. Later, remove the surface compresses. Clean the area with a solvent and dry the tissues.
5. If a puncture to the skin is present (i.e., from an intravenous line), the puncture can be sealed with a drop of super adhesive.

Ecchymosis or Hematoma of the Eye. In treating an ecchymosis or hematoma of the eye (Figure 20–3), commonly known as a "black eye," it is wise to raise and separately inject both the left and the right common carotid arteries. A stronger solution can be employed and the embalmer can control the amount of solution entering the head. The solution that is injected will be strong, so a smaller volume can be used in the event that the eye (or eyes) begin to distend. Do not inject the head of these bodies with a preinjection fluid.

In addition to surface embalming or hypodermic treatment of the eyes, a preservative such as cavity fluid can simply be placed underneath the eyelid. Use cotton to close the eyes. Place a few drops of cavity fluid on the cotton, then glue the eyes closed. This acts as a com-

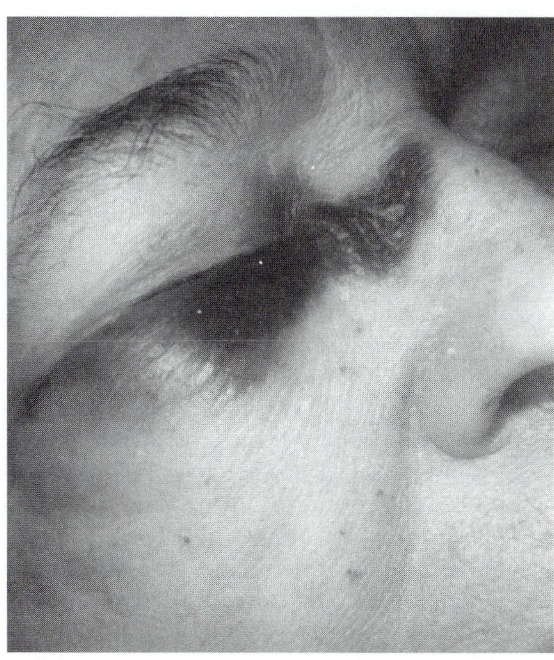

Figure 20–3. Ecchymosis or hematoma of the right eye.

press under the eyelids and assists in preserving the tissues and bleaching some of the discoloration. This method is also good for routine embalming when the embalmer feels the eyelids have not received enough preservative. The eyes can be glued and dehydration need not be a concern. The important factor is preservation. Cavity fluid does not contain dye; over time, fluids with dyes could stain the tissues.

Another approach can be taken to the treatment of swollen black eyes. Inject the tissues around the eyes and the lids with a phenol cautery chemical prior to arterial injection. Wait about 20 minutes for the chemical to cauterize the tissues; then proceed with the arterial injection. This method cauterizes the tissues and does not permit arterial solution to flow into the area. Many phenol chemicals are accompanied by specific directions for their use. Follow the time periods set by the manufacturer. A post-embalming operative correction may be needed to directly incise or puncture and channel the swollen discolored eyelids. This can be done under the eyelids. It will allow a direct outflow of the extravasated blood and accumulated serum.

Postmortem Stain. Postmortem stain, an extravascular blood discoloration, occurs in tissues where livor mortis was present or in surface tissues from which blood could not be drained. With postmortem stain, a period has elapsed between death and embalming. Actually, postmortem stain indicates decomposition or breakdown of the red blood cells. The coloring matter (heme) has moved through the capillaries and into the tissue spaces. Often, postmortem stain occurs with livor mortis in the same tissue regions. When pushed on (or palpated), the skin does not clear.

When embalming bodies with stain, use stronger solutions than used for routine preparation. Keep in mind that stain indicates that the blood has begun to break down. Expect poor distribution of fluid, a tendency for the capillaries to be broken down, and a tendency for the tissues to distend on injection. Thus, the embalming solution used should be of sufficient strength so that a minimum volume effects preservation but at the same time minimizes distension.

Some dye should be added to this solution, because when formaldehyde and the coloring portion of the blood mix to produce a gray hue, the extra dye not only indicates surface distribution of the fluid but also acts to counterstain the adverse discoloration.

Avoid using preinjection solutions in the preparation of these bodies. Bodies dead for long periods require strong, well-coordinated solutions. A preinjection treatment would only fill the vascular system with a weak and often nonpreservative solution and possibly cause distension.

Several factors must be taken into consideration with respect to embalming the body with postmortem stain:

1. A number of hours (approximately 6 or more) have elapsed since death.
2. It is speeded by refrigeration and carbon monoxide death.
3. Pressed on skin does not clear.
4. It is extravascular.
5. It cannot be removed by arterial injection and blood drainage.
6. It is a postmortem chemical change.
7. It is caused by hemolysis and is not blood in the tissues.

▶ TREATMENT OF JAUNDICE

There are three general types of jaundice: toxic jaundice, hemolytic jaundice, and obstructive jaundice. Within each category are a large number of diseases that bring about the antemortem discoloration.

Healthy human blood serum contains approximately 1.0 to 1.5 milligrams of the bile pigment bilirubin (which is yellow in color) per 100 milliliters as a result of the breakdown of red blood cells. Most red blood cells live about 120 days. Because of a variety of diseases that result in *hepatic failure, excessive blood hemolysis,* or *obstruction of the contents of the gallbladder,* the level of bilirubin reaches above 1.5 milligrams per 100 milliliters of blood serum and the tissues of the body

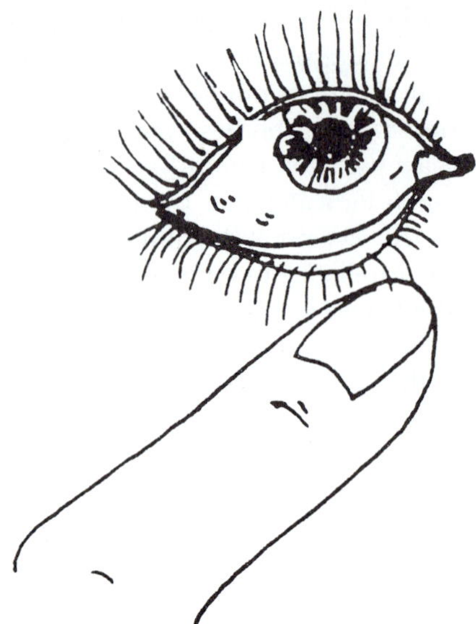

Figure 20–4. Yellow or mild jaundice is often first detected in the sclera (white) of the eye.

begin to take on the yellow jaundiced condition (Figure 20–4).

In embalming, yellow jaundice (bilirubin) can be converted to green jaundice (biliverdin) by the use of strong arterial solutions. The following statement by Mr. Lee Rendon for Champion Chemical Company points out what is thought to be the actual cause of this conversion. Remember that formaldehyde is a chemical *reducing agent* and the conversion of yellow jaundice to green jaundice is an *oxidation* chemical reaction.

> When aldehydes react with proteins, one of the chemical reactions that occurs is said to be that of release of hydrogen ions which, of course, results in a low pH (acid) that is acid in nature. A given amount of formaldehyde or aldehyde can unite with a given amount of protein to form a given aldehyde condensation resin (fixed protein). Once the proteins have received the necessary amount of aldehyde to form these condensation resins, any excess aldehyde tends to become more acid in character and, therefore, causes oxidation changes. From another point of view, aldehydes, in combining with protein or amino acid, increase the local acidity in the tissues by proton release. The hydrogen (H^+) ions which produce the acid condition result from the chemical action between aldehyde and protein. This acid medium, in turn, results in oxidation changes. The yellow (bilirubin) is converted to green (biliverdin). *It is not the formaldehyde* which causes the oxidation (formaldehyde is a reducing agent). It is the chemical reaction (oxidation) as a result of the acid present.

Five methods for treatment of the jaundiced body are discussed in this chapter. Each method employs a different chemical. Many funeral homes do not stock all of the chemicals discussed; however, every embalmer should have at his or her disposal the proper chemicals to clear the mild jaundiced condition.

Each method is based on the assumption that the embalmer uses a small amount of formaldehyde so that yellow jaundice is not converted to green jaundice. *These treatments work best on the body with a mild jaundice.*

As the primary concern of the embalmer in the preparation of the jaundiced body is the clearing of the discoloration present in the face and hands, the preparation of these bodies could entail restricted cervical injection, wherein both common carotid arteries are raised and remain open during injection of the lower body. Then the head is treated separately, much the same as in the autopsied body. Therefore, the embalming solution intended to clear the jaundiced discoloration would be needed only for injection of the head. The embalmer should remember this point when she or he encounters a jaundiced body in which preservation may be a problem. A different, much stronger arterial solution can then be used to inject the trunk region than would be used for the head.

In the embalming of all jaundiced bodies, preservation takes precedence over clearing of the discoloration.

Method 1: Use of a Jaundice Fluid

Almost every chemical manufacturer produces a jaundice fluid. Most of these fluids are very low in formaldehyde. Some even substitute other preservatives for formaldehyde. For the most part, these fluids are not strong preservatives. Therefore, always follow dilutions recommended by the fluid company. Also, inject the volume of fluid (as minimum) recommended in the instructions.

When in doubt about preservation, reinject the body with a stronger preservative solution of standard embalming fluid. Most jaundice fluids contain a large amount of dye and companies recommend that additional dye be added. The dyes not only indicate to the embalmer where the fluid has distributed, but even more important, they serve to counterstain the jaundice and, thus, cover the discoloration.

Method 2: Use of a Preinjection Solution

In the treatment of mild jaundice a preinjection fluid can be injected prior to the arterial preservative. The theory here is to wash out as much of the discoloration as possible. Enough preinjection fluid should be used to thoroughly rid the body of as much blood as possible. After the preinjection solution has remained in the body for a short period, inject a mild arterial solution containing dye. Again, sufficient volume should be injected to satisfy the preservative demands of the body. Dye can be added to the preinjection solution.

Method 3: Use of Mild Arterial Solution

If preinjection fluids are not used and jaundice fluids not purchased, treat the body by injecting a mild arterial solution and adding extra dye to the solution. Run enough solution to satisfy the preservative demands of the body.

Method 4: Use of Cavity Fluids as Arterial Fuids

Some manufacturers state on the labels of their cavity fluids that they may be used as arterial fluids for specific treatments. One of these treatments is the embalming of jaundiced bodies. It is the bleaching chemicals in the cavity chemical that clear the jaundice. Also keep in mind that many cavity fluids are not of high index, so their formaldehyde content is not high. Again, dye should be added to these arterial solutions.

Method 5: Use of Bleaching Coinjection Solutions

Instructions for several coinjection fluids state that they may be used for the treatment of bodies with extravascular discolorations such as postmortem stain, ecchymosis, gangrene, and jaundice. It is the bleaching property of this fluid that acts on these discolorations. The fluid is injected along with a preservative arterial solution. Dilutions are indicated on the labels of these coinjection fluids. They tend to work best on *mild jaundice*. They lighten the dark jaundice but the remaining discoloration must be covered with opaque cosmetics.

In conclusion, it is most important to again state that above all, preservation is most important in the preparation of a jaundiced body. These bodies can always be treated with opaque cosmetics to successfully hide the discoloration. A good foundation even for cosmetic treatment is good preservation.

▶ TREATMENT OF THE PATHOLOGICAL DISCOLORATION OF NEPHRITIS

One of the signs of chronic renal failure is a "sallow yellow color" to the skin resulting from the presence of urochrome in the tissues. This antemortem pathological discoloration takes on the appearance of mild jaundice. Remember that in chronic renal failure, urea in the blood system is converted to ammonia. Ammonia in the tissues and the blood acts to neutralize formaldehyde. The discoloration is generally treated easily by adding additional dye to the arterial solution. Treatment of bodies with renal failure requires strong arterial solutions to establish firming and good preservation.

Chronic renal failure often accompanies diabetes mellitus. One of the major problems for the embalmer in the preparation of bodies with diabetes mellitus is poor peripheral circulation. Again, this calls for stronger arterial solutions with a good coinjection fluid to help increase distribution and diffusion of the chemical. In many of these bodies gangrene has already been established in the lower limbs. A good dye is recommended to indicate fluid distribution.

Should a preinjection solution be used to rid the blood vascular system of the nitrogenous wastes prior to injection of the preservative arterial solution? Here, the embalmer needs to use extreme caution. When it is felt that the circulation and drainage will be good, this preinjection treatment can be used. If, however, there is evidence of poor circulation and drainage may be difficult to establish (if the body has been dead for a long period, gangrene is present, or there is heavy clotting and ischemic necrosis is present), avoid the preinjection treatment and employ a good strong arterial solution, possibly using a coinjection fluid to assist in distribution and diffusion of the preservative.

▶ TREATMENT OF SURFACE DISCOLORATIONS

Surface discolorations may be antemortem or postmortem. They result from the application of some product (e.g., antiseptic such as betadine) to the skin. They can also be the result of a stain applied for surgical or treatment purposes (e.g., gentian violet is used to mark an area where radiation treatment is to be applied), simple discolorations such as marks made after adhesive tape is pulled away, paint, and tobacco stains on the hands.

Blood is, no doubt, one of the most common discolorations and it can be treated very simply by washing the skin surface with cold water. A mild liquid soap is also of help, and an abrasive cloth such as cheesecloth or a gauze pad assists in the removal of dried blood.

Most of the discolorations described above (gentian violet, adhesive tape, surface antiseptics, etc.) respond well to a cleaning with the "dry" hair wash solvents or trichloroethylene (a dry cleaning solvent). Mold, which may occur when the body has been stored for a time, should be scraped away and the area swabbed with a 1% phenol, 1% creosote solution or a mixture of half methyl alcohol and half acetic acid. The majority of surface discolorations respond very well to cleaning with cool water and liquid soap or a mortuary solvent such as the "dry" hair washes.

Surface discolorations should be cleaned away prior to arterial injection. The pores of the skin are easier to clean at this time. After arterial injection the pores close and it is more difficult to completely clean off the discoloration. A second reason is that the embalmer must see the skin to evaluate if arterial solution is present in a particular location. For example, cleaning blood, dirt, and grease from the fingers prior to embalming allows the embalmer to observe the presence of livor mortis in the nail beds. During arterial injection the embalmer can then observe the clearing of the nail beds and the replacement of the livor by the dye of the arterial solution.

▶ TREATMENT OF DISCOLORATIONS RESULTING FROM EMBALMING

Postmortem embalming discolorations and abrasions include dehydration, green jaundice, formaldehyde gray, flushing, razor abrasion, and postmortem bruising. Each should be discussed, because many of these arise as a result of the embalming treatment. A discoloration present prior to embalming, such as yellow jaundice, may be intensified by the embalming. In this case the yellow jaundice is converted to green jaundice.

Dehydration

Dehydration is a drying of the skin. The classic colors of this discoloration are yellow, brown, and black. There are a variety of reasons the dead human body becomes dehydrated. Use of too much and too strong a fluid through a particular area is one reason. Dehydration can also be the result of loss of the superficial layer of skin (e.g., abrasion) or the drying of cut edges of skin (e.g., laceration). Remember that this discoloration cannot be bleached and usually progressively darkens. The application of opaque cosmetics is the best treatment for this discoloration. The embalmer must be able to distinguish this darkening of the tissues from a similar darkening caused by decomposition. Dehydrated skin areas are generally very hard to the touch, whereas a skin area that has decomposed is generally very soft and on touching, skin-slip may be evidenced (Figure 20–5).

Dehydration of the fingers should be mentioned. This condition is frequently seen when the body has been shipped from another location. If strong dehydration chemicals were employed, the ends of the fingers may have wrinkled and darkened because of dehydration. To prevent this from happening, a small amount of tissue builder can be injected into each finger at the conclusion of the embalming. Another area of the hand that frequently darkens as a result of dehydration brought about by the embalming is the tissue between the thumb and the index finger. Again, filling out this area with some tissue builder after arterial injection will hide the discoloration. The arterial solution may also bring about a loss of moisture from the lips. Wrinkling and, possibly, separation can occur. Tissue builder (after arterial injection) can be injected, from the end of each mucous membrane, to round out the lips and restore their natural fullness.

Many embalmers add a humectant coinjection fluid to the arterial solution for the purpose of adding

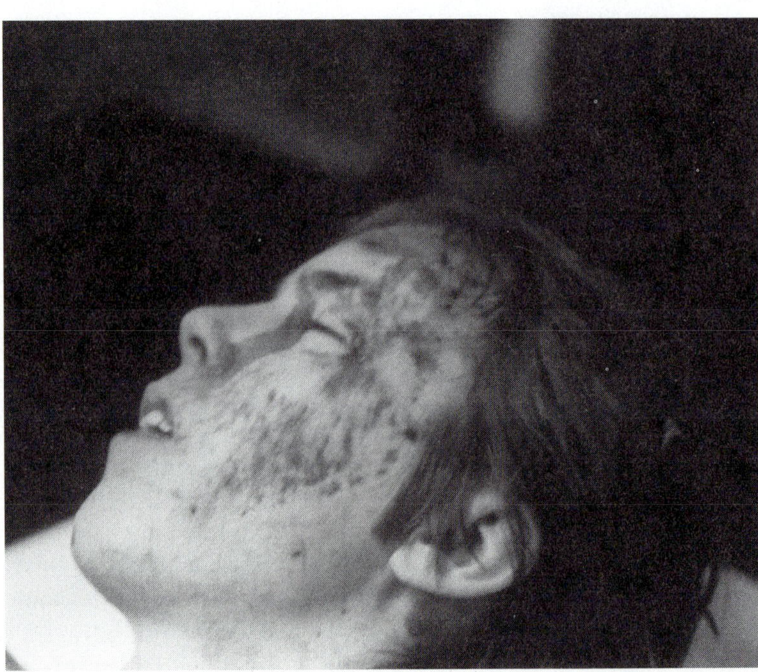

Figure 20–5. Abraded tissues and small lacerations of the left side of the face.

(or retaining) moisture in the tissues of the body. When using a humectant, however, the embalmer should carefully follow the instructions of the manufacturer, because adding this viscous fluid changes the osmotic balance of the arterial solution. The humectant adds large colloid molecules to the solution. Now, the osmotic pressure of the solution can be reversed and can pull the moisture out of the tissues and into the blood drainage. Only a small amount of humectant coinjection should be used and intermittent or alternate drainage employed.

Green Jaundice

The second embalming discoloration is the conversion of yellow jaundice to green jaundice. Refer to the section of this chapter on the embalming of jaundiced bodies. This conversion of bilirubin to biliverdin is an oxidation reaction. Formaldehyde, being a strong reducing agent, is only indirectly the cause of this reaction. The excessive use of formaldehyde is the cause. This gradually brings about an acid condition in the tissues, and it is the acid condition that converts the yellow jaundice to green jaundice. The most important point is the *preservation* of the body. This is more important than clearing the yellow jaundice. Treatment can be accomplished by the use of dye in the embalming solution. If this fails to cover the jaundice condition, an opaque cosmetic treatment will be necessary.

Embalmer's (Formaldehyde) Gray

Embalmer's gray, a graying of the tissues, can be seen about 6 hours after embalming. In essence, it is due to failure of the embalmer to wash as much of the blood out of the body as possible. The remaining blood gravitates and mixes with the preservation fluids in the tissues, and the resulting color is a dark gray. This condition can be avoided by the injection of a large volume of arterial solution accompanied by thorough drainage and complete aspiration of the heart. Be certain the head and shoulders of the embalmed body are kept elevated. This elevation prevents blood present in the heart after embalming from moving into the facial and neck tissues, and, thus, prevents embalmer's gray. The discoloration can create a cosmetic problem, especially when the body has been shipped to another city for final preparation. The firmness of the tissues combined with the dark coloring can create a need for the use of opaque cosmetic treatment.

Flushing

Flushing is seen in those body areas into which the embalmer has been able to distribute arterial solution but has been unable to secure good drainage of blood. Take as an example the body in which the femoral artery is used for injection and the accompanying femoral vein for drainage. If drainage is poor because of clotting in the right atrium of the heart or in one of the internal jugular veins or because of abdominal pressure, arterial solution will quite often flow into the facial tissues. Blood will not be able to rapidly drain from these tissues. The facial tissues and neck look cyanotic. Establishing drainage from another point such as the right internal jugular vein will clear this problem. Some embalmers place a trocar in the right atrium of the heart and drain directly from this point. Relieving gases or edema in the abdominal cavity may solve the problem. If there is edema of the pleural sacs, as seen in some pneumonias, drainage from the jugular will help to remove blood from the facial tissues and the neck. Flushing can result from leaving the drainage closed too long when using intermittent drainage. The establishment of drainage should clear the problem.

Razor Abrasion (Razor Burn)

Another form of dehydration, razor abrasion, occurs when a moist abrasion dries during or after embalming (any abraded area, area of desquamation, or area of skin where superficial layers of tissue have been torn or scraped away will bring about this condition). Air drying alone turns these areas dark brown. With razor abrasion, application of a light layer of massage cream during embalming helps to prevent the nicked area from dehydrating and browning. If cream cosmetics are to be used and a small layer of wax is placed over the area, the discoloration should not darken or be noticed. The darkening may also be considered an advantage, because it indicates that the areas have dried, and an opaque cosmetic can be used to cover the discoloration. Dried tissues accept cosmetics and, when necessary, wax very well. The embalmer can promote the drying of these areas by using a hair dryer for a few minutes. This ensures that there will be no further leakage, and establishes a good surface for cosmetics.

Postmortem Bruising

Postmortem bruising is rare; it occurs if sufficient pressure is applied to tissues to damage capillaries. This condition is particularly noted in persons who have been on blood thinners and in elderly people whose skin is thin. This discoloration is also observed after eye enucleation, because the skin around the eyes is ecchymotic. In fact, the person appears to have had a "black eye" before death. In these situations, the tissues can easily distend when the face is injected. It is wise to raise both common carotid arteries and employ restricted cervical injection. Use a preservative solution that is a little stronger than that normally used so only a minimum of solution need be injected to ensure preservation. Avoid preinjection treatment of the head and facial tissues in these bodies. (Restricted cervical injection is recommended.) A hypodermic injection of a phenol solution may help preserve and reduce the distension. Surface compresses of a phenol solution or other preservatives such as cavity fluid or the autopsy gels may also be used during or following arterial injection to reduce distension, bleach the discoloration, and ensure preservation.

▶ TREATMENT OF DECOMPOSITION DISCOLORATION

Decomposition discolorations are brought about by the action of autolytic and bacterial enzymes, as well as the hemolysis of red blood cells.

Decomposition is evidenced by five signs: odor, desquamation, gas, purge, and color changes. The first external sign of decomposition is a color change, usually a green discoloration of the right inguinal or iliac area of the abdomen. This green discoloration enlarges over a period and outlines on the abdominal wall the ascending, transverse, and descending colon. The green then proceeds upward over the chest area into the tissues of the neck and face. A color change is also evidenced throughout the skeletal tissues. Generally the color changes from yellow to green to blue-black to black. In addition, the blood in the veins begins to break down. This discoloration progresses from the red of the postmortem stain to a black, and follows the course of the particular vein. The pattern thus forms a "spider web" and the veins are described as being mottled.

Both the general progression of color changes resulting from decomposition and the mottling of the veins are discolorations that can be bleached with external compresses such as phenol solutions, cavity fluid, or autopsy gel. These discolorations can be lightened but not to normal skin color. Hypodermic treatment can also be used to lessen the discolorations and to help ensure preservation.

▶ CONDITIONS RELATED TO DISCOLORATIONS*

As previously defined, a discoloration is simply any abnormal color appearing in and on the human body. The discolorations already described involved color changes and possibly some swellings. There were no breaks or tears in the skin surface with the exception of the razor abrasion. In the following conditions, a discoloration is present but, in addition, there is some form of disruption of the skin surface (Figure 20–6). The emphasis is not so much on the pathological origins of these conditions, but rather on the treatment of these conditions from an embalming standpoint. Restorative treatment is not discussed beyond the extent of those treatments begun in the embalming phase of the restoration.

A *skin lesion* is any *traumatic* or *pathological* change in the structure of the skin. The objective of the embalmer is to properly sanitize skin lesions, clean them of debris, remove skin that cannot be used in the restorative treatment, and secure adequate preservation and drying of the tissues. There are four categories of skin lesions: (1) unbroken skin, (2) skin scaling, (3) skin that is broken or separated from the body, and (4) pustular or ulcerative lesions.

Unbroken but Discolored Skin

Skin may remain unbroken but discolored for a variety of pathological and traumatic cases, for example, allergic reaction, inflammation, trauma, and tumors. Generally, a discoloration will result from an increase in blood flow into the tissues of the affected area and some swelling. If this area is to be viewed (face, neck, or hands), a strong arterial solution can be used to help decrease further swelling or surface compresses can be used to help bleach the area and possibly reduce some of the distension. A phenol solution can be injected beneath the skin after arterial injection to preserve, bleach, and reduce the swelling.

Scaling Skin

Exanthematous diseases such as measles and chickenpox can result in small discolored skin eruptions. Dry skin and large amounts of medications can result in extensive scaling of the skin on the face and hands. Some of the skin breaks away, as in the healing of sunburn. The embalmer must make certain that as much of the loose skin as possible is removed. This is necessary for a good cosmetic treatment on the affected area. Sometimes, a razor can be used to shave the loose skin. Take a solvent (e.g., trichloroethylene and the dry hair washes) and, applying pressure, clean off as much of the loose skin as possible. Apply massage cream to the area, leave it on during the embalming process, then wipe off with solvent. This helps to remove skin debris.

All eruptive and scaling skin conditions should be treated as if they were infectious and/or contagious. Thoroughly disinfect these areas prior to any treatments.

If there is any question as to preservation, brush autopsy gel over the affected area for several hours or apply compresses of a surface preservative. The gels

* Conditions discussed relating to discolorations and lesions pertain to those conditions located on the face and/or hands of the deceased or other areas of the body that will possibly be viewed.

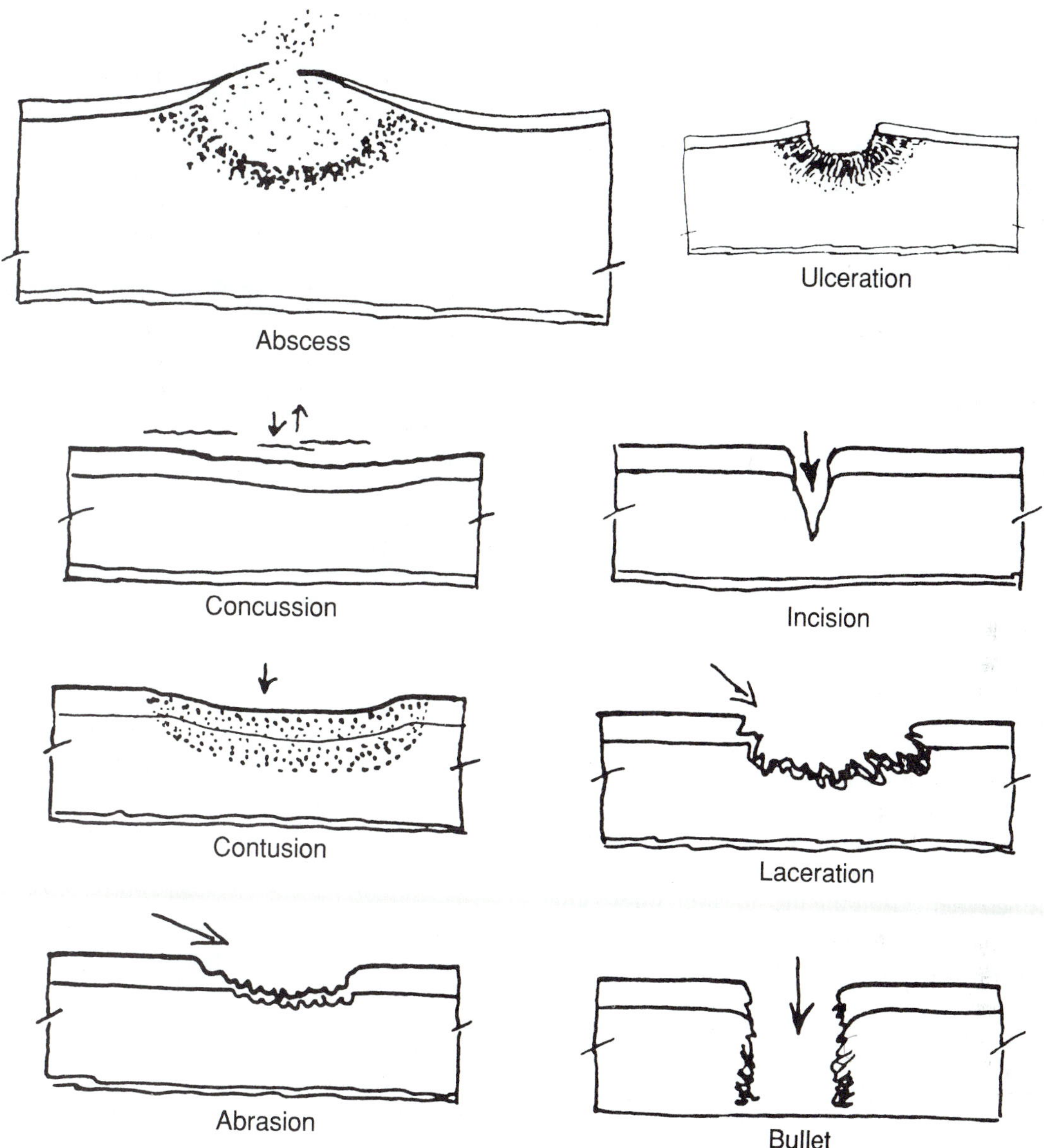

Figure 20–6. Types of skin trauma.

work well because they can be evenly applied and are not harsh bleaching agents. Surface compresses or gels should always be covered with plastic to reduce fumes.

Broken Skin

Three types of broken skin are discussed: abrasions, blisters, and skin-slip.

An **abrasion** is defined simply as skin rubbed off. When the raw skin is exposed to the air and dries, it discolors to a brown (Figure 20–7). An abrasion must be dried before restorative treatment commences. This may be cosmetic application, wax application, or surface glue treatment. When an individual falls at the time of death, the moist abrasion might not be noticed by the family. After drying, however, the abrasion is very noticeable.

The embalming treatment is quite simple. During injection, the surrounding tissues can be protected with massage cream. **Do not apply massage cream to the abrasion.** Let the fluid flow through the broken skin. After embalming use a hair dryer to dry the tissues. The tissues will darken and will be firm and dry and ready for restorative treatment. Abrasions on areas that will be viewed must be dry. If there is a preservation problem and fluid did not reach the abraded tissue, a surface compress of phenol cautery solution will help promote preservation and drying of the tissues. Abraded tissue cannot be bleached with surface packs because it is dehydrated.

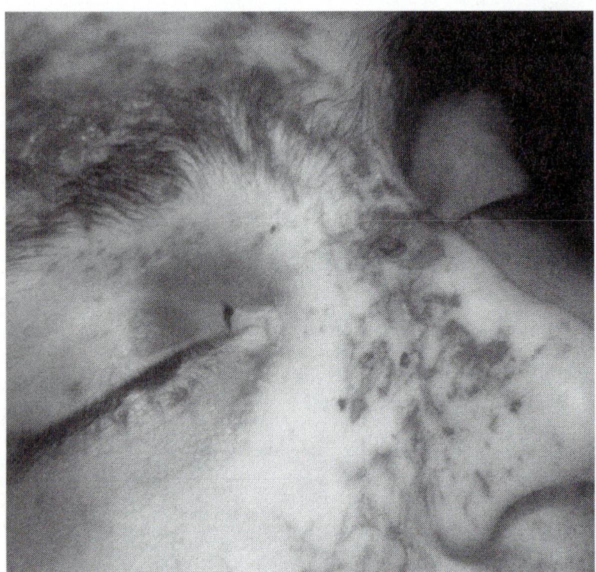

Figure 20–7. Minute lacerations and abrasions, once dried, turn dark brown.

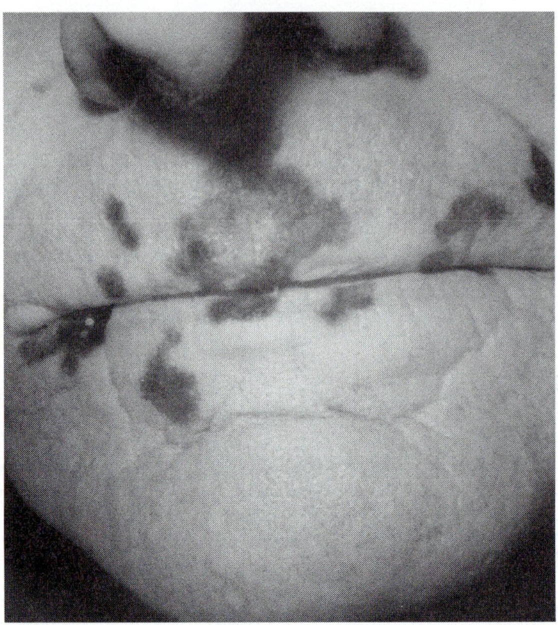

Figure 20–8. Blisters from a herpes infection dried with phenol. Note the dark brown color.

Blisters are elevations of the epidermis containing a watery liquid. The embalmer must make some decisions here. When blisters are present on an area of the face and preservation has been adequate, they could be coated with a preservative gel for a period, then merely treated with cosmetics. On the lip, however, where glue must be applied, blisters can be "glued under," and no treatment is needed except the creation of a new lip line with cosmetics. If the embalmer feels that blisters should be opened and drained, this can be done prior to arterial treatment. Be certain to remove all loose skin. A phenol cautery solution compress can be used to help dry the raw tissue (Figure 20–8), or after embalming, a hair dryer can be used to force-dry the tissue.

Tissues must be dry before they are treated with cosmetics, waxes, or surface glues.

Blisters that have been opened and drained prior to death can pose a problem. If the scab is noticeable, it can be removed. A scalpel may be needed to remove the scab, and this should be done prior to arterial injection. The area can be cleaned with a solvent and disinfectant then force-dried with a hair dryer. Drying may also be accomplished with the use of a concentrated phenol cautery compress.

Blisters are characteristic of second-degree burns. In most second-degree burns, the individual lives for a time during which the blisters are opened and drained as part of the treatment. When present on the face, these lesions should be cleaned of loose skin with a sharp razor. A stronger than average solution should be used to embalm the affected area. Then the lesions would be force-dried with a hair dryer, or phenol solution would be used to dry and cauterize the opened blisters.

TREATMENT

1. **Lance and drain.**
2. **Remove all damaged skin.**
3. **Cauterize.**
4. **Dry.**

Desquamation (Skin-Slip)

Desquamation, separation of the upper layer of skin (the epidermis) from the deeper dermal layer, can be a sign of decomposition. The embalmer's goal is to achieve good preservation and make sure the areas are dried. Remove all loose skin prior to arterial injection. Peel all loose skin away then use a scalpel to cut at the point where freed skin joins attached skin. For exposed areas with desquamation the following protocol is recommended:

1. Apply a topical disinfectant.
2. Open and drain vesicles if present.
3. Remove all loose skin.
4. Apply surface compresses of cavity fluid or phe-

nol solution to the "raw" tissue or coat the "raw" tissue with autopsy gel.

5. Sectional embalming may be necessary. Use a strong arterial solution.
6. Check preservation. Compresses can be continued or hypodermic treatment instituted with cavity fluid or phenol solution.
7. Clean away all preservative chemicals with a solvent (e.g., dry hair washes or trichloroethylene).
8. Dry the area with a hair dryer to ensure no further leakage.

If desquamation is present on the eyelids or in the vicinity of the eye orbit, cotton can be used to close the eye. Saturate the cotton with a few drops of cavity fluid and glue the eyelids closed. This will serve as an additional internal compress to help establish good preservation. Leave it in place and use cosmetics over the affected skin areas when dried.

Desquamation in unexposed body areas can be treated in the following manner:

1. Apply a topical disinfectant.
2. Open and drain any vesicles that are present.
3. Remove all loose skin.
4. Embalm the body with a strong well-coordinated arterial solution.
5. If possible apply a cavity or phenol compress to the raw tissue or paint it with an autopsy gel.
6. Check for preservation. If not complete, hypodermically treat the area with cavity fluid.
7. Paint again with autopsy gel, cover with embalming powder, or do both.
8. Cover the area with absorbent cotton.
9. Use plastic garments over the affected area.

Pustular and Ulcerative Lesions

Examples of pustular or ulcerative lesions are ulcerations, pustules, herpes fever blisters, chickenpox lesions (Figure 20–9), boils, carbuncles, and furuncles. These lesions are pustular and contain dead tissue. Treat these lesions in the following manner:

1. Disinfect the surface of the lesion.
2. Open and drain or remove any material in the lesion; clean the lesion and coat with autopsy gel or compress with cotton saturated with cavity fluid or a phenol cautery solution.
3. Embalm the body.
4. Check for preservation. Hypodermic treatment with a preservative or surface compress may be necessary.
5. Dry the area with a solvent and force-dry with a hair dryer.

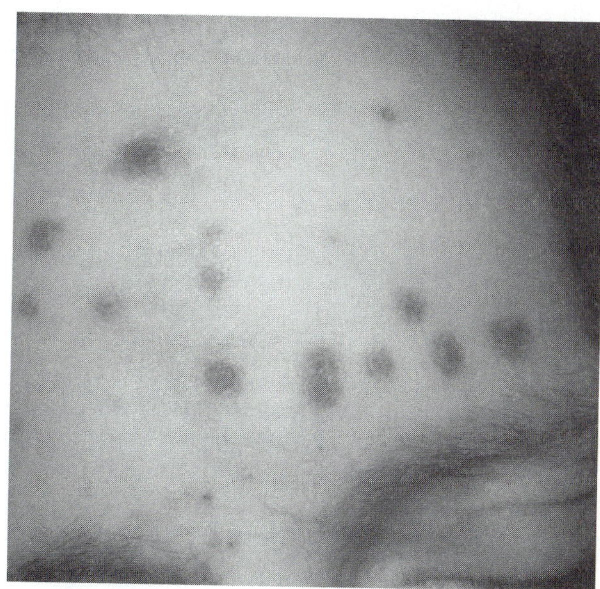

Figure 20–9. Chickenpox lesions on the forehead.

Decubitus Ulcers (Bedsores)

Because of their size and the fact that most occur on body areas that are not visible during viewing, decubitus ulcers bear special mention. These lesions are the result of a constant inadequate blood supply to the tissues overlying a bony part of the body against which prolonged pressure has been applied. These ulcerations can be very large and are most frequently seen over the sacrum, heels, ankles, and buttocks. In addition, bacterial infections often occur at these locations. Not only does the skin break and drain, but an odor is emitted because of the infection, usually staph infections. Be certain proper barrier attire is worn when treating all skin lesions.

Routine treatment of these ulcerations (when present on body areas that are not visible) can be summarized:

1. Disinfect the surface. Remove all bandages and apply a droplet spray.
2. Temporarily pack the area to reduce odors and to promote surface preservation.
   A. Autopsy gel can be painted over the ulceration.
   B. A cavity or phenol solution compress can be placed over the ulcer. When the lesions are located on the sides of the body, it may be helpful to leave taped bandages in place and soak them with cavity fluid.
3. Embalm the body.
4. Hypodermically inject cavity fluid (via infant trocar) into all the areas surrounding the ulceration.
5. Apply new surface compresses of cavity fluid or autopsy gel to the ulceration.

6. Clothe the body in plastic garments (stockings, pants, coveralls, etc.). If plastic garments are not available for the buttocks, make a larger diaper.
7. Spread embalming powder in the plastic garments to control odors.

▶ CONDITIONS RELATED TO DISCOLORATIONS: UNNATURAL CAUSES OF DEATH

The unnatural causes of death are briefly discussed at this point. In most instances, these causes are related to discolorations (Table 20–2). Although it is not a cause of death, refrigeration does result in some special discoloration problems. Suggestions are given for preparation of bodies dead from unnatural causes.

Almost all deaths from unnatural causes are investigated by legal authority, either the coroner or a medical examiner. Some of these deaths may be work related and the subject of workmen's compensation and insurance claims. Investigation by the coroner or medical examiner, in most states, leads to autopsy. The autopsy presents its own set of problems for the embalmer. Many of these deaths occur in the absence of other individuals, and there may be a considerable delay between death and finding of the body.

Because of these two factors (investigation and delay), specific directions as to how the body should be prepared are not given here. In the face of a long delay, two actions are recommended: the use of a strong arterial preservative solution (special-purpose high-index arterial fluids) and injection of the right common carotid artery and accompanying internal jugular vein. Injection of both common carotid arteries (restricted cervical injection) is recommended when problems are anticipated in preservation or circulation.

Preservation must be the most important goal in embalming these bodies. Discolorations can always be masked with opaque cosmetics.

TABLE 20–2. UNNATURAL CONDITIONS RELATED TO DISCOLORATIONS

Burns	First degree—redness of the skin Second degree—blistering and redness Third degree—charred tissue
Carbon monoxide poisoning	Bright red color to the blood Low blood viscosity, intense livor Rapid postmortem staining
Drowning	Low blood viscosity, intense livor Head faced downward, livor and stain Possible abrasions and bruising
Electrocution	Point of contact, burn marks can be present
Exsanguination	Little livor mortis, paleness to skin surfaces
Gunshot wounds	Eyelids can show ecchymosis, swelling of eye area when injury is to face or head
Hanging	Intensive livor in facial tissues; some capillary rupture showing petechial discolorations; no blood present in facial tissues
Mutilation	Loss of blood—little livor mortis Ecchymosis and bruising at affected areas
Poisons	Variable—from generalized conditions such as jaundice and cyanosis to localized discolorations such as caustic burns and petechiae
Refrigeration	Low blood viscosity, intense livor Postmortem stain speeded Dehydration of mucous membranes and skin surface after long exposure to cold air

Refrigerated Bodies

From a discoloration standpoint, intense livor mortis can be expected in bodies that are refrigerated shortly after death. The cooling process helps to keep the blood liquid. When the body has been stored 6 to 12 hours prior to preparation, the dependent tissues can turn a variety of dark hues from red to blue-black. It is important to elevate the head and shoulders of refrigerated bodies to avoid intense livor mortis in the tissues of the neck and face.

Postmortem stain is also prevalent in these bodies. Hemolysis is speeded by cooling. In addition, the capillaries are more porous. Thus, stain can be expected in areas where livor is present if the body has been refrigerated more than 12 hours.

If the body has been refrigerated several days, expect surface dehydration of the body. The lips and fingertips darken because of dehydration, as does the remaining skin, after a long period of refrigeration.

The means of storing bodies have changed in the past several years. Many hospitals and institutions now place the body in zippered plastic pouches or wrap the body in plastic. Years ago, the body was wrapped in cotton sheeting. The plastic bags cause the body to retain some heat and tend to trap moisture, thus slowing the dehydration process. This accelerates decomposition—sometimes extensively!

No treatment for refrigerated bodies is given at this point, but several items should be remembered:

1. No one condition such as refrigeration should dictate the method of embalming. Other factors are equally as important (e.g., manner of death,

time between death and preparation, effects of conditions such as edemas and jaundice, and effects of drugs).

2. Today, if death occurs in an institution, the body is usually refrigerated for some period. Refrigeration slows, but does not stop, postmortem changes such as decomposition and rigor mortis. These processes continue at a slower pace in these bodies.
3. Hemolysis also occurs in blood trapped in superficial nondependent tissues. The tissue looks as if it has already been embalmed; it is a light pink. Close observation and tracer dyes should be used in the preparation of these bodies to ensure the presence of embalming solution in all tissues.
4. Refrigeration can also solidify subcutaneous fatty tissues so that they feel firm to the touch. This can falsely signal that a reaction has occurred between the preservative solution and the body proteins.
5. All chemical reactions slow in colder environments; thus, the reaction between body proteins and preservative solution is not as rapid as that in bodies that have not been refrigerated.
6. Remember that after death, blood is trapped in the large arteries of the body, particularly the aorta. This blood thickens and agglutinates during refrigeration, and, on arterial injection, these large blood masses can be loosened and pushed along with the fluid. The common carotid artery (arteries) is a wise choice of vessels in the preparation of bodies refrigerated for long periods.
7. If the body has been refrigerated longer than 24 hours, expect a high moisture content in some body tissues because the serum portion of the blood leaves the blood vascular system and gradually makes its way to the surface of the body as a result of surface dehydration. This increase in tissue fluids is called postmortem edema.

Hangings

Self-inflicted, accidental, or intentional hanging can result in two different situations. First, extensive discoloration may appear on the face as a result of the pressure placed on the jugular veins in the last moments of life, when blood was able to enter the facial tissues via the common carotids and vertebral routes, but was unable to drain from these tissues. The eyes and tongue may also protrude. The discoloration can be intense enough that the face appears almost black.

Second, no blood is present in the facial tissues because the blood was able to drain from the tissues.

Many cyanotic and blood discolorations in the facial tissues clear after the pressure has been relieved from the neck. Additionally, almost all of these bodies come under the jurisdiction of the coroner or medical examiner and most would be examined by autopsy. During autopsy a great amount of blood is drained from the facial tissues. It is wise in the preparation of bodies dead from hanging on which no autopsy has been performed that both common carotid arteries be raised and the head separately injected (restricted cervical injection).

The strength of the solution depends on the time between death and preparation, pathological conditions, and so on. As in most cases of delay, a medium to strong 2.0 to 2.5% well-coordinated arterial solution should be used.

Expect some postmortem staining if there has been a delay. In addition, there is a possibility of some small capillary hemorrhages. Preinjection fluid should be avoided. Use of a medium to strong arterial solution is advised as is the use of a coinjection fluid. The head should be injected separately, left side first then right side. Use a minimum amount of fluid, for there is a good possibility of swelling. Remember, strong solutions help to bleach discolorations (minimum amounts are needed) and to prevent swelling.

Burned Bodies

Burns may be caused by heat (thermal burns), electrical shock, radioactive agents, or chemical agents. It is not always the local effect of the burn that should concern the embalmer, but rather the systemic effects brought about by major burns: bacterial infections, lack of blood flow to peripheral areas of the body, and kidney failure and the resulting buildup of wastes in blood and tissue fluids.

Many victims of burns will have lived for a period between the injury and their death. The blistering of second-degree burns is rarely seen. These blisters are opened, drained, and treated long before the death. It is the systemic effects that the embalmer must keep in mind. Burned bodies have a very high preservative demand. Circulation may be very difficult to establish, unless the cause was electrical shock. Very strong arterial solutions are used to prepare these bodies. Dye is added to trace the distribution of solution. Sectional injection, if the body has not been autopsied, is often needed. The skin must be dried:

1. Remove all loose skin before arterial injection using a good sharp razor (on visible areas).
2. Apply surface cavity (or phenol) compresses or paint the visible areas with autopsy gel. These gels can be painted over damaged skin areas that will not be viewed. (It is not necessary to

clean these areas as they will be covered with plastic and clothing.)
3. Clean the skin surface with a good solvent.
4. Air-dry or force-dry with a hair dryer.

Burns are classified into three categories:

- *First degree:* The skin surface is red (erythema); only the surface epithelium is involved.
- *Second degree:* The skin blisters and edema is present. Blisters beneath or within the epidermis are called *bullae.* There is destruction of the deep layers of the epidermis and the upper layers of the dermis (Figure 20–10).
- *Third degree:* The tissues are charred. The epidermis, the dermis, and epidermal derivatives such as hair follicles and glandular inclusions are destroyed.

Often, burns (and scalds) affect large regions of the body but not the face or hands. The affected areas may emit an odor. Painting these unseen areas with an autopsy preservative gel helps to ensure preservation and reduce odors. Edema and swelling are often present with second-degree burns. To prevent leakage and again to control odors, use of a *unionall* garment is recommended. This plastic garment covers all of the body except the face and hands. Unionall garments cover the arms and shoulders, areas not covered with other plastic garments such as coveralls or sleeves. Ample embalming powder should be spread in the unionall, especially over the burned areas. The autopsy gel may be left in place. The sprinkled powder adheres to the gel surface. Moisture-absorbent kitty litter can be liberally sprinkled over the burnt tissues to help control odor.

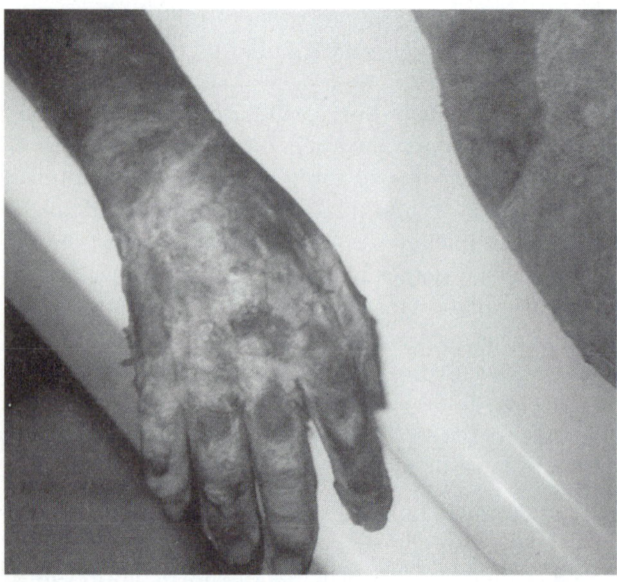

Figure 20–10. Second-degree burns. Burned bodies often have a very high preservative demand because of kidney failure.

The need to achieve preservation cannot be overemphasized in the preparation of burned bodies. Many of these bodies should be embalmed with 100% high-index arterial fluid using no water. Coinjection fluid may be added to help dilute.

Many bodies cannot be viewed because the facial tissues are severely swollen. All the embalmer can do is obtain some preservation and control leakage and odors.

Another problem arises in suture of the incision used for embalming. Application of super glue may help. There is no question that the best vessels to inject and drain in burned bodies are the common carotid artery and the internal jugular vein.

Use restricted cervical injection whenever possible so the maximum preservative solution can be injected. There is one exception. If only the neck area is affected by the burns, it might be wiser to inject and drain from an area of the body not affected by the burn.

Electrocution

Electrocution is related to discoloration because of the burn that results from contact with the electrical source. Many times the palms of the hands are burned. Remember, however, the body is embalmed on the basis of a number of conditions (e.g., time between death and embalming, pathological problems, body size and weight, presence of rigor mortis).

The cause of death, the electrical contact, should present no problem to the embalmer. Restoration of the burn area is a restorative art problem only if the burn exists in a viewable area. Often, these bodies are autopsied, as the death must be investigated by a coroner or medical examiner. For the preparation, the routine autopsy protocol is followed. In some instances the coroner or medical examiner may have excised the area of tissue where the electrical burn occurred. If so, a strong cautery phenol solution should be applied to the raw tissue to dry and firm the area.

Carbon Monoxide Poisoning

The primary concern in discolorations associated with deaths from carbon monoxide poisoning is the classic "cherry-red" color. Students of mortuary science who have not viewed these bodies often mistakenly believe that the entire body turns bright red. The bright red color is found in the dependent areas of the body to which the blood gravitates after death—the areas where livor mortis is present (Figure 20–11).

Most areas of the body where livor mortis is not present appear normal, although some blood is usually

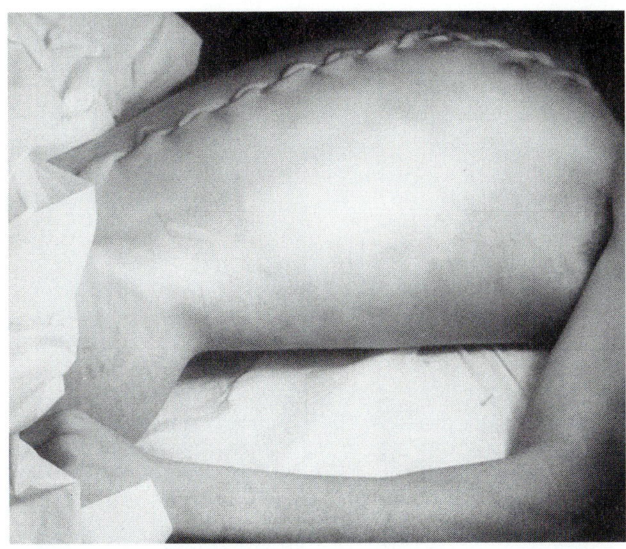

Figure 20–11. Dependent areas are bright red in this unembalmed autopsied body. The cause of death was carbon monoxide poisoning.

trapped in the anterior surface tissues. It looks as if the tissue was well embalmed and fluid dye was employed.

The bright color of the blood is due to carboxyhemoglobin, a component of blood. In addition, if the body is prepared a short time after death, the blood has a very low viscosity, and very few clots are present. Of course, as time progresses so do the problems of distribution.

This blood discoloration is classified both as an antemortem discoloration and as an intravascular discoloration. It should clear during arterial injection and subsequent blood drainage; however, there are usually some time delays between the death and the preparation of the body. Because most of these deaths must be investigated by a coroner or medical examiner, preparation is delayed and the blood rapidly undergoes hemolysis. Therefore, in the majority of these bodies, some, but not complete, clearing of the discoloration occurs.

Solution strength should be based on the postmortem changes, the length of the delay, and the size and weight of the body. Delay and refrigeration necessitate use of a stronger-than-average solution. Extra dye should be used to indicate solution distribution and diffusion. Once circulation is established, the solution strength can be increased further. Individuals who commit suicide by carbon monoxide poisoning often may have been suffering from some disease process. Again, such complications as jaundice, edema, and circulatory problems, as well as drug therapies, influence the strength of the solution used.

With regard to the selection of vessels, if there are no major problems or delays, any vessel is appropriate. Where there has been a delay, pathological problems, and so on, the best vessels are the common carotid artery and the internal jugular vein. If the embalmer feels that large volumes of solution are needed, as in the preparation of obese bodies with generalized skeletal edema, or decomposed bodies, restricted cervical injection is recommended.

Carbon monoxide poisoning in and of itself should not be a big problem for the embalmer. In many cases, the blood is quite thin and there is minimal clotting. If the facial tissues and neck are dependent, however, intense livor and staining can be expected. When some discoloration exists after embalming, a semiopaque or opaque cream cosmetic is advised, as the tissues tend to gray over time. Again, counterstaining with extra dye in the arterial solution helps to overcome this graying.

Most of these bodies are autopsied for medicolegal purposes. In these situations, follow the normal autopsy preparation protocol.

Drownings

In a victim of drowning, the most noticeable discolorations are intense livor mortis and possibly cyanosis. The livor mortis is due to the low temperature of the water, similar to refrigeration; the blood remains liquid and rapidly settles to the dependent tissues. If enough gas is generated to bring the body to the surface, the body floats face downward. Therefore, the livor and the resulting postmortem stain are intense in the facial areas. The cyanosis would be the result of the asphyxia (from the water in the respiratory system).

Each case must be handled on an individual basis. Preparation of some bodies has been delayed months because the drowning occurred in winter but the body was not recovered until spring. These bodies were viewable. Other drowned bodies that have been in the water for a matter of hours have been so decomposed that they could not be prepared for viewing.

In addition to livor, postmortem stain, and cyanosis, some bodies may be dragged by currents along a river or ocean floor and bruised (lacerations). Large abrasions are frequently seen. Cool water preserves the body. Warm water speeds decomposition. In addition, fish and marine animals may desecrate the body.

A constant problem in the preparation of a drowned person is the possibility of **purge,** either lung or stomach purge. Selection of vessels should be based on the condition of the body. If the embalmer has any doubts, use of the common carotid artery and the internal jugular vein is recommended. The ideal is restricted cervical injection. The strength of the fluid again depends on the extent of decomposition, the size of the body, pathological complications, and other factors in the case analysis. Aspiration should be thorough, with a minimum of two to three bottles of cavity fluid used on adult bodies.

Be certain an adequate amount of cotton or cotton webbing is packed into the throat and respiratory passageways. These bodies should be reaspirated, and if gases are evident or the viscera do not appear firm, at least one more bottle of cavity fluid should be injected.

Gunshot Wounds

Death from gunshot wounds poses a number of problems for the embalmer. Some gunshot wounds are barely noticeable. Many embalmers have seen bodies where a pistol was discharged in the mouth but there was no exit wound. In other cases, the bullet exited through a small hole in the forehead. Still others present great amounts of trauma. These deaths must be handled individually. The conditions most likely to be found are ecchymoses and possible swelling of the eyelids. Bones of the face and cranium are often fractured. Purging is quite likely from the nose and the ears (Figure 20–12).

Again, most of these bodies are autopsied. Difficulty arises in reshaping of the cranium when the bones are fractured. Plaster of Paris may prove helpful in realigning and reshaping the cranium after embalming.

To minimize swelling, especially if facial bones are fractured and the eyes are ecchymotic and swollen, use a very strong, well-coordinated arterial solution. The **instant tissue fixation** method of embalming has proven very useful in embalming these bodies. In this method almost 100% arterial fluid is injected in short spurts under high pressure. With this method, the fluid is distributed as far as possible, but only a minimum amount of fluid is needed. As this method is so valuable in the preparation of bodies with gunshot wounds, whether autopsied or not, it is outlined here:

1. Realign the features as best as can be done.
2. Raise the right and the left common carotid arteries and insert tubes directed upward on both the right and left sides. Direct one tube downward on the right side.
3. Prepare a solution for injection into the trunk.
4. Inject the trunk. Be certain that the tubes directed toward the head remain open and that the lower portion of the left common carotid is ligated.
5. Prepare a solution for injection of the head: two bottles of 25-index or stronger fluid, one bottle of coinjection fluid (or one bottle of water), and fluid dye.
6. Set pressure on a centrifugal machine to 20 pounds or more with the rate-of-flow valve closed.
7. Inject the left side of the head first. Open and immediately close the rate-of-flow valve so the fluid is injected in spurts. Do this until you are satisfied that the tissues are preserved.
8. Repeat injection on the right side of the face.

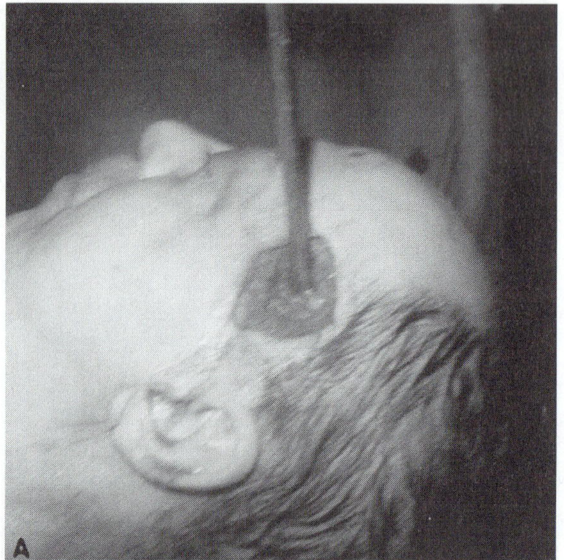

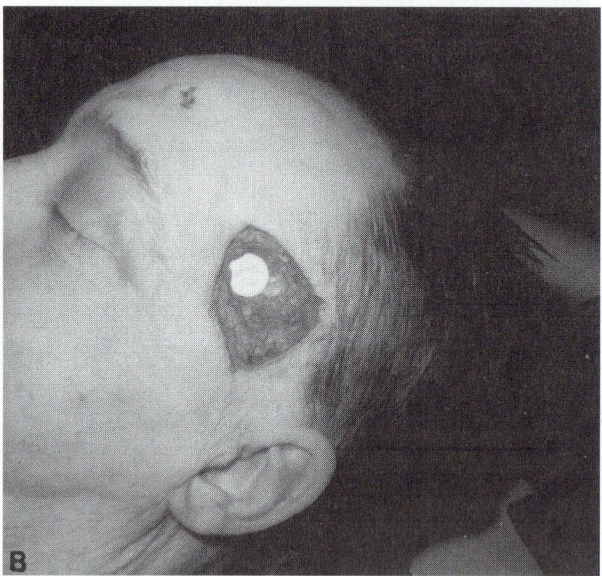

Figure 20–12. Bullet wound. **A.** The bullet entry wound is used to aspirate the cranial cavity. **B.** Wound is closed with a trocar button.

If the eyelids are distended, a phenol-reducing and bleaching agent can be hypodermically injected using "hidden points of entry." It is possible for this solution to leak out of the hypodermic needle punctures; the hidden points provide a location where leakage is least likely to be seen. The following points of entry are suggested:

1. Lower eyelid and surrounding tissues
   A. Inside the mouth

   B. Inside the nostril
   C. Behind the ear or in the hairline
2. Upper eyelid and surrounding tissues
   A. Eyebrow
   B. Hairline

Let the phenol solution remain undisturbed for 20 to 30 minutes; then apply pressure to decrease swelling. Remove excess liquids through the needle punctures.

Surface compresses (of cavity fluid or a surface bleaching compound) may be applied to add weight to help reduce the distension as well as to preserve and bleach tissues. These compresses take more time to work and are much less effective than injection of a phenol solution into the tissues. If there is doubt about preservation, cotton may be used to close the eyelids; it can be saturated with cavity fluid and then the lids glued.

In some cases, the eyes are so distended that the eyelashes cannot be seen. The protocol just explained has been quite successful in treating such distended eyes and reducing and bleaching them to a point at which opaque cosmetics can be applied.

With black eyes or distended eyes, always encourage the use of glasses on the deceased. The lights over the casket or on either end of the casket reflect off the lenses and hide some of the problem areas.

Not all gunshot wounds affect the head or face. When the bullet enters thoracic or abdominal areas, a large amount of blood may be lost. Livor mortis is minimal in such bodies. If the body is not autopsied, use the right common carotid and the accompanying internal jugular vein. If there is drainage and signs of distribution are evident, continue the injection, but use a slightly stronger-than-average arterial solution containing plenty of tracer dye.

There may be abdominal swelling or blood purge through the mouth or nose. The abdominal distension may be blood and fluid draining into the abdomen if a large vein was affected by the gunshot. If the arterial system is intact look for signs of distribution. Blood purging from the mouth or nose during injection may indicate that a vein in the stomach was severed by the gunshot. As long as there are signs of arterial solution distribution, continue the injection. Standard drainage from the selected vein may be very decreased.

If the abdomen begins to swell immediately after the artery is injected and there is no drainage or signs of arterial solution distribution, it is obvious that a large artery has been affected by the gunshot. Stop injection and begin sectional arterial injection. The following order of injection is suggested: legs, arms, left side of the head, right side of the head. The trunk walls may be treated by hypodermic injection with an infant trocar. Several points of entry are needed to reach all of the tissues.

As previously stated, each body with gunshot wounds must be treated on an individual basis. Most of these bodies are autopsied, so the standard autopsy routine can be followed. If the eyes are affected, as has been described, instant tissue fixation may be used to control swelling and maximize preservation.

Poisoning

A variety of discolorations are associated with poisoning deaths. Some poisons act in a very short time. Others have a cumulative effect on the body. The latter poisons may affect the liver, which, in turn, leads to jaundice. Some poisons induce shock; the blood is drawn into the large veins and the body exhibits very little livor mortis.

A large number of poisons act on the nervous and muscular systems. Respiration becomes difficult and the body becomes cyanotic. Other poisons are corrosive and burn areas such as the mouth and hands with which they come into contact. In addition, the corrosive agent destroys tissues of the gastrointestinal tract, causing the rupture of veins and arteries in these organs. Some poisons cause petechiae on the skin surface. Others bring about anaphylactic shock, causing the skin to redden and swell.

Most of these bodies are autopsied. Dyes can be used to counterstain discolorations. Preservation should be the first concern. Areas burned by corrosive poisons need to be cleaned and dried before restorative treatment begins.

Mutilations

The conditions caused by the various types of mutilation could fill an entire book. An automobile accident involves mutilation; a stabbing involves mutilation; accidental deaths can involve mutilation; even some extensive surgical procedures might be classified by laymen as mutilation; the results of poor autopsy technique and some medicolegal autopsies may be viewed as mutilation.

These bodies cannot be embalmed by the "one-point" method of arterial embalming. Most require sectional arterial embalming. In addition, hypodermic and surface embalming is necessary to achieve adequate preservation of the body (Figure 20–13).

In these bodies discolorations usually manifest as ecchymoses and antemortem and postmortem bruises. As with most unnatural causes of death, an autopsy is likely, but even with the autopsy, additional sectional and regional arterial injection may be necessary.

Remember that in the preparation of mutilated remains, arteries remain open when they are severed. An embalmer familiar with the arterial pathways can easily dissect to locate the arteries. These vessels can be used

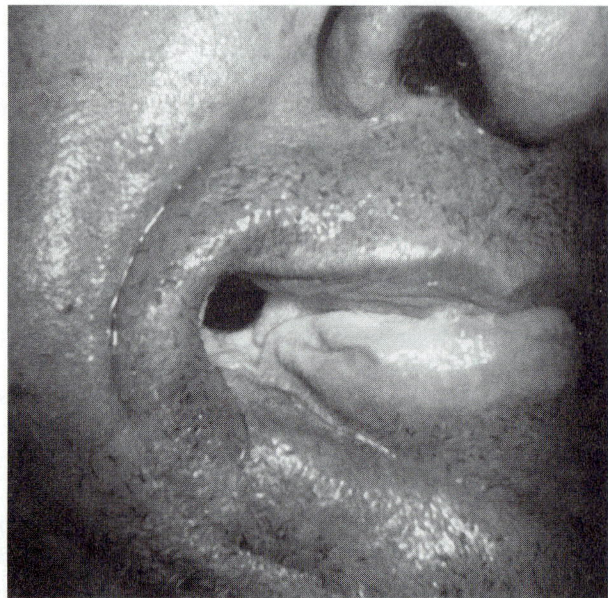

Figure 20–13. Corner of mouth deformed from use of a gastric tube.

for the injection of embalming solution. Drainage need not be a concern as many of these bodies have sustained a major blood loss and drainage will be minimal. Strong arterial solutions should be used. Such cases constitute an excellent example of the type of body for which special-purpose high-index fluids can be used. Use dyes to trace arterial solution distribution.

Exsanguination

Exsanguination is excessive blood loss to the point of death. The blood loss is not always external, as in massive hemorrhage. It can be internal, for example, rupture of a blood vessel caused by ulceration of an area or rupture of an aneurysm in one of the large body cavities. Blood loss can also occur without a break in the blood vascular system, as seen in shock. Here, the blood flows to the large, deep veins of the body, draining the capillaries of needed blood.

Exsanguination deaths are characterized not so much by discoloration as by a lack of color. Whether blood is lost externally, internally, or into the deep veins, very little livor mortis is evident. In cases of shock, the blood tends to congeal in the large veins and drainage may be difficult to establish. The largest vein possible should be employed in the preparation of these bodies. That would be the right internal jugular vein, which leads directly into the right atrium of the heart.

In injecting bodies that have sustained a large blood loss, a slightly stronger arterial solution should be used, for there is likely to be a loss of arterial solution depending on the cause of blood loss. Additional dye should be added to the arterial solution to trace the distribution of arterial solution.

When necessary, sectional arterial embalming should be employed. The most difficult area to embalm, when there has been a "break" in the circulatory system, is the trunk. Legs, arms, and the head pose no difficulty as these can be directly injected. The trunk may absorb some solution, but if an artery such as the aorta has ruptured, the trunk walls will have to be embalmed hypodermically, using a small trocar attached to the embalming machine.

A strong solution should be used for the hypodermic injection. A solution of cavity fluid and water is a good mixture and probably less costly than arterial fluid; however, some embalmers prefer the arterial fluid. This work must be thorough, as areas not reached by the hypodermic treatment stand little chance of contact with fluid by gravitation or diffusion from other areas. Several points will have to be used to introduce the trocar into the trunk. Special emphasis should be placed on the buttocks and shoulder areas.

▶ KEY TERMS AND CONCEPTS FOR STUDY AND DISCUSSION

1. Define the following terms:
   abrasion
   antemortem extravascular blood discoloration
   antemortem intravascular blood discoloration
   blood discoloration
   decomposition discoloration
   discoloration
   drug and/or therapeutic discoloration
   ecchymosis
   embalming discoloration
   formaldehyde gray
   hypostasis
   livor mortis
   pathological discoloration
   postmortem extravascular blood discoloration
   postmortem intravascular blood discoloration
   postmortem stain
   skin lesion
   skin-slip
   surface discoloring agent
2. Discuss the embalming treatments for a body with "mild" jaundice.
3. Discuss the arterial solutions that can be used to help clear livor mortis in embalming a body that still retains heat.
4. Discuss the problems that can be encountered, with respect to discolorations, in the preparation of a drowned body, a body dead from hang-

ing, and a body dead from carbon monoxide poisoning.

5. Discuss the differences between postmortem hypostasis, livor mortis, and postmortem stain.

▶ BIBLIOGRAPHY

Adams J. Embalming the jaundice case—Part IV. *Dodge Magazine*, Jan–Feb, 1995.

Bedino JH. Waterless embalming—An investigation. *Champion Expanding Encyclopedia.* 1993;619–620.

Embalming Course Content Syllabus. American Board of Funeral Service Education, 1991.

Kazmier H. *Essentials of Systemic Pathology.* Dubuque, IA: Kendeil-Hunt Publishing Co; 1976.

Mayer JS. *Color and Cosmetics.* (3rd ed) Dallas: Professional Training Schools, Inc; 1986.

Mayer JS. *Restorative Art.* (6th ed) Bergenfield, NJ: Paula Publishing Co, Inc; 1974.

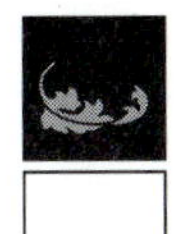

CHAPTER 21
MOISTURE CONSIDERATIONS

There are three objectives of embalming: preservation, sanitation, and restoration of the body. Water plays an important role in achieving these objectives. A properly embalmed body should not show evidence of dehydration. Bodies that have died from conditions that resulted in edema (or high moisture content) should be treated in such a manner that the excess moisture is removed or controlled. Similarly, dehydrated bodies should be treated in such a manner that water is added to the dry tissues. The control of moisture is a major concern for the embalmer. **A major objective of the embalming process should be to establish or to maintain a proper moisture balance in the dead human body.**

Three conditions characterize the dead human body with regard to moisture: normal moisture, dehydration, and edema. It is important that the embalmer recognize that all three of these conditions can occur generally or locally in a body.

In this chapter, bodies with normal water balance are considered first. It is important that this normal water balance be maintained during the funeral. It is the job of the embalmer to prevent bodies with normal tissue moisture from dehydrating. Dehydration is discussed next, as are the methods the embalmer can employ to moisturize tissues. Finally, localized and generalized edema is discussed together with methods that can be employed to reduce moisture.

Embalming analysis involves many components and choices. Examination of the body determines what embalming chemicals are to be used and in what manner these chemicals should be injected. Body moisture plays a very large role in these decisions. Some examples of chemicals and injection techniques the use of which is determined by the moisture condition of the body follow:

- Arterial fluid (index, firming action, etc.)
- Dilution of the arterial fluid
- Volume of arterial solution to inject
- Use of coinjection or humectant fluid and its dilution
- Vessel or vessels for injection and drainage
- Injection and drainage techniques to add, maintain, or remove moisture
- Speed of arterial injection
- Use of special techniques and fluids that add or remove moisture.

FACTORS THAT MUST BE DETERMINED IN THE EMBALMING ANALYSIS

1. Vessels for injection and drainage
2. Strength of the embalming solution
3. Volume of the embalming solution
4. Injection pressure
5. Injection rate of flow

Note: These factors will vary by the individual body and can vary in different areas of the same body.

▶ NORMAL BODY MOISTURE

For the healthy, average, 160-pound male adult, *total body water* constitutes 55 to 60% (for normal to obese bodies) and approximately 65% (for thin bodies) of *total* body weight. For the female adult, the proportions are, on average, 10% less than those for the corresponding male body types. **Edema is said to be established when there is a 10% increase in total body water.**

After death, several factors bring about dehydration. Storage of the body in a refrigerator is one of the leading causes of a postmortem loss of moisture. Dry, cool, or warm air moving across the body promotes dehydration. Between death and embalming, the blood and tissue fluids begin to gravitate into dependent body regions, increasing the moisture levels in the dependent tissues but reducing the moisture in the elevated body areas.

The embalming process itself can either add or greatly reduce moisture. The primary ingredient in embalming fluids is formaldehyde, and formaldehyde dries tissues. During arterial injection the skin becomes dry to the touch. The lips and the area between the thumb and index finger rapidly indicate if the arterial embalming is producing dehydration. This dehydrating effect can be evidenced before arterial injection is completed.

The embalmer must see that a good moisture balance is established or maintained. The well-embalmed body should not show signs of wrinkled, dark dehydrated tissue during the funeral. **Thoroughly embalmed tissues dehydrate LESS than underembalmed tissues.** Today, many bodies are shipped to other locations for funeral services and disposition, so there are delays. It is most important that the body change little in appearance during these delays.

Some embalming techniques can dehydrate a body that was normal at the beginning of the embalming process. Persons who die suddenly (e.g., accidental death or heart attacks) usually have normal moisture levels.

An article published many years ago (by Philip Boehinger in *Esco Review*) cited some interesting relationships dealing with the loss of moisture from the dead human body:

> If a pint of water weighs approximately 1 pound, consider the following: If the embalmer injects 3 gallons of arterial solution, 24 pounds of liquid is injected.
>
> The following liquid losses were estimated: $1\frac{1}{2}$ gallons of drainage = 12 pounds moisture lost; 1 quart of liquid aspirated = 2 pounds moisture lost. Up to 3 pints can be lost per day by dehydration; funerals average 3 days = 9 pounds moisture lost.

One pound of moisture remains (or was added) by the preceding example. This body should not have evidenced any dehydration during viewing. These are conservative figures, but they do present an interesting challenge for the embalmer.

A simple way to maintain the proper moisture level during the embalming process is simply to follow the dilution recommendations on the label of the arterial fluid. Almost all fluid manufacturers recommend dilutions based on the moisture conditions of the body. Many times, they recommend the volume to be injected, the type of drainage, and the rate of flow at which to inject the arterial solution. The temperature of the water is also often stated on the label. For example, a typical fluid label might state the dilution for "normal bodies," the dilution for "dehydrated" bodies, and the dilution for "edematous" bodies.

The dilution rule also applies to the use of coinjection and humectant fluids. Improperly used, these fluids can act in an opposite manner. A humectant can act as a dehydrating chemical as well as a moisturizing chemical.

The following techniques can help to maintain a good balance of moisture in the body:

1. Avoid the use of astringent or hypertonic arterial solutions. Follow dilutions recommended by the manufacturer. Hypotonic solutions penetrate better, and their diffusion and retention will be increased. Strengths of 0.75 to 1.5% help to add moisture to the tissues. Most manufacturers recommend dilutions for dry, moist, and normal bodies.
2. Avoid the use of concurrent or continuous drainage after surface discolorations have cleared. Intermittent or alternate drainage helps to distribute and diffuse the arterial solution. These methods also help the body to retain arterial solution.
3. Avoid rapid arterial injection and drainage. A slower injection helps fluid to penetrate the tissues and reduces "short circuiting" of fluids, so the solution is better distributed. Less tissue fluid is withdrawn from the tissues.
4. The delay of aspiration, if just for a short time, assists in diffusing arterial solution into the tissues. For best results, the final portion of arterial solution should be injected with the drainage closed. If aspiration is then delayed for a short time, the solution will have ample time to properly diffuse into the tissues.
5. If refrigerated prior to embalming, the body should be covered with plastic sheeting to prevent the surrounding air from dehydrating the surface tissues.
6. Strong alkaline or acid fluids can alter the reaction between protein and preservative. Formaldehyde has a drying effect on the tissues. Acid or rapid-acting arterial fluids often produce very firm and dry tissues. Old (outdated) fluids should be avoided. These fluids cause the tissues to dehydrate rapidly.
7. Disinfectants should not dry and bleach the surface tissues.
8. Use of cotton to set features can cause tissues to dry. Massage cream and cream cosmetics help to slow the dehydrating effect of cotton. Nonabsorbent cotton can be used as a substitute.
9. Fumes from the injection of cavity fluids into the neck area can dehydrate the mouth and the nose. These areas can be packed tightly so fumes cannot enter.
10. Short circuiting of arterial solution causes dehydration of the areas in which the solution is

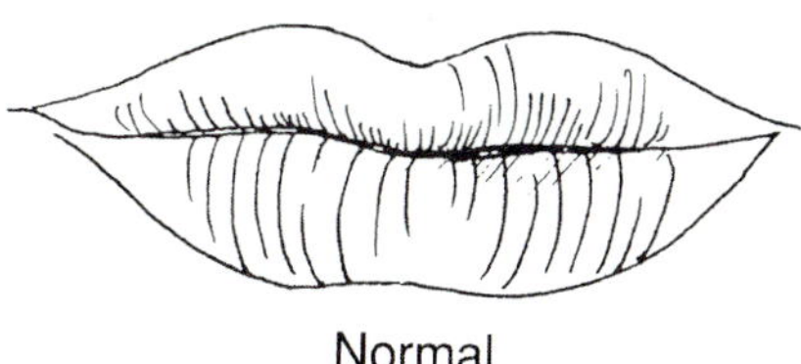

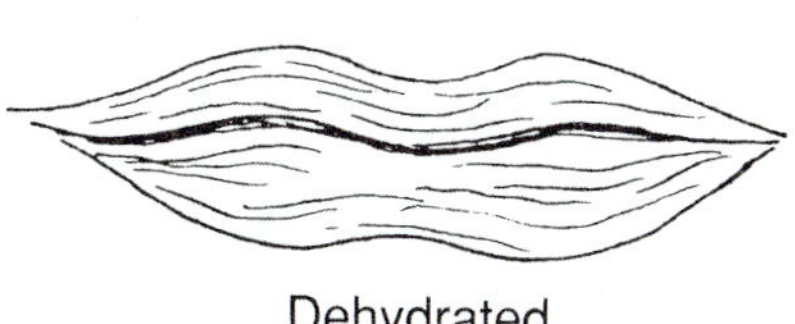

Figure 21–1. Dehydration causes horizontal wrinkles to form on the lips. With the disease processes seen today it is necessary that the body be properly sanitized. A moderate arterial solution by today's standards is 1.5 to 2.0%. Many fluids are reaction controlled and do not release the preservative ingredients until they come into contact with body cells.

circulating. Distribution is uneven and the short circuiting regions are very firm and dry.

11. Warm water solutions increase fluid reaction. Follow the manufacturer's recommendations for water dilution temperatures. Cool solutions slow the formaldehyde reaction, thus allowing better distribution and diffusion of the arterial solution throughout the entire body.
12. After embalming, the body should be covered to prevent circulating air from dehydrating the surface. Application of cream cosmetics and massage cream to the surface tissues helps to reduce moisture loss to the atmosphere (Figure 21–1).

It is important that the embalmer maintain the moisture present in the "normal" body. Because of drainage and the arterial fluid itself (remember that formaldehyde dries tissues), the embalmer must actually *add* moisture to the normal body. This is why so much water is used to dilute arterial fluid. Almost 20 ounces of water is added for each ounce of arterial fluid!

▶ PREPARATION OF THE DEHYDRATED BODY

Antemortem Dehydration

Dehydration may have occurred while the person was alive. A number of disease processes result in a loss of fluid from the body cells and tissues: slow hemorrhage, febrile diseases, kidney diseases, diabetes, some cancers and localized neoplasms, and some first-degree burns. All these antemortem conditions contribute to a loss of body moisture. The classic example of a disease process that can cause dehydration is tuberculosis, especially tuberculosis of the lungs. Drug therapy, intravenous fluid injection, and stomach tube feedings are employed to maintain a normal moisture level in the living person. Therefore, today, tuberculosis may not always produce the characteristic signs of dehydration. Drug therapy and chemotherapy can result in dehydration in the living body.

Postmortem Dehydration—Preembalming

After death, a major cause of dehydration is refrigeration. Dry, cool air moves around the body and gradually draws the moisture in the tissues to the surface of the body and from the surface into the surrounding air. (Refrigerated bodies are discussed in Chapter 19.) Refrigeration keeps the blood in a fluid state. Thus, the blood and tissue fluids slowly gravitate to the dependent tissues of the body. The upper areas of the body lose moisture because of surface evaporation and the gravitation of fluids.

Embalming Treatments to Control Dehydration

The skin on a dehydrated body is very dry. Often, the skin is quite "flaky" and small pieces of tissue easily come loose. These small scaly flakes of skin must be removed from the facial areas or they will create a problem when cosmetics are applied. A liberal application of massage cream helps to control the flaking. The massage cream can be firmly wiped off with a gauze pad saturated with solvent, completely removing the loose skin. A second application of massage cream can then be applied.

The skin of dehydrated bodies is often very dark. A condition similar to a suntan may exist. It may be difficult to trace the distribution of arterial solution through these skin areas. Dehydrated skin is very firm to the touch. The skin feels as if it has already been embalmed. Additional fluid dye is needed to be certain of arterial solution distribution.

Desiccation

Regardless of the antemortem or postmortem conditions that have brought about the condition of dehydration, there is only one positive benefit to the embalmer. Dehydrated bodies tend to decompose more slowly, as water is necessary for decomposition. Likewise, in embalming, the reaction of the preservative with the proteins leads to the drying and firming of tissues. Extreme dehydration is called *desiccation*. Desiccation is a form of preservation; however, desiccated bodies are not viewable.

Often, certain areas are desiccated in bodies that have been frozen or refrigerated for a long period. For example, desiccated lips appear black, very wrinkled, and shrunken. The lips are drawn back and the teeth exposed. When the tips of the fingers are desiccated, the skin becomes parchmentlike and turns a yellow brown. Other body areas easily desiccated are the thin skin areas such as the ears, nose, and eyelids. Arterial injection or hypodermic injection cannot correct this condition.

▶ LOCAL DEHYDRATION PROBLEMS

An abrasion is defined as "skin rubbed off"; the epidermis has been removed. At first, the tissue is quite moist, but as the skin dries a "scab" forms. This is also true of abrasions that occur at the time of death. Such an abrasion may not even be noticed. Air passing over the body during or after embalming dries the abraded skin, which turns dark brown and hardens. This type of discoloration does not respond to bleaching and must be covered with an opaque cosmetic. Abrasions are often incurred after falls on pavement or carpeting.

When the body has been roughly shaved and small nicks have occurred on the skin surface, surface drying, in time, turns these areas into small, dark brown marks. These small discolorations are referred to as razor abrasions. They are easily covered with an opaque cosmetic or waxed.

The drying of the tissues in the preceding two examples is actually desired by the embalmer, for the skin surface is now sealed and there is no leakage from these areas. Opaque cosmetics (or waxes) can be applied over these dried areas. To speed the drying of abraded tissues, following arterial injection, a hair dryer can be used. Massage cream should not be applied to these areas, because it slows the drying of tissues.

▶ ARTERIAL EMBALMING PROBLEMS

Dehydration occurring during the antemortem, agonal, and postmortem periods prior to arterial embalming can result in a thickening of the blood. Satisfactory blood removal is essential to establish uniform distribution and even diffusion of arterial solution. Drainage may be difficult to establish in these bodies. A more important problem, however, may be congealing and clumping of this thick blood in the arterial system. On arterial injection, the heavy arterial blood and any clots may be forced into small arteries, thus cutting the flow of arterial solution into tissues supplied by these small arteries.

Blood should be drained from the best location possible, the right internal jugular vein. Likewise, arterial injection from the right common carotid artery or restricted cervical injection pushes arterial coagula toward the legs. A secondary injection point (e.g., femoral vessels) may be necessary, and if this is not successful, hypodermic and surface treatment of the legs can be used to establish preservation.

It is unwise to inject from the femoral or external iliac arteries if clots are present. The arterial clots can be pushed into the carotid arteries, making embalming of the face a most difficult task. Slow injection will minimize arterial coagula from being dislodged and moved to block smaller arteries.

From an arterial chemical standpoint, preinjection fluids, coinjection fluids, and dilute arterial solutions can be used to prepare the dehydrated body (Table 21–1).

TABLE 21–1. PROBLEMS ASSOCIATED WITH DEHYDRATION

Darkened skin	Corrected by cosmetic application; use fluid dyes to ensure fluid distribution to all body areas
"Flaking" or peeling of skin, especially in facial areas	Apply massage cream and then clean with a solvent to remove all loose skin; mortuary cream cosmetics further reduce skin drying
Firm feel to the skin	Skin feels embalmed; additional dye helps to trace the distribution of fluid
Desiccated lips, eyelids, or fingertips	May need correction with restorative waxes; tissue building; opaque cosmetics needed to hide discolorations
Thickened blood	May be diluted with a preinjection fluid; use right internal jugular as drainage point; inject from the carotids to push arterial coagula toward the lower extremities
Dehydration created by the embalmer; wrinkled lips, fingertips; facial areas	Use correct dilutions for arterial and humectant fluids; areas may be filled out with tissue builder after embalming
Dehydration of large facial area from embalming and passage of air over body	Use massage cream on exposed areas prior to cosmetic application; if skin is discolored, opaque cosmetics will be needed; cream cosmetics further reduce dehydration; fingertips and facial areas may also be treated with tissue builder to reduce dehydration

▶ TREATMENTS THAT MINIMIZE OR PREVENT POSTEMBALMING DEHYDRATION

Every body that is embalmed dehydrates to a certain extent. Formaldehyde solutions not only firm tissues but *dry* them. Drainage removes a large amount of moisture from the body tissues. These factors account for a great amount of dehydration during and after embalming. Some treatments can be used to maintain the level of moisture in or add moisture to these dehydrated bodies:

1. Use a moderate arterial solution. A moderate arterial solution by today's standards is 1.5 to 2.0%. Many fluids are reaction controlled and do not release the preservative ingredients until they come into contact with body cells. Many arterial fluids contain antidehydrants in their formulations. Large volumes of a mild solution can be used to moisturize and to secure preservation. Follow the recommendations of the manufacturers of the arterial fluid. They generally recommend dilutions for dehydrated bodies.
2. Use a coinjection fluid with the arterial solution. The coinjection fluid helps to reduce the astringent dehydrating action of the arterial solution and also adds moisture to the tissues. It is recommended that equal amounts of coinjection and preservative arterial fluids be used.
3. Use a humectant coinjection fluid along with the arterial solution. These fluids are designed to maintain or add body moisture. It is very important that the dilution recommended by the manufacturer be used. If improperly used, humectants can dehydrate the body.
4. Run large amounts of fluid through these bodies to replenish the lost moisture.
5. Intermittent or alternate drainage can be used to help the tissues retain the arterial solution and also to reduce short circuiting of fluids and, thus, achieve more uniform embalming. This type of drainage also helps the arterial solution to penetrate the deeper body tissues (Figure 21–2).
6. Apply massage cream, petroleum jelly, lanolin, or silicone to exposed skin surfaces of the face and the hands during and immediately after arterial injection to retard water loss to the surrounding atmosphere. In the preparation of infants, the arms and legs should also receive treatment. It is not necessary to use a large amount of lubricant. A light layer is sufficient. Cream cosmetics also retard surface dehydration.
7. Avoid excessive massage of the hands, neck, and face. Massage is often necessary to distribute fluid through these regions, but excessive massage not only draws additional fluid into these areas but also removes tissue and arterial solution from these areas.
8. Do not expose reposing or stored bodies to air currents. Forced-air heating and air-conditioning currents quickly dehydrate the exposed areas of the body.

▶ EDEMA

Edema in a body, whether localized or generalized, creates many problems for the embalmer. This condition is one of the most frequently encountered problems in embalming today. **Edema is defined as the abnormal collection of fluid in tissue spaces, serous cavities, or both.**

Interstitial or tissue fluids enter and leave the bloodstream (in a similar manner to embalming fluids) through the walls and pores of the capillaries, the small

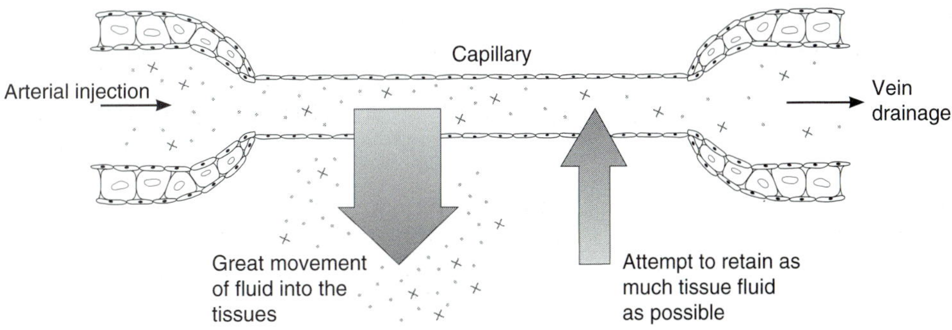

Figure 21–2. Hypotonic arterial solutions help the tissues to retain moisture.

vessels connecting the smallest arteries (arterioles), and the smallest veins (venules). If more fluid leaves the blood vascular system and enters the tissues than is absorbed from the tissues into the blood, the tissues become filled with moisture; this condition is called *edema.*

The condition can be local, for example, when surgery has involved the axillary area and the lymph and venous channels have been obstructed; the arm swells with edema. It may be generalized and present in all the dependent tissues, as in seen in bodies dead from congestive heart failure.

From an embalming standpoint, the embalmer can identify edema in three body sites: within the individual cells, in the intercellular spaces, and within the body cavities.

A number of diseases and conditions can cause edema: diseases that affect cardiac function and result in increased venous pressures, diseases that affect the renal system and result in small amounts of plasma proteins, capillary damage or inflammation and allergic reactions, and obstructive diseases that interfere with venous or lymphatic circulation.

In addition, long-term use of drugs can damage such vital organs as the liver and kidneys and the circulatory system. Failure of these organs or systems can lead to edema. Drugs also act on cell membranes, causing cells to retain or take up moisture, thus creating a condition of edema within the cell.

It is not the purpose of this discussion to explain the disease processes that bring about edema. The embalmer should have an understanding of pathology and microbiology to recognize the relationship between certain conditions and edema. The following diseases/conditions are often associated with edema. The embalmer should be able to relate the cause of the edema with the condition.

- Alcoholism
- Burns
- Cirrhosis of the liver
- Carbon monoxide poisoning
- Congestive heart failure
- Allergic reactions
- Inflammatory reactions
- Extended drug therapy
- Renal failure
- Trauma
- Lymphatic obstruction
- Steroid therapy
- Venous obstruction
- Phlebitis
- Malnutrition
- Hepatic failure and/or obstruction
- Surgical and transplant procedures

▶ CLASSIFICATION OF EDEMA BY LOCATION

Cellular (Solid) Edema

When moisture is retained by the cell, or abnormal amounts of moisture are allowed to pass into the cell, a condition called solid edema results. The tissues appear swollen and, when pushed on by the embalmer, feel very firm. Indentations are not made by pushing on these tissues. Frequently, this condition arises when large doses of corticosteroids have been administered over a long period. This form of edema, often seen in the facial tissues, does *not* respond to embalming treatments. The swelling and distortion remain. The only possible, although not practical, method of reducing the swelling is excision of the deep tissues after arterial treatment is completed.

Intercellular (Pitting) Edema. In intercellular edema, fluids accumulate between the cells of the body. When these swollen areas are pushed on by the embalmer, the imprint of the fingers remains for a short period after the fingers are withdrawn. This form of edema, also known as **pitting edema** (Figure 21–3), responds well to embalming treatments and can be gravitated to dependent body areas. It can be drained from the tissues into the circulatory system and removed with the blood drainage. This edema may be localized, as is frequently seen in bodies dead from cardiac diseases where only the legs are distended, hydrocele (edema of the scrotum) and pulmonary edema (edema of the alveolar spaces in the lung tissue). Or, it may be generalized, as is frequently encountered after death from liver or re-

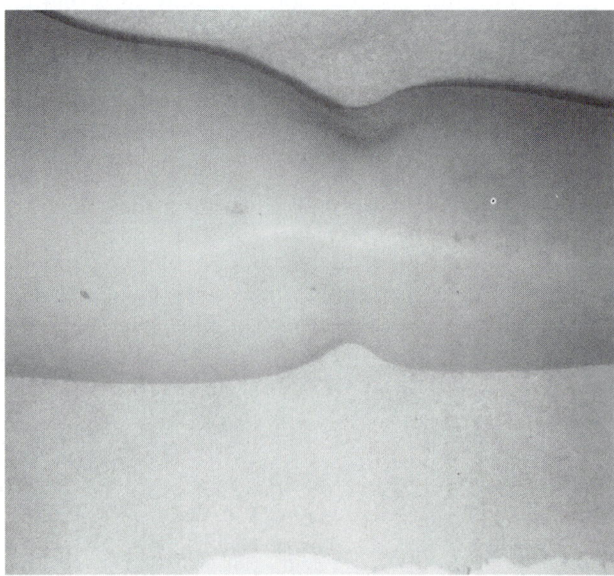

Figure 21–3. Pitting edema of the leg.

nal failure. Generalized edema is referred to as anasarca.

Edema of the Body Cavities

Ascites is edema of the abdominal (or peritoneal) cavity; the edema is found within the cavity and surrounds the abdominal viscera. **Hydrothorax** is edema of the pleural cavity; it may involve one or both pleural cavities. **Hydrocephalus** is edema of the cranial cavity, and **hydropericardium** is edema of the pericardial sac surrounding the heart.

> Edema of the cavities does not dilute the arterial solution. If the body being prepared has ascites it is not necessary to increase the strength of the arterial solution because of the edema in the abdominal cavity. Edema of the cavities does not mix with the arterial solution. The embalmer's concern is that the edema in the abdominal cavity might dilute the cavity fluid when it is injected.

▶ EMBALMING PROBLEMS CREATED BY EDEMA

Generalized edema presents a number of problems for the embalmer. The tissues in which edema is present are swollen. When this involves the face and the hands, measures must be taken to reduce the distortion. Edema of the skeletal tissues has a tendency to gravitate into the dependent body areas, during life as well as after death.

In the bedridden patient, the edema is found largely in the back, buttocks, shoulders, and backs of the legs. The embalmer must understand that this movement or gravitation of edema into the dependent areas eventually leads to the passage of this fluid through the skin. This exit of fluid from the body can dampen the clothing of the deceased and the casket bedding, unless precautions are taken (e.g., use plastic garments to trap and hold the fluids).

Bodies with large amounts of edema also exhibit leakage from intravenous punctures and small openings such as those made with hypodermic needles. Any surgical incisions or openings resulting from other invasive procedures are possible sites of leakage. Another major concern with edema is that the excess moisture in the tissues will hasten the decomposition cycle. A good, moist environment for bacterial growth is provided. Autolytic enzymes will have an ample source of water for their role in decomposition, and embalming fluid is throughly diluted by this excess fluid.

▶ EMBALMING PROBLEMS CREATED BY ANASARCA

1. Affected tissues are swollen with fluid.
2. When edema gravitates or moves from a region, the skin can wrinkle and appear distorted.
3. Fluid can leak from intravenous or invasive punctures, through the skin surface by gravitation, through hypodermic needle punctures, through surgical incisions, and through incisions made for embalming purposes.
4. Arterial fluid is diluted (secondary dilution).
5. Decomposition is speeded.
6. The possibility of separation of the skin layers (skin-slip) is increased.

When the face is affected by edema, the embalmer must first determine whether *solid* or *pitting* edema is involved. This can be done by gently applying digital pressure to the swollen tissues. Solid edema *cannot* be indented by pressure from the fingers. With solid edema, the extra fluids are located within the individual cells of the tissues. This type of edema is seen in allergic reactions and as the result of certain drug therapies, such as the extended use of corticosteroid drugs. Solid edema cannot be removed by arterial or mechanical means. It would not be wise to attempt to reduce the swelling by surgical removal of subcutaneous tissues after arterial embalming. Leakage would be a major problem.

In pitting edema the fluid is in the interstitial spaces (between the cells). Pitting edema can be gravitated. Merely elevating the head helps to drain some of the fluid from the tissue spaces. Solid edema, especially of the facial tissues, is not as frequently encountered as pitting edema. It should also be mentioned the facial tissues are not as frequently affected by edema as are other body tissues, probably because the head is almost always elevated.

When a general facial edema exists in the unautopsied body, the trocar, on aspiration, can be passed into the tissues of the neck to make channels for drainage of the edematous fluids. Pressure can be applied to the face in a downward motion to squeeze the edema from the facial tissues into the neck and finally into the thorax. The carotid incisions can be left open several hours after embalming to drain fluid from the face. Following arterial injection and cavity treatment some embalmers place the body onto the removal cot and secure the body to the cot. The head end of the cot is then fully elevated, thus placing the body in a standing position. The body remains in this position for several hours to encourage as much edema as possible to gravitate from the head, face, and neck.

Edematous arms and hands (especially hands) can be elevated. Leaking intravenous punctures on the backs of hands can be sealed with super adhesive after embalming. Super adhesive is the one type of glue that can be used to seal a moist area. The embalmer may also want to squeeze as much edema as possible out of any intravenous punctures on the back of the hand. Elevation and firm massage of the tissues help to move the edema from the hand to a point above the wrist where it will not be visible. An edematous arm can be wrapped in plastic or a plastic sleeve to cover the swollen areas. It would be unwise to lance and drain the edema after embalming, as closure of the incision may be quite difficult.

▶ ARTERIAL TREATMENT FOR GENERALIZED EDEMA

Generalized edema presents a number of problems for the embalmer. First and foremost is the increased rate of decomposition resulting from the presence of a large amount of body moisture. Water is necessary for decomposition. In generalized edema, vast quantities of water can be found in almost all the dependent skeletal tissues. In addition, the excess moisture causes a great secondary dilution of the arterial fluid, reducing the ability of the embalming solution to dry, sanitize, and preserve. The edema will, in time, seep through the skin, soiling the clothing and the casket interior. The large blebs that can form at edematous sites can break open and release fluids.

The objectives of the embalmer are to (1) inject an arterial solution of sufficient strength and volume to counteract the secondary dilution that occurs in the tissues, and (2) to remove as much of the edema from the tissues as possible. **It is very important that the embalmer know what condition caused the edema.**

For example, generalized edema can be the result of heart disease or renal failure. With renal failure, in addition to the edema, there is a buildup of nitrogenous wastes in the tissues. The nitrogenous wastes have the ability to neutralize the preservative solution. Therefore, very astringent solutions should be used.

Edema also coexists with nitrogenous wastes in bodies dead from second-degree burns, especially when the patient lived several days or weeks after being burned. These bodies demand large amounts of preservation solution.

Edema can be present in all body types. Edema can and does quite often exist in emaciated bodies. The first concern, even in an emaciated body, is to achieve preservation and dry the tissues. Overdehydration of the face and features is best avoided by raising both common carotid arteries at the beginning of the embalming and injecting the head separately.

Frequently in cases such as cancer of the liver, the body with generalized edema may also be jaundiced. Again, of primary importance are the preservation and drying of the tissues. The discoloration is secondary. Only the face and hands will be viewed. The restricted cervical method of injection allows the head to be embalmed separately. A jaundice fluid could be employed for embalming the head and a strong arterial solution in large amounts for the preparation of the trunk.

When arterial methods have not been completely successful, hypodermic injection of cavity fluid (or concentrated arterial solution) via the embalming machine can be used to inject local body areas. A small trocar can be used for the injection. The puncture is easily closed with a trocar button. Application of super adhesive around the trocar button helps to prevent leakage. The body is clothed in plastic garments. This technique works well with edematous legs.

Methods of Arterial Treatment

In treating the body with generalized edema, the embalmer should realize that often large amounts of arterial solution must be injected. Generally, the facial tissues are not affected by the edema, so to control the amount of arterial fluid entering the facial tissues it is wise to use restricted cervical injection. In this method, both right and left common carotid arteries are raised at the start of the embalming. The left artery is opened and a large tube is inserted toward the head; the lower portion of the artery is ligated. A tube directed toward the head is placed in the right artery, as is a tube directed toward the trunk. Both tubes directed toward the head remain open during the injection of the trunk.

In some of these treatments, several gallons of arterial solution are injected. Fluid that enters the head and facial areas exits through the open tubes while the lower portion of the body is being injected (Figure 21–4). After satisfactory injection of the lower portion, the head can then be injected using a strength and quantity of arterial solution desired by the embalmer. In many instances, this solution is much milder than that used to inject the portions of the body where edema was present.

In bodies where the head and facial tissues are affected by edema, the restricted cervical injection is still recommended. The embalmer can inject the head separately with arterial solution of sufficient strength and quantity to ensure proper preservation of the facial tissues. The embalmer may wish to employ a specially prepared arterial solution with osmotic qualities that assist in removing the excess fluids from the facial tissues.

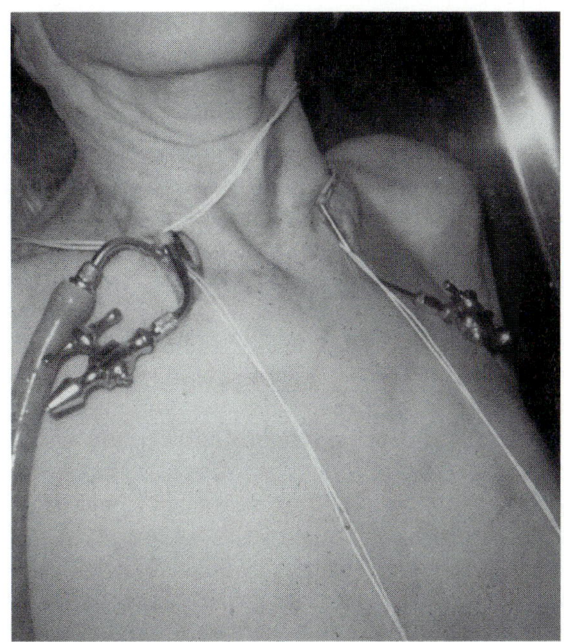

Figure 21–4. Restricted cervical injection allows large volumes of very strong arterial solution to be injected without overembalming the head.

When edema affects the head and facial tissues, the tongue and eyes may be grossly distended. Digital pressure on the scalp (especially the dependent portions) reveals the presence of pitting edema. Elevation of the head and shoulders is necessary. In addition to employing a strong arterial solution for the injection of the head, the embalmer may wish to channel neck tissues during cavity embalming to provide a route for fluids to drain from the face, scalp, and neck into the thoracic cavities. Reaspiration helps to remove some of this excess fluid. Downward massage of the facial tissues also assists in draining the excess fluids from these regions.

Local areas such as the eyes can be treated by a variety of techniques to restore swollen tissues. The first concern for the embalmer should be the complete preservation of these tissues. By injecting the left and right sides of the face separately, the embalmer can control the quantity of arterial solution entering the facial tissues. If the eyelids exhibit large amounts of edema and do not seem to be adequately embalmed, cotton can be placed under the eyelids and saturated with undiluted cavity fluid to ensure their preservation.

If areas of the face appear to lack adequate arterial solution, surface compresses of undiluted cavity fluid can be applied and left in place several hours. If preferred, autopsy gels may be applied to facial surfaces to assist in preservation. These, too, should remain in position, covered with cotton or plastic, several hours. Facial areas can also be preserved hypodermically, but the points of entry must be carefully considered, as the edema may leak through the entry points. Most of this work should be done from within the mouth. When the head has been autopsied, a long hypodermic needle can be introduced from within the margins of the cut scalp areas.

In summary, arterial treatment for facial edema consists of injection of both common carotid arteries with a solution of sufficient strength and quantity to ensure complete preservation. Keep the shoulders and the head elevated. Use fluid dyes to locate areas of the face not receiving adequate arterial solution. These areas can then be treated by hypodermic or surface embalming methods. To drain fluid from the face and neck, channel the neck with the trocar during aspiration of the body cavities. Reaspiration as well as cavity fluid reinjection of bodies with edema is always recommended.

Several types of arterial solutions can be used to treat bodies with generalized edema (Figure 21–5): a very large volume of an average-strength solution; a sufficient volume of a very strong "hypertonic" solution; a special "high-index" dehydrating arterial solution; an average to strong arterial solution accompanied by a salt coinjection (Epsom salts); an average to strong arterial solution accompanied by a vegetable humectant to help draw moisture out of the tissues into the capillaries.

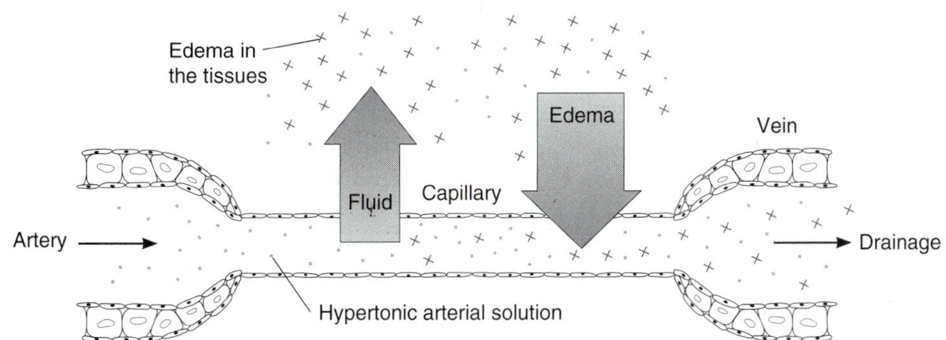

Figure 21–5. Hypertonic arterial solutions and arterial solutions containing large colloid molecules help to draw the edema from the tissues into the circulatory system.

Most bodies with generalized edema exhibit very good circulation. Few clots are found in the drainage from these bodies. There should be good distribution of the arterial solution, probably because the blood was diluted and thinned by the edema during life and after death. Therefore, formation of coagula in the blood vascular system postmortem is minimal.

In the majority of bodies with generalized edema, the embalmer can expect copious drainage and good fluid distribution and, thus, can inject large volumes of arterial solution. There are two means by which the preservative demand (or formaldehyde demand) of the body is met: by injection of strong arterial solution or by injection of a large volume of mild (average) arterial solution.

Injection Site. In the body with generalized edema, it is recommended that both common carotid arteries be raised at the beginning of the embalming. This allows saturation of the trunk without overinjection of the head and separate injection of the head after the trunk has been embalmed (the body can be aspirated prior to injection of the head; features may be set after the trunk has been embalmed and after aspiration).

Drainage Site. The center of blood drainage is the right atrium of the heart. If the right internal jugular vein is used for drainage, instruments can be inserted directly into the right atrium and the head and neck drained from this site. Some embalmers prefer to drain from both the right and the left internal jugular veins when preparing a body with severe facial edema. Continuous drainage encourages removal of edematous fluids from the body.

Rate of Flow. All embalming should begin at a slow rate of flow. Once distribution has been established the embalmer can increase the rate of flow to ensure good distribution to distal body areas.

Interrupted Injection. It is very important in removing edematous fluids from the tissue spaces to allow the embalming fluid, once injected, time to bring about osmotic exchange wherein the edematous fluids move into the capillaries and the preservatives move from the capillaries into the tissue spaces. After injecting $1\frac{1}{2}$ to 2 gallons, stop injection for one-half hour to allow these physical exchanges to occur. Then inject about $\frac{1}{2}$ to 1 gallon and again stop and allow the physical exchange. Massage and squeeze the limbs from their distal portion toward the heart to encourage drainage of the edematous fluids from the veins into the blood drainage. Elevation of the arms and legs also encourages the edematous fluids to move into the large veins. The injection of additional arterial solution after a rest period helps to force edematous fluid out of the vascular system into the drainage.

Arterial Solutions

Arterial Solution 1. A very large volume of a mild or average (standard) arterial solution is used. By today's standards, the strength of this solution would be 1.5 to 2.0% formaldehyde (approximately 8 ounces of a 25-index arterial fluid is used to make a gallon of arterial solution). Continuous drainage is established with the injection of the solution. It is recommended that fluid dye be added to the last gallon to trace the distribution of the arterial solution. It is not uncommon to inject at least 2 to 3 gallons of arterial solution into each leg of the autopsied body with generalized edema. The theory is that injection of large volumes of mild solution ensures good distribution of the solution and instills into the body a large volume of preservative, but at the same time washes as much of the edema as possible out of the tissues. To accomplish the fluid removal, a steady to fast rate of flow is recommended along with continuous or concurrent drainage. If the embalmer feels that preservation is inadequate, it is recommended that he or she add several ounces of a high-index special-purpose arterial fluid to the embalming solution and make use of intermittent drainage to ensure that a sufficient amount of preservative solution remains in the tissues.

Arterial Solution 2. A very strong (or astringent) arterial solution is used. Some of the high-index fluids are accompanied by instructions on their use for embalming bodies with edema. The solutions for edema are generally quite strong, and dilution occurs when the arterial solution mixes with the edema in the tissue spaces. Arterial solution 2 should be used when the embalmer feels that circulation will not be good. As previously stated, circulation is generally good in bodies with generalized edema. There may be long delays, however, between death and embalming, and signs of decomposition may already be noticed. Use of large volumes of mild solution is not advised for these bodies. It is important to establish preservation first, then to dry the tissues. These strong solutions help both to preserve the tissues and to remove the edema. As these solutions are hypertonic relative to the moist tissues, the edematous fluids in the tissues are drawn back into the capillaries and, thus, removed with the drainage. It has been stated that use of these strong or astringent solutions is advised when the body with edema has been dead for a long period. Many of the capillaries are broken, so it is very difficult to inject arterial solution without causing even more swelling than already exists. Therefore, the strongest fluids possible should reach the tissues to establish preservation; injection of a large fluid volume would result in distortion from the swelling caused by the broken circulatory system. The embalmer's goal is delivery of the least amount necessary of the strongest arterial fluid. Knowledge of the cause of the edema is also important (e.g., renal failure, or burns). Kidney wastes in the tissues neutralize preservative and necessitate use of strong solution. Concurrent drainage can be instituted with this solution. The embalmer, however, may wish to use some form of restricted drainage during injection of the last gallon to ensure solution retention. Cavity embalming can be delayed a short time to ensure fluid diffusion and saturation of the tissues. Again, fluid dye is recommended so the embalmer can see where the arterial solution has distributed. Firming may be minimal in these preparations. Firming of the tissues and drying of the skin are not dependable signs of arterial distribution. Areas that do not receive adequate solution should be arterially embalmed separately or treated by surface or hypodermic embalming techniques.

Arterial Solution 3. Some fluid companies manufacture special-purpose high-index fluids designed specifically to preserve and dry tissues with edema. Some companies further describe these arterial fluids as either dehydrating or nondehydrating. For treatment of the body with generalized edema, the dehydrating fluid is preferred. These high-index fluids are especially useful in the embalming of bodies dead from second-degree burns or liver or renal failure. Directions on the bottle should be followed to ensure proper dilution of the arterial solutions. The quantity of fluid injected depends on the size and weight of the body, the dilution effected within the body by the edema present, the amount of edema present, and the distribution of embalming solution. Fluid dyes can be used to trace the distribution of arterial fluid. Use of coinjection fluid depends on the recommendations of the fluid manufacturer. Because these special fluids are strong, have a dehydrating effect, and must be injected in a large volume, it is strongly urged that the restricted cervical injection be implemented (raising both right and left common carotid arteries). If the head and the facial tissues have not been affected by the edema the embalmer will, no doubt, want to use a standard arterial solution to embalm the head. Keep in mind that renal failure also affects the facial tissues; these tissues will contain nitrogenous waste, which neutralizes formaldehyde. Be certain that an adequate amount of sufficient-strength arterial solution is injected into the head.

Arterial Solution 4. Arterial solution 4 works to reduce the presence of edema by the use of dehydrating coinjection chemicals. These coinjection products are designed to be injected with a preservative arterial solution. They are generally added to the last gallon of arterial solution. The amount of chemical to use and the time at which the chemical should be added to the preservative solution will depend upon the severity of the edema. These coinjection chemicals increase the osmotic qualities of the arterial solution either through the addition of salts or large colloidal molecules. These products are especially effective for facial edema. Facial edema responds well for not only is there a chemical drying of the tissues by the coinjection chemical, but elevation of the head allows for gravitation of the edematous fluids from the facial tissues. Firm massage and pressure should also be applied to the facial tissues especially after the chemical has been injected. Aspiration of the cavities can help to relieve additional pressure caused by edema in the thoracic and abdominal cavities. This also helps edema to drain from the facial tissues. Restricted cervical injection is advised when using this method of treatment for facial edema.

The hands respond well to the use of a dehydrating coinjection fluid. They should be well massaged during and after arterial injection. Elevation will assist in the movement of the edematous fluids from the hands to the upper arms. Sectional injection using the coinjection fluid solution may be necessary.

Manufacturers' instructions as to the quantity and methods of use of these fluids should be followed. Overdehydration of the face and hands is always a possibility. Postembalming tissue building can be used to correct this problem.

Arterial Solution 5. Arterial solution 5 works to reduce the swollen condition brought about by the edema. It is made using Epsom salts, which create a hypertonic solution. This hypertonic solution sets up an osmotic gradient that draws the edema from the tissue spaces toward this concentrated salt solution in the capillaries. The embalmer may wish to begin the embalming and clear the blood vascular system with either strong or average arterial solution. Injection continues until the blood drainage clears and the distribution appears uniform. When strong dehydrating solutions such as this arterial mixture are used, it is very important that both common carotid arteries be raised as the primary injection site. In this manner, the head can be separately injected. If the head is grossly distended by the edema, arterial solution 5 should help to remove it. The following arterial solution is suggested.

Fill a container with half a gallon of cool water; add as much Epsom salts as can be dissolved. Thoroughly stir this solution. Next, add 4 to 6 ounces of a high-index (25–35) arterial fluid. Pour this solution into the embalming machine but do not pour any of the undissolved salt that may have settled to the bottom of the container.

Inject this solution into the area affected by the edema. Massage the tissues (after they are injected). Assume that the head and face are grossly distended with edema (often seen after cardiac surgery or aortic repair). First inject the left side of the head; then inject the right side. Massage the swollen tissues downward to encourage the edema to drain through the veins. (Some embalmers allow this solution to remain in place approximately one-half hour and then reinject with a strong arterial solution. Thus the Epsom salt solution remains in the capillaries long enough to draw the edematous fluid from the tissue spaces. This edematous fluid is then flushed away by the reinjection.) Massage plays a very large role in the success of this process. This is an excellent technique to use on an arm or leg grossly distended with edema. Care should be taken to keep the solution thoroughly stirred, for it is easy to clog the delivery lines of the embalming machine. If this should occur, flush the machine with warm water to dissolve the Epsom salt crystals. An aspirator hose can be attached to the delivery line to pull the crystallized materials out of the machine. After using a solution containing Epsom salts, always flush the machine with warm water. This very old technique can be quite effective (Figure 21–6). The Epsom salt solution works best on the facial tissues, especially when the edema is re-

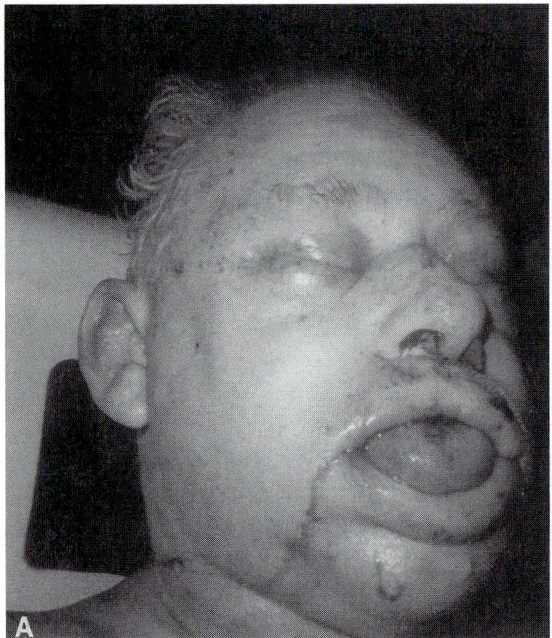

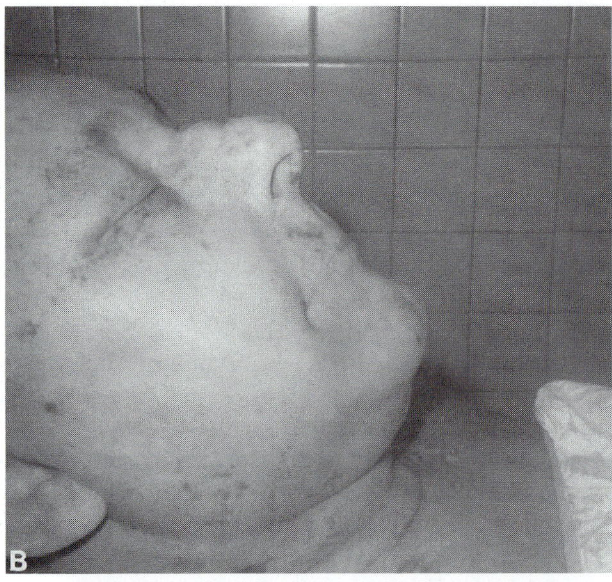

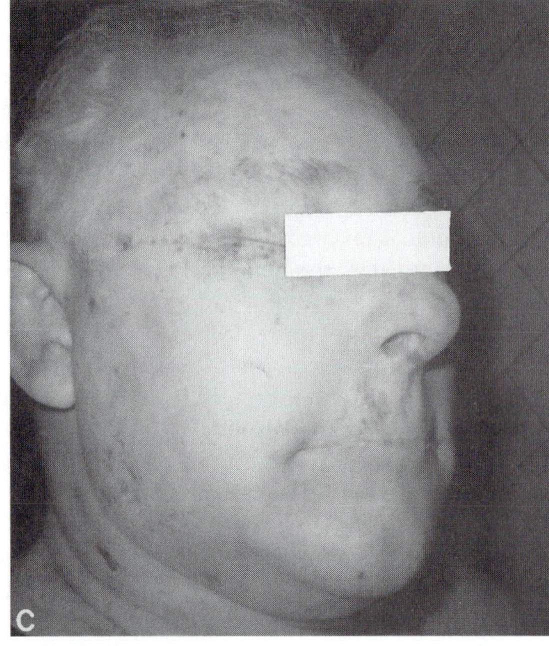

Figure 21–6. Facial edema after repair of an aortic aneurysm. The swelling was reduced by the addition of Epsom salts to the arterial solution. **A.** Facial edema prior to injection. **B and C.** Reduction of the facial edema at completion of the embalming.

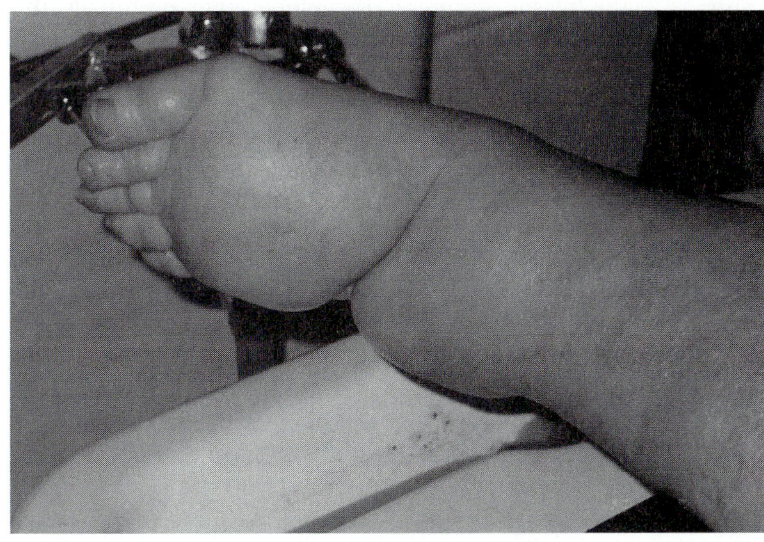

Figure 21-7. Extreme edema of lower extremities.

cent (e.g., recent surgical patients, heart or aortic surgery). This process does not work well when the edema has been present for a long period (e.g., trauma cases, drug therapy cases).

Arterial Solution 6. Arterial solution 6, like the previous solutions, makes use of the osmotic gradient between the fluids in the capillaries and the edematous fluids in the tissue spaces. Arterial solution 6 consists of a preservative arterial fluid and a coinjection humectant. Humectants, when used in small quantities, add or maintain moisture in the tissues. When large quantities of humectants are used, the arterial solution becomes very viscous. The large molecules of the humectant draw the moisture from the tissue spaces into the capillaries. Once there, the edematous fluids exit with the drainage. The humectant must be a *vegetable* and not a lanolin (or animal) humectant. The fluid manufacturers should be consulted for specifics. One suggestion is to use 6 to 8 ounces of 20- to 25-index preservative to make a gallon of arterial solution. To this solution add 20 to 24 ounces of humectant. Inject at a moderate rate of flow, thus allowing time for the exchange to occur. Continuous drainage is necessary. Stopping the drainage could waterlog the tissues if the humectant is forced from the capillaries into the tissue spaces. Before this solution is injected it is best to establish good fluid distribution by injecting a well-coordinated arterial solution of sufficient strength; a 2% arterial solution (or slightly higher) should distribute well. If desired, a coinjection chemical can also be used in equal amounts with the arterial fluid. Fluid dye added to the solution will be a good indicator of fluid distribution. After the blood vascular system is perfused with this first injection, the humectant solution can follow to dehydrate the edematous tissue.*

▶ LOCAL TREATMENT FOR EDEMA

Legs

One of the most frequently affected areas is the legs. When only the legs are affected by edema, it is best to embalm the body with a standard-strength arterial solution. This, of course, depends on the general condition of the body. The important point is not to prepare a strong arterial solution for the entire body based on the fact that edema is present only in the legs (Figure 21-7).

After embalming the body, raise the femoral or iliac vessels and separately inject the legs using one of the arterial solutions just discussed. If the edema is severe, after arterial injection use the trocar to pierce the upper thighs beneath the inguinal ligaments while embalming the cavities. Elevate the legs and, if desired, wrap with an elastic bandage beginning at the foot and moving up the leg. This pushes some of the edema into the pelvic cavity from which it can later be aspirated. The legs should be elevated several hours to make this treatment effective.

The legs can also be injected with cavity fluid using a trocar. This is done *after* arterial injection of the legs. The cavity fluid is placed (undiluted) in the injection machine, and the delivery tube is attached to an infant

* Several articles published in the 1930s indicate success with the removal of edema using glycerine and even corn syrup to make a solution that promotes dehydration of tissues.

trocar. The inside of the calf is a good point of entry. From this point, the lower leg and thigh can be reached. Saturate the leg with the cavity fluid and place a plastic stocking on it to ensure surface preservation. The leg can first be painted with autopsy gel and embalming powder sprinkled inside the stocking. The powder and the gel assist in preservation of the leg. When edema is more extensive and affects the hips and buttocks, plastic coveralls or pants should also be used. When shoulders and trunk walls are affected along with legs and arms, use of a unionall is advised, for it covers all these areas.

Arms

When only the arms and hands are affected with edema (as found after any surgery in the axillary area) the arm can be separately injected after the body has been embalmed. The hand and arm can be elevated to gravitate some of the edema into the upper arm. Wrinkling of the back of the hand now becomes a problem.

A wide piece of duct tape can be placed across the palm of the hand to "pull" the wrinkles from the back of the hand. If distal areas such as the fingers become badly wrinkled, a small amount of tissue builder can be injected into each finger. Some wrinkling may be removed by the injection of tissue builder; good points of needle entry would be between the fingers. If there are intravenous or needle punctures on the back of the hand, the embalmer can remove a considerable amount of edema through these openings by squeezing and then sealing the openings with a drop or two of super adhesive.

Edema of the Trunk

After death, edematous fluid gravitates to the dependent areas. Sectional arterial injection of the trunk is not as easily accomplished as sectional injection of a leg or arm. When edema is present in the dependent trunk areas (e.g., shoulders, buttocks, lateral walls), direct hypodermic injection will serve best to increase the preservation of these regions. If the arterial preservation of the trunk walls appears insufficient, hypodermic injection using a concentrated preservative chemical will help to insure better preservation. An infant trocar can be inserted into the lateral walls on each side of the body. The point of entry can be along the right or left midaxillary line in the soft tissues inferior to the rib cage. From this point of entry, the trocar should be able to reach as far up as the axilla and also as far down as the buttocks. Cavity fluid or very concentrated arterial solution can be injected through the embalming machine. This added embalming measure, of course, is done after arterial injection of the body. Coveralls or a unionall can be placed on the body, and a liberal amount of preservative powder can be sprinkled into the plastic garment. Remember that eventually this edema will pass through the skin of the back and dependent trunk walls. This exit of fluid can occur even before disposition of the body. It is essential to protect the clothing and the interior of the casket by use of the plastic garments.

Ascites (Edema of the Abdominal Cavity)

Ascites can exist almost unnoticed until the embalmer begins to aspirate the cavity or it can severely distend the abdominal cavity, because the edematous fluid is located within the cavity and around the visceral organs. It is unaffected by arterial fluid treatment or blood drainage. Ascites will not dilute arterial fluid, because arterial solution and the edema in the abdominal cavity do not come into contact.

When ascites is present and noticeable, do not mix arterial solutions in the belief that ascites will be a secondary dilution for arterial fluid. Ascites *will* be a diluting factor for cavity fluid. When ascites is present and the abdomen is very tense prior to arterial embalming, the pressure in the abdominal cavity may be sufficient to interfere with arterial distribution. More importantly, the pressure can interfere with blood drainage. This pressure is created not only by the enormous amount of fluid in the abdominal cavity (often several gallons) but also by possible gases in the intestinal tract. The pressure should be removed prior to arterial injection. Several techniques can be used:

1. Using a scalpel, make a small opening in the abdominal cavity and insert a drain tube or a trocar from which the point has been removed. Many embalmers prefer to make this incision in the inguinal or hypogastric area of the abdominal wall. At this lower point more liquid can be removed from the cavity. Attach the aspirating hose to the drainage tube or trocar for delivery of the edematous fluids directly into the drainage or collection system.
2. Insert a trocar keeping the point just under the anterior abdominal wall. Pierce the transverse colon to release gases. Attach the aspirating hose to the trocar.
3. Make a small incision over the area of the transverse colon, exposing the colon (which can be opened). The incision is an outlet for the edema. This technique is most unsanitary and, if possible, should be avoided.

When the distension of the abdomen is not severe enough to restrict the flow of arterial solution or interfere with blood drainage, the ascites can be removed during the normal period for aspiration of the abdominal cavity.

Hydrothorax

In hydrothorax, edema is present in the space between the wall of the thoracic cavity and the lung. This condition is not easy to recognize because the rib cage cannot expand like the abdomen does when edema is present. This condition can be expected in bodies dead from heart disease or pneumonia. Often, there is some distension of the neck, and, very frequently, both the face and neck exhibit a great amount of livor mortis after death. Aspiration of the thoracic cavity removes the fluid. Aspiration is generally done after arterial embalming. The trocar should be directed to the posterior portions of the thorax, where the fluid will have gravitated. It is possible to remove one or more gallons of fluid from the thorax when this condition is present.

If it is necessary to relieve some of this pressure prior to or during arterial injection, a trocar can be introduced from the standard point of trocar entry and guided along the lateral wall of the abdomen into the thoracic cavity. This provides a drainage outlet for the fluid, but does not rupture any large arteries or veins. When hydrothorax is suspected, use the common carotid artery for injection and drain from the right internal jugular vein. This is the best location from which to drain the head and arms. Aspiration should immediately follow arterial injection. Very often distension of the neck will diminish and any swelling that may have occurred in the facial tissues will be reduced.

Hydrocele

In the male, the scrotum can become distended with edematous fluid. Quite frequently, insufficient arterial solution reaches the tissues of the scrotum, which can be a site for decomposition. This condition is treated during aspiration and injection of the body cavities, after arterial injection. During aspiration pass the trocar over the pubic symphysis and pubic bone and enter the scrotum. Place a towel around the scrotum and apply pressure. This forces the edematous fluid through the channels that have been made with the trocar and into the pelvic cavity. The scrotum can then be filled with undiluted cavity fluid to ensure preservation. Care should be taken not to puncture the scrotum with the trocar. It can be difficult to close the puncture and to stop the drainage of edematous fluids. Use super glue or a trocar button for closure. If the leakage cannot be stopped, drain the edematous fluids and the cavity fluids that were injected. Let the drainage continue several hours.

Hydrocephalus

When edematous fluid fills the cranial cavity during fetal development, the head is grossly distended. Some individuals survive after birth and live many years with this condition. In the unautopsied infant, it is necessary to drain some of this fluid, or very rapid decomposition of the brain and fluids of the cranial cavity may occur. Drainage can be established by passing a large hypodermic needle through the nostril and directing it through the anterior portion of the cribriform plate of the ethmoid bone. This process should be done after arterial embalming.

Several ounces of undiluted cavity fluid or phenol solution can be injected in the same manner as the fluid was aspirated. The nostrils should be tightly packed with cotton to protect against leakage. When there has been ossification of the bones of the cranial cavity, it is not always necessary to aspirate and inject the cavity. Leakage must always be considered when the cranial cavity is aspirated.

▶ SPECIAL CONDITIONS

Burned Bodies

Edema accompanies burns, especially second-degree burns. Generally, these victims live days or weeks after the burns. Blistering of the skin is characteristic of second-degree burns. The embalmer, however, very rarely sees the blistering condition. The blisters have been opened and drained and preparations placed on the denuded skin area to encourage cellular growth and skin replacement. Death usually results from renal failure. Because of the skin damage, many waste products that normally leave the body via the skin are retained in the blood. As a result, the kidneys cannot handle the wastes that rapidly build up in the body. These bodies are often so grossly distended with edema that the face is not recognizable.

The first concern of the embalmer is preservation. These bodies have a very high preservative demand. Restricted cervical injection with drainage from the right internal jugular vein is recommended for these bodies when they are not autopsied. Astringent arterial solutions should be injected. Fluid dye can be added to the arterial solution to identify those body areas receiving arterial solution. Areas not reached by the arterial solution are best treated by hypodermic injection of cavity fluid or an astringent arterial solution. These bodies are very difficult to handle as they are often covered with various ointments. Washing the skin surface with a good disinfectant soap removes surface medications and debris.

Long open incisions are the result of one method used to treat burn patients. The embalmer cannot suture these long incisions. The surface can be thoroughly dried after it has been bathed with a soapy solution. Exposure to air also helps to dry the skin surface. These bodies can be placed in a unionall; this plastic garment covers all body areas except the

TABLE 21–2. SUMMARY OF EDEMA

Edema	Definition	Problems	Treatment
Solid	Edema within body cells	Swollen tissues; difficult preservation	Must be excised for reduction Strong arterial solutions; coinjection fluids
Pitting	Edema in tissue spaces, between the cells	Distension; fluid dilution; leakage; difficult preservation	May be gravitated; use strong arterial solutions; may be punctured and drained; use plastic garments to protect from leakage
Anasarca	Generalized edema in all body tissues	Leakage; distension; arterial fluid dilution	Strong arterial solutions; hypodermic and surface embalming; plastic garments; gravitation; puncture and drain
Edema of face	Edema in facial tissues	Swollen tissues, eyelids, and tongue	Restricted cervical injection; strong coordinated arterial solutions; possible use of salt or high-index solutions to reduce swelling; elevate head; channel with trocar neck area for drainage into thorax; surface weights for eyes and lips; surface and hypodermic embalming to ensure preservation with cavity fluid
Edema of hands	Edema in tissues of the backs of the hands	Swollen tissues; possible leakage from intravenous punctures; wrinkles after removal	Sectional injection from axillary artery; surface packs with cavity fluid to ensure preservation; bleach any discolorations; elevate to gravitate edema into arm
Edema of legs	Edema in thighs and lower legs	Dilution of arterial fluid; leakage	Sectional injection of legs from femoral or external iliac artery; use of strong arterial solutions; use of salt solutions or dehydrating solutions to remove edema; hypodermic injection with undiluted cavity fluid; surface treatment using autopsy gel; plastic stockings containing embalming powder and autopsy gel; elevate to gravitate edema into abdominal cavity; puncture and drain.
Pulmonary edema	Edema in the alveoli of the lungs	Purge	Aspiration and injection of lungs
Hydrothorax	Edema in the thoracic cavity	Purge; dilution of cavity fluid; pressure can cause venous congestion of neck and face; facial distension	Aspiration; injection of cavity fluid; careful draining prior to arterial injection
Ascites	Edema of abdominal cavity	Pressure can cause purge of stomach contents; anal purge; dilution of cavity fluid	Aspiration and injection of undiluted cavity fluid; preembalming draining via trocar or drainage tube; reaspiration and reinjection
Hydropericardium	Edema of pericardial cavity	Dilution of cavity fluid Pressure could cause drainage problems	Aspiration and injection of undiluted cavity fluid
Hydrocele	Edema of scrotum	Leakage; dilution of arterial fluid; distension; problems in dressing	Channel with trocar to drain into abdominal cavity; inject via trocar undiluted cavity fluid; surface coating with autopsy gel; use of plastic garments and embalming powder
Hydrocephalus	Edema of cranial cavity	Purge in infant	Drain in infant via ethmoid foramen; inject cavity fluid via ethmoid foramen

hands, neck, and face. The body surface can be liberally covered with embalming powder. In addition, the skin surface can be painted with autopsy gel, or cavity compresses can be applied before the body is clothed in the unionall. Strips of sheeting or gauze can be used to wrap extremities when long incisions are present.

Leakage can be a major problem with these bodies. Allowing the body to drain as much as possible and to air-dry prior to placing plastic garments on the body diminishes the amount of leakage into the plastic garments after the body is casketed. Frequently, these persons have had a tracheotomy. It may be very difficult to close the tracheotomy opening if the neck area was affected by the burns. In these cases, after aspiration of the body, fill the opening with cotton and incision seal powder and liberally apply surface glue over the opening.

Renal Failure

Chronic renal failure brings about an increase in toxic wastes (urea, uric acid, ammonia, and creatine) in the blood and tissues of the body. Retention of these wastes results in acidosis (the tissues become acidic). Over time, there is a decrease in cardiac function leading to congestive heart failure and pulmonary edema. Gastric ulcerations occur and gastrointestinal bleeding can be expected. The patient becomes anemic and the skin turns sallow as a result of the retention of urochrome.

This condition is very important to the embalmer. Bodies with renal failure rapidly decompose. The edema present dilutes the arterial solution. The waste products in the bloodstream and tissues neutralize the formaldehyde. The color can deepen after embalming and become more pronounced, creating a cosmetic problem. Tissues do not firm normally, for the proteins of the body have been altered. Such bodies have a very high preservative demand. It is important that the embalmer use strong arterial solutions. Special-purpose high-index fluids are recommended. Preinjection should be avoided if there has been a delay between death and embalming or if the embalmer feels circulation may be difficult to establish. Restricted cervical injection with drainage from the right internal jugular vein is recommended.

A very strong arterial solution should be used. Dye can be added to the arterial solution not only to trace the distribution of fluid, but also to counterstain the sallow color produced by the urochrome in the tissues. In many bodies that have been in chronic renal failure, other visceral organ damage has taken place. The body may be very jaundiced, and ecchymoses from disease and medications may be seen on the skin surface. Emaciation and protein damage may have occurred in the tissues. The embalmer will have problems with discolorations, firming, and preservation.

The most important objective in embalming these bodies is good preservation. Firming is not always necessary. Tissue can be preserved without being intensely firmed. Discolorations are secondary and can always be treated with cosmetics.

Cavity embalming is very important after renal failure. Frequently, bleeding has occurred in the gastrointestinal tract, providing an excellent medium for bacterial proliferation and a good site for the formation of gas. It may also be a source of purge. Thorough aspiration of the cavities is necessary. The embalmer may note arterial solution in the cavities or hollow viscera where bleeding occurred in life. A minimum of two to three bottles of undiluted cavity fluid should be injected. Several hours later, the body should be reaspirated and reinjected with cavity fluid. Renal failure is a condition that the embalmer must learn to recognize. If it is not detected, the body can rapidly decompose. **Check the death certificate carefully if available for references to renal involvement.** Areas not receiving adequate arterial solution should be sectionally injected. If necessary, undiluted cavity fluid can be injected hypodermically, or compresses of undiluted cavity fluid or autopsy gel can be applied to the surface to ensure preservation.

The embalming complications associated with chronic renal failure can be summarized:

1. Decomposition occurs rapidly.
2. Acidosis alters the reaction between proteins and the preservative.
3. The body appears sallow because urochrome is present in the tissues.
4. Sites of gastrointestinal bleeding may be sites of arterial fluid loss and sources of purge.
5. Edema dilutes the arterial fluid.
6. Uremic wastes in the blood and tissues neutralize preservatives.
7. Skin infections may be caused by uremic pruritis.

See Table 21–2 for a summary of edema.

▶ KEY TERMS AND CONCEPTS FOR STUDY AND DISCUSSION

1. Define the following terms:
   anasarca
   ascites
   concurrent drainage
   dehydration
   edema

hydrocephalus
hydrothorax
hypertonic arterial solution
hypotonic arterial solution
intermittent drainage
osmosis
pitting edema

2. Discuss what treatments can be employed to help restore moisture to a body that is badly dehydrated during embalming.
3. List some of the conditions, both antemortem and postmortem, that cause dehydration.
4. Discuss some of the complications created by the presence of skeletal edema.
5. Discuss the arterial solutions and embalming techniques that can be used to remove edema from the skeletal tissues.
6. Discuss the complications that arise in the preparation of a body dead from renal failure.

▶ BIBLIOGRAPHY

Elkins J. Major body elevation as a technique for the reduction of swelling in the face and hands of embalmed bodies. In: *Champion Expanding Encyclopedia.* Springfield, OH: Champion Chemical Co.; 1985:No. 554.

Henson RW. Controlling the moisture content of the tissues. *Professional Embalmer,* November 1940.

Henson RW. Controlling the moisture content of the tissues. *Professional Embalmer,* October 1940.

Regulating the Moisture Content of Tissues. Wilmette, IL: Hizone Supplements; 1938:11.

Sheldon H. *Boyd's Introduction to the Study of Disease.* 10th ed. Philadelphia: Lea & Febiger;1988.

Shor MM. Can magnesium sulfate be safely used to rid body of fluid in lower extremities? *Casket and Sunnyside,* July 1965.

Sturb CG. Distribution and diffusion. *Funeral Directors Journal,* May 1939.

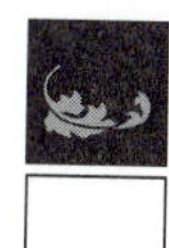

CHAPTER 22
VASCULAR CONSIDERATIONS

The blood vascular system is the distribution route for the embalming solution. Any pathological change that obstructs this delivery system either completely blocks or reduces flow of arterial solution to a body region.

As people age, many degenerative changes can occur in the circulatory system. Although the immediate cause of death may not be heart or blood vessel disease, such a condition can greatly influence the embalming procedure. Likewise, drugs given for the treatment of heart or vascular diseases may have more influence on the embalming procedure than the condition of the diseased vessels.

The embalmer is concerned primarily with intravascular conditions, diseases or tissue changes in the walls of or within the blood vessels. The arteries are the vessels that carry the embalming solution to the capillaries. At the capillaries some of the arterial solution will leave the vascular system to enter the interstitial spaces, where it will come into contact with the body cells and cellular proteins. Arteries have three layers:

- *Intima:* the inner lining of endothelial cells, which continue to form the walls of the capillaries and then the inner walls of the veins and arteries (this endothelial layer of cells lines the entire blood vascular system)
- *Media:* the middle layer composed of muscle cells and elastic tissue
- *Adventitia:* the outer layer composed mostly of connective tissue

The cavity of the vessel is called the *lumen.* Narrowing or obstruction of the lumen is of great concern to the embalmer, because it can decrease or stop flow of arterial solution to a body area. Intravascular problems can also result in breaks or tears in vessels. These can be very small ruptures such as petechiae or major ruptures such as aortic aneurysms.

Table 22–1 lists intravascular arterial conditions that can limit the distribution of arterial solution to various body areas. Arteriosclerosis and arterial coagula are the problems most frequently encountered by the embalmer.

Preinjection fluid should not be used when it is thought it will be difficult to establish arterial solution distribution. Swelling could result later when the preservative solution is injected, as the system would be filled with the preinjection solution. Preinjection fluid should be used only if circulation is thought to be good; in such cases, it maintains the good distribution and drainage. Many persons who had vascular diseases were given blood thinners and anticoagulants. These bodies generally exhibit good arterial solution distribution and few or no clots in the drainage.

▶ ARTERIOSCLEROSIS

Almost any body over the age of 30 may exhibit arteriosclerosis. Most people think of this degenerative condition as occurring in old age. Many persons who die from heart disease in their midfifties exhibit more sclerosis than the 90-year-old. Of the vessels used for embalming, the femoral artery is the most likely to be affected by arteriosclerosis. Thus, use of the common carotid artery as the primary site for injection is recommended.

The embalmer encounters three types of arteriosclerosis (Fig. 22–1):

- *Type 1:* The inner wall of the artery is hardened and thickened but the lumen is well defined and large. These vessels can usually be used for arterial injection. This condition is frequently observed in the autopsied body when the common iliac arteries are exposed.
- *Type 2:* The lumen is quite reduced in size and pushed to one side of the artery. The lumen can usually be identified and a small arterial tube can be used for injection.
- *Type 3:* The artery is completely occluded. If ischemia or gangrene is *not* present in the area supplied (e.g., the leg), the collateral circulation may have increased to supply blood to the limb, *or* there may be minute paths in the occluded

TABLE 22–1. CONDITIONS RESULTING FROM INTRAVASCULAR DISEASE PROCESSES

Vascular Condition or Injury	Description	Embalming Concern
Advanced decomposition	Breakdown of the body tissues	Arteries are one of the last "organs" to decompose. Some circulation may be possible. Expect a large number of intravascular clots. Distribution is very poor. Capillary decomposition causes rapid swelling of the tissues.
Aneurysm	Localized dilation of an artery	If aneurysm ruptures, fluid cannot distribute.
Arteriosclerosis	Hardening of the arteries	Vessel may not be suitable as an injection site. Narrowed arteries may easily trap arterial coagula.
Arteritis	Inflammation of an artery	Artery may narrow, resulting in poor distribution of arterial solution. Artery may also weaken and rupture from pressure of injection.
Asphyxiation	Insufficient oxygen supply	Right side of heart is congested (poor drainage). Purging can result as blood flows back into lungs instead of draining. Tissue is cyanotic. Intense livor mortis is present in neck and facial tissues. Blood may remain liquid. Capillary permeability is increased. Swelling could easily occur.
Atheroma, atherosclerosis	Patchy or nodular thickening of the intima of an artery	Flow of arterial solution may be restricted or occluded. Arterial coagula may be easily trapped during injection. Vessel is poor injection site.
Burns	Local or general damage to tissue from heat	Capillaries constrict resulting in extensive coagulation. Distribution of arterial solution may be reduced. Large burns can result in kidney failure, with retention of nitrogenous wastes, thus increasing the preservative demand of the tissues.
Cerebrovascular accident	"Stroke" caused by a clot or the rupture of a small artery in the brain.	Vasoconstriction may occur on one side of the body, reducing the distribution of arterial solution.
Clots or coagula	Antemortem or postmortem clumping of blood elements	Arterial clots can block or reduce fluid flow to a body region, and may *not* be removed through drainage. Venous clots may often be removed; if clots are unmovable, swelling and discoloration can result.
Congestive heart failure	Decreased heart function	Venous congestion and clotting and cyanosis occur. Legs and feet are edematous. Capillary permeability increases. Tissues can easily swell.
Corrosive poisons	Toxic and corrosive chemicals	If poisons are swallowed, purge can usually be expected. Corrosive action may destroy blood vessels causing loss of solution or blood into the gastrointestinal tract.
Diabetes	An endocrine disease affecting the control of blood glucose levels	Poor peripheral circulation can reduce solution distribution. Gangrenous areas require surface and/or hypodermic embalming treatments. Dehydration frequently occurs. Breakdown of protein results in poor firming of tissues.
Emboli	Detached blood clot	Blockage of a small artery interrupts solution distribution. Venous emboli can block drainage.
Esophageal varices	Swollen, tortuous veins caused by a stagnation of blood and generally seen in the superficial veins	Drainage may be difficult to establish. Rupture and massive purge may occur.
Extracerebral clot (stroke)	A clot, usually in the carotid artery, that stops blood supply to the brain	The clot can occlude the artery, making it impossible for arterial solution to flow to one side of the face. Blockage may occlude the carotid so it cannot be used as an injection site. Resulting stroke may cause vasoconstriction on one side of the body, reducing arterial solution distribution.

Febrile disease	A disease or condition accompained by an elevation of body temperature	Decomposition may be speeded. Dehydration is possible. Blood coagulates and causes congestion. Distribution and drainage may be hard to establish.
Freezing (postmortem)	Cooling of the body to the point where ice crystals form in body tissues	Small vessels and tissues easily swell on injection of solution.
Gangrene (dry)	Poor arterial circulation into an area of the body, causing death of body cells	Distribution of arterial solution into the affected area is impossible to establish. Surface and hypodermic treatment is needed.
Gangrene (moist)	Occlusion of veins draining a body area that becomes the site of bacterial infection	Very strong fluid must be injected into the general area arterially. The affected necrotic tissues require hypodermic and surface treatments.
Gunshot wounds	Entry of a foreign missile into the body	Arterial system may rupture. Multisite injection may be needed. Conditions vary depending on location of wound. Blood loss may result in very little drainage. Bodies are usually autopsied.
Hanging	Asphyxiation resulting from exertion of pressure against the large vessels of the neck	Livor mortis is intense *or* absent in facial tissues. Vessels may be damaged or severed. Restricted cervical injection and jugular drainage are recommended.
Hemorrhage	Loss of blood caused by a break in the vascular system	Blood volume may be quite low so there is little drainage. Livor mortis may be minimal. If hemorrhage is the result of a ruptured artery, arterial solution may be lost to body cavities. Multisite injection may be necessary. If a vein has ruptured, much of the drainage may collect in the body cavity where the hemorrhage occurred. If the stomach or esophageal veins are affected, stomach purge can be expected.
Ischemia	Lack of blood supply to an area, frequently resulting in tissue necrosis	Arterial solution cannot reach the affected tissues. Hypodermic and surface embalming treatments are needed.
Leukemia	Cancer of the tissues that form white blood cells	Purpura are observed over the thorax, arms, and abdomen. Edema may be present. Circulation of arterial solution and drainage may be difficult to establish.
Mutilation	Traumatic tissue injuries	Several arteries may result in difficulty in establishing distribution. Multipoint injections may be needed.
Phlebitis	Inflammation of a vein	Edema may be present in the area. Blood does not easily drain from the area and discolorations may result.
Pneumonia	Acute inflammation of the lung	Broken lung capillaries can result in lung purge. Fever speeds the onset of rigor and decomposition. Congestion may lead to hydrothorax. Distension of the neck can easily occur. Body should be aspirated immediately after arterial injection.
Shock	Sudden vital depression, reduced blood return to the heart	Vasodilation may be present, which can cause swelling. In other types of shock, capillaries constrict and blood congestion occurs in the large veins, making drainage difficult to establish. Capillary congestion may interfere with the distribution and diffusion of arterial solution.
Syphilis	Venereal disease caused by the spirochete *Treponema pallidum*	Aneurysms may occur in arteries. Rupture can make distribution of arterial solution impossible.

(*continued*)

TABLE 22–1. CONDITIONS RESULTING FROM INTRAVASCULAR DISEASE PROCESSES (*Continued*)

Vascular Condition or Injury	Description	Embalming Concern
Thrombosis	Blood clots attached to the inner wall of a blood vessel	Arterial solution distribution may be difficult. If occurring in a vein, drainage may be hard to establish from the affected tissues.
Tuberculosis	Infection of the lungs by *Mycobacterium tuberculosis* that may spread to other organs (e.g., bone, brain, kidney)	When the lungs are affected, cavitation may result; this causes small vessels and capillaries to rupture. There may be a great loss of arterial solution through purging. Purge can be expected. Untreated dehydration and emaciation may be observed.
Tumor	Benign or malignant growth of cells	Pressure may be exerted on the outside of an artery or vein. Distribution to and drainage from an area may be difficult to establish.
Vasoconstriction	Narrowing of a blood vessel	When arteries are affected, as in a "stroke," it may be difficult to supply sufficient arterial solution to the affected side of the body. Multipoint injection may be necessary.

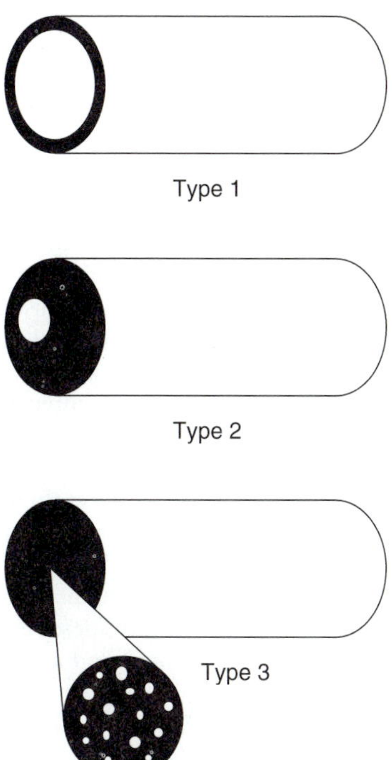

Figure 22–1. Types of arteriosclerosis seen in arteries used for arterial injection.

artery through which the blood can pass. The formation of these paths or canals is called **canalization.** These arteries *cannot* be used for injection.

In the presence of sclerosis, the strength of the arterial solution can be increased if distribution is poor or slow. Use of a stronger solution ensures that sufficient preservative reaches the tissues even if a large amount of solution cannot be injected. Coinjection chemicals may be used to help distribute the preservative solution. Dye can be added to the solution; it will help to indicate what tissues are receiving the arterial solution.

Lowering the hands over the sides of the table and gently but firmly massaging the limbs help to distribute fluid in sclerotic bodies. Begin injection using a very slow rate of flow. After the vascular system is filled, rate of flow can be increased. When multisite injection is used, higher pressures and pulsation can be used to establish local distribution. Once circulation is established, the pressure and the rate of flow can be reduced.

If a femoral vessel must be used, avoid cutting into the artery where an atheroma can be felt. Make the incision a little larger at a point where the vessel is softest. Avoid raising these sclerotic arteries to the surface. Work with them from within the incision. Ligate the arterial tubes in place with an arterial hemostat or thick cotton ligature. Thin linen ligatures may separate and tear the vessel. Use an arterial tube small enough that it easily slips into the lumen.

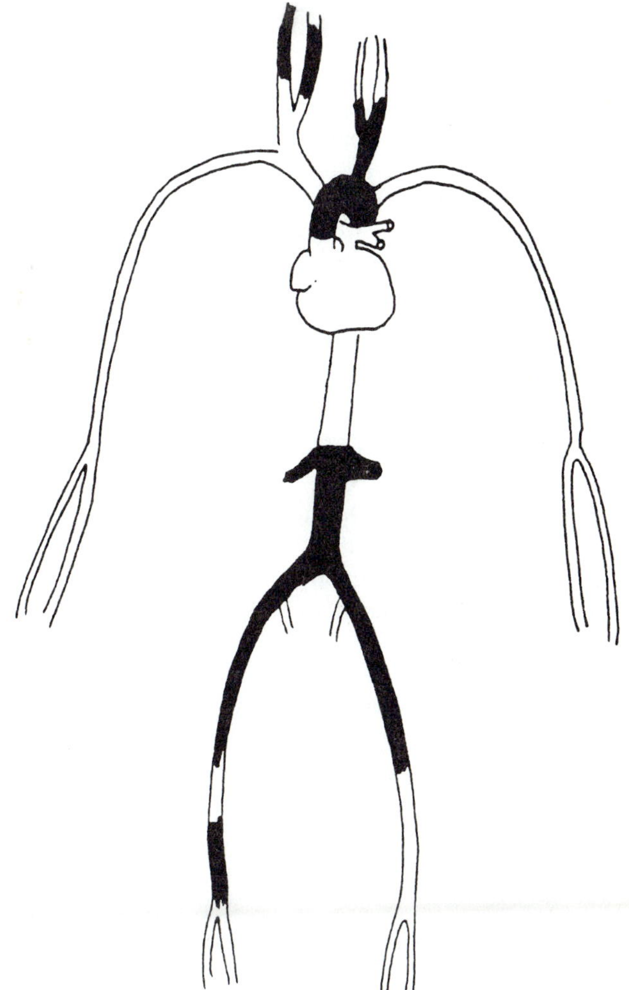

Figure 22–2. Common sites of arteriosclerosis. (Courtesy of H. E. Kazmier.)

A large arterial tube can damage the lumen of the artery and make it unusable as an injection point. If this happens, it will be necessary to hypodermically embalm that portion of the body. A surface preservative and plastic garment can also be applied to the area (Figure 22–2).

▶ AORTIC ANEURYSM

A ruptured aortic aneurysm can seriously affect fluid distribution in the unautopsied body. If surgical repair of the vessel was performed, extreme facial edema can often accompany this surgical repair. In the unautopsied body, determine whether fluid can be distributed from a single-site injection. Inject from the right common carotid artery or use restricted cervical injection.

Often, the femoral vessels in these bodies are sclerotic. Use a strong arterial solution with additional fluid dye as a tracer. Inject slowly. If drainage is established, continue to inject. **If there is no drainage and the abdomen begins to swell, stop the injection** and institute a multipoint injection to embalm the various body areas. The trunk walls may have to be injected by use of an infant trocar with cavity fluid. Often, when the death certificate cites the immediate cause of death as a ruptured aortic aneurysm, it may be possible to embalm the entire body from one injection site.

▶ VALVULAR HEART DISEASES

The following article, "Damage to Aorta May Bring Embalming Problems," written by Murray M. Shor, describes how disease or malformation may prevent the aorta from being the center of arterial solution circulation.

> Because of the position of the aortic semilunar valve, embalmers generally consider the aorta as the center of arterial fluid circulation. In most cases this seems to be true. In the absence of damage to the circulatory system or the heart, it is only after the aorta is filled with fluid that its branches can be expected to receive fluid under any appreciable pressure.
>
> Were it not for the position and construction of the aortic valve, fluid would pass from the ascending portion of the aorta into the left ventricle. Under those conditions the aorta would not be considered the center of embalming fluid circulation. If because of disease or malformation of the aortic semilunar valve fluid did pass into the left ventricle and was confined there by the proper functioning of the mitral valve, the problem would be merely academic. It is when other heart valves are impaired concurrently that embalming problems are created.
>
> ### Anatomy of the Heart
>
> Let us pause here for a brief review of the anatomy of the heart. The functioning valves are the left atrioventricular or mitral, which allows blood to pass from the left atrium to the left ventricle; the right atrioventricular or tricuspid, which opens from the right atrium into the right ventricle; the pulmonary semilunar, a tricuspid valve which opens to allow blood to flow from the right ventricle into the lungs via the pulmonary artery; and the aforementioned aortic semilunar, a tricuspid valve which opens into the aorta from the left ventricle.
>
> During life any one or any combination of these valves can be affected by the same degenerative diseases that affect the arteries. They can also be attacked by bacteria and damaged irreparably or suffer a congenital malformation. In all of these conditions the circulation of blood during life and of the preservative during embalming is substantially altered.
>
> The great strides made by the medical profession in the fields of infant mortality and infectious diseases leave an older population; one more likely to die of degenerative diseases. Also, because of better medical care, some of the infectious diseases that damage the heart, such as diphtheria and rheumatic fever, have been controlled to such an extent that victims of these diseases survive the infectious stage and live many years afterwards, often with a damaged heart valve or valves.
>
> In the United States we have reached a point where one of every two deaths is attributable to cardiovascular disease. Therefore, it behooves the embalmer to become thoroughly familiar with embalming problems associated with these diseases.
>
> In situations where the mitral and aortic semilunar valves are damaged, embalming fluid under pressure will pass from the aorta into the left ventricle and from there into the left atrium. The left atrium receives the pulmonary veins from the lungs. These veins have no valves. Therefore, a fluid in the atrium, under pressure, would pass back into the capillaries of the lung.
>
> ### Lung Purge
>
> During most embalming procedures the pulmonary capillaries also receive fluid from the bronchial arteries, coming from the descending thoracic aorta. When the two fluid masses, one from the bronchial arteries and the other from the pulmonary veins, meet, their collective volume and pressure create a lung purge by virtually squeezing the contents of the hollow portions of the lung out through the trachea.
>
> This event should not cause too much apprehension. The matter thus emanating from the mouth or nostrils is the material the embalmer seeks to remove during routine cavity work.

▶ CONGESTIVE HEART FAILURE

Frequently, death certificates cite congestive heart failure as the primary cause of death. Some complications of the end stage of congestive heart failure are of particular interest to the embalmer:

1. Blood is congested in the right side of the heart.
2. The neck veins are engorged with blood; the facial tissues are dark because of the congestion of blood in the right side of the heart and the veins of the neck.
3. Lips, ears, and fingers are cyanotic.

4. Generalized pitting edema may be present. Edema of the legs and feet is pronounced in most bodies. Ascites may be present.
5. Blood may be more viscous because of an increase in red blood cells (polycythemia).
6. Salt is retained in the body fluids.

The carotid artery is used for injection and the right internal jugular vein for drainage, or restricted cervical injection is employed. This helps to ensure good drainage from the head and the right atrium of the heart. The first gallon of arterial solution is made mild to clear the blood congestion and discolorations. If edema is present, the subsequent gallons should be stronger to meet the preservative demand of the body. If the ascites is severe, some of the fluid can be drained with a trocar or drain tube inserted into the abdominal cavity.

Lowering the arms over the table at the start of arterial injection helps to establish good distribution so the discolorations of the hands and fingers can be cleared. The facial tissues may need to be massaged to clear the blood discolorations. It may be necessary to inject both common carotid arteries. When there is extensive discoloration of the face some embalmers prefer to drain from both the right and left internal jugular veins.

Begin injection at a high enough pressure and rapid enough rate of flow to establish good distribution. Continuous drainage should be used to clear the congested blood. Pressure and rate of flow may be increased as the embalming progresses; the pressure and rate of flow should be sufficient to move arterial solution through the entire body. In the presence of generalized edema, distribution and drainage can be expected to be good.

The liver may be enlarged and its functions decreased. This should improve drainage, as the level of clotting factor in the blood will be low.

Pulmonary edema, often observed in cases of congestive heart failure, may cause lung purge. The purge should be allowed to continue during the embalming process. Cavity treatment and repacking of the nasal cavity with cotton after embalming should correct this condition.

Thorough aspiration is necessary to remove distension in the neck tissues resulting from the engorgement with blood. Remove (as much as possible) the edema that led to the ascites. This edema dilutes cavity fluid. It is best to reaspirate and, if necessary, reinject the cavities several hours after the first treatment. Bodies dead from congestive heart failure should be aspirated immediately after arterial injection to help reduce distension in the neck and facial tissues.

▶ VASODILATION AND VASOCONSTRICTION

Sometimes, the dye used to trace the distribution of arterial solution indicates that one side of the body has received a large amount of solution and the other side a small amount. This difference is often evident down the midline of the body. This unequal distribution of arterial solution frequently occurs after death from cerebrovascular accident. The vessels on one side of the body have undergone vasoconstriction. In an effort to supply more oxygen to the tissues in life, the vessels on the opposite side of the body have undergone vasodilation. Multisite injection may be necessary, but in most bodies injection of a sufficient quantity of solution should overcome the problem. This condition may be seen when the deceased has suffered a stroke.

▶ ARTERIAL COAGULA

At death, some blood remains in the arteries, especially in the large aorta. During the postmortem period, this blood can congeal (Figure 22–3). Injection of the arterial solution may loosen and push coagula into the smaller arteries. By injecting the common carotid arteries these coagula would be moved toward the legs.

If the femoral artery is used as the primary injection point, coagula can be moved into the common carotid arteries and stop the flow of arterial solution into the facial tissues. When the femoral artery is injected upward arterial coagula, most frequently, flow into the left subclavian artery, and it becomes necessary

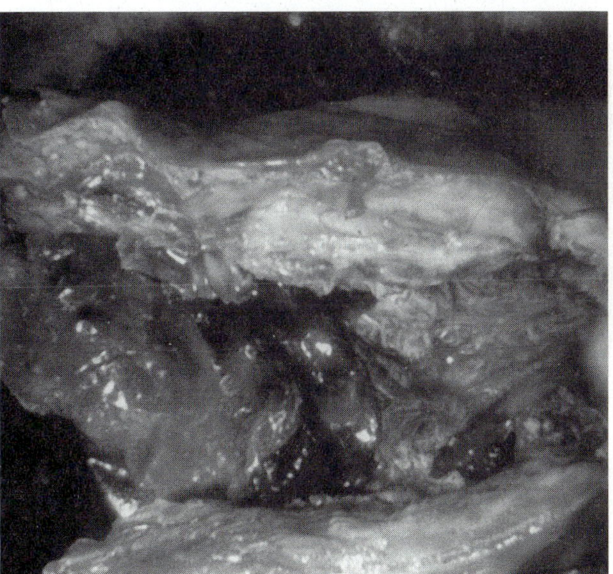

Figure 22–3. Dark areas are large dots in this sclerotic segment of the aorta.

to raise and inject the axillary or brachial artery of the left arm. When the common carotid is used as the primary injection site, arterial coagula are moved into the iliac and femoral arteries. The femoral arteries can be raised to embalm the legs; should this prove unsuccessful, the legs can be treated by hypodermic or surface embalming, or both.

If embalming is begun at a slower rate of flow and the use of preinjection fluids (which may loosen arterial coagula) is avoided, the arterial solution can pass *over* but not loosen coagula.

▶ VENOUS COAGULA

As veins enlarge toward the drainage site, venous coagula do not pose as serious a problem as arterial coagula. Failure to move the coagula, however, can block a vein, and this blockage can lead to tissue distension and discoloration. Massage from distal points toward the heart. Use the right internal jugular vein for drainage, as coagula in the right atrium can be easily reached with angular spring forceps and removed. Intermittent drainage helps to increase venous pressure and loosen coagula from the veins. Multisite injection and drainage may be warranted. When this condition is encountered in a localized area, use a stronger arterial solution to ensure that a minimum amount of arterial fluid delivers the maximum preservative.

▶ DIABETES

A variety of problems arise in the embalming of a diabetic. Of primary concern to the embalmer is the establishment of good fluid distribution. Diabetics tend to develop arteriosclerosis, especially in the smaller vessels, and poor peripheral circulation can be anticipated (Figure 22–4). These persons are also subject to increased bacterial and mycotic infections; all these conditions require use of a strong arterial solution. The first gallon can be slightly milder than subsequent gallons. To assist in establishing distribution and clearing of blood discolorations, the first gallon of arterial solution can be milder than subsequent injections. Some embalmers prefer to use a coinjection fluid to assist in the clearing of discolorations. Restricted cervical injection is suggested, and the embalmer should use moderate to high pressure to help distribute the solution. Massaging the extremities and using intermittent drainage also facilitate fluid distribution. High pressure and pulsation promote flow to the peripheral tissues (fingers, toes, ears, nose, and lips). Fluid dye can be used to trace the distribution of solution in the tissues.

The tissues of the diabetic may exhibit abnormal pH values. This may result in difficult tissue firming.

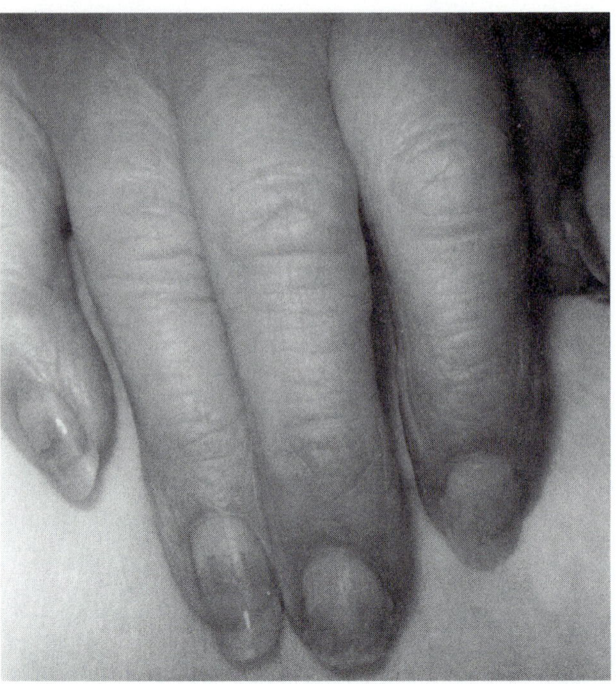

Figure 22–4. Discolored fingertips of a diabetic. Poor peripheral circulation often is seen in the diabetic.

Use of a moderate to strong solution accompanied by a coinjection fluid and dye should meet the preservative demands.

Many obese individuals are diabetic. Restricted cervical injection and drainage from the right internal jugular vein ensure tissue saturation. A large volume of solution can be injected without concern that the face may be overembalmed. The large volume of solution also promotes better fluid distribution.

Cavity embalming should be thorough. Mycotic infections are often found in the lungs of diabetics. A minimum of 16 ounces of cavity fluid should be used for each major body cavity. Abscesses, necrosis, and gangrene may be present in the pancreas and liver. Arterial solution may not have reached these tissues. The cavity fluid is the only preservative that will be available to halt the decomposition that occurs in the tissues of these diseased organs.

Gangrene may also be present in distal tissues such as the fingers and toes. These areas will *not* receive arterial solution when the body is injected. Cavity fluid should be injected into these areas by hypodermic injection or injection with an infant trocar. The surface of feet affected by gangrene should be painted with autopsy gel or cavity fluid compresses should be applied and the leg clothed in a plastic stocking.

Diabetics are also subject to decubitus ulcers. These lesions should be disinfected topically and the tissue around them injected hypodermically with cavity fluid or a phenol cautery solution. Surface compresses of autopsy gel, cavity fluid, or phenol cautery solution should be applied to the necrotic surface tissues.

Restricted cervical injection allows the injection of a milder arterial solution into emaciated and dehydrated facial tissues. Coinjection chemicals and humectants may be used to help restore some moisture. After arterial preparation, tissue builder can be used to restore emaciated and sunken facial tissues.

▶ EXTRAVASCULAR RESISTANCE

Pressure on the outside of an artery or vein is referred to as **extravascular resistance,** and may restrict the flow of arterial solution into a body region or may restrict drainage through a vein.

A slightly stronger well-coordinated arterial solution should be used as distribution may be limited. Multisite injection may be necessary if extravascular resistance is present. Use of higher embalming pressures may promote distribution. Stopping the injection and allowing time for drainage may help to prevent blood discolorations: inject–drain without injecting–inject. Use concurrent drainage throughout the entire operation. Massage and manipulate the tissues to promote both fluid distribution and blood drainage.

Sources of extravascular resistance and suggestions on how to overcome the resulting problems are listed here:

- *Rigor mortis:* Relieve as much rigor as possible by manipulation prior to arterial injection.
- *Ascites:* Relieve the abdominal pressure by draining prior to or during arterial injection.
- *Gas in cavities:* Puncture the abdomen and relieve gases prior to or during arterial injection.
- *Bandages:* Remove tight bandages prior to injection.
- *Contact pressure:* Massage these areas.
- *Tumors:* Excise, with permission, if absolutely necessary. Sectional injection may be necessary.
- *Swollen lymph nodes:* Sectional injection may be necessary.
- *Hydrothorax:* Drainage may be possible prior to injection, but can be difficult.
- *Visceral weight:* Above- and below-heart injection and drainage points can be employed.

▶ KEY TERMS AND CONCEPTS FOR STUDY AND DISCUSSION

1. Define the following terms:
   aneurysm
   arterial coagula
   arteriosclerosis
   canalization
   embolus
   extravascular
   extravascular resistance
   intravascular
   intravascular resistance
   lumen
   vasoconstriction
   vasodilation
   venous coagula
2. Describe the vascular problems created by diabetes.
3. Discuss the problems created by congestive heart failure.

▶ BIBLIOGRAPHY

Day DD, Poston G. Embalming the diabetic case. In: *Champion Expanding Encyclopedia.* Springfield, OH: Champion Chemical Co.;1985:No. 560, pp. 2254–2257.

Mulvihill ML. *Human Diseases: A Systemic Approach.* 2nd ed. Norwalk, CT: Appleton & Lange;1987.

Sheldon H. *Boyd's Introduction to the Study of Disease.* 9th ed. Philadelphia: Lea & Febiger;1984.

Shor MM. Damage to aorta may bring embalming problems. *Casket and Sunnyside,* June 1960.

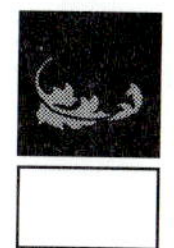

CHAPTER 23 EFFECT OF DRUGS ON THE EMBALMING PROCESS

The contemporary professional embalmer practices this art and science in an age that has often been referred to as the *Chemotherapy Era.* **(Chemotherapy is the treatment of disease with chemical agents and drugs.)** The aims of modern medicine are to cure disease and alleviate pain via the long-sought-for "magic bullet" of Dr. Paul Ehrlich. Today, there is not a single case on which the embalmer works that has not been injected, dusted, or made to ingest some type of chemical substance or substances (drugs) prior to death. In many cases, particularly those received from medical facilities and institutions, many different types of drugs were used prior to the patient's death. Although the Chemotherapy Era began with Ehrlich's "magic bullet" for the treatment of syphilis, today we live in an age of *multiple-agent* chemotherapy.

The way antibiotics are used today exemplifies the multiple-drug approach common to the medical profession. It is very unlikely nowadays that a single antibiotic is prescribed for the treatment of an infection. Usually, two or more antibiotics are administered. In cancer chemotherapy, the multiple-drug approach is also common. It is not unusual for an oncologist to administer both a *cytotoxic* drug (one that kills the cancer cell directly) and an *antimetabolite* (one that slowly "starves" the cancer cell by depriving it of a needed nutrient). One result of this multiple-agent approach has been an increase in the number and types of embalming problems.

Before the embalming problems caused by chemotherapeutic agents are discussed, "normal" embalming must be defined. There is *no* "ideal case." It is probably impossible to find a person who has not been treated by one or more doctors with one or more drugs prior to death. So, in addition to the problems caused by the pathological processes resulting in death, the chemotherapeutic agent or agents administered for various intervals prior to death have physiological effects. The longer the drug was taken before death, the more intense are the embalming problems likely to be encountered.

Another problem may arise from the chemical reaction between the administered drugs and the components of the embalming fluid. For example, are there any components of arterial embalming fluid that form insoluble precipitates when they react with antibiotics? If so, the circulatory path may become blocked, thus preventing the preservative components of the arterial fluid from reaching the tissues for preservation.

▶ THE CHEMISTRY OF PROTEINS

To discuss the chemistry of embalming, it is essential to understand the chemistry of proteins. These materials form the physical structures of the body. They give the body form. *The professional embalmer must achieve the absolute preservation of these structures.* This means that the proteinaceous materials forming portions of the various tissues and organs of the human body must be rendered chemically inert. Essentially, these structures must be frozen in time and space!

Proteins are labile substances. The molecules break down quite rapidly even without bacterial action. There exist proteins that break down other proteins. These specialized proteins, called *enzymes*, are endowed with a physicochemical structure that allows catalytic activity. These enzymes can speed up decomposition reactions. It must be realized that even if a cadaver were completely sterile, the proteolytic enzymes in the cells and tissues of that body would still be fully active and capable of causing the breakdown of tissue proteins.

One goal of embalming must be to render the proteins resistant to attack by catalytic enzymes. There are two ways to do this: (1) The proteins themselves can be treated so that they are no longer susceptible to the action of proteolytic enzymes. (2) The enzymes themselves can be so changed or inactivated that they cannot exert catalytic action on other proteins. Modern embalming chemicals are formulated to do both.

To determine how both of these goals can be achieved in a so-called "ideal" case, a brief mathematical formula is helpful.

What this means in terms of actual chemicals used to embalm a case should be discussed from a practical standpoint.

AVERAGE BODY PROTEIN

The average body = 150 pounds = 65.3 kilograms.
A 65.3 kg body contains 10.7 kg of protein = 10,700 grams of protein.

FORMALDEHYDE DEMAND

100 grams of soluble protein requires 4.4 grams of formaldehyde for preservation.
The average body contains 10,700 grams of protein.
Therefore,

$$\frac{10{,}700}{100} \times 4.4 = 470.8 \text{ grams of formaldehyde needed.}$$

SOLUTION NEEDED

Given: Standard 30-index arterial fluid contains 16 ounces of 30% formaldehyde = 142.08 grams of formaldehyde.
Need: 470.80 grams of formaldehyde.

$$\frac{470.80}{142.08} = 3.31$$ sixteen-ounce bottles of a 30-index fluid needed, or approximately 53 ounces of arterial fluid

For a nonideal case (as practically all cases today are), the conclusion that some of the formaldehyde will be lost in embalming seems obvious. For example, many chemotherapeutic agents are nephrotoxic and, therefore, cause a breakdown of kidney function. As the kidneys are the main organs responsible for elimination of nitrogenous wastes, these waste materials (ammonia, urea, uric acid, etc.) are retained by the body. There is no better way to neutralize formaldehyde than to react it with ammonia, and this is exactly what happens in the body. If there has been a buildup of nitrogenous waste materials as a result of chemotherapy-induced kidney dysfunction, a standard dilution of arterial embalming fluid will not be sufficient. A large proportion of the formaldehyde in the embalming fluid will be neutralized when it encounters the nitrogenous wastes in the body. The remainder is insufficient to preserve the tissues, and the body starts to decay.

Normally, arterial embalming fluids are supplied as 16-ounce concentrates. These are diluted with water and additives prior to injection into the body. An embalming fluid containing 30% formaldehyde supplies 142 grams of formaldehyde per bottle. To embalm the "average" or "ideal" body containing 10.7 kilograms of protein, 470 grams of formaldehyde is needed, that is, a minimum of three bottles of arterial embalming fluid. (If the body has been dosed with drugs, more than double this amount of formaldehyde may be necessary!)

▶ THE CHEMOTHERAPY CASE

All chemotherapeutic agents are toxic. This is the one axiom universally applicable to all drugs. Cellular and tissue changes occur when drugs are used. It does not matter what drug is administered; even the seemingly innocuous aspirin tablet has its effects. Drug-induced changes may be relatively minor, perhaps limited to slight skin discolorations, which, in the deceased, readily respond to cosmetic treatment. When drugs cause major problems, such as acute jaundice, or saturate the body tissues with uremic wastes, the fixative action of the preservative chemicals in the arterial embalming fluid is seriously impaired.

The chemotherapeutic agents common to modern medicine exert their effects in many ways. They may impair function of the liver, the circulatory system (heart and blood vessels), the kidneys, the lungs, and the skin. These drugs can inactivate the embalming fluid by causing the buildup of nitrogenous wastes or decreasing the permeability of the cell membrane (Figure 23–1).

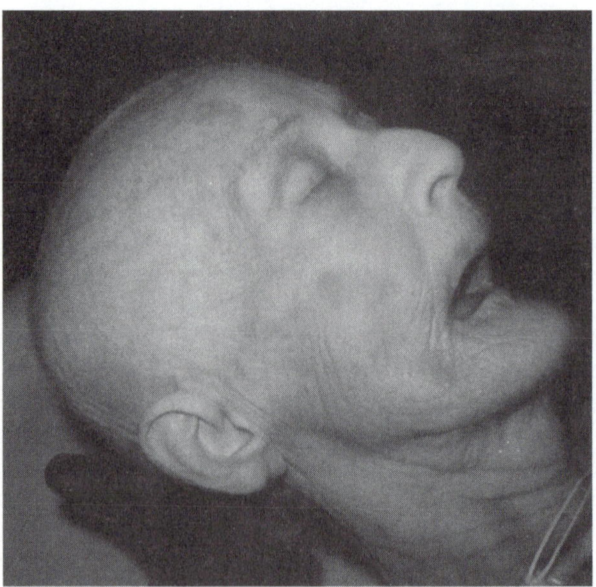

Figure 23–1. Chemotherapy patient showing weight loss and hair loss.

Because the *liver* is the main detoxification center, every drug eventually enters the hepatic circulation. While in the liver, the drug may be changed to an innocuous form by hepatic enzymes, or the drug may cause profound changes in the liver itself. When the liver is damaged, the embalmer may have to cope with a jaundiced body.

All drugs ultimately pass through the kidneys. Even those that accumulate in other body areas must pass at least once (and often more) through the kidneys. If the drugs cause extensive changes in this organ, renal insufficiency follows, resulting in the buildup of nitrogenous wastes in body tissues. Saturated with urea, uric acid, ammonia, creatinine, and other wastes, the tissues become spongy and difficult to preserve. In such cases, preservation is almost impossible to achieve unless the treatment is modified.

Drugs also change the biochemical constituents of the blood. Some drugs damage even the connecting blood vessels themselves extensively. The circulatory system may become impaired as a result of extensive clot formation, lysis of the blood cells, or extensive damage to the walls of the arteries and veins.

The effects on *skin* are closely associated with the changes in the circulatory system and may include the formation of widespread areas of discoloration stemming from lysis and release of blood pigments from red blood cells. Lesions on the skin surfaces may also result from use of the nitrogen mustards.

Pharmacologically, the dividing line between the beneficial effects and toxic effects of drugs is very slender. The professional embalmer must learn to cope with these effects.

▶ INACTIVATION OF PRESERVATIVE AGENTS BY DRUGS

The problems likely to be confronted while embalming a body administered chemotherapy do *not* result from the reactions of formaldehyde or other preservative aldehydes with the drug or drugs. Much too little drug is present, even after aggressive therapy. **It is the physiological effect of the drug that is culpable.** A drug that causes nephrotoxic changes enhances the accumulation of nitrogenous waste products in the body. These waste products, which result indirectly from the physiological effect of the drug, are responsible for the inactivation or, more specifically, the neutralization of the formaldehyde:

$$4NH_3 + 6CH_2O \rightarrow (CH_2)_6N_4 + 6H_2O$$

This neutralization reaction, whereby formaldehyde is converted to hexamethylene, is probably at the root of at least 90% of the contemporary embalmer's problems.

A change in permeability of the cell membrane is another effect of most systemically administered drugs. It is through this membrane that everything must pass, either to enter or to leave the cell. Preservative chemicals such as formaldehyde must pass through this membrane if they are going to inactivate the intracellular enzymes that decompose the proteins there.

If a chemotherapeutic agent reduces or destroys membrane permeability, preservative solutions may not be able to enter the cell. The antibiotic tetracycline is a case in point. Although most antibiotics exert their effects on bacteria they also have an effect on the human cell. They are chelating agents and tend to lodge in the cell membrane, causing calcium to form an impenetrable layer around the cell. "Chelating" means they have an affinity for metallic ions, particularly calcium and magnesium. Antibiotics appear to act selectively on cell membranes. After they are entrenched in the membrane, they start chelating or sequestering calcium and magnesium ions. [There is generally no shortage of calcium in the body; it is present in all biological fluids (secretions, excretions, etc.).]

Eventually, as more calcium and magnesium ions become lodged in the chelate in the cell membrane, the permeability of the membrane changes; the membrane becomes less permeable. It becomes increasingly more difficult for some chemicals to enter such a cell. Because the goal of embalming is to inactive the intracellular enzymes present, it is essential that the preservative enter the cell. If it does not, the proteolytic enzymes inside the cell can proceed to break down the proteinaceous materials in the cell, and the tissue is subject to decomposition and lysis of its structural features. In essence, it turns into a puddle of fluid.

To study these effects, Fredrick (1968) devised a histological method based on a chemical method of Gomori (1939). Gomori observed that if an enzyme were supplied with a substrate, it would release a material (phosphate) that could be precipitated in situ. Using this technique, one is able to determine the location of active enzymes.

There has recently come into use a group of antibiotics that exert their effects in the kidney, hampering its ability to dispose of nitrogenous wastes—the aminoglycosides, represented by kanamycin and, most recently, gentamicin. These antibiotics cause nitrogenous waste products to be retained, and if the so-called standard dilution of arterial fluid is used, embalming will fail.

▶ COMBINATION ANTIBIOTIC CHEMOTHERAPY

Today, it is routine procedure for physicians to prescribe two or more antibiotics at the same time. This, of course, intensifies the embalming problems. The embalming problems resulting from synergistic combination chemotherapy are not new, only more intense. Use of a combination such as gentamicin and a synthetic penicillin (e.g., methicillin) makes preservation and firming difficult to achieve. These bodies are usually saturated with ammoniacal and other nitrogenous wastes. The arterial fluid in such cases must be very concentrated if any embalming is to be accomplished.

▶ CORTICOSTEROIDS AND ANTIINFLAMMATORY DRUGS

If antibiotics are the most widely used drugs, then cortisone and its derivatives constitute a close second. The antiinflammatory drugs have many uses (e.g., itching caused by allergies) and are the drugs of choice for arthritic and rheumatic conditions. Corticosteroids are also widely used in the chemotherapy of cancer.

With regard to specific embalming problems caused by these drugs, the chief effect is blockade of the cell membrane. **Corticosteroids decrease the permeability of this membrane** and thereby block passage of liquids into the cell. On a gross macroscopic level, liquids are retained by the cells and tissues, resulting in an increase in cell turgor and waterlogging of tissues.

The use of cortisone for the treatment of chronic diseases (over long periods) may result in **gastrointestinal ulcerations with possible perforations of the gut.** Prolonged use in the treatment of ulcerative colitis has also resulted in dehydration of the body.

Corticosteroids have been shown to exert a "protective" effect on proteolytic enzymes. This is demonstrated by the difficult task one has in trying to denature these enzymes in cortisone-treated bodies. Even if these enzymes are extracted from such cortisone-treated tissues and are obtained in an almost pure form, they are still difficult to inactivate. They retain the "protective" effect originally conferred by the corticosteroids. This means that more undenatured proteolytic enzymes remain in the body after embalming. Such bodies tend to "go bad" (decompose) very rapidly after an apparently trouble-free embalming.

What has so far been described with respect to corticosteroids can also occur as the result of the use of oral contraceptives by women. Progesterone and its derivatives have chemical structures similar to that of cortisone. It has long been known in pharmacology that similar chemical structures elicit similar biological reactions. Many of the embalming problems observed after use of corticosteroids are identical to those encountered in bodies of young women who died while taking oral contraceptives.

Another problem encountered when corticosteroids have been administered for some time prior to death is of a more insidious nature. These persons have been shown to have disseminated tuberculosis. The antiinflammatory action of the corticosteroids results from their suppression of immunity. In cases of "arrested" (or so-called "cured") tuberculosis in which large doses of cortisone were administered before death, it is not uncommon to find that because immunity was suppressed the mycobacterium was reactivated and spread throughout the body. Such cases offer hidden hazards to the embalmer's health and sanitation precautions should be observed.

To secure preservation in these bodies, some permeability should be restored to the cell membranes so that preservatives can enter the cells. This can be done through the use of adjunct fluids. Preinjecting such a body restores some of the permeability; and the surface-active chemicals in such preparations facilitate entry of the preservative components of the arterials into cells. At the same time, a stronger-than-normal arterial injection should be used together with a coinjection fluid. (It is also possible to use some coinjection fluids as a preinjection.)

▶ CANCER CHEMOTHERAPEUTIC AGENTS AND THEIR EFFECTS

Various drugs are used to treat malignancies, but generally they fall into two main classes. *Cytotoxic* drugs act directly on the tumor cells to bring about their death. *Antimetabolite* drugs substitute for an essential metabolite required by the cancer cell for growth. It is not unusual for both types to be given to the cancer patient. This multiple-agent chemotherapy creates tremendous problems for the professional embalmer.

Cytotoxic drugs (e.g., nitrogen mustards, alkylating agents) kill both malignant and normal cells. (A "magic bullet" for cancer has not yet been found.) When cells die, proteins break down and large amounts of nitrogenous wastes are released. Therefore, the tissues in these bodies, besides containing a small amount of protein as a result of the extreme cachexia associated with cancer, are saturated with nitrogenous waste products. Achievement of preservation under these conditions is a herculean task in itself, but the embalming problems that arise from the coadministration of antimetabolites must be added. These are sure to cause symptoms of extensive vitamin deficiency. Such bodies may exhibit everything from scurvy to brittle ricketslike bone disease. If radiation therapy has been administered, there may be extensive skin and circulatory problems (e.g., purpura and body clots).

▶ RADIOACTIVE ISOTOPES AND THEIR EFFECTS

Because radioactive materials are used for cancer therapy, it is not amiss to discuss the radiation-treated body. An embalmer should not attempt to embalm a radiation-treated body unless a radiation safety officer has certified the body as safe because of the possibility of gamma radiation. The main radioisotopes used to diagnose and treat malignancies are cobalt-60, iodine-131, phosphorus-32, radium-226, gold-198, and strontium-89. Beta rays are stopped much more readily than gamma rays, which are similar to x-rays and require lead shielding. In addition, tiny needles or "seeds" of gold-198, as well as radon needles, are implanted in tissues to treat metastatic tumors in the abdomen and lungs. These bodies, if declared safe, may be embalmed as would any cancer case.

A second source of radiation exposure is an occupational accident. Radioactive materials are measured in *millicuries*. A millicurie (mCi) is defined as that amount of radioactive material in which 37 million atoms disintegrate each second. Medical institutions must "tag" bodies, warning that radioactive isotopes are present in the body or that the body has had a high exposure to radiation by accident. The medical institution is not permitted to release the body until the level of radioactivity has dropped below 30 millicuries, for unautopsied bodies. Autopsied remains are not to be released until the radiation level drops to 5 millicuries or below. It is necessary for the embalmer to follow any instructions issued by the radiation protection officer. If embalming is permitted when radiation levels are above the figures cited, the preparation should occur at the hospital under the strict supervision of the radiation officer.

When radiation levels are below 30 millicuries for unautopsied remains and 5 millicuries or below for autopsied remains, standard embalming procedures can be used which would be determined by the conditions present in the dead human body. There are certain recommended precautions the embalmer should exercise. These precautions can be summarized in the words *protection, time of exposure,* and *distance.* During the preparation of bodies that have been exposed to high doses of radioactivity, the embalmer should wear rubber gloves, if possible two pairs, and a heavy rubber apron. In addition, of course, standard Universal Precautions attire should also be worn. The shortest time of exposure should be employed. Time of exposure can be shortened, when possible, by working in pairs; two embalmers can work together performing different tasks (e.g., one embalmer raises vessels and a second sets features). This helps to reduce the exposure time. Having instruments ready and fluids mixed, as soon as the body is observed, again reduces the time spent in preparation. It would be most wise to avoid raising vessels in a body region where tissues have been seeded with the radioactive isotope; for example, if seeds are present in tissues of the neck, use of the femoral vessels would reduce contact with the seeds.

Distance also plays a large role in reducing exposure to radiation. For every 3 feet of distance from the body, exposure is reduced by a substantial amount. When not actually performing a procedure, the embalmer should stand at a distance from the body (e.g., during injection of the arterial solution when massage may not be necessary). There should be a constant flow of water under the body. New tables allow the body to be positioned on slats, which allow water to flow beneath the body without coming into contact with the body. The constant flow of water is necessary to dilute and flush away all drainage matter as it exits the body. Care should be taken to cover the area around the preparation table with sheeting, which can be destroyed by incineration or placed in a biohazard container after the embalming; this ensures that all waste matter is removed from the areas surrounding the preparation table. Gloves should be frequently flushed with soap and water during the embalming procedure. Any spillage should be removed immediately with the use of forceps or tongs and new sheeting or a portion of the sheeting draped onto the floor.

Final cleanup should include the following:

- Instruments should be thoroughly flushed with running water, then soaked in a good soap or detergent and rinsed well with running water.
- Disposable waste matter should be collected in a suitable biohazard container and disposed of (if permitted) by incineration.
- Gloves (if they are to be reused) should be thoroughly washed before being removed from the hands, then placed in a container of soap and water and allowed to soak. Next they should be removed and dried and stored in a suitable place until the radioactivity has decayed to a safe level.
- Gowns, towels, clothing, and so on should be monitored and stored for suitable decay before being sent to the laundry (consult the radiation officer of the medical facility for assistance in this matter).

- If the embalmer suffers any introduction of material from the body into lesions on his or her hands, the injured area should be washed with copious amounts of running water and a physician or radiation safety officer consulted.

The embalmer should follow any instructions that have been made by the radiation safety officer with regard to preparation of the body. An example would be if the officer stated that aspiration and injection of the cavities should not be carried out until a certain time. Strengths of arterial solutions, volume of fluid injected, and so on do not directly affect radiation exposure. Some examples of radioactive isotopes employed in disease diagnosis and treatment are cobalt-60, iodine-131, radium-226, gold-198, and strontium-89. A more detailed discussion of radioactive isotopes can be found in the text *Thanatochemistry*, 2nd ed., by James M. Dorn and Barbara Hopkins, published by Prentice-Hall Inc., Upper Saddle River, New Jersey 07458, 1998.

▶ TRANQUILIZERS AND MOOD-ALTERING DRUGS

It is not easy to discuss prescribed legal drugs without venturing into the field of drug abuse. No matter what the drug is, if it is taken beyond the period prescribed, or if more than the dose prescribed is taken, it becomes "abused." For example, if amphetamines are prescribed for dietary or psychiatric reasons and are taken longer than necessary to alleviate the condition, they become illegal or abused drugs. It should be realized that such components of the drug culture as benzedrine, dexedrine, and methedrine were all at one time (and some still are) rigorously and ethically prescribed by physicians to treat specific ills. The same holds true for such tranquilizers as phenothiazine and its derivatives.

There are roughly five classes of tranquilizers and mood-altering drugs. In general, they have one common characteristic: they result in a loss of weight of the abuser. Embalming these bodies is very frustrating because of the lack of protein (most of the protein stores have been depleted). A person on a "trip" does not care about nutrition.

- *Sedatives:* barbiturates [amobarbital (Amytal), secobarbital (Seconal), etc.]; meprobamate (Quanil, Miltown, etc.)
- *Stimulants:* amphetamines (Benzedrine, Dexedrine, etc.); cocaine; phenmetrazine (Preludin)
- *Tranquilizers:* phenothiazines [chlorpromazine (Thorazine), prochlorperazine (Compazine), etc.]; reserpine (Serpalan, Serpasil); chlordiazepoxide (Librium); diazepam (Valium)
- *Narcotics:* opiates (opium, heroin, morphine, etc.)
- *Antidepressants:* methylphenidate (Ritalin); imipramine (Tofranil)

The continued use (or abuse) of tranquilizers can also result in such embalming problems as jaundice because of the destructive effect of these drugs on liver cells. In addition, tranquilizers may cause hemolysis of the red blood cells and thereby add to the jaundice problem because pigments are released from these red blood cells. Also common to abusers of all five classes of drugs is the depletion of protein stores resulting from their neglect of nutrition. Protein depletion results in the release of large amounts of nitrogenous waste products. If kidney function is impaired (particularly in heroin addicts in whom both constipation and anuresis occur), these waste materials cannot exit the body. They are retained in the tissues and rapidly neutralize formaldehyde (or any aldehyde).

▶ PROBLEMS CAUSED BY ORAL DRUGS THAT CONTROL DIABETES

A group of chemotherapeutic agents with broad-spectrum effects comprises those drugs used to control diabetes, the oral diabetic agents. Use of such drugs as tolbutamide (Orinase) and chlorpropamide (Diabinese) to control adult (type II) diabetes is increasing. These drugs certainly are more convenient (for those who can use them) than the daily (or more frequent) self-injections of insulin.

Tolbutamide was used widely until recently, when it was replaced with another second-generation sulfonylurea called chlorpropamide. Both may cause jaundice. Most of the sulfonylureas can induce changes in the voluntary muscles (site of glycogen storage and breakdown) and the liver (main glycogen storage organ of the body). Continuous use of oral diabetic agents has been linked with circulatory problems, which can result in poor distribution of the arterial chemicals. (This has been observed to be the result of extensive clot formation in the cadaver.) Acidosis sometimes occurs as a result of the altered carbohydrate metabolism and leads to the formation of high concentrations of lactic acid in muscle tissue. Such bodies firm very rapidly unless an alkaline coinjection is used with the arterial embalming fluid.

In general, although oral diabetic agents may cause a large variety of embalming problems, they do not cause as severe embalming problems as do other drugs.

▶ NEUTRALIZING CHEMOTHERAPEUTIC AGENTS

It must be understood that chemotherapeutic agents cause embalming problems not through their reactions with embalming chemicals but through their physiological effects on the body prior to death (Table 23–1). No drug, no matter how often, how long, or in what concentration it is used, could ever be administered long enough during life to react significantly with the components of an arterial chemical injected after death. As has previously been stressed, **it is the physiological reaction the drug induces that causes the problem.** For example, the embalming problem created by the aminoglycoside antibiotics is produced not by the reaction between formaldehyde and kanamycin (even if a few grams of the antibiotic were present), but rather by the reaction between formaldehyde and the nitrogenous waste products released into the tissues through the action of the antibiotic.

Once absorbed into the bloodstream, a drug is rapidly diluted. An average body contains about 6 liters (1 liter is equivalent to 2.1 pints) of blood. This volume of blood circulates once per minute. It comes into contact with 35 additional liters of liquid. (Fifty-eight percent of the body weight of an average 150-pound man is water.) *Therefore, there is a total of 41 liters of liquid (including blood volume) in the average body.* Any drug, usually given in milligram doses, would be so diluted as to have no significant effect in a direct chemical reaction with formaldehyde or any component of embalming fluid. Refer to the section on renal failure for embalming treatments for bodies with high levels of nitrogenous wastes in the tissues and bloodstream.

▶ POSSIBLE SOLUTIONS TO CHEMOTHERAPY PROBLEMS

The problems arising from chemotherapy vary in severity, but can be divided into a few broad categories. Several preventive and ameliorative treatments are available that have been shown to work in the majority of cases. **The professional embalmer must consider each case as unique.** Just as a physician does not prescribe the same dosage of a medication for all patients, so must the embalmer vary procedures (and preservative fluids) to meet the requirements of the particular case.

FACTORS THAT MUST BE DETERMINED IN THE EMBALMING ANALYSIS

1. Vessels for injection and drainage
2. Strength of the embalming solution
3. Volume of the embalming solution
4. Injection pressure
5. Injection rate of flow

Note: These factors will vary by the individual body and can vary in different areas of the same body.

TABLE 23–1. PROBLEMS CAUSED BY CHEMOTHERAPEUTIC AGENTS[a]

Drug	Problem
Antibiotics (penicillins, synthetic penicillins, aminoglycosides, tetracyclines)	Cottonlike circulatory blockages (fungal overgrowth); jaundice; bleeding into skin; poor penetration
Corticosteroids (cortisone)	Cell membranes less permeable; retention of fluids; mild to severe waterlogging of tissues; "protects" proteolysis enzymes, resulting in more rapid breakdown of body proteins
Cancer chemotherapy (antimetabolites, cytotoxic agents, radioisotopes)	Emaciation and dehydration; extensive purpura; jaundice; low protein (because of anorexia and vomiting); perforation of gut; brittleness of bone; nitrogenous waste retention
Tranquilizers (phenothiozines)	Dehydration; weight loss and emaciation; low protein; kidney dysfunction and retention of nitrogenous waste products
Stimulants (amphetamines, cocaine)	Weight loss; emaciation; low protein; mucous membranes bleed easily; other problems as for tranquilizers
Sedatives (barbiturates, meprobamate)	Emaciation; dehydration; low protein; difficult to firm
Oral antidiabetic agents (tolbutamide)	Muscle atrophy; mild to severe jaundice; some emaciation and edema
Circulatory drugs (antihypertensives, anticlotting agents)	Blood clots; impairment of circulation; poor distribution of fluids; purpura; urine retention and spongy nitrogenous waste-filled tissues

[a] Table has been adapted and summarized from many published works. It is neither complete nor exhaustive. It is designed to point out categories of chemotherapeutic agents in use now. It is hoped that this table will stimulate both the student of embalming and the licensed professional to read about the latest developments in journals and trade magazines. As new chemical agents are introduced so frequently by the medical profession, it is impossible to publish up-to-the-minute tables. Keeping up with the literature is of the utmost importance.

In Table 23–1, five different embalming treatments are recommended to combat most chemotherapy-derived problems. Obviously, these cannot solve all the problems the professional embalmer will face. They do, however, serve as a springboard for further research and, therefore, offer the embalmer an opportunity for experimentation and learning—both the marks of professionalism.

▶ CONCLUSION

Mistaken ideas about the specificity of a particular chemotherapeutic agent are quite common. For example, one may believe that a drug known to have a pronounced effect on a particular organ will be found only in that organ. This is not so. That a drug shows a more dramatic effect on a particular tissue does not mean that the effect is limited only to that tissue.

In general, no matter what chemotherapeutic agent is used, it is concentrated, metabolized, and detoxified in the liver and excreted via the kidneys (and, sometimes, the lungs and skin). But before it reaches these organs, it passes through other tissues of the body, which is contrary to the "magic bullet" concept. Actually, there is no magic bullet! It is impossible for a drug to bring about a single reaction in a single organ or tissue. It should not be surprising then that a single drug can cause a plethora of embalming problems. Simultaneous use of two or more drugs, as is common in medical practice today, intensifies the problems.

In the body, a drug is subject to great dilution. The problems it causes do not result from its direct reaction with components of the embalming fluid, but from the chronic physiological effects it produces.

On the basis of both laboratory studies and field work, five embalming treatments for the problems encountered in bodies that have undergone chemotherapy have been recommended. It is the responsibility of the embalmer to modify the treatment to suit the particular case.

▶ CONCEPTS FOR STUDY AND DISCUSSION

1. It is known that elderly persons present chemotherapy-derived embalming problems because the ability of the body to circulate, detoxify, and excrete drugs decreases with age. Discuss, on this basis, the possible effects of an aminoglycoside antibiotic such as gentamicin when the "usual" dilution is used.
2. If approximately 58% of the human body is composed of water, is it defeating the purpose to embalm the body that has undergone chemotherapy, particularly if there is little protein (as in the drug addict) in that body, by further diluting the embalming fluid with water before it is injected? Discuss how use can be made of this intracellular water as a diluent for concentrated arterial fluid. As this "tissue" water is known to be high in calcium, should it be conditioned with a water softener or conditioner?
3. It is a fact that a body treated with antibiotics usually contains all types of fungi. Certain fungi may pose a hazard to the embalmer. Discuss the possibility of contracting *Candida*, *Cryptococcus*, and *Histoplasma* infections from cadavers. What can be done to protect the embalmer?
4. It has been shown that to embalm an "average" body, at least three to four 16-ounce bottles of a 30% formaldehyde arterial solution are necessary. Discuss whether enough preservative is contained in this amount of arterial fluid to embalm a body treated with corticosteroids. What adjunct embalming chemicals should be added to the arterial injection?
5. A young housewife is killed in an automobile accident. The embalmer is told that she has been taking a fertility drug (progesterone) because she was childless and wanted a family. What types of embalming problems can be expected?
6. A chronic diabetic is brought to the preparation room. The embalmer discovers that instead of insulin, the man had taken tolbutamide (Orinase) two times daily for the past 3 years. What embalming fluids should be used on this case, taking into consideration dilution of arterial chemicals, rapidity of firming, and use of preinjection fluid, water conditioners, and other fluids?
7. After arterial injection, the drainage is observed to contain small wads of greenish "cotton." The patient had been taking massive doses of penicillin prior to death. What could these "cotton wads" be?
8. A radiation safety officer has certified the release and permission to embalm a body which contains implanted seeds containing a radioisotope. Discuss the personal protective hygiene practices the embalmer should use during the preparation of this body.
9. Discuss why an embalmer cannot use one type and one concentration of arterial embalming fluid in all cases.
10. A particular drug exerts its effect on only one specific organ. Therefore, after a patient

treated with cortisone for an arthritic condition dies, high concentrations of cortisone will be found only in the joints. Discuss the fallacy of this type of thinking.

▶ BIBLIOGRAPHY

Brozek J. *Body Composition.* New York: New York Academy of Sciences; 1963.

Dorn J, Hopkins B. *Thanatochemistry.* 2nd ed., Upper Saddle River, NJ: Prentice-Hall, Inc.; 1998.

Fedrick JF. An alpha-glucan phosphorylase which requires adenosine-5-phosphate as coenzyme. *Phytochemistry* 1963;2:413–415.

Fredrick JF. *Embalming Problems Caused by Chemotherapeutic Agents.* Boston: Dodge Institute for Advanced Studies; 1968.

Gomori G. Microtechnical demonstration of phosphatase enzymes in tissue sections. *Proc Soc Exp Biol Med* 1939;42:23–26.

Goodman L, Gilman A, eds. *The Pharmacological Basis of Therapeutics,* 4th ed. New York: Macmillan; 1970.

Goth, A. *Medical Pharmacology.* 6th ed. St. Louis, MO: CV Mosby; 1972.

Julian RM. *A Primer of Drug Action.* San Francisco: Freeman; 1975.

Long YG. *Neuropharmacology and Behavior.* San Francisco: Freeman; 1972.

Merck, Sharpe, & Dohme. *Merck Index.* 10th ed. Rahway, NJ: Merck & Co.; 1983.

Physician's Desk Reference (PDR). Oradale, NJ: Medical Economics; 1984:No. 38.

Windholz M, Budavari S. In: *Merck Index.* 10th ed. Rahway, NJ: Merck & Co.; 1983.

Yessell ES, Braude MC. *Interaction of Drugs of Abuse.* New York: New York Academy of Sciences; 1976.

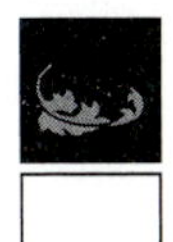

CHAPTER 24 SELECTED CONDITIONS

▶ PURGE

Purge is defined as the postmortem evacuation of any substance from any external orifice of the body as a result of pressure. This condition can occur prior to, during, and after embalming. Purge is generally described by its source—stomach, lung, and so on. The pressure responsible for the purge can develop in several ways:

1. Gas: Gas in the abdominal cavity or in the hollow intestinal tract can create sufficient pressure on the stomach to force the contents of the stomach through the mouth or nose. This abdominal pressure can also push on the diaphragm with sufficient force to cause the contents of the lungs to purge through the mouth or nose. Gas can originate from early decomposition or from partial digestion of foods or may be true tissue gas formed by *Clostridium perfringens.*
2. Visceral expansion: When bodies have been dead for several hours and arterial solution is injected too fast, the hollow visceral organs (intestinal tract) tend to expand. Because the abdomen is a closed cavity this expansion creates sufficient pressure to push on the stomach walls and create a stomach purge. The expansion also pushes on the diaphragm and squeezes on the lungs, possibly resulting in lung purge.
3. Arterial Solution:
   A. Injection of arterial solution at a fast rate of flow, especially in bodies dead for long periods, causes expansion of the viscera (see item 2).
   B. If an area of the stomach, upper bowel, or lung is ulcerated, the arterial solution can leak through the ulcerated vessels, fill the stomach, esophagus, or lung tissue, and the trachea, and develop into a purge.
   C. If esophageal varices break, sufficient blood and arterial solution can exit to create purge.
   D. Gastrointestinal bleeding accompanies a variety of diseases and the long-term use of many drugs. If a sufficient amount of arterial solution and blood leak from these tissues during injection, anal purge results.
   E. Purge can occur when leakage of arterial solution from an aneurysm in the thoracic or abdominal cavity develops sufficient pressure to push on the lungs or stomach.
   F. Sufficient injection pressure can cause leakage from recent surgical incisions. The arterial solution lost to the stomach or abdominal cavity builds up enough pressure to create purge.
4. Ascites and hydrothorax: When edema fills the thoracic or abdominal cavity prior to death, a great amount of pressure builds up and, on injection of arterial solution forces purge.

CONDITIONS PREDISPOSING TO PURGE

- Decomposition
- Long delay between death and embalming
- Drowning or asphyxia
- Recent abdominal, thoracic, or cranial surgery
- Tissue gas
- Hydrothorax or ascites
- Peritonitis or bloodstream infections
- Esophageal varices, ulcerations of the gastrointestinal tract, or internal hemorrhages

Protecting Skin Areas from Purge

When purge occurs prior to or during arterial injection from the nose or mouth, the surrounding tissues of the face should be protected by an application of massage cream. Stomach purge contains hydrochloric acid and can desiccate and discolor the skin. If arterial fluid is contained in the purge material, the dye from the fluid can stain the skin, making cosmetic application difficult. Cover the facial tissues and neck area with the massage cream. Only a light coating is needed. Be certain the inside of the lips is covered as well as the base of the nose. Tightly packing the throat, nostrils, and anus prior to embalming should greatly reduce the possibility of a purge during or after embalming.

General Preembalming and Embalming Treatments

When the abdomen is distended from gas or edema (ascites) prior to embalming, a trocar should be introduced into the upper area of the cavity. Piercing the transverse colon helps to relieve gas pressure. The stomach can also be punctured, as it can contain a great quantity of liquid. If ascites is present, removing some of the edema from the abdominal cavity will relieve the pressure that can cause purging during embalming. (The aspirating hose should be attached to the trocar.)

A nasal tube aspirator can be inserted into the nasal cavity and the throat to remove purge material.

Time Period Treatments

Two factors are necessary for purge to occur. First, there must be a substance to purge, such as stomach contents, blood, arterial fluid, and respiratory tract contents. Second, there must be pressure on an organ such as the stomach, rectum, or lung to evacuate the material.

Preembalming Purge

Stomach or Lung Purge. Preembalming purge generally consists of the stomach contents (Table 24–1). If esophageal varices have ruptured or if a stomach ulcer has eroded a blood vessel, blood can also be expected in the purge. As the stomach contains acid, this purge usually is brown. Stomach purge is often described as "coffee grounds" in appearance. Removal of this material at the beginning of embalming decreases the possibility of a postembalming purge. A nasal tube aspirator can be used to remove purge from the throat and nasal passages. Some embalmers prefer to disinfect the oral cavity and nose and tightly pack the passage with cotton. Others prefer to let the purge continue during embalming and make a final setting of the features after embalming. When restricted cervical injection is used the body can purge during injection. After arterial injection the body can be aspirated, the features set, nasal and throat passages tightly packed, and the head separately embalmed.

Anal Purge. Preembalming anal purge material should be forced from the body by applying firm pressure to the lower abdomen and flushed away with running water. It is recommended that this purge be allowed to continue during embalming. Quite often, fecal matter is difficult to aspirate from the body. The anal orifice can be tightly packed with cotton saturated with cavity fluid *after* cavity treatment.

Brain Purge. Preembalming brain purge results from a fracture of the skull, a surgical procedure in the cra-

TABLE 24–1. POSTMORTEM PURGE

Source	Orifice	Description	Contents	Time
Stomach	Mouth/nose	Liquid/semisolid "Coffee ground" appearance Foul odor Acid pH	Stomach contents Blood Arterial solution	Preembalming Embalming Postembalming
Lung	Mouth/nose	Frothy Blood remains red Little odor	Respiratory tract liquids Residual air from lungs Blood Arterial solution	Preembalming Embalming Postembalming
Esophageal varices	Mouth/nose	Bloody liquid	Blood Arterial solution	Preembalming Embalming Postembalming
Brain	Fracture in skull Nose Fractured ethmoid Fractured ear Temporal bone Surgical opening	White semisolid	Brain tissue Blood Arterial solution	Preembalming Embalming Postembalming
Anus	Anal orifice	Semisolid/liquid	Fecal matter Blood Arterial solution	Preembalming Embalming Postembalming
Embalming solution	Mouth/nose Anus/ear	Color of arterial solution injected	Arterial solution	Embalming
Cavity fluid	Mouth/nose Anal orifice	Color of cavity fluid Blood present is brown in color	Cavity fluid	Postembalming

nial cavity, or a trauma such as a bullet penetrating the bone of the skull. It is possible for gas (a type of purge) to build up in the cranium and travel along the nerve routes to distend such tissues as the eyelids. Numerous foramina in the eye orbit communicate with the cranial cavity. Brain purge from the nose is rare and is usually the result of a fracture of the cribriform plate in the floor of the anterior cranial cavity. The ear can also be the site of brain purge, usually as a result of a fracture of the temporal bone. It is best to let these purges continue during the embalming procedure.

Embalming Purge

During arterial injection, the injected solution can expand the viscera. Pressure on the stomach or diaphragm results in expulsion of the contents of the stomach and/or the respiratory tract. Also during arterial injection, arterial solution can be lost to the respiratory tract, stomach, or esophagus as a result of ruptured capillaries, small arteries, or veins. Ulcerated or cancerous tissues eassily rupture because of the pressure of the solution being injected.

Tuberculosis of the lungs, cancer, pneumonia, and bacterial infections of the lung can cause fluid loss through weakened capillaries. A second cause of lung purge during embalming is congestion in the right atrium of the heart, which easily occurs if disease has involved the valves of the heart. Assume that drainage is being taken from the right femoral vein but has been very difficult to establish. Blood continues to push into the right atrium but cannot be drained away. The pressure builds to the point where the blood flows into the right ventricle and into the pulmonary arteries, squeezing the lung tissues and forcing a purge. Rupture of small veins can also produce a bloody lung purge.

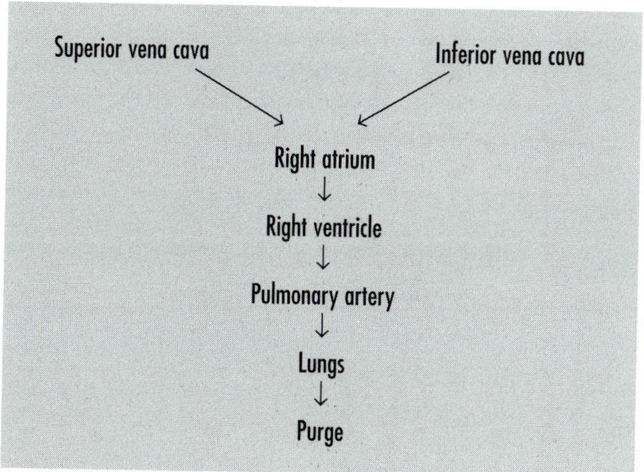

During embalming purge may simply be composed of the contents of the stomach, lung, or rectum or, as already explained, arterial solution. As a large amount of arterial solution is lost in the drainage and possibly as purge, be certain that a sufficient volume of arterial solution is injected to replace these losses. It is not always necessary to turn off the machine and begin a multipoint injection when purge contains arterial solution. When arterial solution is present in purge during arterial injection and ***drainage is occurring,*** inject a sufficient volume to satisfy the preservative demands of the body. When arterial solution is present in purge during arterial injection and ***drainage has stopped,*** a major fluid loss is occurring and distribution is not taking place. Evaluate the body and use sectional arterial injection where needed.

Rarely does anal purge contain arterial solution; however, long-term use of some drugs can cause gastrointestinal bleeding, rectal and colon cancers can erode tissues, and ulcerative colitis can destroy vessels. These conditions make possible a loss of arterial solution as well as blood drainage into the colon and rectum. If a sufficient amount of blood or arterial solution accumulates in the lower bowel, purge containing arterial solution can exit from the anal orifice.

It is usually during arterial injection that brain purge occurs. As already stated, for brain purge to occur, an opening must be present in the skull as a result of fracture, surgery, or trauma. Arterial solution escapes through small leaking arteries within the cranium, building up pressure that forces blood, arterial solution, and tissues of the brain through the openings.

Postembalming Purge

Purge that occurs prior to or during arterial injection can easily be controlled by the embalmer. It is the postembalming purge that should be of utmost concern to the embalmer. After cavity embalming, possibility of purge should be minimal. Many times, purge from the mouth, nose, or anal orifice after cavity embalming is simply cavity fluid that has been injected into these orifices. Tightly repack the nostrils with cotton, and replace moist cotton in the mouth with dry cotton.

Reaspirate prior to dressing whenever possible. If there appears to be a buildup of gas in the abdominal cavity, consider reinjection. Treat postembalming anal purge by forcing as much of the purge material from the body as possible. Then, pack the rectum with cotton saturated with a phenol solution, autopsy gel, or cavity fluid. Clothe the body in plastic pants or coveralls as added protection.

A purge that occurs from the mouth or nose after the body has been dressed and casketed may be temporarily stopped by removing the trocar button and passing a trocar through the viscera to relieve the pressure that has accumulated. The body should be reaspirated and reinjected.

Prevention of Postembalming Purge

1. Thoroughly aspirate the body cavities. Inject (in the adult body) at least 16 ounces (one bottle) of cavity fluid into the abdominal cavity, 16 ounces into the thoracic cavity, and, if possible, 16 ounces into the pelvic cavity.
2. Inject additional cavity fluid into obese bodies, bodies with ascites, bodies that have recently undergone abdominal surgery, and bodies which evidence decomposition.
3. If the abdominal trunk or buttock walls do not appear to have received sufficient fluid, hypodermically inject these areas with cavity fluids. Gases can form in unembalmed tissues and gradually move into the body cavities.
4. Reaspirate, especially those bodies that exhibit abdominal gas. This gas is easily detected when the trocar button is removed.
5. Reaspirate all bodies that have been shipped from another funeral home.
6. Pack the throat and nose with cotton. Nonabsorbent cotton should be used, because absorbent cotton may act as a "wick" to draw cavity fluid into the throat or upper nasal passages. Apply massage cream or autopsy gel to the nonabsorbent cotton before it is inserted into the nostrils or throat.
7. Remove moist cotton if purge has occurred during embalming. Be certain the mouth is completely dry.
8. When purge has been expelled from the skull as a result of fracture, decomposition, or surgical procedure (brain purge), the cranial cavity can be aspirated by passing an infant trocar or large hypodermic needle through the surgical opening, body fracture, or cribriform plate. To aspirate through the cribriform plate, insert the needle through the nostril. Direct the needle toward the anterior portion of the cranial cavity. The brain can be injected with a small amount of cavity fluid. This is best done with a large hypodermic needle and syringe.
9. A body that has had "tissue gas" in an extremity or cavity may need to be reaspirated and reinjected several times before dressing.
10. Inject a cavity fluid supplement (phenol solutions used for external bleaches) along with the cavity fluid into "problem" body cavities. (Labels of these products will indicate cavity injection.)
11. Tie off or sever the trachea and esophagus. This can be done through the incision used to raise the carotid artery.

▶ GASES

Five types of gas may be found in the tissues of the dead human body: (1) subcutaneous emphysema, (2) air from the embalming apparatus, (3) gas gangrene, (4) tissue gas, and (5) decomposition gas (Table 24–2).

In the dead human body, gases move over time to the higher body areas. When the body is in the supine position with the head elevated, the gas will move into the unsupported tissues of the neck and face. The *source* of the gas can be in the *dependent* body areas. Gas can be detected in three ways in the body. It distends weak unsupported tissues such as the eyelids and the tissues surrounding the eye orbit, the temples, the neck, and the backs of the hands. In a firmly embalmed body, distension of veins is a possible sign that gas has formed. Pushing on the tissues where the gas is present may elicit a crackling sound that is both heard and felt. This is called **crepitation.** The area under the skin feels as if it is filled with cellophane.

Types of Gas Found in Tissues

Subcutaneous Emphysema. The most frequently encountered gas condition is caused by antemortem subcutaneous emphysema, brought about by a puncture or tear in the pleural sac or the lung tissue. As the individual gasps for air, more and more air is drawn into the tissues. Subcutaneous emphysema frequently follows compound fracture of a rib, tracheotomy, lung surgery, or projection of an object (such as a bullet) into the pleural sac. A rib can be broken and the pleural sac or the lung itself torn if CPR is not administered with care, permitting a large amount of air to escape into the tissues.

This condition is *not* caused by a microbe and does not continue to intensify after death. The gas, however, moves from dependent areas to the upper body areas such as the neck and face. No odor accompanies this condition; skin-slip or blebs do not form on the skin surface. In the male, the scrotum can distend to several times its normal size. It is best to remove the gas from the tissues *after* the body is embalmed.

COMMON CONDITIONS CAUSING ANTEMORTEM SUBCUTANEOUS EMPHYSEMA

- Rib fractures that puncture a lung
- Puncture wounds of the thorax
- Thoracic surgical procedures
- CPR compression causing a fractured rib or sternum to puncture a lung or pleural sac
- Tracheotomy surgery

TABLE 24–2. GASES THAT CAUSE DISTENSION

Type	Source	Characteristics	Treatment
Subcutaneous emphysema	Puncture of lung or pleural sac; seen after CPR; puncture wounds to thorax; rib fractures; tracheotomy	No odor; no skin-slip; no blebs; gas can reach distal points, even toes; can create intense swelling; rises to highest body areas	Gas escape through incisions; establishment of good arterial preservation; channeling of tissues after arterial injection to release gases
"True" tissue gas	Anaerobic bacteria (gas gangrene), *Clostridium perfringens*	Very strong odor of decomposition; skin-slip; skin blebs; increase in intensity and amount of gas; possible transfer of spore-forming bacterium via cutting instruments to other bodies	Special "tissue gas" arterial solutions; localized hypodermic injection of cavity fluid; channeling of tissues to release gases
Gas gangrene	Anaerobic bacteria, *C. perfringens*	Foul odor, infection	Strong arterial solutions; local hypodermic injection of cavity chemical
Decomposition	Bacterial breakdown of body tissues; autolytic breakdown of body tissues	Possible odor; skin-slip in time; color changes; purging	Arterial injection of sufficient amount of the appropriate strong chemical; hypodermic and surface treatmetns; channeling to release gases
Air from embalming apparatus	Air injected by embalming machine (air pressure machines and hand pumps are in limited use today)	First evidence in eyelids; no odors; no skin-slip; amount depends on injection time	If distension is present, channeling after arterial injection to release gases

Air from the Embalming Apparatus. The injection of air from the embalming machine is NOT a frequent problem today. Most machines automatically shut off when the tank has been emptied. This condition is most likely to occur when an air pressure machine or hand pump is used for injection. Air is forced into the closed container that contains the embalming solution. The pressure from the air forces the fluid into the body. The problem is of most concern if the face is being injected. The eyelids are one of the first areas to distend, even if a very small amount of air is accidentally injected.

Gas Gangrene. Gas gangrene is a fatal disease caused by contamination of a wound infection by a toxin-producing, spore-forming, anaerobic bacterium. This bacterium can be found in soil and the intestinal tract of humans and animals. *Clostridium perfringens* is the most common of the *Clostridium* bacteria responsible for this condition. The organisms grow in the tissue of the wound, especially muscle, releasing exotoxins and fermenting muscle sugars with such vigor that the pressure build up by the accumulated gas tears the tissues apart.

The gas causes swelling and death of tissues locally. The exotoxins break down red blood cells in the bloodstream and, thereby, damage various organs throughout the body. The bacteria enter the blood just before death (the incubation period is 1–5 days). Because of the destructive action of the exotoxins and enzymes produced, tissue involvement and spread are very rapid. Gas gangrene usually occurs after severe trauma, especially farm or automobile accidents and close-range shotgun discharges, where the wound may be contaminated with filth, manure, or surface soil. Gas gangrene is particularly likely after compound fractures; the bone splinters provide foreign bodies that enhance the infection as well as permit entrance of embedded debris or dirt.

The gangrenous process begins at the margins of the wound. The skin, dark red at first, turns green and then black, and there is considerable swelling that extends rapidly over the body. The tissues are filled with gas, sometimes to the point of bursting. The affected tissue decomposes, blisters and skin-slip form on the surface, and there is no line of demarcation. A very foul odor permeates the surroundings.

Gas causes the tissue to crackle when touched. The danger involved, as an embalming complication, lies in the fact that if death occurs shortly after injury, the gas gangrene may not be visible; it may be totally internal. If embalming treatment is not sufficient to control the spread of the organisms or their by-products, the symptoms of gas gangrene may show up several hours after embalming. In addition, if the postmortem examination is delayed, internal spread will be extensive and could create disastrous postembalming complications.

Tissue Gas. Tissue gas is caused primarily by *Clostridium perfringens.* It may begin prior to death as gas gangrene. After death, the condition may result from contamination of tissues by the gas bacillus, which has translocated from the intestinal tract. Contaminated hypodermic needles have also been known to transfer C. *perfringens* to tissues of the extremities. Contaminated autopsy instruments have spread this condition from one body to another. This condition may also be spread when embalming instruments (cutting instruments, i.e., scalpels, scissors, trocar, suture needles) are not thoroughly disinfected. These organisms are very resistant to most disinfectants. Thus, the condition can occur after the body has been embalmed if all the tissues of the body and the visceral organs have not been adequately sanitized and preserved (Figure 24–1).

The gas is ordinarily formed more rapidly and with greater intensity in dependent tissues and organs. These areas are frequently congested with blood and later poorly saturated with arterial solution and, therefore, provide an ideal medium for bacterial growth. Being lighter than the liquids it displaces, the gas rises to the highest receptive parts of the body. In addition, the gas is larger in volume than the liquid it displaces and, thus, tears and distends the tissues.

Distension is usually greatest in soft tissue areas such as the eyelids, neck, and scrotum of the male. The gas spreads rather rapidly through the tissue, causing blebs to form on the surface. As the condition progresses, the blebs grow and burst, releasing the gas and putrefactive fluids and causing skin-slip.

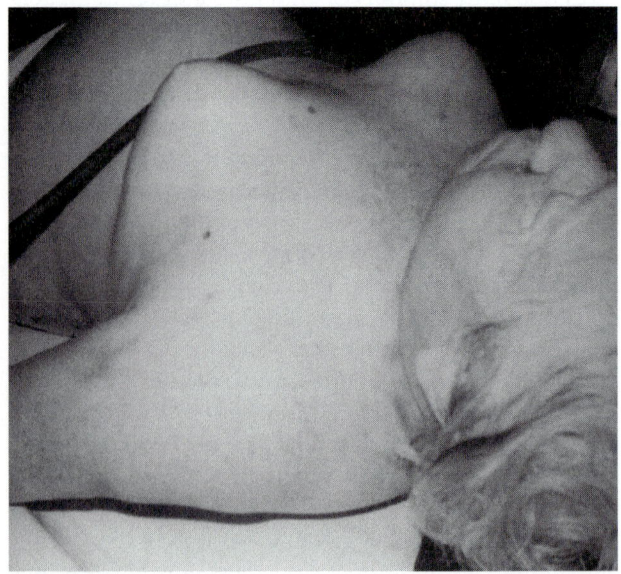

Figure 24–1. Body distended within 2 hours of death by tissue gas.

CONDITIONS PREDISPOSING TO TISSUE GAS

- Recent abdominal surgery
- Presence of gangrene at the time of death
- Intestinal ulcerations or perforations
- Contaminated skin wounds or punctures
- Intestinal obstruction or hemorrhage
- Unsatisfactory embalming
- Contact with contaminated instruments

Decomposition. In the dead human body two factors are responsible for decomposition: bacterial enzymes and autolytic enzymes. Gases are formed that accumulate in the visceral organs, body cavities, and the skeletal tissues. These gases are responsible for the odor of decomposition. As the gases accumulate in the body cavities, sufficient pressure is produced to cause purge. The gases produced by decomposition are not often as intense as tissue gas or gas gangrene. Likewise, decomposition cannot be spread from body to body by contaminated instruments. The generation of gas ceases when the tissues are properly embalmed. Gases can be removed by cavity aspiration and postembalming channeling of the tissues.

Embalming Protocol

Subcutaneous Emphysema. Because subcutaneous emphysema does not involve microbes, treatment involves merely removal of the gas from the tissues. There are no foul odors, blebbing, or skin-slip with this condition. During arterial injection, some of the gas in the tissues may relocate, most likely into the neck and facial tissues.

Restricted cervical injection should be used for the arterial injection. Fluid strength should be based on the postmortem and pathological conditions. A slightly stronger solution should be used to embalm the head, because if gas should relocate into the head after embalming (if the tissues are firm), sufficient resistance will be exerted to prevent distension. In restricted cervical injection, two incisions are made at the base of the neck. These incisions provide an exit for the gas in the tissues. The incisions can also be used as points from which to channel the neck so air can be pushed from the facial tissues.

Decomposition Gas, Gas Gangrene and True Tissue Gas. Decomposition gas, gas gangrene, and true tissue gas all have a bacterial origin. It is very important to saturate the tissues of the body with a very strong arterial solution. Restricted cervical injection should be used so large quantities of sufficient-strength arterial solution can be injected into the trunk. Chemicals specifically made for the treatment of decomposing bodies and tissue gas should be used, for example, special-purpose arterial fluids, coinjection chemicals, and cavity fluids that can be injected arterially.

If the gas appears to have originated in an extremity, sectional arterial embalming should be done. If the condition is well advanced, 100% chemical should be injected into the localized area. A coinjection chemical can be added for each ounce of arterial chemical. High pressure may be needed to inject the solution into the affected area. Often tissue gas is not noticeable at the time of death. As the organism responsible is anaerobic, after death the human body becomes an ideal medium.

Gases can form very rapidly after death. These postmortem changes can be devastating enough that a viewing of the body by family and the public would be impossible. It is imperative that the preparation be started as soon after death as possible. If the gas source is an extremity or an area such as the buttocks, a *barrier* can be made by hypodermic injection of undiluted cavity fluid in addition to sectional embalming.

Clinical Application

The source of the tissue gas appears to be a gangrenous condition of the left foot. The lower portion of the leg has turned a deep purple black. The leg is swollen and gas can be felt beneath the tissues. Injection is begun using a high-index special-purpose arterial fluid and employing restricted cervical injection as the primary injection point. Drainage is taken from the right internal jugular vein. The left femoral artery is then raised and the left leg arterially injected. Pulsation and high pressure are used to distribute the solution. A trocar is introduced from the medial side of the middle of the thigh. Cavity fluid is injected through the embalming machine throughout the area above the knee. In addition, the trocar is thrust into the deep tissues of the lower leg. Undiluted cavity fluid is injected. A barrier has now been formed with cavity fluid in an attempt to contain the *C. perfringens* and prevent it from migrating to other body areas.

In treatment of a body with true tissue gas, six-point injection can be employed with a strong arterial solution to ensure good preservation. The incisions for the arterial injection can remain open several hours, providing an exit for the gas.

Cavity treatment should be very thorough. Gas rises to the anterior portions of the viscera and cavity. Carefully aspirate the cavity, including the walls, to provide exits for the gas if it can be felt in the trunk walls. Inject a minimum of 16 ounces (or more) into each cavity. The trocar puncture can remain open to allow the escape of gases, later to be closed after reaspiration and reinjection.

Such bodies can be reaspirated and reinjected several times to ensure that bacterial activity has ceased. The treatments so far suggested are radical, but tissue gas is a very serious problem.

Tissue gas can form in bodies that have not been thoroughly embalmed. *C. perfringens* is a normal inhabitant of the gastrointestinal tract, which after death rapidly moves to other body areas.

Removal of Gas from Tissues

Regardless of the source of the gas, the method of removing it is the same. There is only one effective way to remove gas from distended tissues and that is to lance and channel the tissues and release the gas. Arterial injection and subsequent blood drainage may remove gases in the circulatory system, but do little to remove gas trapped in the subcutaneous tissue. The incision made to raise any vessels is an escape route for gas from the body.

Remember that in bodies with true tissue gas, release of the gas from the tissues does not stop its generation. The microbe causing the gas must be killed. Although gas accumulates in the superficial body tissues, the source of the gas may be located in a distal extremity or in dependent tissues.

Trunk Tissues. Gases in trunk tissues can be removed by trocar after arterial injection. During aspiration of the cavity, the trocar is channeled through the thoracic and abdominal walls. If the scrotum is affected, it too can be channeled by passing the trocar over the pubic bone.

Neck and Face. After arterial embalming, the trocar can be used to channel the neck to remove gas. Insert the trocar into the abdominal wall, after making certain the trocar can reach the neck tissues. Pass the trocar beneath the rib cage and under the clavicle to reach the neck. The trocar can also be inserted into the neck by passing under the clavicle. Make a large half-moon incision at the base of the neck lateral from the center of the right clavicle to a point lateral from the center of the left clavicle. Reflect this flap and, with an infant trocar or scalpel, channel the neck tissue. Squeeze the neck tissues. Force the gas toward the openings. The half-moon incision can also be used for restricted cervical injection. If restricted cervical injection is used, this incision prevents more gases from entering the neck and facial tissues. If possible, leave these incisions open several hours or until the body is to be dressed and casketed (see page 528).

Eyelids and Orbital Areas. After embalming, the eyelids can be opened and slightly everted. Using a large suture needle, make punctures along the undersurface of the lids. Deep channels can also be made from this location to the surrounding orbital areas. By digital pressure move the gases from the most distal areas toward the punctures. A bistoury knife or large hypodermic needle can also be inserted from within the hairline of the temple area to remove gases in the orbital area and the temple. Cotton should be used for eye closure. It absorbs the small amount of liquid that may seep from the punctures. It may be best not to seal these punctures, for they are an escape route for any further gas that may accumulate in the orbital area. The closed eye can be glued after the gas is removed. In the autopsied body the orbital area can generally be channeled by carefully reflecting the scalp. A bistoury blade can be used to dissect into the orbital areas. All this can be done from beneath the skin surface through the tissues exposed by the cranial autopsy.

Facial Tissues. Gases present in the cheeks and facial tissues can easily be removed after arterial injection and cavity embalming (Figure 24–2). Aspiration of the thoracic cavity and channeling of the neck tissues may help to remove some of the gas in the facial tissues. Open the mouth and insert a bistoury knife into the tissues of the face; run it deep to the facial bones to make channels for the gas to escape. This channeling provides escape routes for the gas. Digital pressure is needed to force the gas from the tissues to the exits. Begin at the distal points of the face and work the gas to the points where the bistoury knife or large hypodermic needle has been inserted. Any liquid leakage will drain into the mouth and throat areas. The lips can be glued. This is a radical treatment, but is the only way to provide an escape route for the gas. In the autopsied body, reflect the scalp with a bistoury knife or large hypodermic needle, and make channels into the facial tissues from the temple areas (Figure 24–3). This may be sufficient to release the accumulated facial gases.

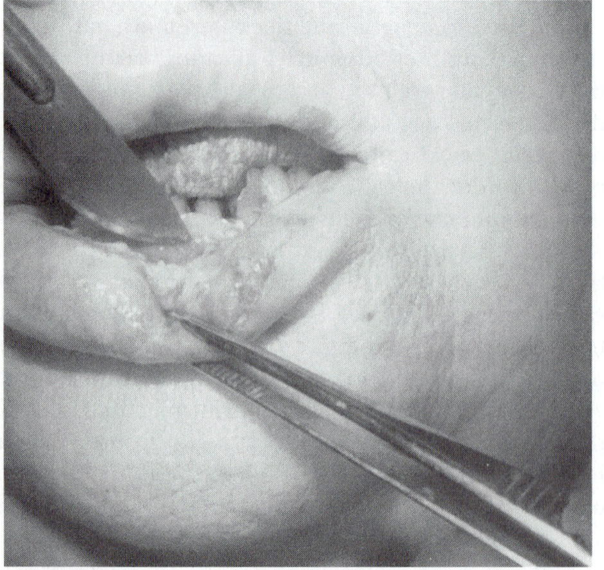

Figure 24–2. Lips are lanced to allow gas to escape (a postembalming treatment).

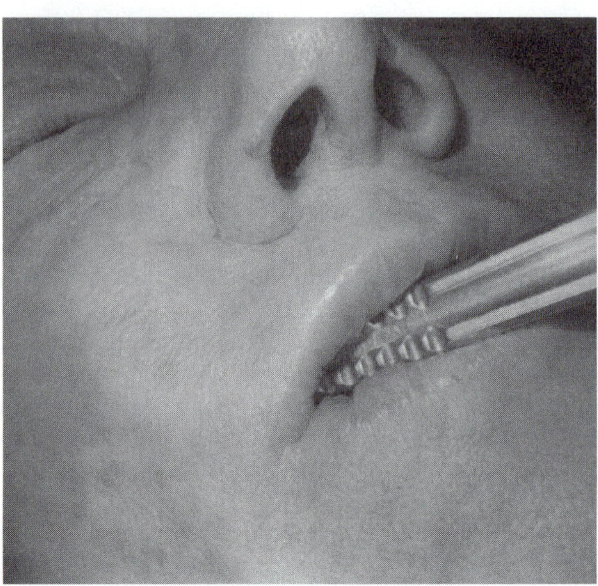

Figure 24–3. A scalpel is used to cut channels through which gas in the tissues can escape (postembalming treatment).

Instrument Disinfection

Tissue gas and gas gangrene involve a spore-forming bacillus, *C. perfringens,* which can easily be passed from one body to another via contaminated instruments. Great care should be taken in the disinfection of cutting instruments and suture needles. Wash instruments in cool running water using a good disinfectant soap. Then, soak them in a very strong disinfectant solution for several hours. Be certain that the disinfectants used in the preparation room are active (most disinfectants have a specific shelf life). Place disposable scalpel blades in a sharps container. Care should be given to disinfection of the trocar and suture needles. Consult Chapter 3 for specific disinfectant recommendations.

▶ BODIES WITH FACIAL TRAUMA

In the preparation of bodies with facial trauma, the embalmer's goal is maximum tissue preservation with a minimum amount of swelling. If good preservation can be established, the restorative and cosmetic procedures will be easier to perform and will provide satisfactory results.

Traumatic injuries vary greatly; however, facial trauma can be classified into two categories: injuries in which the skin is broken and injuries in which the skin is not broken.

Unbroken Skin	**Broken Skin**
Depressed fractures	Abrasion
Swollen tissues (hematoma)	Laceration
Ecchymosis	Incision
Simple fracture	Compound fracture

Traumatic injuries also vary with respect to their location on the head. A laceration of the cheek may be simple to restore; however, a lacerated upper eyelid may involve swelling and discoloration, as well as torn skin, resulting in a much more serious problem.

It is not within the scope of this text to detail the restorative treatments for each type of facial trauma and describe how treatment varies with location. It is the intent of this text to give a general outline of embalming protocol for traumatic facial injuries. Most of these injuries involve delay, for there usually is an inquiry by the coroner or medical examiner. Quite frequently, when an autopsy is performed, refrigeration may precede or follow the postmortem examination.

This discussion is concerned only with preparation of the head. If the body has been autopsied, the head is separately embalmed by injecting first the left common carotid artery and then the right common carotid. In the unautopsied body, restricted cervical injection can be used (right and left common carotid arteries are raised at the beginning of the embalming). Insert two arterial tubes into the right common carotid, one directed toward the trunk of the body and the other directed toward the right side of the head. Open the left common carotid artery, tie off the lower portion of the artery, and insert one tube into the artery directed toward the left side of the head. Leave both arterial tubes directed toward the head *open*. Inject the trunk first, then the left side of the head, and, finally, the right side. Drainage can be taken from the right internal jugular vein. Some embalmers prefer to drain from both the right and the left internal jugular veins when they inject the head.

General Considerations

Begin the preparation of these bodies by spraying the body with an effective topical disinfectant. Next, run cool water over the facial areas and hair to remove debris and blood. If glass was involved in the trauma, watch for small shards of glass that can easily rip gloves and cut the embalmer's fingers. Some glass can be flushed from the wounds with water, and forceps may be needed to pick glass pieces from broken tissues.

Align fractures. Incisions may have to be made prior to embalming to prop or align simple and depressed fractures. Next, align lacerated or incised skin areas. This is accomplished with a drop or two of super adhesive, or single (bridge) sutures of dental floss can be sewn with a small curved needle. Remove loose skin that cannot be embalmed by arterial means (this includes loose scabs). Apply surface preservative and bleaching compresses at this point or, if preferred, wait until the arterial injection is completed. Compresses of cavity fluid or phenol help to bleach, preserve, and dry the tissues. Phenol solutions work much faster than formaldehyde. Good tissue may be protected with a very small amount of massage cream.

Instant Tissue Fixation

Prepare a strong arterial solution. These solutions can vary depending on the arterial fluid chosen. Two examples are given here:

Solution 1	1 bottle (16 ounces) of 25- to 35-index arterial fluid
	1 bottle (16 ounces) of coinjection chemical
	Several drops of arterial fluid dye
Solution 2	1 bottle (16 ounces) of 25-to 35-index arterial fluid
	$\frac{1}{4}$ gallon water
	Several drops of arterial fluid dye

These solutions are very strong because the index of the fluid is high and there is little dilution.

Set the pressure gauge on the centrifugal injection machine at 20 psi (or higher) with the rate-of-flow valve closed.

After running some of the arterial solution through the machine to evacuate all air from the delivery hose, attach the delivery hose to the left common carotid artery. Now, open the rate-of-flow valve and allow the fluid to surge into the left side of the face. As soon as the fluid starts to flow, shut the valve off. Pause a few moments and repeat the process. The dye rises to the skin surface immediately so the embalmer is able to see what tissues are receiving fluid. In the autopsied body, the internal carotid artery may have to be clamped.

This method allows the embalmer maximum distribution, using a minimum amount of arterial solution. Keep in mind the strength of this solution. The dye helps to prevent postmortem graying of the tissues and also serves as a tracer for the fluid. Drainage is minimal and is not a concern. This method can also be used to inject the legs and arms when problems exist in the extremities.

In the unautopsied body, the trunk would generally be embalmed first and the facial area last. A suitable solution for preservation of the trunk and limbs can be used for injection. In the autopsied body the legs and arms are embalmed first, and the instant tissue fixation method is used to embalm the head.

▶ BODIES THAT REQUIRE REEMBALMING

There are occasions when it may be necessary to reembalm a body:

- Fluid was not distributed to all areas.
- Too little solution was injected.
- The concentration of the fluid was too low to meet the preservative demands of the body.
- The injected solution was neutralized by the body chemistry (often seen in bodies dead from renal failure or edema).
- Rigor mortis was mistaken for embalming fluid tissue fixation.

Instant tissue fixation and waterless embalming techniques are good methods to use when a body must be reembalmed. Use multisite injection (if necessary) to inject the legs, arms, and head at high pressure but a pulsed rate of flow, as described for bodies with facial trauma.

In the unautopsied body cavity embalming will have been completed, so begin by aspiration before arterial injection. In this manner the drainage can be taken from the heart. It is not necessary to drain from each site of injection. As only a minimum amount of fluid is used in the instant tissue fixation process, drainage should not be a big concern. After injection, thoroughly aspirate and then inject a minimum of two or three bottles of concentrated cavity fluid into the cavities. It is always suggested that these bodies be reaspirated prior to dressing.

▶ RENAL FAILURE

A more common complication associated with embalming today is due to kidney failure. Improvements in medicine and long-term drug therapy have increased the life span of persons with terminal diseases. The embalmer must check the death certificate carefully for references to renal failure or dysfunction. If the death certificate is not available, the embalmer should look for the signs of renal failure when making the preembalming analysis. Also, during and after embalming, if tissues fail to respond (by firming), the embalmer may suspect renal failure.

It has been estimated that six times more preservative chemical is needed to preserve tissues of bodies dead from the complications of renal failure. The embalmer can use some of the following signs to determine whether renal failure has affected a body:

- Sallow color to the skin as a result of urochrome buildup
- Uremic puritis (scratch marks on the extremities)
- Increase in the amount of urea, uric acid, ammonia, and creatine (urea and ammonia can be detected by their odor)
- Acidosis
- Edema (retention of sodium by the kidneys leads to increased retention of water)
- Anemia
- Gastrointestinal bleeding (blood in the gastrointestinal tract and purging)

As can be seen, a variety of signs indicate renal failure. The embalmer should realize that renal failure may be only a contributory cause of death, as it often accompanies other life-threatening diseases. Thus, the cancer or heart patient will display the bodily changes associated with these diseases, as well as the signs associated with kidney failure.

The importance of this disease to the embalmer lies in the fact that these bodies rapidly decompose. The acidity of the tissues leads to rupture of lysosomes, which contain the autolytic hydroenzymes that begin the decomposition cycle. Edema present provides the moisture needed for the hydrolytic enzymes to act, blood in the intestinal tract provides an excellent medium for the growth of putrefactive microorganisms, and the abundant ammonia in the tissues readily neutralizes formaldehyde.

Embalming Protocol

Preparation of the body affected by renal failure calls for the use of strong arterial solutions. Preinjection fluid should be avoided, because if circulation is impaired, tissues can easily swell. Begin with at least a 2.0% formaldehyde-based arterial solution. The use of a 30- to 35-index fluid is advised. Many fluid manufacturers make high-index arterial fluid specifically for bodies dead from uremia. Follow the dilution instructions of the manufacturer. After surface blood discolorations have cleared and circulation is established, arterial solution in subsequent injections can be increased in strength. Use dye to indicate the distribution of arterial solution. If edema is extensive, inject a sufficient amount of fluid to dry some of the edema.

Some embalmers prefer to use an "average-strength arterial solution" made from a 20- to 30-index fluid. After surface blood discolorations are cleared and circulation is established, they add several ounces of a high-index formaldehyde-based arterial fluid to the arterial solution. This increases the strength of the solution being injected.

Two theories are held with respect to arterial solutions: (1) solution of one strength is used throughout the embalming procedure; (2) average solution is used at the beginning, and then strength is increased gradually until the desired tissue firmness is obtained.

When both edema and renal failure are present (in addition to side effects of drug therapy, effects of the immediate cause of death, and postmortem changes that have occurred if embalming was delayed), it is easy to understand why these bodies are so difficult to prepare and why fixation of the protein can be so difficult. It is most important to saturate these tissues with a strong preservative arterial solution. If this is not done the body will soften in a few hours, blebs can form, desquamation can develop, and the body can discolor and show signs of decomposition within a day or so.

To inject these strong solutions without overembalming the facial tissues, restricted cervical injection is advised. A large volume of very strong arterial solution can be injected into the trunk, and later a milder solution can be used to embalm the facial tissues.

The cavities should be thoroughly aspirated. Inject a minimum of one bottle of concentrated cavity fluid into each cavity. During arterial injection purge is possible from gastrointestinal ulcerations, so a large amount of blood and arterial solution may be present in the contents aspirated from the abdominal cavity. These bodies should be aspirated immediately after arterial injection. It is also advised that these bodies be reaspirated and reinjected.

Some of the dependent areas press against the embalming table. These pressure point areas often do not receive sufficient arterial solution. These dependent areas are high in moisture, and so hydrolytic changes occur and the putrefactive bacteria flourish. Coveralls and possibly a unionall may be needed to prevent leakage if pitting edema is present. Preservative–deodorant powder should always be sprinkled inside the plastic goods.

▶ ALCOHOLISM

The preparation of the body that has suffered from chronic alcoholism can present a number of problems for the embalmer.

Many of these bodies exhibit jaundice as a result of liver failure. The primary goal is good preservation. Liver failure can also cause edema in the skeletal tissues or the cavities (ascites, hydrothorax). In addition, hepatic failure depletes the blood of clotting factors; therefore, good drainage can be expected if the body is prepared a reasonable time after death. Both the common carotid artery and the femoral artery are good primary injection sites; however, if skeletal edema is extensive and a large volume of strong arterial solution must be injected, restricted cervical injection is recommended. Injection should proceed at a moderate rate of flow so the tissues can assimilate the arterial solution without swelling. A moderate rate of flow also helps to prevent purging and rupture of weakened esophageal veins.

Purge is often seen in these bodies. Bloody purge may exit the mouth or nose during arterial injection. Later, it turns into a fluid purge. A good sign that fluid is being distributed to the tissues is blood drainage. Inject a large volume of arterial solution to compensate for the fluid lost through purge. Arterial fluid dye is used to trace fluid distribution and to counterstain jaundice.

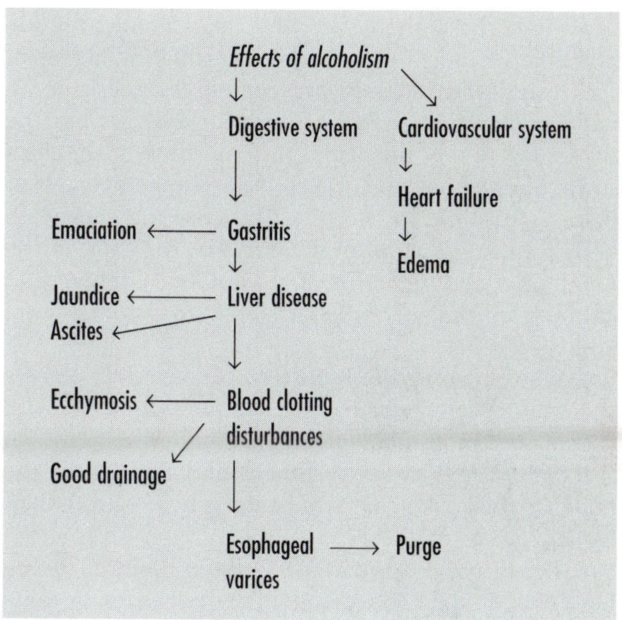

Because of the effect of long-term alcohol abuse on tissues, firming may be difficult to establish. These bodies should be injected with a moderate to strong preservative arterial solution. Do not use weak solutions even when the tissues may be emaciated or jaundiced. Add sufficient arterial fluid to firm the tissues.

Ecchymoses on the back of the hands can be treated by hypodermic injection of cavity fluid or phenol cautery solution after arterial injection. Before, during, and after arterial injection, compresses of cavity fluid, autopsy gel, or phenol solution may be applied to the skin surfaces to bleach and firm the ecchymotic areas.

Most of these bodies require tissue building after arterial injection. Tissues may be built up by injection of a restorative humectant in the last gallon of arterial solution.

At the beginning of the embalming, if ascites is present and the abdomen very distended, puncture and drain the abdomen of this serous fluid prior to or during arterial injection. By keeping the point of the trocar just beneath the surface of the anterior abdominal wall, no large vessels will be punctured. Cavity embalming should be thorough, and, of course, reaspiration is recommended.

▶ OBESITY

Preparation of the obese body has been discussed elsewhere in this book. Some of the items discussed are reviewed here. The first concern is positioning. The shoulders of an obese body should be raised high off the table. The body should occupy three levels: the head is highest, then the chest, and, finally, the abdomen. Keeping the head high facilitates raising of the vessels and helps to prevent purge. Keep the elbows as close to the body wall as possible. It may be necessary to tie the arms into position with cloth straps after embalming to keep the elbows high and as close as possible to the body. Just moving the heavy body on the preparation table can be difficult. Movement of a body is easier if it rests on a sheet or is clothed. Unclothed bodies are easier to move on a wet table.

When turning the body from side to side, place a sheet under it. It is much easier to move the body with this sheet. Some embalmers place undergarments on the large body, casket the body, and then dress the body in the casket. Others prefer to dress and then casket.

Try to use a standard-size casket. Position the elbows close to the body. Because the neck is usually quite short, keep the head straight and tie the feet together. Later, when the body is placed in the casket, tilt the shoulders and head slightly to the right.

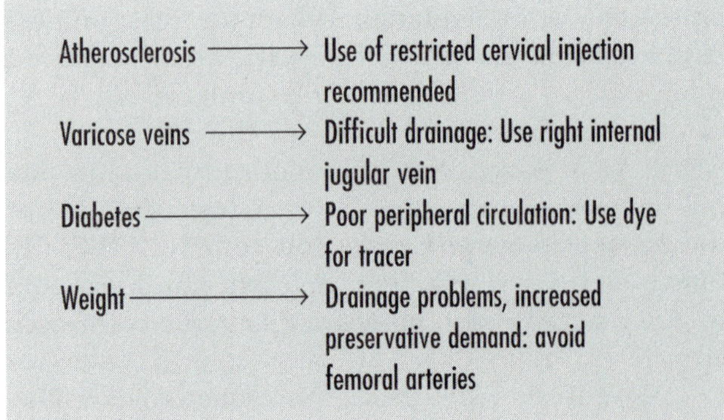
Atherosclerosis → Use of restricted cervical injection recommended
Varicose veins → Difficult drainage: Use right internal jugular vein
Diabetes → Poor peripheral circulation: Use dye for tracer
Weight → Drainage problems, increased preservative demand: avoid femoral arteries

The preceding scheme illustrates some of the complications associated with obesity.

Restricted cervical injection affords the use of the largest arteries, which should be free of arteriosclerosis. These vessels are not as deep as the femoral arteries. The right internal jugular vein can be used for drainage. It is the largest vein the embalmer can use in the unautopsied body.

Because of the short neck, drainage forceps are easier to use than a drain tube. The forceps can be inserted directly into the right atrium of the heart through the right internal jugular vein. If varicose veins are present, large clots may be observed in the drainage. The internal jugular vein allows passage of these clots out of the body.

If the obese person was also a diabetic, begin the embalming with the arms lowered over the sides of the table. Leave them in this position until the arterial solution reaches the tissues of the hands. Massaging the hands and radial and ulnar arteries promotes the flow of fluid into these peripheral areas.

This body will demand large volumes of solution. The solution can be an average dilution unless edema or other complications are present that call for stronger arterial solution mixtures. If restricted cervical injection is used, large volumes of solution can easily be injected without overembalming the facial tissues. Some embalmers prefer to increase the strength of the solution toward the conclusion of the embalming, before the head and face are injected. This increased solution strength helps to dry and firm tissues. A well-firmed body is much easier to dress and lift. Sufficient pressure should be used to overcome the resistance, particularly the resistance exerted against the large vessels by the weight of the viscera. Massage, manipulation, and intermittent drainage assist in fluid distribution.

If the legs do not receive sufficient arterial solution, try raising the external iliac artery at the level of the inguinal ligament. The vessels here are more superficial than the femoral artery. It is often observed that the arteries in obese bodies are quite small in size.

Purge is always a problem with obese bodies. Weight of the viscera pushing against the stomach can easily create sufficient pressure to cause a stomach purge. These bodies also retain heat for extended periods after death and gases easily form in the gastrointestinal tract. Again, restricted cervical injection allows the trunk to be embalmed first; then the cavities can be aspirated, the features set, and the head embalmed. Purge is thus easily dealt with. This order of embalming also eliminates the need to set features twice if the mouth becomes filled with purge material.

▶ MYCOTIC INFECTIONS*

Mycotic infections are fungal infections that may have been present as an antemortem condition or occurred as the result of a postmortem invasion. Fungi may be saprophytic or parasitic; that is, they obtain their nourishment from dead organic material or from a living organism. Fungal infections are not rare in humans and frequently are serious. Often, skin and mucous membranes are affected by the fungal infection, as in athlete's foot and thrush. The more destructive parasitic fungi produce widespread chronic lesions.

In some fungal infections, the inflammatory response and tissue damage are the result of hypersensitivity to the fungal antigens. Fungi that are ordinarily saprophytic, such as *Aspergillus, Mucor,* and *Candida,* proliferate in patients receiving prolonged antibiotic, immunosuppressive, or steroid therapy and in those with predisposing diseases such as diabetes mellitus, leukemia, and AIDS. Although there are many types of fungal infections, discussion is limited to those specific to embalming.

Candidiasis (Moniliasis)

Candida species are commonly found in the mouth, intestinal tract, and vagina of healthy individuals. *Candida albicans* is the most common cause of candidiasis. A common form of the disease known as thrush affects the oral mucosa (tongue, gums, lips, and cheeks) and the pharynx and is seen most often in debilitated infants (especially premature) and children. The lesions, white patches on the mucosa, comprise an overgrowth of yeast cells and hyphae and a nonspecific acute or subacute inflammation of the underlying tissue. Similar lesions occur on the vulvovaginal mucosa, particularly in diabetic and pregnant women and women on birth control pills. The skin, especially moist skin (e.g., perineum, inframammary folds, and between the fingers), may be affected.

Candida may produce lesions of the nails (onychia) and around the nails (paronychia), particularly in people whose hands are always in water (e.g., cooks). Occasionally, esophageal, bronchopulmonary, and widely disseminated forms of candidiasis are observed. Invasiveness is promoted by the lowered resistance of the host, as may occur in various debilitating illnesses and with intensive antibiotic, immunosuppressive, or steroid therapy. Candidal endocarditis has been reported in drug addicts, as a result of the intravenous injection of narcotics, and in patients who have undergone cardiac surgery.

Oral candidiasis can occur at any age during the course of a debilitating disease. It can also occur under dentures and orthodontic appliances and can complicate other erosive mucosal diseases (e.g., pemphigus vulgaris). The moist folds at the corners of the mouth provide a friendly environment for a troublesome candidal infection.

Oropharyngeal candidiasis is a specific complication of AIDS, because individuals with AIDS are immunosuppressed. Mouth lesions can spread down the trachea and esophagus and produce extensive gastrointestinal infections.

Aspergillosis

Most species of the genus *Aspergillus* are saprophytic and nonpathogenic. Some are found as harmless invaders of the external auditory canal, nasal sinuses, and external genitalia and as secondary invaders in lung abscesses.

In involvement of the ear, the external auditory canal may be partially filled with foul moist material spotted with black granules. The lung appears to be the most common site of serious infection. Pulmonary lesions manifest as bronchopneumonia, abscesses, small infarcts (resulting from thrombosis caused by vascular invasion), or masses of *Aspergillus* mycelia ("fungus balls") in a newly formed cavity or a preexisting inflammatory (e.g., tuberculosis) or carcinomatous cavity. Chronic granulomatous reactions to the organisms in the lungs are also possible.

A primary fatal disseminated infection is relatively uncommon. Generalized aspergillosis is more frequent as a secondary complication and tends to occur in patients with debilitating diseases and in those who have received steroid, antibiotic, or immunosuppressive therapy. Aspergillosis occurs in various tissues and organs and is characterized by abscesses, necrotic and necrotizing lesions, and sometimes chronic granulomatous inflammation.

Phycomycosis

Phycomycosis is an infection of the lungs, ears, nervous system, and intestinal tract caused by a fungus commonly encountered as a saprophyte or contaminant. The lesions may display an intense necrotizing and suppurative inflammation process. Although this infection is commonly called mucormycosis, it may be caused by several members of the group Phycomycetes, including *Mucor, Rhizopus,* and *Absidia.* These fungi invade vessels and cause thrombosis and infarction. Phycomycosis is especially seen in patients with uncontrolled diabetes mellitus, leukemia, AIDS, and other debilitating dis-

---

* This section on mycotic infections is taken from *Pathology of Human Disease* and *Synopsis of Pathology,* 10th ed. See the Bibliography at the end of the chapter.

eases and in those receiving antibiotics, corticosteroids, chemotherapeutic agents, and irradiation. The resulting lesions are similar to those mentioned earlier.

Histoplasmosis (Reticuloendothelial Cytomycosis)

Histoplasmosis is caused by the oval, yeastlike organism *Histoplasma capsulatum.* Histoplasmosis occurs worldwide, although infection is particularly common in the Mississippi Valley of the United States. Positive diagnosis depends on identification of the organisms in cultures of sputum, blood, or bone marrow or in biopsied tissue from the lymph nodes. This infection may spread throughout the body.

Histoplasmosis is not generally spread between individuals. It appears to be contracted from soil contaminated with fecal material of chickens, pigeons, starlings, other birds, and bats. In South Africa, most of the recognized benign pulmonary infections seem to have been acquired from contaminated caves (cave disease). Histoplasmosis is endemic in many parts of the world, particularly near large rivers and in high-humidity warm-temperature regions. The lungs are believed to be the usual portal of entry of the organisms. Histoplasmosis can be classified into four forms: acute pulmonary, chronic pulmonary, acute disseminated, and chronic disseminated.

The acute pulmonary form may be asymptomatic or symptomatic. The basic reaction in the lungs and lymph nodes consists of foci of tuberculoid granulomas that tend to heal. Most cases of histoplasmosis are benign, asymptomatic pulmonary infections, with positive histoplasmin skin tests and healed calcified nodules in the lung and peribronchial lymph nodes, often resembling the healed primary complex of tuberculosis. The symptomatic pulmonary infections may be either mild and "flulike" or more severe, resembling atypical pneumonia. Usually the prognosis is good. Multiple pulmonary infiltrations, with or without hilar lymphadenopathy (involvement with the entrance to the glands), may be indicated in x-rays of the chest and, in the more prolonged cases, tend to calcify and simulate healed miliary tuberculosis. In some cases, a localized pulmonary tuberculoid granulomatous lesion with caseation necrosis, calcification, and fibrotic border (histoplasmoma) may occur, appearing in an x-ray of the chest as a "coin" lesion. This lesion is sometimes removed surgically because of the clinical suspicion of lung cancer.

The *chronic pulmonary* form is progressive, forming granulomatous inflammation with caseation necrosis and cavitation, and frequently is misdiagnosed as pulmonary tuberculosis, or it may occur as a secondary complication of tuberculosis. It is seen most commonly in otherwise healthy males over the age of 40. The prognosis is poor. Occasionally, either the acute primary complex or the chronic pulmonary type is disseminated, spreading through the blood to involve many organs. Involvement of the lymph system, liver, spleen, and bone marrow dominates the clinical picture. The organs involved are packed with macrophages stuffed with organisms, so the histologic picture resembles that of visceral leishmaniasis. Jaundice, fever, leukopenia, and anemia lead to a condition that mimics acute miliary tuberculosis.

The *acute disseminated* form may be either benign or progressive. The acute progressive form is rapidly fatal, and is usually encountered in young children or immunosuppressed (AIDS) adults. The spleen, lymph nodes, and liver are enlarged. There is a septic-type fever with anemia and leukopenia. Bone marrow smears may reveal the organisms or granulomas. Occasionally, the organisms may be found in mononuclear cells in blood smears.

The *chronic disseminated* form may occur in the elderly and otherwise healthy individuals and may be fatal. In the more protracted form, which occurs in otherwise healthy individuals, the clinical features vary according to the organ most severely involved. For instance, involvement of the heart valves leads to endocarditis, and involvement of the adrenal glands leads to Addison's disease. Other organs that can be affected are the gastrointestinal tract, spleen, liver, lymph nodes, lungs, bone marrow, and meninges. In some cases, infection and ulceration of the colon, tongue, larynx, pharynx, mouth, nose, and lips are initial manifestations.

Other Mycotic Infections

Several other mycotic infections may be encountered but are rare. These include dermatomycosis, cryptococcosis, North American blastomycosis, and protothecosis. More than 100,000 species of fungi are known, of which approximately 100 are human pathogens. For the most part, they occur as secondary complications of other diseases.

Significance of Mycotic Infections to Embalming

Mycotic infections are frequently encountered, especially in those with debilitating or immunosuppressive diseases and diabetes mellitus. The widespread use of immunosuppressive drugs, combined with modern medical advances that keep patients alive but debilitated, has led to a considerable increase in the incidence of fungal infections. In the modern hospital, they are one of the most important and lethal examples of opportunistic infection.

The greatest danger presented is to the embalmer and to others who work directly with the dead human bodies. Many fungal infections produce superficial lesions on the skin and mucous membranes. As many of the fungi involved are saprophytic, they continue to multiply until they are effectively arrested. Other fungal infections involve the oral/nasal cavity, larynx, pharynx, esophagus, and lungs. These may also be saprophytic and continue to multiply in untreated or poorly embalmed dead human bodies.

In all fungal infections or unidentified lesions, careful handling of the remains is essential. When moving the remains, do not compress the abdominal or thoracic cavity. Such compression causes air and fungal organisms (including spores) to be expelled into the environment. The spores may lay dormant in the environment until conditions conducive to fungal growth arise. The spores and fungal organisms may also be inhaled by embalming personnel, establish colonies in the lungs and throat, and cause further infections.

Bodies with superficial lesions should never be handled with bare hands. A cut or break in the skin of the hands of embalming personnel represents a portal of entry for fungal and other organisms. Should the organisms enter the bloodstream, they can spread throughout the body and cause serious infections. In addition, the embalmer's clothing may harbor fungal organisms and spores, as well as other infectious organisms, which could be spread to other persons with whom the embalmer comes into contact.

Most, if not all, fungal organisms form spores. These spores may be resistant to weak disinfecting agents. Therefore, the spores may lay dormant in an improperly cleaned and disinfected preparation room and on improperly disinfected instruments. These spores could contaminate subsequent remains embalmed in that preparation room. The greater danger, however, lies in the possibility that unsuspecting embalming personnel might inhale airborne spores or contract them through cuts or breaks in the skin. Spores may enter the ventilation system and be spread to other areas.

Embalming personnel should wear protective garments in the preparation room (gloves, apron and/or impermeable disposable coveralls, oral/nasal mask, goggles, head and shoe coverings). Personal or bed clothing should be removed carefully and disposed of properly. The body should be thoroughly bathed with a proper disinfectant solution as soon as it is undressed. All superficial lesions should be treated immediately, and the mouth, nose, and eyes properly disinfected. All of these procedures must be accomplished before any embalming procedure is initiated (this would be true of all cases).

FACTORS THAT MUST BE DETERMINED IN THE EMBALMING ANALYSIS

1. Vessels for injection and drainage
2. Strength of the embalming solution
3. Volume of the embalming solution
4. Injection pressure
5. Injection rate of flow

Note: These factors will vary by the individual body and can vary in different areas of the same body.

Once the external disinfection has been completed, embalming procedures may be carried out as prescribed by the preembalming analysis. Routine arterial injection of a solution of sufficient strength and thorough cavity treatment should control internal fungal infections. Oral, nasal, vaginal, and anal cavities may be packed with disinfectant-soaked cotton as an added precaution. For autopsied bodies, careful handling of drainage is recommended.

Students of funeral service education are taught that every body should be treated as though it were infectious, because it very well may be. This has been sound advice for many years and is especially important today in light of the fact that it is not always known what diseases the deceased may have had or may have come into contact with. Whether the body is a seemingly routine case or a victim of a severe infectious disease (e.g., hepatitis or AIDS), the protection of personal and public health rests solely in the procedures used by the embalming personnel.

▶ KEY TERMS AND CONCEPTS FOR STUDY AND DISCUSSION

1. Define the following terms:
   crepitation
   esophageal varices
   instant tissue fixation
   lung purge
   mycotic infection
   postembalming purge
   preembalming purge
   purge
   renal failure
   stomach purge
   "true" tissue gas
2. Discuss the measures that can be taken to prevent postembalming purge.

3. Discuss the difference between subcutaneous emphysema and "true" tissue gas.
4. Outline the embalming of a body with tissue gas in the tissues of the right leg.
5. Discuss the problems encountered in embalming a body dead from chronic alcoholism.
6. List some mycotic infections encountered by the embalmer.
7. Discuss the problems encountered in preparation of the obese dead human body.
8. Discuss the complications encountered in embalming bodies dead from renal failure.

▶ BIBLIOGRAPHY

Anderson WAD, Scotti M. *Synopsis of Pathology.* 10th ed. St. Louis, MO: CV Mosby; 1980.

Boehringer PR. Uremic poisoning. *ESCO Rev* 1964: second quarter.

Boehringer PR. *Controlled Embalming of the Head.* Westport, CT: ESCO Tech Notes: 1967;57.

Grant M. Selected embalming complications and their treatment. In: *Champion Expanding Encyclopedia.* Springfield, OH: Champion Chemical Co.; 1987:No. 573.

Mulvihill ML. *Human Diseases.* 2nd ed. Norwalk, CT: Appleton & Lange; 1987.

Robbins SL. *Pathology.* 3rd ed. Philadelphia: 1967.

Sheldon H. *Boyd's Introduction to the Study of Disease.* 9th ed. Philadelphia: Lea & Febiger; 1984.

Tissue gas cause and treatment. In: *Champion Expanding Encyclopedia.* Springfield, OH: Champion Chemical Co.; 1971:No. 420.

Walter JB. *Pathology of Human Disease.* Philadelphia: Lea & Febiger; 1989.

CHAPTER 25
EMBALMING FOR DELAYED VIEWING

In 1989, the American Board of Funeral Service Education Curriculum committee on Embalming changed the definition of **embalming** from "the preservation of the dead human body" to "the **temporary preservation** of the dead human body." Standard embalming practices never guaranteed a *permanent* or *indefinite* preservation of remains. Embalming for funeralization is not the same as preparation of tissues, organs, or organisms for museum or laboratory study. Objectives of embalming for funeralization not only involve preservation of the body but the creation of a natural appearance of the body. This natural appearance would not be possible using preservation methods such as mummification, desiccation, freeze drying, vulcanization, or even embalming for dissection. In time, all organic matter will be reduced; we even see this with the desiccated mummies of ancient Egypt. Embalming slows this reduction process, because embalming removes tissue moisture. In time—perhaps many years—a gradual breakdown of the embalmed body will take place, rather than a putrefactive process involving liquefaction and odors. This process might be compared to a rose preserved by drying; over time, the flower parts gradually break apart.

In preparing any remains, concern should be with the preservation of the entire body, not just those areas that will be viewed. A standard for each preparation should be that the preservation of the body last more than several days or "until the burial." Standard embalming and preservation practices should conceivably keep the remains intact for months or years with no special treatments. Three major factors affect the degree and length of preservation:

1. Condition of the body at the time of the preparation.
2. Embalming thoroughness and chemical formulations.
3. Aftercare.

A unique and interesting opportunity to study many hundreds of embalmed and entombed bodies was afforded Professor John Pludeman, a Funeral Service Instructor at the Milwaukee Area Technical College in Milwaukee, Wisconsin, in 1996. His discussion is included here because it pertains to the past and present of long-term embalming.

> In recent years, funeral service professionals have begun to question the need for long-term preservation of human remains. Funeral directors, mortuary college professors, and other funeral service professionals have engaged in serious discussions on the subject. Because of the ethical, moral, and legal issues related to preservation of human remains, the issue raises important questions worthy of consideration. Frequently debated questions include:
>
> - How long should modern embalming preserve human remains?
> - What are the purposes and benefits of long-term preservation?
> - What does the consumer have a right to expect in terms of long-term preservation?
>
> The answers to these important questions of today may be partially answered by looking to the past. In the United States, it was not so many years ago that nearly all human remains were embalmed as a matter of standard practice. Society, the surviving relatives, and the funeral director correctly assumed that preservation was a customary and proper part of the traditional funeral.
>
> More recently, diverse societal attitudes and cultural changes have raised questions about the value of the funeral altogether, not to mention the value of embalming and long-term preservation. As a result, the funeral director can no longer assume that embalming and preservation will be authorized by the deceased's relatives. Further, certain federal regulations forbid the funeral director from making statements guaranteeing long-term preservation.
>
> Several years ago I managed a very unique project involving the demolition of an 85-year-old mausoleum that was in ruins. The massive project first required the disinterment of all human remains entombed within. Once completed, more than 650 casketed human remains and about 350 cremated remains were reinterred in another, well-maintained

cemetery. Because the mausoleum entombment records were vandalized and incomplete, every casket was opened to confirm occupancy and reestablish identities. By observing large numbers of embalmed human remains that had been preserved and entombed over an 85-year period, the following anecdotal information was derived about the subjects of this study.

- Between 1900 and 1960, nearly 99% of human remains were embalmed.
- In most cases, there was strong evidence of successful long-term preservation, lasting many decades.
- There was much evidence of thorough preservation through the use of adequate embalming chemicals and implementation of proper embalming methods of the day.
- In numerous cases, the deceased were very well preserved and distinctly recognizable. Facial features, hands, jewelry, and clothing remained intact.
- Some remains were completely desiccated but still recognizable while others were only skeletons. In either case, there was no odor present.
- Less than 15% (approximately 35) of all 650 disinterments were in a state of active decomposition. The majority of these cases were in sealer caskets and it appears that moisture was trapped inside the casket and could not escape, or the crypt accumulated water and it seeped into the casket.
- There was consistent evidence of extreme care given the deceased in respectful final preparation (dressing, positioning, cosmetizing, hair dressing, etc.).
- Funeral directors achieved these admirable accomplishments without the assistance of modern embalming machines, advanced embalming chemicals, eye caps, needle wire injectors, hydroaspirators, and so on.

If the previous observation and examples are an indication of successful long-term preservation from the past, does this not set a certain professional standard for the present?

Most ancient and modern funeral customs around the world include the remains of the deceased as a ceremonial focal point. Some societies believe in expedient disposition of the remains, usually through cremation, while other societies have recognized the benefits of long-term preservation to accomplish their funeral objectives.

Should the professional embalmer of today strive to achieve short-term or long-term preservation? What are the purposes and benefits of long-term embalming? Are the family and the public concerned about preservation beyond the funeral and final disposition? Are they entitled to a certain degree of preservation because they requested and paid for embalming by a professionally licensed funeral director?

Today, consumers are better informed, better educated, and demand value in exchange for the money they spend. So when faced with the decision of paying for the cost of embalming, some may question just how long embalming will preserve their loved one. If the funeral director is asked this question directly, his response may be influenced by a Federal Trade Commission (FTC) requirement that prevents the funeral director from representing that preservation will delay the natural decomposition of human remains.

There exists yet another consumer-related argument for long-term preservation, which involves the offering of protective funeral merchandise. Considering the many well-constructed, durable, highly protective caskets, burial vaults, crypts, and mausoleums offered to the consumer, what is it these products are protecting if long-term preservation is not possible? And will the consumer be willing to select these products if they perceive long-term preservation as an unlikely possibility?

The mausoleum disinterment project mentioned earlier demonstrates another important principle of protection for the deceased: A thoroughly embalmed, well-preserved body is fundamental to long-term protection of that body. Without initial preservation, no casket, crypt, or other product will retard decomposition and protect the body in the efficient manner that embalming can accomplish. Consequently, caskets, burial vaults, crypts, and other protective devices offer added protection of the deceased and then provide good value.

Long-term preservation accomplishes a number of objectives. Families have the assurance of a professionally prepared loved one and the peace of mind that it affords. Also, there will be greater value, function, and purpose of the protective products surrounding the deceased.

How long will quality embalming preserve the deceased? Because the extent of preservation and the rate of decomposition is subject to many intrinsic and extrinsic environmental factors, the degree of long-term preservation cannot be accurately predicted. However, a generally accepted consensus states that long-term preservation should far surpass the period of the funeral and ideally continue as long as the grieving process of the mourners. Because many people grieve the loss of a loved one their entire lives, it would then be reasonable to expect preservation to last numerous decades.

▶ GENERAL CONCEPTS

Three groups of embalming chemicals can be used in the preparation of bodies for extended preservation and delayed viewing: (1) preservative embalming chemicals, (2) supplemental embalming chemicals (injectable chemicals such as humectants, co- or preinjection chemicals, dyes, and other preservative chemicals), and (3) accessory embalming chemicals (noninjectable chemicals such as mold retardants, embalming powders and gels, and autopsy compounds). In addition, many funeral homes have the luxury of a refrigeration unit. This is particularly helpful when the decision about embalming is delayed several days. It is also helpful to have a refrigeration unit for the remains that will have a delayed viewing. However, it should be understood that any remains can be properly and thoroughly embalmed without the use of accessory and supplemental chemicals. Refrigeration is also not necessary for a delayed viewing of the body.

Some special considerations for the preparation of a remains for delayed viewing include the following.

- Restricted cervical injection allows the injection of large volumes of arterial solution without overinjecting the facial tissues; one solution strength can be used for the face and another strength for the trunk and limbs.
- Intermittent or restricted drainage is a good strategy.
- Delay aspiration and cavity treatment. This helps the arterial solution to thoroughly saturate the body tissues and organs.
- Place the remains on "body bridges or blocks" so that as little body surface as possible makes contact with the surface it is laying on. This is important during embalming and storage of the body.
- Avoid excessive elevation of the head. This can cause fluids to drain from the face and neck, bringing about a sunken appearance.
- Because some "drain off" of fluid can be expected, it is recommended to do some feature tissue building prior to storage. If the body is well-preserved, use regular feature builder to fill out the areas of the cheeks, temples, lips, finger tips, and so on. If these are slightly soft a mixture of 1 : 1 humectant and cavity fluid can be injected.
- Hypodermically treat all areas of ecchymosis including the tops of the hands; left untreated over time they will turn black. Use a phenol cautery solution or cavity fluid; this will bleach the tissues and ensure good preservation.
- Apply liberal amounts of massage cream to the face, neck, hands, and wrist areas. These areas can also be covered with cotton or plastic to help prevent further evaporation of the massage cream.
- Spray the remains with a mold retardant (there are some specific mold retardants available, but any topical embalming spray should prevent the growth of mold) initially, and at regular intervals, during storage.
- Do not place the remains in a closed, sealed environment; it encourages mold growth.
- The remains must be inspected on a regular basis once in storage. If problems develop they can be corrected immediately (Figure 25–1A–H).

Embalming for delayed viewing can adversely effect the remains:

- Overdrying or desiccation of tissue
- Development of mold on the surface of the remains
- Insufficient preservation, requiring re-embalming

Desiccation (an overdrying of tissue that causes dehydration or a leathery appearance to the remains) can

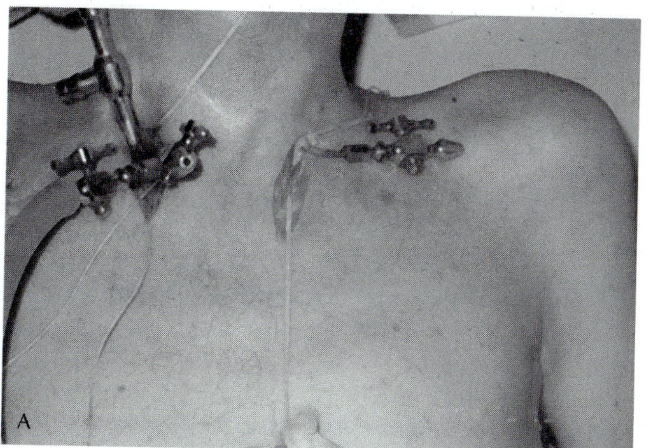

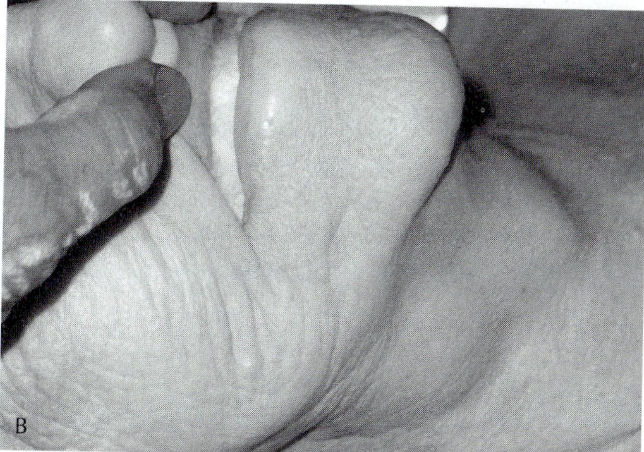

Figure 25–1. A. Preparation using restricted cervical injection. **B.** After embalming, soft areas such as the lips require treatment using cotton within the mouth saturated with cavity fluid, lips are sealed with super glue. (*Continued.*)

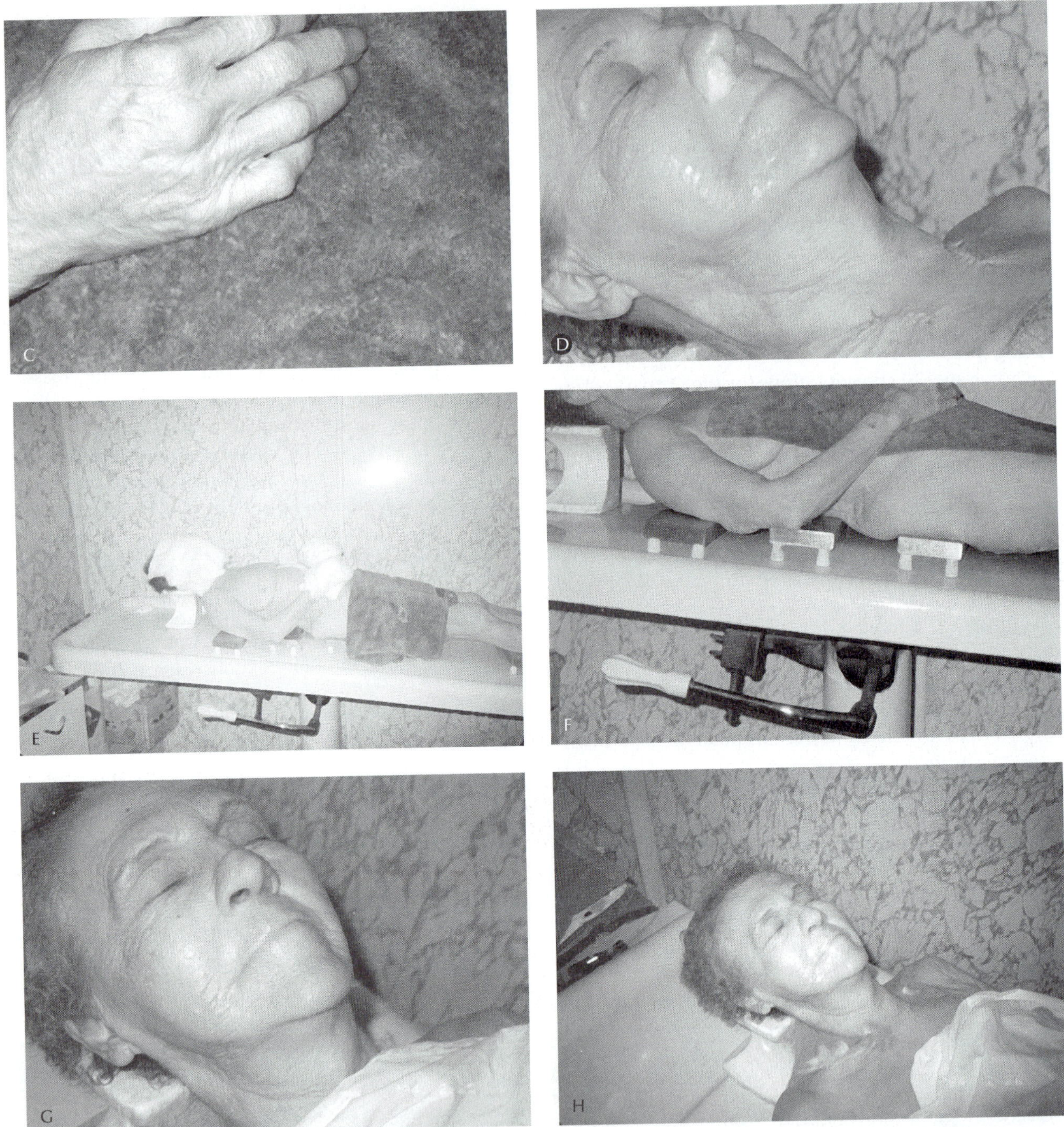

Figure 25–1. *(Continued)* **C.** Each finger tissue built after embalming. **D.** Massage cream placed on facial tissues; vasoline used to cover lips and eylids. **E.** Loose cotton covering face and hands. **F.** Body stored on body bridges. **G.** Face at end of 1 week; no dehydration, eyes and lips closed. **H.** Face at end of 2 weeks; no dehydration, eyes and lips closed.

also make it difficult to keep the eyes and mouth properly closed (Figure 25–2). Closure should be done preferably with a "super glue"; this will help to retain the closure for the dúration of storage. Use of liberal amounts of massage cream throughout the storage period will also help to reduce dehydration. Mold formation can be prevented by the topical use of a mold-retardant chemical. The remains should never be placed in a closed, dark environment as this promotes the growth of mold. During the time of storage if any area exhibits inadequate preservation, it should be treated by hypodermic injection of undiluted preservative chem-

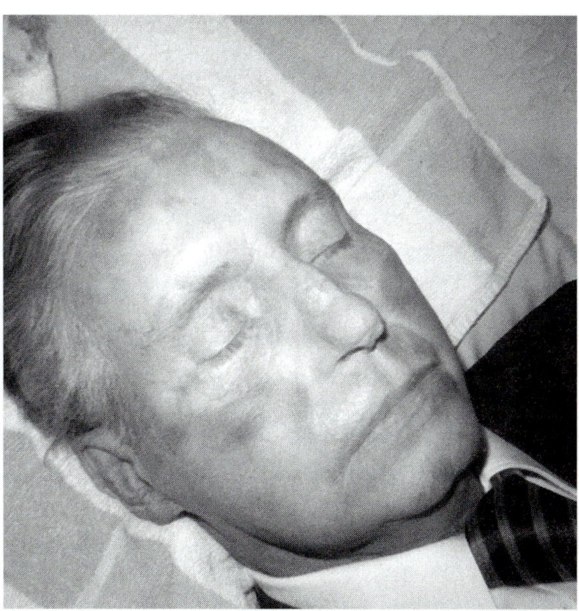

Figure 25–2. Extreme dessication 3 days after embalming.

ical or reinjected using undiluted preservative chemical. This should be done as soon as problems are identified.

▶ RE-EMBALMING

There are times when an embalmer will find it necessary to re-embalm remains that have previously been arterially preserved, including when the body has been inadequately preserved during the initial preservation or will have a delayed date of final disposition.

The re-embalming of any remains will always involve a six-point injection for nonautopsied cases. The previous aspiration and cavity injection will have disrupted the circulatory system within the body cavities making it unusable for re-injection. The arterial solution of choice is a waterless or undiluted solution sufficient to preserve all body tissues. This may require not only arterial injection but hypodermic injection of other areas of the body including the hips and buttocks. Autopsied remains may need to be fully opened with additional arterial injection and hypodermic treatment of the side walls, hips, buttocks, and head areas (see page 428).

Embalming for Delayed Viewing up to 14 Days

Embalming for delayed viewing or interment can be defined as a preparation of a remains that will allow the initial viewing up to 14 days after death. Initial viewing may be delayed for a number of reasons. Examples include:

- The family of the deceased needs to make travel arrangements.
- There is difficulty in locating the family of the deceased.
- There are legal reasons (i.e., the remains are in the custody of the coroner or medical examiner).
- The remains are being shipped to a foreign country.
- Family members are waiting for someone to be released from the hospital or awaiting the imminent death of another family member in accident cases.

In embalming any remains, it is important to base choice of arterial fluids and amounts of solution to be injected on the condition of the remains, length of time since death, and refrigeration status. This is done through an analysis of the remains prior to making any selection of fluids. Some important factors to be considered include:

- Edema or emaciation
- Kidney or liver failure
- Trauma
- Infectious diseases
- Obesity
- Signs and/or degree of decomposition present

The United States Army Regulation 638-2 *Care and Disposition of Remains and Personal Effects* in Appendix D—Armed Service Specifications for Mortuary Services (Care of Remains of Deceased Personnel and Regular and Port of Entry Requirements for Casket and Shipping Cases) in Section D-5 (5) under *Treatment of Remains* (see the Selected Readings section) states that:

> Frequently, final disposition of processed or reprocessed remains may not be effected for a period of 10 days or more; remains may be transported over long distances or subjected to hot, humid conditions. At all times the remains must be free of putrefaction and infectious agents. This requires the thorough disinfection and uniform preservation of all body tissues. Employment of continuous injection and intermittent drainage will enhance chemical distribution and penetration. Use of humectants (moisture retention chemicals) in the arterial injection solution will help to achieve greater tissue penetration and to restore normal body moisture content.

This description adequately states the desired results of all remains, not just those that will be subject to delayed viewing. The military takes an aggressive methodology toward the preparation of its deceased members as described in section D-6 *Preparation of Remains*, Processing Viewable Remains: "a thorough pre-embalming case analysis shall be made in order to determine the best embalming techniques to be used to obtain optimum results." It goes on to state the specific preferred method of treatment:

> Whenever possible, a six-point arterial injection with multi-site drainage shall be accomplished. The arterial chemical injection solution shall contain a 2 to 3 percent concentration, by volume, of aldehyde or aldehyde derivative preservative agents, with equal parts of a humectant chemical also being added to the injection solution. The thoracic, abdominal, and pelvic cavities shall be thoroughly aspirated and injected with full strength cavity chemicals having a 30-index (percent) or greater, using a minimum of 16 ounces for each cavity.

Embalming for Delayed Viewing for Greater Than One Month

In some rare instances it may be necessary to keep remains for longer than one month. Any of the examples presented earlier on delayed viewing can be applied to a situation that grows into greater than a 1-month period of time. Some suggested formulations for this type of delayed viewing include (see the Selected Readings section):

- 64 ounces of a humectant arterial fluid
- 64 ounces of a water corrective
- 64 ounces of a clot disperser or vascular lubricant
- 32 ounces of mold retardant or
- 8 ounces of phenol cauterant or
- 16 ounces of phenol cavity fluid
- 32 to 48 ounces of water
- dye, if desired

If your arterial fluid has *no humectant, make the following substitutions:*

- 48 ounces of water corrective
- 48 ounces of clot disperser or vascular lubricant
- 32 ounces of humectant or fabric softener (e.g., Downey)

When no signs of decomposition exist in the remains, use the following solution (1 gallon of solution):

- 32 ounces arterial humectant fluid
- 32 ounces coinjection
- 16 ounces of water corrective
- 16 ounces humectant
- 32 ounces tepid water

For remains showing early or intermediate signs of decomposition use the following solution:

- 32 ounces high index fluid
- 32 ounces coinjection fluid
- 32 ounces water corrective
- 16 ounces of humectant
- "0" ounces of water

Many funeral homes in the United States do not use supplemental chemicals or they might use only one or two such formulations. Excellent results are possible without the use of supplemental chemicals; many preservative arterial fluids contain humectants and high amounts of dye. Restricted cervical injection is the preferred method of injection for treatment of these bodies. The use of intermittent drainage and delaying aspiration of the cavities will allow for more thorough distribution and diffusion of the preservative chemicals.

The body must be thoroughly analyzed after embalming to insure that all areas are well preserved. This can be thought of as a quality assurance inspection. By carefully inspecting the remains and taking whatever additional steps are necessary to preserve the body, we can assure the viewing for the family will be as if the remains were embalmed yesterday.

Storage for Delayed Viewing

Refrigeration is not necessary for storage of remains for delayed viewing, but a cool location is preferred. Carefully inspect the body prior to placing it in storage. Some storage suggestions include the following.

- Lay a large sheet of thick plastic down, place body bridges on top of the plastic sheet, and lay remains on top of body bridges.
- Cover the remains with a cotton hospital gown or sheet, but do not cover the face or feet.
- Prepare a chemical wetting agent by mixing two-thirds of a gallon of humectant, 4 ounces mold retardant (thymol or phenol), and 1 gallon of water. Semisaturate the body covering with the wetting agent. Reserve the rest in a spray bottle.
- Loosely cover the remains with the plastic sheeting, trapping a moderate amount of air inside the sheeting.
- Place in a cool area.
- Check the remains every 3 to 4 days; aspirate or sponge out any liquid that has collected inside the plastic, spray the gown or sheet with the wetting agent, and reapply massage cream to facial and hand areas.
- Follow these guidelines until day of final viewing.
- Thoroughly wash and dry (so that no evidence of moisture exists) the remains, dress or redress, and cosmetize.

Or this method may also be used if the body has already been dressed and casketed:

- Remove the clothing from the remains, inspect the body for any problems, and treat accordingly.
- Spray the interior of the casket and the remains with a mold retardant.

- Use a firm board over the top of the soft mattress, or, in a casket with a metal spring bed, remove the mattress.
- Place a large sheet of plastic over the top of the board or metal bed, place body blocks down, lay pieces of cotton saturated in a chemical cauterant on top of the body blocks, place the remains on the body blocks, and cover with the plastic.
- **Do not seal the casket** as this will enhance the growth of mold; prop open the lid of the casket.
- Treat the remains hypodermically to prevent desiccation of the nose, eyes, mouth, and fingertips using 1 : 1 solution of humectant and cavity fluid. The objective is to preserve normal feature shape and guard against overdrying (dessication).
- Apply massage cream to the facial areas, arms, and hands.
- Place premium-grade cotton over the face, arms, hands (cotton should be placed between the fingers and entirely around the palm surface). All these surfaces should be sprayed liberally with the humectant/cavity fluid solution.
- Cover the genital area and the feet (between the toes also) with cotton saturated with a cauterant chemical.
- Check the remains at least once a week. Resaturate the cotton areas as needed, and spray the body surface periodically with an embalming disinfectant to protect against skin slip and mold. Reapply massage cream as needed.
- When the remains are ready to be viewed thoroughly wash and dry the remains, including the hair; avoid the use of the hair dryers as it tends to dry tissue, not just hair.
- Gently rub massage cream into facial areas and allow to sit for a few minutes. Wipe away, apply cosmetics, redress, and recasket.

Without all the accessory chemicals, you can still properly store remains for a delayed viewing through this simple method:

- Thoroughly wash and dry the body; a dry external surface will assist in preventing mold development while in storage.
- Wrap the remains in plastic sheeting.
- Fill in the tips of the fingers, the eye area including temples, and cheeks with feature builder.
- Coat the hands, face, and neck with a massage cream; cover with cotton and saturate with a commercially available fabric softener.
- Check the remains every few days to determine the ongoing condition of the body and reapply the fabric softener.
- If mold develops, it can be scraped off using a spatula or scalpel blade.

It should be stressed that it is not necessary to prepare all remains in this manner. However, to successfully make remains presentable for a delayed viewing, extra time and effort will be required on the part of the embalmer. Attention and correction of any problems during the storage time is essential to avoid the possibility of nonviewable remains.

Anatomical Embalming

Today, medical schools around the country continue the practice of embalming bodies donated for anatomical purposes. Anatomical donation in the past has precluded the traditional funeral for the family. This in some cases has caused families not to proceed with donation. To address this issue some state Anatomical Boards have created stipulations that allow funeral homes to initially embalm the bodies so that the families may have a visitation and funeral. In these situations the Anatomical Board provides the directions for the embalming of the body. After the funeral, the body is delivered to the medical school and is re-embalmed. The majority of schools use a combination of pressure injection and gravity injection overnight to thoroughly perfuse the embalming fluid. Gravity injection is done through large "percolators"; some will hold as much 8 gallons of solution. These are raised to a height of 6 to 9 feet above the body creating the pressure for the perfusion. The use of large arterial tubes helps to increase the rate of perfusion.

Most schools inject between 4.5 and 9 gallons of preservative, depending on the size of the body. Some medical schools use arterial embalming fluids available commercially from embalming fluid companies; other schools use special anatomical formulations. Formulations for anatomical embalming contain some or all of the following ingredients: formaldehyde, phenol, methanol, glycerine, formol, ethylene glycol, and isopropyl alcohol. Depending on how the body will be used, some schools drain the blood while others do not. There is no aspiration of bodies for medical schools (Figure 25–3).

Many of the bodies used by medical schools are kept for 2 years or more. At the University of Pittsburgh they currently have an embalmed body for 5 years and have in the past had one for 9 years. Dessication and mold are two major concerns in keeping bodies for long time periods at medical schools. Some schools feel it is not necessary to submerge and soak the bodies after embalming; rather they can be maintained indefinitely by using body bags with an anti-mold agent and humectant. Some schools refrigerate the bodies—not for preservation but for mold growth prevention.

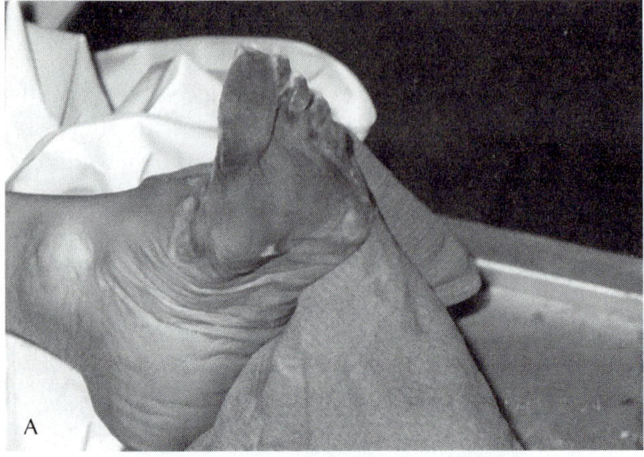

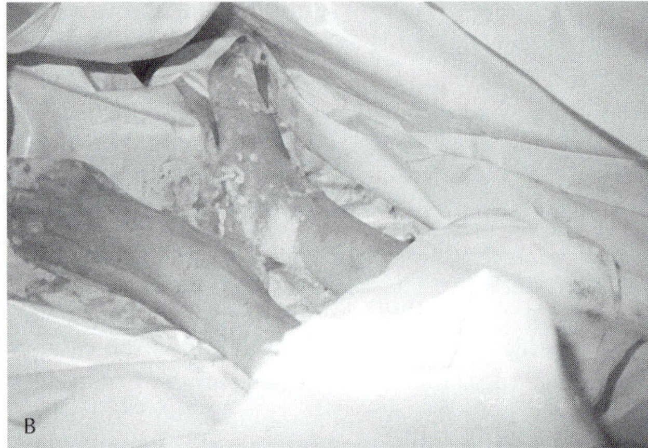

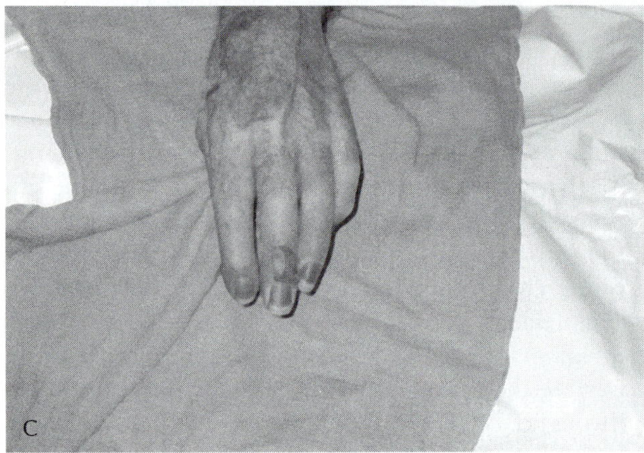

Figure 25–3. A. Excessive dehydration 2 years after preparation. **B.** Mold on foot and ankle 2 years after preparation. **C.** Loose epidermis of finger tips 4 years after preparation.

Preparation for Shipping

As discussed in Chapter 1, the transportation of human remains not only within the United States but internationally is a steadily increasing practice. The condition of the remains is of primary concern to the receiving funeral home and from an ethical standpoint must be prepared by the shipping funeral home as if it were being prepared for a local family.

The responsibilities of the shipping funeral home and embalmer are to remove the remains from the place of death, thoroughly embalm and prepare the remains for an extended period of time (i.e., 5 or more days would not be an unusually long period of time), and secure the necessary legal documents for shipping and interment. This should be done as quickly as possible to relieve anxiety for the receiving funeral home and family. There are many individual funeral firms today that specialize in the shipping of human remains. There are also several nationwide services that will contract with locally owned services to handle the arrangements. In this situation the responsibilities of the receiving funeral home are to counsel the family on an appropriate time frame for the funeral and burial. This will be done by communication with the shipping funeral home. It is inappropriate for a receiving funeral home to set a time and date for a service before the shipping funeral home has the remains.

Once the remains have arrived in the funeral home, the embalmer should inspect the body noting any problem conditions. The embalming process for shipping is based on the condition of the remains as they enter the preparation room from the place of death. The decision on arterial embalming solution should be based on these factors. All areas of the body need to be treated to guard against decomposition during the transportation, viewing, and the funeral. To achieve this, arterial injection supplemented by hypodermic injection and/or surface treatments may be necessary. If additional treatments are required, it may be necessary to communicate this to the receiving funeral home. This information should be contained on the embalming case report form but it is also advisable to relay the information over the phone. The communication of "a condition report" should be done by the embalmer to, at least, a funeral director at the receiving funeral home, **not** to secretarial help or an answering service. Both parties should clearly know the names of the person they spoke to in the event that questions come up later.

After embalming, the remains should be thoroughly bathed and dryed so that no moisture is evident on the body. The nails, nose, and mouth should be cleaned. The nose and ears should have any hair removed. For women, facial hair should also be removed prior to embalming. Pack **all** external body orifices. Minimally, plastic pants or coveralls should be placed on all remains that are to be shipped—use additional plastic garments should any leakage be anticipated. An embalming powder should be placed inside the plastic garments to absorb any moisture and prevent mold or mildew.

Unless requested, restorative and cosmetic treatments are the responsibility of the receiving funeral home. Many embalmers who provide embalming for shipping **do not** glue the mouth and eyes shut. It would be advisable to check with the receiving funeral home to determine what they want done prior to shipping the remains. A light layer of massage cream can be applied to the face and hands.

Today, it is very important to prepare an embalming case report for all embalming cases regardless of the shipping status. This document can help protect all parties involved in case of a legal dispute. It is of particular importance when shipping because the receiving funeral home has no firsthand knowledge of the condition of the remains prior to embalming, what was done during the course of embalming, and what follow-up treatment might be needed upon arrival.

The body should be placed in underclothing, hospital gown, or pajamas and wrapped in a clean sheet prior to placement in the shipping container. The inside of the container should have a large sheet of plastic laid down and the body placed inside of it. This will prevent the wooden bottom of the combination unit from becoming soaked with body fluids in the event that the body develops leakage during transportation. The body should then be securely tied in place. The head should be placed on a styrofoam head block or other elevation device. When the lid of the container is in place it should not touch the nose or forehead. **The lid of container must be nailed or screwed in place.** This prevents it from collapsing inside the container and causing damage to the remains. The "head" end should be clearly marked on the outside of the container along with the name of the deceased, the consignee (receiving funeral home and phone number), and the transportation arrangements. The necessary legal documents and embalming case report should be placed in a sealed envelope and placed on top of the container in the document envelope.

When the body is to be shipped in a casket, the remains should be secured in place with padding along the elbows and at the feet to prevent sliding during transit prior to shipping. Plastic should be placed around the head and neck to prevent any soilage should purge occur. The pillow should be turned over or have a piece of plastic covering it. Cover the face and hands to prevent any make-up from damaging the interior of the casket. If the casket has a moveable bed it should be lowered to its lowest position. If the casket is a sealing type it should **not** be cranked all the way shut to allow for any air pressure changes inside the cargo hold of the plane. The crank for the casket should be wrapped and placed on the outside of the casket so that it can be used by the receiving funeral home to open the casket. This is important as there are many different casket companies and some have a crank that is unique to a particular casket. The casket will be placed in an air tray and the information placed on the outside as suggested above.

▶ BIBLIOGRAPHY

Army Regulation 638-2. Care and Disposition of Remains and Disposition of Personal Effects. Headquarters, Department of the Army, Washington, D.C., 9 February 1996 (unclassified).

"Basic factors relating to the embalming process." *Champion Expanding Encyclopedia,* September, 1981.

Hirst T. Diagnose your cases before you start embalming. *American Funeral Director,* March, 1930.

Mayer R. The secret is in its strength. *The Director,* April, 1992.

Peterson K.D. The two year fix: Long-term preservation for delayed viewing. *The Director,* April, 1992.

Sanders, C.R. Preventing restorative problems caused by delayed interment. *The Dodge Magazine,* March–November, 1997 and January, 1998.

Shor M. Condition of the body dictates the proper embalming treatment, not cause of death. *Casket and Sunnyside,* November, 1972.

Strub C.G. Embalmed body may become "disembalmed." *Casket and Sunnyside,* 1966.

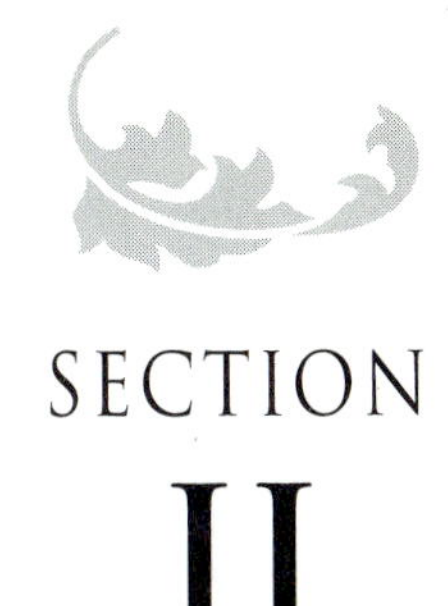

The Origin and History of Embalming

SECTION

II

Edward C. Johnson • Gail R. Johnson • Melissa Johnson

A statement in 1875 by the N. Y. State Supreme Court is still relevant, concise, and conceptually complete:

> The decent burial of the dead is a matter in which the public have concern. It is against the Public Health if it does not take place at all and against a proper public sentiment should it not take place with decency.

Winston Churchill stated in his gifted style:

> Without a sense of history, no man can understand the problems of our time, the longer you can look back, the further you can look forward—the wider the span, the longer the continuity, the greater is the sense of duty in individual men and women, each contributing their brief life's work to the preservation and progress of the land in which they live, the society of which they are the servants.

Esmond R. Long, M.D., a medical historian, wrote:

> Nothing gives a better perspective of the subject than an appreciation of the steps by which it has reached its present state.

So it is with the subject of embalming. The authors of this chapter trust that this brief exposition of the origin and history of embalming will impart to the reader a sense of the tradition and technical advances achieved over the nearly 5000 years that the art and science of embalming have been practiced. There is a clear indication that both tradition and new technical advances will continue to be maintained in the future.

Embalming, one of humankind's longest practiced arts, is a means of artificially preserving the dead human body.

I. **Natural means of preservation:** obtained without the deliberate intervention of humans
   1. Freezing: By this method bodies are preserved for centuries in the ice and snow of glaciers or snow-capped mountains.
   2. Dry cold: A morgue located on the top of St. Bernard Mountain in Switzerland was so constructed to permit free admission of the elements. True mummies were produced as a result of the passage of the cold, dry air currents over the corpses.
   3. Dry heat: Natural mummies are produced in the extremely dry, warm areas of Egypt, southwestern America, and Peru.
   4. Nature of the soil at the place of interment: There are recorded instances of the discovery of bodies in a good state of preservation after long-term burial in a peat bog that had a high tannin content or in soils strongly impregnated with salts of aluminum or copper.

II. **Artificial means of preservation:** secured by the deliberate action of humans
   1. Simple heat: Simple heat is the means employed to preserve bodies in the Capuchin Monastery near Palermo, on the island of Sicily. The Monastery is connected to a catacomb or underground burial vault composed of four separate chambers. Treatment of the bodies consists of slow drying in an oven that is heated by a mixture of slaked lime. The desiccated bodies, quite shrunken and light in weight, are placed in upright positions along the walls of the catacombs.
   2. Powders: In powder methods, the body is placed on a bed of sawdust mixed with zinc sulfate or other preserving powder.
   3. Evisceration and immersion (used by the Egyptians and others)
   4. Evisceration and drying (the Guanche method)
   5. Evisceration, local incision, and immersion (employed in Europe, particularly in France, during the period AD 650–1830)
   6. Simple immersion (in alcohol, brine, or other liquid preservatives)
   7. Arterial injection and evisceration (used by the Hunter brothers and others)
   8. Cavity injection and immersion (method of Gabriel Clauderus)
   9. Arterial injection (mode of treatment of Gannal, Sucquet, and many others)
   10. Arterial injection and cavity treatment (method in daily use by all present-day em-

balmers; generally taught in schools and colleges of embalming today)

11. Artificial cold (by a system of refrigeration to reduce the body temperature to inhibit bacterial activity; in use in most hospitals and morgues today)

▶ PERIODS OF EMBALMING HISTORY

Embalming originated in Egypt during the period of the first dynasty. It is estimated to have begun about 3200 BC and continued on until AD 650. The motive of Egyptian embalming was religious in that preservation of the human body (intact) was a necessary requirement for resurrection, their religious goal. During this nearly 4000-year period of embalming practice there obviously existed a number of variations of technique. Egyptian embalming began to decline with the advent of Christianity, as the early Christians rejected the practice, associating embalming with various "pagan religious rites." When the Arabs conquered Egypt they, too, rejected the practice of embalming.

The second period of embalming history extends from AD 650 to 1861 and its principal geographical area of practice and growth was Europe. This era is termed the *Period of the Anatomists,* as the motive was to advance the development of embalming techniques for the preservation of the dead to permit detailed anatomical dissection and study.

The third or modern period of embalming history extends from 1861 to the present day. It is during this period that embalming knowledge, which had been transferred from Europe to America during the previous period, finally reverted to its original use, principally for funeral purposes. Embalming again became available to all who requested it. Motives in this period are diverse, with sentiment probably predominant, as the average person desires to view the decedent free of evidence of the ravages of disease or injury. Public transportation is another reason to embalm, as the procedure prevents a dead body from becoming offensive during a protracted period of travel and is required by many public transport agencies.

Although the value of embalming to the public health is disputed and debated, it is most apparent that a decaying, unembalmed body is surely a health menace to those exposed to its effluvia. From earliest Egyptian times embalmers have been closely associated with the medical profession. In fact, most embalmers in the United States were doctors of medicine until the later portion of the 19th century.

▶ ESTABLISHMENT OF EMBALMING SCHOOLS

The incentive for embalming in the period AD 650 to 1861 was the preservation of anatomical material to further the study of and research in anatomy. Those who made the early strides in embalming were the anatomists, but about the time of J. N. Gannal (early 19th-century France) and Thomas H. Holmes (late 19th-century United States), general public interest was aroused in the preservation of the dead. This interest and the later demand for preservation for funeral purposes of all human dead grew far beyond the means and desires of the few, trained embalmers in the medical profession. During the late 19th century in the United States, schools of embalming instruction were established by experienced embalmers. Many funeral directors and doctors attended the schools to study embalming and to seek employment. By the beginning of the 20th century in the United States, separation of the fields of embalming and medicine was complete. This brought about the advancement of both professions, particularly that of embalming, because it placed a complex art in the hands of specialists who are still striving to acquire more knowledge and skill in preserving the human dead.

How, then, and why did the practice of embalming develop?

▶ EGYPTIAN PERIOD

During the early predynastic period, well before 3200 BC, the Egyptians had a very simple culture. When death occurred, the unembalmed body was placed in the fetal position (arms and legs folded), wrapped in cloth or straw mats, and placed in a shallow grave scooped out of the desert sand west of the Nile River. A few pieces of pottery and other artifacts were placed in the grave with the body, which was positioned on its side. The body was preserved by drying, from the contact with the arid, porous sand and the total absence of rainfall or other moisture. From time to time, desert winds uncovered the bodies in their shallow graves, and cemetery guards or relatives saw that the bodies were indeed preserved (Figure 1).

As Egyptian civilization grew, towns and villages sprang up and commerce and industry created a substantial middle and upper class of landlords and other well-to-do persons, as well as a supreme class of tribal and area rulers. When members of this group died, the old practice of simple burial in the desert sands no longer sufficed. Graves were dug deeper and were lined with wooden boards or with stone slabs so that the body,

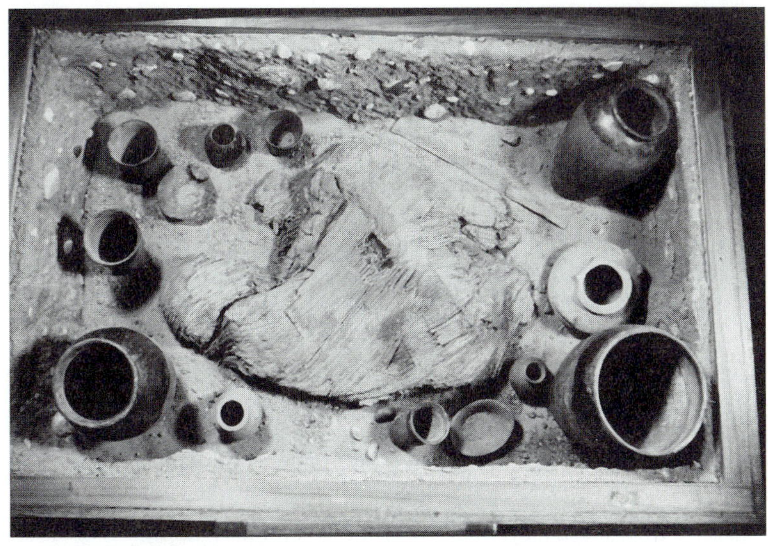

Figure 1. Predynastic (3200 BC) Egyptian burial site, west of the Nile. The unembalmed corpse is in the fetal position, wrapped in straw matting. *(Courtesy of the Royal Ontario Museum.)*

still in the fetal position, remained untouched by the sand. With these more prosperous or noble individuals were buried more valuable artifacts such as jewelry and furniture.

Then, as now, there existed members of society who were criminals, and some devoted themselves to grave robbing. When the cemetery custodians or family survivors of such elaborate burials noted the opening and desecration of burials, they also noted and were appalled that the corpse was no longer preserved, but had begun to decay. One attempt to forestall decomposition was the enclosure of the body within a solid stone coffin cut from a single mass of stone. The body of the coffin was without seams and the cover fit tightly. These burials were subsequently plundered and again the custodians or relatives contemplated the remains which, to their horror, had on many occasions completely decomposed to a skeletal status. Without a scientific knowledge of the process of putrefaction, they expressed the belief that the stone coffin ate the soft tissues. To this day, massive bronze and copper caskets are termed *sarcophagi* from the Greek *sarco* for "flesh" and *phagus* for "eater." The Egyptians, not wishing to revert to their simple burial-in-the-sands method, found it necessary to devise some system of preserving the human body—embalming.

It is not too difficult to understand how Egyptian embalming was first developed when it is kept in mind that Egypt has a basically warm climate. The culture was such that hunting and fishing provided some of the food requirements. Thus, a hunter or fisherman might have a successful catch and secure more birds, fish, or game than he or his family could consume immediately. Such animals, fish, or birds could, like the human body, quickly decay and become worthless for food. The hunter, however, knew how to prepare his catch and to preserve it. He eviscerated and bled his catch and then, by one or another method such as salting, sun drying, smoking, or cooking, preserved it for future consumption. *(This procedure for the preservation of food was common knowledge and it requires little imagination to recognize the ease with which the basic food preservation process could be adapted with refinements to the preservation of the dead human body.)*

Variation in Embalming Methods

The actual methods of embalming employed by the Egyptians varied from dynasty to dynasty according to custom and to the technique of the individual embalmer. History provides views of four contemporary writers on the subject who have frequently been quoted.

The earliest account is that of the Greek historian Herodotus, who lived about 484 BC:

> There are certain individuals appointed for the purpose [the embalming], and who profess the art; these persons, when any body is brought to them, show the bearers some wooden models of corpses; the most perfect they assert to be the representation of him whose name I take it impious to mention in this matter; they show a second, which is inferior to the first and cheaper; and a third which is cheapest of all. They then ask according to which of the models they will have the deceased prepared; having settled upon the price, the relations immediately depart, and the embalmers, remaining at home, thus proceed to perform the embalming in the most costly manner.
>
> In the first place, with a crooked piece of iron, they pull out the brain by the nostrils; a part of it

they extract in this manner, the rest by means of pouring in certain drugs; in the next place, after making an incision in the flank with a sharp Ethiopian stone, they empty the whole of the inside; and after cleansing the cavity, and rinsing it with palm wine, scour it out with pounded aromatics. Then, having filled the belly with pure myrrh pounded, and cinnamon, and all other perfumes, frankincense excepted, they sew it up again; having so done, they "steep" the body in natrum, keeping it covered for 70 days, for it is not lawful to leave the body any longer.

When the 70 days are gone by, they first wash the corpse, and then wrap up the whole body in bandages cut out of cotton cloth, which they smear with gum, a substance the Egyptians use instead of paste. The relations, having then received back the body, get a wooden case in the shape of a man to be made; and when completed, they place the body in the inside and then, shutting it up, keep it in a sepulchral repository, where they stand it upright against the wall. The above is the most costly manner in which they prepare the dead.

For such who choose the middle mode, from a desire of avoiding expense, they prepare the body as follows: They first fill syringes with oil of cedar to inject into the belly of the deceased, without making any incision, or emptying the inside, but by sending it in by the anus. This they then cork, to hinder the injection from flowing backwards, and lay the body in salt for the specified number of days, on the last of which they release what they had previously injected, and such is the strength it possesses that it brings away with it the bowels and insides in a state of dissolution; on the other hand, the natrum dissolves the flesh so that, in fact, there remains nothing but the skin and bones. When they have done this they give the body back without any further operation upon it.

The third mode of embalming, which is used for such as have but scanty means, is as follows: after washing the insides with syrmaea, they salt the body for the 70 days and return it to be taken back.

The second writer is Diodorus Siculus, who lived about 45 BC:

When anyone among the Egyptians dies, all his relations and friends, putting dirt upon their heads, go lamenting about the city, till such time as the body shall be buried. In the mean time they abstain from baths and wine, and all kinds of delicate meats, neither do they during that time wear any costly apparel. The manner of their burials is three-fold: one very costly, a second sort less chargeable, and a third very mean. In the first, they say, there is spent a talent of silver ($1,200); in the second, 20 minae ($300); but in the last there is very little expense ($75). Those who have the care of ordering the body are such as have been taught that art by their ancestors. These, showing to the kindred of the deceased a bill of each kind of burial, ask them after which manner they will have the body prepared. When they have agreed upon the matter, they deliver the body to such as are usually appointed for this office. First, he who has the name scribe marks about the flank of the left side how much is to be cut away. Then he who is called the cutter or dissector, with an Ethiopian stone, cuts away as much of the flesh as the law commands, and presently runs away as fast as he can. Those who are present pursue him, cast stones at him, curse him, thereby turning all the execrations which they imagine due to his office upon him.

For whosoever offers violence, wounds, or does any kind of injury to a body of the same nature with himself, they think him worthy of hatred; but those who are called embalmers are worthy of honor and respect; for they are familiar with their priests and go into the temples as holy men without any prohibition. So soon as they come to embalm the dissected body, one of them thrusts his hand through the wound into the abdomen and draws out all the viscera but the heart and kidneys, which another washes and cleanses with wine made of palms and aromatic odors.

Lastly having washed the body, they anoint it with oil of cedar and other things for 30 days, and afterwards with myrrh, cinnamon, and other such like matters, which have not only a power to preserve it for a long time, but also give it a sweet smell; afterwards they deliver it to the kindred in such manner that every member remains whole and entire, and no part of it changed. The beauty and shape of the face seems just as it was before, and may be known, even the hairs of the eyebrows and eyelids remaining as they were at first. By this method many of the Egyptians, keeping the dead bodies of their ancestors in magnificent houses, so perfectly see the true visage and countenance of those that died many ages before they themselves were born that in viewing the proportions of every one of them, and the lineaments of their faces, they take as much delight as if they were still living among them.

The third account is given by Plutarch, who lived between AD 50 and 100:

The belly being opened, the bowels were removed and cast into the River Nile and the body exposed to the sun. The cavities of the chest and belly were then filled with the unguents and odorous substances.

The fourth description is by Perphry, who lived about AD 230 to 300:

When those who have care of the dead proceed to embalm the body of any person of respectable rank, they first take out the contents of the belly and place them in a separate vessel, addressing the sun, and utter on behalf of the deceased the following prayer, which Euphantus has translated from the original language into Greek: "O thou sun, our lord, and all ye gods who are the givers of life to men, accept me, and receive me into the mansions of the eternal gods; for I have worshiped piously, while I have lived in this world, those divinities whom my parents taught me to adore. I have ever honored those parents who gave origin to my body; and of other men I have neither killed any, nor robbed them of their treasure, nor inflicted upon them any grievous evil; but if I have done anything injurious to my soul, either by eating or drinking anything unlawfully, this offense has not been committed by me, but by what is contained in this chest." This refers to the intestines in the vessel, which is then cast into the River Nile. The body is afterwards regarded as pure, the apology having been made for its offenses, and the embalmer prepares it according to the appointed rites.

Differences in Translations

As may be observed, there were differences in embalming methods as described by the foregoing writers. This may be, in part, due to inaccuracies in copying and translating of the original manuscripts. Egyptologists generally dismiss the accounts of Plutarch and Porphry as unreliable because the intestines either were removed and placed in containers that were kept near the body or were replaced in the body. As to the accounts of Herodotus and Diodorus, they were given the seal of approval for their general verity. Scientific proof is lacking, however, with regard to the corrosiveness of oil of cedar, and it is believed that the covering of the corpse with natron took place before the filling of the trunk cavities with the spices and other substances.

Present-day translations of the *Book of the Dead*, a textbook guide for the Egyptian embalmer, do not agree on the 70-day period for the covering with natron. One of the chronologies of the most costly method states that the 1st to the 16th days were occupied with the evisceration, washing, and cleansing of the body; from the 16th to the 36th days, the body was kept under natron; from the 36th to the 68th days, the spicing and bandaging took place; and from the 68th to the 70th days, the body was coffined.

Steps in Egyptian Preparation

Step 1: Removal of the Brain. The brain was generally removed by introducing a metal hook or spoon into the nostril and by forcing it through the ethmoid bone to the brain. As much as possible was scooped out in this way. In some mummies the brain was not removed. A few craniums had the brain removed through the eye socket. There is one case on record in which the evacuation of the cranium was accomplished through the foramen magnum, after excision of the atlas vertebra. After the body was removed from under natron, the cranium was usually repacked with linen bandages soaked in resin or bitumen. One writer tells of removing 27 feet of 3-inch linen bandage from the cranium of a mummy. Sometimes the cranium was filled with resin believed to have been introduced while molten with the aid of a funnel.

Step 2: Evisceration. Many bodies were not eviscerated. The earliest incision was made vertically in the left side, extending from the lower margin of the ribs to the anterior superior spine (crest) of the ilium. This incision would measure between 5 and 6 inches in length. At a later period the incision became oblique, extending from a point near the left anterior spine (crest) of the ilium toward the pubis. A variant incision extended vertically from the symphysis pubis toward the umbilicus. In the very late 26th dynasty (665–527 BC) some bodies were eviscerated through the anus. The incision was usually made with a flint knife called Ethiopian stone because of its black color. All the viscera, with the exception of the kidneys and usually the heart, were removed, washed, and immersed in palm wine or packed in natron. (*Their disposition will be referred to later.*)

Step 3: Covering with Natron. Natron is a salt obtained from the dry lakes of the desert and is composed of the chloride, carbonate, and sulfate of sodium and the nitrate of potassium and sodium. Because of its corrosive action on the body the embalmers had to affix the toes and fingernails to the body during the macerating period. This was accomplished by tying the nails on with thread or copper or gold wire. Alternatively, metal thimbles were fit over the ends of the fingers and toes for the same purpose. The body was then ready for the natron treatment. Early Egyptologists believed that the bodies were placed in a solution composed of natron dissolved in water, as described by Herodotus. Present-day authorities, in studying the original writing of Herodotus and other prime sources, detect a flaw in the translation of the text that is responsible for the misrepresentation. Present-day research, where the embalming process was recreated, indicates conclusively that only application of the concentrated dry salt over the body to some depth could dehydrate and preserve it. Experiments with different concentrations of the natron solution and immersion of specimens therein were largely unsuccessful in preventing decay.

Step 4: Removal from Natron. At the end of the 20th day of immersion in natron, the body was washed with water and dried in the sun.

Step 5: Wrapping and Spicing. The body was coated within and without by resin or a mixture of resin and fat. The skull was treated as in Step 1. The viscera, when removed from the body and not returned to the body, were placed in four canopic jars, the tops of which were surmounted by the images of the four children of Horus. Each jar held a specific portion of the viscera. The jar topped with the human head represented Imset and contained the liver. The jar covered with the jackal's head represented Duamutef and contained the stomach. The jar topped with the ape's head represented Hapy and held the lungs. The fourth jar, surmounted by a hawk's head, represented Qebeh-Snewef and contained the intestines. No mention is made of the disposition of the spleen, pancreas, or pelvic organs (Figure 2).

The canopic jars varied in size and material. They were from about 9 to 18 inches in height and 4 inches in diameter and were made of alabaster, limestone, basalt, clay, and other materials. The canopic jars were usually placed in a wooden box and kept near the body. When the viscera were placed in these jars, images in miniature of the jars were returned to the cavity, which was padded in straw, resin-soaked linen bandages, or lichen moss. On return to the body cavity, the viscera were usually wrapped in four separate parcels to which were attached specific images, as mentioned above. Originally, the incision was not sewn but merely had the edges drawn together. Sometimes the edges were stuck together by resin or wax; however, there are recorded instances in the 18th, 20th, and 21st dynasties (1700, 1250, and 1000 BC) of closure effected by sewing that closely resembles the familiar embalmer's stitch of today. The incision was covered, whether sewn or not, by a plate of wax or metal on which was engraved the eye of Osiris (Egyptian god of the dead).

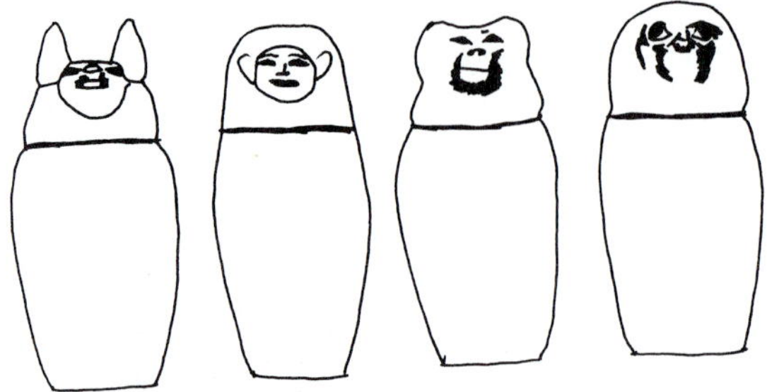

Figure 2. Canopic urns—containers of the viscera removed during embalming preparation and not returned to trunk of body. From left to right are the jackal's head, Duamutef (contained stomach); the human head, Imset (contained liver); the ape's head, Hapy (contained lungs); and the hawk's head, Qebeh-Snewef (contained intestines). *(Courtesy of Paula Johnson De Smet.)*

Ancient Restorative Art

It was during this part of the preparation in the 20th dynasty (1288–1110 BC) that a little known process was performed. Most present-day embalmers feel that the restoration to normal of emaciated facial features of a corpse is of comparatively recent origin. On the contrary, the Egyptian embalmers performed this operation, but on a much more extensive scale. Not only were the facial features restored, but the entire bodily contours were subcutaneously padded to regain their normal shape. The methods and materials used varied.

The mouth was usually internally packed with sawdust to pad out the cheeks, while the eyelids were stuffed with linen pads. Then, working from the original abdominal incision by burrowing under the skin of the trunk in all directions, the packing material was forced into these channels. In places such as the back and arms that could not be reached from the original incision, additional local incisions were made through which to pass the padding material. In later periods, the cheeks and temples were padded with resin introduced through openings in front of the ears. This material, introduced while warm, could be molded to conform to the desired contour. The packing materials most commonly used were resin, linen bandages, mud, sand, sawdust, and butter mixed with soda. It was also during this stage of preparation that repair of bodily injuries took place. Broken limbs were splinted, and bed sores were packed with resin-soaked linen bandages and covered with thin strips of antelope hide.

There is a case of a crooked spine having been straightened. Eyes were sometimes replaced with ones of stone or, as in one instance, with small onions. The bodies that were to be gilded (covered with golden leaf) were then treated. Some were completely covered with a gold leaf; on others, only the face, fingernails, and toenails, or genitals were gilded, as there was much variation on this matter. After the complete covering of the body with a paste of resin and fat, the bandagers set to work. It is believed that there were individuals who specialized in wrapping certain parts of the body such as the fingers, arms, legs, and head. Each finger or toe was first separately swathed; then each limb. The body was first covered with a kind of tunic and the face covered with a large square bandage followed by the regular spiral bandages. Pads were placed between the bandages to aid in restoration and maintenance of the bodily contour. Lotus blossoms have been found between the layers of linen bandages. Some authorities claim that the living saved cloth all their lives to provide bandages for use as mummy wrappings. The bandages varied from 3 to 9 inches in width and up to 1200 yards in length and were inscribed at intervals with hieroglyphics indicating the identity of the enswathed person. Authorities believed that only one of ten mummies was prepared by the first method. The others were prepared by the cheaper methods, as described by the earlier writers. Another means of embalming used then was simple covering of the entire body with natron or molten resin. This latter process, while preserving the body, destroyed the hair and most of the facial features, fingers, and toes.

During the last 1000 years of Egyptian embalming practice, the emphasis gradually changed from producing a well-preserved body capable of withstanding decay for all eternity to creating an increasingly elaborate external appearance of the wrapped body. Wrapping patterns became quite elaborate and cartonage and plaster were employed to present a sometimes fanciful external recreation of the deceased. During the terminal centuries of Egyptian embalming, portraits on a flat surface were painted and placed over the head area, which more faithfully resembled the dead.

The Receptacles

The wrapped mummies were usually additionally encased and placed in boxes or coffins. An additional encasement, termed *cartonage,* was made of 20 or 30 sheets of linen cloth or papyrus saturated in resin, plaster of Paris, or gum acacia and placed over the wrapped body while wet. To ensure a tight fit, the material was drawn together in the back of the body by a kind of lacing not unlike present-day shoelacing. The cartonage, when dry, was as hard as wood and was covered with a thin coating of plaster, then painted with a representation of a human head and other designs. Two or more wood cases of cedar or sycamore might encase the cartonage and each other. These coffins or mummy cases were of different shape, depending on the period when they were made. The outer wooden case was, at times, rectangular in shape with a cover resembling the roof of a house. Early coffined embalmed bodies were placed within the coffins lying on their side. The exterior of the coffin contained the representation of a pair of eyes on one side near the head of the coffin (Figure 3). This indicated the position of the body facing outward at this point. Coffins shaped like the human form were termed anthropoid or mummiform (Figure 4). If the deceased was a member of a great family he might be enclosed within a stone sarcophagus that was a stone coffin or vault fashioned of marble, limestone, granite, or slate.

Even in Egyptian times the tombs of the dead were plundered for their valuables. Many mummy cases were broken open and the mummies themselves were damaged. The embalmers were called on to repair the damaged mummies and to rewrap and recoffin them. This

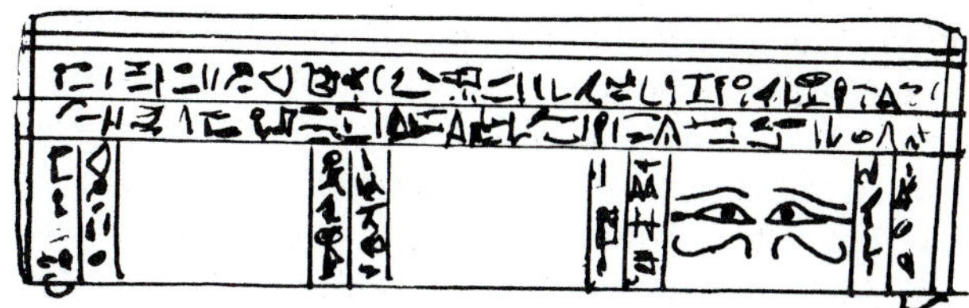

Figure 3. Wooden coffin. The body, placed inside, lies on its left side with the head at the end where eyes are drawn thus looking outward. *(Courtesy of Paula Johnson De Smet.)*

may explain, in part, the so-called faking of mummies. In the Field Museum of Natural History in Chicago there are numerous x-ray pictures of unopened mummy cases and unwrapped mummies. Some of these pictures show damage that may have occurred prior to or during the course of embalming. One x-ray

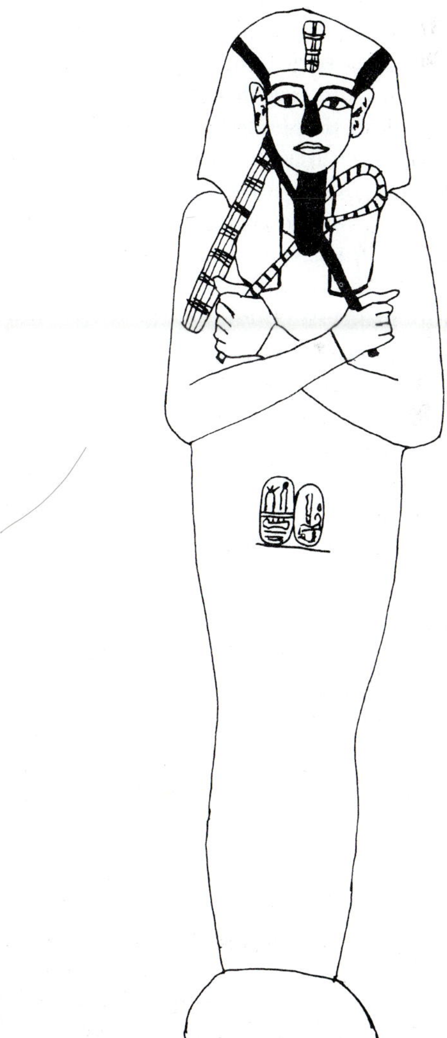

Figure 4. Wooden anthropoid or mummiform coffin. *(Courtesy of Paula Johnson De Smet.)*

photo of a young child displays the complete absence of the arms and bilateral fractures of the femurs at about their midpoint, with the lower broken portion entirely missing. Museum authorities advance the theory that this was done to fit the child into a smaller mummy case. Another x-ray photo reveals a wrapped mummy lacking arms and the trunk of the body. The head was connected to the legs by a board and the body has been represented by padding of straw or lichen moss.

Additional faking may be the result of a curious custom of the early middle ages of using bits of mummies as good luck pieces and as a drug for internal consumption. This demand created a brisk business for the Arabs of North Africa, and as the supply of natural mummies was difficult to maintain, the Arabs began to produce their own from the bodies of the lepers and criminal dead.

Animals were also embalmed, wrapped, and coffined in a manner similar to humans. The variety of animals so treated was large and included baboons, monkeys, full-grown bulls, gazelles, goats, sheep, antelopes, crocodiles, cats, dogs, mice, rats, shrews, hawks, geese, ibis, snakes, and lizards. X-ray examination of these wrapped packages discloses an occasional falsity. Some of these false mummies are composed of straw or rags wrapped in the form of the animal they were to represent. G. Elliot Smith, in his article on the Significance of Geographical Distribution of Practice of Mummification, states that knowledge of the Egyptian method of embalming was carried westward as far as the Canary Islands. He bases his decision on the similarity of the embalming procedures carried on in these areas of the world and the knowledge that the Egyptian method preceded those in all other known parts of the world.

▶ THE PRACTICE OF BODY PRESERVATION OF VARIOUS ETHNIC GROUPS AND PLACES

Jews. The Jews did not embalm but simply washed and shaved the body and swathed it in sheets, between the folds of which were placed spices such as myrrh and aloes. The purpose of herbs and spices was to disguise the odor of decay of the body, not to preserve it.

Ancient Persians, Syrians, and Babylonians. Sometimes, the ancient Persians, Syrians, and Babylonians immersed their human dead in jars of honey or wax. Alexander the Great was said to have been so treated to preserve his body during the long journey from the place of death in Babylon in 323 BC (during a military campaign) to Egypt.

Ancient Ethiopians. The ancient Ethiopians eviscerated and desiccated their dead in a manner similar to the Egyptian method. The bodily contours were restored by applying plaster over the shrunken skin. The plaster-covered corpse was then painted with lifelike colors and given a coating of clear resinlike substance believed by some authorities to be a fossil salt and by others to be a type of amber, somehow rendered fluid at the time of application.

Canary Islands. (from at least 900 BC). In the Atlantic Ocean, about 4° south of the Madeira Islands, on the northwest coast of Africa, there is a cluster of 13 islands known as the Canary Islands. These islands were not subdued by any European nation until the Spaniards overran them in the late 15th century. The original inhabitants, known as Guanches, are thought to have been descendants of the lost continent of Atlantis. It is believed that only prominent and influential families had the dead embalmed. The Guanche's method of embalming their dead is very similar to the Egyptian method.

The Guanche embalmers were both men and women who performed the services for their own sex. These embalmers were well paid, although their touch was considered contaminating and they lived in seclusion in remote parts of the Islands. On the death of a person, the family bore the body to the embalmers and then retired. The embalmers placed the body on a stone table and an opening was made in the lower abdomen with a flint knife called *tabona.* The intestines were withdrawn, washed, cleaned, and later returned to the body. The entire body, inside and outside, was very thoroughly saturated with salt and the intestines were returned to the body along with numerous aromatic plants and herbs.

The body anointed with butter, powdered resin, brushwood, and pumice, was exposed to the sun, or, if the sun was not hot enough, the body was placed in a stove to dry. During the drying period the body was maintained in an extended position; the arms of men were placed along the sides of the body, while women's arms were placed across the abdomen.

The embalmers maintained a constant vigil over the body during this period to prevent it from being devoured by vultures. On the 15th or 16th day the drying process should be complete and the relatives would claim the body and sew it in goatskins. Kings and nobles were, in addition, placed in coffins of hollowed juniper logs. All bodies were deposited in caves in the hilly regions of the islands.

In another method of preparation described, a corrosive liquid believed to be juice of the spurge or euphorbia plant, was either introduced through the belly wall or poured down the throat; this was followed by the drying process described above. The mummies produced by these processes were called *xaxos* and the method of embalming was believed to have been introduced from Egypt about 900 BC. In T. J. Pettigrew's *History of Egyptian Mummies,* there is a description of a xaxos as found by a sea captain in 1764. The author points out the "flesh of the body is perfectly preserved, but it is dry, inflexible and hard as wood . . . nor is any part decayed. The body is no more shrunk than if the person had been dead only two or three days. Only the skin appears a little shriveled and of a deeply tanned, copper color." The xaxos were extremely light in weight, averaging about 6 to 9 pounds for bodies up to $5\frac{1}{2}$ feet in length.

Peru. Preservation of the body in Peru was practiced for at least a thousand years before the Spanish conquest in the early 16th century. It had for its motive a religious belief in the resurrection of the body. Most authorities agree that the Peruvians had no process of embalming, but that their mummies were a product of the extremely dry climate of the region. There are reports that the Incas or ruling classes were embalmed, and because only mummies of the common people have been discovered, this report may be true. The manner in which the Inca rulers are believed to have been prepared was by evisceration. The intestines were placed in gold vases, the cavity filled with an unspecified resin, and the body coated with bitumen. The bodies were said to have been seated on their thrones, clothed in their regal robes, hands clasped on the breast, and head inclined downward. There is mention of the use of gold to plate or replace the eyes.

The usual Peruvian mummy, of which there are many specimens in the Field Museum at Chicago, was often found buried with the face toward the west, together with provisions of corn and coca contained in earthen jars. The mummies themselves were wrapped in cloth and tied with a coarse rope. The outer covering was of matting and followed a roll of cotton which, in turn, enveloped a red or varied-color wool cloth wrapped about the body. The innermost wrapping was a white cotton sheet. The corpse was found in a squatting position, knees under chin, arm over breast, with the fists touching the jaws. The hands were usually fastened together, and on most mummies there was a rope passed three or four times around the neck. In the mouth there was usually a small copper, silver, or gold disk. The greater part of the mummies was well preserved, but the flesh was shriveled and the features were disfigured. The hair was preserved, with the women's hair braided. Nearly all types of animals and birds have been found mummified, including parrots, dogs, cats, doves, hawks, heron, ducks, llamas, vicunas, and alpacas wrapped in the manner of human mummies.

Ecuador. The Jivaro Indians of the Marano River region of South America had a method of preserving heads by shrinking them. Technically, this process does not come under the heading of embalming, but a brief general description of the process is of interest.

The bones of the skull were first removed through long slits in the scalp. The skin of the head, with the hair attached, was boiled in water containing astringent herbs. On completion of this process, hot stones of gradually diminishing size were inserted into the space formerly occupied by the skull bones. When the shrinking process was completed, the stones were removed and the incisions were sutured as were the mouth and eyes. The finished shrunken head is about the size of a man's fist, with the features rather clear and retaining their proper proportions. It has been stated that this same process has been applied to an entire human body with equal success, although no such specimens have been found.

Mexico and Central America—Aztecs, Toltecs, and Mayans. On the basis of information received from Alfonso Caso, Mexico's outstanding anthropologist, there is no evidence of the employment of any artificial means of preservation of the body in the pre-Spanish era in these regions. There are accounts of finding mummies wrapped in matting and buried in the earth or in caves, but it is the opinion of Caso and others that such mummification was the result of the natural climate of the region.

North American Indians. Although no proof exists to substantiate claims that some of the Indian tribes embalmed their dead, there are quotes from two accounts of embalming means as recounted by H. C. Yarrow in his *Study of Mortuary Customs of North American Indians* from 1880, collected from earlier publications. On page 185 of the *History of Virginia* (by Beverly, 1722), this statement is found:

> The Indians are religious in preserving the corpses of their kings and rulers after death. First they neatly flay off the skin as entire as they can, slitting only the back; then they pick all the flesh off the bones as clean as possible, leaving the sinews fastened to the bones, that they may preserve the joints together. Then they dry the bones in the sun and put them into the skin again, which in the meantime has been kept from shrinking. When the bones are placed right in the skin, the attendants nicely fill up the vacuities with a very fine white sand. After this they sew up the skin again, and the body looks as if the flesh had not been removed. They take care to keep the skin from shrinking by the help of a little oil or grease, which saves it from corruption. The skin being thus prepared, they lay it in an apartment for

> that purpose, upon a large shelf raised above the floor. This shelf is spread with mats for the corpse to rest easy on, and screened with the same to keep it from the dust. The flesh they lay upon hurdles in the sun to dry, and when it is thoroughly dried, it is sewed up in a basket and set at the feet of the corpse, to which it belongs.

Another account appeared in Volume XIII, page 39, of *Collection of Voyages* (Pinkerton, 1812), concerning the Werowance Indians:

> Their bodies are first bowelled, then dried upon hurdles til they be very dry, and so about most of their joints and neck they hang bracelets or chains of copper, pearl and such like, as they are used to wear. Their innards they stuff with copper beads, hatchets and such trash. Then they lap them very carefully in white skins and so roll them in mats for their winding-sheets.

The Indians are known to have wrapped their dead in cloth or leather and to have suspended the bodies in a horizontal manner in trees or buried them in the earth, in caves, or in the ground covered by rocks. This may have had a religious significance, but more likely it was done to prevent vultures or animals from devouring the dead.

Aleutian Islands and Kodiak Archipelago. It is believed that the inhabitants of the Aleutian Islands and Kodiak Archipelago practiced preservation of their dead from at least AD 1000, although the custom did not prevail on the mainland. The internal organs were removed through an incision in the pelvic region and the cavity was refilled with dry grass. The body was placed in a stream of cold running water, which was said to have removed the fatty tissues in a short time. The corpse was removed from the water and wrapped in the fetal posture, knees under the chin and arms compressed about the legs. This position was accomplished by use of force, breaking bones if necessary. In this posture the body was sun-dried and, as a final gesture, was wrapped in animal skins and matting.

▶ PERIOD OF THE ANATOMISTS (AD 650–1861)

With the Arabic conquest of Egypt and the fall of the Roman Empire, European and Mediterranean civilizations declined virtually to the vanishing point. The old world of law and order as the Romans and others knew it was replaced by anarchy. Geographical areas were ruled by bands of armed men with little stability of control. The Dark Ages were to continue until the year 1000 when a gradual elimination of unstable leaders left a few more wise and capable individuals in charge of substantial geographical divisions of Europe. With a return to a more normal civilized existence came the establishment of schools and colleges in what is today Sicily, Italy, France, and England and later in Germany, Holland, Belgium, and Switzerland. The schools were, in part, the product of the Catholic Church, which throughout the Dark Ages had maintained and served as a sanctuary for work in the fields of medicine, nursing, teaching, copying of manuscripts, and establishment of orphanages and poorhouses.

The medical schools that were established used some texts originally written during the glory era of Egypt. In Alexandria, on the Mediterranean at the mouth of the Nile, there existed the greatest center for teaching that history had known. The Library, before its destruction, was said to have contained more than half a million manuscripts on subjects varying from astronomy to mathematics to engineering to medicine. It was here that a famous teacher and practitioner of medicine, Claudius Galen (130–200 AD), born in Pergamum, Asia Minor, taught and wrote on the subject of anatomy. His textbook on anatomy described human anatomy principally from dissections of animals such as the pig or monkey. It must be obvious today that there are substantial differences or variations between the anatomical structure of the pig or monkey and those of the human being. Galen and others were not encouraged to dissect the human body as it was considered a mutilation and a crime under Egyptian law. Nevertheless, Galen's teachings and writings on human anatomy were to be considered as the unchallengeable authority for the next 1000 to 1200 years.

With the emergence of Europe from the Dark Ages came a craving for learning that had to that time been suppressed. The medical schools lacked the authority to legally acquire dead human bodies for dissection and anatomical study until the 13th and early 14th centuries. Such authority was granted in 1242 by Frederick II, King of the two Sicilies, and again in 1302 for the delivery of two executed criminals to the medical school at Bologna, Italy, each year for dissection. Such dissections were public affairs, often conducted in open areas or amphitheaters always during the cold months of the year because the dissection subjects were not preserved. The dissection itself was rapid, frequently confined to a 4-day period. In the actual procedure, the anatomy professor, who was seated, read from Galen's text on anatomy while pointing out (with a wand) the body structures mentioned by Galen. An assistant, a barber–surgeon, did the actual dissection as the lecture progressed. Obviously, there were frequent contradictions between Galen's description of a body part and its actual appearance as disclosed by the dissection. These most evident discrepancies encouraged the more intelligent student and medical practitioner to steal bodies from cemeteries and gallows for personal study and research. Every part of such a purloined cadaver was probed speedily for knowledge of its structure or function until it became too loathsome to conceal and had to be disposed of. In many cases the soft tissues were thrown away and the bones boiled to secure the skeleton.

Military Religious Campaigns

During the period from 1095 to 1291 a series of military religious campaigns mounted by the Christian nations of Europe (termed *Crusades*) were conducted to recapture the Holy Land from the Moslems. The campaigns were successful early on, but with the passing of time the Christian occupation forces in the Holy Land became complacent and less martial and eventually were expelled from the entire conquered territory. Many prominent members of the nobility, including King Louis XIX of France, died far from home during the crusades. To allow the return to their homeland of their remains it was necessary to develop what became a gruesome procedure, as no certain means of embalming was available during the campaigns. The procedure consisted of disemboweling and disarticulating the body, cutting off all soft tissues, and then boiling the bones until they were free of all soft tissues. The bones were then dried and wrapped within bull hides and returned to their homeland by the couriers who maintained the communication lines.

In 1300 Pope Boniface VIII issued a Papal Bull (a directive) that prohibited the cutting up of the dead for the purpose of transport and burial under penalty of excommunication. For a brief period, this Papal Bull was interpreted by some members of the medical profession to ban anatomical dissection. For example, in 1345 Vigevano stated that dissection was prohibited, and Mondino (1270–1326) said sin was involved in boiling bones. In any case, such interpretations were rare and were seldom given any regard by the majority of anatomists.

As the years passed it became obvious that some system of preservation, even temporary, had to be contrived to permit a more careful and intensive study of body structure. Early efforts at preservation followed the ancient regimen of drying the parts, for moisture was and is the enemy of preservation. Preservation by drying of cadavers or their components was first sought by exposure to the natural heat of the sun. Later, use of controlled heat in ovens was employed to accomplish desiccation. Eventually, while probing the nature and extent of the hollow blood vessels, it was noted that warm air forced through the blood vessels removed blood and eventually dried out the tissue.

Reports of preservation attempts from the 15th century did not include injections of the blood vascular system. Such early injections into hollow structures of the body were made to trace the direction and continuity of blood vessels or to inflate hollow organs so as to reveal their size and shape or to make internal castings of areas under study. As early as 1326, Alessandra Giliani of Italy injected blood vessels with colored solutions that hardened; Jacobus Berengarius (1470–1550) employed a syringe and injected veins with warm water; Bartolomeo Eustaschio (1520–1574) used warm ink; Regnier De Graaf (1641–1673) invented a syringe and injected mercury; Jan Swammerdam (1637–1680) injected a waxlike material that later hardened. The great artist Leonardo Da Vinci (1452–1519), who is said to have dissected more than 30 corpses to produce hundreds of accurate anatomical illustrations, injected wax to secure castings of the ventricles of the brain and other internal areas.

Early Instruments for Injection

Early instruments for injection were crude and usually made in two parts: a container for the injection material and some form of cannula. The cannula was often contrived from a hollow straw, feather quill, hollow metal, or glass tube which was attached by ligature to an animal bladder (stomach or intestine). The cannula was inserted into the hollow opening being studied and the bladder tied onto its free end. The bladder, in turn, was filled with a liquid and then tied to retain the bladder full. Entrance of the liquid material into the hollow area was secured by squeezing the bladder until it emptied.

As early as 1521 Berengarius wrote of using a forerunner of the modern syringe. Early syringes similar to the hypodermic syringes employed today were constructed. They were filled and then attached to a cannula in position within the opening to be injected. To refill the syringe the operator had to detach the syringe from the cannula, refill it, and then reattach it. Bartholin (1585–1629) developed the first continuous-flow syringe. It could be recharged during use without halting the injection process.

During the entire time from the end of the Egyptian embalming activity through the Dark Ages and into early medieval period, some members of the elite, clergy, nobles, tradesmen, and landowners were embalmed, a procedure ordinarily neither contemplated by nor available to the average European. The embalming procedure, not surprisingly, was virtually identical to the Egyptian technique described by Herodotus and others, with the exception that far less time was consumed in its execution.

One of the best accounts of nonanatomical embalming for burial purposes is related by the Dutch physician Peter Forestus (1522–1597), who wrote about embalming. His account, in German, is contained as an appendix in the 1605 edition of Peter Offenbach's treatise on *Wound Surgery*. Forestus specifically described the embalming process and the materials used in five named cases between 1410 and 1548, two of which he personally performed:

1410	Pope Alexander V of Bologna, Italy
1511	Lady Johanna of Burgundy, Holland
1537	Bishop Magoluetus of Bologna, Italy
1582	Countess of Hautekerken of The Hague, Holland
1584	Princess Auracius of Holland

As these cases are essentially similar, only one embalming report is cited in its entirety.

Most of the above embalmings were performed in the room of the residence where the death occurred, a practice rather commonly followed later (well into the 20th century) in many countries including the United States.

The following is the full description of the Forestus embalming of the Countess of Hautekerken. The others listed are quite similar with some individual variations such as opening the cranium and removing the brain and making long and deep incisions in the extremities to press out the blood, then filling the incisions with the powdered mixture.

> I personally was bidden to embalm the Countess of Hautekerken, who was a daughter of a nobleman of Egmont (Holland) and who died of childbirth on January 9, 1582 at The Hague (Holland) before Johannes Heurnius (1543–1604), my good friend, and professor at Leyden in Holland was asked. Preceding all things, before the embalment was begun, there was made the following preparation . . . I took $2\frac{1}{2}$ lbs. aloes; myrrh, $1\frac{1}{2}$ lbs.; ordinary wermut, seven handsfull; rosemary, four handsfull; pumice, $1\frac{1}{2}$ lbs.; marjoran, 4 lbs.; storacis calamata, 2 loht; the zeltlinalipta muscata, $\frac{1}{2}$ loht. Mix all and reduce to a powder. Lay open the trunk of the body, remove all the viscera, afterwards take such sponges which were previously immersed in cold fresh water, afterwards dipped in aqua vita, and wash out the interior of the body by hand with the sponge. This having been done, fill the cavities (of the body) with a layer of cotton moistened in aqua vita; sprinkle over it a layer of the previously mentioned powders; place another layer of the moistened cotton and a layer of powder one over the other until the abdomen together with the chest is entirely full. Afterwards sew the above (abdominal walls) again together. Wrap around (the body) with waxed cloth and other things. Now having heard this you understand this embalment was performed by me, the aforementioned Heurnius and Arnold the Surgeon on January 10, 1562, in the dwelling of the wellborn Count and Countess Von Wassenaer in The Hague.

Ambroise Pare (1510–1590)

Born in France, Ambroise Pare was military barber–surgeon and eventually surgeon to French kings Henri II, Francois II, and Charles IX. He was famous for rediscovery and improvement of use of ligature to control bleeding after amputations, podalic version (changing the position of an unborn infant within the uterus) to facilitate delivery, and designing of artificial limbs. Pare, like many surgeons of the period, embalmed the bodies of prominent military leaders and noblemen killed during military campaigns as well as similarly prominent civilians dying of natural causes.

In one of his books written in 1585 and entitled *Apology and Account of His Journeys into Diverse Places,* Pare described embalming a follower of the Duke of Savoy, a Monsier de Martiques who died following a gunshot wound through the chest received in battle. The embalming was followed by coffining and transportation to the home of the deceased.

In his book *The Works of Ambroise Pare,* translated into English and published in London in 1634, he devotes a portion of the 28th chapter On the Manner Howe to Embalme the Dead:

> But the body which is to be embalmed with spices for very long continuance must first of all be embowelled, keeping the heart apart, that it may be embalmed and kept as the kinsfolkes shall thinke fit. Also the braine, the scull being divided with a saw, shall be taken out. Then shall you make deepe incisions along the armes, thighes, legges, backe, loynes, and buttockes, especially where the greater veines and arteries runne, first that by this means the blood may be pressed forth, which otherwise would putrifie and give occasion and beginning to putrefaction to the rest of the body; and then that there may be space to put in the aromaticke powders; and then the whole body shall be washed over with a spunge dipped in aqua vita and strong vinegar, wherein shall be boyled wormewood, aloes, coloquintida, common salt and alume. Then these incisions, and all the passages and open places of the body and the three bellyes shall be stuffed with the following spices grossely powdered. Rx pul rosar, chamomile, balsami, menthe, anethi, salvia, lavend, rorismar, marjoran, thymi, absinthi, cyperi, calami aromat, gentiana, ireosflorent, assacederata, caryophyll, nucis moschat, cinamoni, styracis, calamita, benjoini, myrrha, aloes, santel, omnium quod sut ficit. Let the incisions be sowed up and the open spaces that nothing fall out; then forthwith let the whole body be anointed with turpentine, dissolved oyle of roses and chamomile, adding if you shall thinke it fit,

> some chymicall oyles of spices, and then let it be againe strewed over with the forementioned powder; then wrap it in a linnen cloath, and then in cearecloathes. Lastly, let be put in a coffin of lead, sure soudred and filled up with dry sweete hearbes. But if there be no plenty of the forementioned spices, as it usuall happens in besieged townes, the chirurgion shall be contented with the powder of quenched lime, common ashes made of oake wood.

The procedure described by Pare was the most prevalent in use from the end of the Egyptian system to well past the discovery of arterial injection.

Discovery of a New Technique

Anatomical dissection, nonpreservative injections, and study continued until inevitably the technique of arterial injection of some preservative substance into the blood vascular system to secure an embalmed subject was stumbled upon. Contrary to popular belief, three men, all Dutch and all friends, were involved and must be recognized for their contributions to the technique: Jan Swammerdam (1637–1680), the original inventor or discoverer; Frederick Ruysch (1638–1731), the great practitioner who refined the technique; and Stephen Blanchard (1650–1720), the person who openly published the method.

Swammerdam was educated in medicine but devoted the greatest part of his life to the study of insects and small animals. He perfected a system of injection to preserve even insects through tiny cannulas made of glass and manipulated by the aid of microscopes designed by Leeuwenhoek (the inventor of the microscope). His preservatives were said to have included various forms of alcohol, turpentine, wine, rum, spirits of wine (purer form of alcohol), and colored waxes. This injection technique was transmitted to Ruysch who applied it to human subjects, both entire bodies and portions thereof. His superb collections of anatomical specimens provided great teaching aids. His embalming of complete human remains included individuals such as British Admiral Sir William Berkley, who was killed during a sea battle off Holland in 1666, and whose body was recovered from the sea in a decomposing condition. Ruysch was requested by the Dutch government to embalm the body so that it might be returned to England for funeral and burial. It is said that the body was normal in appearance and color after his treatment.

In another episode the Russian Czar Peter the Great, during one of his visits to western Europe, visited the medical school of Leiden, Holland, and Ruysch's home, where his museum was situated. During the visit with Ruysch, it is related that some domestic problem required Ruysch's attention and he left Czar Peter alone for a few minutes. Czar Peter began to explore the various rooms and, in opening one door, discovered an infant apparently asleep. Tiptoeing into the room he contemplated the beautiful pink child, then bent down and kissed it, only to discover by its cold exterior that it was one of Ruysch's many preparations. Czar Peter purchased one entire museum collection from Ruysch which some historians report was lost or destroyed. The truth is that it is still on exhibit in Leningrad today. Ruysch personally never did make a full disclosure of his technique or preservative. There are many who conjecture that his preservative was alcohol, turpentine, or even arsenic.

Blanchard, an anatomist of Leiden, published a book in 1688 entitled *A New Anatomy with Concise Directions for Dissection of the Human Body with a New Method of Embalming.* Pages 281 to 287 and several diagrams of syringes and instruments constitute the appendix describing his method of embalming. He mentions the use of spirits of wine and turpentine. In one of his embalming treatments, he began by flushing out the intestinal tract by first forcing water from the mouth to the anus. Then he repeated the flushing with spirits of wine and retained it in place by corking the rectum. He opened large veins and arteries and flushed out the blood with water, then injected the preservative spirits of wine. **(This technique described in the book appears to be the earliest mention of injection of the blood vessels for the specific purpose of embalming.)**

Ludwig De Bils (1624–1671)

Ludwig De Bils was a Flemish anatomist and resident of Leiden who was also an embalmer. As with Ruysch, he never divulged his embalming methods and is said to have gone to great lengths to prevent accidental discovery of his method by visitors to his museum. Gabriel Clauderus, while viewing De Bils' specimens, shrewdly moistened his forefinger and applied it to the skin of an embalmed body and, tasting the moistened finger, disclosed a salty flavor which led Clauderus to suspect that the principal ingredient in De Bils' fluid was salt. De Bils wrote several books on the subject of embalming but failed to disclose his methods.

Gabriel Clauderus (Late 17th Century)

Gabriel Clauderus, a physician from Altenburg, Germany, was a contemporary of De Bils. In 1695 he published a book, *Methodus Balsamundi Corpora Humani, Alique Majora Sine Evisceratione,* in which he described his method of embalming, which omitted evisceration. His fluid was made from 1 pound of ashes of tartar dissolved in 6 pounds of water, to which was added $\frac{1}{2}$ pound of sal ammoniac. After filtration it was ready for use and was denominated by Clauderus as his "balsamic spirit." He injected this fluid into the cavities of the body and then immersed the cadaver in the fluid for 6 to 8 weeks. The treatment was concluded by drying the corpse either in the sun or in a stove.

England's Customs and Achievements

Although the British Isles are geographically grouped with Europe, they developed different customs and their scientific achievements advanced at a pace different from that in continental Europe.

Some individuals regard the Company of Barber–Surgeons of London to be the first group licensed to embalm. A brief examination of the background of this organization reveals that from about 1300 to 1540 the Company of Barbers and the Guild of Surgeons were separate entities. In 1540 they received a charter from Henry VIII consolidating these two groups under the title of the Company of Barber–Surgeons and granting them the right to anatomize four executed criminals each year. In 1565 Queen Elizabeth I granted the same privilege to the College of Physicians. In 1745 the Surgeons and Barbers ended their joint relationship and again became two separate organizations. During the Barber–Surgeons period they were permitted to be the sole agency for embalming and for performing anatomical dissections in the city of London, although there is no record of any of the bodies for anatomy being embalmed.

This was never a well-respected or enforced monopoly. In their 200-year existence there were fewer than ten complaints, and in several of the cases cited in the College of Barber–Surgeons records, no fines or other punishment is noted. In several cases no conclusion of the case appears. Most complaints were lodged against members for performing private anatomical dissections not on the premises of the College. The more influential members such as William Cheselden and John Ramby simply ignored the rule and even withdrew from the organization as William Hunter did. **(The barber–surgeons made no progress in the development of licensing of embalmers as such and even today in the British Isles, no license or permit is needed from any governmental agency to perform embalming and never has been so required.)**

William Hunter, M.D.

William Hunter (1718–1783) was born in Scotland and studied medicine at the University of Glasgow and at Edinburgh. He finally settled in London where he specialized in the practice of obstetrics and taught anatomy. He became one of the great teachers of anatomy in English medical history and received many awards and appointments to honor societies, climaxed in 1764 by his appointment as Physician-Extraordinary to Queen Charlotte of England. He was the author of many brilliant treatises on medical subjects, perhaps the greatest being his *Anatomy of the Gravid Uterus.* His private collections of anatomical and pathological specimens, together with his lecture and dissecting rooms, occupied a portion of his home. All of this, plus a large sum of money, were donated to the University of Glasgow after his death.

Hunter was in the habit of delivering, at his private school at the close of the anatomical lectures, an account of the preparation of anatomical specimens and embalming of corpses. He injected the femoral artery with a solution composed of oil of turpentine, to which had been added Venice turpentine, oil of chamomile, and oil of lavender, to which had been added a portion of vermillion dye. This mixture was forced into the body until the skin exhibited a red appearance. After a few hours during which the body lay undisturbed, the thoracic and abdominal cavities were opened, the viscera were removed, and the fluid was squeezed out of them. The viscera were separately arterially injected and bathed in camphorated spirits of wine. The body was again injected from the aorta and the cavities were washed with camphorated spirits of wine. The viscera were returned to the body, intermixed with powder composed of camphor, resin, and niter, and placed in the eyes, ears, nostrils, and other cavities. The entire skin surface of the body was then rubbed with the "essential" oils of rosemary and lavender. The body was placed in a box on a bed of plaster of Paris for about 4 years. When the box was reopened, and if desiccation appeared imperfect, a bed of gypsum was added to complete the process.

One of Hunter's admonitions to his students, which is still applicable to attainment of the finest results, was to begin the embalming process within 8 hours of the death in the summer and within 24 hours in the winter.

Until the wartime aerial bombing of the Royal College of Surgeons Museum in 1941, the embalmed body of the wife of eccentric dentist Martin Van Butchell, a pupil of William Hunter, was on exhibition. There was a letter in Van Butchell's handwriting describing the embalming process. It is reproduced here verbatim:

> *12–Jan.–1775:* At one half past two this morning my wife died. At eight this morning the statuary took off her face in plaster. At half past two this afternoon Mr. Cruikshank injected at the crural arteries five pints of oil of turpentine mixed with Venice turpentine and vermillion.
>
> *15–Jan.:* At nine this morning Dr. Hunter and Mr. Cruikshank began to open and embalm my wife. Her diseases were a large empyema in the left lung (which would not receive any air), accompanied with pleuropneumony and much adhesion. The right lung was also beginning to decay and had some pus in it. The spleen was hard and much contracted; the liver diseased, called rata malphigi. The stomach

was very sound. The kidneys, uterus, bladder and intestines were in good order. Injected at the large arteries oil of turpentine mixed with camphored spirits, i.e., ten ounces camphor to a quart of spirits, so as to make the whole vascular system turgid; put into the belly part six pounds of rosin powder, three pounds camphor and three pounds niter powder mixed rec. spirit.

17–Jan.: I opened the abdomen to put in the remainder of the powders and added four pounds of rosin, three pounds niter and one pound camphor. In all there were ten pounds rosin, six pounds niter and four pounds camphor, twenty pounds of powder mixed with spirits of wine.

18–Jan.: Dr. Hunter and Mr. Cruikshank came at nine this morning and put my wife into the box on and in 130 pounds of Paris plaster at eighteen d. a bag. I put between the thighs three arquebusade bottles, one full of camphored spirits, very rich of the gum, containing eight ounces of oil of rosemary, and in the other two ounces of lavender.

19–Jan.: I closed up the joints of the box lid and glasses with Paris plaster mixed with gum water and spirits wine.

25–Jan.: Dr. Hunter came with Sir Thos. Wynn and his lady.

7–Feb.: Dr. Hunter came with Sir John Pringle, Dr. Heberden, Dr. Watson and about twelve more fellows of The Royal Society.

11–Feb.: Dr. Hunter came with Dr. Solander, Dr.——, Mr. Banks and another gentleman. I unlocked the glasses to clean the face and legs with spirits of wine and oil of lavender.

12–Feb.: Dr. Hunter came to look at the neck and shoulders.

13–Feb.: I put four ounces of camphored spirits into the box and on both sides of neck and six pounds of plaster.

16–Feb.: I put four ounces oil of lavender, an ounce of rosemary and $\frac{1}{2}$ ounce of oil of camomile flowers (the last cost four Sh.) on sides of the face and three ounces of very dry camomile flowers on the breast, neck, and shoulders.

The body was said to resemble a Guanche or Peruvian mummy and was very dry and shrunken.

John Hunter, M.D.

John Hunter (1728–1793) was born in Scotland, the younger brother of William Hunter, in whose anatomy classes he first proved so adept. After studying under the great surgeons of his time he was appointed to hospital staffs and lectured on anatomy. A region of the body he described was named in his honor: "Hunter's canal." He served as a surgeon in the British army during the campaign in Portugal (1761–1763) and, on his discharge from the service, settled in general practice in London. There he continued the collection and study of anatomical and natural subjects. He was a most brilliant and prolific writer on all phases of medicine and surgery and later founded his own private anatomy classes, which were unexcelled for the number of students who later distinguished themselves in medicine. Among these students were Jenner, Abernathy, Carlisle, Chevalier, Cline, Coleman, Astley Cooper, Home, Lynn, and Macartney.

In 1776 Hunter was honored by appointment as Surgeon-Extraordinary to the King of England. In 1782 he constructed a museum between his two homes in London to house his anatomical and natural history collections. These eventually contained nearly 14,000 items, and at his death were purchased by the British government for the Royal College of Surgeons. The main exhibit hall, measuring 52 by 28 feet, was lighted from above and had a gallery for visitors.

Many stories are told of body stealing for dissection and for securing specimens for collections. None would better illustrate this than John Hunter's acquisition in 1783 of the body of the Irish giant O'Brien, at a cost to him of about $2500.00. O'Brien, about 7 feet 7 inches in height and dreading dissection by Hunter had, shortly before his death, arranged with several of his friends that his corpse be conveyed by them to the sea and sunk in deep water. The undertaker, who it was said had entered into a pecuniary agreement with Hunter, managed that while the escort was drinking at a certain stage of the journey to the sea the coffin should be locked in a barn. Confederates, which the undertaker had concealed in the barn, speedily substituted an equivalent weight of stones for the body. At night, O'Brien's body was forwarded to Hunter who took it immediately to his museum, where it was dissected and boiled to procure the bones. The skeleton was on exhibit until May 1941, when three fourths of the museum of the Royal College of Surgeons, London, was destroyed by German bombers. Joshua Reynold's portrait of John Hunter displays the huge skeletal feet of O'Brien in the background.

Matthew Baillie

Baillie (1761–1823) was a nephew of William and John Hunter. He was educated by his uncles and became famous as a physician and writer on medical subjects. He modified the Hunterian method of embalming so as to provide as good preservation as ever in a shorter period. Using a solution of oil of turpentine, Venice turpentine, oil of chamomile, and oil of lavender (to which was added vermillion dye) he injected the femoral artery. He allowed several hours of elapse before he opened the body as in a postmortem examination and made a small incision in the bowel below the stomach, into which he inserted a small piece of pipe through which he introduced water to wash out the contents of the bowels. Then, ligating the rectum above the anus and the small bowel below the stomach, he filled the intestinal tract with camphorated spirits of wine. The lungs were filled with camphorated spirits of wine via the trachea. The bladder was opened and emptied of its contents and a powder of camphor, resin, and niter was dusted over the viscera and the incision was closed. The eyeballs were pierced and emptied of their contents and repacked to normal with the powder mixture, as were the mouth and ears. The body was rubbed with oil of rosemary or lavender and placed on a bed of deep plaster.

Europe's Access to Cadavers

Continental European countries such as France, Germany, and Italy did not encounter the problems in supplying medical schools with cadavers as existed in Great Britain. Medical schools had access to bodies unclaimed for burial, a situation not present in the British Isles until after passage of the **Warburton Act in 1832.** The problem in continental Europe was different, consisting of securing a means to preserve cadavers for dissection with nonpoisonous chemicals. In France, for example, medical schools in the north had scheduled anatomical dissection classes during the cold months of the year as the cadavers were unembalmed.

By the late 18th and early 19th centuries, France and Italy had a number of different techniques and chemicals for embalming proposed by members of the medical or scientific communities.

Baron Leopold Cuvier (1769–1828) of France was a comparative anatomist whose classification of mammals and birds forms the groundwork for present-day systems. Cuvier advocated the use of pure alcohol as a preservative agent.

Francois Chaussier (1746–1828) of France recommended immersion of an eviscerated body in a solution of bichloride of mercury for preservation.*

Louis Jacques Thenard (1777–1857) of France was a brilliant teacher of and researcher in chemistry. He discovered the nature of hydrogen peroxide and made a study of human bile and the preservative action of bichloride of mercury. In 1834 he advocated introduction of an alcoholic solution of bichloride of mercury into the blood vessels to preserve cadavers for anatomical dissection.

G. Tranchina (also spelled Tranchini or Franchini) of early-19th-century Naples, Italy, openly advocated and successfully used arsenical solutions, arterially injected, to preserve bodies for both funeral and anatomical purposes. Tranchini's method of embalming varied, but the fluid was usually composed of 1 pound of arsenic dissolved in 5 pounds of alcoholic wine. He usually injected 2 gallons of this solution into the femoral artery without drainage of blood. At other times he injected the same amount into the right common carotid artery, sending the fluid first toward the head and then downward toward the body, allowing some drainage through the jugular vein. This was followed by incision of the abdomen, opening and emptying of the bowels, and moistening of the bowels with the injecting solution. The lungs were filled with the fluid via the trachea. A body prepared in this manner is said to have completely dried in 6 weeks.

J. P. Sucquet of France (mid-19th century) was one of the earliest proponents of the use of zinc chloride as a preservative agent. He injected about 5 quarts of a 20% solution of zinc chloride in water through the popliteal artery and also introduced some of this solution into the abdomen. One body prepared in this way was buried for 2 years, then disinterred and found to be in an excellent state of preservation. About 1845 an agent representing Sucquet sold the U.S. rights to his method and chemical to Chas. D. Brown and Joseph Alexander of New York City.

Jean Nicolas Gannal (1791–1852), a chemist in France (Figure 5), began his life's work as an apothecary's assistant. From 1808 to 1812 he served in the medical department of the French Army, including the Russian campaign under Napoleon. After his discharge from the army he reentered the field of chemistry and was appointed assistant to the great French chemistry teacher Thenard. He later became interested in industrial chemistry and did research on methods of refining borax and improving the quality of glues and gelatins. In 1827 he was awarded the Montyon science prize for developing a method of treating catarrh and tuberculosis with chlorine gas. In 1831 he was asked to devote his time to devising an improved method of preserving cadavers for anatomical purposes. Close application to the problem resulted in success, which was recognized in 1836 by the award to Gannal of a second Montyon science prize.

His experiments included the use of solutions of acids (acetic–arsenous–nitric–hydrochloric), alkali salts (copper–mercury–alum), tannin–creosote–alcohol, and various combinations such as alum, sodium chloride, and nitrate of potash, and acetate of alumina and the chloride of alumina, the latter of which obliterated the lumen of blood vessels. His perfected method of embalming cadavers for anatomical purposes comprised the injection of about 6 quarts of a solution of acetate of alumina through the carotid artery without drainage of any blood. No evisceration or other treatment was used, although occasionally the bodies were immersed in the injecting solution until ready for dissection. Gannal used practically the same solution for

*_**Bull. Hist. Med.**_ 1957; 30(5, Sept–Oct.): "Medicine in 16th Century New Spain," by Saul Jarcho, contains frequent mention of corrosive sublimate as a disinfectant for wounds.

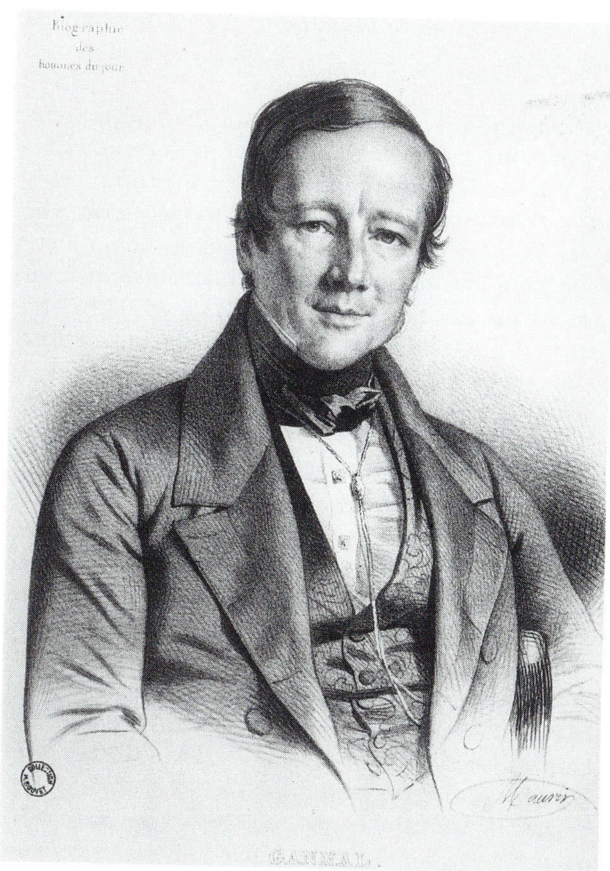

Figure 5. Portrait of J. N. Gannal at age 40. *(Courtesy of Ordre National de Pharmacien.)*

embalming bodies for funeral purposes, although he did add a small quantity of arsenic and carmine to the solution. He injected about 2 gallons of this mixture, first upward and then downward in the carotid artery in less than one-half hour. No special treatment was given to the trunk viscera. In his book *History of Embalming*, he cited case histories of bodies he had embalmed and subsequently disinterred from 3 to 13 months after burial. Gannal states that in every such case the body was found in exactly the same state of preservation and appearance as when buried.

Gannal was involved in several precedent-making events. In mid-April 1840, a Paris newspaper published the following article:

> The young boy found murdered in a field near Villete not having been recognized and the process of decomposition having commenced, the Magistrates ordered it to be embalmed by M. Gannal's simple method of injection through the carotid arteries, so that this evidence of the crime may remain producible. This is the first operation of the kind performed by order of the Justices, and it was completed in a quarter of an hour.

In his translation of Gannal's *History of Embalming* (1840) (Figure 6), Harlan mentions that the Paris police have access to Gannal's embalming process to preserve bodies in the Paris morgue where murder has been suspected.

Gannal was indirectly responsible for the passage of the first law prohibiting the use of arsenic in embalming solutions in 1846 (to which the use of bichloride of mercury was also prohibited in 1848).

There are several versions of the story. In one, Gannal had omitted stating that a portion of arsenic was added to his alumina salts embalming chemical, and when this solution was analyzed and arsenic found, the medical community was enraged and compelled the law to be decreed. The other tale, never documented, relates that Gannal was retained to embalm the corpse of a member of the nobility who died suddenly. The members of the nobleman's family accused the decedent's mistress of poisoning him with arsenic.

HISTORY

OF

EMBALMING,

AND OF

PREPARATIONS IN ANATOMY, PATHOLOGY

AND NATURAL HISTORY;

INCLUDING

An Account Of A New Process

For Embalming.

BY J. N. GANNAL.

Paris, 1838.

Translated From The French, With

Notes And Additions.

By R. Harlan, M.D.

PHILADELPHIA:

PUBLISHED BY JUDAH DOBSON,

NO. 106 CHESNUT STREET.

. . . . . .

1840

Figure 6. Title page of Harlan's translation of the *History of Embalming*.

Under French law she was arrested and tried, the burden of her defense on her shoulders. Gannal followed the progress of the trial in the Paris newspapers and noted that the accused mistress was unable to prove her innocence. Finally, at the last possible moment, Gannal appeared at the trial and requested permission to testify in her behalf. He states that in his opinion the arsenic found in the body tissues of the deceased came there during the embalming with his embalming solution, as it contained arsenic. She was freed and the legal community petitioned for the abolition of arsenic in embalming solutions.

Gannal had two sons, Adolphe Antoine and Felix, who became physicians and continued the embalming practice after his death. They embalmed many famous people including De Lessups, who constructed the Suez Canal. The sons died in the early 1900s.

Richard Harlan (1796–1843) of Philadelphia, Pennsylvania, graduated from the Pennsylvania Medical College in 1818 and was placed in charge of Joseph Parrish's private anatomical dissection rooms in Philadelphia. After engaging in various projects in company with other Philadelphia physicians he became a member of the city health council. In 1838 he traveled to Europe and spent a portion of his time in Paris visiting various medical facilities and meeting local savants, among whom was J. N. Gannal. After being presented with a copy of Gannal's *History of Embalming*, he became so fascinated with it that he requested and received permission to publish an American edition translated into English. **The book, published in Philadelphia in 1840, became the first book devoted entirely to embalming procedures that was published in the United States in English** (Figure 6).

Other Physicians and Anatomists

Girolamo Segato. A physician of Florence, Italy (17th century), Segato is known to have converted the human body to stone by infiltrating the bodily tissues with a solution of silicate of potash and succeeded this treatment by immersion of the body in a weak acid solution. The exact modus operandi is unknown.

Thomas Joseph Pettigrew. A London physician and surgeon, graduate of Guys Hospital, and fellow of the Royal College of Surgeons, Pettigrew (1791–1865) was one of the great historians of the science of embalming. His treatise *History of Egyptian Mummies,* published in London in 1834, is a masterpiece revealing Pettigrew's ability to accurately observe and minutely describe objects and processes of interest to students and practitioners of the art of embalming. This volume is to this day considered one of the fine works on Egyptian embalming methods and customs. In 1854 he withdrew from the practice of medicine and devoted his entire energy to the study of archaeology.

Dr. Falconry. A French physician of the mid-19th century, Falconry employed a means of preservation of cadavers for anatomical purposes that is of interest because of its simplicity. The corpse was placed on a bed of dry sawdust to which about a gallon of powdered zinc sulfate had been added. No injections, incisions, baths, or any additional treatment was used. The bodies so treated were said to have remained flexible for about 40 days, after which time they dried and assumed the appearance of mummies.

Thomas Marshall, M.D. Marshall was a London physician who published an account of a means of embalming in the *London Medical Gazette* in December 1839. His technique consisted of generously puncturing the body surface with needles or scissors and repeatedly brushing the body surface with strong acetic acid. A diluted acetic acid solution was introduced into the cavities of the body. The author claimed that the acetic acid would restore normal color even to gangrenous tissue.

Dr. John Morgan (Circa 1863). A professor of anatomy at the University of Dublin, Morgan made use of two principles that are widely recognized as necessary to achieve the best embalming results: (1) the use of the largest possible artery for injection and (2) the use of force or pressure to push the preserving fluid through the blood vessels. Also noted are his use of a preinjection solution (the earliest mention found) and his controlled technique of drainage. Morgan cut the sternum down its center, opened the pericardium to expose the heart, made an incision into the left ventricle or into the aorta, and inserted a piece of pipe about 8 inches long. This injecting pipe was connected by 15 feet of tubing to a fluid container that was maintained 12 feet above the corpse, thereby producing about 5 pounds of pressure (Figure 7).

The tip of the right auricular appendage was clipped off to allow blood drainage. The first injection was composed of $\frac{1}{2}$ gallon of a saturated salt solution to which was added 4 ounces of niter. After this solution was allowed to "rush" through the circulatory system, a clamp was fastened over the auricular appendage when the drainage stopped. Several more gallons of a solution of common salt, niter, alum, and arsenate of potash was injected until the body was thoroughly saturated with the fluid. No special treatment of the internal organs or viscera was mentioned.

At this time there was virtually no embalming of the dead for funeral purposes available for the largest percentage of deaths. Many books were written regard-

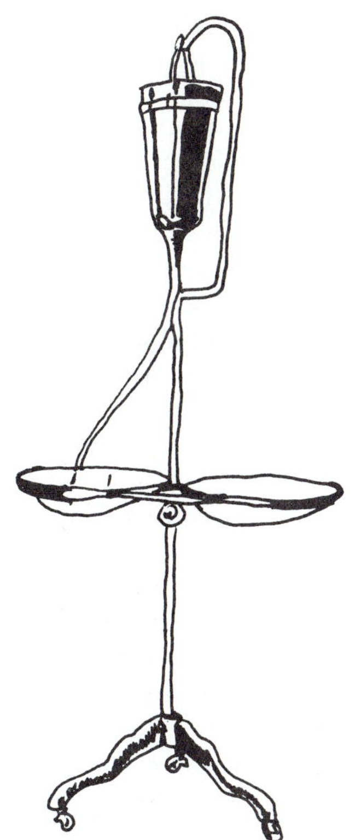

Figure 7. Gravity fluid injector. The jar filled with arterial chemical could be elevated several feet above the corpse, thus creating pressure for injection. *(Courtesy of Paula Johnson De Smet.)*

From Europe to the Colonies

The transfer of embalming knowledge from Europe to the colonies in what today is the United States was accomplished by several means.

Anatomical study in the colonies as early as 1676 in Boston and again in 1750 recorded that "Drs. John Bard and Peter Middleton injected and dissected the body of an executed criminal for the instruction of young men engaged in the study of medicine." In 1752 the *N.Y. Weekly Postboy* carried an advertisement offering anatomy instruction by Dr. Thomas Wood. From 1754 to 1756, William Hunter, physician and student of the famed anatomy teacher Alexander Monroe I of Edinburgh, Scotland (and a relative of the Hunter Brothers), lectured on anatomy at Newport, Rhode Island. Doctors William Shippen and John Morgan of Philadelphia studied medicine in Europe and anatomy under British anatomists. On their return to the United States between 1762 and 1765 they became engaged in teaching medical subjects, especially anatomy, in Philadelphia.

In 1840 the translation of Gannal's book *The History of Embalming* into English was to provide the first text in English printed in the United States devoted to embalming. In the mid-1840s the acquisition of Sucquet's embalming technique and chemicals as a franchise by Dr. Charles D. Brown and Dr. Joseph Alexander of New York City added to the increasing amount of embalming knowledge transferred to the United States.

ing the dangers to the living of exposure to the dead buried or entombed (unembalmed) in churches or in city cemeteries. There was also concern for those who handled the dead.

Bernardino Ramazzini. The founder of occupational medicine, Ramazzini (1633–1714) wrote the *Diseases of Workers* in 1700, and an enlarged edition of that text was published in 1713. The latter edition contained a chapter on the Disease of Corpse Bearers.

Numerous publications varying in size from leaflets to bound books were printed inveighing against existing burial practices. A few relevant titles are *Considerations on the Indecent and Dangerous Custom of Burying in Churches and Churchyards etc.*, 1721, London, A. Batesworth; *Blame of Kirk Burial, Tending to Persuade Cemeterial Civility,* 1606 NP, Rev. William Birnie; *Gatherings from Graveyards, Particularly Those of London etc.*, 1830, G. A. Walker, surgeon, London; and *Sepulture, History, Methods and Sanitary Requisites,* 1884, Stephen Wickes, Philadelphia. The astonishing accounts contained in these or similar works should convince even the most skeptical opponent of embalming of the sanitary value of the embalming process.

▶ MODERN PERIOD

By the year 1861 and the onset of the Civil War, the transfer of embalming knowledge from Europe to the United States was virtually concluded. A small group of medically trained embalmers existed together with printed information such as Harlan's translation of Gannal's textbook and various European embalming formulas and techniques that had been acquired.

Until the Civil War, however, little or no embalming was performed for funeral purposes. Most preservation, such as it was, for brief periods was provided by ice refrigeration when available.

With the outbreak of the Civil War in April 1861, there began the raising of troops by the North and South to prosecute the war. Little if any embalming was available to the Southerners during the war. Virtually all embalming was done by Northerners. As Washington, D.C. was the capital city of the North, it became a center for troop concentration both to protect the city and to serve as a marshalling point for the armies moving against the south.

Northern troops composed of individual companies from small geographical areas and regiments from individual states as disparate as Vermont and Maine, Minnesota and Wisconsin, and Ohio, Pennsylvania, and New York crowded into the Washington, D.C. area. Civilian embalmers Dr. Thomas Holmes, William J. Bunnell, Dr. Charles Da Costa Brown, Dr. Joseph B. Alexander, Dr. Richard Burr, Dr. Daniel H. Prunk, Frank A. Hutton, G. W. Scollay, C. B. Chamberlain, Henry P. Cattell, Dr. Benjamin Lyford, Samuel Rodgers, Dr. E. C. Lewis, W. P. Cornelius, and Prince Greer are known to have embalmed during the Civil War. There are others who, to this day, remain anonymous.

None of the embalming surgeons, as they were called, were ever employed in the military as embalmers. Some had been or would become military surgeons but did not perform embalming while in the military service.

Civil War Times

At the beginning of the Civil War, as in all previous wars fought by the United States, there was no provision for return of the dead to their homes. In the Seminole Indian Wars (during the 1830s), the Mexican War (1846–1848), and the campaigns against the Indians up to the outbreak of the Civil War, the military dead were buried in the field near where they fell in battle. It was possible for the relatives to have the remains returned to their home for local burial under certain conditions:

1. The next of kin was to request the disinterment and return of the body in a written request to the Quartermaster General.
2. On military authority confirmation that the burial place was known and disinterment could be effected, the family was advised to send a coffin capable of being hermetically sealed to a designated Quartermaster Officer nearest the place of burial.
3. Such Quartermaster Officer would provide a force of men to take the coffin to the grave, disinter the remains, and place them in the coffin and seal it. The coffined remains would then be returned to the place of ultimate reinterment.

During the early days of the Civil War and less frequently as the war dragged on, some family members of the deceased personally went to hospitals and battlefields to search for their dead and bring them home for burial. Civil War embalming was carried out with a variety of chemicals and techniques. Arterial embalming was applied when possible. An artery, usually the femoral or carotid, was raised and injected without any venous drainage in most cases. Usually, no cavity treatment was administered. When arterial embalming was believed impossible because of the nature of wounds or decomposition, other means of preparation of the body for transport were resorted to. In some cases the trunk was eviscerated and the cavity filled with sawdust or powdered charcoal or lime. The body was then placed in a coffin completely imbedded in sawdust or similar material. In other cases, the body was coffined as mentioned without evisceration.

Chemicals employed during the Civil War were totally self-manufactured by the embalmer and included, as basic preservatives, arsenicals, zinc chloride, bichloride of mercury, salts of alumina, sugar of lead, and a host of salts, alkalies and acids. An example of fluid manufacture of one of the most popular embalming chemicals, zinc chloride, was the immersion of sheets of zinc in hydrochloric acid until a saturated solution was obtained. The resulting zinc chloride solution was injected without further dilution. Many of the injection pumps employed were quite similar to what would be described as greatly enlarged hypodermic syringes. Many required filling of the syringe, attachment of a cannula, emptying of the syringe, unfastening of the syringe, and refilling. It was an extremely slow process! A few pumps were designed to provide continuous flow, aspirating the embalming chemical continuously from a large source into the pump during the injection process. Others, such as the Holmes invention, were designed to fit over a bucket that could hold a gallon or more of liquid.

On May 24, 1861, 24-year-old Colonel Elmer Ellsworth, commander of the 11th N.Y. Volunteer Infantry, was shot to death in Alexandria, Virginia, as he seized a confederate flag displayed atop the Marshall House Hotel. He became the first prominent military figure killed in the war. His body was embalmed by Dr. Thomas Holmes, who had set up an embalming establishment in Washington, D.C. Colonel Ellsworth had funeral services in the White House, in New York City, and in Albany, New York, with burial in his home town of Mechanicsburg, New York. His funeral set a pattern to be followed by prominent members of the military, culminating in President Lincoln's historic funeral services. Colonel Ellsworth's embalming and viewable appearance were widely and favorably commented on in the press and did much to familiarize the previously uninformed public with embalming.

The Army issued only two sets of orders relative to fatal casualties in the early stages of the war. On September 11, 1861, War Department General Order 75 directed the Quartermaster Department to supply all general and post hospitals with blank books and forms for the preservation of accurate death records and to provide material for headboards to be erected over soldiers' graves. On April 3, 1862, Section II of War Department General Order 33 stated:

> In order to secure as far as possible the decent interment of those who have fallen, or may fall in bat-

tle, it is made the duty of commanding generals to lay off lots of ground in some suitable spot near every battlefield, as soon as it may be in their power, and to cause the remains of those killed to be interred, with headboards to the graves bearing numbers, and when practicable the names of the persons buried in them. A register for each burial ground will be preserved, in which will be noted the marks corresponding with the headboards.

This was the origin of what was to become the National Cemetery System.

Embalming Surgeons of the Civil War

Dr. Thomas Holmes (1817–1900). Holmes was born in New York City in 1817 and educated in local public schools and New York University Medical College, though the records of the period are incomplete and document only his attendance, not his graduation. He did practice medicine and was a coroner's physician in New York during the 1850s as numerous newspaper stories attest. He apparently moved to Williamsburg (now Brooklyn) and experimented with a variety of chemicals for embalming and techniques. When the Civil War broke out he opened an embalming office in Washington, D.C. and Colonel Ellsworth became his first prominent client. Holmes subsequently embalmed Colonel E. D. Baker, a prominent politician and soldier killed in battle. This case brought more publicity both for Holmes and for embalming (Figure 8).

Holmes ultimately prepared about 4000 bodies (including 8 generals), and patented many inventions relating to embalming during his lifetime. One in particular, a rubber-coated canvas removal bag, was far ahead of its time (Figure 9).

When the war ended, Dr. Holmes returned home to Brooklyn and only occasionally practiced embalming. He operated a drugstore and manufactured a variety of products as diverse as embalming fluid and root beer! He invested heavily in a health resort and lost the investment. He wrote little about embalming, did not teach, and had no children. After a serious fall in his home he became periodically psychotic and occasion-

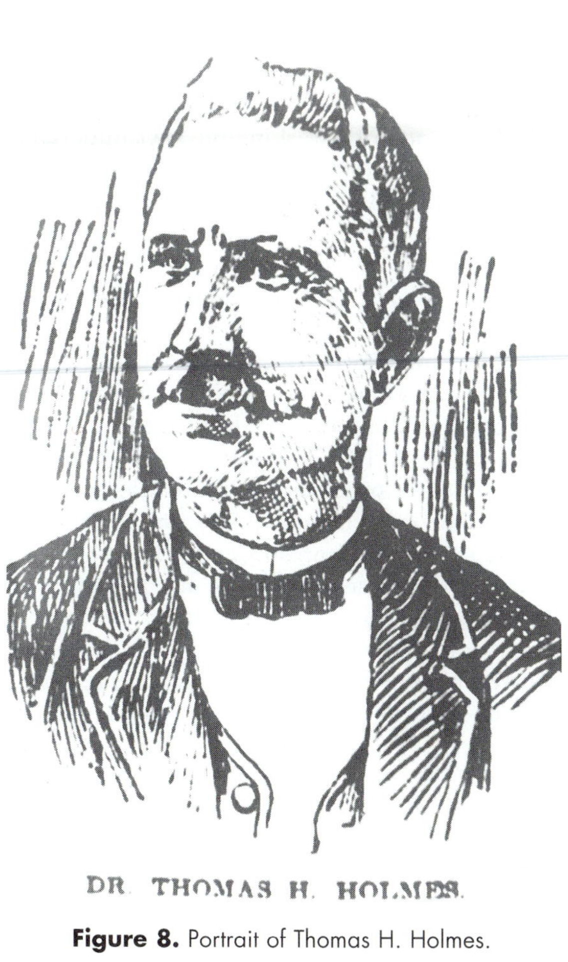

DR. THOMAS H. HOLMES.

Figure 8. Portrait of Thomas H. Holmes.

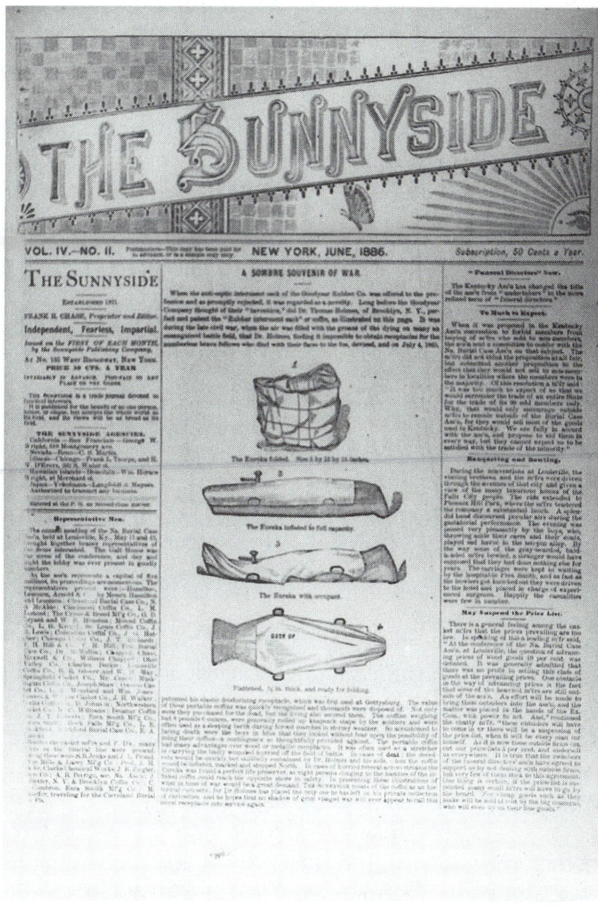

THE SUNNYSIDE

VOL. IV.—NO. II. NEW YORK, JUNE, 1886. Subscription, 50 Cents a Year.

THE SUNNYSIDE

Independent, Fearless, Impartial.

A SOMBRE SOUVENIR OF WAR.

The Eureka inflated to full capacity.

The Eureka with occupant.

Banqueting and Bowling.

May Suspend the Price List.

Figure 9. Front page of *The Sunnyside,* June 1886, featuring an article on Holmes's removal bag, citing its all-around utility as a sleeping bag and stretcher, its ability to be inflated as a raft, and, of course, its use as a corpse removal bag or coffin.

ally required confinement. When he died in 1900 it was said that he wanted no embalming.

William J. Bunnell (1823–1891). Bunnell was born in New Jersey, moved to New York City, and in the 1850s became acquainted with Dr. Holmes and married his sister. Dr. Holmes found him employment as an anatomy technician for some New York medical schools while teaching him embalming. When war broke out, Bunnell did not work directly with Dr. Holmes but formed his own Embalming Surgeon's organization with Dr. R. B. Heintzelman from Philadelphia as his active partner. Holmes and Bunnell did occasionally work together during the war at Gettysburg and at City Point, Virginia. After the war, it was reported that Bunnell was practicing medicine briefly in Omaha, Nebraska, and eventually opened an undertaking establishment in Jersey City, New Jersey. He became a marshall at the funeral of General Grant and became prominent in undertakers associations. His son, George Holmes Bunnell (1855–1932), followed his father in the business and was given assistance by his uncle, Dr. Holmes, George H. Bunnell had twin sons: Milton became a funeral director, and Chester became a physician.

Charles Da Costa Brown, Joseph B. Alexander, and Henry P. Cattell. Brown, Alexander, and Cattell were all active in the firm of Brown and Alexander, Embalming Surgeons. It is not known whether Brown and Alexander met in New York City in the late 1850s or in Washington, D.C. in early wartime. Cattell (Figure 10) is believed to have been the stepson of Dr. Charles Brown's brother, as his mother married a Brown in 1860. In any event, he entered the employment of the firm that embalmed Willie Lincoln, son of President Abraham Lincoln, and later embalmed the President himself in 1865. After the war Dr. Brown abandoned embalming, returned to New York City, practiced dentistry, and became very active in the Masonic Lodge. He died in 1896 and is buried in Greenwood Cemetery in Brooklyn.

Alexander died in 1871 in Washington, D.C. H.P. Cattell halted his embalming practice after the war, became a lithographer, and then entered the Washington, D.C., police force. None of his family was ever aware that he had embalmed President Lincoln. He died in 1915 and is buried in Washington, D.C.

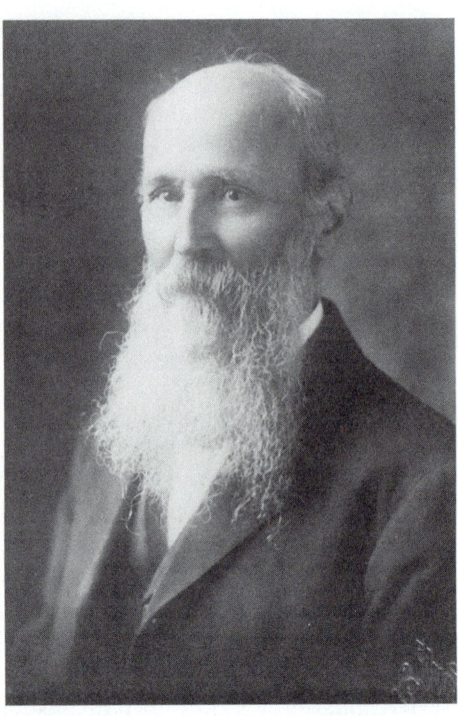

Figure 10. Portrait of Henry P. Cattell, an associate of Brown and Alexander, the embalming surgeons who embalmed Willie Lincoln in 1862 and President Lincoln in 1865.

Frank A. Hutton. Little is known of Hutton's personal biography. Born in or near Harrisburg, Pennsylvania, about 1835, he was a pharmacist by occupation. He had military service in the 110th Pennsylvania Volunteer Infantry ending in June 1862, was discharged in Washington, D.C. and became a partner in the firm of Chamberlain and Hutton, Surgeons. This partnership did not last long and Hutton withdrew in February 1863. He formed the firm of Hutton and Company with E. A. Williams, son of a Washington, D.C. undertaker as his partner. Hutton advertised in the Washington City Directory, taking a full page space to extol his embalming expertise. He was also issued Patent 38,747 for an embalming fluid on June 1, 1863. The formula included alcohol, arsenic, bichloride of mercury, and zinc chloride.

During mid-April 1863, Hutton became embroiled in an argument with a client over charges for shipping his son's body to him. The client complained to Colonel L. C. Baker, provost marshall of the capitol, who, on April 20, 1863, arrested Hutton and seized the contents of his office as evidence. Hutton was confined in the Old Capitol Prison for about 10 days and then released. No details of his release or trial have been found. He subsequently relocated his quarters and continued in business with a much diminished clientele. Hutton is said to have returned to Harrisburg after the war ended and died there within a year.

Daniel H. Prunk (1829–1923). Born in Virginia in 1829, Prunk and his family migrated to Illinois where he attended college. After attending medical school in Cincinnati he began medical practice in Illinois and, in April 1861, moved to Indianapolis where he joined the 19th Indiana Volunteer Infantry as an assistant surgeon in September 1861. He was transferred to the 20th Indiana Volunteer Infantry in June 1862, and was arrested in November of that year and incarcerated in the Old Capitol Prison in Washington, D.C. for about 3 months for conduct unbecoming an officer. He was then dismissed from the service. From July to October 1863 he was acting assistant surgeon at the 2nd Division Army Hospital at Nashville, Tennessee, and subseqently requested permission to provide embalming services in Nashville. The request was initially refused but finally granted late in 1863. He eventually had embalming establishments located not only in Nashville but also in Chattanooga and Knoxville in Tennessee; at East Point, Atlanta, Dalton, and Marietta in Georgia; and at Huntsville in Alabama (Figure 11).

In 1865 Dr. Prunk was licensed by the Army to practice embalming and undertaking. (He was also engaged in a wholesale grocery business, cotton trading, and money lending.) He made his own embalming fluid by dissolving sheets of zinc in muriatic acid (hydrochloric acid) until a saturated solution of zinc chloride was obtained to which a quantity of arsenious acid was added. The fluid obtained was injected quite warm without dilution or blood drainage.

Prunk sold all his embalming establishments in 1866 and returned to Indianapolis to practice medicine. It seems that he never engaged in embalming after his return to Indianapolis. He made one of the earliest written statements regarding the necessity of cavity treatment in a letter written in 1872, to Dr. J. P. Buckesto of San Jose, California

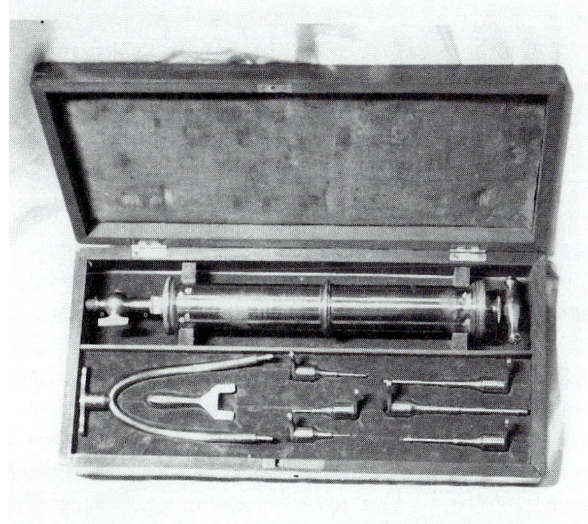

Figure 11. Injection syringe and cannulas of Daniel H. Prunk, Civil War embalming surgeon. *(Courtesy of the Illinois Funeral Directors' Foundation.)*

> If I were going to ship a corpse from San Jose to New York City, we have advised for sometime the puncturing of the stomach to give vent to gases which accumulate at this time. In a subject with a large abdomen, where the bowels are discolored, the introduction of a couple of quarts into the peritoneal cavity by making a puncture near the umbilicus and throwing a thread of strong silk around it like a drawstring on a button cushion which can be readily closed after you are thru injecting.

Dr. Richard Burr. Although little biographical information other than his rumored origin in Philadelphia is available concerning Burr (who apparently practiced during the period 1862–1865), he has achieved immortality as the embalmer photographed by the Civil War photographer Brady in front of his embalming tent while injecting a subject (Figure 12). W. J. Bunnell complained about Burr's unprofessional conduct, alleging that, among other things, he set Bunnell's embalming tent on fire! He was also one of the men against whom complaints had been issued regarding inflated prices and poor services, which resulted in all embalmers being excluded from military areas by order of General U. S. Grant in January 1865. **This resulted in establishment of the first set of rules and regulations for the licensing of embalmers and undertakers in the United States.**

The final Army order for embalmers contained some of the suggestions made by Dr. Barnes, chief of the Army Medical Service in December 1863, to the effect that a performance bond should be posted by any embalmer desiring to practice. In addition, the requirement stipulated by the Provost Marshall General ordered the embalmer to furnish a list of his prices as charged for work or merchandise to the Provost Marshall General, the medical director of the department, and the Post Provost Marshall.

U.S. Army General Order 39 concerning embalmers (March 15, 1865) read as follows:

1. Hereafter no persons will be permitted to embalm or remove the bodies of deceased officers or soldiers unless acting under the special license of the Provost Marshall of the Army, department, or district in which the bodies may be.
2. Provost marshalls will restrict disinterments to seasons when they can be made without endangering the health of the troops. They will grant licenses only to such persons as furnish proof of skill and ability as embalmers, and will require bonds for the faithful performance of the orders given them. They will also establish a scale of prices by which embalmers are to be governed, with such other regulations as will protect the interest of the friends and relatives of deceased soldiers.

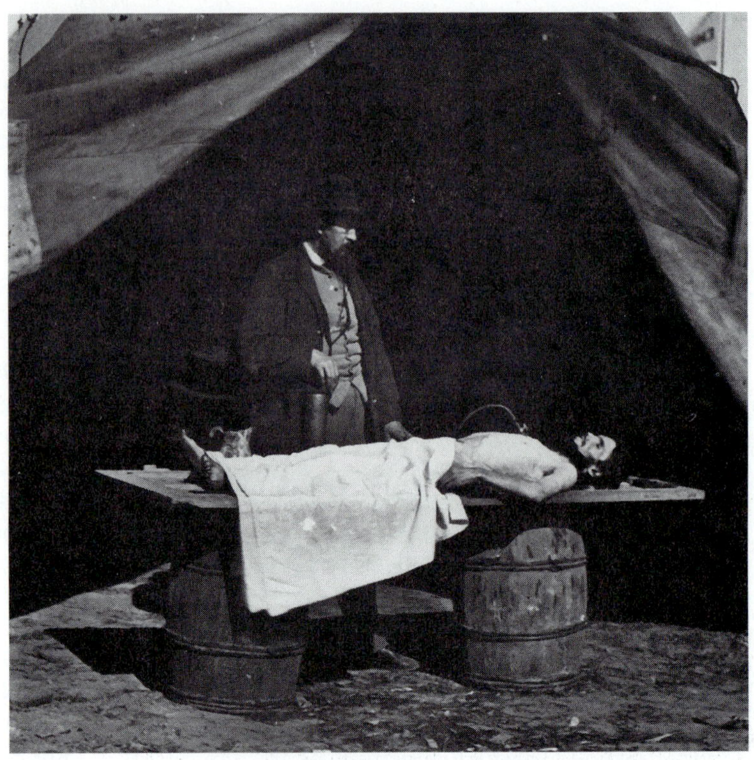

Figure 12. Richard Burr embalming near a battlefield during the Civil War. *(Courtesy of Library of Congress.)*

3. Applicants for license will apply directly to the Provost Marshall of the Army or department in which they may desire to pursue their business, submitting in distinct terms the process adopted by them, materials, length of time its preservative effect can be relied on and such other information as may be necessary to establish their proficiency and success. Medical directors will give such assistance in the examination of these applications as may be required by the Provost Marshall.

In the Army of the Cumberland the following additional requirements were stipulated:

1. No disinterments will be permitted within the department between the 15th day of May and the 15th day of October.
2. The following scale of prices will be observed from and after this date: At Nashville and Memphis: for embalming bodies each at $15.00 to disinter, furnish metallic burial cases, well boxed, marked and delivered to the express office each at $75.00, zinc coffins and the above listed services each at $40.00. An additional charge of $5.00 may be made for embalming and also for either of the above styles of coffins at Murfreesboro, Chattanooga, Knoxville, and Huntsville, Alabama, or in the field.
3. No person will be permitted to operate as an embalmer under any license issued to him until he shall have filed a bond in this office in the penal sum of $1000 conditioned for the faithful observance of this order, and for the skillful performance of such works he shall undertake by virtue of his license. [Such licenses were not transferable from one individual to another.]

By 1864 the Armory Square Military Hospital in Washington, D.C., had all its deceased patients routinely embalmed and the grave recorded so that the body could be disinterred and sent to family or friends when requested.

C. B. Chamberlain. Chamberlain is said to have Philadelphia as his origin. Although very little is known of the man, he definitely was an early partner of F. A. Hutton. He and Hutton apparently were not compatible, and he formed a new partnership with Ben Lyford. They both can be documented as practicing embalming surgeons on the scene at Gettysburg after the battle. Chamberlain is listed in the Washington, D.C., City Directory as late as 1865 as a partner in Chamberlain and Waters Embalmers at 431 Pennsylvania Avenue. He is mentioned by F. C. Beinhauer, Pittsburgh undertaker, as being in the Pittsburgh area prior to and during the Civil War. Joseph H. Clarke also mentioned Chamberlain as a teacher of embalming in the post–Civil War period.

G. W. Scollay. Judging from the various patents issued to him, Scollay was apparently from St. Louis, Missouri. Very little personal information about him has been uncovered. He appeared to be an active embalming surgeon at the Gettysburg battlefield and in the area near Richmond. He has a listing in the 1865 Washington, D.C., City Directory as a member of the firm of Scollay and Sands—Embalmers of the Dead. Frank T. Sands was a prominent undertaker in Washington, D. C. Scollay patented two methods of embalming in the post–Civil War period, one in January 1867 and the other in October 1869. Both patents involved the use of gaseous compounds injected via the blood vascular system, one of the earliest recommendations for choice of gas rather than a liquid as a preservative introduced into the blood vascular system. In 1860, Scollay patented a two-piece cast glass coffin and, during the war, produced a number of different "sanitary" coffins.

Benjamin F. Lyford. Born in Vermont in 1841 and receiving public school education there, Lyford attended and graduated from Philadelphia University's 6-month course of medical studies. He first appears on the Civil War scene as a partner of C. B. Chamberlain, who provided embalming after the Battle of Gettysburg. Later he had altercations with Provost Marshall General Rudolf Patrick of the Army of the Potomac. This series of disagreements stimulated him to accept appointment on July 13, 1864, as assistant surgeon of the 68th Regiment of Infantry—U.S. Colored Troops. He reported to the unit in Missouri and subsequently served in Memphis. For a time he served as commanding officer of a small cavalry and artillery contingent in southern Alabama.

He returned to his regiment stationed near New Orleans, Louisiana, and went to leave in New Orleans. He was arrested inside a bordello in full uniform and faced court martial charges. Apparently found innocent of the charges, he was discharged from the Army on February 5, 1866, traveled to San Francisco, and opened an office for medical practice. One of his early patients was a wealthy widowed landowner who had an attractive daughter whom he fell in love with and married. The mother owned large tracts of land in Marin County across the bay north of San Francisco. Lyford built a health resort and dairy as well as his own home on this property and prospered.

In 1871 Lyford patented An Improvement in Embalming, which was a very complicated system consisting of the introduction through the blood vessels of specially distilled chemicals (including creosote, zinc chloride, potassium nitrate, and alcohol) while the body was enclosed in a sealed container. The container, had the air within it alternatively evacuated to create a vacuum and reversed to create pressure. Finally, the body was eviscerated and the trunk cavity filled with an arsenical powder. His final recommendation was the use of cosmetics to color the features; he was one of the first to make this recommendation. In 1870, a local newspaper carried a story describing a body he had successfully embalmed. Lyford died in 1906 without issue and had a large well-attended funeral.

Dr. E. C. Lewis, W. P. Cornelius, and Prince Greer. This most interesting account of the Civil War embalming surgeons relates the method of the transmission of embalming technique from a medically trained practitioner to an undertaker, who, in turn, trained a layman in the skill. Dr. E. C. Lewis was a former U.S. Army surgeon, W. P. Cornelius (1824–1910) was a successful undertaker in Nashville, Tennessee, and Prince Greer was a former orderly, body servant, and slave of a Colonel Greer of a Texas cavalry regiment who died in the fighting in Tennessee.

Thomas Holmes wrote:

> In the forepart of the war a young ex-Army doctor named E. C. Lewis called at my headquarters in Washington and wished me to instruct him in the embalming profession and sell him an outfit to go to the western Army and locate at Nashville. He offered as security a property holding in Georgetown, DC for any amount of fluid I would trust him for. I made a bargain with him and he used many barrels of fluid. I was often surprised at his large orders. (*Note:* Dr. Lewis' headquarters were at Mr. Cornelius' undertaking establishment in Nashville.)

Cornelius stated:

> It was during the year 1862 that one Dr. E. C. Lewis came to me from the employ of Dr. Holmes and proposed to embalm bodies. It was new to me but I at once put him to work with the Holmes fluid and Holmes injector. He was quite an expert, but like many men could not stand prosperity and soon wanted to get into some other kind of business, which he did. When Lewis the embalmer quit, I then undertook the embalming myself with a colored assistant named Prince Greer.

Cornelius explained that Prince Greer had earlier brought the body of Colonel Greer of a Texas cavalry regiment to Cornelius for shipment back to Texas. After shipping back the body Prince Greer remained at Cornelius' premises and was asked what he wanted to do to earn his room and board. Prince Greer indicated he would do anything.

Cornelius continued:

> Prince Greer appeared to enjoy embalming so much that he himself became an expert, kept on at work embalming during the balance of the war, and was very successful at it. It was but a short time before he could raise an artery as quickly as anyone and was al-

ways careful, always of course coming to me in a difficult case. He remained with me until I quit the business in 1871.

Prince Greer is the first documented black embalmer in U.S. history.

Public and Professional Acceptance

With the ending of the war and the assassination of President Lincoln, the Civil War's last major casualty, the public had been familiarized with the term *embalming* and obtained personal knowledge of the appearance of an embalmed body. This knowledge was acquired by the hundreds of thousands who viewed not only President Lincoln but other prominent military and civilian figures as well as the ordinary soldiers embalmed and shipped to their homes.

Despite the end of the war and the establishment of peace there was no wide adoption of embalming by civilian undertakers of the United States. There were many reasons for this apparent reluctance to adopt a worthwhile new practice. Undertakers in the United States at the end of the Civil War were an unorganized, largely rural group of individuals lacking a professional body of knowledge and skills. Specifically, they lacked textbooks of instruction on embalming, instructors and schools of embalming, professional journals, and professional associations. Until these necessities became available embalming would not flourish.

The first step taken was to attempt the sale of embalming fluid to undertakers. Some Civil War embalming surgeons, such as Dr. Thomas Holmes, engaged in this endeavor on returning home. Holmes had a large local market (metropolitan New York City) for his preservative chemical, which he had named *Innominata,* and he promoted it well. Holmes, like other embalming chemical salesmen, realized quickly that the undertakers were interested in the preservative qualities of such chemicals but the clients were without knowledge of embalming techniques. Holmes therefore promoted the use of his Innominata as an external application, to wash the body and to saturate cloths to place over the face. His fluid was also poured into the mouth and nose to reach the lungs and stomach. Holmes' early practices were duplicated by other purveyors of embalming chemicals.

In these early post–Civil War years some instruction of undertakers in arterial embalming was imparted by the occasional knowledgeable traveling salesman who sold embalming chemicals. C. B. Chamberlain is reported to have done this in the late 1860s and early 1870s.

Examples of chemical embalming fluid patents include one issued to C. H. Crane of Burr Oak, Michigan, in September 1868. It was a powdered mixture of alum salt, ammonium chloride, arsenic, bichloride of mercury, camphor, and zinc chloride. It could be used as a dry powder or dissolved in water or alcohol to form an arterial solution and was named Crane's electrodynamic mummifier. In 1876 he sold the patent rights to this or a similar formulation to a Professor George M. Rhodes of Michigan. Another early embalming chemical manufacturer in 1877 was the Mills and Lacey Manufacturing Company of Grand Rapids, Michigan, whose embalming fluid featured arsenic as its preservative.

Instruments and chemicals available in the post–Civil War period included rubber gloves at $2 per pair (1877); anatomical syringes and three cannulas in a case for $20 to $22; surgical instruments in cases for $4 to $5; Rulon's wax eyecaps and mouth closers at $1 each; and Segestor embalming fluid for $4.50 per dozen pint bottles (1873). Professor George M. Rhodes was said to have sold 10,000 bottles of his dynamic Electro Balm in 1876 with more than 3000 undertakers using the product. Egyptian Embalmer Fluid (1877) sold for $6.50 per dozen pint bottles and was also available in 5- and 10-gallon kegs as well as $\frac{1}{2}$ and 1-gallon carboys at $3.00 per gallon.

Until the first quarter of the 20th century, embalming was most frequently carried out in the home of the deceased or, in some communities, in the hospital where death occurred. There were early attempts in some funeral homes in the 1870s to provide both a preparation room and chapel space for the wake and services. In issues as early as 1876 of both *The Casket* and *The Sunnyside,** there were accounts of the installation of preparation rooms. For example:

> Maynard Funeral Home, Syracuse, N.Y., had a morgue fitted with marble slabs and running water for storing bodies.
>
> Hubbard and Searles Undertaking establishment at Auburn, N.Y., could provide seating for 100 persons at a service and had a cooling room with cement floor and marble slabs (2 × 8 feet) and running water connection.
>
> Knowles Undertaking establishment at Providence, R.I., had a preserver room and a corpse room where surgical procedures and postmortems were made.
>
> The Douglas Undertaking Co. of Utica, N.Y., had a room for funeral services and a cooling vault in the cellar which had walls three feet thick and also contained shelves for body storage.

* The most significant impetus to spreading embalming knowledge was the founding of the professional journals *The Sunnyside* in 1871 and *The Casket* in 1876. Both, from their inception, carried advertisements for various embalming chemicals.

Dr. Auguste Renouard. In 1876, Dr. Renouard (1839–1912) became a regular contributor to *The Casket* of articles on all phases of embalming knowledge, which greatly implemented interest in embalming. He was born on a plantation in Point Coupee Parish, Louisiana, and received his early schooling locally. He is said to have attended the McDowell Medical School in St. Louis, Missouri, and, at the outbreak of the Civil War, to have returned to Louisiana to enlist in the Confederate Army. Despite his claim to military service in the confederate forces, no documented evidence has been found in some 50 years of searching. In the postwar period he secured employment as a pharmacist in various cities such as New York, Memphis, and Chicago, where he was married. His son, Charles A., was born shortly before the Chicago fire of 1871. Losing everything in the fire, Renouard traveled to Denver, Colorado, and secured employment as a bookkeeper for a combination furniture store and undertaking establishment. Because of its altitude, Denver at this time was regarded as a health resort for treatment of lung diseases.

The undertaking section of the firm returned many bodies to the east and south for hometown burial, and Renouard became interested in the procedures employed at his firm for shipment of the bodies. After studying the existing rudimentary system he suggested to his employer that he be permitted to prepare the bodies for shipment by arterial embalming. This consent was given and it almost immediately produced a volume of letters from the receiving undertakers inquiring about the procedure used to create such beautiful corpses, which resembled a person asleep. Renouard graciously replied, explaining his chemicals and technique to the extent that it assumed the proportions of a correspondence course. Additionally, there were a number of individual undertakers who traveled to Denver to receive personal instruction in embalming from Renouard.

The publisher of *The Casket* urged Dr. Renouard to write a textbook on embalming and undertaking for use by undertakers. In 1878 he published *The Undertaker's Manual,* which contained 230 pages of detailed instruction on anatomy, chemistry, embalming procedures, instruments, and details of undertaking practice (Figure 13). **This was the first book published specifically as an embalming textbook in the United States and would be followed by a horde of others.** In 1879, notices appeared in *The Casket* that undertakers in states such as Connecticut and Pennsylvania were agents for the sale of Auguste Renouard's chemical formulas and techniques (Figure 14).

In 1881 the doctor was requested to open a school of embalming in Rochester, New York, but, for a variety of reasons, this did not become a reality until early 1883. In 1880 the state of Michigan was the first to form an undertakers' association, which, in 1881, changed its name to Funeral Directors Association. Other states quickly followed the Michigan lead and organized state associations. **The various state associations met in 1882 in Rochester and organized the National Funeral Directors Association, another important step toward professionalism.** Renouard provided demonstrations of embalming in Rochester at the first national convention of the Association. This set a pattern for many years of an obligatory embalming demonstration at state and national conventions. During the 1882 gathering, agents of an English firm (Dotridge Brothers, Funeral Supply Firm) offered Renouard a 5-year contract to teach embalming in London at $5000 per year, which he rejected.

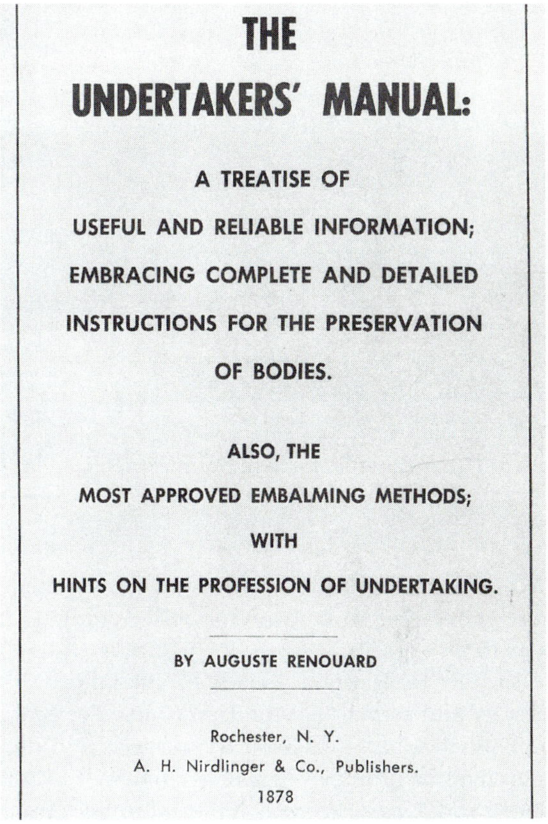

THE

UNDERTAKERS' MANUAL:

A TREATISE OF

USEFUL AND RELIABLE INFORMATION;

EMBRACING COMPLETE AND DETAILED

INSTRUCTIONS FOR THE PRESERVATION

OF BODIES.

ALSO, THE

MOST APPROVED EMBALMING METHODS;

WITH

HINTS ON THE PROFESSION OF UNDERTAKING.

BY AUGUSTE RENOUARD

Rochester, N. Y.

A. H. Nirdlinger & Co., Publishers.

1878

Figure 13. Title page of Auguste Renouard's first edition of *The Undertaker's Manual.*

The Rochester School of Embalming headed by Dr. Renouard under the auspices of the Egyptian Chemical Company opened in 1883 and he continued his affiliation with this school until December 1884. He then entered into an agreement with Hallett and Company Undertakers in Kansas City, Missouri, to locate his school, the School of Embalming and Organic Chemistry, on the company's premises. By mid-1886 he terminated his school in Kansas City and returned to Denver. He then began to travel to distant points such as Ft.

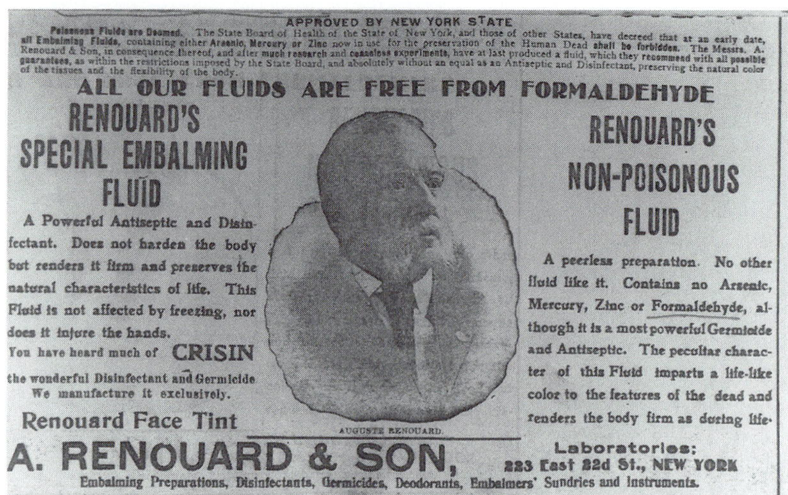

Figure 14. Auguste Renouard's advertisement for embalming fluid.

Worth, Texas, and Toronto and Montreal, Canada, providing embalming instruction for periods ranging from 3 days to 2 weeks.

In 1894 Dr. Renouard made his final move to New York City and established the U.S. College of Embalming. The school had no fixed term classes and the student remained until he was able to embalm. In 1889 the doctor's son, Charles A., was reported to be a shipping clerk with the firm of Dolge and Huncke—Embalming Chemical Manufacturers. Early in 1899 Charles opened the Renouard Training School for Embalmers in New York City and, in February 1900, Auguste Renouard closed the U.S. College of Embalming and joined Charles at his school. Charles provided several months of embalming instruction in London, England, on behalf of the O. K. Buckhout Chemical Company of Grand Rapids, Michigan. In 1906 Auguste traveled to England and continental Europe where he was most graciously received and entertained.

Auguste Renouard died in his home in 1912. A monument paid for by voluntary subscription of his former students was an example of the esteem in which he was held by those he instructed. **He can, without question, be regarded as the first major figure to provide embalming instruction for undertakers in the United States.** His son Charles continued the Renouard Training School for Embalmers until his death in 1950.

Joseph Henry Clarke. Born in Connersville, Indiana, Joseph Henry Clarke (1840–1916) received his early education in pharmacy and enrolled as a student in a medical college in Keokuk, Iowa. His studies, however, were interrupted by the Civil War. He volunteered for service with the Union Army but was rejected because of physical defects. He was permitted to serve as a civilian and later held the position of assistant hospital steward in the 5th Iowa Infantry. After the death of his father, he returned home before the end of the war to support his family. He married and secured employment as a casket salesman. During the course of his travels he became acquainted with a fluid manufacturer and became sufficiently interested in embalming to sell embalming fluids as a sideline. His interest in embalming grew as he realized the need to demonstrate the method of use of the fluid he hoped to sell to his patrons. This, in turn, led to his study of and experimentation with embalming chemicals to solve problems relating to preservation of the dead. He enrolled in an anatomy course conducted by Dr. C. M. Lukens of the Pulte Medical College in Cincinnati, Ohio, which broadened into a lifetime friendship and professional partnership in the founding of the Clarke School of Embalming at Cincinnati in 1882 (Figure 15).

The school lacked permanence because Mr. Clarke traveled most of the year giving courses of instruction, each course varying in length from 2 to 7 days. His second course of instruction away from Cincinnati was presented in New York City. One class member was Felix A. Sullivan, who would later become a well-known teacher and writer in the embalming field. Sullivan and Clarke became rivals and bitter enemies. One major clash occurred when General and ex-President Ulysses S. Grant died on July 23, 1885, at Mt. McGregor, New York. Clarke had been advised by the Holmes Undertaking Company (no relation to Thomas Holmes) of Saratoga, New York, that the company would be retained to handle the funeral of General Grant and that they wanted Clarke to do the embalming. Clarke was in Baltimore on the day of Grant's death, but he became ill and went to his Springfield, Ohio, home where he was bedridden for 3 to 4 weeks. The embalming was accordingly performed by one member of the Holmes Undertaking Company family and a Dr. McEwen using Clarke's proprietary embalming chemical (Figure 16).

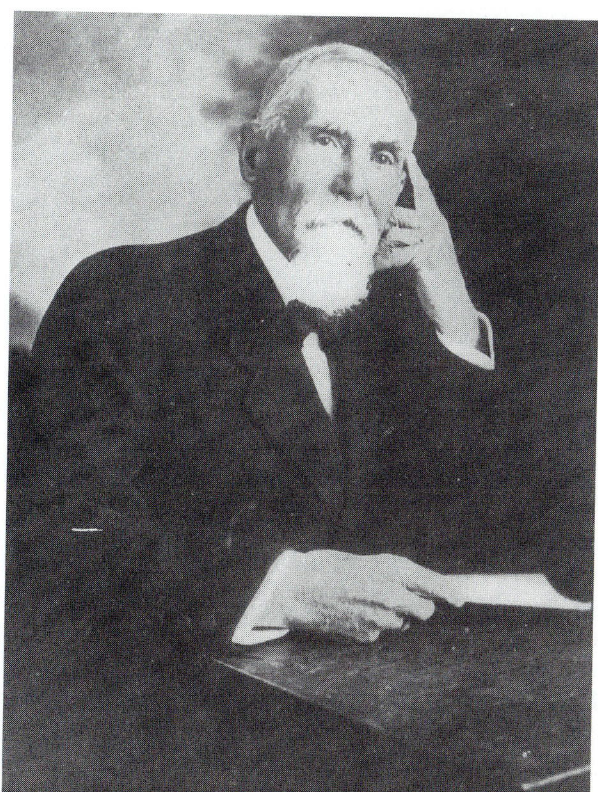

Figure 15. Portrait of Joseph Henry Clarke, founder of the Cincinnati College of Embalming.

After the body had been embalmed Rev. Stephen Merritt, clergyman and undertaker of New York City and also General Grant's religious adviser, arrived together with Felix A. Sullivan and announced that they were to take charge. The Holmes personnel withdrew from the premises and Sullivan proceeded to reembalm the body. He claimed he withdrew all previously injected arterial fluid and replaced it with the chemical made by the company he represented. Clarke rebuffed these claims in the professional journals. A reporter from the *New York Times* wrote that Mr. Holmes (of Saratoga, New York) was too drunk to carry out the necessary preparation of the body. The *New York Times* was subsequently sued for libel and lost the case, and Mr. Holmes was awarded several thousand dollars in damages.

The name of the embalming school was changed in 1899 to the Cincinnati College of Embalming and was established on a permanent basis. Mr. Clarke conducted only occasional lecture tours at that time. He was ably assisted in the management of the school by his son, C. Horace Clarke. In 1907 Charles O. Dhonau became associated with him and later took over operation of the school. Mr. Clarke was a capable teacher, lecturer, and author of several texts on embalming, and he held several patents in the embalming field. He retired

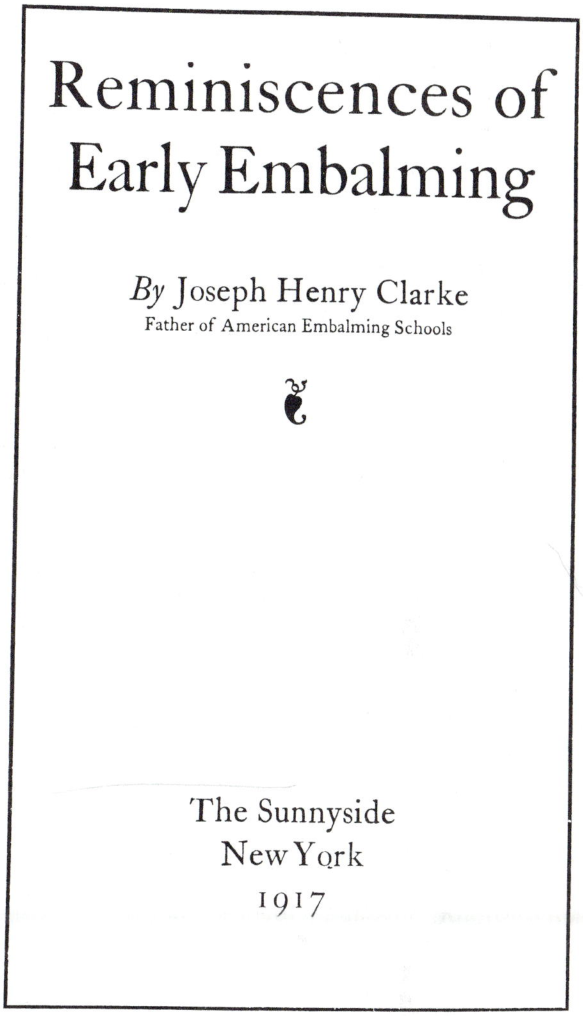

Reminiscences of Early Embalming

By Joseph Henry Clarke
Father of American Embalming Schools

The Sunnyside
New York
1917

Figure 16. Title page of an article by Joseph Henry Clarke for *The Sunnyside*.

in 1909 to San Diego, California, where he died in 1916.

Felix Aloysius Sullivan (1843–1931). Sullivan was born in Toronto, Ontario, Canada, in 1843, the son of a Scotch immigrant undertaker and an Irish mother. He unquestionably had the most interesting, controversial, riotous, and successful career as a practitioner, writer, teacher, and lecturer of embalming and related subjects. His career was so full of incidents that it would be impossible to recount all but a few highlights.

After the usual parochial school education and some experience working with his father, Sullivan, together with several other friends, crossed the border into the United States and enlisted in a New York cavalry regiment during the Civil War. Military records verify his service but reveal he deserted the service near the end of the war. He claims to have assisted in embalming while in the service, but the claim can neither be affirmed nor denied as it lacks proof.

After the Civil War he followed various occupations and traveled. He eventually drifted to New York City where he secured employment with various casket companies and finally became a funeral director for hire. He studied anatomy and other medical sciences and, by 1881, became an embalmer of some local repute. He was hired to go to Cleveland, Ohio, to reembalm President Garfield, who died from an assassin's bullet, and seems to have been successful in this venture. Sullivan attended Clarke's embalming class in New York City in 1882 to learn how such a class of instruction was conducted. Sullivan, together with W. G. Robinson, opened the New York School of Embalming in 1884 and a year later was again involved in the embalming of a president, this time President Ulysses Grant (see previous information on Clarke's career). He then entered and left a long list of employers. In 1887 he was in Chicago when the anarchists who bombed the police in 1886, killing and wounding police and civilians, were condemned to die. One exploded a dynamite cap in his mouth in jail and the others were hung. He prepared all bodies and was praised for his plastic surgery on the "mad bomber."

Sullivan continued his erratic employment or work habits, working for one firm, quitting, and then working for another. By 1891 he was again a lecturer/demonstrator, this time for the Egyptian Chemical Company. By 1892 he reached the height of his career as a lecturer, speaking and teaching in more cities to larger classes than anyone previously had. He was expelled from the State Funeral Directors convention in 1893 in St. Louis, Missouri, and a resolution was passed to forbid ever inviting his return. Sullivan settled in Chicago and opened a school of embalming. Local papers relate his arrest there together with a female companion (not his wife) on charges of adultery and wife and child desertion. When he finally settled the charges he underwent a cure for alcoholism and resumed teaching in a succession of shortlived appointments at various schools.

In 1900, the O. K. Buckhout Company of Michigan, a manufacturer of embalming chemicals, had Charles A. Renouard under contract to lecture, and sent him to London, England, to present a 3-week course of instruction that was very well received. Renouard returned home to attend similar engagements in the United States. The Buckhout Company had to find someone to continue the successful course of instruction in England, and the position was offered to Sullivan, who immediately accepted. Sullivan began teaching in London on October 8, 1900, a career that would extend to 1903. He lectured throughout the British Isles and helped to organize the British Embalmers Society as well as a journal entitled the *British Embalmer*.

He related that when Queen Victoria died in 1901 he was consulted about the possibility of embalming her. He recommended against it since it was impossible to guarantee perfect results. When he returned to the United States, he purchased an embalming school in St. Louis, Missouri, but the venture proved unprofitable. He then moved to Denver and Salt Lake City and eventually back to St. Louis, where he died. Sullivan wrote hundreds of articles plus eight books, taught thousands to embalm, and probably received more gifts from his classes than any other teacher before or since his time.

Increase in Embalming Schools

Some early "graduates" of embalming courses of instruction gave up regular employment at an undertaking establishment to provide embalming service to a number of undertakers who had no staff member trained to embalm. **This is how the terms, *embalmer to the trade* or *trade embalmer* originated.**

Many undertakers and/or their assistants were eager to learn to embalm but were unable to absent themselves from their business or employment to take advantage of such training. Some, however, managed to attend the 3- to 5-day schools, sponsored by the embalming chemical companies, in their city where they were taught the basic skills by the itinerant instructors. Others augmented their meager knowledge by enrolling in home study courses offered by many of the established schools of embalming.

Schools of instruction in embalming increased in number and activity by the beginning of the 20th century. Many manufacturers of embalming chemicals entered into the business of teaching embalming to maintain and increase the market for their products. Although the repair of injuries to the dead caused by disease or trauma had been dealt with since Egyptian times, it was not until 1912 that a systematic treatment for such cases was developed by a New York City embalmer, Joel E. Crandall (1878–1942). From this time on the schools of embalming slowly began to adopt instruction in this special phase of embalming treatment. Today, the subject area is commonly referred to as **restorative art.** It would be impossible to list in this text every personality who became an embalming professor or every school that was established, but a few should be mentioned.

Carl Lewis Barnes. Born into a family that operated an undertaking establishment in Connellsville, Pennsylvania, Barnes (1872–1927) studied medicine in Indiana, opened an embalming school there (Figure 17), and moved it to Chicago. He manufactured embalming

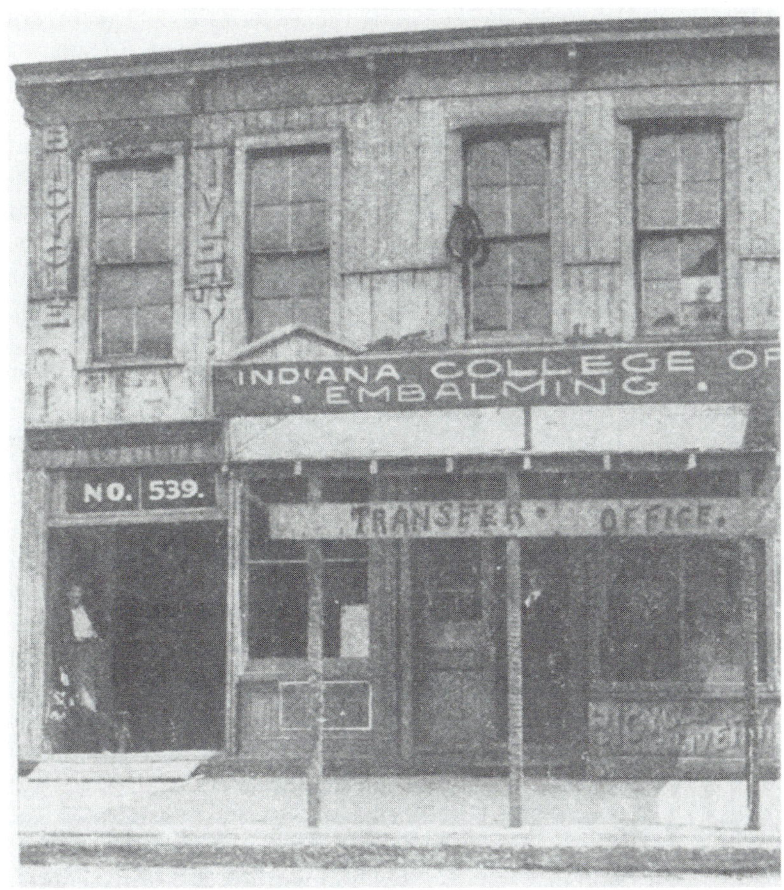

Figure 17. Old Indianapolis College of Embalming, Indianapolis, Indiana.

chemicals, wrote many books and articles on the subject, and had the largest chain of fixed-location schools in history in New York, Chicago, Boston, Minneapolis, and Dallas. While serving overseas as a medical colonel in the U.S. Army in World War I, his business failed. He never reopened the schools, continuing the practice of medicine until his death (Figure 18).

Albert H. Worsham. Worsham (1868–1939) attended Barnes' school and was on the faculty from 1903 to 1911 when he opened his own school in Chicago, with his wife Laura and brother Robert as faculty members. He lectured widely and was noted principally for contributing to the early foundation of postmortem plastic surgery.

Howard S. Eckels. Eckels (1865–1937) was a manufacturer of embalming chemicals and the founder of Eckels College of Embalming in Philadelphia, Pennsylvania. *(The school and chemical plant were in the same building, which was not an uncommon arrangement.)* Eckels wrote many articles and books, was successfully sued for plagiarism, and was not adverse to engaging in prolonged debates in the press. After his death his son John managed the school well into the post–World War II period when it closed after a period of affiliation with Temple University.

William Peter Hohenschuh. Born in Iowa City, Iowa, the son of an undertaker, Hohenschuh (1858–1920) took over the family business on the death of his father and began to teach embalming, which he had learned by correspondence from Auguste Renouard in the mid-1870s. Hohenschuh was active in the Iowa State Association and was elected president to the National Funeral Directors Association. He operated an embalming school in Chicago and, in 1900, in partnership with Dr. William S. Carpenter (1871–1944), opened the Hohenschuh–Carpenter School of Embalming in Des Moines, Iowa. He also operated a funeral home. In 1930 Dr. Carpenter moved the school to St. Louis and merged it with the Moribund American College of Embalming owned by F. A. Sullivan. After Dr. Carpenter's death his daughter Helene Craig and her son Golden Craig operated the school as well as the American Academy in New York City. This continued well into the post–World War II period.

Clarence G. Strub. Born in Iowa March 1, 1906, Strub attended the University of Iowa in Iowa City, Washing-

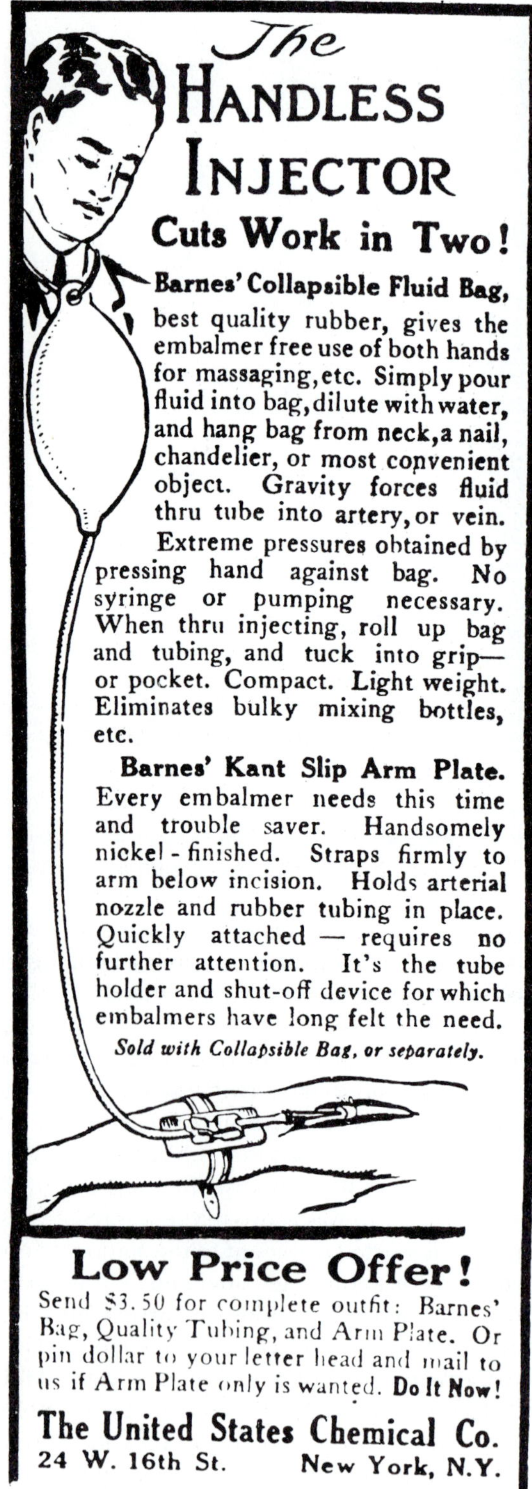

Figure 18. Advertisement for Barnes' handless injector.

ton University in St. Louis, Missouri, and the Hohenschuh–Carpenter College of Embalming in Des Moines, Iowa. He became an instructor at Hohenschuh in 1929. In 1930, the school was moved to St. Louis where it merged with the American College of Embalming and operated under the name of the St. Louis College of Mortuary Science. In 1934 he became a member of the staff of the Undertaker's Supply Company of Chicago and conducted clinics and demonstrations throughout the United States and Canada. He taught embalming and funeral management at the University of Minnesota and the Wisconsin Institute of Mortuary Science and was the director of research for the Royal Bond Chemical Company for many years (Figure 19).

His greatest contributions to embalming lie in his ability to write clearly and simply, explaining embalming theory and practices. During his career he published well over 1000 articles, as well as many teaching outlines and quiz compendia. His little text, *The Principles of Restorative Art,* was the true prototype of all present-day texts on the subject. He also authored the monumental textbook *Principles and Practice of Embalming,* published by L. G. "Darko" Fredericks, which became the standard embalming text used by most colleges of mortuary science. Strub also wrote several technical movies such as the *Conquest of Jaundice* and *The Eye Bank Story,* as well as many purely children's stories and movies. He was the architect of the Eye Bank System in Iowa, which set the national pattern, as well as the curator of the state of Iowa's anatomical donation program. He died in Iowa City, Iowa, on August 6, 1974.

Women Embalmers. Women as well as men were trained as embalmers and not only practiced embalm-

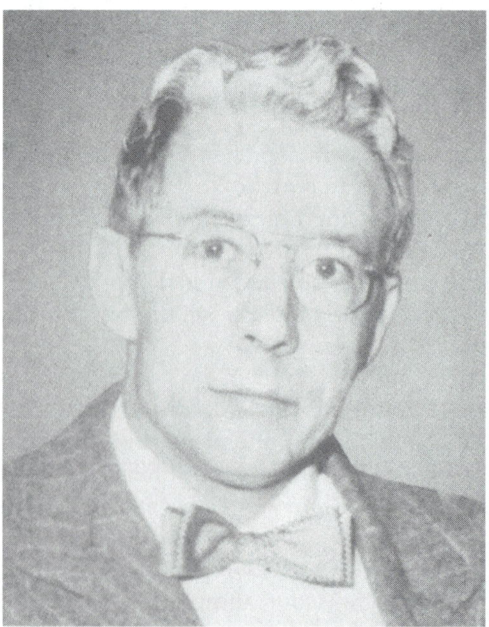

Figure 19. Photograph of Clarence G. Strub.

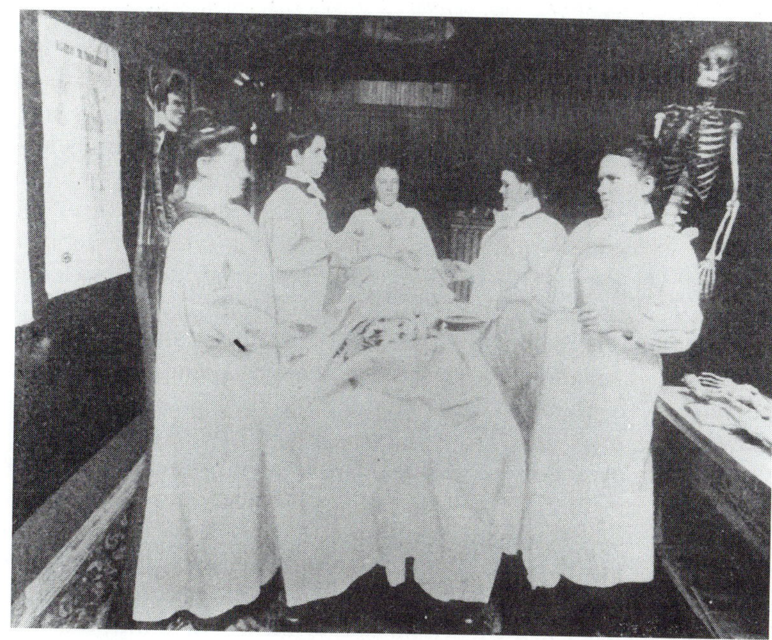

Figure 20. Anatomy class at Odou Institute of Embalming, New York, circa 1900 (Professor Odou at center of group).

ing but founded schools of instruction. Among these women were **Mrs. E. G. Bernard** of Newark, New Jersey, who founded the Bernard School of Embalming; **Mme. Linda D. Odou,** who founded the Odou Embalming Institute in New York City (Figure 20); and **Lena R. Simmons,** who founded and operated the Simmons School of Embalming in Syracuse, New York, until her son Baxter took over the management.

▶ MORTUARY EDUCATION

Each course in a college of mortuary science employs a basic course content. Now overseen by various committees of the American Board of Funeral Service Education, the basic course content in embalming is a foundation for uniform performance standards in the preparation of all bodies embalmed in the United States. This basic course content also allows the Conference of Funeral Service Examining Boards to administer a uniform objective examination to those candidates for a license. As an introduction to this chapter we are going to take an overview of the development of the basic course content in embalming, as it lays the foundation for professional performance standards.

Mortuary colleges, as we know them today, are relatively recent in origin. The development of mortuary education has followed the general pattern common to all professional fields. It emerged slowly from a period in which knowledge was transmitted from preceptor to student by means of observation and informal discussion, to its present academic status.

Following the American Civil War, when funeral homes first came into existence, the pioneers in funeral service experimented with materials, equipment, and methods for their use. There were no channels for wide distribution of the knowledge they gained through trial and error. Training was conducted solely by means of apprenticeship.

As the scope of funeral service expanded and as embalming came into wider use, commercial companies were organized to supply the needs of the embalmer and funeral director. Research was directed to developing better products, and this resulted in a rapid increase in knowledge of what today is termed *mortuary science.* During the latter decades of the 19th century, the establishment of trade journals made possible a wider distribution of this knowledge. These same companies employed skilled lecturers and demonstrators to instruct funeral directors in the use of these products and in improved methods of embalming. These early "classes," lasting from a few hours to a few days, provided the first formal vocational instruction.

As the public health and welfare aspects of funeral service became more widely recognized, state licensing laws were established. For the first time educational requirements were formulated and a definite course of training was legally prescribed. At about this same time educators established the first schools of embalming to train students in a relatively new art. Over the years, these pioneers in mortuary education expanded and improved the scope of training, often keeping far ahead of requirements prescribed by law and by licensing authorities.

A system for national accreditation of mortuary schools was first introduced in 1927 by the Conference of Funeral Service Examining Boards, a national association of state licensing boards. Higher standards governing qualifications of faculty, the curriculum, and teaching facilities were established and enforced. Details of the development of mortuary schools can be found in Part II of this textbook.

The National Council on Mortuary Education was established in 1942 by the National Funeral Directors Association and the National Association of Embalming Schools and Colleges. After World War II, with the termination of restrictions on assembly, a formal meeting was held in December of 1945 in Cleveland, Ohio. Officers for the Council were Chairman, Ralph Millard; Vice-Chairman, Jacob Van't Hof; and Secretary-Treasurer, R. P. MacFate. The Council was attended by 62 school administrators, faculty members, state board authorities, and various funeral service association officers. The program committee comprised John Eckles, Jacob Van't Hof, and Otto Margolis. This meeting gave a fresh impetus to progress toward educational competence and professional status in funeral service. In March of 1947 the First National Teacher's Institute was held in Cincinnati, Ohio. Forty-four representatives from 14 schools met to lay the foundation for the course content in Chemistry and Mortuary Administration. Charles O. Dhonau of the Cincinnati College of Embalming presided over the meeting. In November of 1947 the Second Teacher's Institute was held in Pittsburgh, Pennsylvania (Figure 21). More than 75 individuals from 23 schools and associations were present. Adopted at this meeting was the first basic course content syllabus for anatomy and embalming and the Mortician's Oath (drafted by R. P. MacFate). The Oath remains unchanged (except for one word) and has been administered to all graduates of a mortuary college since 1948. Dr. Emory S. James of Pittsburgh, was chair of the anatomy course content committee. The committee on the basic course content in embalming consisted of R. H. Hannum (Cleveland), L. G. Frederick (Dallas), R. Victor Landig (Houston), J. E. Shea (Boston), and E. L. Heidenreich (Wisconsin). The formulation and analysis of the embalming basic course content was brought about through the efforts of mortuary colleges, state boards, state associations, and the profession in general. The task was difficult because it meant resolving many individualistic teaching procedures into one common, sound educational basis. Once the basic course content was established it was immediately recognized there would be an imperative need to review and update the curriculum every few years. Revision of the course content has continued over the years and is currently overseen by the American Board of Funeral Service Education. In their July 1994 meeting in Denver, Colorado, a glossary of terminology was appended to the basic course content in embalming. In a meeting in Denver as late as July of 1995, the basic course content in embalming was again reviewed, amended, and prepared for editing and input by the member schools of the American Board of Funeral Service Education. This basic course content is an example of a professional performance standard in the field of embalming in America.

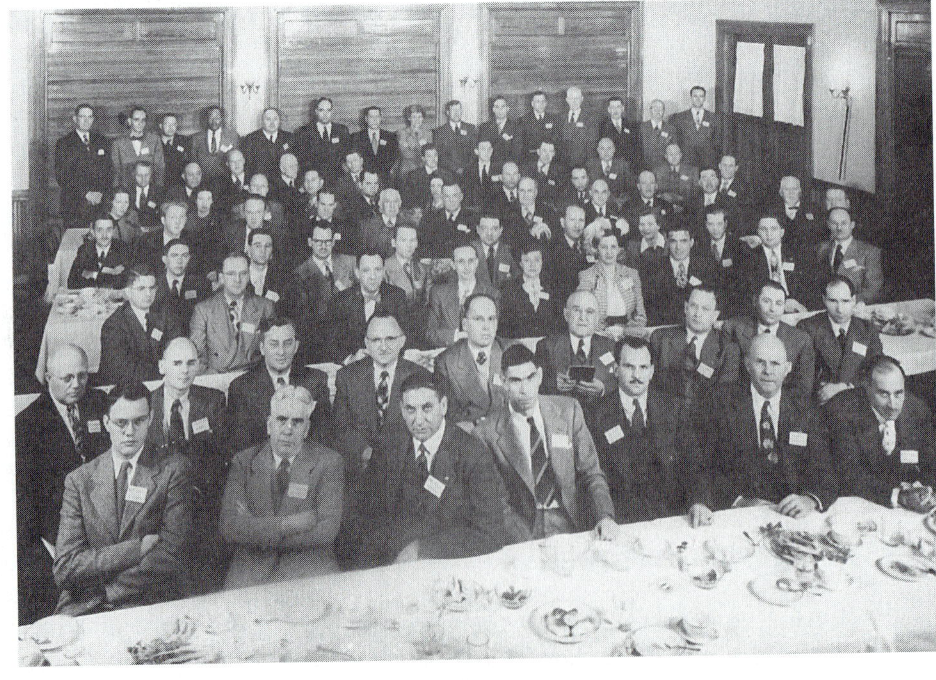

Figure 21. Educators from across the United States gathered for the Second Teachers Institute held in Pittsburgh, Pennsylvania, November 8 and 9, 1947. At this meeting the first curriculum in anatomy and embalming was established and the Mortician's Oath was adopted. *(Courtesy of the Pittsburgh Institute of Mortuary Science, Pittsburgh, Pennsylvania.)*

▶ CONCERN FOR TREATMENT

Early embalming reports concerning arterial injection indicated some concern for special treatment of the trunk viscera. Most such treatments consisted of removal, treatment, and replacement of viscera in the trunk cavity together with some preservative material, either powdered or liquid. Other reports, such as those of the Gannal–Sucquet era, indicate dependence for total preservation solely on the arterial injection unaccompanied by any special treatment for the trunk cavities. Gabriel Clauderus had advocated preservation based on introduction of his preservative chemical into the trunk cavity followed by immersion of the entire body in the preservative.

It was not until the mid-1870s that a "modern" system of treatment for the cavities was designed. The inventor of the trocar, Samuel Rodgers (listing Los Angeles, New York City, and San Francisco as his residence) secured two patents for the trocar, one in 1878 and the second in 1880. The 1878 patent described the trocar much as it exists today. The 1880 patent was issued for a system of embalming that consisted of introduction of his trocar, thrust through a single point in the navel into all the organs of the trunk to distribute a preservative fluid throughout the trunk viscera. The simplicity of this treatment and its modest success made it appealing to those who, for whatever reason, did not adopt arterial embalming, which required greater knowledge of anatomy and surgical skill. The inevitable result was a confrontation between "belly punchers" (cavity treatment advocates) and "throat cutters" (arterial embalmers) concerning the merits of their respective means of preservation.

It slowly became evident that neither system was always completely successful and that combination of the two systems, arterial injection followed by cavity treatment, offered the greatest promise of embalming success. Although Rodgers did not mention aspiration prior to injection of preservative chemicals in his process, Auguste Renouard did specifically recommend this in his *Undertaker's Manual.* Rodgers' method of a single-entrance opening into the trunk cavity was a brilliant concept not followed by all his contemporary "authorities." Espy's and Taylor's books of embalming instruction, for example, advocated multiple (three to four) points of insertion through the trunk wall for the trocar. Rodgers formulated an embalming preservative chemical named *Alekton,* which was believed to have phenol as its principal preservative. He also recommended cavity treatment followed by hypodermic injections using his trocar, inserted into the limbs of the corpse.

Since the introduction of arterial injection of the blood vessels in the late 17th century no other system of corpse preservation explored had ever been seriously used. In 1884 a British physician, Dr. B. W. Richardson, devised what he termed **needle embalming.** The process consisted of inserting a trocar (the needle), such as Rodgers' invention, at the medial corner of the eye socket and forcing it into the brain area, where the injection process was repeated. After removal of the trocar from the brain area, cavity treatment, aspiration, and injection were carried out. This process was most often referred to as the **eye process.** Rodgers in his early patent had proposed insertion of his trocar through the nose to inject preservative chemicals into the brain area, but did not suggest that this process would preserve the entire body as Richardson contended. It eventually was to be called the **nasal process.** Professor Sullivan, ever alert for any new procedure to interest his students, adopted Richardson's eye process and exploited its simplicity to the maximum.

Carl Barnes offered a variation of the procedure by inserting the trocar through the neck and into the brain via the foramen magnum. T. B. Barnes, his brother and school instructor associate, inserted the trocar between dorsal vertebrae into the spinal canal. In this method, Dr. Eliab Meyers drilled a hole through the center of the vertex of the skull, permitting direct access for a small trocar into the superior sagittal sinus. The process, regardless of point of access, is said to have delivered the preservative chemical eventually into blood vessels within the cranium and then to the rest of the body.

A dramatic test demonstration of the process is both described and illustrated in Barnes' textbook, *The Art and Science of Embalming.* A severed head of a dissection room subject had trocars inserted into the brain area through the eye socket route. Rubber tubes connected the carotid arteries and jugular veins with collecting bottles. As fluid was injected through the trocars into the brain area, fluid flowed into the collecting bottles via the carotid arteries and jugular veins. The process achieved moderate popularity until about 1905 when it became extinct. Not all teachers of embalming were advocates of it, and J. H. Clarke was a vigorous critic.

A variation of the process was the short-lived attempt to insert the trocar into the left ventricle of the heart and inject the arterial system. The great difficulty encountered in positively locating the left ventricle quickly discouraged this procedure. The intentional application of an electric current directly to a corpse for the intended purpose of simulating the effect of lightning or accidental electrocution on the blood—destruction of blood coagulation—has been attempted many times without any appreciable success.

One early experimenter was Charles T. Schade of McAlester, Oklahoma, who as early as 1909 conceived the idea of applying an electric current, powered by dry cell batteries, to the body surface, in the belief that this would cause small muscles to contract and hence force blood out of the areas of discoloration. No effect was noted concerning the ability of an electric current applied externally to a corpse to prevent normal postmortem blood coagulation or promote dissolution of any existing intravascular clots. Similar attempts to accomplish this desirable effect have been attempted through the years down to the present both in the United States and England without success. Those who have experimented have concluded that the dead human body does not conduct an electrical current well enough to accomplish the intended purpose.

▶ PROFESSIONALISM IN EMBALMING

Toward the end of the 19th century and on into the 20th century a number of events were to occur that would accelerate embalming toward the level of professionalism. A convergence of two movements became apparent about 1897, with the appearance of advertisements by embalming fluid companies stating that their fluid contained formalin. For some years there had been arguments to eliminate arsenic and other poisons from inclusion in embalming fluid formulas for the same medicolegal reason that the French prohibited arsenic in 1846 and bichloride of mercury in 1848. Now that a powerful disinfectant, **formalin,** was available and reasonably priced, the opportunity to eliminate poisonous chemicals was at hand. The state of Michigan led the way in 1901 and was followed by other states.

The second movement was to require regulations for both licensing and governing those who practiced embalming, and in 1893–1894 the state of Virginia became the first state to do so. Formalin content fluids were not a total blessing and were not as favorably received as might have been expected. Embalmers of the period were unaccustomed to the very different characteristics of the new preservative. For example, bodies embalmed with arsenic were said to have been relatively supple, making dressing and positioning relatively easy. Many of the poisonous chemicals had bleaching qualities and left the body quite white. Only a few left any undesirable coloration, such as those reported to contain copper, which tended to produce a bluish color in the skin. Then too, little or no problem was reportedly encountered to the penetration of all the body tissues, with or without blood drainage. There was also the proven ability of such poisonous chemicals to preserve the body tissues. There were, of course, some negatives such as the possible absorption of poisonous chemicals through the embalmer's unprotected skin, various skin irritations, and thickened and cracked fingernails.

Embalmers beginning to experiment with the formalin-based embalming fluids had to learn that they must remove the blood in all cases and began to use low-formalin-content or nonformalin fluids to wash the blood out before injection of the preservative formalin-based solutions. They also learned that they had to position the body properly before injection and the hardening effected by formalin or they would encounter serious problems later in trying to properly position hands together. To their astonishment, embalmers also discovered that formalin reacted with the bile pigments present in the skin of jaundiced bodies to produce an unsightly green-colored skin.

The opponents of formalin fluids were highly critical of the formaldehyde fumes, which irritated mucous membranes, claiming these effects were more dangerous to health than the poisonous chemicals. Reason and science prevailed and the embalming fluid formulas were improved to overcome most of the early problems. With the eventual transfer of the site of embalming from the family home bedroom to the funeral home preparation room, proper ventilation tended to eliminate most of the irritation problem. Chemicals became more diverse. For example, different formulas were developed for specific uses, such as arterial and cavity, preinjection, coinjection, and for special purposes as in decomposing cases. The delivery of embalming fluids in concentrated form, to be added to water to create the desired dilution strength, was a distinct contrast to the former embalming chemical packaging which was delivered in containers already combined with water ready to inject. Thus, the embalmer had to become more experienced and intelligent in the mixing of the formalin embalming solution than he had formerly.

▶ UTILIZATION OF NEW DEVICES

Over the years of embalming in bedrooms of the home of the deceased, little in the way of improvements was instituted in injection pumps or aspirating devices. With the transfer of the majority of embalming preparations to the funeral home, however, new devices could be used. In the last quarter of the 19th century most embalming pumps or injectors were based on the gravity bowl, the hand pump, or the rubber bulb syringe. The gravity bowl was simply a container suspended above the body and connected to the arterial tube by a length of rubber tubing. The height of the bowl above the body determined the pressure. Its main advantage was that it did not require the constant pumping by the embalmer and, therefore, left hands free to perform other tasks. The hand pump could produce either pressure or vacuum for injection or aspiration into or from a glass container.

When the preparation of the body was moved to the funeral home, water pressure was used to create suction to aspirate. Special aspirators, such as the Penberthy, Worsham, and Slaughter, generated suction by water pressure and were made to attach to preparation room sink faucets, connected by rubber tubing to the trocar. Later in the 1950s special electric motor-driven aspirators were devised and were found to overcome the aggravation encountered by low water pressure during high-water-use periods. *Most communities today have requirements relating to the need for preventing suction of aspirated material into the water system.*

At a New York state convention in 1914, a battery-powered electric pump, the Falcon Electric Embalmer for injecting embalming chemicals, was demonstrated but was not widely adopted. Some new instruments devised to simplify or improve certain embalming procedures were developed in the 1920s and 1930s. A new method of jaw closure was devised involving "barbed tacks" driven into the mandible and maxillae by a spring-propelled hammer. Wires attached to the "tacks" were then twisted together to secure the desired degree of jaw closure. A plastic, threaded, screwlike device called the **trocar button** became the most useful waterproof seal for trocar punctures, bullet wounds, and even for intravenous needle punctures (when surgically enlarged). A metal dispensing device that was attached directly to any standard 16-ounce bottle of cavity fluid (by screwing it into the bottle opening in place of the cap) simplified cavity fluid injection. The dispenser was connected to the trocar by a length of rubber hose and injection was accomplished by gravity after the cavity fluid bottle was elevated and inverted.

It was not until the mid-1930s that electric-powered injection machines were available and in use. Some were simply electric motors with fittings to produce pressure or vacuum-connected to suitable containers by rubber tubing. One of the first "self-contained" embalming fluid injection machines put on the market in the 1930s was the Snyder/Westberg device. It was originally designed to hold $\frac{1}{2}$ gallon of embalming fluid. The machine was compact, durable, and trouble free, and was originally designed with motor and the fluid container side by side. Model II was designed so that the fluid container was placed above the injection motor; thus, the fluid was "gravity fed" to the pump. This arrangement has become standard on all self-contained units. In 1937 the Slaughter Company developed an all-metal fluid injection tank equipped with a pressure gauge; in 1938 the Flowmaster electric-powered injection machine was announced; in 1939 the Frigid Fluid Company developed a pressure injector consisting of a metal container for holding embalming fluid complete with exit connection with shut-off and a carbon dioxide gas cylinder to create the necessary pressure to inject the fluid. **In mid-1939 the Turner Company announced the availability of the Porti Boy, which was to become the all-time most popular injection machine.** Several improvements over the years included a pulsator device, a larger fluid tank, and the ability to produce extreme high-pressure injections. By the 1960s, extreme high-pressure injection machines such as the Sawyer were available and in use.

▶ AVAILABILITY OF MORE MATERIALS

With the end of World War II, metal and other materials became available to produce various new embalming devices. The concept of using externally generated agitation to assist in blood removal became popular. Some embalming tables had such pulsating devices built in as an integral part of the structure. Other pulsating devices were devised to be attached to existing operating tables or were handheld devices to be applied to the body over the course of the major blood vessels. Disillusionment with this development came after a short period of use. The vibrations produced by such devices made it impossible to keep instruments, and even the body itself, from sliding downward toward the foot of the table.

Another innovation was the development of a conventional embalming fluid by the Switzer Corporation of Cleveland that contained a large quantity of fluorescent dye. The dye was to act as a tracer or indicator of the degree of circulation or penetration of the embalming fluid when viewed under an ultraviolet light illuminator furnished with the embalming fluid. Although the system did indeed disclose the extent of the distribution of the embalming chemical and its fluorescent dye, it never was proof positive that areas of the body beneath the skin were thoroughly embalmed.

In the wake of Hiroshima and Nagasaki and other major disasters such as airline crashes, earthquakes, mudslides, and building collapses, a search was instituted for some new means of quickly processing (preserving) huge numbers of dead. Over the years, different means of processing (preserving) the victims of such tragedies were devised, tested, and found unsuitable for a variety of reasons. Experiments were conducted with processes using ultrasound, radiation, atomic bombardment, and ultracold. No process tried seemed to be capable of preserving a tremendous number of bodies in a brief period. The search continues!

Indisputably the greatest change in embalming procedures began in the 1980s by the intervention of federal government agencies. The Federal Trade Commission (FTC) adopted rules concerning the necessity for embalming and the securing of consent for same. The Occupational Safety and Health Administration

(OSHA) adopted rules relating to embalming procedures, funeral home personnel protection, and similar public health and hygienic measures. The Environmental Protection Agency (EPA) issued rules concerning the use and control of formaldehyde and chemicals used by embalmers.

Although it has been generally conceded that formaldehyde-based fluids performed well as preserving and fixing agents for the embalming process, chemical research for an improvement in embalming chemicals has always been active.

During the 1930s, Hilton Ira Jones of the Hizone Company performed extensive research on glyoxal, a chemical that seemed to display much promise for use in an embalming formula. World War II, however, reduced the available supply and thus the research in this direction.

Another chemical, glutaraldehyde, was thoroughly researched and developed into an embalming formula by the Champion Company.

At the time of publication of this textbook edition, several embalming fluid companies have formulations that replace formaldehyde in embalming solutions.

Since the intervention of OSHA in embalming procedures, the search has intensified to find a substitute for formaldehyde and thus eliminate the vexatious problems of monitoring formaldehyde fume levels and wearing filter masks as required by OSHA regulations.

It is astonishing what has been achieved in the embalming field in nearly 5000 years of growth of knowledge, skill, and experience. Naturally, what the future holds is unknown, but those working in the field feel it will be as exciting and rewarding as the past millenia.

▶ KEY TERMS AND CONCEPTS FOR STUDY AND DISCUSSION

1. List and describe the natural means of preservation.
2. List and describe the artificial means of preservation.
3. Describe the three periods of embalming history.
4. Describe the procedures employed in each of the five steps used by the Egyptians in the preparation of mummies.
5. Explain the contributions made to the development of embalming by each of the following:
   A. William Harvey
   B. Marcello Malpighi
   C. Jean Nicholas Gannal
   D. Gabriel Clauderus
   E. John Hunter
   F. Richard Harlan
   G. John Morgan
   H. Thomas Holmes
   I. Frederick Ruysch
   J. Joseph Henry Clark
6. Explain the following terms:
   anthropoid (mummy) form coffin
   canopic jars
   cartonage
   evisceration
   natron
   needle embalming
   preinjection fluid
   sarcophagus
   trade embalmer
   trocar

▶ BIBLIOGRAPHY

Beverly R. *History of Virginia.* 1922:185.

McClelland EH. *Bibliography on Embalming* (mimeo copy). New York: National Association of Mortuary Science (limited to 100 copies); 1949.

McCurdy CW. *Embalming and Embalming Fluids—With Bibliography of Embalming.* Wooster, OH: Hearld Printing; 1896

Oatfield H. *Literature of the Chemical Periphery—Embalming.* Advances in Chemistry Series No. 16 (a key to pharmaceutical and medicinal chemistry literature). Washington, DC: American Chemical Society.

Pinkerton J. *Collection of Voyages.* (Vol. 13), 1812.

Surgeon General's Catalogue. Washington, DC: U.S. Army; 1883–1884.

Townshend J. *Grave Literature* (a catalogue of some books relating to the disposal of bodies and perpetuating the memories of the dead). New York (private collection); 1887.

Egypt

Aliki. *Mummies Made in Egypt.* New York: Thomas J. Crowell; 1979.

Arcieri GP. *Note E Ricordi—Sulla Preservatione Del Corppo Umano.* Rivista Di Storia Delle Scienze Medicine E Naturoli, No. 1. Florence; 1956.

Bardeen CR. Anatomy in America. *Bulletin of University of Wisconsin,* No. 115. September 1905.

Budge EAW. *The Mummy.* Cambridge: University Press; 1893.

Choulant L. *History and Bibliography of Anatomical Illustration.* New York: 1962 (reprint).

David AR, ed. *Manchester Museum Mummy Project.* Manchester, England: Maney and Sons; 1979.

Harris JE, Weeks KR. *X-Raying the Pharaohs.* New York: Charles Scribner's Sons; 1973.

Hemneter E. *Embalming in Ancient Egypt.* Ciba Symposia, Vol. 1, No. 10, Summit, NJ: Ciba Pharmaceuticals; January 1940.

Herodotus. *History.* (translated by George Rawlinson). New York: Dial and Tudor Presses; 1928.

Liebling R, et al. *Time Line of Culture in the Nile Valley and Its Relationship to Other Countries.* New York: Metropolitan Museum of Art; 1978.

Martin RA. *Mummies.* Anthropology Leaflet No. 36. Chicago, IL: Chicago Natural History Museum Press; 1945.

Mendelsohn S. *Embalming.* Ciba Symposia, Vol. VI, No. 2. Summit, NJ: Ciba Pharmaceuticals; May 1944.

Moodie RL. *Anthropology Memoirs.* Vol. III: *Roentgenologic Studies of Egyptian and Peruvian Mummies.* Chicago, IL: Field Museum Press; 1931.

Pettigrew TJ. *History of Egyptian Mummies.* London: Longman, Rees; 1834.

Pons A. *Les Origines de L'Embaument et L'Egypte Predynastique.* Montpelier, France: Inprimerie Grollier; 1910.

Smith GE, Dawson WR. *Egyptian Mummies.* New York: Dial Press; 1924.

Steuer RO, Saunders JB de CM. *Ancient Egyptian and Cnidian Medicine.* Berkeley/Los Angeles: University of California Press; 1959.

Peru*

Garcillaso de la Vega. *Royal Commentaries of Peru.* (translated by Paul Rycant). London; 1688.

Prescott WH. *History of the Conquest of Peru.* (2 vols.). Philadelphia: JB Lippincott; 1882.

Rivero ME, Von Tschudi JJ. *Peruvian Antiquities.* (translated by Francis L. Hawks), New York: George Putnam; 1853.

Von Hagen VW. *Realm of the Incas.* New York: New American Library of World Literature; 1957.

Alaska and Aleutian Islands

Quimby GI. *Aleutian Islanders.* Anthropology Leaflet, No. 35. Chicago: Natural History Museum; 1944.

North American Indians

Yarrow HC. *Study of Mortuary Customs Among the North American Indians.* Washington, DC: U.S. Government Printing Office; 1880.

Ecuador—Jivaro Indians

Cottlow LN. *Amazon Head Hunters.* New York: Signet Book/Henry Holt; 1953.

Flornoy B. *Jivaro.* New York: Library Publishers; 1954

* Also see Moodie in list under Egypt.

Canary Islands

De Espinosa A. *The Guanches of Tenerife.* London: Hakluyt Society; 1907.

Hooton EA. *The Ancient Inhabitants of the Canary Islands.* Harvard African Studies, Vol. II. Cambridge, MA: Harvard University Press; 1925.

Europe (Early Period)

Bradford CA. *Heart Burial.* London: Allen & Unwin; 1933.

Castiglioni A, Robinson V. *The Anatomical Theater.* Ciba Symposia, Vol. III, No. 4. Summit, NJ: Ciba Pharmaceuticals; May 1941.

Clauderus G. *Methodus Balsamundi Corpora Humane Aliaque Majora sine Evisceratione et Sectione Hucusque Solita.* Altenberg, Germany: G. Richterum; 1679.

De Villihardouin G, DeJoinville J. *Memoirs of the Crusades.* New York: EP Dutton; 1938.

Dionis M. *Cours D'Operations de Chirurqie.* Paris: d'Houry; 1746.

Garrison FH. *Introduction to the History of Medicine.* Philadelphia: 1929.

Greenhill T. *Nekrokadeia—Or the Art of Embalming.* London: printed for the author; 1705.

Guichard C. *Des Funerailles et diverses Manieres.* Lyon, France: D'ensevelir; 1582.

Guichard C. *Funerailles.* Lyon, France: Jean de Tovrnes; 1581.

Guybert P. The charitable physitian showing the manner to embalm a dead corpse. In: *The Charitable Physitian.* London: Thomas Harper Printer; 1639.

Pare A. *How to Make Reports and to Embalm the Dead* (translated). London: Cotes & Young; 1634.

Pilcher LS. The Mondino myth (reprint). *Med Library Hist J.* 1906; 4(4, Dec.).

The Art and Science of Embalming Dead Bodies (taken from the 29th book of Peter Forestus and translated from the Latin into German), contained in *A New Medical Treatise* by Petrum Offenbach, M.D. Frankfort: Zacharian Palthenium; 1605.

Treece H. *The Crusades.* New York: Random House; 1962.

Walsh JJ. *The Popes and Science.* New York: Fordham University Press; 1908.

Walsh JJ. *The 13th—Greatest of Centuries.* New York: Catholic Summer School Press; 1907.

Wellcome HS. *The Evolution of Antiseptic Surgery.* London: Burroughs Wellcome; 1910.

Young S. *The Annals of the Barber Surgeons of London.* London: Blades East & Blades; 1890.

Europe (Late Period)

Bailey JB. *The Diary of a Resurrectionist 1811–1812.* London: Swan-Sonnenschein; 1896.

Ball JM. *The Sack em Up Men.* London: Oliver & Boyd; 1928.

Bayle DC. *L'Embaumement.* Paris: Adrien Delahaye; 1873.

Blanchard S. *Anatomia Reformata—Balsamatione, Novus Methodus.* Leiden: Boutesteyn & Lughtmans: 1687.

Cole FJ. *A History of Comparative Anatomy.* London: MacMillan: 1944.

Coliez A. *Conservation Artificielle des Corps.* Paris: Amedee Legrand; 1927.

Cope Z. *The History of the Royal College of Surgeons.* Springfield, IL: Charles C Thomas; 1959.

Dawson WR. Life and times of Thomas J. Pettigrew. *Med Life.* (3 issues) 1931;38 (1–3, Jan./Feb./March).

DeLint JG. *Atlas of the History of Medicine,* Vol. I. London: HK Lewis; 1926.

Eriksson R, ed., translator, *Andreas Vesalius 1st Public Anatomy at Bologna—1540.* Uppsala: Almquist & Wikselle; 1959.

Gannal JN. *Histoire des Embaumements.* Paris: Ferra Librairie; 1838.

Gannal JN (as translated by R. Harlan): *History of Embalming.* Philadelphia: Judah Dobson; 1840.

Gerlt-Wernich-Hirsch. *Biographisches Lexikon Der Herrvorragenden Arzte Aller Zeiten und Volker.* Berlin: Urban & Schwarzenberg; 1932.

Laskowski S. *L'Embaumement, la conservatione des Sujets et les Preparations Anatomiques.* Geneva: H. Georg; 1886.

Mann G. The anatomical collections of Fredrick Ruysch at Leningrad. *Bull Cleve Med Library.* 1964;11 (No. 1, Jan.).

Nordenskiold E. *The History of Biology.* New York: Tudor; 1928.

Paget S. *John Hunter.* London: T. Fisher University; 1898.

Peachy GC. *The Homes of Hunter in London.* London: Bailliere, Tindall & Cox; 1928.

Pettigrew JT. Fredrick Ruysch. In: *Pettigrew's Medical Portrait Gallery.* London: Whitaker; 1840.

Ramazzini B. *De Morbio Artificum* (ed 2, 1713). *Diseases of Workers* (translated by WC Wright). New York: Hafner; 1964.

Richardson BW. *The Art of Embalming.* In *Wood's Medical and Surgical Monographs.* Vol. III. New York: 1889.

Sigerist HE. *The Great Doctors.* Garden City, NY: Doubleday; 1958.

Singer C. *Studies in the History and Method of Science.* (2 vols.). Oxford, England: Clarendon Press; Vol I.—1917, Vol II.—1921.

Sucquet JP. *De L'embaumement et des Conservation pour l'etude de l'anatomie.* Paris: Adrien Delahaye; 1872.

Sucquet JP. *Traits due Visage Dans L'embaumement.* Paris: Adrien Delahaye; 1862.

United States

Barnes CL. *The Art and Science of Embalming.* Chicago, IL: Trade Periodical; 1905.

Clarke CH. *Practical Embalming.* Cincinnati, OH: C. H. Clarke; 1917.

Clarke JH. Reminiscences of early embalming. *The Sunnyside,* 1917.

Crane EH. *Manual of Instructions to Undertakers.* 8th ed. Kalamazoo, MI: Kalamazoo; 1888.

Dodge AJ. *The Practical Embalmer.* Boston: A. Johnson Dodge; 1908.

Eckels HS. *Practical Embalmer.* Philadelphia: H. S. Eckels Co.; 1903.

Espy JB. *Espy's Embalmer.* Springfield, OH: Espy Fluid Co.; 1895.

Gallagher T. The body snatchers. *Am Heritage,* June 1967.

Johnson EC. Civil war embalming. *Funeral Directors Rev,* June/July/August; 1965.

Johnson EC, Johnson GR. A Civil War embalming surgeon—The story of Dr. Daniel H. Prunk. *The Director* (NFDA publication), January 1970.

Johnson EC, Johnson GR. *Alone in His Glory.* Unpublished manuscript, Civil War Mortuary Practices.

Johnson EC, Johnson GR. *Prince Greer—America's First Negro Embalmer.* Liaison Bulletin, International Federation of Thanatopractic Association, Paris, April 1973.

Johnson EC, Johnson GR. The undertakers manual. *Canadian Funeral News,* Calgary, July 1980.

Johnson EC, Johnson MDH Rhodes—Conscientious caretaker of Arlington National Cemetery. *Am Funeral Director;* January 1984.

Johnson EC, Johnson GR, Johnson Williams M. Dr. Renouard's role in embalming history. *Am Funeral Director* 1987. August 1987.

Johnson EC, Johnson GR, Johnson M. Dr. Thomas Holmes—Pioneer embalmer. *Am Funeral Director* July/August 1984.

Johnson EC, Johnson GR, Johnson Williams M. History of modern restorative art. *Am Funeral Director* January–April 1988.

Johnson EC, Johnson GR, Johnson Williams M. The trial, execution and embalming of two Civil War soldiers. *Am Funeral Director* December 1986.

Johnson M. *A historic precedent to the FTC rules of 1977 (Civil War licensing for embalmer requirements).* NFDA Bulletin, 1979.

Johnson M. Lena R. Simmons—The grand dame of early embalmers. *Am Funeral Director* January 1977.

Johnson M. *Lina D. Odou—Embalmer.* July 1977.

Keen WW. *Addresses and Other Papers.* Philadelphia: Saunders; 1905.

Mendelsohn S. *Embalming Fluids.* New York: Chemical Publishing; 1940.

Mills and Lacey Mfg. Co. (no author stated). *Practical Directions for Embalming the Dead.* Grand Rapids, MI: Stevens, Cornell and Dean; 1881.

Myers E. *Champion Textbook on Embalming.* Springfield, OH: Champion Chemical Co.; 1908.

Renouard A. *Undertakers Manual.* Rochester, NY: A. Nirdlinger; 1878.

Renouard CA, ed. *Taylor's Art of Embalming.* New York: H. E. Taylor; 1903.

Samson H, Crane ON, Perrigo AB, Hatfield MD. *Pharmaceutical, Anatomical and Chemical Lexicon* (the NFDA official textbook). Chicago, IL: Donohue & Henneberry; 1886.

Strub CA, Frederick LG. *The Principles and Practice of Embalming.* 4th ed. Dallas, TX: L. G. Frederick; 1986.

Sullivan FA. *Practical Embalming.* Boston: Egyptian Chemical Co.; 1887.

The Faculty of the Cincinnati School for Embalming, Lukens CM and Clarke JH. *Textbook on Embalming.* Springfield, OH: Limbocker; 1883.

War Department. General Order 33, April 3, 1862.

War Department. General Order 39, March 15, 1865.

War Department. General Order 75, September 11, 1861.

Wightman SK. In search of my son (Civil War). *Am Heritage,* February, 1963.

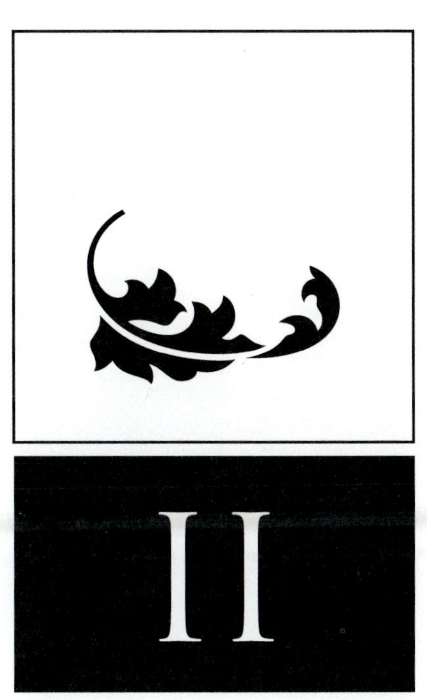

RESTORATIVE ART AND MORTUARY COSMETOLOGY

Restorative Art

SECTION I

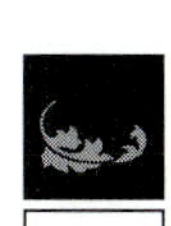

RESTORATIVE ART—PART 1

Restorative art is defined as, "care of the deceased to recreate natural form and color." Two divisions are seen in this definition: first, the re-establishment of natural contour or form to the visible surfaces. Examples would include reduction of swollen tissue, elevation of sunken tissue, closure of broken tissue, replacement of missing skin, and alignment, elevation or depression of fractured bones. Second is establishment of normal skin color. Examples would include bleaching and/or covering of a discoloration, replacement of natural skin color lost through the embalming process, and application of ornamental cosmetics for women. This phase of restorative art is often referred to as mortuary cosmetology. This portion of the text will concentrate on the restoration of surface contours and skin surfaces. A practical approach to restorative work is taken in this text. For detailed study of the bones, muscles, tissues and vascular systems of the head and hands and an in-depth study of physiognomy of the face refer to anatomical publications or texts devoted entirely to restorative art. Throughout this portion of the text and the section on mortuary cosmetology the term *embalmer* will be used rather than *restorative artist* or *cosmetologist*. In all states the embalmer is licensed to perform all three tasks: embalming, restorations, and cosmetic application.

Since the mid-1930s funeral service professionals and the public have come to expect the body to be prepared so that viewing is possible by family and friends. Damage from traumatic injuries, tissue and organ donations, the effects of disease, therapeutic drug and surgical treatments, or early postmortem changes should not be evident when proper restorative treatments have been performed. The practitioner has chemicals and techniques available today which allow the body to be viewed even when there will be an extended period of time between preparation and disposition of the body.

▶ CONSERVATIVE APPROACH

The funeral director and the embalmer should always take a conservative approach to restorative work and its end results. Statements of assured physical improvement should be limited and no guarantees should be made. No more restorative work should be performed than is necessary, unless the embalmer is certain improvement can be made in the appearance of the body. Discuss with the family changes which may have occurred through extended illness, traumatic injury, autopsy examination, organ donation, or postmortem interval between death and preparation of the body. If there has been a long illness the family will be aware of facial and body appearance; however, the family may not be aware of the condition of the body if death was traumatic or if changes occurred during the postmortem interval prior to embalming. Assure the persons making arrangements that everything possible will be done to improve the appearance of the body, but a final decision about public viewing by family and friends will rest with those making the arrangements. The funeral director making the arrangements should make every effort to see the body prior to meeting with the persons making the arrangements. If this is not possible (e.g., the body is at a medical examiner's office or at a central embalming facility) a verbal description of the body should be given to the funeral director. Unusual conditions should be discussed with the arranging party for instructions, e.g., obesity, extreme height, facial tumor, or crippling arthritic deformities. Distinguishing markings and characteristics should also be discussed with the arranging party to inquire if they should be altered or removed. Examples would include moles, facial scars, facial hair, visible birthmarks, goiter, or visible tattoos.

▶ PERMISSION

Permission for embalming and restorative work should be obtained by the funeral director from the party in charge of arrangements. These permissions, if first obtained by oral agreement, should be confirmed and signed in writing. Embalming and restorative treatments are interdependent and interrelated—many restorative treatments are actually performed during the embalming of the body. The closure of the mouth and eyes accomplishes a restorative function; embalming injection techniques can swell sunken tissues of the face or reduce swollen tissues and some fluid dyes can restore the skin to natural color.

▶ PHOTOGRAPHS

A recent photograph of the deceased should be obtained from the persons making funeral arrangements. Photographs provide information about facial characteristics and hairstyle of the deceased, and with men the photo can provide valuable information about facial hair such as moustache, beard or sideburns.

Desirable Characteristics of the Photos

1. The photo should be recent.
2. The individual should appear in normal good health in the photo.
3. Shadows should not appear on the face.
4. Snapshots are preferred over professional portraits which may have been retouched.
5. Hairstyle of the deceased should be visible.
6. Symmetry and asymmetry of the facial features can be observed.
7. Shape of the attached mucous membranes (lips) can be observed.
8. A photo in three-quarter profile shows the fullness of the cheeks and the jaw line.
9. Projection of the mouth and lips can be noted in a three-quarter profile photo.
10. A frontal view photo will depict length and width relationships and distances can easily be measured.
11. A profile view photo will show projections and recessions of the face.

Photographs should be studied and interpreted by holding the picture upside-down. In this manner the embalmer is not distracted by the features of the subject and a better comparison of features can be made when the photo is held in this position. A Polaroid photo is often taken as a part of the embalming report when a body is to be embalmed then shipped to another city for final preparation, dressing, and casketing. This photo will alert the receiving funeral home of any pre-embalming problems present in the face. Permission for confidential photos for the embalming report can be included in the embalming permission form.

▶ VIEWING

The presentation of the casketed body is as important as any embalming, restorative, or cosmetic treatment of the deceased. Local customs, church affiliation, and ethnic background are all factors contributing to the position of the deceased in the casket. When restorative work has been performed or there is concern about facial swelling or extreme weight loss some of the following suggestions may be of value in posing the deceased in the casket:

1. The body is generally viewed with the head tilted about 15 degrees to the right; the head is elevated on the pillow to decrease the angle between the chin and the chest. Local and ethnic customs may dictate that the head be kept perfectly straight so the deceased appears to be looking directly upward (see Figure 1).

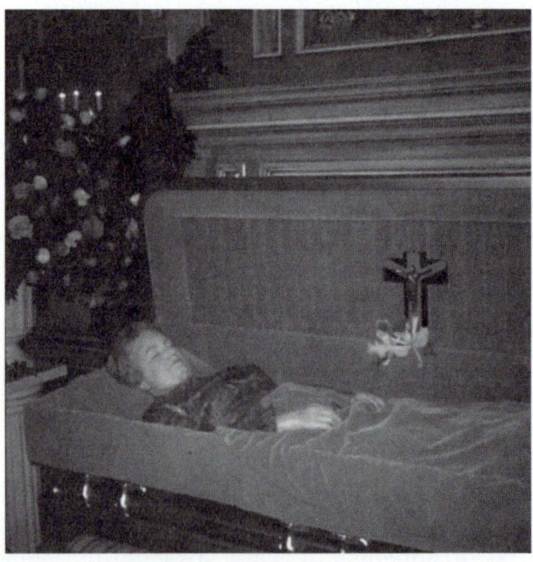

Figure 1. Local and ethnic custom can dictate body casket position.

2. For obese bodies keep the head in a straight position and elevate the left shoulder to tilt the deceased slightly to the right. By keeping the head straight and the chin high there will be less bulging of the neck, making it appear smaller.
3. If a full couch casket is used and there is a problem on the right side of the head or face, or if hair has been shaved from the right side of the head, reversing the body in the casket can hide these problems. Keeping the head in a straight position can also help to hide right side problems when the body is turned in the full couch casket (see Figure 2A–C).
4. When there are extensive facial problems the casket can be covered with a "casket veil." These veils help to give a smoother look to areas where wax has been used and they prevent persons from touching restored areas.
5. Profiles change the least; if a kneeler is to be used, place it at the head of the casket. The person kneeling sees the profile of the deceased rather than the bilateral view.
6. When facial problems exist, especially problems with the eyes, encourage the use of glasses (if worn by the deceased). Glasses actually reflect light and help to hide problems and they also help to distract from problem facial areas.
7. Stanchions with roping can be used to keep persons a short distance from the casketed body. These are often used when the body is viewed in a public place such as a church or public building.

Clothing

It is generally unnecessary to recommend any specific clothing color. For women it is generally recommended, if the family is using their own clothing, that

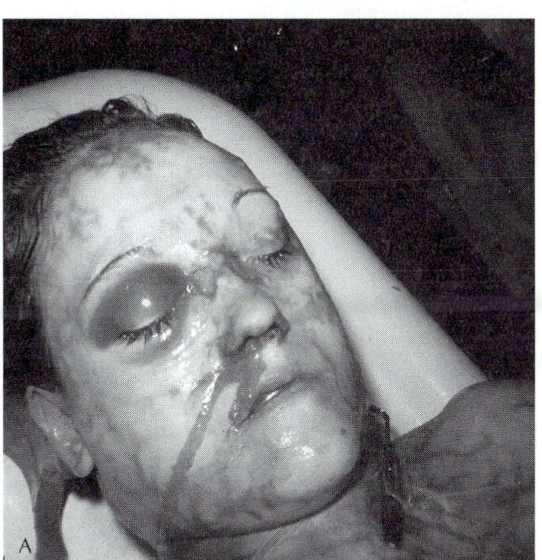

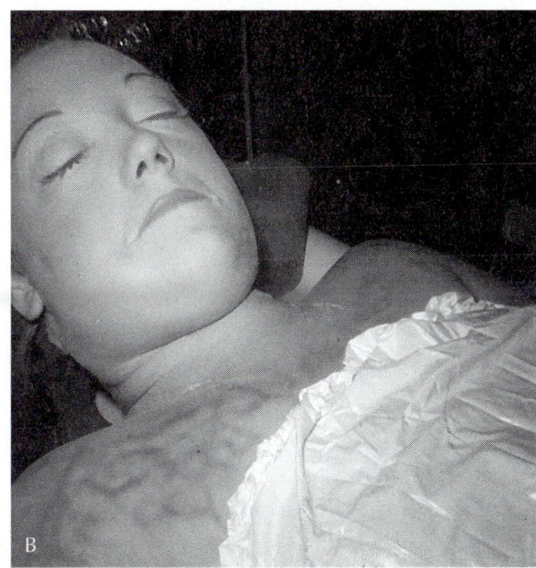

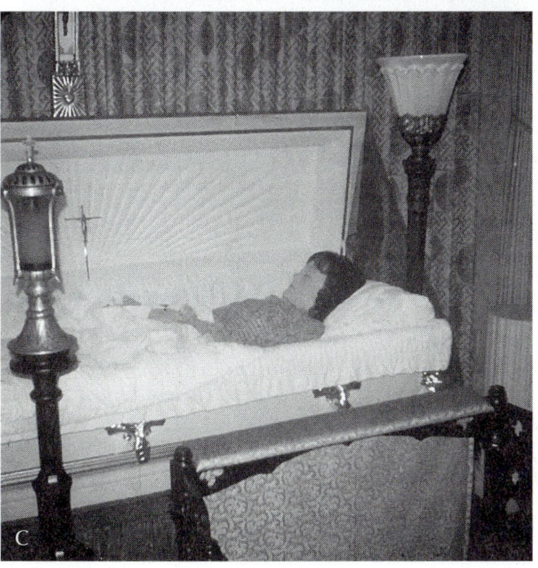

Figure 2. A. Early decomposition; note ecchymosis of right eye. **B.** Opaque undercoat cosmetic applied; normal cream cosmetics applied over the opaque undercoat. **C.** Body reversed in full couch casket; kneeler at head so profile is seen by the person kneeling.

the garment have sleeves of sufficient length to cover the arms. For men proper measurements should be taken so shirts, suits, and sportcoats fit properly. Care should be taken when dressing men that the collar of a shirt be properly seen when a tie and coat are also used. Likewise a small amount of the shirt cuff should be seen when the deceased is dressed in a suit or sportcoat.

When the deceased has jaundice, it is helpful if clothing of cold colors are avoided, such as blue, green, or violet. Yellow is also not recommended. In addition, black and white should be avoided for they provide too much contrast with the skin tone. All warm colors from peach through pink, even to maroon, are recommended. Gray is also excellent for this type of body. Casket interior color can also enhance the cosmetic appearance of the deceased. A white casket interior provides the most difficult background for a cosmetized body because it provides too much contrast. For bodies with a normal skin color, after they have been cosmetized, grays and other dark tones provide the best background for display of the body.

Lighting

Illumination of the casketed body not only provides light to view the deceased; it also contributes to the cosmetic color effect on the deceased. It is ideal to apply the cosmetics to the deceased using the same lighting that will be used to display the casketed remains. When colored lights (pink or red lights) are used to illuminate the cosmetized body they have the effect of decreasing the red tones that are present in the skin cosmetic, because there is a general increase in the overall reddish or pink appearance. Red lights have a tendency to fade reds in the facial cosmetic. When red or pink bulbs are used it becomes necessary to increase the amount of red used in the warm (red) areas of the face, such as the cheeks, lips, and ears. If these bodies were to be viewed under normal lighting, they would appear overcosmetized and theatrical, but when viewed under red lighting they will appear quite normal. Colored lights do have value, particularly when you want to create the illusion of the presence of reddish tones in the face. This is of particular value with jaundiced bodies.

Use of a standard incandescent bulb with shaded lamps, which have eggshell or ivory glass globes or shades will compliment the cosmetized body. The combination of the incandescent bulb with the eggshell shade adds yellow to the face. A great deal of yellow is found in the natural skin complexion, especially in the elderly. Many funeral homes also use point lighting over the casket to add color to the cosmetized body. The color magenta (magenta adds a small amount of blue to the cosmetic, and this helps to emphasize facial reds) works well for point lighting. The body and casket should be lighted evenly. Lighting which is too strong and uneven will have a tendency to create unnatural shadows on the face.

▶ CLASSIFICATION OF CONDITIONS AND TREATMENTS

Some degree of restorative treatment is necessary in the preparation of each body which is to be viewed by the public. Proper support, closure and sealing of the eyelids and mouth could be considered a restorative treatment. Application of some cosmetic treatment, if only to reinstate the warm areas of the cheeks and lips, is a form of restoration. More than one restorative treatment may be performed in the preparation of a body for viewing. For example, a typical preparation of an elderly female may involve some of the following restorative treatments:

1. If there has been a loss of weight, cotton or a mortuary mastic will be needed to fill out sunken areas of the mouth, even if teeth or dentures are present. If there are no dentures the entire reshaping of the mouth contour will be necessary. Cotton and/or eyecaps will be necessary to help shape, support, close, and raise sunken eyes.
2. Eyelids and lips need to be sealed.
3. Dyes may be added to the arterial solution to help restore a natural coloring to the skin.
4. Restorative fluids can be added to the arterial solution to assist in swelling sunken areas of the face and hands.
5. After arterial injection tissue building can be done to hands and face to restore emaciated or dehydrated areas.
6. Ecchymosis or purpural hemorrhage may be present on the back of a hand as a result of use of medication, and these areas need to be bleached and covered with an opaque cosmetic.
7. A small fever blister on the lips may need to be removed, and the area dried and waxed.
8. Facial hair needs to be removed prior to embalming.
9. Cosmetics need to be applied to face and hands to restore their natural coloring.
10. The hair needs to be washed and properly styled.

Here we see with just a "normal" preparation a variety of minor restorations are needed. Facial trauma, and tissue changes from disease or decomposition can result in the need for major restorative work (see Fig. 3A–B).

Classification of tissue conditions and restorative treatments may seem like an academic exercise for the

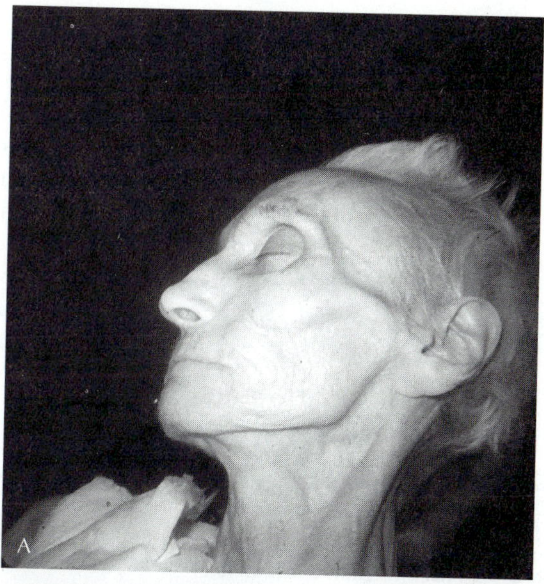

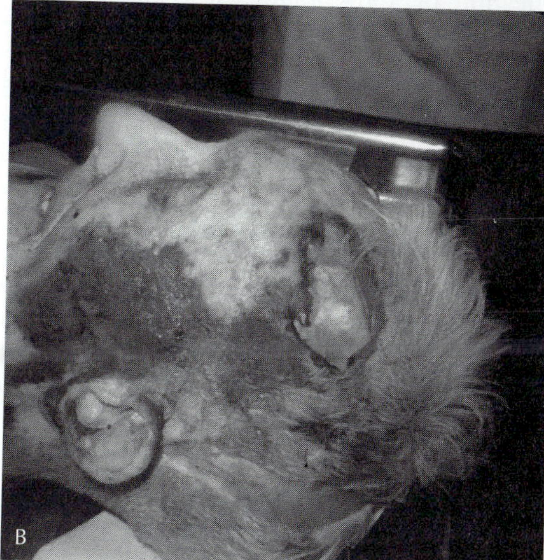

Figure 3. A. Emaciation of the face, an antemortem condition. **B.** Facial trauma; note facial abrasions and lacerations. The body has also been autopsied.

classroom. By recognizing the various problems present and treatments available, guidelines for treatment can be established. Restorative work uses very few treatments to correct a large number of adverse tissue conditions. Embalmers making a preembalming restorative analysis of the body need to first recognize the problems needing correction, and second to formulate a strategy or guideline for the correction of the problems.

Conditions Requiring Restorative Treatment

1. Pathological (disease)—tumor; ecchymosis discoloration; edema
2. Trauma (injury)—abrasions; torn tissue; fractures
3. Post-mortem changes—skin slip; gasses in the tissues; discolorations
4. Embalming—swollen tissue; dehydrated (wrinkled) areas (e.g., lips)

Changes can occur in the antemortem and postmortem time periods which will necessitate restorative treatments. In the antemortem time period two groups can be listed.

Antemortem Time Period

1. Pathological conditions: Disease processes which result in visible manifestations. These include a loss of weight in the facial tissues; loss of hair; increased growth of hair in areas such as the forehead or on the faces of women; discolorations; tumors; skin eruptions; and swelling of the face or hands. Drug and surgical treatments can result in visible body changes necessitating restorative treatments, e.g., visible scars, incisions, discolorations, swelling, loss of hair, etc. The effects of some drugs or surgical procedures create greater restorative problems than the disease processes themselves.
2. Injury: Trauma restoration is the procedure most associated by the public with the embalming process. Degree of trauma is widely variable, so it is absolutely necessary for the funeral director to see the extent of the injury before assuring the family that the deceased can be viewed. The difficulty here is that often when a death is the result of trauma, the body will first be autopsied or examined by the medical examiner or coroner, so it can be hours or even days until the extent of the damage from trauma or autopsy can be seen by the embalmer. Trauma does not always result in immediate death. It may be days, weeks, or even years until the death finally occurs. Medical treatments, as in the disease category above, may create more need for restorative work than the traumatic injury itself. An example would be a traumatic injury to the head, which might simply result in a small bruise and possibly a discoloration of the eyes. However the treatment may involve shaving and invasive surgery of the head, along with drug therapy, which may have a variety of visible side effects.

Postmortem Time Period

1. Preembalming changes:
   a. Discoloration resulting from the movement of blood to dependent parts of the body (e.g., if the body dies with the head in a dependent po-

sition the resulting discoloration may require treatment with opaque cosmetics to conceal the discoloration).

b. Compression from surface contact. If the face were dependent or in such a position that the face or hands were pressed against a solid object such as a floor or wall, their soft tissues could be flattened, thus the contour of the skin surface would need to be corrected.

c. Gasses. If CPR was attempted, the rupture of the plural sac could result in air entering the subcutaneous tissues. These gasses will frequently move into elevated areas such as the neck and face.

d. Decomposition changes. These changes are the most obvious postmortem tissue changes requiring restorative treatment. Discolorations, gasses in the tissues, and separation of the epidermis from the dermis can all create major problems.

e. Dehydration of the face and hands. This postmortem loss of body moisture can result in fingers and features such as the lips, eyelids, and ears discoloring to deep browns or black and shrinking in size to a point where they cannot be rehydrated.

f. Organ and tissue donation: Donation of the whole eye, inner ear, pituitary gland and mandible would all require restorative treatments to the head and/or facial tissues.

2. Embalming Changes:

a. Swelling: As a result of injecting embalming solution under pressure there is the possibility of distension of unsupported tissues and glands of a particular face or neck area (e.g., eye, neck, submaxillary and parotid glands, cheeks). Bodies where decomposition has begun or where the tissues have been frozen distend easily during arterial injection.

b. Discolorations: Livor mortis, if present in the face, can often be converted to a stain if too strong an arterial solution is employed. Yellow jaundice can be converted to a green discoloration by the use of strong formaldehyde solutions. Harsh formaldehyde solutions and inadequate aspiration of the heart can create a graying of the face. The shoulder and head area of the embalmed body should always be elevated to help prevent "formaldehyde gray"—a graying of the tissues resulting from a mixing of blood not removed during the embalming process with formaldehyde. The use of fluid dye can help to prevent graying of the tissues.

c. Dehydration: Excessive dehydration of the facial tissues can result if these areas are overembalmed using solutions which are too strong or if an excess of solution is run through these areas. Improper storage of the body following embalming can also cause dehydration necessitating restorative treatments.

d. Overembalmed tissues: Too strong an arterial solution or too much arterial solution injected into the face can result in a number of conditions which may make restorative treatment quite difficult to perform, including separation of lips and eyelids, inability to tissue build the face or features, and wrinkling of the face and features.

▶ CLASSIFICATION OF RESTORATIVE TREATMENTS

Wax and Non-wax Treatment

Classification of a restoration as a wax or non-wax restoration simply means that wax will or will not be employed in the restoration. Wax plays a major role in replacing missing skin, and in creating a skin-like surface over those areas of the face where the skin is broken. It can also be used to recreate skin contours in large depressed areas in the natural skin surface. Typical wax restorations include: abrasions; second and third degree burns; repair where fever blisters have been removed; a treatment for skin slip; replacing torn skin; use of wax as a filler for deep wound restoration; covering an area where inter-dermal suturing was performed or where edges of torn tissues were glued; and repair to close separated lips and eyelids.

Today there are some excellent surface glues and opaque paints which can be used as wax substitutes for some restorations (e.g., replacement of missing or abraded skin). Mortuary mastics (mortuary putty) can be used as a deep filler as well as a surface filler for deep wound restorations.

Moist or Dry Tissue Condition

Tissue conditions can be classified as either dry or moist. Examples of dry conditions might be treatments for swollen or emaciated tissues, simple fractures, hair which needs to be replaced, discolorations, and separated lips or eyelids. These non-broken skin conditions would almost always be considered dry tissue conditions. When the skin is dry, cosmetics, waxes and glues can be more easily applied to the surface.

Examples of moist conditions might include skin slip, lacerated tissues, compound fractures, second and third degree burns, blisters, scabs, pustules, and abrasions. Broken skin conditions may be moist or dry, depending on the amount of dehydration which has occurred. Frequently embalming solution will be seen exiting from moist skin areas (e.g., abrasions, lacerations) during arterial injection. This indicates the area is receiving good preservation treatment. Massage cream should be placed on the surrounding "good tissues," **not** over the moist tissues. This will protect the "good" tissues and allow faster drying of the problem area. Moist tissue must be dried. Following arterial injection, treatments with an electric spatula or hairdryer, or chemical compresses of phenol solutions or concentrated formaldehyde, can be used to dry moist tissue. When chemical compresses have been used, after their removal, the tissues need to be cleaned with a solvent and then air-dried with a hair dryer. Dehydrated tissues cannot be bleached. Once the skin is dry, opaque cosmetics, waxes and surface glues can adhere to the affected surface. Condensation can occur on the surface of bodies which have been refrigerated. This can make cosmetic application difficult, especially cream cosmetics.

Time Periods for Restorative Treatments

Restorative treatments can be divided into three time periods: 1) before the arterial injection of the body (preembalming), 2) during the arterial injection, and 3) a postembalming period, during which most restorative and cosmetic treatments are done, including the final grooming and dressing of the body. This time period can begin with a period of rest during which tissues dry and firm.

Knowing in which time period a particular procedure should be performed results in more orderly and satisfactory work. Body conditions and personal preference guidelines of the embalmer can and will vary. The treatment periods outlined below serve only as guidelines.

Guidelines for Restorative Treatments Made in the Preembalming Period. *Objectives:* It is in this time period that a restoration analysis, along with the embalming analysis, is made. Conditions of the body are evaluated and a plan is designed for restorative treatments. General treatments performed in this time period will include: alignment of bone structure; alignment of torn tissues and deep cuts; posing and alignment of the mouth and eyelids; removal of loose or torn epidermis; drainage of skin eruptions; removal of surface discolorations; and cleaning of all skin areas of the face and hands.

Treatments performed during this time period:

1. Surface sanitizing of the body and external orifices
2. Removal of tubes or devices which in any way mark the face; removal of any facial bandages
3. Washing of the skin surface and hair with warm water and soap (borax can be used to assist in cleansing); cleaning of the fingernails and removal of any old nail polish
4. Removal of surface stains caused by adhesive tape, gentian violet, etc.; solvents such as dry hair washes or tricholoroethylene remove most stains; blood can be removed by using cool water with laundry bleach added
5. Shaving of facial hair
6. Positioning of face and hands; alignment of features
   a. Place cotton in the nostrils to expand them if they have become depressed.
   b. Cotton is placed behind the ear to expose the lobe, important when earrings are to be worn by the deceased.
   c. Hands can be laid at the sides or hang off the table until fluid distribution is established. Later a towel can be placed on the abdomen to position the hands and cup the fingers.
7. Mouth and lip closure
   a. Lips may be held together with thick petroleum jelly or mortuary compound. Later this can be removed and the mucous membranes sealed with lip adhesive or super glue.
   b. Prognathism of the upper teeth may require gluing of the lips to hold the membranes together during embalming. Cotton can be placed over the lower teeth or dentures when the upper teeth protrude. This will bring the lower lip into alignment with the protruding upper lip. (Rubber-based glue is recommended for temporary gluing; super glue is recommended for permanent sealing.)
   c. Sunken facial areas may be raised by inserting cotton or mortuary mastic in the buccal cavity.
   d. Scabs, oozing scabs and fever blisters should be removed from the lips or face and a cotton compress of phenol or formaldehyde can be placed over the raw tissue to sanitize, preserve, and eventually dry the exposed tissues.
   e. Correct misalignment of the mandible. If the lower jaw has separated from the mandibular fossa of the temporal bone, the mandible should be massaged back into position at this time. Lip closure cannot be made if the mandible is not in proper alignment.
8. Closure of the eyelids
   a. Sunken eyes can be elevated by closure with cotton, or a combination of cotton and an eyecap.
   b. When a glass eye is present the lids may need to be glued or the artificial eye removed and a closure made with cotton or eyecaps.
   c. Eyelashes should be cleaned and properly aligned. A brush moistened with water or a solvent such as dry hair wash can be used to clean the lashes.

d. Enucleated eyes–
   i. Remove any packing from the orbit.
   ii. Gently clean the orbit with cotton.
   iii. Very loosely place a cotton pack saturated with autopsy gel in the orbit using enough cotton to establish the contour of the closed eyelid.
   iv. Gently abut the lids to give a natural closure to the eye.

9. Glass shards should be removed with the embalmer wearing heavy gloves. Some shards can be flushed loose with water, and others will need to be removed with spring forceps.
10. Align lacerated and cut tissue edges.
    a. Small bridge sutures of dental floss can be used.
    b. A drop or two of super glue along the laceration can be used to align surface skin edges.
    c. Deep lacerations can be pulled into alignment with deep sutures using dental floss.
11. Remove torn epidermal tissue and visible desquamation.
12. Open and drain blisters, pustules, boils, or similar skin eruptions.
13. Remove loose skin from opened blisters and skin eruptions. Remove loose scabs.
14. If a tumor of the face is pushing a feature out of alignment it may be necessary to excise the tumor at this time. Some embalmers prefer to do all excisions in this time period.
15. Apply surface compresses over blood discolorations to begin bleaching the affected areas.
16. Apply surface compresses of phenol or concentrated formaldehyde to raw surface areas (e.g., moist abrasions, desquamation, burned areas, opened pustules and blisters, areas where tissue has been excised).
17. Align simple and compound fractures and if possible, raise depressed fractures.
18. Apply massage cream to face and hands over intact tissues. Cream should not be applied to surfaces where wax, opaque cosmetics or surface glue is to be used.
19. Apply compresses to swollen areas caused by trauma. Use compresses of phenol or concentrated formaldehyde to bleach bruised tissues. Place weighted compresses over the affected areas to help reduce swelling during arterial injection.

Guidelines for Restorative Treatments Made During Arterial Injection. During this time period very few restorative and cosmetic treatments are performed. However, this phase of embalming is significant because this is when the embalming solution is introduced. For most restorative and cosmetic treatments the surface tissues must be dry and firm. Well preserved tissues are the key to successful restorative treatments.

Objectives: To establish good preservation so the tissues will be firm and dry. In addition, adequate preservation will help to insure the facial features will be maintained in their posed positions. The contour of the facial areas can be altered by the injection of the arterial solution. Normal facial contours can be maintained by use of the proper arterial solution and its correct introduction into the facial tissues; some previously swollen facial areas can actually be reduced. Likewise, emaciated and sunken facial areas can be restored to a normal contour by arterial solutions containing chemicals designed to restore tissue contour by slightly swelling these sunken areas. Dyes in the arterial solution will add color to the skin surface and serve as an internal coloring.

Treatments performed during this time period:

1. Establish good even preservation to the tissues of the face and hands.
2. Surface compresses of concentrated formaldehyde (cavity fluid) or phenol compounds can be placed over areas where skin has been removed to help dry and firm these tissues.
3. Massage areas of the face and hands which have been compressed to help to expand these tissues (e.g., if face was dependent or pushed against an object, or if hands were placed over one another).
4. Control swelling of facial tissues.
5. Reduce swollen facial tissues caused by edema by the use of mechanical embalming techniques and arterial chemicals.
6. Distend slightly emaciated facial areas by the use of additives to the arterial solution designed for this purpose.
7. Arterial solutions firm and set the facial tissues and features. Successful embalming will produce a dry skin surface.
8. Cosmetic dyes in the arterial solutions give a lifelike effect to the skin surface.
9. Clearing of intravascular blood discolorations (e.g., livor mortis).
10. Strong arterial solutions and supplemental fluids will bleach and lighten blood discolorations (e.g., hematoma, postmortem stain, ecchymosis, purpura).
11. Facial tissues can be moisturized by supplemental fluids added to the arterial solution.
12. External application of massage cream moisturizes dry skin, prevents tissue dehydration, and cleanses the skin. Application by massage assists in relieving rigor mortis in the facial tissues, which will help promote distribution of the arterial solution.

Guidelines for Restorative Treatments Made After Arterial Injection (Postembalming). This time period occurs after arterial injection and cavity embalming have been completed. This phase usually begins with a period of rest, during which the tissues firm, the chemicals are given time to work, and it gives moist tissues an opportunity to dry. This is the time when the majority of restorative treatments are performed.

PERIOD OF REST. This time period can be very brief after arterial and cavity embalming, simply long enough to suture all embalming incisions, evaluate what areas need additional hypodermic and surface preservative treatments, and perform final washing and drying of the body. In the preparation of bodies with facial trauma this may be a longer period of time, during which surface compresses will be placed over areas to bleach and reduce swollen tissues. With an extremely emaciated body, some embalmers attempt to distend the facial tissues using the arterial solution and a restorative chemical, then, allowing a long period of rest between arterial injection and cavity aspiration the features of the face are able to thoroughly "set." Many funeral establishments will allow several hours of time between the completion of the embalming and the start of restorative and cosmetic treatments.

Objectives: The following are reasons for a period of rest:

1. To allow drying of areas where superficial tissues are missing (e.g., from desquamation, abrasions)
2. To allow tissues of the face and hands time to dry before the application of cosmetics
3. To allow time for the tissues of the face and hands to firm
4. To allow time for surface bleaching compresses to bleach discolorations (e.g., from ecchymosis, bruises, purpura)
5. To allow time for hypodermically injected bleaches to lighten discolorations
6. To allow time for surface preservative compresses to penetrate and preserve underlying tissues
7. To allow time for hypodermically injected solutions to preserve injected tissues
8. To allow time for surface compresses placed over swollen tissues to reduce the distended area
9. To allow maximum drainage to occur and gasses to escape
10. To observe if any additional treatments are necessary

Following a brief or extended period of rest the majority of restorative and cosmetic treatments are performed. A careful examination of the body is necessary to check for evidence of gas formation, lack of preservation, and any previously unnoticed leakage.

Objectives:

1. Hypodermic injection of preservatives, bleaches, reducing agents, etc.
2. Hypodermic tissue building of face and hands
3. Suturing of disconnected tissues
4. Gluing of disconnected tissues
5. Gluing (sealing) of eyelids and lips
6. Application of surface glues over sutured areas and to replace skin
7. Application of surface waxes
8. Rebuilding of missing features or facial areas
9. General cosmetic treatments
10. Cosmetic treatments for discoloration
11. Facial expression changes made by tissue building and cosmetic shaping
12. Nail treatments
13. Hair grooming and restoration
14. Swelling reduction by use of heat, channeling, aspirating, gravitation, aspiration, and excision
15. Excision of tumors and reconstruction of the affected area
16. Eye enucleation restoration
    a. Drying of the orbit
    b. Deep filling of the orbit with a moisture absorbent material such as mortuary mastic or incision seal powder
    c. Replacement of the missing eye with a material such as cotton, mortuary mastic, or wax
    d. Placement of an eyecap over the filler material
    e. Closure and sealing of the eyelids

It can be seen from these examples the majority of restorative treatments are performed during this postembalming period. It will be necessary to allow additional rest periods when certain treatments are performed to allow tissues to dry and chemicals to properly act on the tissues. It is necessary that the funeral director, when making arrangements, allow sufficient time for cosmetic and restorative treatments to be properly performed.

▶ SUMMARY

In 1965 G. Joseph Prager published in his *Manual of Restorative Art* the following summary which incorporates a general sequence of procedures for most restorative treatments:

1. Obtain permission for incisions or excisions necessary for restoration.
2. Cleanse the body thoroughly and remove all stains and foreign matter.

3. Straighten and replace fractures or missing bones.
4. Temporarily suture all disconnected tissues in visible areas.
5. Embalm the body.
6. Make incisions and excisions required for restoration; suture disconnected tissues.
7. Reduce swelling, bleach discolorations, and fill sunken areas as required.
8. Apply sealing compound to exposed subcutaneous tissues and fill cavities with a suitable foundation for wax surfacing.
9. When tissues are firm and dry perform the wax restoration.
10. Replace eyelashes.
11. Apply corrective cosmetics.
12. Replace eyebrows and cranial hair.
13. Reproduce skin pores in waxed areas.

▶ ESTABLISHMENT OF GOOD PRESERVATION

When facial conditions such as the following exist in the unautopsied body, the common carotid arteries should be used for arterial injection: trauma to the head (cranium) or the face; evidence of early or advanced decomposition; extensive pathological lesions; bruising, abraded, lacerated or burnt tissue; ecchymosis, hematoma, or lacerations of the eyelids; eye enucleation; facial or cranial tumor which must be excised; cranial or facial swelling from edema. This method of injection is called restricted cervical injection; it allows the best control over the amount and the strength of arterial solution entering the head and facial tissues.

Restricted cervical injection is performed by raising the right and the left common carotid arteries (some embalmers also prefer to raise both right and left internal jugular veins as sites for drainage from the head). In the right common carotid a large tube is inserted toward the head and another tube is inserted toward the body trunk. Into the left common carotid artery a large tube is inserted toward the head and the inferior portion of the artery is tied off with a ligature. It is a matter of personal preference if the head or the trunk is injected first—most embalmers prefer to inject the trunk first. If the trunk of the body is injected first; be certain to leave both arterial tubes directed toward the head open. This prevents the arterial solution from being retained in the facial tissues. The trunk can be injected with an arterial solution suitable for its existing conditions, and the head injected with a solution suitable for conditions present there (see Figure 4).

Arterial solution for injection into the head and face for these restorative cases requires the use of a strong preservative solution. This is done to insure firm

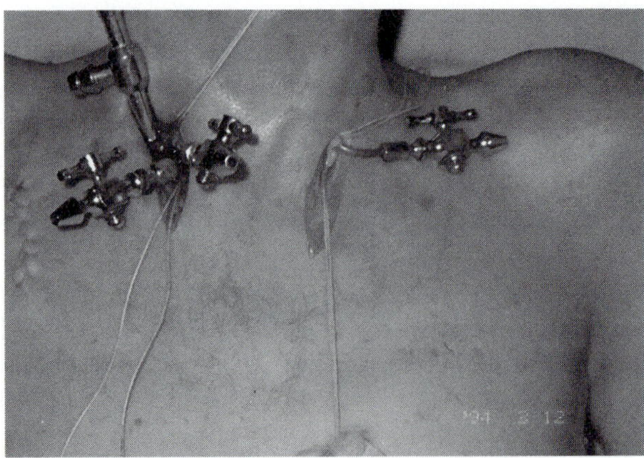

Figure 4. Restricted cervical injection.

and dry facial tissues. Swelling can be controlled with stronger arterial solutions because less volume of the solution is used to preserve the tissues. Concentrated arterial solutions also help to bleach blood discolorations, reduce facial swelling (edema), and dry moist tissues such as burns, desquamation or abraded tissues. Dye may be added to the solution to assist in prevention of graying of the tissues and as a fluid tracer.

Instant tissue fixation is an embalming technique in which a minimal amount of concentrated arterial solution is injected by a series of pulses under high pressure. The object of this technique is to achieve maximum preservation using as little embalming solution as possible, to keep any swelling to a minimum. The left side of the face is injected first, then the right side.

Below are formulas for arterial solutions used to embalm the head and face when conditions such as extensive facial trauma or early decomposition exist.

1. 16 ounces of a high index arterial fluid (25 index or higher)
   16 ounces of co-injection chemical
   $\frac{1}{2}$ ounce dye
2. 16 ounces of a medium index arterial fluid (16 to 22 index)
   16 ounces of a high index arterial fluid (30 to 35 index)
   16 ounces of co-injection chemical
   $\frac{1}{2}$ ounce fluid dye
3. Chemical companies make a special purpose high-index arterial fluid for difficult cases. Directions for use by the manufacturer should be followed.

Some embalmers prefer not to use the solutions described above. They prefer to use a standard arterial solution and add several ounces of a high index arterial fluid. The primary goals of the embalmer are to establish well-preserved, firm, dry tissues, and to control facial swelling. Arterial treatment may need to be supple-

TABLE 1. CHEMICALS USED IN RESTORATIVE TREATMENTS

Chemical	Use	Application
Tissue builder	Raises sunken, emaciated tissues, rounds out wrinked lips and fingers	Hypodermic injection
Tissue builder solvent	Cleans hypodermic syringe after any chemical is injected	Not injected into body tissues; use to flush out syringe
Trichloroethylene, dry hair washes (solvents)	Cleansing of skin; assists in removal of scaling skin; loosens scabs; dries skin surface; prepares skin for waxes, glues and opaque cosmetics; removes surface stains, adhesive tape; can be mixed with a cream cosmetic to make an opaque undercoat; smoothes wax; cleans cosmetics from hair, eyebrows and eyelashes	Applied on the skin surface with cotton, gauze or soft cotton, or brush
Cautery, bleaching, reducing agents (may contain phenol)	Bleaches tissue, bleaches blood discolorations, cauterizes broken tissue, preserves localized tissues; dries and firms tissues, reduces swollen tissues	Surface compress over affected area; chemical can also be injected by hypodermic syringe; may be painted or swabbed over the area
Formaldehyde (undiluted cavity fluid)	Used as a substitute for a phenol cautery preservative	Surface compress or hypodermic injection
Preservative gel	Preserves, bleaches, firms tissues	Surface compress or painted over area to be treated
Acetone	Fingernail polish remover; removes surface stains; loosens scabs, smoothes wax; cleans hair	Applied by cotton pad; gauze or cloth
Sodium hypochlorite	Used with water to clean blood from skin surface, hair, etc.	Gauze pad or soft cloth

mented by local hypodermic and surface embalming. A bleaching-cautery chemical, or concentrated cavity fluid can be used to make surface compresses. The phenol-cautery solutions work much faster than the formaldehyde compresses, but the formaldehyde compresses penetrate deeper into the tissues. These surface compresses can be applied in all three restorative time periods. They should be covered with thin plastic to contain fumes and prevent the chemicals from dehydrating. Preservative or autopsy gels can be painted over affected areas to preserve and dry tissues. The gels should also be covered with plastic. When gels or chemical compresses are removed, the area needs to be cleaned using a solvent such as trichloroethylene. These chemical compresses or gels will bleach blood discolorations, and preserve, dry and firm tissues. Concentrated phenol or formaldehyde can also act as a cautery to sear torn or excised tissues.

Hypodermic preservative treatment is usually done after the arterial injection. Injection into tissues should be done from hidden points of entry such as within the nostrils, mouth or hairline, between the fingers or on the palm side of the fingers, because chemicals such as formaldehyde or phenol compounds can leak. Commercial bleaching and cautery restorative chemicals for hypodermic injection usually contain phenol. As a substitute undiluted cavity chemical may be used as a bleaching, preservative, and reducing agent. Hypodermic injection of an arterial chemical should be avoided if it contains a tissue dye; in time this dye can stain tissues and create a discoloration.

Broken skin areas need to be dried before wax or cosmetic treatments can be done. Examples include skin slip, torn skin, moist abrasions, and second degree burns. Chemical cautery agents will assist in drying these tissues. In addition these problem areas can be dried by the use of heat or by passing dry air over the affected areas by using an electric spatula or hair dryer. If time permits, allowing air to pass over the raw tissues will dry these skin areas. Intact tissues can be protected with a coating of massage cream, this prevents stains from chemicals and dehydration.

Tables 1 and 2 list the chemicals, materials, and instruments used in restorative procedures.

TABLE 2. RESTORATION MATERIALS AND INSTRUMENTS AND THEIR USES

Material, Instrument	Discussion or Technique
Airbrush	A pressured atomizer used for the application of a liquid transparent or opaque cosmetic onto the skin surface.
Armature	A framework, commonly of metal or wood, used to provide support for a wax restoration. Examples would include pipe cleaners, lengths of wire, various small pieces of screen, or dowel rods of wood or metal. If a feature such as an ear were to be built on the body, the armature would be secured to the scalp or bony structures, and the modeled ear would then be built upon this framework.
Basket weave suture	A network of stitches which crosses the borders of a cavity or excision to anchor fillers and to sustain tissues in their proper position. A framework for attachment of wax or mortuary mastic where tissues or a feature is being rebuilt; also serves to hold the margins of the cavity or excision in a uniform position. The sutures are usually made into the subcutaneous areas of the skin.
Bridge suture	A temporary suture consisting of individually cut and tied stitches employed to sustain the proper position of tissues. Dental floss can be used for these temporary sutures. They are usually put into place during the preembalming time period.
Cotton	A highly absorbent natural white fibrous substance, it has numerous uses in restorative work; also available in a non-absorbent form.
Cotton (webbed)	A non-woven, lint-free absorbent fabric made from cotton. Can be used as a replacement for absorbent cotton.
Cyanoacrylate sealer (Super glue)	A strong and fast-acting bonding adhesive (viscosity can vary), used to seal lips and eyelids, lacerations and incisions, and bony fractures; primarily composed of alpha cyanoacrylate
Deep filler	A material used to fill cavities or excisions and to serve as a foundation for the superficial wax restoration. Examples include "wound filler," wax, mortuary mastic, plaster of Paris, cotton and sealer, cotton and plaster.
Electric spatula	An electrically heated blade used to dry moist tissues, reduce swollen tissues, and restore contour to natural form. Massage cream should be liberally applied to a skin surface before using the spatula (This is not necessary when it is used to dry and/or cauterize deep tissues).
Gauze	A light, open mesh variety of muslin or similar material; used over a mortuary mastic to prevent the mastic from separating from the edges of a cavity; used with a sealer to replace missing skin; by gently pressing onto a waxed area it imparts a pore-like effect to the wax.
Hypodermic syinge	Used for the subcutaneous injection of liquid tissue builder, bleaches, and preservatives. A needle gauge of 17 works well for all of the liquids listed, but some embalmers prefer a higher gauge needle for lip treatments. Syringes and needles should be cleaned with tissue builder solvent after each use.
Intradermal suture	A suture used to close incisions such that the ligature remains entirely under the epidermis. It may be a double or single suture.
Inversion suture (worm or draw suture)	Parallel stitches are made in the surface edges of an incision and the skin from the stitch to the opening of the incision is inverted as the sutures are drawn tight. The suture is easily concealed with wax or surface glue; used to tighten loose skin.
Ligature	Thread, cord, or wire used for tying vessels, tissues or bones. Cotton is the softest and weakest, linen is very strong, and for restorative work dental floss is often used.
Lip-eye cement	Fast setting liquid adhesive designed to bond the eyelids and lips.
Massage cream	A soft, white, oily preparation used as a protective coating for external tissues; a base for cream cosmetics and a wax softener; an emollient. It can also be used as a skin cleanser; to soften and loosen scabs; loosens and helps in the removal of loose scaling skin. Substitutes would include lanolin or baby oil. Massage cream should not be applied over an area where an opaque undercoat is going to be applied.
Mastic compound	A soft, putty-like substance; an absorbent sealing adhesive that can be injected under the skin or applied to surface tissues to establish skin contour. A substitute for incision powder. May be used as a deep cavity filler.

TABLE 2. RESTORATION MATERIALS AND INSTRUMENTS AND THEIR USES (*Continued*)

Material, Instrument	Discussion or Technique
Needle injector	An instrument used to impel specially designed metal pins (with wires attached) into bone. Normal use would be as a method of mouth closure. It can also be used in trauma situations as a means of joining fractured bones.
Petroleum jelly	A semi-solid, yellow mixture of hydrocarbons obtained from petroleum. It can be applied to the mucous membranes of the lips prior to embalming to hold the lips in a closed position. This technique also helps to remove horizontal wrinkles from the lips. Similar products to help affix free margins such as the eyelids and lips in a closed position are available through embalming suppliers.
Plaster of Paris	Calcium sulfate; a white powdery substance which forms a quick-setting paste when mixed with water. Drying time can be speeded by using warm water or slowed by mixing with cold water. Uses include repair of fractured bones, use with cotton as a deep filler, and as a means of attachment for the calvarium to the base of the skull in autopsied bodies.
Pneumatic collar	A plastic collar which surrounds the neck and is inflated with a rubber bulb pump; the collar places external pressure on the neck tissues and helps to reduce swelling.
Powder	Any solid substance in the state of fine, loose particles as produced by crushing or grinding. Talc or cornstarch is a common ingredient. Powder may be applied with an atomizer, puff, or brush. a. White drying—used for drying cream cosmetics; may be mixed with soft waxes to give more firmness to the wax; used for drying cream cosmetics placed over or within wax. b. Tinted powders—contain a coloring agent; these will alter the color of complexion cosmetic when applied over the cosmetic. Do not apply this powder over a waxed area; apply a white drying powder first followed by a tinted powder. If used as a transparent cosmetic a very light coating of massage cream should first be applied to the skin, then the powder applied.
Rubber cement	A viscous adhesive consisting of vulcanized rubber dispersed in an organic solvent; used for the attachment of hair patches to the scalp or face.
Sealer (collodion, liquid sealer, surface sealer)	A quick-drying liquid; available in a variety of viscosities; creates a firm, thin transparent coating through which moisture cannot pass. Used over sutured areas to prevent leakage; may be used as a replacement for epidermal skin. Surfaces must be dry for a sealer to adhere.
Spatula	A flat, blunt, knife-like instrument used for mixing cosmetics and modeling, a palette knife. The blade must be clean each time it touches the wax being modeled. The blade can be warmed by holding it between the thumb and index finger. The blade can be dipped in a solvent to make wax adjustments over delicate areas.
Undercoat	An opaque coloring applied to an area which, when dry, will be covered with wax or another cosmetic colorant. May be liquid or aerosol. Surface to which it is applied should first be cleaned with a solvent to remove any oils or grease. Surface to which it is applied should also be free of any moisture.
Wax	A restorative or surfacing material composed of beeswax, spermaceti, paraffin, starch, etc. and a coloring pigment which will soften at body temperature and will reflect light in a manner similar to normal skin. Most waxes need to be warmed prior to application. This can be done by mixing the wax with a spatula in the palm of the embalmer's hand. Cream cosmetic or colored powders can be added to neutral colored waxes to alter their color. Examples include: a. Lip wax—a soft restorative wax, usually tinted, used to surface the mucous membranes or to correct lip separations. b. Surface restorer (soft wax)—a surface filler wax used to fill shallow depressions; softer and more pliable than wound filler. c. Medium wax—a derma surgery or restorative wax. d. Firm wax (wound filler)—the most viscous type of wax; a putty-like material used to fill large cavities or model features.
Worm suture	See Inversion suture.

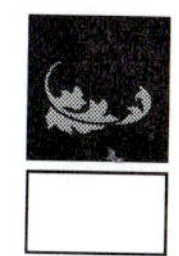

RESTORATIVE ART—PART 2

▶ DEEP CAVITY RESTORATION

In this section we will look at deep cavity restoration. It is an extensive and radical restoration and it outlines the basic order of steps which must be followed to achieve a natural looking restored area which will not change over the period of time the body is viewed (Figures 5, 6A–K, and 7A–E).

The following case presentation will assume there is a cancerous growth on the lower right lateral cheek of the deceased. It is not possible to remove the growth from inside the mouth. Therefore, the cancerous protrusion must be removed by excising the tumor directly from the surface of the face. The tumor should be removed after arterial embalming if it is not distorting another feature of the face. If it is distorting another feature of the face it should be excised prior to arterial injection and several bridge sutures can be made across the cavity to align the margins. The cavity can be filled with a compress of a preservative-cautery chemical during the arterial embalming of the body.

Protocol	Discussion
1. Obtain permission from the persons in charge of disposition of the body.	Permission from the arranging party will assure the embalmer in writing that the tumor is to be removed and the resulting excised area restored. (Other options might include using a full-couch casket, turning the body and viewing the deceased from the left side; leaving the malignant growth on the face and covering it with a clean bandage.)
2. Sanitize and clean the affected area.	Cleansing the area with a surface disinfectant will destroy pathogenic surface bacteria and deodorize the tissues. If radiation treatments were given, marker stains such as gentian violet may be present on the intact skin surface. Cleaning with a solvent will remove these stains.
3. Protect undamaged skin areas.	Cover the undamaged skin areas surrounding the tumor with massage cream; this prevents chemicals from staining or drying the intact tissues.
4. Embalm the body.	If unautopsied, restricted cervical injection will insure good distribution of arterial solution to the tissues of the face. If autopsied, simply inject left and right sides of the face. Arterial solution should be strong enough to insure very firm and dry tissues.
5. Excise the tumor.	Cut around the tumor in a circular fashion holding the scalpel at an angle as if you were attempting to cut under the tumor. This is described as undercutting. The circular cut should be made in the undamaged tissue surrounding the growth. Excise as much of the tumor as possible. Dissect until undamaged tissues and bone are reached. Excise all diseased tissue. The excised material should be collected in a plastic container, treated with a preservative, and placed within the casket for burial or cremation with the deceased (see Figure 6A–K). (Text continues on page 508.)

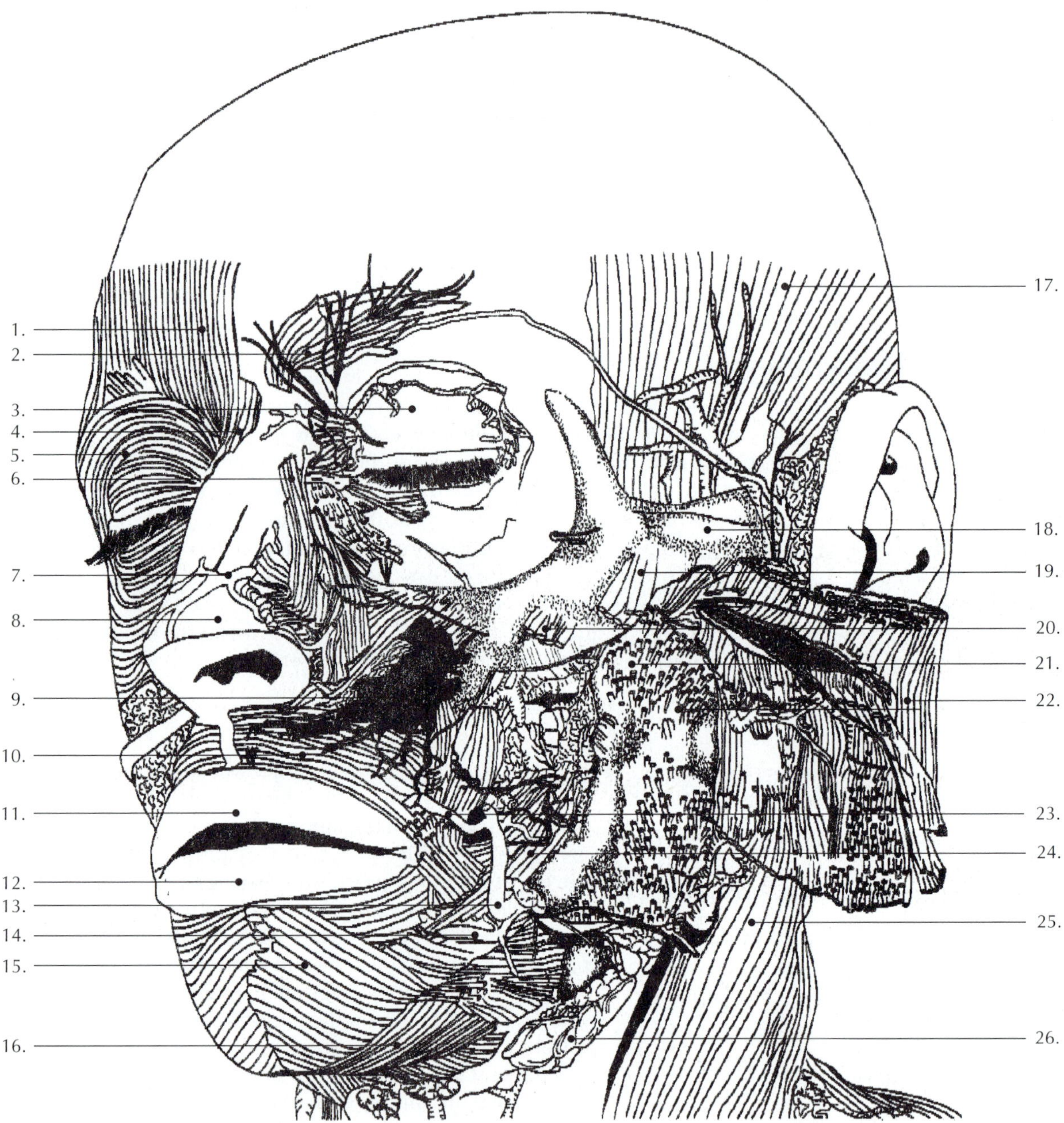

Figure 5. Three-quarter profile of the face dissected. The orbicularis oculi muscle has been removed from the left side of the face exposing the tarsal plate of the upper eyelid. The skeleton of the nose has been exposed. The masseter muscle has been separated from its origin on the zygomatic bone and its insertion on the mandible, then retracted posteriorly. Key to the illustration: 1. frontalis muscle; 2. corrugator muscle; 3. superior tarsus; 4. procerus muscle; 5. orbicularis oculi muscle; 6. quadratus labii superior, angular head; 7. nasal branch of the angular artery; 8. cartilage of the nasal wing; 9. infraorbital nerve plexus; 10. orbicularis oris muscle; 11. superior mucous membrane; 12. inferior mucous membrane; 13. facial artery; 14. inferior labial artery; 15. quadratus labii inferior; 16. triangularis muscle; 17. temporalis muscle; 18. zygomatic arch; 19. zygomatic muscle; 20. zygomatic head of the quadratus labii superior muscle; 21. coronoid process of the mandible; 22. masseter muscle (reflected); 23. superior labial artery; 24. buccinator muscle; 25. sternocleidomastoid muscle; 26. submaxillary gland. *(Drawing courtesy of: Jude Waples, Oakville, Ontario, Canada).*

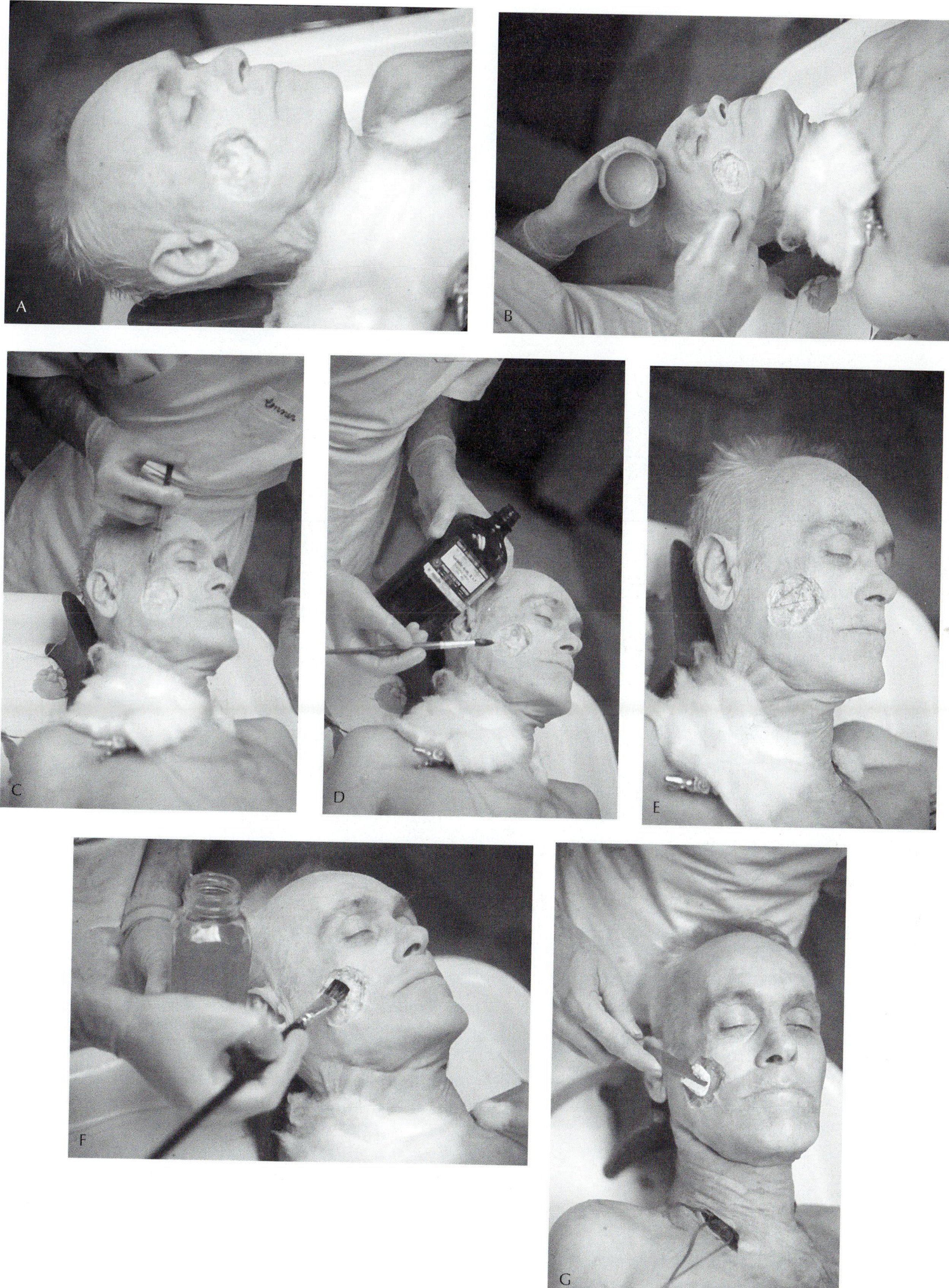

Figure 6. A. Tumor excised after embalming **B.** Massage cream protects intact tissues. **C. and D.** Phenol treatments to dry the cavity. **E.** Basket weave suture applied. **F.** Sealer applied. **G.** Deep-filler (mortuary mastic) applied.

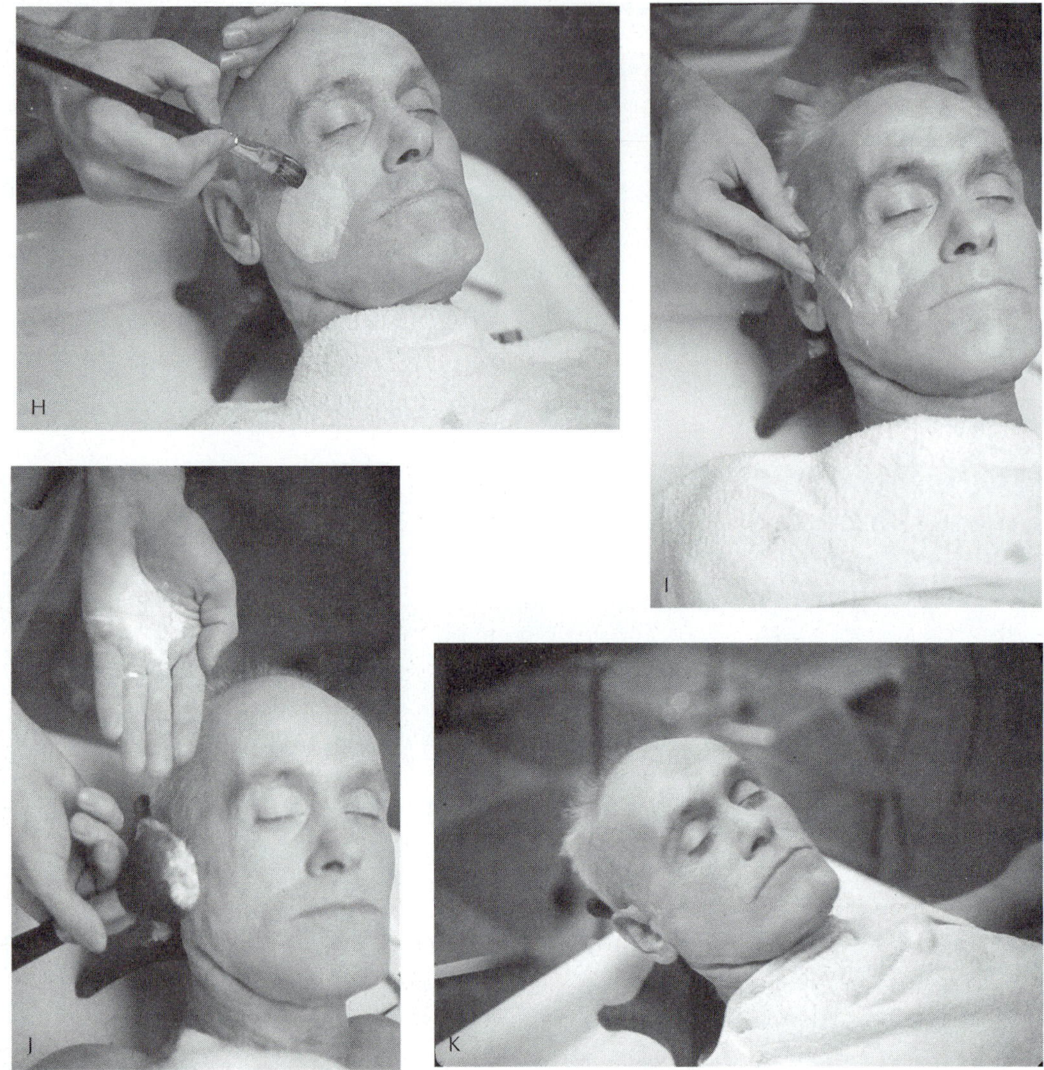

Figure 6 (*Continued*). **H.** Gauze placed over filler and sealer applied. **I.** wax adjustments. **J.** Cosmetics applied. **K.** Completed restoration.

Protocol	Discussion
6. Apply surface compresses to the surrounding subcutaneous walls; hypodermically inject the surrounding tissues from within the cavity.	Inspect the subcutaneous tissues to be certain the cavity is clean. If tissues appear moist inject the surrounding tissues hypodermically with a preservative-cautery solution or undiluted cavity fluid. Pack the floor and walls of the cavity with cotton saturated with the same chemical. Cover the area with a thin layer of plastic.
7. Allow a period of rest.	If a phenol compound is applied to the raw tissues it will work much faster than a compress of formaldehyde. The phenol should dry and firm the tissues very rapidly depending on the strength of the chemical. Formaldehyde may require two to four hours. It is very important that the tissues be dry and firm for this will prevent leakage and possible separation of the wax from the intact tissues.

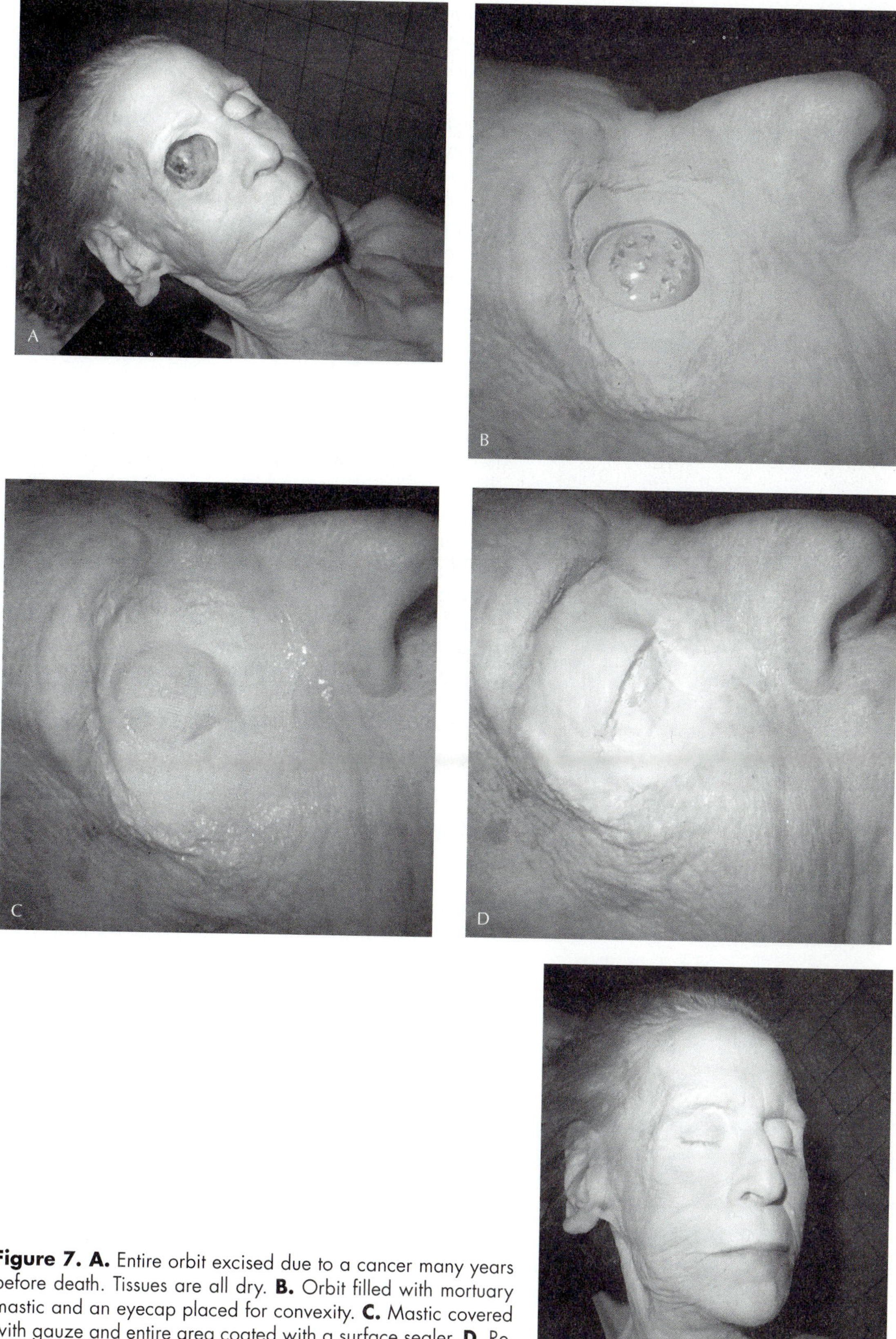

Figure 7. A. Entire orbit excised due to a cancer many years before death. Tissues are all dry. **B.** Orbit filled with mortuary mastic and an eyecap placed for convexity. **C.** Mastic covered with gauze and entire area coated with a surface sealer. **D.** Rebuilding of the lids (upper first) with surface wax. **E.** Completed.

Protocol	**Discussion**
8. Dry the subcutaneous surfaces.	Remove the compresses; some digital pressure can be applied to the surrounding intact tissues in an attempt to force out any leakage. The walls of the cavity can be swabbed with cotton or gauze saturated with cleaning solvent. If the walls seem moist they can be force dried with a hair dryer or electric spatula. Time permitting, a fan blowing over the area can dry the tissue. Be certain the surrounding intact skin surface is protected with a coating of massage cream. Drying is important for it will prevent any leakage and wax separation.
9. Apply sealer to the cavity walls.	A sealer can be applied to the base and walls of the cavity. Several coats of sealer will help to prevent the accumulation of moisture within the cavity. The glue may be force dried by using a hair dyer. This step can be omitted if the cavity is completely dry.
10. Fill the lower area of the cavity with a deep wound filler.	A variety of deep fillers may be used including mortuary mastic, deep-wound filler wax, cotton dipped in plaster of paris, alternating strips of cotton or cotton webbing saturated with surface glue, and auto repair mastic.
11. Apply a basket weave suture just beneath the top of the rim of the cavity.	Suture with dental floss or a linen thread using a sharp needle. Begin the suturing by tying the ligature in place; do not use a knot; leave about three inches of thread. When you are ready to end the suture, end at the same point as you began by tying two ends of suture thread together. Do not pull the basket weave sutures too tight or they will cause the marginal skin to "pucker." This lattice work of sutures helps to hold the margins of the cavity in alignment and holds the deep filler and surface wax in position.
12. Apply the surface restorer wax.	A softer surface restorer wax can be placed over the deep filler and at the same time pushed into the threads of the basket weave suture. Mound the surface wax in the center of the excision then feather it to the margins of the cavity and extend it slightly over into the surrounding intact tissues. Smoothing of the wax can be done with a soft brush dipped in solvent or wax thinner. View the results from a variety of positions and adjust if necessary. Some cosmetic colorant may be added to the surface wax to obtain a good skin tone match (See Figure 7A–C).
13. Apply the surface cosmetics over the waxed areas; complete with white drying powder.	A cream cosmetic can be placed over a waxed surface. This step can be done if it is necessary to make a better match of the waxed area to the surrounding intact tissues. Never apply a tinted or colored powder directly to a wax surface.
14. Reinstate the pores.	Gently "dabbing" the waxed area with a soft powder brush will create the effect of skin pores. Other methods include gently pressing with moist lintless gauze or paper toweling, or lightly tapping a stippling brush over the area.
15. Seal the cosmetics.	This can be done with a light spray of commercial hair spray.

To better match the cosmetized skin colors of the undamaged tissues with the restored waxed area it is recommended that the undamaged areas of the face be cosmetized first. It may be possible to mix some of the cosmetic cream into the wax before it is applied. Neutral or straw-colored waxes are recommended rather than using colored waxes.

▶ RESTORATIVE TREATMENTS FOR DISCOLORATIONS

The majority of discolorations present on the visible body areas cannot be completely removed, but most can be altered so less cosmetic treatment will be needed. Those which can possibly be removed would include surface stains (discolorations) and antemortem and postmortem intravascular blood discolorations. Surface discolorations can be removed with a solvent or by washing with soap and water. Intravascular blood discolorations can be cleared through arterial solution injection and subsequent drainage. Blood, some pathological, decomposition, and chemotherapeutic (drug) discolorations can be altered or lightened by arterial injection and drainage and surface and hypodermic bleaches. Phenol and formaldehyde are the primary chemicals used in most mortuary bleaches. Bleaching of a discoloration does not return the skin to its normal color, but the discoloration will be less intense. Phenol and formaldehyde in addition to being bleaches are also preservatives. Use of these chemicals helps to insure preservation of the area and prevents decomposition from occurring. Surface compresses provide a more uniform bleaching of the skin surface; hypodermic injection of a discolored area such as an eyelid does not always insure an even distribution of the chemical. Often both surface and hypodermic treatments are necessary, particularly when there is swelling accompanying the discoloration. Dehydrated and dessicated tissue or scabs over abraded tissues will not respond to bleaching.

For discussion in this text discolorations are divided into three categories: 1. Surface discolorations; 2. Discolorations associated with non-broken skin conditions; and 3. Discolorations associated with broken skin conditions.

Surface Discolorations

Surface stains (discolorations) result from an external agent on the surface of the skin or hair. Common examples include blood, dirt, nicotine stains, adhesive tape, betadine, and gentian violet. These discolorations need to be removed in the pre-embalming time period. Simply washing the discoloration with a soft washcloth using warm water and a liquid soap will loosen and remove a large number of discolorations. Adding sodium hypochlorite to the water will ease the cleaning of blood stains. A cleaning solvent (trichloroethylene) will remove most medicinal stains including adhesive tape. Whenever a solvent has been used to clean the face or hands it should be followed by a light coating of massage cream to prevent dehydration. Finger-nails should also be cleaned at this time. Acetone will assist in removing nail polishes and other paint products.

Non-Broken Skin Discolorations

Discolorations associated with non-broken skin conditions can be local or general. Common local examples include blood discolorations such as ecchymosis, purpura, hematoma, vascular nevus or birthmark, small areas of dehydrate tissue, or postmortem stain. General discolorations would include jaundice, decomposition, or dehydration.

Blood decomposition discolorations will respond to mortuary bleaches. Most mortuary bleaches can be used for several functions–to bleach, preserve, and cauterize tissues and to reduce liquid and semi-solid swellings. Many of these preservative-cautery-bleaching chemicals contain phenol (carbolic acid) and depending upon the strength of the phenol present they work very rapidly. A substitute preservative-cautery-bleach can be undiluted cavity chemical. These chemicals can be applied three ways—as a compress on the surface of the body; as a compress under the surface of the skin, e.g., under eyelids, inside lips and mouth or inside the nares; or by hypodermic injection into or beneath the skin. Hypodermic injection makes it possible for cosmetic treatment to begin immediately. If preservative (bleaching) gels are used they can be painted onto a surface. A surface compress or gel may be placed over the discoloration before, during, or after embalming the body. After the compress (or gel) is removed it will be necessary to clean the area with a solvent and thoroughly dry the tissues before the application of cosmetics. If the bleach is to be injected by hypodermic syringe this is usually done in the postembalming time period. These bleaches should be injected into areas of the face and hands keeping in mind that some leakage will occur for a short time, therefore hidden needle entry points should be used.

Dehydrated tissues do not respond to bleaching. Even the arterial injection of embalming solution does little to alter dehyrated tissues. Severely dehydrated areas will appear dark brown to black. If the area affected is the lips or eyelids and this severe condition exists it may become necessary to excise these tissues or build new features upon them. Areas where the dehydration is less severe—perhaps the fingers or lips—can often be restored by hypodermic tissue building and the discoloration covered with opaque cosmetics.

A frequently encountered discoloration is ecchymosis on the back of the hands. Simple treatment of this discoloration is to inject a preservative-cautery-bleaching chemical (or undiluted cavity fluid) between the fingers into the discolored area. Insert the needle and make several channels through the discolored tissues being careful not to pass the needle back through the surface of the skin. Slightly withdraw the needle and proceed to inject sufficient chemical that a slight swelling of the discoloration is noted. With gloved fingers or a cloth, press on the raised areas to distribute the chemical throughout the discolored tis-

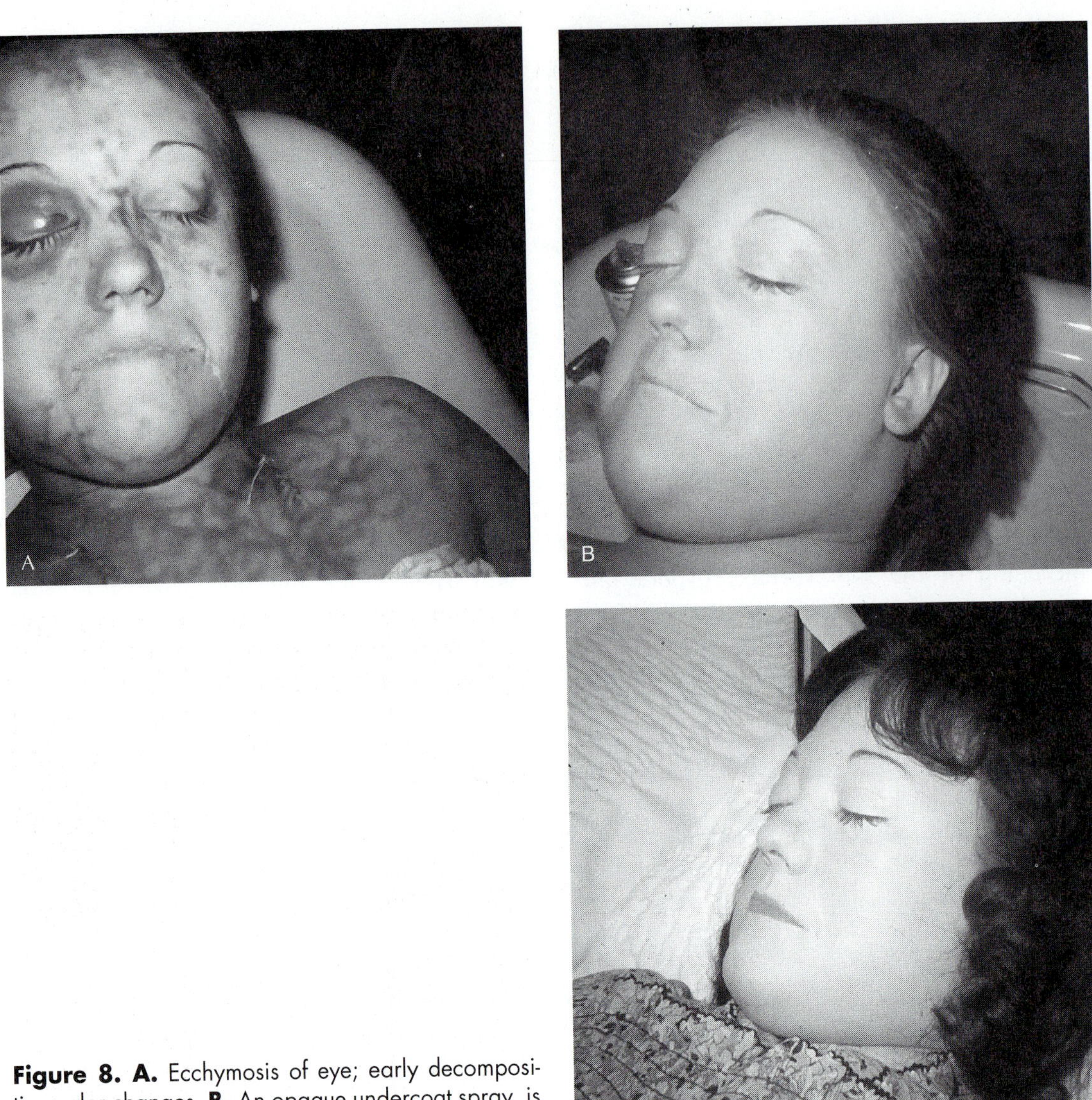

Figure 8. A. Ecchymosis of eye; early decomposition color changes. **B.** An opaque undercoat spray is applied. **C.** Cream cosmetics applied over the undercoat.

sues. If a towel or large piece of cotton is placed under the hand it will absorb any chemical that may leak—this leakage will stop in a short time. A semi-opaque or opaque cosmetic can be applied over the discoloration.

Large discolorations such as jaundice, decomposition, or postmortem stain can be altered by the embalming technique. Special arterial fluids are available to assist in bleaching this type of discoloration. These treatments are followed by the application of opaque or semi-opaque cosmetic treatments. In some situations the embalmer may want to place a fluid compress over the entire face during and/or after the arterial injection (Figure 8A–C).

Superficial Broken Skin Conditions and Discoloration

Superficial disconnected (broken) skin conditions include abrasions, razor abrasions, desquamation, torn epidermis (possibly associated with ecchymosis and purpura), second degree burns, blisters and pustules (which need to be opened and drained), and loose scabs. These conditions all involve the epidermis and possibly upper areas of the dermis. Deeply torn tissue conditions (e.g., lacerations, surgical incisions, compound fractures) are discussed in another section of this chapter. Discolorations such as livor mortis, postmortem stain, bruising, and ecchymosis may also be associated with broken skin conditions (Figure 9A–D).

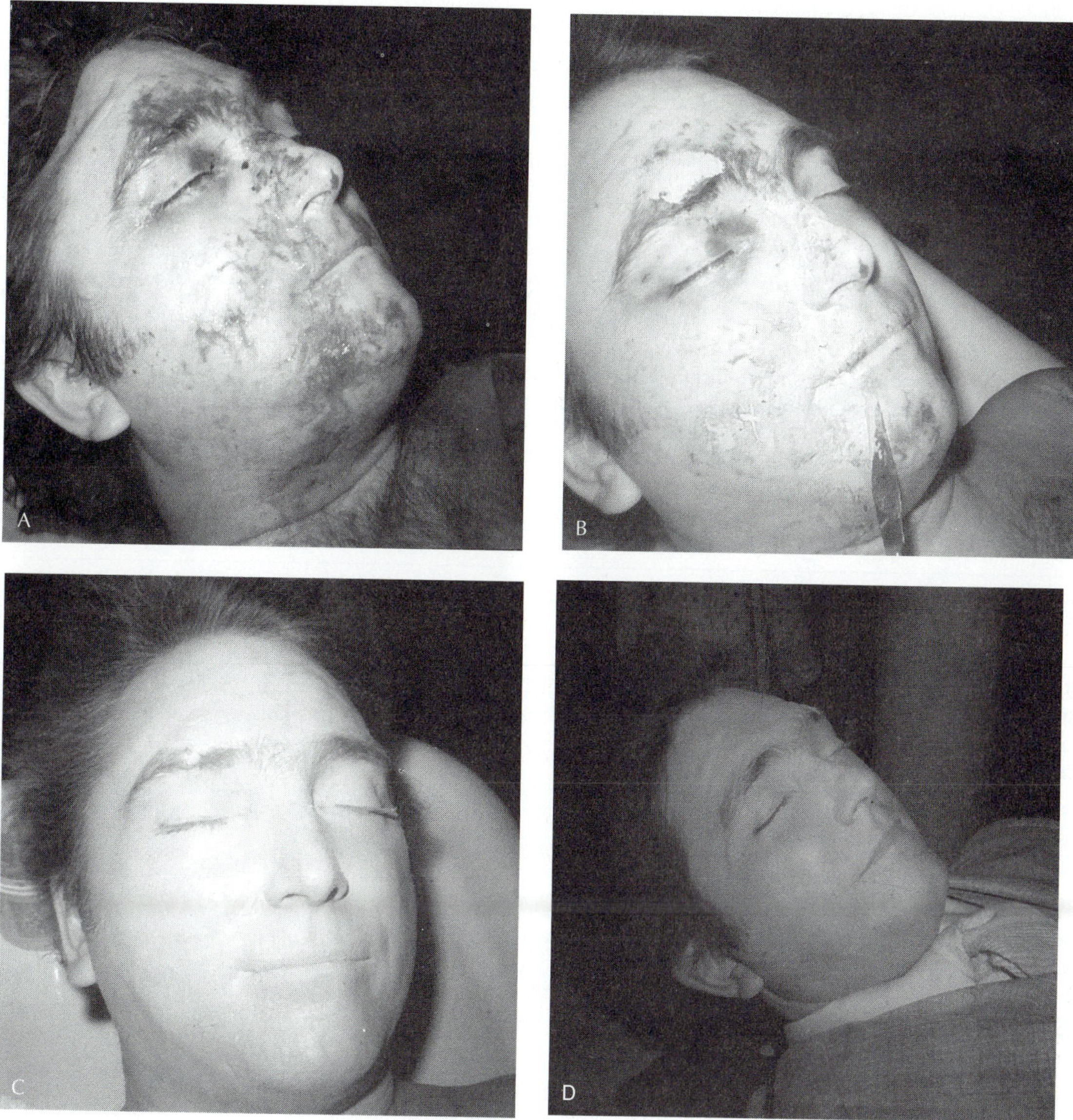

Figure 9. A. Multiple small lacerations and abrasions. **B.** Wax adjustments after embalming. **C.** Opaque undercoat sprayed over tissues. **D.** Cream cosmetics applied over the undercoat.

Dehydration can also be present over the broken skin areas. Dehydrated tissues can vary in color from light yellow to black. Wax, undercoat paints, and cosmetics can be applied over these dried tissues.

Depending upon the specific condition the following treatments will be necessary to restore the face or hands where superficial broken skin conditions exist (Tables 3–5).

1. Disinfect and clean the area with solvent; protect unaffected tissues with massage cream but do not apply massage cream over the affected tissues; establish a restoration plan.
2. Remove all loose tissues using a sharp scalpel or scissors.
3. Establish good preservation through:
   a. Direct injection of a strong arterial solution into the affected region
   b. Application of surface compresses of a concentrated cautery chemical, undiluted cavity fluid, or preservative gels before, during, or after arterial injection
   c. Postembalming subcutaneous hypodermic injection of a concentrated cautery chemical or undiluted cavity fluid beneath the affected areas and in the immediate surrounding area

TABLE 3. TREATMENTS FOR LOCALIZED DISCOLORATIONS—NON-BROKEN SKIN CONDITIONS

Surface discolorations and stains can be removed by the use of solvents and thorough washing in the pre-embalming time period. Discolorations from trauma, pathological disorders, therapeutic treatments, postmortem changes as well as antemortem and postmortem blood changes need to be treated through the entire embalming process. This chart gives the order for treatment of these discolorations:

1. Ecchymosis, purpura, petechia
2. "Black eye," no swelling
3. "Black eye," with swelling
4. First-degree burn
5. Postmortem stain

No broken skin exists with these conditions. However, there are situations where they will be accompanied by a broken skin condition (eg, ecchymosis caused by an IV puncture). Bodies will also contain one or more of these conditions in addition to the necessary "routine" restorative treatments such as tissue-building, sealing of the features, and the application of cosmetics.

	Ecchymosis, purpura (1)	Black Eye no swelling (2)	Black Eye swelling (3)	First degree burn (4)	P.M. Stain (5)
I. Evaluate condition; sanitize tissues, remove debris (e.g., glass shards, dirt, blood)	x	x	x	x	x
II. Excise loose tissues by scalpel, razor, or scissors **A. Trauma**—dehydrated margins, torn skin **B. Pathological**—open pustules, boils, blisters, remove scabs, fever blisters **C. Postmortem**—remove all desquamation and loose skin					
III. Massage cream applied to protect unaffected skin; **not applied** over discolorations or moist tissues	x	x	x	x	x
IV. Align margins of separated tissues with temporary bridge sutures or dabs of super glue (eg, lacerations)					
V. Apply surface compresses, of a preservative-cautery-bleach chemical; undiluted cavity fluid; surface gels	o*	o*	o*	o*	o*
VI. **Embalm the body**—for facial problems use a strong arterial solution; unautopsied restricted cervical injection	x	x	x	x	x
VII. Hypodermic injection into affected tissues and/or surface compress of a preservative-cautery-bleach undiluted*	o	o	o	o	o
VIII. **REST PERIOD FOR CHEMICALS TO WORK**					
IX. **Excise** tumors or necrotic areas; **reduce** swellings: **tissue building** of sunken and emaciated areas			o		
X. Dry subcutaneous tissues of an excised area with compresses and hypodermic injection of the walls					
XI. Dry tissues—swab with a solvent; let air pass over tissues; hair dryer; electric spatula	x	x	x	x	x
XII. Permanent sutures or super glue to close separations					
XIII. Apply surface sealer glue**					
XIV. Cosmetize unaffected areas of the face and/or hands	x	x	o	x	x
XV. Apply opaque paint to the affected area	x	x	o	x	x
XVI. Apply a surface restorer wax to affected area***					
XVII. Blend surface cosmetic over area being treated	x	x	o	x	x

KEY

O—optional treatment—order can vary.

*—compresses may be placed **under** eyelids or **under** lips.

**—a protection against moisture and a replacement for skin; may be used in lieu of step XVI

***—cream cosmetic can be applied **over** the wax, **under** the wax, or mixed **into** the wax

TABLE 4. TREATMENTS FOR TRAUMATIC AND POSTMORTEM BROKEN SKIN CONDITIONS

The following conditions represent situations where the surface layers of the skin have been broken. If there is a period of time before embalming some of these conditions may dry by exposure to the air. They will appear dry and firm, possibly requiring only cosmetic treatment. When loose pieces of tissue exist be certain to remove all separated tissue.

1. Abrasion (dry) (small lacerations)
2. Abrasion (moist)
3. Razor Abrasion (burn)
4. Desquamation (skin slip)
5. Third degree burn

These are all broken skin conditions. The tissues immediately surrounding one of these problem areas will often be discolored. In trauma cases a variety of restorative problems may exist in addition to the routine restorative treatments such as tissue building and the application of cosmetics.

	Abrasion, small lacerations (1)	Abrasion, moist (2)	Razor abrasion (3)	Skin slip (4)	Third degree burn (5)
I. Evaluate condition; sanitize tissues, remove debris (e.g., glass shards, dirt, blood)	x	x	x	x	x
II. Excise loose tissues with scalpel, razor, or scissors					
A. Trauma—dehydrated margins, torn skin	x	x			x
B. Pathological—open pustules, boils, blisters, remove scabs, fever blisters					o
C. Postmortem—remove all desquamation and loose skin				x	
III. Massage cream applied to protect unaffected skin; **not applied** over discolorations or moist tissues	x	x	x	x	x
IV. Align margins of separated tissues with temporary bridge sutures or dabs of super glue					
V. Apply surface compresses, of a preservative-cautery-bleach chemical; undiluted cavity fluid; surface gels	o	o	o	o	o
VI. **Embalm the body**—for facial problems use a strong arterial solution; unautopsied restricted cervical injection	x	x	x	x	x
VII. Hypodermic injection into affected tissues and/or surface compress of a preservative-cautery-bleach undiluted*		x		x	x
VIII. **REST PERIOD FOR CHEMICALS TO WORK**					
IX. **Excise** tumors or necrotic areas; **Reduce** swellings: **Tissue building** of sunken and emaciated areas					
X. Dry subcutaneous tissues of an excised area with compresses and hypodermic injection of the walls					
XI. Dry tissues—swab with a solvent; let air pass over tissues; hair dryer; electric spatula	x	x	x	x	x
XII. Permanent sutures or super glue to close separations					
XIII. Apply surface sealer glue**	o	o	o	o	o
XIV. Cosmetize unaffected areas of the face and/or hands	x	x	x	x	x
XV. Apply opaque paint to the affected area	x	x	x	x	x
XVI. Apply a surface restorer wax to affected area***	o	o	o	o	o
XVII. Blend surface cosmetic over area being treated	x	x	x	x	x

KEY

O—optional treatment—order can vary.
*—compresses may be placed **under** eyelids or **under** lips.
**—a protection against moisture and a replacement for skin; may be used in lieu of step XVI
***—cream cosmetic can be applied **over** the wax, **under** the wax, or mixed **into** the wax

TABLE 5. TREATMENTS FOR BROKEN SKIN CONDITIONS—PATHOLOGICAL AND TRAUMATIC

The following problems represent conditions where it will be necessary to open the skin as part of the restoration. Failure to do so may result in leakage from the lesion. Conditions exhibiting deep trauma to the tissues are also listed here. Frequently these problems will be accompanied by surrounding discolored tissues.

1. Pustules, blisters, boils
2. Scab
3. Torn skin
4. Laceration, surgical incision
5. Second degree burn

If there is a period of time between death and embalming some of these conditions may exhibit drying and dehydrated margins. Trauma cases will frequently have several conditions requiring restorative treatments in addition to the routine treatments such as tissue-building, sealing features, and the application of cosmetics.

	Pustules, blisters, boils (1)	Scab (2)	Torn skin (3)	Laceration (4)	Second degree burn (5)
I. Evaluate condition; sanitize tissues, remove debris (e.g., glass shards, dirt, blood)	x	x	x	x	x
II. Excise loose tissues with scalpel, razor, or scissors					
A. Trauma—dehydrated margins, torn skin			x	x	x
B. Pathological—open pustules, boils, blisters, remove scabs, fever blisters	x	x			x
C. Postmortem—remove all desquamation and loose skin					
III. Massage cream applied to protect unaffected skin;	x	x	x	x	x
not applied over discolorations or moist tissues				x	
IV. Align margins of separated tissues with temporary bridge sutures or dabs of super glue					
V. Apply surface compresses, of a preservative-cautery-bleach chemical; undiluted cavity fluid; surface gels	o	o	o	o	o
VI. **Embalm the body**—for facial problems use a strong arterial solution; unautopsied restricted cervical injection	x	x	x	x	x
VII. Hypodermic injection into affected tissues and/or surface compress of a preservative-cautery-bleach undiluted*	o	o	o	o	o
VIII. **REST PERIOD FOR CHEMICALS TO WORK**					
IX. **Excise** tumors or necrotic areas; **Reduce** swellings: **Tissue building** of sunken and emaciated areas				x	
X. Dry subcutaneous tissues of an excised area with compresses and hypodermic injection of the walls					
XI. Dry tissues—swab with a solvent; let air pass over tissues; hair dryer; electric spatula	x	x	x	x	x
XII. Permanent sutures or super glue to close separations				x	
XIII. Apply surface sealer glue**			o	o	o
XIV. Cosmetize intact areas of the face and/or hands	o	o	o	o	o
XV. Apply opaque paint to the affected area	o	o	o	o	o
XVI. Apply a surface restorer wax to affected area***	x	x	o	o	o
XVII. Blend surface cosmetic over area being treated	x	x	x	x	x

KEY
O—optional treatment—order can vary.
*—compresses may be placed **under** eyelids or **under** lips.
**—a protection against moisture and a replacement for skin; may be used in lieu of step XVI
***—cream cosmetic can be applied **over** the wax, **under** the wax, or mixed **into** the wax

4. Dry the tissues.
   a. Surface compresses preserve and dry tissues.
   b. Clean with a solvent.
   c. Use a hair dryer or electric spatula to dry the surface tissues.
5. Restore the area using wax, opaque paint, or surface glue.
   a. *Method 1:* Apply an opaque undercoat paint; after it dries apply a cream cosmetic over it to match the surrounding cosmetized skin (Figure 10A–C).
   b. *Method 2:* Apply a surface sealer to replace the missing skin; after the sealer dries an opaque cosmetic can be applied over the sealer.
   c. *Method 3:* Apply an opaque undercoat paint; after it dries apply a thin layer of surface restorer wax over the area.
      i. Cream cosmetics may be mixed into the wax.
      ii. Cream cosmetics may be applied over the wax.
   d. *Method 4:* If the area is small (e.g., razor abrasion, fever blister, etc.) apply the cosmetic to the face including powder; make small adjustments with surface wax in which some of the cosmetic has been mixed.
   e. *Method 5:* Apply a surface sealer; when it has partially dried, apply a white powder with an atomizer or dropped from a brush. This will produce a skin-like color over the area where the sealer was applied.

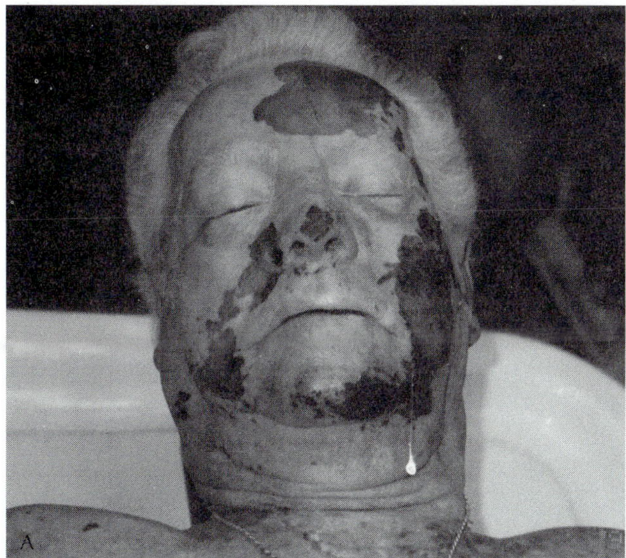

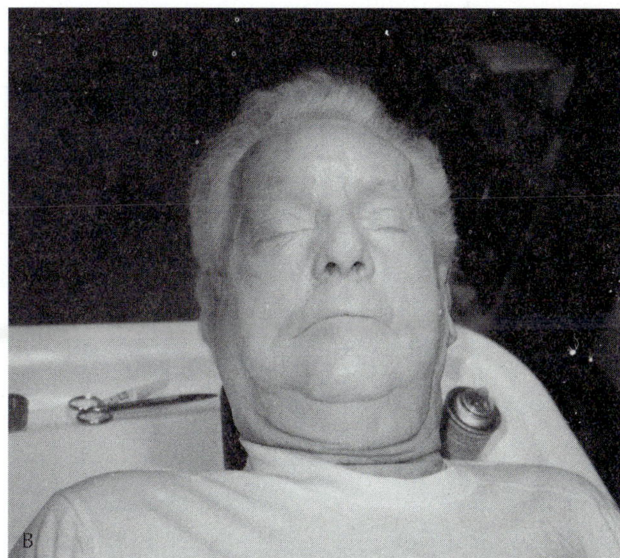

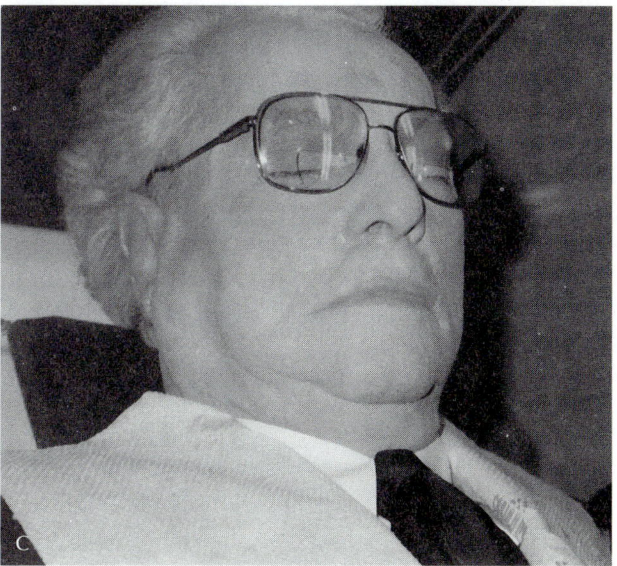

Figure 10. A. Desquamation (skin-slip); damaged skin removed and tissues dried. **B.** Dried skin surface painted with an undercoat paint, with cream cosmetics applied over it. **C.** Body dressed, glasses used.

▶ ESTABLISHING FORM—CORRECTING EMACIATED, DEPRESSED, AND COMPRESSED TISSUE

There are a variety of reasons why a body area such as the face or hands will require a reestablishment of form. Examples include absence of teeth or dentures or a mild or extreme loss of weight. The emaciated body will exhibit unnatural depressions in various parts of the face and hands. Embalming itself can bring about dehydration to areas like the fingers and the lips making them appear slightly shrunken or wrinkled. For persons dying in a position in which the face, or a portion of the face or hands, is pushed against an immovable solid object, these contact areas will appear crushed. Trauma to the face or skull can cause a depressed fracture, resulting in a depression of the surface tissues.

There are natural depressions on the surface of the cranium and the face. These include the temple area and zygomatic arch depression in the cranium and the buccal depressions in the face (which extend obliquely downward from either the medial or lateral margins of the cheekbones). The deepest part of these depressions is located over the area of the teeth. These natural depressions have a tendency to deepen when there has been a loss of weight. Similarly, areas of the face containing fatty tissue may need to be rebuilt, areas including the cheeks, chin, and jawline (Figure 11).

Correction of emaciated, depressed, or compressed tissue can be made using these restorative treatments:

1. Embalming treatment—use of restorative co-injection fluids
2. Support inserted under sunken tissues
   a. Dentures

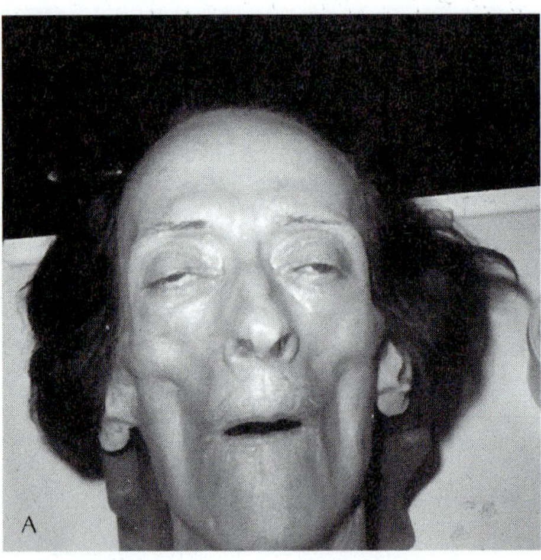

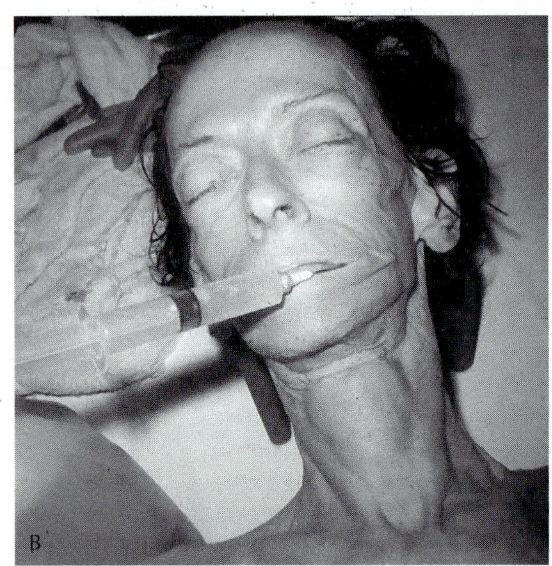

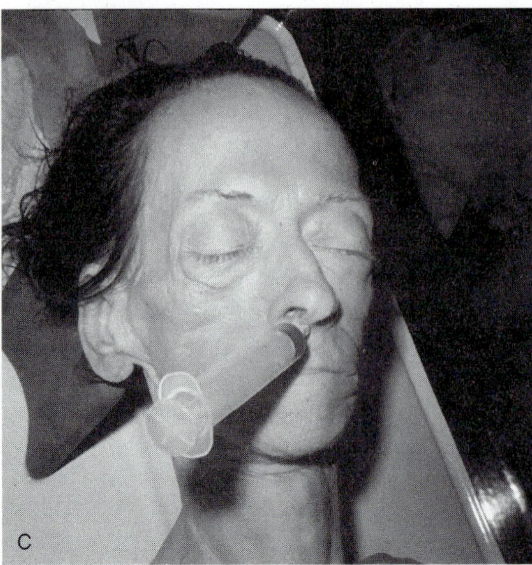

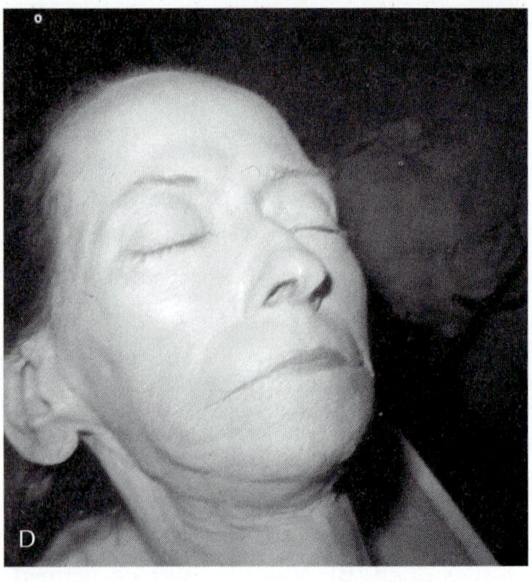

Figure 11. A. Emaciation of the face. **B. and C.** Hypodermic tissue building after embalming. **D.** Cosmetics applied.

   b. Mouth formers; eyecaps
   c. Absorbent or non-absorbent cotton, kapoc, webbed cotton
   d. Mortuary mastics or feature posing mastic
3. Subcutaneous injection of hypodermic tissue builder
4. Subcutaneous injection of a mortuary mastic compound
5. Build upon the skin surface over the depressed area
   a. Lip wax or surface restorer wax
   b. Thick surface sealer (glue)
   c. Mortuary mastic + surface sealer + gauze + surface sealer
6. Excise damaged tissues and rebuild the area

Embalming Treatment

A restorative co-injection chemical can be added to the arterial preservative solution. When accompanied by restricted drainage, it is possible to distend sunken areas of the face, neck, and cranium. Directions of the individual chemical manufacturer should be followed. It is important to delay aspiration of unautopsied bodies for a period of several hours when using this treatment. It is not always possible to have complete control using this process; raising of the sunken areas is not always uniform. Some tissues will rapidly respond to this process and others will not respond at all.

Crushed or compressed tissues can be treated by firm vigorous massage during arterial injection. This may help to fill out the depressed tissues. If there is little response from this treatment the areas can be filled out with tissue builder after embalming. If the condition is severe, it may be necessary to apply a surface restorer wax over the area to rebuild the surface contour.

Mouth and Eyelid Support

Posing of the features is usually done in the preembalming time period. If dentures are absent, several types of supports or a combination of supports may be used. A mouth former of plastic or metal can be placed on the exposed portions of the mandible and maxillae within the mouth, or it can be placed over the few remaining teeth if the majority are missing. Absorbent or non-absorbent cotton and kapoc can be used to support the mouth when teeth and dentures are missing. For the eyelids, plastic eyecaps, cotton, or kapoc can be used to keep the eyelids closed and elevated.

A feature-posing mortuary mastic compound can also be used as a support for missing teeth. The compound can be injected through the nozzle of a caulking gun. The compound alone can be used to fill out a sunken mouth or injected over the teeth (if present) or a mouth former. The mastic can also be used with eyecaps to elevate sunken eyelids. An advantage of the mastic compound is that the material does not dehydrate the tissues as cotton can.

Treatments for Sunken Eyes: Emaciated Borders of the Eye Socket

Raising sunken eyes with tissue builder is not always a successful process. Embalmers are divided on the entry point for the needle; some prefer the inner canthus of the eye and others prefer the outer corner of the eye. Once entered, direct the needle along the bony side wall, being careful not to puncture the eyeball. Tissue builder is injected very slowly behind the eyeball. There is a tendency for the builder to flow into the upper eyelid and the supraorbital tissues giving the closed eye an unnatural appearance. Many find that using cotton as a method of eye closure is a more effective method of correcting sunken eyes. If cotton or a combination of cotton and eyecaps is used to raise the eyelids, the embalmer should also fill in the sharp bony inferior rim of the eyesocket. This can easily be done by tissue building; insert the needle through the nostril and direct it to the inferior rim of the eyesocket. Slowly inject a small amount of tissue builder and with digital pressure distribute it along the inferior rim. This will help to remove the sharp margin of the lower eyelid.

Treatments for Underembalmed Eyelids

If the eyelids feel soft to the touch and appear underembalmed, use one of these two methods:

1. Close the eyes using absorbent cotton saturated with several drops of undiluted cavity fluid, then seal the eyelids and act as an internal preservative compress and the glue will prevent separation of the lids. Cosmetics can be placed over the closed eyelids. It is recommended that cream cosmetics be used with this procedure.
2. A method which takes longer is to set and close the eyelids using caps or cotton and seal the eyelids with super glue. Place a preservative compress over the closed eyelids or coat the lids and surrounding area with preservative gel. Cover the compress or gel with a small sheet of thin plastic to prevent evaporation of the chemical and to help to control any fumes. Leave the preservative in place for several hours. Remove the chemical, clean the eyelids with a solvent, and if necessary dry the tissues with a hair dryer. Proceed to cosmetize the eyelids.

Treatments for Nasal Distortion and Tissue Erosion

If the anterior nares are depressed, cotton or mortuary mastic can be placed within the nares to hold them in correct position. These corrections should be made in the preembalming time period.

Plastic tubing (nasogastric tube) inserted through the nostrils and remaining in place for a long period of time may cause an erosion of the nasal tissue where the posterior, inferior portion of the wing of the nose attaches to the cheek. Often tissue is missing and the area appears brown and dehydrated. The tissues are generally dry. If they are moist a preservative surface compress can be applied in the preembalming time period. When the tissues are completely dried, a surface restorer wax can be used to fill in the missing tissues. If the discoloration is pronounced, the area can first be sprayed with an opaque undercoat paint. When it has dried the area can be restored using wax.

Treatment for Earlobe Distortion

The earlobe may be depressed against the cranium and neck due to the body being wrapped in a sheet or improper placement on the headrest. The ear lobes should be freed and properly positioned. A pledget of cotton coated with massage cream placed behind the lobe will hold it in position during the embalming process. This small correction is very important if earrings are to be worn by the deceased. A small amount of tissue builder injected into the lobe after embalming can also help to project the lobe (Figure 12).

Treatment for Underembalmed Ear Tissue

If the tissues of the ear have received insufficient arterial solution, preservation is best accomplished by applying a preservative surface compress or coating the ear with a preservative gel. When sufficient time has been allowed for these chemicals to work, the tissues should be cleaned with a solvent and thoroughly dried. If badly discolored the ear can be sprayed or painted with an opaque undercoat. After this has dried surface cream cosmetics can be applied.

Treatment—Hypodermic Tissue Building

Hypodermic tissue building is done in the postembalming time period. Many embalmers still prefer to use hidden points of entry—inside nostrils and mouth or within the hairline or eyebrows. These points were used in past years to conceal possible leakage. Most quality tissue builders today leak only for a few moments following their injection. A 17 gauge needle works quite well (though some embalmers prefer a slightly smaller diameter). The 17 gauge will not clog and is easy to clean. Tissue builder solvent should only be used for cleaning syringes; it should not be used as a dissolving agent if too much builder is injected into the tissues. A good rule to follow is to always inject a minimum of tissue builder, because more can always be added. Syringes should be stored containing about 5 ccs of tissue builder solvent. Never attempt to clean a needle and syringe using water. Water is what causes the tissue builder to gel in the tissues. Tissue builder solvent is good for cleaning needles and syringes after use with undiluted cavity fluid, mortuary bleaches, or cautery agents.

Treatment—Hypodermic Tissue Building of the Fingers

Tissue building of the fingers is often overlooked. It is especially necessary when the body is to be kept for any extended period of time, because it helps prevent dehydration of the fingertips. Tissue builder should also be injected into the area between the thumb and index finger; quite often this area will dehydrate as a result of the embalming process. Tissue builder can be injected into the back of the hand between the ten-

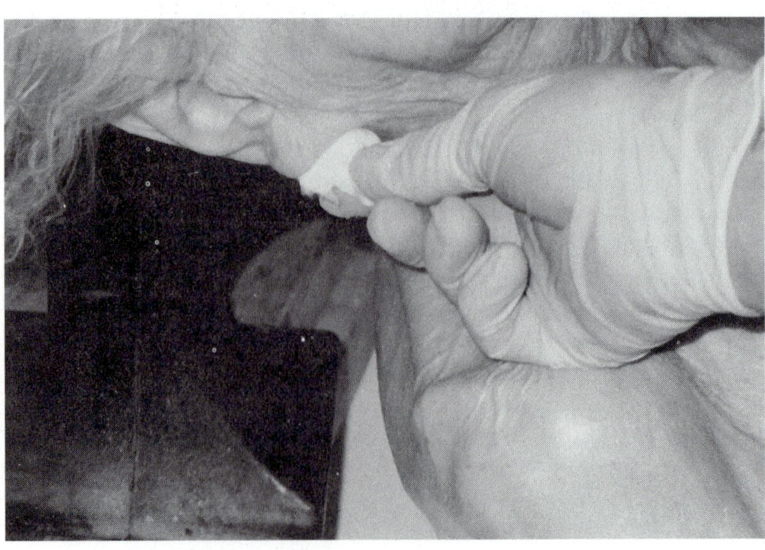

Figure 12. Earlobe supported by cotton.

dons to compensate for weight loss and to help hide the discoloration produced by the lumbrical muscles (Figure 13).

Treatment—Hypodermic Tissue Building of the Cheeks, Mouth, and Orbit

Tissue builder injected into the anterior cheek and the angulus oris eminence (at the corners of the mouth) can help to produce a more pleasing expression. Some filling of the upper anterior cheek area may be required for almost every body because gravity has a tendency to cause the fleshy cheek areas to sag. The cheeks can be filled by inserting the needle through the respective nostril. The inferior bony margin of the eye can also be reached by inserting the needle through the respective nostril. If this margin is sharp due to a loss of weight, it can be filled in by injecting tissue builder into the area and distributing it with finger pressure. The inferior lateral cheek area, especially over the teeth, may be depressed. This area can be filled out in the pre- or postembalming period using cotton or mortuary mastic placed over the back teeth (see Figure 11).

Treatment—Depressed Fractures of the Cranium, Forehead, and Cheek

Trauma cases are so unique that each needs to be individually evaluated. A frequently encountered condition is the depressed fracture of the cranium or the face. If the body has been autopsied, this will provide easy access to the cranial cavity. If necessary the floor of the cavity can be properly aligned and held in position by wooden splints, plaster of Paris, or strips of cotton dipped in plaster. The bone alignment should be done

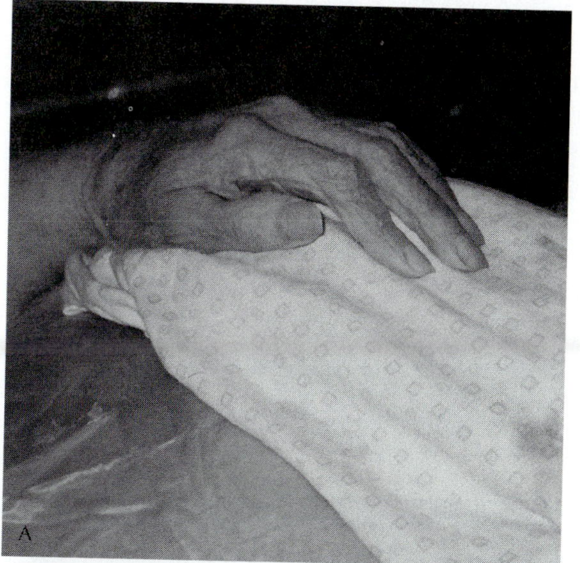

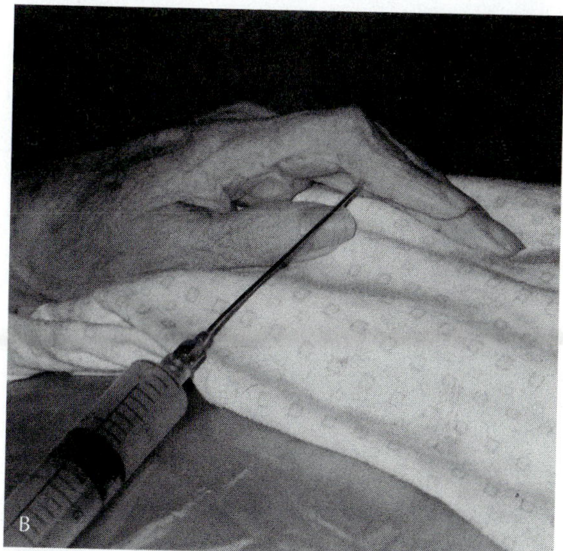

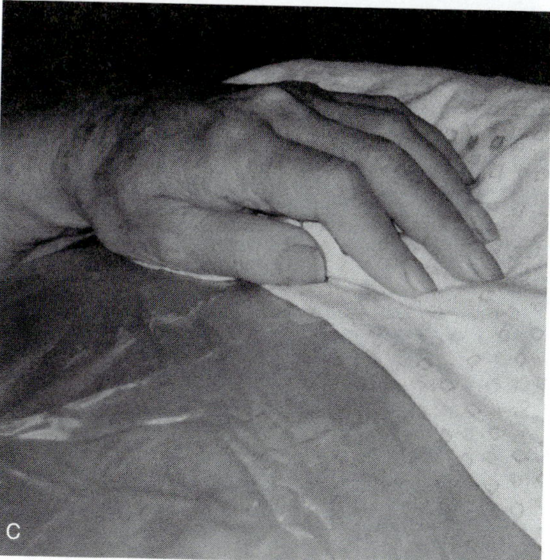

Figure 13. A. Wrinkled, dehydrated fingers. **B.** Tissue builder injected into each finger and area between thumb and index finger. **C.** Completed.

prior to arterial injection. After arterial injection the cranium can be filled with packing, and the fractured bones of the calvarium placed in position over the packing. These bone fragments may be held in position by plaster of Paris or possibly super glue. If a portion of the frontal bone has been depressed or crushed, the autopsy allows access to prop the bone in the correct position. If the skin of the forehead is not torn and the frontal bone is crushed, after arterial injection pack the cranial cavity, place the scalp into its normal position, insert the nozzle of the mastic gun into the area where the frontal bone is missing, and inject sufficient mastic to create an evenly contoured forehead. Restorative wax could also be used to fill in the missing area of bone before the scalp is reflected into position. If the head has not been autopsied, an incision can be made in the hair, the nozzle of the mastic gun inserted, and the depressed area raised with mastic compound after arterial embalming. (Figure 14A–F). Similarly if the cheekbone (maxilla) has been crushed and the surface skin is not broken, an inscision can be made inside the mouth or inside the nostril to admit the nozzle of the mastic gun, the mastic compound can be injected into the area of crushed bone to raise the cheek to a normal position. The mastic compound treatments are done in the postembalming time period.

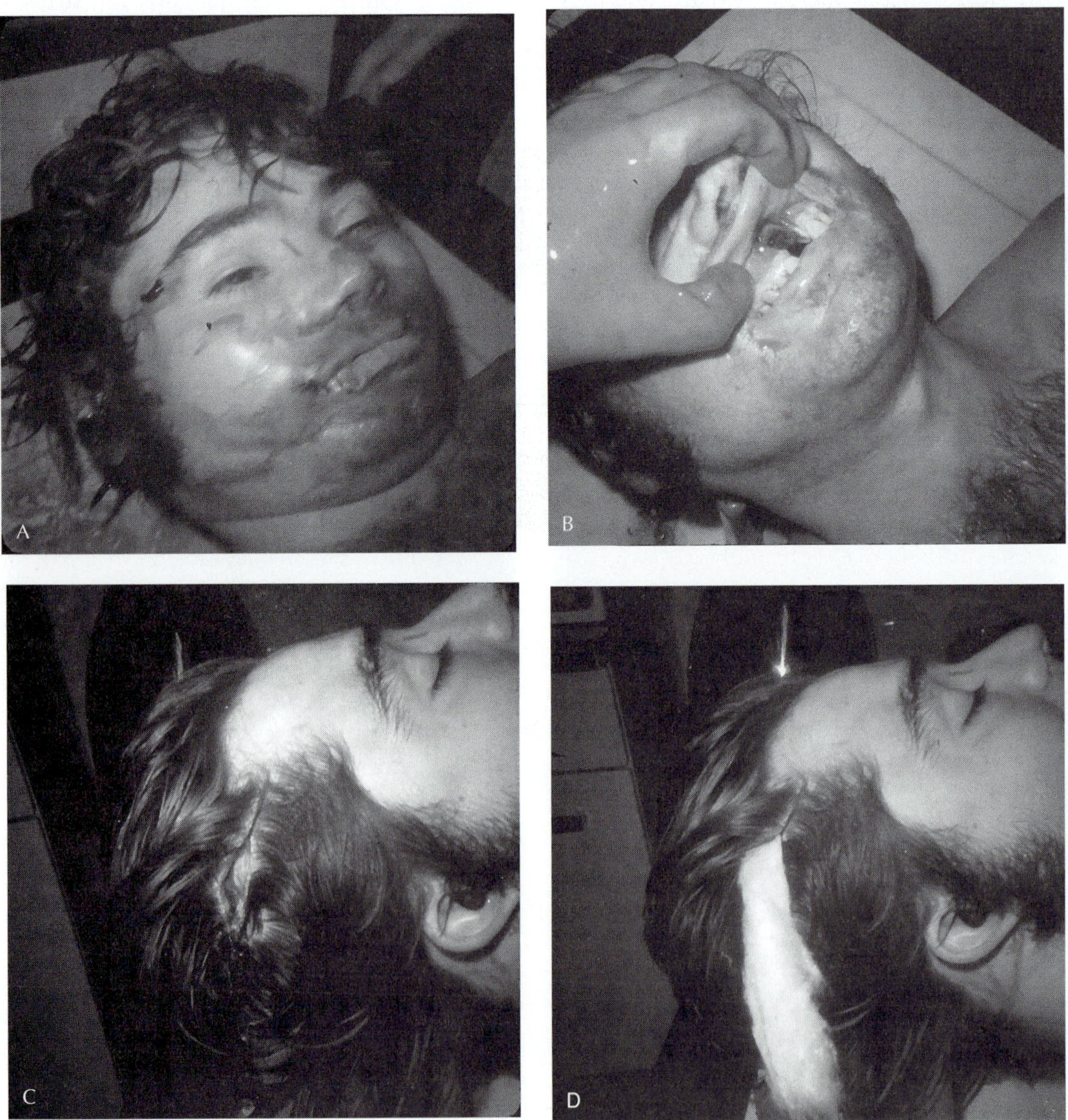

Figure 14. A. Self-inflicted gunshot into mouth; depressed frontal bone (no autopsy). **B.** Midline fracture of the mandible. **C.** Incision made in scalp after embalming. **D.** Depressed frontal bone raised with kapoc.

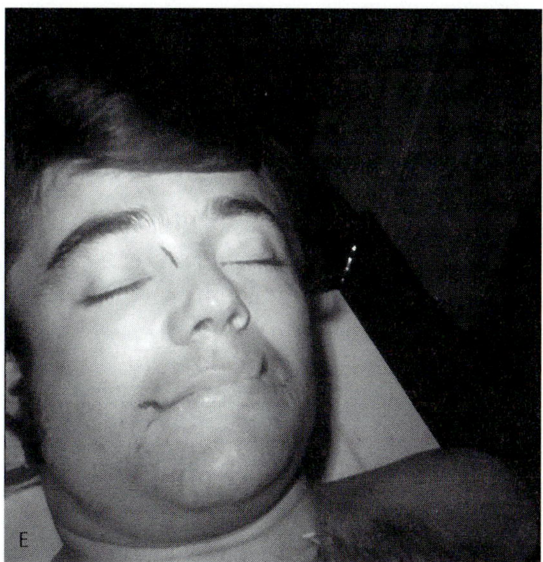

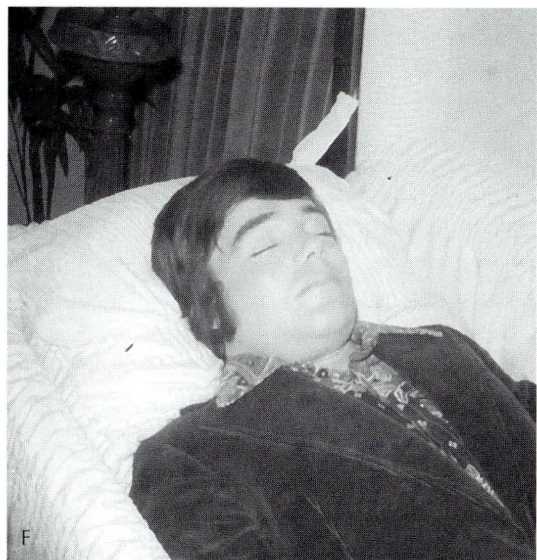

Figure 14 (*Continued*). **E.** Small lacerations waxed, not sewn. **F.** Completed. Instant tissue fixation method of embalming treatment was used.

Treatment—Dehydrated Lips

Wrinkled mucous membranes of the lips is usually caused by dehydration. The lips can become dried in the period before death, in the period between death and embalming, as a result of the embalming, or in the period between embalming and disposition of the body. Depending on the severity of the condition, correction can be made by cementing, tissue building, or waxing. Massage cream, lanolin spray, or a baby oil applied to the lips during the preparation of the body and during the interval between embalming and application of cosmetics will help to delay some drying. During embalming, the application of petroleum jelly or an adhesive emollient cream to the lips may help to gently "pull out" small wrinkles in the mucous membranes. After the embalming of the body the following steps can be taken incorporating all three treatments:

1. Part the lips, then using a spring forceps with cotton, dry the buccal cavity so it is free of all liquids such as blood, arterial solution, or purge.
2. Make any adjustments within the buccal cavity by adding or removing cotton or mortuary mastic to achieve good curvature and projection of the mouth and lips; raise any depressed cheek areas.
3. If the tissues of the mucous membranes or the integumentary lips appear soft and underembalmed, place a thin layer of cotton over the teeth, dentures, or mouth former, and saturate it with undiluted clear cavity fluid. This will serve as an internal preservative compress, and it will remain in the buccal cavity. A surface preservative compress or preservative gel may also be used; these will need to remain in place for several hours. When the compress or gel is removed the tissues need to be cleaned with a solvent and dried before cosmetics can be applied.
4. Clean the lips with a solvent to remove any loose skin or scabs, massage cream, or emollient creams used to hold the lips together during embalming.
5. Observe any broken skin areas on the mucous membranes; these can be dried by placing a small compress of phenol or undiluted cavity fluid over the area for a period of time; or dry them with a hair dryer.
6. Tissue build the mucous membranes and/or integumentary lips.
7. Seal the lips using a small amount of super glue placed behind the weather line.
8. Apply wax if necessary.
9. Cosmetize the face and lips.

If tissue builder is used to restore dehydrated wrinkled lips, inject the upper mucous membrane first inserting the needle from right and left corners of the mouth. Some embalmers prefer to inject from the center of the upper lip at or behind the weather line; it is then necessary to direct the needle in two directions. A third method of rounding out the upper mucous membrane is to insert the needle through the right nostril to inject the left side of the lip and the left nostril to inject the right side. Great care should be taken when filling out the mucous membranes because only a small amount of filler is needed to round them out. A finger placed firmly on the integumentary lip at its juncture with the mucous membrane will help to force the tissue builder into the mucous membrane portion of the lip. When injecting from the corners of the mouth push the needle to the center of the mucous membrane, then carefully inject the filler as the needle is withdrawn. If the integumentary portions of the lips need filling this can be done from the corners of the mouth.

Some wrinkled lips may be corrected by gluing the mouth closed. A super glue is recommended. The glue should be placed behind the weather line of the upper or lower mucous membrane. Be certain the mouth is free of any liquids prior to sealing. The mucous membranes must be cleaned with a solvent so they are free of any moisture or oils before gluing.

Some embalmers prefer to correct wrinkled lips by waxing the lip. They may or may not first seal the lips with glue. The upper lip should be waxed first. It may not be necessary to apply wax to both lips. A cosmetic may be mixed into the wax prior to application, either a "mortuary red" or a lipstick red. The color can also be applied by brush to the lips after they have been waxed. Wax can be smoothed and feathered into the margins of the mucous membranes using a solvent or acetone applied with a small brush.

Treatment—Surface Restorations for Sunken, Crushed, or Eroded Tissues

With each of the conditions listed in the title of this section it will be necessary to establish the form of the area. Sunken and crushed (or depressed) tissues need to be elevated and eroded tissue needs to be replaced. In addition to establishing form it may also be necessary to replace missing skin. Elevation of the tissue may come about during the arterial embalming of the face or hands. Firm massage of an area may help to bring about some swelling. There may be ruptured capillaries in the tissues and leakage of fluid into the tissues could possibly swell the area. It is possible that this could be an advantage for the embalmer.

Tissue elevation can also be done after embalming by tissue builder. If a large area has been crushed or depressed, the nozzle of a mortuary mastic gun can be placed deep into the tissues and the mastic injected to bring about the elevation. Some depressed areas can be corrected, after embalming, simply by application of surface wax. Substitutes for wax might include alternate layers of surface glue and strips of cotton or a layer of mortuary mastic then a layer of surface glue followed by a covering of gauze and then another application (or several) of surface glue.

Replacement of skin can be made with (1) wax, (2) a thick application (with a spatula) of a cream cosmetic, (3) surface glue (several applications), (4) alternate layers of surface glue and cotton, (5) mortuary mastic painted with a surface glue over which a single layer of thin white gauze is placed, then the gauze is painted with surface glue.

Frequently, the angulus oris sulcus will be very long and this can make the mouth look too long. Filling in the sulcus with a surface wax can conceal the depressed tissues. A cream cosmetic can be mixed with the wax or applied over the wax to blend with the surrounding skin cosmetic. Pronounced wrinkles in the lips can be concealed by placing a thin lip wax over the affected area. Tubes inserted into the mouth may leave deep erosion marks on the lateral corners of the mouth. During embalming these areas can be firmly massaged to attempt making the tissues swell. If the tissues do not fill out, after embalming seal the lips with glue, then rebuild the corners of the mouth with a surface restorer wax.

The deep mark of a rope or similar material on the neck following a trauma such as hanging can be treated by placing wax over the affected area. This treatment may need to be done after the body has been dressed and positioned in the casket. If the mark is low enough the clothing may cover the injury to the neck. If it is not, a surface correction may need to be made. This can be done thusly: wax the tissues; cover the depressed tissues with several layers of a surface glue; apply a thin layer of mortuary mastic; coat the mastic with a surface glue; place a thin piece of gauze over the mastic and glue; and paint the gauze with surface glue. Cosmetics can be applied over the wax, or the glue.

Treatment—Autopsied Neck Restoration and Tongue Excision

Several restorative problems are associated with the complete autopsy. If the neck organs have been removed this area will need to be rebuilt. After embalming the autopsied body and prior to suturing, the neck can be filled out using cotton. Frequently the tissues of the neck will lack sufficient preservation. The cotton being used as a filler for the neck area may be saturated with undiluted cavity fluid or preservation gel and tightly packed into the neck area to replace the missing organs. This will serve not only to correct the depressed skin areas of the neck, but will also provide an internal compress for preservation of the tissues. If the tongue has been removed at autopsy, cotton saturated with undiluted cavity fluid, a cautery chemical, or autopsy gel can be inserted through the neck (if the neck organs have been removed) to reach the floor of the mouth, or it can be inserted through the mouth. Tightly pack the oral cavity before arterial injection.

The internal compress assists in preservation and its pressure helps to reduce the loss of embalming solution from severed vessels. The cotton compress within the oral cavity does not have to be removed after embalming. Mortuary mastic could also be used to pack the oral cavity if the tongue has been removed at autopsy, but it is not a preservative.

Treatment—Cranial Autopsy, Temple Area

Mastic compound is a good filler for the temple area when a cranial autopsy has been performed. It will remove the depression formed if the temporalis muscles have been severed or removed. With the calvarium in place fill in the temple areas with the mastic (a soft surface restorer wax could be used as a substitute). Next, replace the scalp over the calvarium. The mastic is easily molded by pressure from moistened gloved fingers. This mastic compound (or incision seal powder) can also be placed along the scalp margins as the closure sutures are made. This will help to prevent any postembalming leakage from the cranial autopsy. The inversion suture is recommended for closure of the scalp incision, beginning on the right side of the head and ending on the left. The following protocol can be followed:

1. After arterial embalming dry out the base of the cranial cavity.
2. Paint the inside of the cavity with a preservative gel.
3. Pack the foramen magnum and the base of the cavity with autopsy compound and cotton to absorb any leakage.
4. Attach the calvarium.
5. Fill the temple areas with mortuary mastic.
6. Paint the outside of the calvarium with an autopsy gel.
7. Place mortuary mastic or incision seal powder along the inside of the scalp as the suturing proceeds.
8. Suture closed using a worm (inversion) suture.
9. The inversion suture, properly done, leaves only a thin line on the scalp surface, which is easily waxed.

Treatment: Infant Cranial Autopsy

A problem with the infant cranial autopsy can be depressions in the cranial surface at the locations of the fontanels. Treat these depressions after embalming by tightly packing the cranial cavity with cotton or other filler material, then filling the fontanels with mortuary mastic compound. This compound can easily be smoothed by simply moistening the gloved fingers with water. The large cartilage segments forming the crown of the head can be held in position by bridge sutures made with dental floss after the cranial cavity is packed. If preservation of the scalp has been insufficient the entire cranium can be painted with a preservative gel before the scalp is reflected back into position for suturing. A suggested protocol follows.

1. After arterial embalming, paint the floor of the cranial cavity with autopsy gel.
2. Place incision seal powder or autopsy compound in the base of the skull to absorb any moisture.
3. Tightly fill the cranial cavity with cotton or similar material.
4. Align the pieces of cartilage into their proper positions and if necessary suture them into position using dental floss.
5. At the fontanels place mortuary mastic over the cotton and blend over the cartilage (a soft surface restorative wax or several layers of thick surface glue may be used as substitute).
6. If the scalp needs additional preservative treatment, paint the inside of the scalp with autopsy gel and reflect the scalp into its normal position. If the scalp appears well preserved a light layer of massage cream can be painted on the inside of the scalp to control dehydration.
7. Suture the scalp closed using thin suture cord or dental floss; an inversion suture is recommended, beginning on the right side of the head and ending on the left; as the suturing proceeds, place incision seal powder or mortuary mastic along the inside scalp margins to prevent leakage (Figure 15).

Treatment—Eye Enucleation Restoration

This restoration is presented in the embalming portion of the text. Please refer to Chapter 18.

▶ ESTABLISHING FORM—REDUCTION OF SWOLLEN TISSUES

Swellings of the face may be general or localized. General swelling of the face may be the result of edema, gasses, or extensive trauma to the facial tissues. General swelling can also be the result of the long-term use of corticosteroid drugs or an allergic reaction. Local swelling may be due to a tumor, disease such as exopthalmic goiter causing the eyes to protrude, or trauma. Distended and discolored eyes are frequently seen in cases of cranial trauma or surgery.

The following list summarizes these antemortem and postmortem causes of swelling.

1. Pathological—tumor, edema
2. Trauma—impact to head or face, surgery

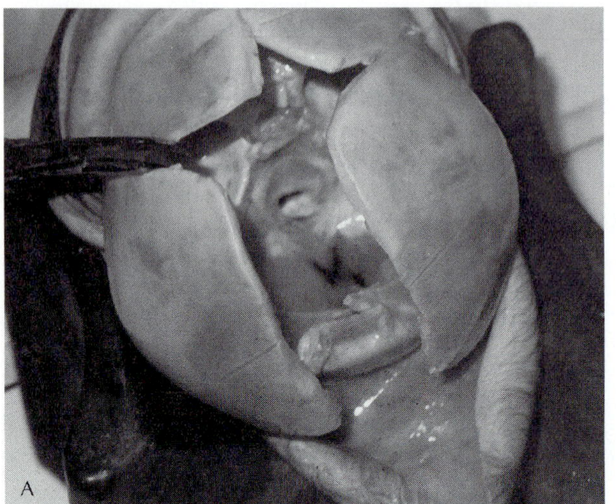

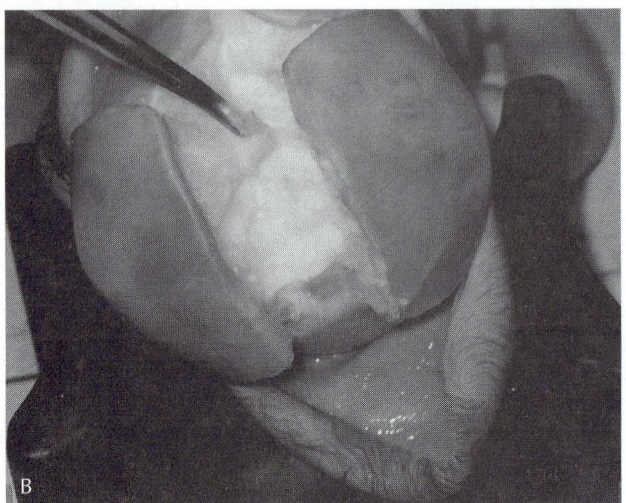

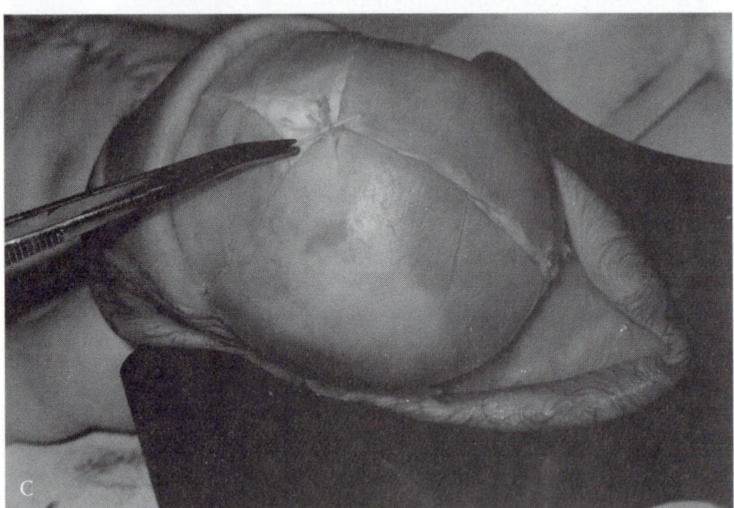

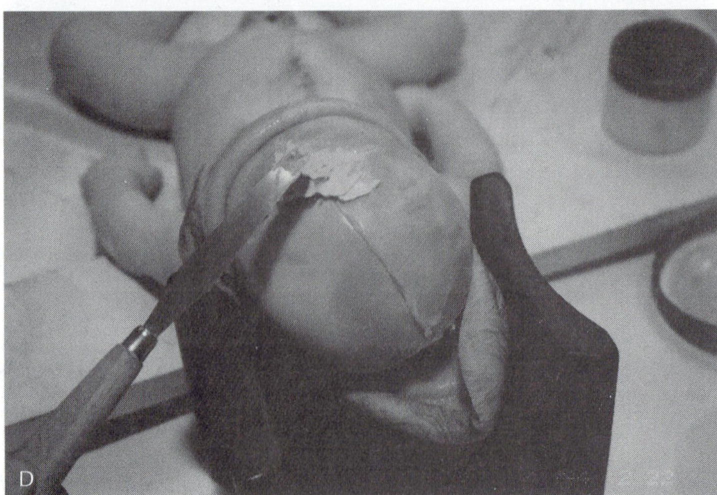

Figure 15. A. Infant skull showing fontanels. **B.** Cranial cavity tightly packed after embalming. **C.** Skull cartilage tied into position. **D.** Fontanels filled with mortuary mastic before suturing the scalp.

3. Decomposition gasses
4. Medical procedures—e.g., tracheotomy, heart-lung procedures (allowing air to enter the tissues)
5. Embalming treatment—poor drainage from the face and neck; overly rapid injection of solution into facial tissues; glandular swelling in the face and neck; escape of embalming solution in areas with broken capillaries as a result of facial trauma

The actual types of distension created by the listed causes can be one or a combination of the following:

1. Liquid swellings—edema, blood, embalming solution
2. Gasses—decomposition, subcutaneous emphysema, true tissue gas caused by *Clostridium perfringens*
3. Solid—neoplasm, goiter, swollen facial glands
4. Semi-solid—pus

The embalmer must first determine the type of swelling before reducing the distended tissue. Restorative treatments for reducing swellings of the face and neck include the following methods. All of these treatments, with the exception of the embalming treatment, are done in the postembalming time period.

1. Embalming treatment—(1) Use of a strong embalming solution (hypertonic), (2) special purpose arterial fluids for edema, (3) dehydrating co-injection fluids. These solutions and fluids are designed to dry moist tissues. Type of swelling reduced: liquids.
2. Gravitation—To move downward from an elevated position. Elevation of a body part (e.g., head or hands) to remove a liquid swelling. Type of swelling reduced: liquids.
3. External pressure—Weight applied to a surface: examples include compresses of fluid or water, pneumatic collar, water collar, small sandbags, elastic bandage, or digital pressure. Type of swelling reduced: liquids, gasses, semi-solids.
4. Channeling—to make passages through tissues for the movement of gasses or liquids. Depending on the body area this can be done with a scalpel, trocar, or large hypodermic needle. May be combined with external pressure, gravitation, or aspiration. Type of swelling reduced: liquids, gasses.
5. Reducing chemicals—Chemicals used to constrict or dry tissues, usually containing phenol or a phenol derivative. May be combined with other reducing techniques such as external pressure, channeling, incising, and aspiration. Type of swelling reduced: liquids, semi-solids.
6. Aspiration—To draw out liquids or gasses by means of suction. This may be done using a large hypodermic needle and syringe or infant trocar and hydroaspirator. It may be done along with channeling. Type of swelling reduced: gasses, liquids, semi-solids.
7. Incise—To make a clean cut into tissue or skin. This would be done with a scalpel, bistury, or hypodermic needle; after incising a localized swelling, pressure would be applied to express or drain the contents. Type of swelling reduced: liquids, gasses, semi-solids.
8. Excise—To remove by cutting. This treatment would be used to reduce a localized area. Type of swelling reduced: solids.
9. Heat—To reduce a localized swollen area by increased temperature. This is done using an electric spatula. It may be applied to the skin surface to restore contour or natural form by drying moist tissues. The skin must be thoroughly coated with massage cream. It may also be applied directly to moist tissues under the skin. Type of swelling reduced: liquids, semi-solids.
10. Wicking—The use of an absorbent material to draw moisture away from an area. The material (e.g., absorbent cotton) is inserted under the skin surface directly in contact with the moisture; the exposed end is outside the surface of the skin. Type of swelling reduced: liquids.

Restorative Treatments for Liquid Swellings

In recent years generalized edema of the face has become a frequently encountered postmortem condition. This condition often accompanies extensive chemotherapeutic drug therapy, cardiac and vascular surgery, and organ transplantation. Diseases causing the axillary lymph nodes to swell or impairment to the vascular circulation of the arm can result in accumulation of edema in the arm and hand. There are several treatments for edema (liquid) swellings.

Embalming treatment—the area affected by the edema can be injected using a concentrated embalming solution. In addition to strong preservative solutions, co-injection chemicals designed to reduce edema can be added. Directions for these co-injections should be carefully followed. Epsom salts can also be used as an additive to the preservative solution to dry tissues where edema is present. When the face is swollen as a result of edema, and the body is not autopsied, restricted cervical injection and continuous drainage is recommended. If the facial edema is recent, e.g., a result of recent surgery, the edema will respond best to this treatment. When the face is swollen as a result of trauma, which may have occurred several weeks before death, these swellings do not respond as well to the chemical embalming treatment. Elevation of the head accompanied by external massage of the face and neck during and following arterial injection will assist in removal of the edema.

Elevation and gravitation—elevation of the head and shoulders will help to gravitate edema from the facial tissues. Elevation of a distended hand after embalming can gravitate edema from the hand into the forearm. Removal of large quantities of edema from the face, hands, or a local area such as the eyelids may result in wrinkled tissues or broad flat areas. This can be seen particularly in the eyelids and hands. With the hands it is prudent to limit the amount of edema removed so the hand looks more presentable. After the edema is removed, tissue building may help restore a more natural appearance to the hands.

For treatment of extreme facial edema some embalmers have taken the embalmed body, placed it on a removal cot, secured the body well with straps, then stood the cot in an upright position. Allowing the body to remain in this erect position for several hours promotes gravitation of the edema from the facial tissues.

Elevation and gravitation can be started in the preembalming time period and continued through the embalming and postembalming treatments. Thorough aspiration of the cavities is important, because this relieves internal pressure from the neck and face. Channeling the neck and the submandibular areas with a trocar by lowering the head and passing the trocar under the clavicles may help to provide passages for the facial fluids to drain into the thoracic cavity. External pressure applied by firm massage, working from the face to the neck, will help to promote drainage of the edema from the face or neck into the thorax. Time is necessary for gravitation to be effective, but when combined with aspiration, channeling, and external pressure, the time period may be shortened. In addition to the above methods after embalming, the embalmer may make a semilunar incision beginning above the center of the right clavicle and extending to a point above the center of the left clavicle. The flap formed can be lifted and the tissues of the neck and lower face channeled using an infant trocar. These channels will provide passage for the edema to the incised area. Cotton can be placed under the flap of tissue which acts as a wick to draw the edema from the face and neck. Several hours time should be allowed for exit of the edema. When completed, the tissues under the flap can be filled with incision seal powder and the incision tightly sutured with a baseball suture or an inversion suture. The incision should be covered with surface glue.

External pressure—generalized facial edema can be treated to a limited degree by external pressure. This can be in the form of weighted compresses (e.g., cotton saturated with diluted cavity fluid) or by firm digital pressure (e.g., a rolling motion of the embalmer's fisted hand, rolling in a downward direction toward the neck). The pressure rolling may be done during injection of embalming solution and would be repeated many times in the postembalming time period. Methods discussed in the previous sections can be combined with external pressure and aspiration of the cavities.

A swollen neck will respond better than the face to external pressure. After arterial injection several devices can be used to put pressure on the swollen neck tissues: water collar, pneumatic collar, or wrapping with an elastic bandage. These external pressure devices should be combined with aspiration of the cavities and channeling of the neck with the trocar passing under the clavicles. If these treatments are not successful surgical excision may be necessary to treat a swollen neck.

Restorative Treatments for Solid and Semi-solid Swelling

Excision (surgical reduction) is usually reserved for treatment of localized solid swellings such as a tumor or swollen glandular tissue, and is sometimes also used to reduce swollen neck tissues. This section discusses the reduction of swellings caused by distended muscles and glands of the neck.

If there is general swelling of the neck and the glandular tissues (parotid, submandibular and sublingual glands) an extensive excision of swollen tissues may be required. Two approaches can be used to accomplish this: method A uses two incisions and method B uses a single incision. These excision reductions are performed in the postembalming time period.

Method A

1. Make a vertical incision on each side of the neck from a point behind and slightly below the ear, directed downward toward the superior border of the trapezius muscle.
2. Using a scalpel, dissect the skin away from the underlying structures in the area of the distension. Work over as far as the median line from the respective sides, upward and in front of the ear, removing the parotid gland if necessary.
3. Excise all structures necessary to return the neck to its normal size and shape. Grasp the tissues with lock forceps and dissect from the lower border of the mandible downward to the clavicle. Remove tissues in layers and avoid removing more than necessary. (Excised tissues

should be retained in a plastic bag, preserved and buried or cremated with the body.)

4. Pack the cavity with cotton saturated with a phenol cautery solution or with undiluted cavity fluid. This will preserve and dry the remaining tissues (Figure 16).
5. Allow at least 1 to 4 hours for chemical action (this will depend on the product used and its concentration), then remove the internal compresses and dry out the pocket with absorbent cotton.
6. Place mortuary mastic compound to help reshape the neck and to prevent leakage; if not available, place incision seal powder within the cavity.
7. Insert a long, straight needle on the left side through the subcutaneous tissues at a point posterior to the angle of the mandible. Direct the needle through the neck. Reinsert the needle in the subcutaneous tissue on the right side at the same position. Direct the needle back through the neck to the original point of entry. Tie the ends of the ligatures tight enough to give form to the angle of the jaw.
8. Suture the incision using an inversion suture. The amount of skin turned under should be proportionate to the amount of reduction that was necessary.
9. The incision is hidden in normal casket repose. To further minimize the possibility of leakage paint the closure with a surface glue.

Method B. Method B involves the use of a single incision. A semilunar incision is carefully made beginning approximately one or two inches above the center of the right clavicle directed downward over the first or

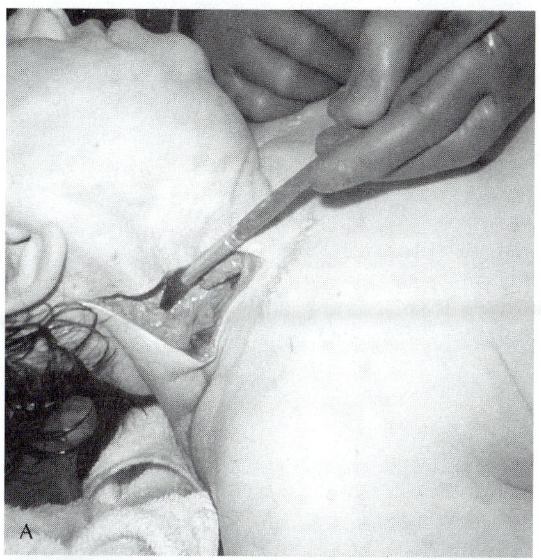

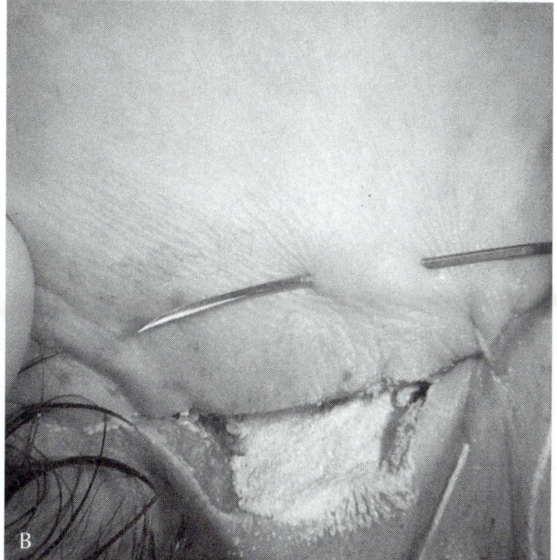

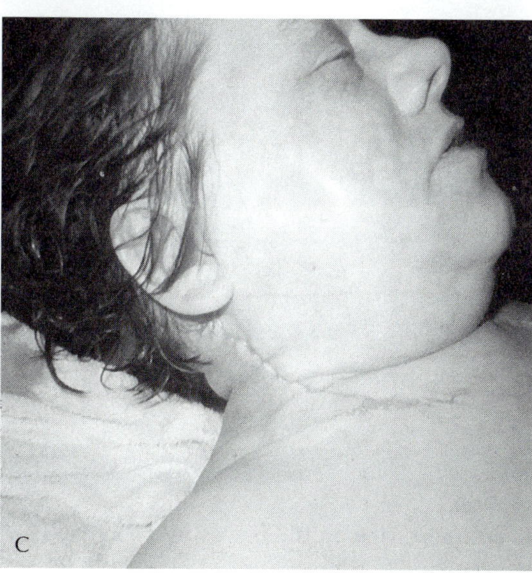

Figure 16. **A.** Surgical neck reduction. Phenol applied after excision of swollen tissues. **B.** Worm (inversion) suture used to roll under excess skin. **C.** Completed reduction, glue applied over incision.

second ribs across the sternum and upward passing through the center of the left clavicle and continuing about one or two inches above the clavicle. This will create a large flap of skin. The skin is carefully dissected from the subcutaneous tissues. The flap is lifted and with a scalpel in an orderly fashion from superficial to deep the swollen muscles and glands are excised (Figure 17). After sufficient tissue is removed the cavity can be packed with cotton compresses saturated with phenol cautery solution or undiluted cavity fluid. These compresses can be left in place from one to four hours. When the tissues appear dry remove the compresses. Insert mortuary mastic compound to re-form the neck. This material will also help to prevent leakage. If the mastic is not available incision seal powder can be liberally spread throughout the cavity. The incision can be aligned using one or two temporary bridge sutures. An inversion suture or a tight baseball suture can be used to close the incision. Coat the incision with surface glue and cover it with a piece of plastic to prevent leakage.

Treatment: Goiter Excision

With permission, after embalming, a goiter can be removed through a semilunar flap incision made from the center of the right clavicle to the center of the left clavicle. Lift the skin flap formed by the incision and dissect through the subcutaneous tissues until the enlarged lobes of the thyroid gland are reached. Using a scalpel or double pointed scissors carefully excise the glandular tissue. If reshaping of the neck is necessary

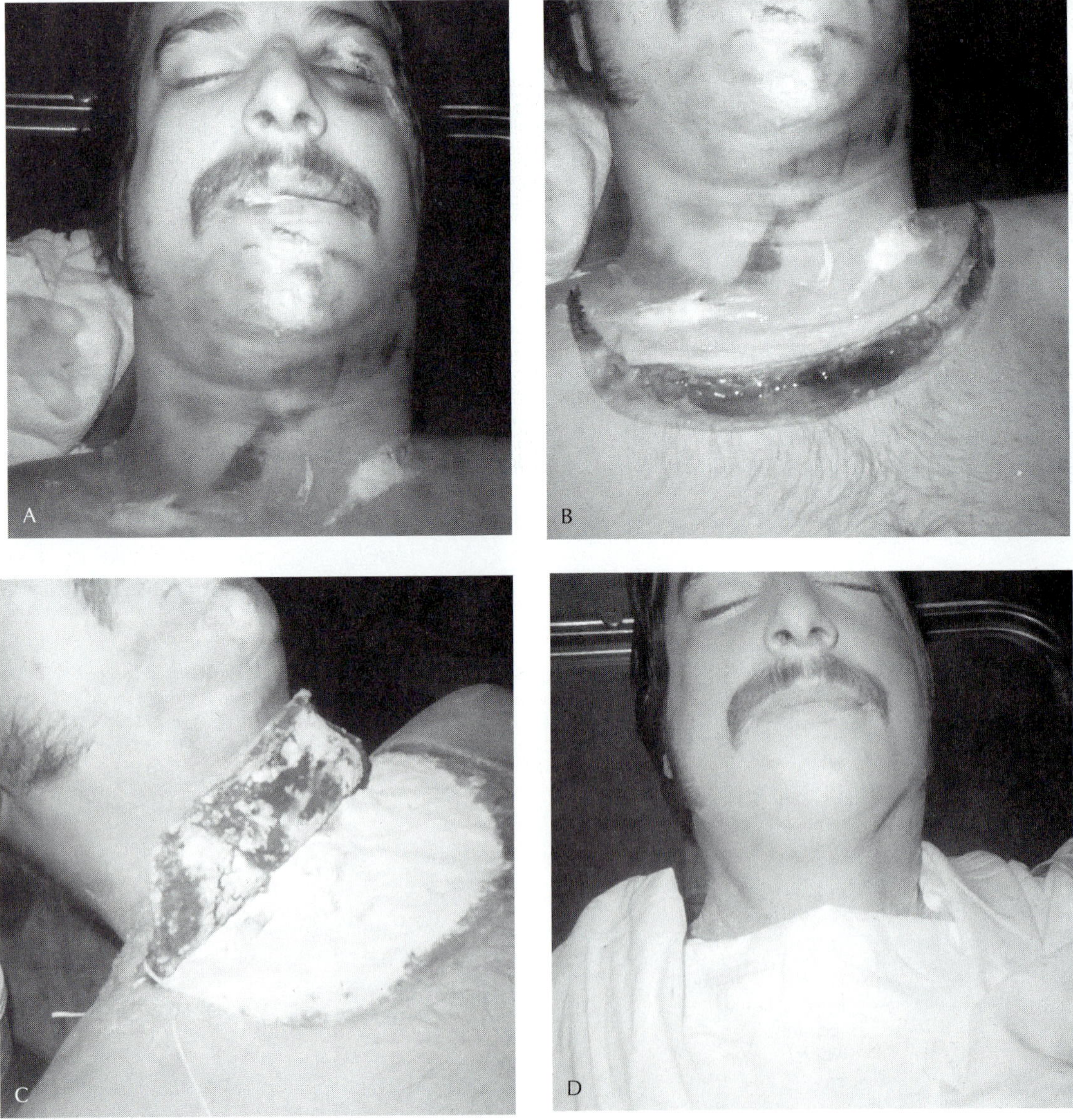

Figure 17. A. Swollen neck, auto accident, no autopsy. **B.** Semilunar incision. **C.** Tissues removed; incision seal powder applied. **D.** Reduced neck.

mortuary mastic compound can be injected into the region where the tissue was excised. The neck can be shaped by light pressure applied to the skin surface. Dry the subcutaneous marginal tissues and apply a liberal amount of incision seal powder or mortuary mastic compound along the margins of the incision. A tight baseball or inversion suture can be used to close the incision. Apply surface glue to the closed incision. If leakage is a concern, place a piece of plastic over the surface glue.

Treatment: Submandibular Swelling

Glandular swelling can be a problem when there is a long delay between death and embalming of the body. There may be a lengthy delay between death and embalming when there is an autopsy. During arterial injection of the head there is frequently a tendency for the glandular tissues to swell (parotid, sublingual, and submandibular glands). Very firm external digital pressure applied immediately following injection will help to reduce the swollen glands. If this is unsuccessful the head can be lowered, and entering through the neck (if the neck organs have been removed) the glandular tissues can be removed or incised using an infant trocar or bistoury, again followed by very firm external digital pressure applied to the swollen tissues. If the swelling remains, a scalpel or bistoury can be inserted up through the neck and the swollen glandular tissues excised. Care should be taken not to pierce the skin. Reshaping of the neck can be done with cotton saturated with cavity chemical.

Treatment: Solid/Semi-solid Reduction by Incising

When the skin surface over a tumor or facial swelling is undamaged and the tumor is in such a position that it can be excised from inside the mouth, this approach should be given first consideration. If skin over a tumor or swelling is broken and discolored it may be best to excise the swelling as well as the damaged skin.

The following protocol was used to reduce a very large growth on the left side of the face in the lateral cheek in front of the ear. The ear was unaffected. When pressed, the swelling did not appear to be solid tissue; it felt like liquid and semi-solid material. The approach for incising, aspirating, and draining was from within the mouth (buccal cavity). Whenever possible, localized tumors of the face should be incised or excised from inside the buccal cavity. This approach leaves the surface skin intact, and any leakage occurs within the mouth and drains into the throat.

1. The body was disinfected, washed, and positioned.
2. The face was shaved and features set.
3. Arterial embalming of the body was performed.
4. The lips were parted and a scalpel inserted into the left cheek wall, puncturing the wall and entering the growth.
5. An infant trocar with the point removed attached to the hydroaspirator, was inserted into the growth through the opening made by the scalpel.
6. The contents of the swelling were aspirated.
7. A long hypodermic needle was inserted through the opening made by the scalpel into the cavity of the collapsed swelling and 3 ounces of undiluted cavity chemical was injected.
8. Thirty minutes were given for the chemicals to work, during which time the cavities were aspirated and injected. The trocar was inserted under the left clavicle from within the thoracic cavity, through the neck tissues, and into the collapsed area of the swelling to provide a drainage channel.
9. The temples and anterior cheek areas were filled with tissue builder.
10. Through the mouth the cavity fluid was aspirated from the collapsed swelling with a blunt infant trocar, and cotton grasped by spring forceps was inserted through the mouth to dry the treated area and the buccal cavity. This was repeated several times.
11. Cotton was placed over the teeth on the left side of the buccal cavity to absorb any accumulated cavity fluid.
12. The excess loose tissues over the collapsed swelling were rolled inward and secured with super glue, giving the appearance of a straight line. An inversion suture using a small circle needle and dental floss joined the two sides of the inverted tissue.
13. Surface glue was painted over the suture and allowed to dry.
14. Opaque paint was lightly sprayed over the entire area of discolored tissues and allowed to dry.
15. Cream cosmetics were applied to the face over the painted area; the face was dried using white talcum powder.
16. Hair spray was lightly sprayed over all areas of the cosmetized face.

Restorative Treatments for Facial Swelling from Gasses

There are three causes for gasses in the body tissues: antemortem subcutaneous emphysema, gas resulting from decomposition, and gas from the growth of the bacterium *Clostridium perfringens,* also known as tissue gas. Gas or air in the tissues tends to move in the postmortem period from the dependent tissues gradually into the more elevated areas of the body. Often these are the upper chest walls, neck, and facial tissues. Methods used to release gasses include incising and channeling combined with external pressure and aspiration. The eyes and mouth should not be sealed with glue until every effort has been made to remove as much gas as possible.

Antemortem subcutaneous emphysema is the presence of air in the subcutaneous tissues, and it often remains in the deceased body. It is brought about by surgery or trauma when there has been a rupture of the pleural sac or an air passageway. It is frequently seen when CPR has been administered and a rib has fractured and pierced a lung or the pleural sac. Patients who die following surgery where a tracheotomy has been performed often exhibit gas or air in the tissues. After death these gasses in the subcutaneous tissues have a tendency to move to the most elevated areas, often the face. Palpation of the affected tissue will move the gas and often a "crackling" sound can be heard as the gas moves. This is called crepitation. The condition can be quite severe and the unsupported tissues of the face and upper chest can be greatly distended. There is no odor, desquamation, or blebs on the skin surface with this condition. The distension does not intensify during the injection of arterial fluid; it is the movement and relocation of the gas which gives the impression that the amount of gas is increasing.

If the tissues of the face and the chest are affected they can be treated with the following procedures.

1. Prior to embalming: Using the common carotid artery as an injection site creates an exit point for gasses in the immediate vicinity. Some embalmers use a semilunar incision made from the center of the right clavicle to the center of the left clavicle. This provides a large opening for the exit of gasses. Applying firm external pressure with the hands moves the gasses toward the incision.
2. Cavity embalming: During aspiration of the cavities the trocar can be directed over the ribs and into the tissues of the chest wall. This channeling will provide passages allowing gasses to move into the abdominal cavity and then be aspirated. Channels can also be made into the tissues of the neck as passages for the gasses to be drawn back into the thoracic cavity. Firm external pressure directing the gas from the face to the neck and chest will help to move the gas into the channels while aspirating the thoracic cavity.
3. Postembalming: The lips can be separated and a scalpel or bistoury inserted to incise the tissues and the buccal cavity. Channels can be made into the anterior and lateral cheek areas to release the gas. Passages for the gas can also be made within the hairline of the temples. From within the nostrils a large hypodermic needle can be inserted to reach the lower eyelids and the inferior orbit. The eyelids can be gently everted and the tissues of the conjunctiva of the lids incised to release gas. Pressure is then exerted to move the gas from the lids to the openings. To prevent leakage cotton can be used to close the eyelids; the cotton can be saturated with cavity fluid to insure good preservation of the lids. If the embalmer wishes, the cotton compresses can be removed after several hours, and the eyes dried and closed with an eyecap and glued.

Gasses from decomposition will also move to the high points of the body, especially the face. Thorough embalming is necessary to arrest the generation of the gas. Restricted cervical injection and use of a strong preservative solution are recommended to achieve the most complete preservation of the face and at the same time control facial swelling. It may be necessary to aspirate the cranial cavity if the body has not been autopsied. This can be done by passing a large hypodermic needle through a nostril and piercing through the ethmoid foramen located in the cribriform plate of the ethmoid bone. Undiluted cavity chemical should be injected after aspiration is completed. This treatment can help stop further generation of gasses in the cranial cavity. Gasses in the cranial cavity can move through the various cranial foramina to enter the facial tissues and create swelling, especially around the eye.

After thorough embalming, including multi-site injection and the supplemental treatments of hypodermic injection and surface compresses, any gasses present in the facial tissues can be removed by the methods previously discussed—incising and channeling combined with external pressure and aspiration. The embalmer may need to re-aspirate and re-inject the cavities several times prior to dressing and casketing the body.

True tissue gas is a rare condition caused by the bacterium *Clostridium perfringens*. The tissues rapidly fill with an immense amount of gas. In only a few hours the face may become unrecognizable. There will be a very strong odor of decomposition, skin blebs will develop, and desquamation will occur. The origin of the gas may be in the dependent tissues, but as with the previous conditions, the gas rapidly moves into the elevated body areas, especially the tissues of the face.

The preparation of a body with true tissue gas necessitates the use of multi-site injection, very strong preservative solutions, special purpose tissues gas fluids, and localized hypodermic injection. After thorough embalming, incising, channeling, and multiple aspiration of the body cavities may be necessary to remove the gasses trapped in the tissues. Incisions should remain open for several hours to allow all gas to escape. All cutting instruments used on the body should be thoroughly sanitized because this bacterium can easily be passed from one body to another. Special care should be taken to disinfect the trocar used to aspirate and inject the cavities of these bodies.

Restorative Treatments for Localized Swellings

Hematoma of the Eye—Chemical Bleaching and Reduction. A large blood discoloration is called an ecchymosis, and when the area is also swollen it is called a hematoma. The discoloration and swelling is caused by an extravasation of blood into the tissues. The most common cause for this condition is trauma. The following treatments can be used to bleach the bluish-black discoloration and reduce the distension. Prior to any treatment of a "black eye" the unaffected tissues of the face should be coated with massage cream to protect them from the effects of the chemicals which will be used. No massage cream should be placed over the discolored tissues (Figure 18A–D).

1. During arterial injection a bleaching chemical or cavity fluid external compress may be placed over the swollen eyelids to retard further distension and begin the bleaching process.
2. After the arterial embalming, a hypodermic injection of a bleaching-cautery agent or undi-

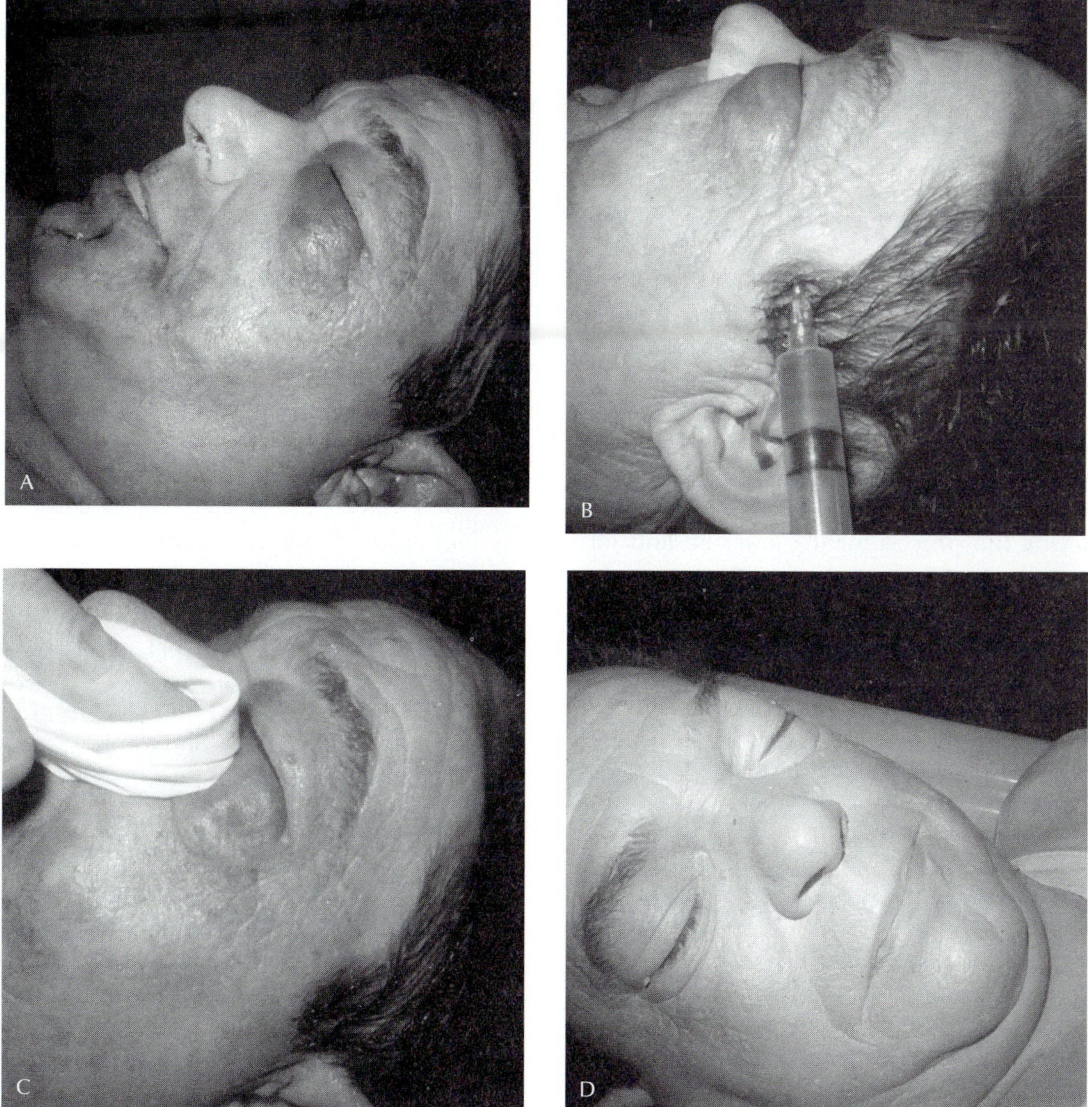

Figure 18. A. Hematoma of the eyelids. **B.** Injection of a phenol cautery agent into the lids. **C.** Firm pressure applied as the phenol solution is pressed out of the tissues. **D.** Completed.

luted cavity fluid may be made directly into the eyelids and affected surrounding tissues. Entry points can include the lateral corner of the line of closure, inner side of the eyelids, eyebrow, and the respective nostril. Insert the needle and in a "fanning" motion make a series of channels through as much tissue as possible. Each time the needle is withdrawn from its furthest point slowly inject the chemical. There will be additional swelling as this is done.

3. About 2 cc of the concentrated chemical can be deposited behind the center of the eyeball. This can be done by inserting the needle at the medial or lateral canthus of the eye and slowly directing the needle along the bony margin of the respective wall until the back of the eyeball is reached. Care should be taken not to puncture the eyeball.
4. Using a cotton compress or webbed cotton pad apply firm pressure to the skin surface where the chemical has been injected and attempt to distribute the chemical under the skin.
5. Using cotton, pose the eyelids, saturating the cotton with the same bleaching chemical or cavity fluid. This places a bleaching-reducing chemical between the eyelids and the eyeball.
6. Allow 30 minutes to one hour for chemicals to work.
7. Remove the cotton from between the lids and the eyeball and replace it with dry cotton to help absorb any liquids.
8. Using cotton or a cloth begin to apply external pressure to the swollen upper lid and supraorbital tissues. Press the chemical and blood out through the points where the needle entered. Repeat this process for the lower lid and surrounding area.
9. If necessary, after as much liquid as possible has been expressed from the tissues, compresses of the bleaching solution or undiluted cavity chemical may again be placed on the lids, especially where they attach to the supraorbital and infraorbital areas, to help establish good form. These can remain in place for several hours.
10. Remove the compresses and clean the lids with a solvent and dry them with a hair dryer.
11. Pose the lids using cotton or eyecaps. The tissues should be quite firm at this point.
12. Seal the lids together with super glue.

Hematoma of the Eye—Heat Reduction and Chemical Bleaching. This treatment uses a heated electric spatula and a bleaching-cautery chemical for restoration of a "black eye."

1. Apply massage cream to the unaffected facial tissues.
2. Prior to arterial injection, place cotton under the swollen eyelids, saturated with a bleaching chemical or undiluted cavity chemical.
3. Apply a cotton compress saturated with the same bleaching chemical or undiluted cavity chemical to the surface of the swollen eyelids. This will help to preserve and bleach the tissues.
4. Embalm the body.
5. Remove the compresses over and under the distended eye.
6. Apply a thick coating of massage cream over the distended eye.
7. Preheat an electric spatula to its maximum setting.
8. Draw the heated blade across the swollen tissues of the lower and upper lids, moving from medial to lateral sides. After each pass, lift the spatula and wipe the blade clean with a dry cloth. The heat will dehydrate the tissues and reduce the swelling. Do not touch the heated spatula to the eyelashes.
9. Repeat the process reapplying massage cream to the swollen tissues each time.
10. Clean the eyelids with a solvent to remove all of the massage cream.
11. Pose the eyelids with cotton or eyecaps and glue eyes shut with super glue.
12. Apply an opaque cosmetic to match the normal complexion coloring.

A variation of this treatment is to apply the electric spatula to the underside of the eyelids to reduce the swelling.

Hematoma of the Eye—Reduction by Excision. A third treatment for swollen eyelids is surgical reduction. In the majority of cases the eyeball proper is not protruding. The capillaries in the eyelids have ruptured and the result is both a distension and a discoloring of the eyelids. The following outline describes a surgical treatment for the reduction of this distension by tissue excision from the eyelids.

1. Apply massage cream to the unaffected surrounding tissues.
2. Apply a cotton compress saturated with a bleaching chemical or undiluted cavity chemical to the distended eyes.
3. Embalm the body.
4. Remove the compresses and elevate the upper eyelid. An incision is made through the conjunctiva, where the eyelid and eyeball meet along its entire length.

5. Using spring forceps, enter the incision and remove the congested tissue from around the eyeball.
6. If the frontal or temporal regions are engorged with blood, channel these areas with a scalpel or large hypodermic needle and massage the free blood toward the incision.
7. Make a series of small incisions along the undersurface of the upper eyelid. Be careful not to cut through the surface skin of the eyelid.
8. Place absorbent cotton or cotton webbing between the eyeball and the upper eyelid and express as much liquid as possible by applying external pressure to the surface of the eyelid. This process can be repeated many times if necessary.
9. Turn back the lower eyelid and make an incision through the conjunctiva along the border of the lower lid and excise the congested tissues.
10. Repeat the incisions along the undersurface of the lower eyelid; do not cut through the surface skin of the lower eyelid. Place dry cotton between the eyeball and the lower eyelid and express as much liquid as possible by external pressure.
11. Place an eyecap over the eyeball and on top place a pledget of cotton saturated with a bleaching chemical or undiluted cavity chemical.
12. Apply compresses externally to aid reshaping. Small compresses of cotton saturated with cavity fluid are tamped firmly into position at the inner and outer corners of the eye, giving a proportionate depth to the corners and creating a convex surface to the closed eyelid.
13. Compresses can also be applied along the attached borders of the upper and lower eyelids.
14. The compresses may remain in place for several hours.
15. Remove external and internal compresses and dry the external lids with a solvent.
16. Pose the lids with an eyecap and/or cotton.
17. Seal the lids with super glue.
18. Apply an opaque undercoat cosmetic to the discolored tissues.

▶ RESTORATIONS FOR SEPARATED FEATURES

Separated lips and eyelids will be considered in this section. Conditions causing separation before and after embalming will be discussed.

Eyelid Separation—Prior to Embalming

Eye closure difficulties can be found in bodies with sunken eyes or the presence of a glass eye. Posing and closure of the eyes can be done prior to, during, or following arterial injection. Where a condition exists making closure difficult, it is best to attempt to close the eyelids prior to arterial injection. First the eyelids should be exercised. This can be done by inserting the rounded handle of an aneurysm needle or spring forceps under the eyelid. Move the instrument under the lids along the attached margins of the lids, and gently raise and stretch each lid being careful not to tear the tissues. After exercising attempt to close the eyelids using cotton or an eyecap to support the lids.

Sunken Eyes. If the body is extremely emaciated the eyes will be sunken deep into the orbits. After the lids have been exercised cotton can be used for eye closure. The cotton will help to raise the eyelids and keep them together. A combination of eyecaps and cotton can also be used: a cap over the eyeball: or a layer of cotton, and a cap on top of the cotton. Sealing (gluing) is usually not done until after the embalming of the body but with sunken eyes it may help to seal the eyelids prior to embalming.

Glass Eye. When a glass eye is present there is frequently atrophy of the eyelids and closure may be difficult. The lids should be exercised and an attempt made to close the eyelids prior to arterial embalming. It may not be possible to raise the eye with a cap or cotton, so simply use the glass eye. To keep the lids closed it may be necessary to glue the lids shut at this time. Using super glue the lids can even be glued directly to the glass eye. In some cases a better closure may be made by removing the glass eye and setting the lids with a cap and/or cotton. If closure is not possible at this time, set the eye after arterial embalming. After embalming the lids can be exercised and if necessary the levator palpebrae superioris muscle and connecting tissues at the attached margin of the upper eyelid can be incised, and this will help to lower the upper lid.

Exophthalmic Goiter. This rare thyroid condition creates a protrusion of the eyes. It may be very difficult to insert any cotton or an eyecap under the lids. It may be necessary to simply seal the lids closed. This could be done prior to arterial injection. If super glue is being used the sealing could be done prior to or following arterial injection.

Eyelid Separation—Postembalming

Eyelids which have separated slightly because of dehydration may be treated by exercising the lids and sealing the free margins with super glue. The super glues adhere better to the eyelids than the rubber-based glues, and they react faster and assure a more secure closure.

Frequently in the case of an embalmed body shipped to a funeral home there has been a delay and the eyelids may show a marked degree of separation, if they had not been glued prior to shipment. The lids can be stretched, and if absolutely necessary the muscle (levator palpebrae superioris) high under the attached margin of the upper lid can be incised and the lid stretched to obtain closure. Closure can be maintained by an application of super glue to the free margins of the lids.

Prevention of eyelid separation can be accomplished by securing the lids with glue at the conclusion of embalming. Massage cream to retard dehydration can be placed under the lids by applying a light coating of the cream to an eyecap. A light coating of massage cream placed on the surface of the eyelids and later the use of cream cosmetics will retard dehydration. Well-embalmed tissue will not dehydrate as fast as underembalmed tissue. If the eyelids, at the conclusion of arterial embalming, appear to have insufficient arterial solution cotton can be used for closure and the cotton slightly saturated with undiluted cavity chemical. The eyelids, after being set, should be sealed with super glue. In several hours the lids and surrounding areas will feel firm and well preserved.

Lip Separation—Prior to Embalming

When teeth or dentures are present and the jaw is elevated to close the mouth, usually the lower lip rests on the inferior margin of the upper teeth. A difficult lip closure prior to embalming is usually caused by physical abnormalities of the jaw or teeth. Lip separation after embalming is more common, caused by dehydration of the mucous membranes or loosening of the wires used for mouth closure.

Disarticulated Mandible

A dislocated jaw can make mouth closure and lip contact almost impossible, caused when the condyle of the mandible has slipped out of the mandibular fossa of the temporal bone. When raising the mandible to close the mouth, the upper and lower teeth do not come into contact. The jaw will be thrust forward and instead of the teeth coming into contact, the lower teeth will be extended outward and actually above the upper teeth. The embalmer needs to take a firm grip on the mandible and attempt to push downward and backward to slip the condyle into the mandibular fossa. Several attempts may be necessary before this is accomplished. The jaw must be put into its proper place before the body is embalmed. When the jaw is in proper position the upper and lower teeth should come into contact or the lower teeth should slip slightly behind the upper teeth. This same relationship should exist when dentures are used. The mouth can now be secured by needle injector or suture. Lip closure should be possible and the lips can be glued after the embalming of the body.

Dental Prognathism

Dental prognathism, or protrusion of the upper teeth, can make lip closure very difficult. A simple method of correction is to:

1. Close the mouth by needle injector or suture.
2. Stretch the lips as far as possible to attempt to bring the lips into contact.
3. Place a strip of cotton over the lower incisor teeth. This should nearly bring the lips into contact.
4. Coat the lips with an adhesive lip cream to hold the lips in contact. If the lips will not stay in contact a rubber-based lip glue or super glue can be applied to hold them in position during embalming.
5. After embalming the lips should be opened to ascertain if the buccal cavity is dry (free of purge material, embalming solution, or blood). Expression adjustments can be made with cotton or a posing mastic.
6. Reseal the lips with glue.

Slight Lip Separation after Mouth Closure

Some embalmers actually prefer to embalm the body with a slight separation of the lips (about the thickness of a nickel). This slight separation allows the lips to round out during the arterial injection. If this is not desired, first check if a needle injector was used to close the mouth. If it was, be certain the head of one or both needle injector barbs is not placed on the gum where the inner mucous membrane of the lip joins the gum. If so, the head of the barb may be pulling on the mucous membrane and not allowing the lips to come into contact. Using a hemostat pull the mucous membrane over the head of the barb. This will give more extension to the lip. An adhesive lip cream will assist in holding the lips together.

Lip Separation—Postembalming. A slight separation of the lips can be corrected by one of the following treatments:

1. The lips should be parted and using cotton attached to spring forceps, thoroughly dry the buccal cavity. In addition to assuring dryness of the cavity, the cotton passed over the inner tissues of the lips will help to exercise them. After the buccal cavity has been dried and the lips ex-

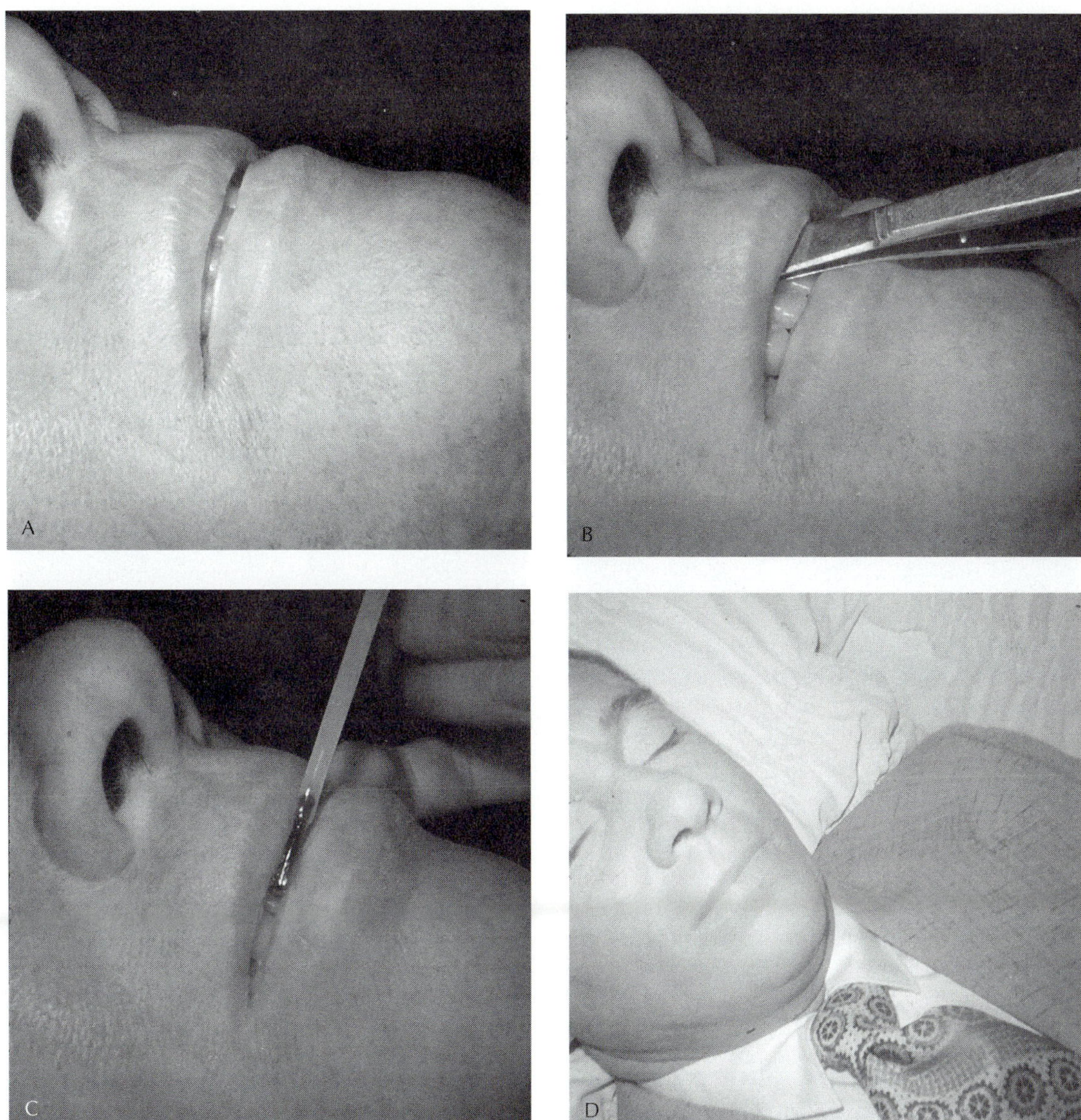

Figure 19. A. Slight lip separation in a body shipped by air. **B.** Lips exercised with the handle of forceps. **C.** Glue applied. **D.** Completed.

ercised, if the separation is small an application of super glue just behind the weather line should firmly seal the lips together (Figure 19A–D).

2. Inject tissue builder into the upper mucous membrane to expand the lip sufficiently to make contact with the lower lip. It may be necessary to tissue build both the upper and lower mucous membranes to bring the lips into contact.
3. A third treatment for closing small separations is to apply a thin layer of wax to the upper mucous membrane. If there is sufficient separation both mucous membranes may need to be waxed.

Of the three methods described, securing the lips with super glue is generally the simplest and most satisfactory treatment. Some embalmers may want to combine two of these methods, e.g., tissue building one or both mucous membranes followed by gluing of the membranes.

▶ RESTORATIONS FOR BROKEN TISSUES

In this section treatments for deeply torn or disconnected tissues in visible areas of the head, face, neck, arms, and hands are discussed. Examples include trauma such as lacerations, compound fractures, and penetrating wounds; visible surgical incisions and tracheotomy; and postmortem treatments such as the autopsy scalp incision and visible incisions related to embalming treatments. Small lacerations and surgical incisions of the eyebrow, eyelids, surrounding orbital tissues, and laceration of the lips are included in this section.

There are three objectives for performing these restorative treatments: 1) to realign and keep aligned the severed margins of the wound or incision, 2) to prevent any leakage from the wound or incision, because leakage could loosen and possibly free any cosmetic or wax treatment over the problem area, and 3) to hide the presence of the wound or incision by making the skin surface and contour appear natural (Figure 20A–D).

The separations discussed in this section are cuts extending deeper than the skin level. Three treatments are used to close these separations: suturing, gluing, and waxing. These treatments are generally done in the postembalming time period. A suggested sequence of treatment is as follows:

1. Using a moist cloth or moist cotton carefully clean blood and debris from the cut and the surrounding tissues; use thick gloves if glass shards are present.
2. After cleaning the wound, evaluate the depth and extent of the separated tissues, apply massage cream to the surrounding unaffected tissues, and excise dehydrated margins.

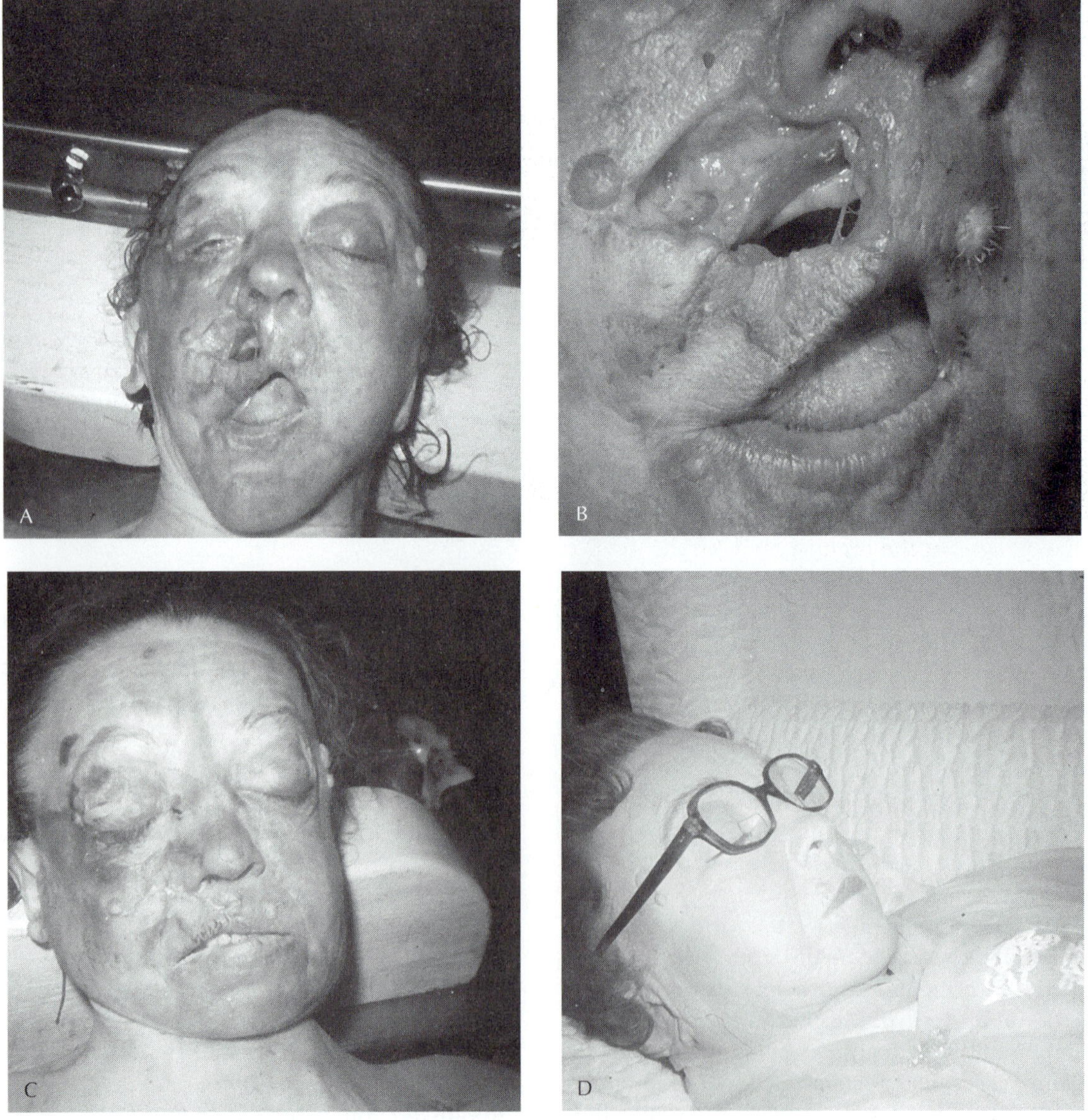

Figure 20. A. Deep laceration of cheek and hematoma of both eyelids. **B.** Deep laceration of cheek. **C.** Following embalming, laceration is sutured. **D.** Laceration waxed; eyes reduced by injection of phenol; discolorations undercoated before cream cosmetics were applied.

3. Align bony tissues if necessary.
4. Align deep tissues and suture into position using individual bridge sutures.
5. From within the wound hypodermically inject the walls using a cautery chemical or undiluted cavity fluid. A compress saturated with the same chemical can be placed between the separated tissues.
6. Align the surface margins using individual bridge sutures of dental floss.
7. Embalm the body.
8. Check for thorough preservation and dryness of the tissues, and if inadequate renew compresses.
9. Remove the compresses and clean the wound with a solvent. A hair dryer or electric spatula can be used to dry the walls of the wound.
10. Place incision seal powder or a thin ribbon of mortuary mastic into the deep areas of the wound.
11. Close the wound:
    a. Using a single or double intradermal suture
    b. Using an inversion suture, if excess skin is present
    c. Using a small baseball suture made with dental floss, which can be covered with wax or surface sealer
    d. Using subcutaneous sutures placed about $\frac{1}{4}$ inch below the surface of the wound and super glue to close the skin surface
    e. If the wound is not too deep seal edges with super glue
    f. If the deep wound is small enough and suturing may cause the skin to "pucker" (e.g., small lacerations of the eyelid or lip) fill the separation with a surface restorer wax
12. Replace surface skin:
    a. If the laceration or puncture has been waxed, simply blending the wax into the surrounding area will cover the problem area. Cream cosmetics can be mixed into the wax or applied over it to blend in with the surrounding intact tissues. Apply white drying powder and using the powder brush "stipple" lightly over the waxed areas to reproduce the pores of the skin.
    b. If the laceration or puncture was closed with super glue or sutured
        i. and the area is discolored, spray or paint an opaque undercoat over the discolored area and the glued laceration or puncture. Once dry, make a wax adjustment along the laceration or puncture and blend the wax into the surrounding tissues. Cream cosmetics can be applied over the wax.
        ii. and the area is not discolored, apply several thick layers of surface sealer over the laceration or puncture. Allow the sealer to dry and apply cream cosmetics over the sealer and the surrounding tissues.
        iii. and the area is or is not discolored apply a transparent or opaque cosmetic, and dry the cosmetic with a white drying powder. Apply a thin layer of matching surface restorer wax over the margins of the laceration or puncture and gently feather the wax into the surrounding areas. Powder can again be applied over the wax in a "stippling" fashion to give a porous effect to the wax (Figure 21A–E).

Autopsy Scalp Incision

First the base of the cranium needs to be dried and packed with an absorbent material. The calvarium may need to be anchored to the skull, and this can be done by suturing or with calvarium clamps. An inversion suture can be used to close this incision. Linen thread is stronger than cotton thread, and a 7-twist linen suture thread is strong enough that the thread does not have to be doubled. The suturing should begin on the right side of the head and end on the left side. If the incision is not uniform (e.g., a right angle second incision is present at some point along the autopsy incision) it will be necessary to align the margins using temporary bridge sutures before the primary autopsy incision is closed. A small baseball suture could substitute for an inversion suture. Tie the first stitch into position rather than relying on a knot to anchor the ligature.

Compound Fractures

Compound fractures should be realigned before arterial embalming. Rigor is often present in trauma cases and this needs to be manually broken up before the fractured bone is placed back into its correct position. It may be necessary to temporarily hold the bones into position during arterial embalming. This can be done by placing a bandage of gauze or strips of cloth over the area to hold the bones in position until the tissues firm. To reset the bones it may be necessary to use a flat bladed instrument to force the bones into re-alignment. The blade is placed between the fractured ends of the bone and used to forcefully retract the ends of the bones into alignment. After the bone is reset and the body embalmed the broken skin can be sutured. The 12-step protocol outlined above can be followed (Figure 22).

Lacerations and Surgical Incisions

Conditions associated with trauma and surgical procedures are widely variable. The embalmer must see the existing conditions before a treatment plan can be

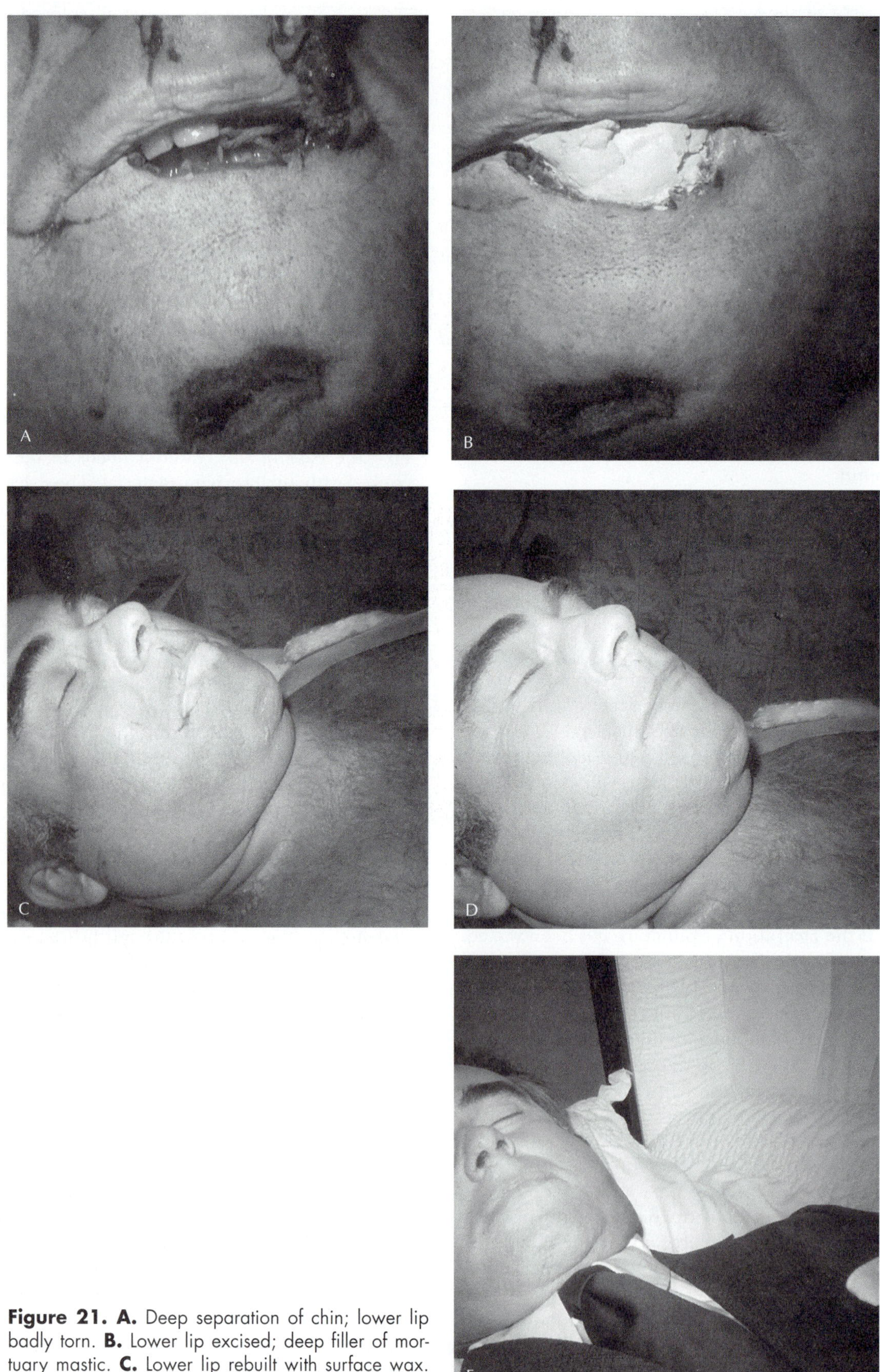

Figure 21. A. Deep separation of chin; lower lip badly torn. **B.** Lower lip excised; deep filler of mortuary mastic. **C.** Lower lip rebuilt with surface wax. **D.** Chin waxed; lip color applied. E. Completed.

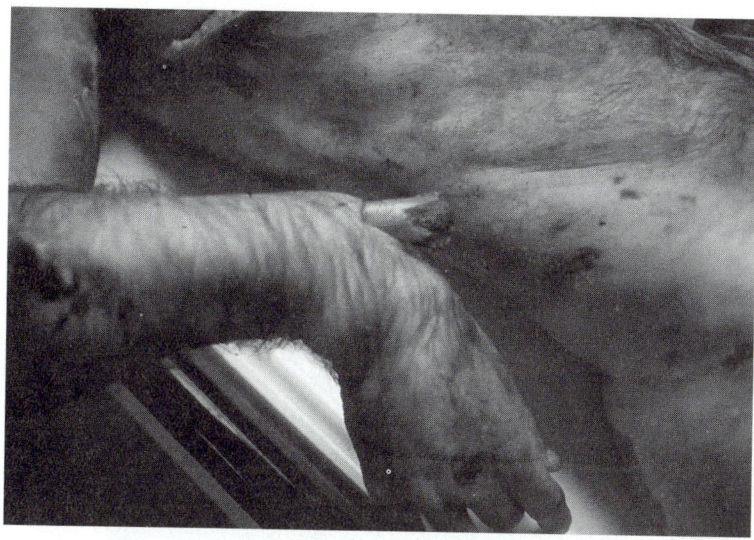

Figure 22. Compound fracture of the wrist.

made. It is important that the marginal tissues be re-aligned prior to embalming. For this reason, surgical staples and sutures should remain in place until arterial embalming is completed. The staples can be removed by grasping them, one at a time, in the center with a hemostat and with a right to left motion of the instrument they can be freed. Surgical sutures, if they are thin enough and there is no leakage from the incision, can be left in place and the incision covered with wax or with a surface sealer. Cosmetics can be applied over the wax or sealer. If there is any concern about leakage, after embalming the surgical sutures can be removed, the incision cleaned, cautery chemicals applied, the incision dried and sealed with super glue or re-suturing, and surface treatments performed as previously outlined.

Tracheotomy

Restorative treatments for the tracheotomy should be done after arterial and cavity embalming is completed. About 2 ounces of a cautery chemical or undiluted cavity fluid can be gently poured or injected into the tracheotomy opening. This will help to disinfect and preserve any materials in the air passageways. The passages can be filled with incision seal powder or mortuary mastic to help prevent any leakage. Finally the tracheotomy can be tightly packed with cotton to almost the surface of the skin. A final layer of incision seal powder or mortuary mastic can be applied and the incision closed by suturing. The suture can be covered with surface sealer glue or wax to hide the sutures. If the tracheotomy has been present for a length of time the edges will appear very firm and slightly swollen. Suturing will not be possible because the margins cannot be drawn together and the tissues easily tear. The aperture can be closed after the opening is packed as described above by (a) waxing over the opening with a surface restorer wax; (b) alternating strips of cotton or webbed cotton with surface sealer glue; or (c) applying several layers of a thick surface sealer glue.

Penetrating Wounds

These wounds are defined as deep wounds which penetrate an organ or cavity. Because these trauma wounds are so variable it is necessary to view the body and the damage produced by the wound. A penetrating wound could be as small as the entry point for a small caliber bullet or a thin bladed knife. With shooting victims both entry and possibly exit wounds must be evaluated. Frequently the exit wound damages more tissues than the entry wound. The coroner or medical examiner may also enlarge these wounds if the tissue surrounding the wounds is excised for use as evidence. Most of these wounds would be cleaned and packed with a cautery chemical in the preembalming time period. After arterial and cavity embalming the wound can be filled with incision seal powder or mortuary mastic to prevent leakage and closed by suture or super glue. If the margins of the wound cannot be drawn together the wound can be filled with: 1) a surface restorer wax, 2) mortuary mastic then covered with surface sealer glue, gauze, and another coating of sealer, or 3) filled with alternate layers of sealer glue and cotton (Figure 23A–E).

If the penetrating wound involves the cranium and if no autopsy was performed it may be necessary to aspirate the cranial cavity to evacuate any blood or fluids which may have accumulated there during the arterial injection. A small trocar can be inserted through the wound or the nostril. The injection of several ounces of undiluted cavity fluid or cautery chemical into the cranium will help to assure good preservation of the contents of the cranial cavity. It is very important to seal the portion of the wound penetrating the bone. This may be done with a trocar button, cotton saturated with plaster of Paris, mortuary mastic, or packing with cot-

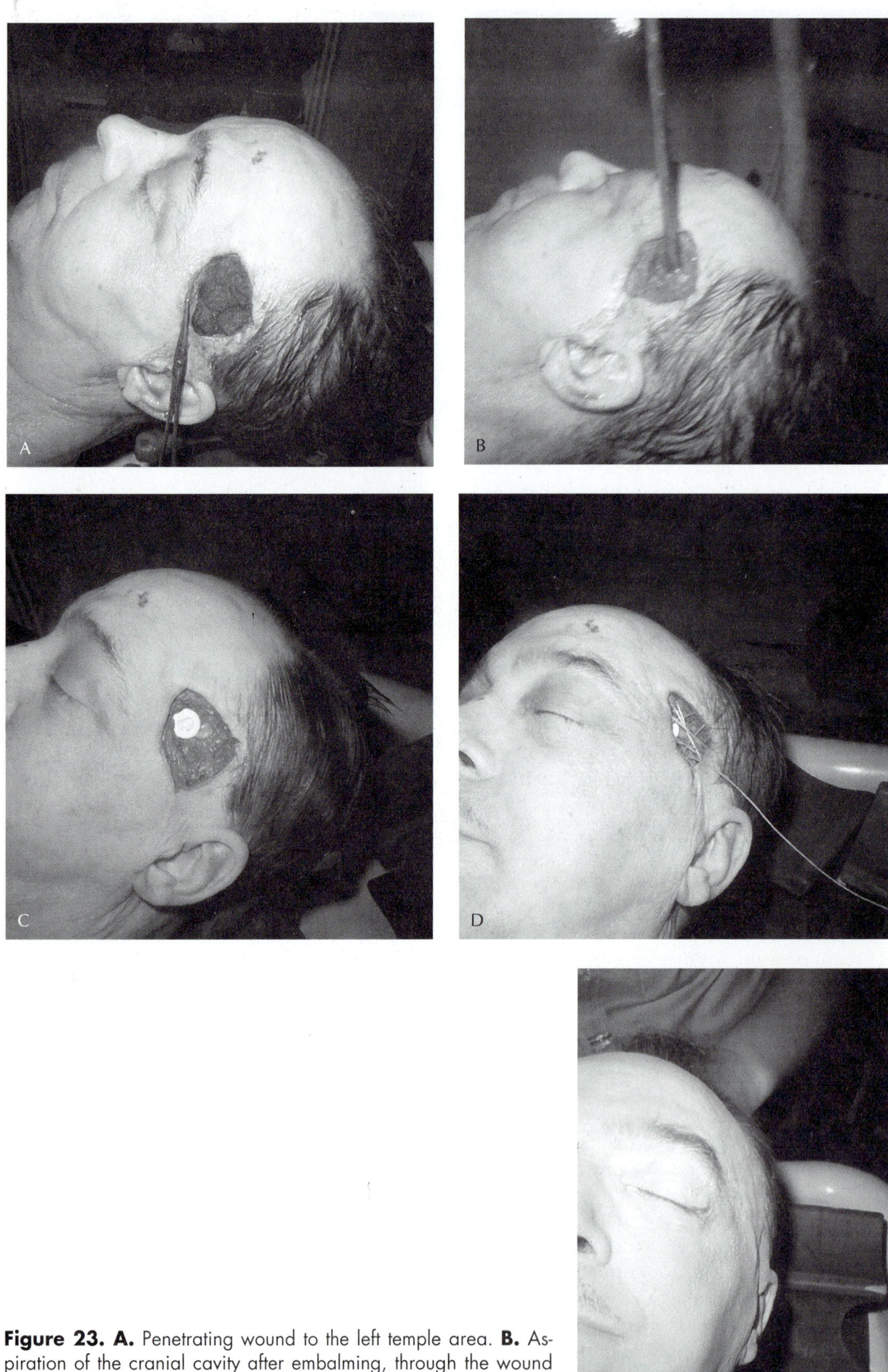

Figure 23. A. Penetrating wound to the left temple area. **B.** Aspiration of the cranial cavity after embalming, through the wound entrance. **C.** Trocar button used to close wound to the cranium. **D.** Basket weave suture applied. **E.** Area waxed.

ton. Hair replacement may be necessary with a penetrating cranial wound. Often hair can be taken from the back of the scalp and attached over the visible wound area using rubber cement or wax for attachment. A hair patch can also be cut from a matching wig. If this is done, cut the material to which the hair is sewn to a size that will cover the wound. Using super glue attach the piece of wig to the scalp. The attached hair can then be combed into the surrounding natural hair.

Small Laceration or Surgical Incision of the Lip or Eyelid

The suturing of a small laceration or surgical incision may cause a puckering of the skin. It may be best to let the small disconnected tissues dry and then wax over the separation with a surface restorative wax. These separations can be dried by heat or with chemicals. Air drying and the use of a hair dryer may sufficiently dry the tissues that wax can easily be applied over the small wound.

▶ HAIR TREATMENTS

The widespread use of chemotherapeutic and radiation treatments has greatly increased the number of bodies where cranial hair is absent. Today, very natural looking wigs and toupees are available at relatively low prices. Often in life, the individual undergoing these treatments has already made use of these cosmetic hair replacements. These hairpieces can be styled by a hair-

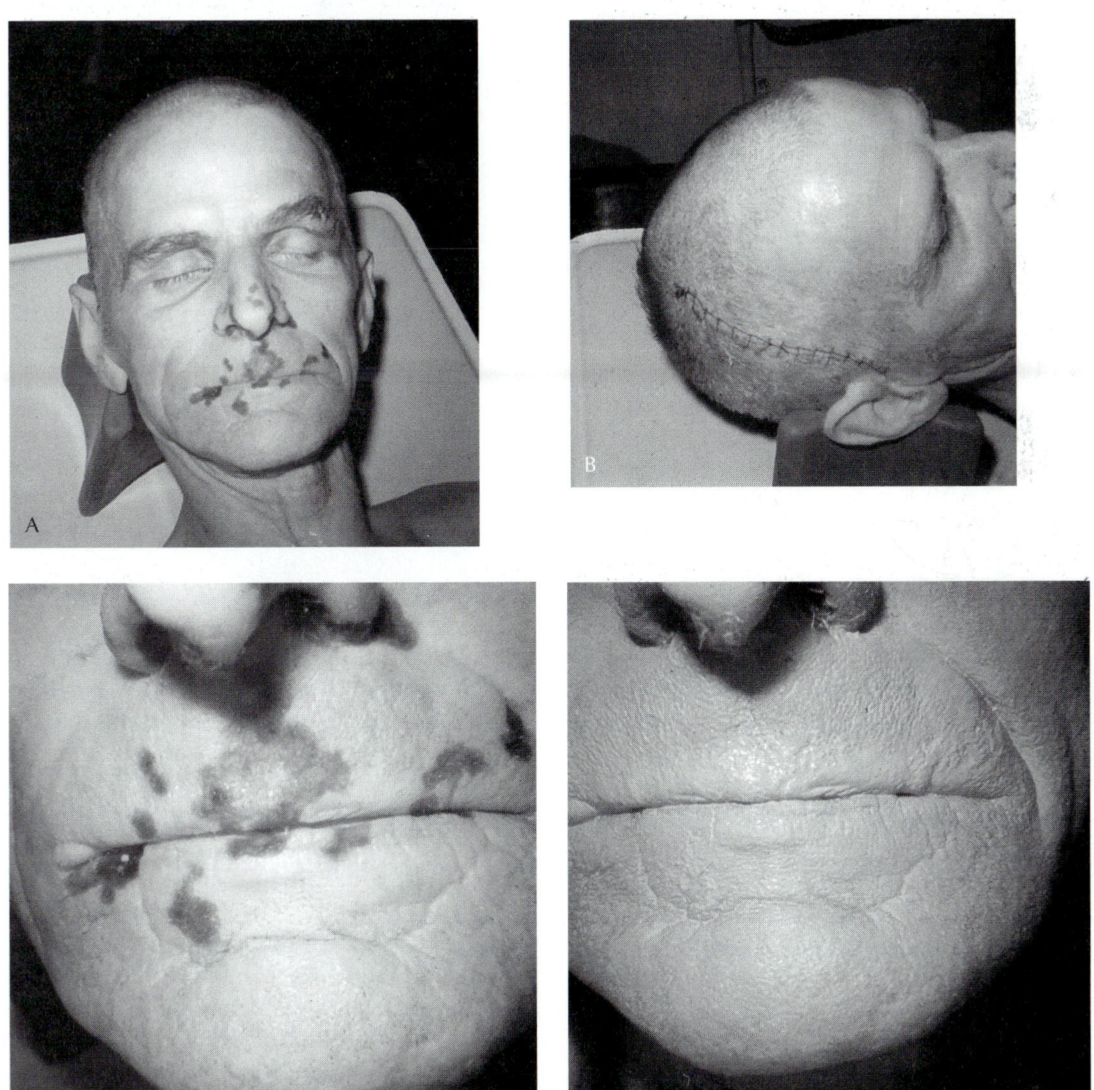

Figure 24. A. Crainotomy performed; vitamin B deficiency—note lesions around mouth. **B.** Craniotomy, right side. **C.** Mouth lesions. **D.** Lesions undercoated. (*Continued.*)

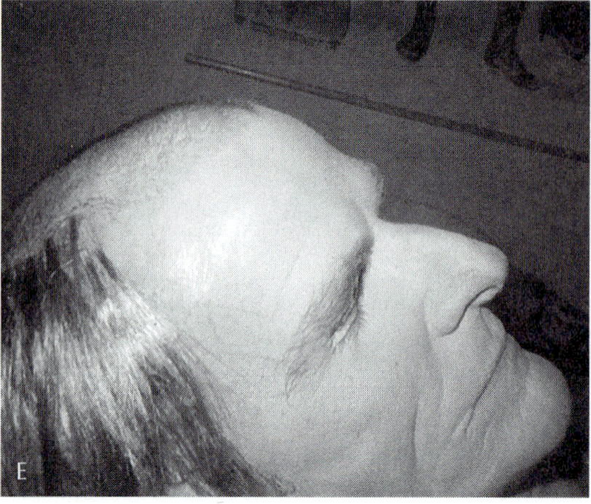

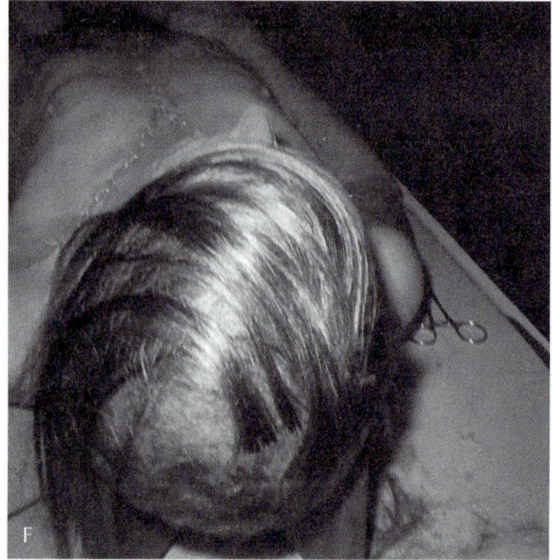

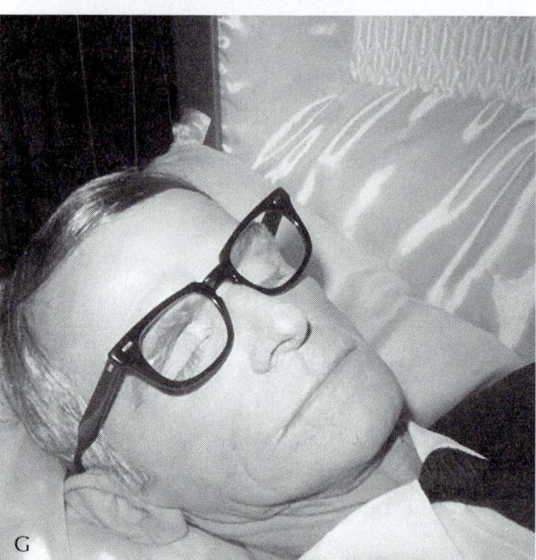

Figure 24 (*Continued*). **E.** Sideburn rebuilt using rubber based glue for attachment. **F.** Cranial hair attached. **G.** Completed.

dresser or barber and easily attached by the embalmer. The cranium should be thoroughly washed and sanitized during the embalming process. After embalming the cranium can be wiped with a solvent to insure the removal of all oils. The wig or toupee can be placed on the head and if necessary held in position using drops of super glue on the cranium. If a wig or toupee is not available, a scarf or bandage could be used for women and a bandage or a hat for a man. For infants a bonnet might be used.

If the left side of the cranium has been shaved, position the deceased straight—do not turn the head to the right, and comb some of the hair along the center of the cranium to the left to cover some of the nude scalp. A wig can also be cut and attached with super glue on the left side of the cranium, trimmed, and the wig and remaining hair blended together (Figure 24A–G).

When hair replacement is necessary it may be possible to use hair from the back of the deceased's head. The skin surface must be clean, so use a solvent such as trichloroethylene to remove all oils and debris. Short stubble need not be shaved; often it can aid in making a good attachment. A wig, toupee, or skein of artificial or real hair can be used as a hair source. Attachment can be made using rubber cement, hot wax, or surface restorer wax. Rubber cement makes the firmest attachment. As with most restorative work, use the least amount of hair necessary for each hair patch, because it makes for a much better attachment. Place the hair ends to be attached over the glue or wax, then with a rounded instrument press the patch ends into the wax or glue and roll the instrument away, because lifting it may pull the hair and the attachment material away. Overlaying of the hair patches is usually necessary: eyebrows would be rebuilt from lateral to medial; sideburns would be rebuilt from inferior to superior; and cranial hair would be rebuilt in the opposite direction of its growth. Rebuilt hair restorations are trimmed and thinned after all attachments are completed.

Eyebrows and eyelashes can often be corrected by lightly drawing them in using a brown eyebrow pencil. Moisten the point of the pencil and lightly sketch in the missing hair. Often this will give the illusion of the presence of hair. A moustache can also be thickened with the use of an eyebrow pencil. Artificial eyelashes can be purchased, but they usually need to be slightly trimmed. They will need to be inserted under the free margin of the upper eyelid prior to gluing the eyelids closed. Eyelashes can also be constructed by attaching hair to a plastic eyecap which has been cut in half. Glue would be placed along one of the free margins of the cap and the hair attached. The cap is then inserted deeply under the upper eyelid.

Details for the construction of full heads of hair, beards, moustaches, eyebrows and eyelashes can be found by consulting publications on stage and theatrical makeup.

▶ BIBLIOGRAPHY

Embalming Course Content Syllabus. American Board of Funeral Service Education; 1996.

Johnson, Edward C. *Restorative Art,* Worsham College of Mortuary Science: Chicago, IL; circa 1955.

More Thoughts on Postmortem Restorations, No. 434. Champion Expanding Encyclopedia, Springfield, OH: The Champion Company; February 1973.

Prager, G. Joseph, *Manual of Postmortem Restorative Art.* Cincinnati, OH; 1965.

Principles of Restorative Art, No. 428–433. Champion Expanding Encyclopedia, Springfield, OH: The Champion Company; June 1972–January 1973.

Restorative Art Course Content Syllabus, American Board of Funeral Service Education; 1998.

Strub, Clarence G. *The Principles of Restorative Art,* 2nd ed. St. Louis, MO: The Embalmers Monthly, July 1933.

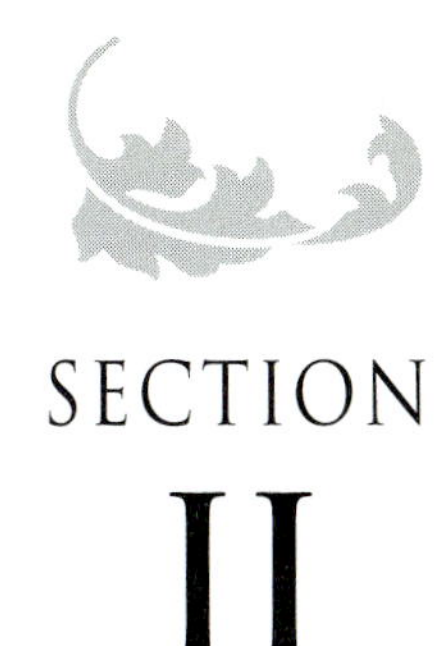

Mortuary Cosmetology

C. Richard Sanders

SECTION II

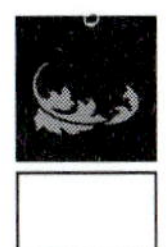

PRELIMINARY PROCEDURES

This section on mortuary cosmetology will study the procedures used to establish a receptive cosmetic surface foundation and the methods and materials used in the technical application of postmortem cosmetics. When preparing the body for viewing, our main objective is to create a natural illusion of peaceful repose. This memory image is achieved through use of well developed cosmetic skills.

If we deny the family the opportunity to view the dead body, it may be difficult for them to accept the reality of death, particularly if the death was sudden or from traumatic injuries. It also makes it difficult for the family and friends to understand the full value of the funeral ceremony. The illusion of repose derived from purely mechanical cosmetic procedures cannot mimic the natural appearance that we associate with the living.

The over-application of cosmetics causing an artificially made-up appearance and the use of a single type of cosmetic for all cases are the primary reasons for the negative attitude towards viewing and embalming. The rising number of bodies being placed under refrigeration is creating technical problems concerning the professional care of the unembalmed body. The body placed in the funeral home refrigerator should receive the same considerations as the body to be arterially embalmed. Pre-refrigeration treatments are as essential as pre-embalming treatments.

▶ BASICS OF MORTUARY COSMETOLOGY

Attaining perfection in mortuary cosmetology depends that a high degree of attention be given to disinfection, cleansing and pre-cosmetic surface treatments. Cosmetic flaws and factors governing control over facial characteristics can best be corrected during the pre-cosmetic surface preparations. Epidermal conditioning is the primary step in establishing a stable, receptive cosmetic surface foundation. Treating the face and hands with an emollient cream will have a positive effect to facilitate application of postmortem cosmetic media. It is recommended that the embalmer use cosmetics formulated to restore and replace the natural color of the living. Successful mortuary cosmetology depends on the following fundamental factors:

1. Understanding of the role memory-image plays in alleviating the trauma of bereavement.
2. Effective employment of cosmetic coordination of arterial embalming, refrigeration, and use of surface cosmetics.
3. Familiarity with the tactical uses and blending characteristics of complexion colors.
4. Complete knowledge concerning the properties, uses, and limitations of various cosmetic types.
5. Development of manual dexterity and artistic creativity which are the driving forces behind all fine craftsmanship.

▶ VALUE OF PHOTOGRAPHS

A photograph of the deceased is an invaluable reference to have on hand when cosmetically treating the face and hands. Analysis of facial characteristics in the photograph will give the embalmer a better understanding of how to apply the toning cosmetics in accentuating the predominant facial lines and natural markings. If it becomes necessary to totally mask the entire epidermal surface of the face and hands, the photograph of the subject will become an essential aid in accurately duplicating the natural lines and markings on the opaque skin surface. Two or three recent photos of the deceased, selected by the family, are considered the best reference for comparison between the facial features in life and the features seen after death. It is important to find out the dates the photos you plan to use were taken, and avoid using older pictures. During the advancement in age the contours of the facial features continually change and this aging process can easily be seen in a series of photos made over a period of years. Avoid using a retouched "vanity photo" as a guide. Commercially produced portraits make the subject appear artificially more youthful and erase the age and character lines needed in establishing a true-to-life appearance. Recent pictures also give the hair stylist valuable information in grooming the hair for both men and women. Examination of the photos under magnification often reveals character lines, wrinkle details, and natural markings invisible to the naked eye.

Care of Photographs

Pictures of the deceased are of great value to the family, particularly professional portraits, which may be irreplaceable. These pictures can easily to soiled or damaged if they are not protected. Place them in a clear plastic insert of the type used in photograph albums to protect them from damage. Also, by placing smaller photos in the plastic insert, they can be arranged together in a logical sequence of different views and can be referred to more easily than they would be separately (Figure 1).

▶ PRE-COSMETIC TREATMENTS

Preembalming Disinfection

The total disinfection of the epidermal tissues of the face and hands is the first step in preparing a stable, receptive cosmetic surface foundation. The embalming disinfectant spray chosen should be able to be used freely on the delicate mucous membranes of the eyes, nose, mouth, and ears without risk of causing dehydration or coarsening of the epidermal texture. It should be specifically formulated for preservation purposes and be designated for use in all general disinfection and deodorizing procedures. The use of disinfectant spray assures a sterile epidermal surface and helps to retard skin-slip and mold growth.

Preembalming Cleansing

The body should be washed completely with undiluted germicidal soap, paying particular attention to the face and hands. The hair should also be washed thoroughly with the germicidal soap—this will disinfect the hair, leaving it clean and soft for styling. The hands and fingernails should be carefully scrubbed, making certain that the epidermal surfaces around the cuticle and underneath the nails are clean and free from all soil and stains. It is important that all cleansing treatments be performed before the arterial injection, because the fixation of the tissue will tend to promote retention of dirt in the pores of the skin, making removal difficult. Alignment and cleansing of the eyelashes and eyebrows also should be done before arterial injection because the hair follicles will become permanently set, making correct alignment impossible after injection is completed. After all cleansing is completed, a second application of the embalming disinfecting spray should be applied to all body surfaces, paying particular attention to the face, arms, and hands. The mechanical action of washing the body can cause dilution of the disinfectant spray applied in the initial disinfecting treatment.

Epidermal Conditioning

After all disinfection and cleansing treatments have been completed, the epidermal surfaces of the face, neck, and hands should be treated with a skin conditioning cosmetic massage cream. The emollient cream should be formulated with skin conditioners to penetrate into the deeper layers of the epidermis and dermal layer. Carefully apply the cosmetic massage cream, paying particular attention to the eyes, nose, lips, cheeks, and ears, and with your fingertips gently work the emollient cream into the epidermal surfaces. This breaks up rigor mortis, making feature posing easier. Before posing the features, all unnatural and downy hair growth should be removed from the face of infants and females. After the shaving is completed, cleanse the lather from the face and reapply a liberal coat of the massage cream. This procedure prevents any razor abrasions from turning brown. When a scaly skin condition must be treated, before shaving the body, massage a liberal amount of massage cream over the affected area. Leave the cream on the skin surface for approximately ten minutes, then remove the cream with a gauze pad. It may be necessary to repeat the procedure two or three times to completely remove the roughened skin. Use of heavy pore-blocking creams for cosmetic massage treatment is not recommended. If the massage cream is not fully absorbed, it fills the pores in the skin, and an undesirable effect will result when the cosmetics are applied.

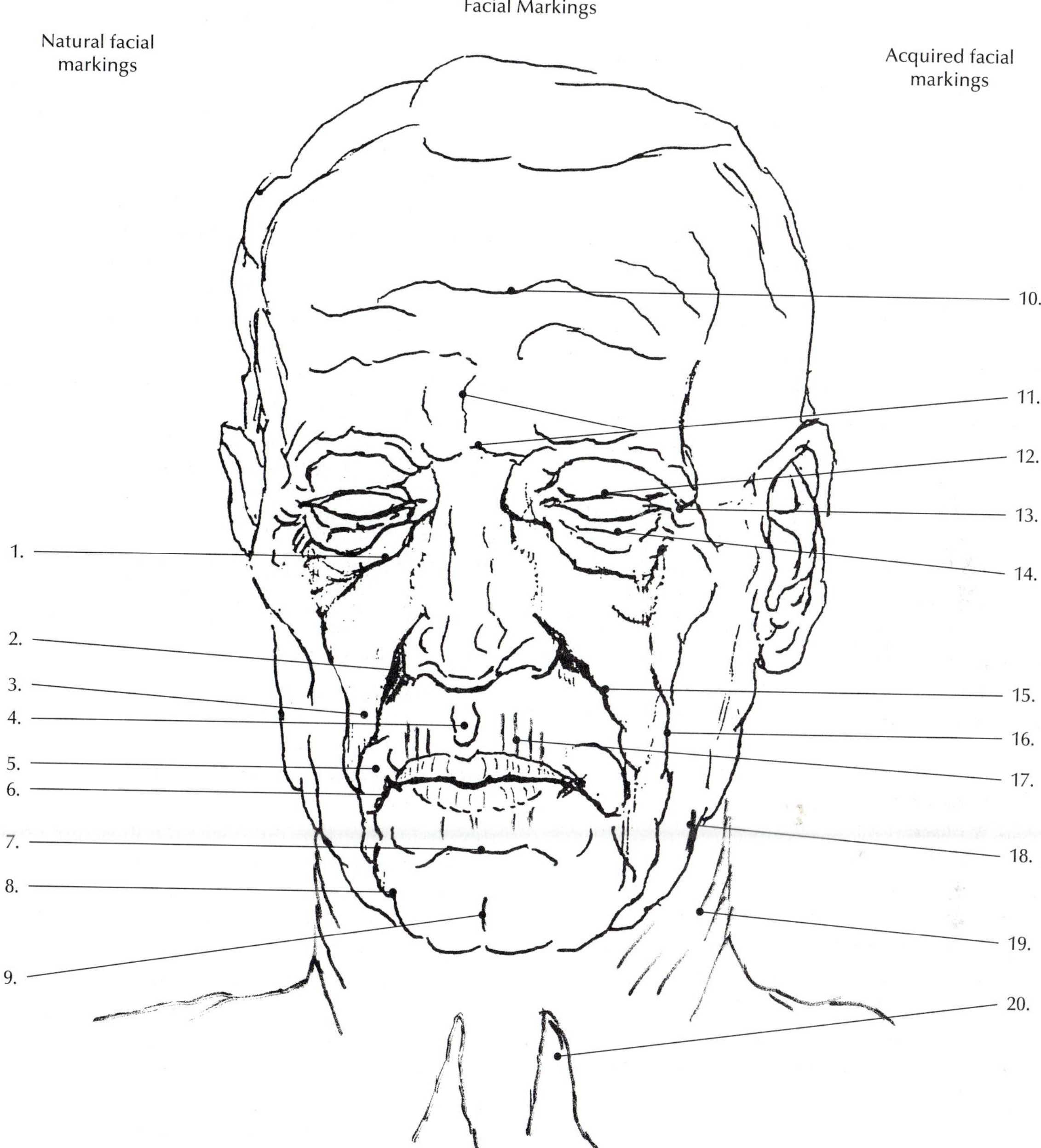

Figure 1. Classification of facial markings. *(Figure adopted from G. Joseph Prager, Manual of Restorative Art, 1965.)*(See the glossary for detailed description of each marking). **Natural facial markings:** 1. oblique palpebral sulcus; 2. nasal sulcus; 3. nasolabial fold; 4. philtrum; 5. angulus oris eminence; 6. angulus oris sulcus; 7. labiomental sulcus; 8. submental sulcus; 9. dimple. **Acquired facial markings:** 10. transverse frontal sulci; 11. interciliary sulci; 12. superior palpebral sulcus; 13. optic facial sulci; 14. inferior palpebral sulcus; 15. nasolabial sulcus; 16. buccofacial sulcus; 17. labial sulci; 18. mandibular sulcus; 19. platysmal sulci; 20. cords of the neck.

▶ FUNERAL ARRANGEMENTS

The funeral director making the arrangements should check the body before meeting with the family to determine if there are any difficult cosmetic or restorative treatments required. It is not uncommon to have the funeral arrangements completed before the body is removed to the funeral home for preparation. Having the deceased's photos on hand will a valuable source of information regarding the individual's shape, weight, and height for use in determining the casket size required. Also, when setting the hour for the family to view the deceased for the first time, the funeral director should allow ample time, for the embalmer/cosmetician to do his or her work without being rushed.

▶ POSING THE FEATURES

Every effort should be made to ensure the correct posing of the features due to their profound impact in establishing a true-to-life appearance. Because the body has been in a horizontal position for an extended period of time before embalming, the soft facial tissues fall downward, gravitating towards the back of the neck. Loss of muscle tone in elderly people will also cause unnatural sagging of the facial tissues. To correct this unnatural contour, bring the chin up and elevate the head slightly backwards so the facial tissues, after the mouth has been closed, can be filled out into their natural appearance. One of the most influential factors in establishing this natural appearance is reflecting the true age of the individual. The slightest amount of swelling in the facial tissues during arterial injection can cause the characteristic facial lines to disappear, making the elderly individual look many years younger. The astringent action of the embalming chemicals, particularly when strong arterial solutions are used, can cause excessive wrinkling of the facial tissues, making a younger person appear prematurely aged. Overinjection, excessive tissue firming, and overfilling of the facial tissues in feature building treatments, impairs recognition to a high degree, and invariably results in a faulty memory-image. These conditions cannot be corrected after the arterial injection is completed or through any corrective cosmetic or restorative procedures.

The Mouth

The mouth is the dominant feature of the face; it varies greatly in width, contour, and length. Any distortion of the contour or change in its proportions produces a drastic change in the appearance of the face. Every precaution should be taken to avoid any alteration of the mouth. The anatomical structures of the mouth and lips are divided into three major categories: (1) mucous membranes, (2) upper integumentary lip, and (3) lower integumentary lip (see Chap. 11).

Mucous membrane: The mucous membrane is composed of soft moisture-retaining tissue, varying in color from a deep to a light shade of red, with the intensity of color dependent on the age of the individual. The membrane lines the entire inner surface of the mouth and lips, extending to the convex (external) surfaces of the upper and lower integumentary lips. The thickness of the external mucous membrane covering the lips is greater at the center than towards the corners of the mouth. In the female, the outer lip membrane appears fuller than in the male, and assumes a more sharply defined "Cupid's bow" shape. In advanced age, particularly if the teeth have been extracted, the mucous membrane tends to recede, drawing the lip inward, with less red tissue visible.

Upper integumentary lip: The upper lip is the flesh above the red surface of the mucous membrane. Its superior limit is formed by the base of the nose and its lateral boundaries are determined by the nasolabial fold. The upper lip is divided into its left and right sections by the indentation of the philtrum.

Lower integumentary lip: The lower lip is located below the red surface of the mucous membrane. The center of the lower lip is crescent shaped and conforms to the contour of the incisive fossa. This line deepens as it reaches the upper limits of the chin.

Posing the Mouth. When posing the mouth the embalmer/cosmetician should keep in mind that the slightest downturn at the corners of the mouth conveys an impression of sadness, whereas an upturn lifts the corners of the mouth into a pleasant facial expression, reminiscent of peaceful repose. A flat, unnatural width of the mouth will also cause a drastic change in facial expression.

The first procedure in posing the mouth is the total disinfection of the mucous membrane lining the oral cavity. To disinfect the mouth, make a cotton swab by wrapping a piece of cotton around the end of a pair of angular forceps. Saturate the cotton with disinfectant solution. Disinfect and cleanse the oral cavity and underneath the upper and lower lips, removing all foreign matter. During the disinfecting treatment, the massaging action of the forceps will help relieve rigor mortis in the lips. Then, using cosmetic massage cream, the cheeks should be massaged upwards. This will relieve muscular tension in the nasolabial fold which may be distorted because the body has been under refrigeration in a horizontal position. Massaging the area around the cheeks and lips also helps relieve rigor mortis in the facial tissues and prepares the mouth for trouble-free posing. The cosmetic massage treatment restores normal texture to the epidermal tissues, making the surface more receptive to cosmetics.

When fitting dentures, keep in mind that poorly fitted dentures can cause gross distortion of the face—if they do not fit correctly they should not be used. A plastic mouth former should be substituted. Insert the dentures so they fall into place easily and naturally. View the face with the jaws closed. If the appearance is natural, remove the dentures, apply a small amount of adhesive stay cream to the inside surfaces of the dental plates and position them. Secure the maxillary and mandible in position. If there are no dentures, or if the extraction of teeth has caused structural changes in the conformation of the gum line, the use of a plastic mouth former in conjunction with mastic compound or cotton will establish a natural facial appearance. Avoid excessive tightening of the upper and lower jaws when closing the mouth. This will invariably result in compressing the lips too firmly together, causing the mouth to appear unnaturally wide. Ideal closure is achieved when the upper and lower lips are just barely in contact with one another—not compressed. This light preliminary closure pressure leaves room for the expansion of the mucous membrane. During arterial injection, the lips will fill out to their natural contours. Remember, the slightest distortion around the mouth and lips can cause profound changes in the natural expression of the individual.

Nasolabial fold and sulcus: The nasolabial fold is the most expressive structure of the face and determines the fullness or leanness of the cheeks. It varies widely in depth, width, length, and contour. Because this fold determines so much of the facial expression, distortion of the contour, or even a slight variation in proportion produces a drastic change in the appearance of the face. This sulcus runs downward from the wing of the nose to the corner of the mouth. The contour of the cheeks, lips, and chin are determined somewhat by the length, depth, and arc of the nasolabial fold. In the preembalming treatments, after the mouth has been closed and before aligning the mucous membranes of the lips, the nasolabial fold should be posed in its natural shape and contour. To shape the fold, inject mastic compound in the buccal cavity using the compound injector with round attachment, along a line drawn from the wing of the nose to the outer edge of the mouth (see Figure 2). Make certain that this critical line is raised to the level of fullness natural for the individual. Inject just enough mastic compound underneath the upper lip to establish a natural expression. An alternate procedure is to impregnate a strip of cotton the length of the fold with adhesive stay cream. Using angled forceps, place the treated cotton under the upper lip along the line of the fold, molding it to the desired fullness with your fingertips. If further adjustment becomes necessary after embalming, feature builder may be hypodermically injected into the cheek tissues along the line of the fold until the natural contour and proper relative depth has been established.

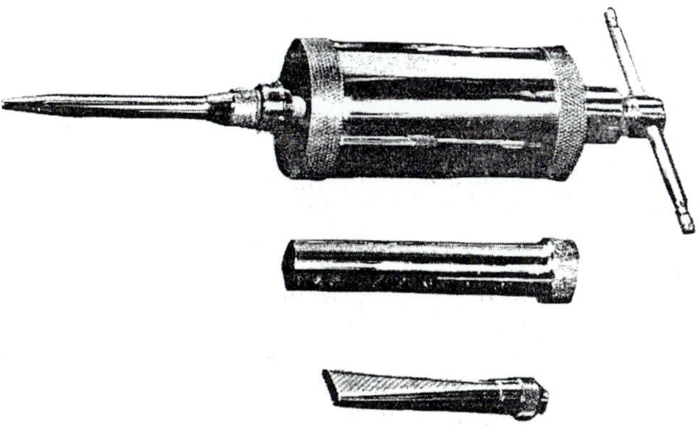

Figure 2. Heavy compound injector with attachments.

Philtrum: Although the philtrum seldom becomes a critical feature-posing problem because of its natural stability, its width and depth should be observed before embalming so that its normal contour may be maintained. This small oval groove which runs vertically down the center of the upper lip from the nasal septum to the edge of the mucous membrane is actually a very sensitive element of facial expression. Even the slightest distortion such as exaggerated depth or excessive prominence in the ridges can cause an astonishing change of facial expression. Discrepancies in proportion appearing after embalming can easily be corrected by placement of a small amount of mastic compound under the groove and molding by gentle finger pressure to the desired contour. Laminates of cotton impregnated with adhesive stay cream may also be used in establishing the natural contour of the philtrum. Fortunately, instances requiring these procedures are few.

The Nose

Swab the inside of the nostrils and crease around the flare of the nose with embalming disinfectant. Trim the hair in the nose to conform to the inside diameter of the nostrils. Saturate a pledget of cotton with humectant, place the treated cotton inside the nostrils, and shape the nose into its natural contour. Before cosmetizing, remove the cotton plug and inject mastic compound to the back of the nostril, using the compound injector with the round attachment. This treatment seals the passageways and aligns the nostrils in their proper contour.

The Eyelids

The eyes and mouth together comprise the sum total of facial expression. In death, the eyes are closed, and the deceased appears to all but the most intimate family members to be sleeping. However, it is through the application of cosmetics to the eyelids that a natural appearance of the eyes is established. The upper eyelid is two to three times larger than the lower eyelid, therefore it is the most prominent of the two when the eyes are closed. When the eye is closed, the upper lid and its lashes become the most prominent feature. The lower lid itself is barely visible when the eye is shut.

The eyes should be thoroughly disinfected and cleansed before attempting closure. During the disinfecting procedures, using the cotton-swabbed forceps, flex the upper and lower eyelids. This procedure will help remove rigor mortis from the levator superioris and make natural eye closure more easy to accomplish. Light massage with cosmetic massage cream, worked well into the external eyelids and surrounding orbital area, will further assist in removing muscle rigor. After completing the disinfecting and cleansing treatments, place a small amount of adhesive stay cream on the underside of the eye cap and insert it over the eyeball. Also apply a small amount of adhesive stay cream in the inner canthus of the eye. This will bring the inner corner of the eye into proper closure. Never overlap the upper eyelid over the lower eyelid. This will create an unnatural expression, detracting from the illusion of natural repose. After the eyelids are closed, use the swabbed forceps and apply a small amount of the embalming disinfecting solution to the eyelashes and eyebrows. This will help straighten and align the hairs into their natural position. If the eyelashes are improperly aligned before arterial injection the follicles will become fixed by the arterial chemical, and it will be impossible to position them in correct alignment. Apply a light coat of cosmetic massage cream and align the natural contours of the eyebrows and eyelashes. Before applying the basic cosmetic application all massage cream should be removed from the eyebrows and eyelashes with mortuary solvent.

The Ear

Disinfect and cleanse the external parts of the ear (auricle) with embalming disinfectant; using a cotton swab thoroughly cleanse the area under the inside rim of the helix and the crease along the backside of the ear and lobe. The earlobe is composed of soft tissue, therefore with the body in a horizontal position, the earlobe sags downward at a right angle towards the side of the neck. To correct this unnatural positioning of the lobe, take a small piece of cotton impregnated with adhesive stay cream, and place it behind the earlobe. This will position the earlobes in their natural contours. For the female subject wearing earrings this procedure assures the earlobes will be in a natural position for their display.

▶ POSING THE HANDS

The hands are often given only perfunctory attention when posing and cosmetizing the body. The hands are a powerful medium of expression both in life and in death and posing them should be given careful consideration.

After disinfecting treatments have been completed, the hands and fingers should be thoroughly cleansed with undiluted soap, making certain that the epidermal surfaces and fingernails are completely clean. Scrub the fingernails and cuticles with a stiff-bristled hand brush until every trace of soil above and below the nail is removed. Dried blood, grease, tobacco stains and any stains caused by application of medicines should be removed before embalming. This is necessary because the protein-fixing action of the arterial solution will permanently bond the soil into the nailbed and cuticle, so it is imperative that the hands and nails be scrupulously clean before arterial injection.

Manual manipulation of the wrist and fingers is an important preembalming treatment in achieving correct hand alignment and natural contour. After manual manipulation is completed apply cosmetic massage cream, working it into the tissues on the back of the hand, around the fingernails and fingertips. On female subjects also apply cream to the arms. The face, arms, hands, and legs of infants should be given thorough cosmetic cream massage before arterial injection. This helps to relieve rigor mortis and makes the delicate epidermal tissues of the infant more pliable and receptive to all cosmetic media. The contour of the relaxed hand during life is convex, with the fingers bent slightly inward towards the palm. This gives the hand a graceful semi-oval contour with the thumb and forefinger in natural parallel contact. The third, fourth, and fifth fingers of the hand should also appear in gentle contact with each other and parallel to the forefinger. To simulate the naturally-curved contour of the reposed hand, place a pad of cotton or cloth saturated with humectant under the palm, molding the hand into a semi-oval contour over the pad. This will help sustain the natural contour of the hand. The three most commonly used poses when aligning the hands in a natural, relaxed manner are:

1. Crossed hand position (right or left hand placed over the top of the opposite hand)—used primarily where religious tradition cells for this position
2. Left forearm and hand resting on the upper abdomen at the mid-line with the right forearm placed on the abdomen just below the left forearm parallel to it
3. Left forearm positioned at a right angle to the body with the center of the hand resting over the diaphragm at the mid-line. The right forearm is set with the elbow bent at an angle of about 60 degrees, and the hand resting at the mid-line on the lower abdomen.

Note: These three basic positions represent traditional customs for posing the hands and arms. However, reasonable variations may be made at the discretion of the embalmer/cosmetician or funeral director. The hands and arms should never be placed in a parallel position at the sides of the body. This produces a stilted effect, an attitude which detracts from the desired memory-image. Moreover, in this position the hands cannot be seen, obscuring their sensitive and expressive beauty in natural repose.

▶ PRE-REFRIGERATION CONSIDERATIONS

There is an increasing number of refrigeration units being installed in funeral homes. One of the main reasons why the need for refrigeration of the remains is on the increase is the fact that federal law now requires the written or oral authorization from the next of kin before embalming can be done. The person responsible for this authorization may not live nearby, or may be difficult to contact for some other reason. Also, the increase in direct cremation without embalming means more bodies being kept under refrigeration. Some other reasons for delays in embalming or disposition are: (1) medical examiner's investigation; (2) donation of body parts; (3) private autopsy; and (4) religious beliefs. If we are to maintain high standards in funeral service, there are important pre-refrigeration treatments that should be performed when preparing the body that is going to the placed, unembalmed, in the funeral home refrigerator (see Chap. 2).

Once the body is removed to the preparation room, the outer covering should be removed. All external body surfaces should be disinfected with embalming disinfecting spray. Bandages and rubber drains should be disinfected, removed, and disposed of. All surgical incisions should be thoroughly disinfected. All exposed parts of the body should be washed with undiluted germicidal soap, paying particular attention to the face and hands. After all basic disinfecting and cleansing treatments have been completed, a liberal application of cosmetic massage cream should be applied to the face, neck, and hands. Massage the cream gently into the tissues before shaving. When the shaving is completed, coat the area again with massage cream. Special consideration should be given to the eyelids and lips. When the unembalmed body is held in refrigeration for an extended period of time, the delicate tissues in these two areas have a tendency to separate and turn brown (leatherizing) from progressive dehydration. The eyes, nose, and lips should receive special treatment before posing the features.

The Mouth: Thoroughly disinfect all surfaces inside the mouth. All liquids should be removed by aspiration using the nasal tube aspirator. Before closing the mouth, if there are dentures, they should be disinfected and positioned in place; coat the inside portion of the dental plate with adhesive stay cream. If there are no dentures or teeth use a plastic mouth former. Close the mouth using the needle injector or suture method.

Lip Surfaces: Saturate thin strips of cotton with humectant and place layers of the saturated cotton underneath the upper and lower lips. This will help set the lips in a natural contour and will retard dehydration. In the final treatment, seal the upper and lower lips with a layer of adhesive stay cream.

The Nose: Swab the insides of the nostrils and nasal sulci around the flare of the nose with disinfectant. Cleanse the inside of the nostrils and coat the passageways with adhesive stay cream. Saturate a section of cotton with humectant and place inside the nostrils. Shape the nose into its natural contour. You will have some measure of preservation from the embalming disinfectant and the treated cotton will prevent drying out of the tissues.

The Eyes: Disinfect the eyes; using the swabbed forceps, pass the swab underneath the upper and lower eyelids. This will flex the eyelids bringing them together and insuring a natural looking closure. Apply a liberal amount of adhesive stay cream under both eyelids. Coat the front and back surfaces of the eye caps with adhesive stay cream, place the eye caps in position, and close the lids into their natural closure. This treatment will retard dehydration of the eye membranes.

The Ears: Using the swabbed forceps, disinfect the inner and outer surfaces of the ears. Take two pieces of cotton impregnated with adhesive stay cream and place one behind each ear lobe. This will position the ear lobes in their natural contour.

After the features have been posed, a second application of cosmetic massage cream is recommended. When placing the unembalmed body in the refrigerator, one of the most important procedures is to elevate the shoulders and head and place the arms and hands in a relaxed position over the abdomen.

The Hands: The hands and fingernails, like the important areas of the face, should receive thorough treatment with embalming disinfectant spray and cleansing with germicidal soap. The undersides of the fingernails, in particular, need careful attention. Place the hands and fingers over a pad of cotton saturated with humectant and form the treated cotton under the palm, cupping the hands into a natural curved contour. Apply a substantial layer of cosmetic massage cream over the hands and fingernails.

Positioning the Unembalmed Body

The first step before placing the body in the funeral home refrigerator is to position the body in correct alignment. One of the most important considerations is to elevate the head and shoulders and place the arms and hands in a normal position over the abdomen. The head should be placed on a disposable headblock in a secure fashion. The forearms and hands should never be placed parallel to the body along its sides because this will cause postmortem staining in the hands and underneath the fingernails. Before placing the body on the storage tray or in the cremation container, place a lightweight disposable body pouch in an open position over the body. Then take a cotton sheet large enough to encase the body, place it over the pouch in a centered position, and place the body on the sheet in the pouch. Place the head on the disposable head block and position the arms and hands over the abdomen. Place pieces of lightweight plastic sheeting (plastic food wrap) over the facial area and the hands. Wrap the sheet around the body and zip up the pouch. Should it become necessary to take the body out of the refrigerator for viewing or embalming, you have saved valuable time and avoided complicating your work in establishing a natural appearance.

Preparing the Unembalmed Body for Viewing

If you are required to cosmetize the unembalmed refrigerated body, the following procedures are recommended:

1. The body should be removed from the refrigerator and allowed to remain at room temperature for a few hours before applying the cosmetic medium.
2. Take the cotton plugs out of the nose. With the compound injector, inject mastic compound into the back of the nostrils to where it is not visible, sealing the nasal passageways. Leave the treated cotton behind the ears, making sure it is not visible.
3. Prepare the epidermal surface by carefully removing all cosmetic massage cream with solvent.
4. Spray several coats of embalming disinfectant over the epidermal surface of the face and hands. This will seal, preserve, and prevent moisture from seeping through the epidermal tissues.
5. Brush apply the cosmetic medium (liquid or cream) and blot the surface with a gauze pad as you go along. The pad will absorb extra moisture and help blend the cosmetics into the tissues.
6. The final procedure is to apply a thin layer of drying powder. All excess powder should be removed from the eyelashes, eyebrows, hairline, and epidermal surfaces of the face and hands. Tinted powders should be avoided since they will change the color and consistency of the cosmetics you have applied.

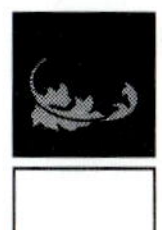

COSMETIC APPLICATION

The art of color blending and the influence of textural values should be fully understood if we are to achieve perfection in embalming cosmetology. A natural appearance can only be achieved when the applied cosmetic medium approximates the true complexion color radiating from beneath the skin surface. The professional embalmer/cosmetician should have a good working knowledge of basic complexion tones and know how to make pre-cosmetizing evaluations based on existing skin color. There are two factors to take into consideration when determining the composition of epidermal coloring: hemoglobin and melanin.

▶ HEMOGLOBIN

The most obvious characteristic of hemoglobin is its bright blood-red color appearing in the arteries as a rich scarlet and as a deep crimson in the veins. Skin coloring, therefore, is influenced by the amount of blood present in the superficial capillaries. These tiny vessels are so numerous and well distributed throughout the body that they are capable of holding enough blood near the epidermal surface to provide a radiating pink overtone under normal conditions. When more heavily charged with blood, these same capillaries will produce the ruddy, purplish-red complexion typical of an individual with high blood pressure. Under anemic conditions and instances where less than normal blood volume flows through the superficial capillaries, a pale complexion results. The pale, colorless skin coloring seen after death is caused by the absence of these radiant pink overtones present in healthy individuals. All living color includes microscopic amounts of red, blue, green, brown, yellow and translucent flesh tones. For postmortem work these colors must be present in embalming cosmetics before any true approximation of living skin coloring can be realized through surface cosmetizing.

▶ MELANIN

The amount of melanin present in the epidermis is an important element in determining complexion coloring, ranging from light tan through browns all the way to deep brown-blacks. It also determines the depth or intensity of complexion color at different ages and among various ethnic groups. Fair-complected individuals show only a faint trace of melanin, while darker-complected persons display an abundance of this skin coloring pigment. Exposure to the ultraviolet rays in sunlight stimulates production of melanin, producing a superficial suntan safeguarding underlying tissues against burn injury. An uneven distribution of melanin produces freckles on the skin, which appear more abundantly and deeper in color when exposed to sunlight. Duplication of freckles is an important aspect of embalming cosmetology, particularly when heavy opaque cosmetics are used. Failure to restore the individual characteristics produced by melanin pigmentation may cause inaccurate representation of the facial features, and is frequently a source of frustration and anger for the family. In persons of advanced age, increased melanin production causes "liver spots" to appear on the face, neck, arms, and hands. Also, the skin color undergoes changes when moisture content changes in the underlying structures, primarily the blood vessels, and lymphatic system, and also when the melanin in the skin undergoes chemical changes. In selecting the proper cosmetic medium and color, consideration should be given to these factors: (1) complexion; (2) environment; (3) sex; (4) age; and (5) lighting.

Complexion

An important step in restoring the natural looking appearance of the deceased is the determination of complexion coloring.

Environment

Environmental effects on complexion color should be considered when selecting the basic complexion color. The individual confined primarily to indoor activity does not, as a rule, have the sun-browned complexion of an outdoorsman, farmer, construction worker, or sportsman. For this reason it is advisable that the embalmer/cosmetician know something about the vocation and activities of the deceased in order to achieve a faithful and natural looking complexion color. True complexion values are often distorted by the pallor of death, but a few pointed inquiries concerning the employment and recreational activities of the deceased can help the embalmer/cosmetician give each case the touch of realism needed to restore lifelike skin tones. During the arrangement interview, the funeral director should ask detailed questions about the facial characteristics, grooming habits, and general appearance of the deceased. This information is important to the embalmer/cosmetician in perfecting his or her work, will give the family confidence in the funeral home's professional staff, and assure the family that the deceased is being well cared for.

Sex

For the female, it is desirable to accentuate her feminine characteristics by using cosmetic color distribution in accordance with current fashion trends and customs. For males and children, color distribution is more natural, and should maintain traditional masculine values in appearance.

Age

The age of the individual is a significant element in determining complexion color. The process of aging modifies skin color, skin texture, and the configuration of facial tissues. Shadows fall differently with emaciation due to advanced age. Aging also changes feature contours, causes wrinkles, and accents the prominence of cheekbones, brows, and jawbones. In contrast, infants display a fresh, vibrant red-pink color. Changes in infant complexion occur at about the age of two, when the skin takes on an aura of brown tones. Few further complexion changes other than those caused by sun exposure take place until the child is about six years old, when hereditary factors give the complexion its permanent identity.

Lighting

The same color and intensity of lighting to be used in the reposing room and chapel should also be used when applying cosmetics in the preparation room. Keep in mind that cosmetics applied to appear natural under brilliant light in the preparation room will look pale and dull under the more subdued funeral home lighting. The importance of light equalization between working areas and viewing rooms cannot be too strongly stressed. Having the correct lighting is a dominant factor in cosmetic color control.

SUMMARY OF COSMETIC APPLICATION

A. Disinfect all tissues; thoroughly wash the face and hands; remove all facial hair
B. If necessary clean the face and hands with a solvent and thoroughly dry the skin
C. Apply surface or hypodermic treatments to discolorations which can be bleached
D. For discolorations, apply an undercoat spray or liquid paint
E. Apply the base cosmetic
F. Adjust or alter the base cosmetic to achieve the correct foundation color
G. Reinstate the highlights and shadows of the face and hands
H. Apply the warm colors (reds) to the face and hands
I. Blend the cosmetic colors
J. Apply a drying powder to the cosmetics
K. Clean eyelashes, eyebrows and hairline
L. Seal the cosmetic by a light application of hair spray

Base Color

The fundamental function of the base color application is to replace the reds missing from the complexion due to blood drainage and bleaching action of embalming chemicals. Natural complexion color can be achieved only when the base cosmetic closely approximates the characteristic color values the individual possessed in life. The base complexion cosmetic is applied strictly as a background color.

Warm Color

The warm colors, namely reds, pinks, and some deeper flesh tones, appear in specific areas of the face, namely the chin, lips, nose, cheeks, ears, and forehead (see Figure 3). Distribution of warm color seldom extends beyond these limits. The most common exceptions are individuals with a lack of color in these areas and those with exceptionally ruddy complexions. The color of the cheeks in the elderly recedes below the tops of the cheekbones, while in younger subjects the color glow rises higher, actually vanishing near the lower eyelids (see Figures 4 and 5).

Color Blending

After the correct base complexion color is established, warm color distributed, and eye make-up and color correctly applied, these applications can be toned down with the brown toning cosmetics. Blending of the brown subdues the brilliance of the warm color just enough to allow a natural glow to emerge, reducing the reds to more lifelike values. The application of the ton-

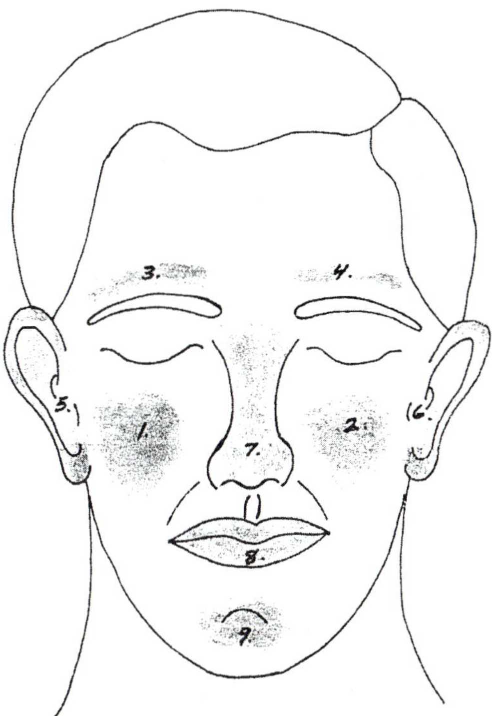

Figure 3. Distribution of warm color.

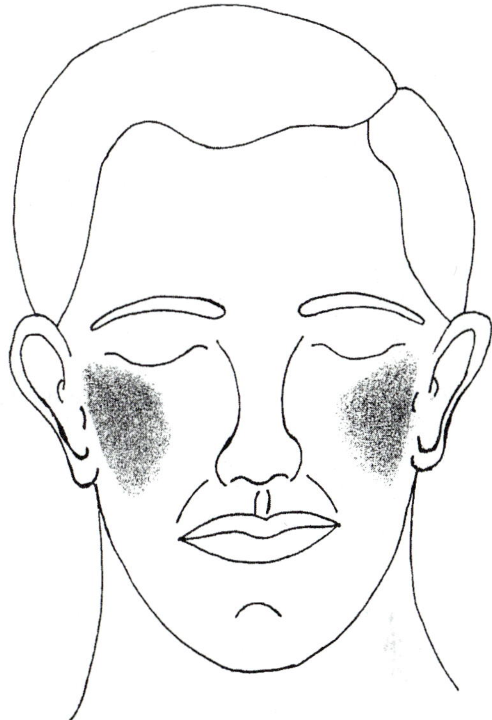

Figure 5. Youthful warm color on cheeks.

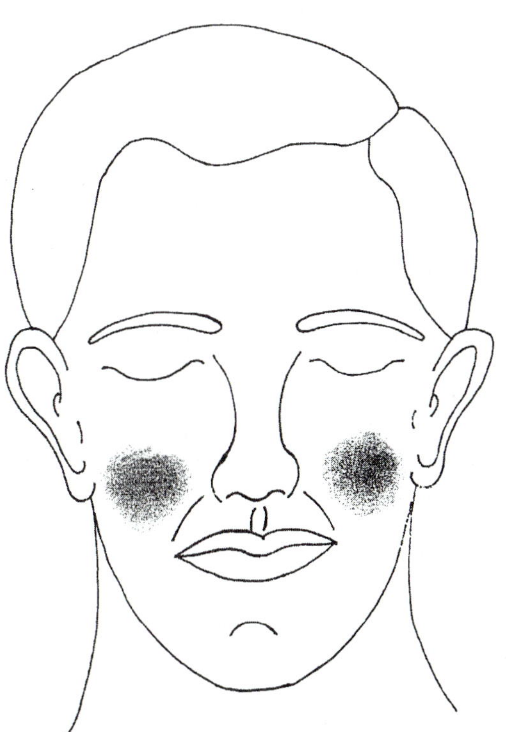

Figure 4. Aged adult warm color on cheeks.

ing medium should be made very lightly, so lightly in fact, that one should be unable to discern exactly where it has been applied. This will bring out the true complexion color, effectively simulating the radiant glow of the blood as it flows under the translucent sheath of skin. Working with the brown toning cosmetics goes a long way towards producing the perfect cosmetic finish. The complexion toning colors are light brown, dark brown, and black. The first consideration is to determine the color intensity category of the deceased; light, medium, or dark. Observe the amount of brown pigmentation in the skin, how deep the color appears in the face and hands. Choose the toning cosmetic from one of the three toning colors (light brown, dark brown, or black) to match the natural complexion of the individual. The correct matching shade should be applied over the basic and warm color application, using the classification of light, medium, or dark to select the correct toning color. All facial lines, wrinkles, freckles, and natural markings should be emphasized with one of the toning colors.

▶ GUIDE FOR COSMETIC APPLICATION

Brush Application

Transparent and opaque liquid cosmetics should be brush applied and dispensed directly from the container. For brush application treatments, the liquid cosmetic medium is applied in short straight strokes confined to a small area. Immediately after application, the liquid cosmetic should be either blotted with a gauze pad or brushed out over the surface and blended such that there is no line of demarcation visible. This should be done quickly, because the vehicle in which the pigment is suspended evaporates almost immediately, limiting the time for distribution. The blotting and brush application procedures insure uniform distribution of color, preventing streaking and blotchy patches of uneven color.

Stipple Application

This method of applying color is done by tapping it off the end of the brush in a delicately controlled "pecking movement." The stipple application procedure is used in applying transparent, semi-opaque, and opaque cream cosmetics. Opaque liquid cosmetics may also be stipple applied to achieve a more natural effect. The cream cosmetics are best applied from the palm of the hand where they are pre-warmed and maintained at a good working consistency. Massage cream may be mixed with the cream cosmetic or applied directly to the skin surface. Begin stipple application with a small amount of cream held in the palm of the hand. Spread the cosmetic out in a fine film with the flat edge of a $2\frac{1}{4}''$ spatula. Keep the thinly spread color restricted to the lower portion of the palm. Pick up a small amount of the cream with the brush. Apply with a light stippling movement—the pressure required is hardly more than the weight of the brush itself being allowed to drop in a controlled descent to the skin surface. Continue with this method until the cosmetic has been stippled out into an even distribution over the desired area.

Finger Application

The finger application method is used in applying tinted emollient cream, semi-opaque complexion cream, and opaque cream. Before applying the cosmetic medium, pre-condition the skin surface by massaging cosmetic massage cream into the tissues of the face and hands. Omit the use of massage cream when an opaque cosmetic is being used. Remove surplus massage cream with a lint-free gauze pad before applying the basic cosmetic medium. Place an ample amount of the cream cosmetic in the palm of the hand, allowing body heat to soften the material to an easy spreading consistency. Pick up a small amount of the cream with the tip of your index or middle finger. Position a dab of cream about the size of a penny on the middle of each cheek, in the center of the forehead, and on the high point of the chin. Wipe the finger clean, then using the tips of all three middle fingers, massage the cream gently into the tissues with a circular motion. Concentrate on producing a smooth, evenly distributed color. When properly massaged into the skin, the cosmetic finish takes on a uniform glow, free of a streaky or greasy looking surface. Treat the hands and fingers in the same manner as the face.

Spray Application

Opaque undercoats (and some transparent tints) are available in aerosole spray containers. The professional embalmer/cosmetician should be thoroughly familiar with the pressure controls and spray patterns used for application of cosmetics. The spray nozzle should not be held closer to the working surface than 6 inches, however, when there is increased nozzle pressure, the container should be moved away up to 10 to 12 inches from the skin. The standard rule is the stronger the pressure, the greater the distance between the spray source and skin surface. Before commencing the basic spray application, position a protective cover carefully over the hair. Coat the hairline, eyebrows and eyelashes with a light application of cosmetic massage cream. This will prevent discoloring and avoid troublesome, time-consuming cosmetic removal. The epidermal surface should be clean, dry, and free of all oily or heavy deposits of massage cream. Moisten a gauze pad with mortuary solvent, and wipe the skin surface very gently until all massage cream is gone, creating a clean, dry surface foundation. Begin spray application just below the line of the mandible. Spray the basic cosmetic on the neck area, testing for proper color value, then proceed up the sides of the face, treating the chin, nose, eyes, ears, and forehead. Movement of the spray stream should be positive, swift, and smoothly executed so no cosmetic build-up or runs appear. Be particularly careful in spraying around the corners of the eyes, the sides of the mouth, the nostrils, and the ears because the irregular configuration of tissue at these points makes them very susceptible to runs. Lift the nozzle well above the skin surface when approaching these areas. When excessive cosmetic build-up occurs, the most practical corrective treatment is to stipple out the surplus, distributing the excess cosmetic into the surrounding areas such that no line of demarcation is visible.

Removal of Cosmetics

When there has been a failure to achieve a properly color-coordinated and natural looking cosmetic result or, as frequently happens, an excessive amount of basic color has been deposited, it may become necessary to remove the entire application. The following methods and materials are used in removing cosmetic media from the epidermal surface of the face and hands.

Gauze Pads: The use of $4'' \times 4''$ gauze pads is recommended for removal of cosmetic massage cream, as opposed to cotton or other material that may leave lint particles on the surface of the skin. The gauze pad is lint-free, absorbent, and useful in many cosmetic procedures. It has an excellent surface with just enough texture in the weave to remove even heavy massage or stay creams from the face and hands. It is also used for blotting and smoothing out liquid surface cosmetics. The pads also are used to good advantage in precosmetic surface treatments and restorative procedures.

Massage Cream Removal of Cosmetics: Cosmetic massage cream removes all cosmetics from the skin surface with the exception of the resin base, adhesion-type opaque liquid and opaque spray cosmetics, which require special solvents. Cosmetic removal is accomplished by applying a liberal coating of massage cream over the epidermal surface of the face and hands, rubbing the cream well into the hairline, eyebrows, and eyelashes. Allow the cream to remain on the skin surface for a few moments, long enough to soften up the cosmetic for easy removal with the gauze pad. To remove the lubricant film left by the massage cream, moisten a clean gauze pad with mortuary solvent and gently wipe the skin surface until all of the film is removed, establishing a receptive cosmetic foundation.

Solvent Removal of Cosmetics: Liquid opaque and opaque spray cosmetics often require special thinner-solvent furnished only by the manufacturer of the cosmetic, but mortuary solvent will serve as a substitute. Brush apply the solvent, limiting the application to small areas, wiping away the cosmetic with gentle pressure on the gauze pad. Repeat this treatment until no trace of cosmetic color or greasy deposit appears on the skin surface. Apply cosmetic massage cream to re-establish the foundation for the new application of the basic complexion color. To prepare the skin for acceptance of transparent liquid tints or liquid opaques, make certain the tissue is totally free of greasy deposits by cleansing with mortuary solvent. Applying transparents or opaques in liquid form on an oily foundation results in patchy, uneven coverage, with total cosmetic rejection where substantial amounts of grease remain on the skin.

▶ BASIC COMPLEXION MATERIALS

Although there is an infinite variety of cosmetic materials, basic complexion materials may be classified as follows:

1. Transparent liquid tints
2. Liquid powder tint
3. Tinted emollient cream
4. Semi-opaque emollient cream
5. Opaque cream
6. Liquid opaque
7. Spray cosmetics

Liquid Transparent Tint

The orange or red pigment in liquid transparents is suspended in a water-alcohol solution combining ultrathin consistency with fast evaporation of the vehicle. It is generally used as a base color for the face and hands when no restorative or special treatments involving opaque cosmetics are required. They are compounded to simulate the basic natural coloring of the body. This cosmetic has been traditionally used in the profession for many years. The major disadvantage of alcohol-based cosmetic solutions is their tendency to dehydrate the delicate surfaces around the eyelids and mucous lip surfaces due to their volatility and rapid evaporation.

Liquid Powder Tint

Liquid powder tints consist of a talc and clay base suspended in an aqueous-alcohol solution combined with a humectant, which helps the powder adhere to the cosmetized surface in a very thin, delicate, and barely visible matte film. The tonal values available for the liquid powder tint are usually confined to shades of red, but in a much wider range than is offered by the transparent liquids. When totally dry, they leave a smooth nonreflecting finish on the epidermal surface with the pores visible. The liquid powder tints tend to dry to a lighter tonal value than their counterparts in the transparent liquids.

Method of Application. A brush application procedure is used when working with the transparent and liquid powder tints. It is not necessary to mix the transparent tints before use because they are held in permanent suspension and will not settle. The liquid powder tints must be mixed well before using since the powder in the solution is not in permanent suspension. Both the transparent and powder tints are applied using the same procedure. These liquid cosmetics are to be applied to a clean, dry surface. To insure uniform adhesion and even distribution, degrease and condition the epidermal surface with a lint-free gauze pad moistened with mortuary solvent. Apply the tint in small areas, blotting excess liquid immediately with the gauze pad, leaving a uniformly distributed color film over the epidermal surface. Halt tint application about $\frac{1}{4}''$ below the hairline, blotting briskly before the film dries into a visible edge or runs under the hairline, where it might produce a change in the hair color. Every precaution should be taken to prevent contamination of facial hair. When required, tint removal is accomplished by using cosmetic massage cream, followed by de-greasing and cleansing with a gauze pad saturated with mortuary solvent.

Tinted Emollient Cream

These cosmetics are compounded with an oil base similar to that used in cosmetic massage cream. There is, however, one important difference: tinted emollient creams are totally free of zinc stearate which gives cosmetic massage cream its characteristic cloudy white color. Tinted emollient cream cosmetics become transparent when applied lightly over the skin surface, allowing the natural complexion to show through, imparting a delicate glow. These tinted creams are excellent basic complexion colors and retard dehydration of the skin.

Semi-opaque Emollient Cream

The semi-opaque emollient creams are virtually identical to the tinted emollient creams except that they are more opaque. Consequently, they allow less of the natural complexion to show through and reduce the conspicuousness of light colored blemishes and mask the unsightly putty-grey pallor of the face and hands, without creating a total blanket of artificial color. These semi-opaque creams allow just enough of the natural undertones to show through to give the illusion of normal skin coloring. Application techniques are the same as those used for the tinted emollient creams. Do not over-apply except to conceal more prominent blemishes.

Method of Application. The tinted emollient and semi-opaque emollient creams may be brush applied, stippled, or rubbed onto the skin with the tips of your fingers. Uniform distribution and excellent surface texture results when the creams are applied over a well-massaged foundation prepared with cosmetic massage cream. Warming the cream in the palm of the hand eases application and helps achieve an even coating. Tinted emollient cream should be worked into the surface to simulate deep pore penetration. Correctly applied, these cosmetics impart a smooth, natural lifelike glow of color. Avoid heavy coatings which tend to leave a greasy-looking appearance. If accidental overapplication occurs, smooth out the finish by stippling a light coating of cosmetic massage cream over the tinted emollient cream until smooth and uniformly blended.

Opaque Cream

The opaque cream cosmetic is a heavily pigmented oil based cosmetic, used primarily to completely mask unsightly blemishes, discolorations, and restored surfaces on the face and hands. Although the objective is to conceal imperfections, it is equally important to avoid an artificial, overly made-up appearance. Opaque cream cosmetics work well over restored surfaces and are compatible with most all other cosmetic media. Light applications yield greater transparency. Opaque creams may also be used as a base cosmetic when applied very lightly. The opaque cream cosmetics are available in soft and firm base consistencies.

Method of Application. Stippling and finger application are the methods normally used when working with opaque creams. These cosmetics, when stippled over the base complexion medium in a very light application (so lightly that it is hardly apparent that it has been applied), establish an excellent and natural skin tone. It is the minimal amount of opaque cream that produces the most natural looking result. Work the cream into the surface so that it blends with the normal pigmentation of the skin. Apply the opaque cream from the palm of the hand and never from the container itself to avoid overapplication.

Liquid Opaque

The liquid opaque medium is normally formulated with a resin base and used most commonly throughout the profession. Drying time is about 10 minutes. Once the liquid opaque is thoroughly dried it will seal the epidermal surface and not rub off, and it also retards dehydration very effectively.

Method of Application. Just about every method of application may be used when working with the liquid opaques. They may be brush applied, stippled, finger blended and airbrushed (when properly thinned). Start application with a base complexion color slightly lighter than what you would normally select when working with other types of cosmetics. Select the closest color match for the background complexion application. After warm area (reds) are treated, follow with the toning color. Blend toning color gradually over the warm color application and into the base complexion color until the natural complexion tone emerges. Use liquid opaques very sparingly, a little goes a long way because of their high opacity and masking qualities. If lightly applied a natural transparent effect can be attained. Total removal of the liquid opaque medium calls for the use of a special solvent formulated for the specific brand of cosmetic. Brush apply the solvent over the treated epidermal surface and using a gauze pad, rub off the solvent and cosmetic until the epidermal surface is clean and dry.

Spray Cosmetics

There are two types of aerosol spray cosmetics available for mortuary use: transparent cosmetic spray and opaque pigmented spray. The transparent aerosol sprays are used as a basic complexion colorant. The opaque pigmented aerosol is used for covering discolorations, restored surfaces, and total masking (undercoating) procedures on the face, arms, and hands.

Supplemental Complexion Color

The glowing undertones of color and textural control created by the arterial injection produces more true color radiance, skin translucence, and textural quality than can be created by even the most skillful cosmetizing. The use of harsh unpredictable arterial chemicals will reduce moisture content in the skin and underlying tissues. This in turn will cause noticeable darkening of the skin, and it takes on a putty-grey color as the chemical reaction with the hemoglobin occurs. Cosmetic application time can be reduced substantially by letting premium quality injection chemicals do their part of the job. Although the complexion coloring can be enhanced through the initial arterial injection, it is necessary to treat the warm areas, lines, wrinkles, and natural markings cosmetically to achieve a natural lifelike appearance.

Arterial Dyes

There are circumstances that require adding chromatic color to the arterial solution to prevent fading of the initial complexion color after the initial arterial injection has been completed. When it is necessary to increase the strength of the arterial chemical for thorough preservation, the increased volume of formaldehyde can cause fading in the epidermal tissues. Under these conditions additional chromatic should be added to the arterial solution to compensate and stabilize the chromatic color in the tissues of the face and hands.

Warm Color Application

The illusion of natural repose is accomplished when the warm color application is blended into the correct background color of the complexion. Even though natural complexion color can be substantially enhanced by the use of advanced chemical formulae for the arterial injection, there is still no injectional chemical available that will color the warm areas of the face and hands. Surface cosmetics must still be used to supplement the underlying red skin tones in the warm areas of the face and hands. The need for surface cosmetizing becomes evident when we realize that in life the warm-toned areas of the face draw their color from the presence of strong reds in the blood (hemoglobin), reflected as a rosy glow through the translucence of the underlying epidermal layers. In analyzing warm color distribution, we see that nature does not normally vary the locations of warm color in the face. Areas of more intense color are uniformly distributed in nearly all individuals. Corrective shaping is usually only needed to create optical dimensional variations, most commonly when it is aesthetically advantageous to widen or narrow the face (see Figures 6 and 7). This is done by shifting the centers and scope of warm color cheek application to create the illusory effect. Women are usually given

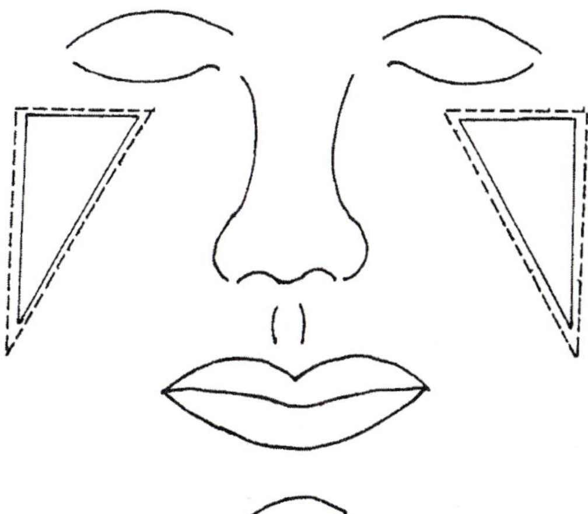

Figure 6. Widening the face.

stronger color treatment of the warm areas—particularly in the cheeks—although this usually is not due to any natural deficiencey. Rather, it stems from the fact that more cheek color has become a familiar personal trait through regular use of artificial cheek color throughout adult life. Questioning of family members will usually reveal the type and color intensity of the facial cosmetics favored by the deceased. Other variations in color distribution include simulating the facial tones of naturally florid or ruddy complexions and duplicating the deeply sun-tanned skin tones of those with outdoor occupations or hobbies. The embalmer/cosmetician should always make a thorough evaluation of facial color characteristics in each individual before attempting treatment. The use of heavy-bodied opaque cosmetic media is frequently indicated for treating jaundice discolorations, diseased or abnormal skin conditions and cosmetizing restored surfaces. Whenever opaque base complexion color is called for, it is advis-

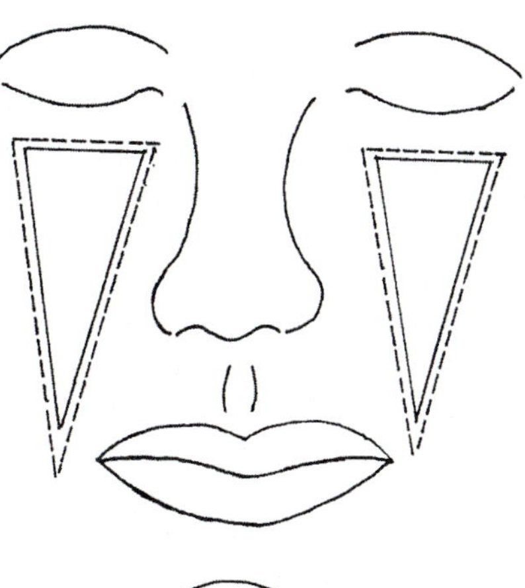

Figure 7. Narrowing the face.

able to choose *more vivid, more intense reds* for the warm facial areas because the brilliance of these colors will be considerably subdued as they are blended into the basic complexion colorant. A second application of warm color is almost invariably necessary to complete this operation successfully. Always blend the reds gradually into the surrounding tissues of each warm area so that no line of demarcation remains visible. When correctly blended, the warm color application will appear as a radiant glow emanating from an unseen subcutaneous source, more like a subtle radiance of pink undertone than a solid flesh-like color. This effect can only be achieved by using warm color in limited quanities, skillfully distributed into the surrounding tissues and carefully blended to a controlled vanishing point.

Method of Warm Color Application

The six dominant features of the face represent nine warm color areas; the chin, lips and nose have only a single warm color area to be treated while the cheeks, ears, and forehead require double area treatment. Proper color application to each of the nine facial areas should be made whether the basic complexion medium is transparent or opaque. To define "warm color" more specifically, it should be understood to mean those portions of the face and hands where high color accents appear normally in life. To begin our discussion on warm color distribution we will first review the three single distribution features of the nine warm color areas of the face.

The Chin. Red toning distributed over this prominent facial feature should be uniformly blended into a color value which cannot be readily identified as red, but merely imparts a vibrant quality to the skin coloring. A small touch of warm color may be placed at the center of the chin and feathered out to remove every trace of a line of demarcation. Allow just enough central toning to give the chin its normal gently rounded conformation. Above all, avoid excessive color on the chin.

The Lips. In evaluating lip color, careful comparison will show that it is identical to that of the cheeks, differing only in the intensity of the red common to both. For this reason the lips should receive a heavier deposit of color and the cheeks a much thinner application of the same shade. Keep in mind the fact that the lips contain a large number of blood-filled capillaries which reflect strongly through a single layer of skin in the living body, while the cheeks, with far fewer capillaries, are seen through a triple-thick epidermal covering, and therefore appear rosy rather than truly red. When applying lip color, confine the color to the central and immediately adjacent areas of the mouth, following the normal lip outline carefully. Do not apply color to the extreme corners of the mouth unless you wish to create an illusion of increased width in this expressive facial feature. Stopping color about $\frac{1}{8}''$ from each corner usually produces a more natural effect. If the mouth appears too wide in proportion to the other facial features, it may be necessary to block out color from the corners. The well defined red area should be limited to the central parts of the lips and distributed gradually in to the basic complexion color on both sides of the mouth. Lips that are too thin impart an undesirable expression to the face. To correct, extend the color above and below the lip outlines, but widen the color bands with care or even more objectionable distortion may result. Lips appearing too full and too short tend to give the face a pouting look. This effect can be corrected by outlining the lips with opaque cosmetic medium (opaque cream or liquid) and re-shaping the fullness and length to the desired dimensions. After the coloring is re-applied, an unnatural line of demarcation may appear where the opaque medium meets the lip edge, and this line, if not corrected, will look artificial. Stippling one of the toning creams (light brown, dark brown, or black) very lightly over the opaque medium where it surrounds the lips will blend it smoothly into the basic complexion color. This treatment will remove the opaque line of demarcation and blend the toning color evenly in, producing a more natural look.

The Nose. Apply warm color to the wings, septum, sides, and bridge of the nose. Terminate the color where a horizontal line drawn between the corners of the eyes would intersect the bridge of the nose. Any color which reaches beyond this imaginary line during the distribution and blending treatments should be immediately subdued or removed. All coloring applied to the sides, wings, and septum of the nose should be used sparingly and fully blended into the surrounding facial tissues so that only the slightest trace of color remains visible. The tip of the nose should always be kept free of strong color.

The Cheeks. The cheeks represent two warm color areas which must be given carefully balanced symmetry in color and tonal values. The slightest variation in color intensity or an abnormal excess of color will produce noticeable facial distortion. Considerable variation in color location, distribution, and brilliance occurs in each specific age group. The following is a general guide in determining warm color distribution by age.

Infant. Unlike the warm color areas typical in the older individual, rosy color in the infant complexion is uniformly distributed over the entire facial expanse with the greatest red intensity centered on the cheeks. When treating infants, blend all red color (pink tones) into the basic complexion color until a uniform radiant glow spreads outward from a rosy red center at the highest contour of the cheek. No trace of linear demarcation will appear if the warm color is properly blended to its vanishing point.

Children. Warm-color distribution on children's cheeks should begin adjacent to the wings of the nose, making certain that equal color values are distributed on both sides. The color should be carried to the center of each cheek and then blended downward to the nasolabial fold. The red colorant must be very uniformly distributed and brought close to the nose without allowing it to extend beyond the uppermost terminus of the nasolabial fold. Color should be carefully feathered out to avoid any visible line of demarcation.

Juveniles and Adolescents. Typical warm color distribution in this group begins high on the cheeks and disappears before it reaches the lower eyelid. Color is applied in a triangular pattern with the apex tangent to the upper margin of the cheekbone and extending toward the ears. It is important to note that the stronger red color values should be confined to the area above the middle of the cheek and not permitted to extend below that point. Reduced color, however, may be drawn downward in blending distribution and kept close to the nose as it spreads to the area below the nasolabial fold. Blend all color to its vanishing point, taking care to achieve symmetrical color values on both sides of the face.

Young Adults. In this group warm color appears high on the cheekbones with the uppermost limits of tonality disappearing into the lower eyelid region. Heightened color should extend slightly beyond the outermost corners of the eyes. It may then be gradually spread downward in a triangular shape and made to vanish at the top limit of the nasolabial fold, establishing uniform tonal values on both sides of the face. Strong reds should be used very sparingly. It's far easier to add a touch of red where needed than to remove excess color.

Middle Aged Adults. Warm color distribution in this age group appears well centered in the cheeks. Color deposit should be confined to below the edge of the cheekbone and then gradually extended to a point just beyond the middle of the cheek. Application of warm color is best made in the standard triangular pattern with the apex of the triangle terminating at the point where a horizontal line extending from the earlobe crosses the cheek. No warm color should appear below this imaginary line. It is advisable to start blending slightly above this line in order to finish at the proper level without showing a line of color demarcation. Uniform distribution and color balance must be achieved on both sides of the face for natural looking results.

Advanced Age. Warm color application in cases of advanced age should be confined to a triangular area below the edges of the cheekbones and extending well into the hollow of each cheek. The tip of the color triangle should terminate at the upper margin of the jawbone. Blend the color so that the most vivid glow is located in the hollow of the cheek rather than high upon its prominence. This lowering of the cheek color is a normal characteristic of old age. This pattern of color should always be considered in treating male cases and those female cases who do not use rouge.

Cheek Color in Females. Because most women use rouge throughout adult life to heighten cheek color, more vivid facial cosmetizing becomes a routine complexion characteristic in the average female case. The position and extent of heightened color varies with personal preference. Under ideal circumstances the professional embalmer/cosmetician can duplicate such an individual's color values by using a color photograph of the deceased as a guide. When no photograph is available, you may use a carefully selected cheek color to create a natural effect. The most common position of cheek color in the adult woman is centered at midcheek (regardless of age) and distributed uniformly over the surface. Avoid excessive color accents. Powder lightly to reduce brilliance where necessary. A compressed dry rouge can be used *after* a drying powder has been applied.

Cheek Color Summary. Uniform rosy to pink coloring is a typical characteristic of the infant complexion. It is distributed over a broader area than in more mature individuals. At ages beyond the infant stage, children have cheek color centered and adjacent to the lower eyelid. Youthful cheek color is characterized by its elevated location on the cheekbones, fading into normal complexion color at the outer corners of the eyelids. At middle age and beyond, the warm color of the cheeks tends to recede, descending gradually to the hollow of the cheek where it remains during advanced age. Balanced color is a critical factor in treating all of the double-area features of the face. Both left and right surfaces must be given identical color intensity to achieve a natural look.

The Ears. Warm color should be applied uniformly to both ears. Distribution of colorant should not extend beyond the tragus. Less color is used on the ears of elderly subjects, and more color on infants and youthful subjects. Color intensity should remain in the midrange of warm color, approximately the same color as the adjacent values at the sides of the face.

The Forehead. Deposit above each eyebrow a half-inch wide band of warm color about equal in length to the curved linear dimension of the eyebrow itself. Distribute warm color evenly across the forehead, blending the red colorant upward towards the hairline and outward over the temples, towards the ears. Impart equal color values on each side. In this procedure the highest color values are placed immediately above the eyebrows with gradual reduction in intensity as the distribution approaches the hairline and sides of the head. Blend warm tones carefully into the basic complexion color so that no line of demarcation is visible. Create a subtle radiance or blush-like glow of color on this broad and prominent area rather than an identifiable red tone. Use *less* red on females than on males.

▶ WARM COLOR COSMETIC MEDIA

There are six cosmetic media commonly used in treating the warm areas of the face and hands. They are comparable in color range to basic complexion media and vary widely in composition, hiding ability, and drying time. They are classified as follows:

1. Transparent liquid
2. Tinted emollient cream
3. Opaque cream
4. Opaque liquid
5. Soft paste
6. Cake cosmetic

Transparent Liquid

Transparent liquid media are brush applied but may also be sprayed or atomized. When spraying, the nozzle should be held close to the skin with color deposit limited to a small area. The transparent tints impart a natural-looking diffuse color radiance which simulates natural warm color in a wide range of complexion types. It is non-masking and has a rapid drying time and is an excellent medium for cosmetizing the hands and fingers. The transparent liquids should be used only over a transparent-liquid complexion base. If it is applied over any other type of cosmetic base, streaking and uneven distribution of color will result. Transparent liquids are formulated to produce a close approximation of natural color translucence on the skin. The transparents have minimal hiding power and are not intended for concealing blemishes. Color deposit can easily be removed with a gauze pad moistened with mortuary solvent.

Tinted Emollient Cream

This cosmetic medium may be used over an emollient cream base complexion application or to add warm color tone over a transparent liquid complexion base. Tinted emollient creams are non-dehydrating and offer superior skin conditioning qualities. They are best applied by stipple brush or fingertip application. When thoroughly massaged into the epidermal surface they produce superb results.

Opaque Cream

This oil-based cosmetic medium is an excellent non-dehydrating skin conditioner as well as a versatile color toning medium. The opaque creams are fully compatible when used over any base complexion cosmetic. Application is made by stipple brush or fingertip method. When lightly applied, the opaque cream produces a transparent effect, allowing the texture, pores, and underlying color to show through. When laid on in a heavier coating they effectively conceal surface discolorations, blemishes, and restored areas.

Opaque Liquid

The opaque liquids leave a fine-textured film with a flat, velvety finish after about five minutes of drying time. This type of cosmetic medium will not fill in the pores or alter the natural texture of the skin. Streak-resistant application is easily achieved with this cosmetic medium, which also offers superb masking capacity. The opaque liquids are fully intermixable, non-caking, and fast drying. This cosmetic may be brush applied without the risk of creating a painted effect.

Soft Paste

The soft paste rouges have a special smooth-textured consistency enabling them to be applied with great ease and precision control. They are evenly smoothed on the skin from a small portion in the palm of the hand by stipple brush or fingertip application techniques. Because of the intensity of the reds in soft paste rouges, they should be applied very sparingly. This type of cosmetic is used mainly when stronger color accents are required to produce natural-looking rouging effects on female subjects. The soft paste colors also prove extremely useful when accenting the warm color after the cosmetic application has been completed. (Commercial lipsticks would be included in this category.)

Cake Cosmetic

Cake cosmetics of good quality will produce a satisfactory result if carefully applied. The application procedure found to be most effective consists of stippling on the cake compound with a soft camel hair brush. Application may also be made with a powder puff or damp sponge. Cake cosmetics may be safely used over other warm color cosmetic media to intensify color after the cosmetic treatment has been completed and dried with a white drying powder.

▶ APPLYING COSMETICS TO THE EYE

One of the most critical aspects in the art of mortuary cosmetology is the cosmetic treatment of the eyes, eyebrows, and eyelashes. The procedures performed at this phase are crucial to the success of our effort to create the illusion of peaceful repose and lifelike appearance. In order to achieve a natural-looking result, we must consider the fact that the living individual is most commonly seen in an erect position. This posture, because of the protuberance of the eyebrows, creates a shadow effect which greatly influences the typical facial expression of the individual. In death, the individual is seen only in a reclining position with light falling directly on those facial areas which would normally remain shaded. This effect must be compensated for if we are to achieve a natural, lifelike countenance for the deceased. The eyelashes accent the margins of each eyelid with a line of short, closely set hairs curving outward and upward from the upper lid, and outward and downward from the lower lid. When the eye is correctly closed, the upper lid and its lashes become the dominant feature of the upper half of the face, with the lower lid just barely visible. Most eyelashes are naturally dark in color. When cosmetizing the eye it is important to pay special attention to the edges of the eyelids, where the lashes are rooted. There is a line of natural color (purple) where the upper lash enters the ridge of the eyelid. Beneath the border of the lower lid is the orbital pouch, a puffy structure that follows the curvature of the orbit under the lower eyelid (see Figure 8). The surface of the pouch is slightly darker in color than the surrounding skin. In cases of advanced age or serious illness, the orbital pouch sags and becomes flabby and discolored. Overaccenting the orbital pouch will result in a major distortion of the facial expression. It must, however, be cosmetically treated when it is a familiar characteristic of the individual, particularly in aged individuals.

Method of Color Application

In applying the basic complexion coloring, the area surrounding the eyes should receive a light, evenly distributed application of base complexion color. When applying the eye shadow it should be used very sparingly, so sparingly in fact, that it should never be apparent that any color has been applied. Stipple brush application, is an effective procedure when simulating the eye shadow. To duplicate the shadow effect apply a small amount of the correct shade above the upper eyelid (see Figure 9). Stipple this color out until it blends into the base color beneath the eyebrows and follow the natural curvature of the lid. Treat the lower eyelid, following the inner perimeter of the orbital ridge to conform to the natural curvature of the lower lid. The chromatic value of the eye shadow used is determine by the age and complexion coloring of the individual. There are four shades of eye shadow: (1) light brown, (2) dark brown, (3) purple, and (4) light blue. After applying the correct color, apply the purple colorant to the upper eyelid along the lash line, and blend the purple into the lash where it enters the ridge of the eyelid (see Figure 10). The color is applied very sparingly, so much so that it should not be evident that it has been applied. The purple is smoothly blended along the lash line so there is no line of demarcation. The purple shading produces a rounded contour of natural color. It is not necessary to treat the lower eyelid.

Shaping the Eyebrows

When the eyebrow is well formed, there is little shaping required. Usually all that is necessary is to lightly trim the eyebrow with barber shears, using a tapered barber comb as an aid. Corrective shaping is required when the line of the brow is unnatural. Such a condition could be caused from a long illness, old age, chemotherapy, or poor grooming. The line of the eyebrow can also be reshaped with $5\frac{1}{2}''$ forceps. It is recommended that all corrective shaping be accomplished after the embalming treatments have been completed. Before trimming the eyebrow, rub massage cream well into the surface surrounding the eyebrow. This treatment will help prevent small indentations from turning brown, which is sometimes caused by nicking and

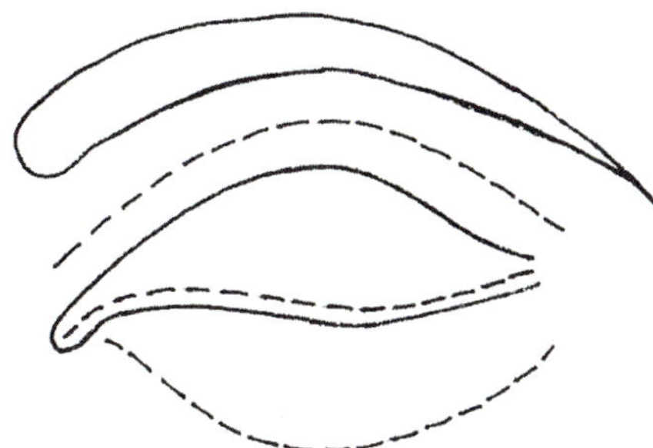

Figure 8. Shaded area under eyebrow, along upper eyelash line, and orbital pouch.

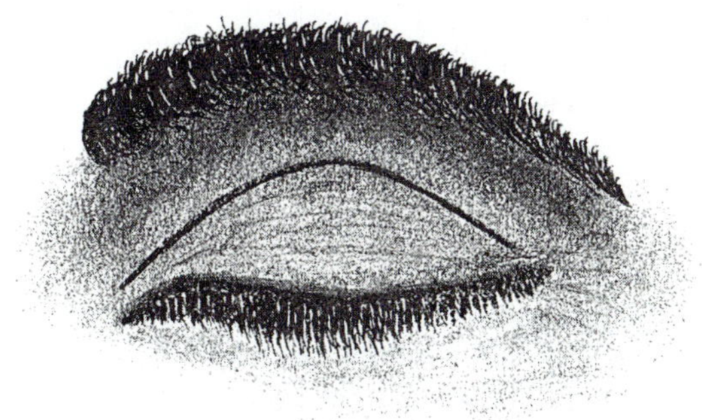

Figure 9. Eye shadow application.

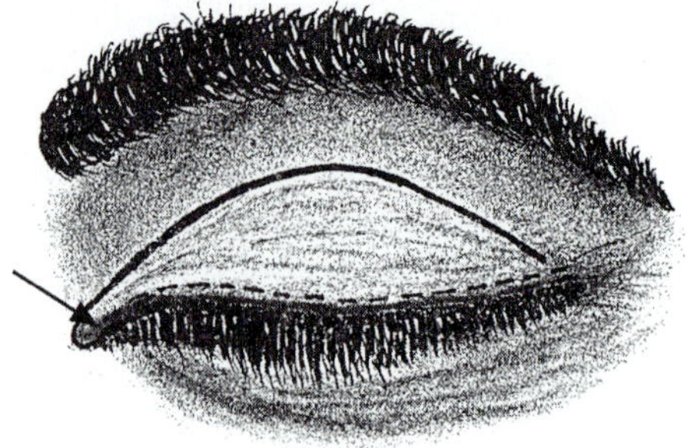

Figure 10. Purple colorant along lash line.

pinching the skin with the tips of the forceps. Further shaping can be done with an eyebrow pencil. There will be times when you need to use an eyebrow pencil to create the appearance of hair where there is none. In such instances, inscribing short individual lines on the skin surface with the sharpened point of the eyebrow pencil, following the normal growth pattern and curvature of the eyebrow, will establish a natural looking result. Using this procedure you can also fill in a sparsely-thin eyebrow, re-establishing the thickness and contour.

Eyebrow Pencil

Two factors affect the effectiveness of the eyebrow pencil. First is the need to restrain the tendency towards excessive use. The second consideration is the selection of the proper color. When using the pencil for its normal function (to darken hairs), be careful to darken only the hair—not the skin underneath. Use the correct color, rather than using the same shade for all cases. A black pencil should never be used unless necessary because it may be too conspicuous. Use short, quick, light strokes and follow the natural direction of the hair growth. The object is to darken the hair but not the skin underneath. Always apply the color very lightly, building it up to the desired degree. The pencil can also be used to effectively remove all traces of cosmetic powder by lightly stroking the hair with the pencil.

Removing Cosmetics from Facial Hair

Since the skin is normally visible within the eyebrow or hairline, it is necessary to apply the base complexion cosmetic so that it colors skin around and underneath these areas. Therefore, in the final cosmetic procedure, it is necessary to remove the base cosmetic contaminating the surface of the hair. To remove this unwanted cosmetic, select a cream cosmetic of the correct shade to match the hair color and place a small amount in the palm of your hand. Pick up a small amount of mortuary solvent on the tip of the brush, just enough to liquify the cream, then stroke a thin layer of the cream lightly over the surface of the hair. Apply no more pressure than the weight of the brush itself.

▶ LIP COSMETICS AND THEIR USE

The professional embalmer/cosmetician must contend with three types of surfaces when applying color to the lips: the natural lip, the discolored lip, and the restored or waxed lip. When applying color to the mucous lip surface certain procedures should be followed to insure a natural appearance and to prevent troublesome build-up of lip cosmetics. There are several different types of lip coloring cosmetics used in surface coloring techniques: cream lip tint, liquid lip tint, soft paste, opaque liquid, and lipstick.

Widening the Mouth

Extend the topmost margin of the upper lip towards each corner of the mouth an equal distance on each side, retaining the existing thickness and contour at the middle portion (see Figure 11). The bottom margin of the lower lip should be broadened gradually beginning at a point approximately $\frac{1}{8}''$ from the corners of the mouth and terminating at its widest point at the center. The broadest band of color now appears at the middle of the lower lip giving the illusion of a larger mouth.

Shortening the Mouth

When it is necessary to shorten the width of the mouth, do not extend the color to the natural corners of the mouth; instead, terminate the color a bit short. The length you choose will depend on the characteristics of the case at hand. Restraint should be exercised or an unrealistic distortion will result. A small amount of surface restorer wax may be placed at the corners of the mouth to move the terminus of the lips inward on each side to create the illusion of a smaller mouth. When applying the lip color, retain the natural contour of the outer limits of the lips as faithfully as possible (see Figure 12).

Waxing the Mucous Lip Surface

The effects of age, disease, dehydration, emaciation, postmortem refrigeration, lip lesions caused by high fever prior to death and traumatic injuries can damage

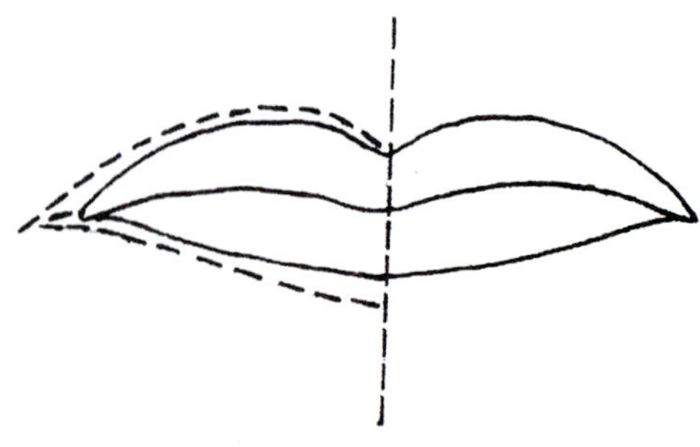

Figure 11. Widening the mouth.

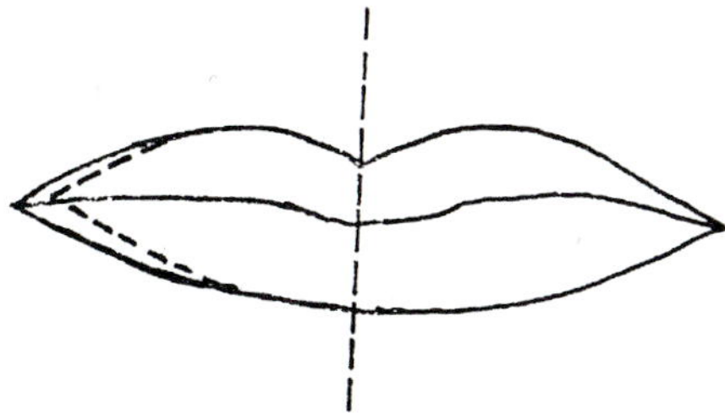

Figure 12. Shortening the mouth.

the mucous lip surface and seriously detract from the illusion of natural repose. The condition must be corrected before a natural looking effect can be achieved. Quality lip wax should work well on soft and slightly moist tissues, and be effective in contouring the lips and simulating lip surface lines. It should have plasticity, firmness, and stability.

Preparing the Mucous Lip Surface

Preparation of a clean, dry and firm operational field is the first step. If the lip tissue is soft, flabby or in any stage of putrefaction, it is important to correct this condition before proceeding. Fill a 10 cc hypodermic syringe with a solution of equal parts of cavity and humectant chemical, and inject both the upper and lower lips. Insert a 1″ hypodermic needle (22 gauge) just below the visible line of the lip (the point of entry is made in the center of the upper lip), directing needle thrust to the corner of the lip. Slowly withdraw the needle, injecting the solution at the same time. Keep the needle well within the rounded portion of the mucous lip surface. Repeat the same procedure for the lower lip, entering the needle just below the visible margin (weather line) in the center. This will preserve and firm the mucous tissues of the lips and establish the natural rounded contour at the same time. Allow a minimum of 30 minutes for firming.

To prepare the lip surfaces for waxing, using swabbed forceps saturated with mortuary solvent, remove all traces of soil, massage cream, and cosmetics. After cleansing operations are completed, the lips should be examined for the presence of scabs, fissures, dried, cracked or peeling skin and traumatic injury. Loose edges of lacerated tissue should be trimmed away close to the lip surface. Fragmented tissue should be repositioned and sutured or cemented in correct alignment. Missing tissue areas should be trimmed to form a neat, well-defined perimeter. Moist lesions on the mucous membrane surface should be dried with a cauterant chemical and sealed with a surface sealant.

Application of Lip Wax

When re-surfacing the mucous lip tissues, place a small amount of surface restorer wax in the palm of your hand where normal body heat will warm it to the right consistency for spatula application. Treat the upper lip first; it is formed by three compound curves which take the shape of a "Cupid's bow." This serpentine curve is more accentuated in the female but is also well defined in the male physiognomy. The dip at the center of the upper lip gives fullness and accentuates the "Cupid's bow" effect. Deposit more wax at the center of the lip to retain the effect of fullness and to create a naturally proportioned curvature. Failure to do this may result in loss of characteristic expression around the mouth. Pick up a small amount of wax from the palm of your hand on the edge of the spatula blade. Start application at the lower margin of the upper lip. Pull the chin downward, separating the upper and lower lips. Place the deposit of wax slightly under the lower margin of the upper lip. Spread the wax upward using very light pressure to form the natural curve of the upper lip with the blade of the spatula. Use the same procedure to wax the lower lip. Again, pull down the chin and apply the wax, tapering the deposit to form a smooth curvature underneath the upper lip, simulating the line of closure and making certain that the full rounded contour is retained.

Establishing the Line of Closure

To perfect the line of closure, apply an ample amount of cosmetic massage cream to the bristles of a small brush. Smooth the bristles into a sharp-edged chisel point between your fingers. Using a horizontal stroke, pass the sharp edge of the brush from the left corner to the right corner of the mouth along the line of closure. Repeat this procedure until you have established a natural looking line of closure.

Simulation of Lip Surface Lines

The final and most important phase of lip waxing, other than applying the lip coloring, is duplicating the lip lines by inscribing them into the wax surface (see Figure 13). The procedure itself is a simple one when done with restraint and a light touch. When we study lip lines, we observe that the lines are spaced further apart at the center of the lips and become more condensed towards the corners of the mouth. The fine vertical lines visible on the red surface membranes are less pro-

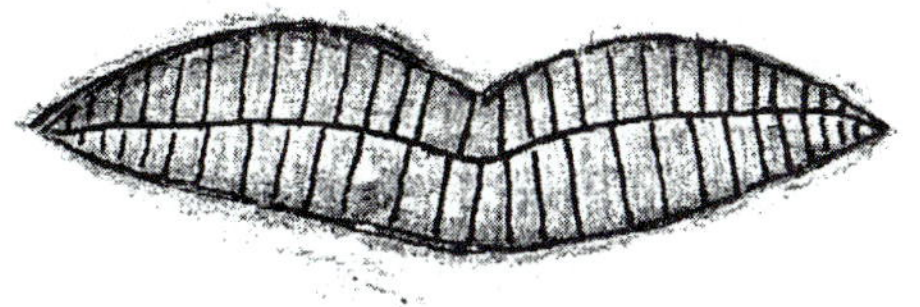

Figure 13. Simulation lip lines.

nounced in youth and become deeper and heavier with advanced age.

To duplicate lip lines and wrinkles, sharpen the end of a round brush handle in a rotary pencil sharpener to a needle-sharp point. Using very light vertical strokes, start at the center of the upper lip, and inscribe the fine lines into the wax surface. (The edge of a spatula moistened with solvant could also be used.) After scribing the lip lines into the surface of the wax it is necessary to remove the ridges (caused by the scribing tool) into a more smooth and natural contour. To accomplish this, dip a small brush in mortuary solvent and using only the weight of the brush, smooth out the lines using a vertical stroke with the brush. This will dissolve the surplus wax particles and shape the lines into their natural contours. Allow the wax to harden before applying the lip cosmetics.

Application of Cream Cosmetics Over Waxed Lips

Mix the lip cream color to the desired shade. Place the mixture in the palm of your hand and spread the cream in a downward direction with the edge of the spatula, forming a thin film of cream on the palm. Dilute the cream using a lip brush dipped in mortuary solvent, and outline the contours of the lips. With the basic shape established, apply the color to the waxed surface with the lip brush diluting the cream with the mortuary solvent before each application. Brush it on very lightly, following the delineated limits of the outline. Build the color up to the desired value with two or three more coats of the lip color. Bring the base complexion color down to meet the outer limits of the upper and lower lips. Remove any visible line of demarcation by stippling with one of the toning shades along the outline of the lips.

▶ COSMETIC POWDER APPLICATION

The principal function of the powder application is to set and dry the various cosmetic media we have applied. When powdering the skin where heavy opaque cosmetics have been applied, a very thin layer of white drying powder should first be evenly distributed. If the powder is applied heavily, it will cake on the surface. If a light layer is applied first and then a heavier layer, as the second application, a smooth and even distribution will be achieved. The general application procedure is to apply a light layer of powder, allow the powder to remain on the surface for a few minutes to set and dry the cosmetics, then remove the surplus. Always apply the powder very lightly. After the correct shade of powder is applied and the powder treatments are completed, there should be no visible traces of powder left on the skin surfaces. The normal skin texture exhibits a slight sheen on both the male and female subject. During the powder treatment, this natural sheen is eliminated, creating a dull matte finish. This dull finish would actually be characteristic of a person who wore makeup in life.

Matte Finish: A non-reflective finish will be the result any time powder is used over mortuary cosmetics. There is no type of powder that does not have the tendency to dull cosmetically treated epidermal surfaces. We must try to duplicate the manner in which the subject applied their own powder, if a natural appearance is to be created. All other skin textures, with the exception of infants and children, require a sheen finish.

Sheen Finish: All normal adult male and female skin textures have a sheen finish. This is because all skin contains natural oils. Since males tend not to wear makeup, a slight sheen must be maintained for their complexion, particularly males with a dark complexion. To create the sheen finish after the powder has dried and set the cosmetics, all visible traces of powder should be removed using the powder brush. The skin is then patted with a gauze pad dampened with water. This treatment removes the dulling effect of the powder and re-establishes the natural sheen of the skin.

Hair Spray: Aerosol hair spray can be used to lightly spray over the surface of cosmetic media after powder treatments have been completed. Lacquer hair spray is particularly effective for adult males with dark complexions in establishing a sheen finish. Non-lacquer spray dries with a matte finish. The use of either type of hair spray will help seal the skin surface and prevent cosmetics from rubbing off.

Method of Powder Application

There are three basic procedures used in applying cosmetic powder over the epidermal surfaces of the face and hands. Cosmetic powder can be applied with a powder brush, powder blower, or powder puff. Whichever method you select, the powder should be applied very lightly in thin layers and evenly distributed.

Brush Application: A powder brush is the most common tool used in application procedures. Brush application consists of scooping up some of the powder on the bristles, holding the brush about two inches above the epidermal surface, and lightly tapping the handle with your index finger, to deposit a light layer of powder. When the brush load is too heavy, tap the brush over the palm of your hand to remove surplus powder before making the application. Allow the powdered surface to dry for approximately five minutes, then remove all excess powder with a clean brush.

Powder Blower Application: The powder blower gives the most control over the amount of powder being deposited. It is excellent for applying drying powder overrestorative media. When using the powder blower, a fine layer of powder can be atomized, eliminating overuse of powder. Even when using the powder blower it is necessary to remove some excess powder with the powder brush after application.

Powder Puff Application: This method of applying powder goes back many years in funeral service, to the time when dry rouge was the most commonly used mortuary cosmetic. The application is made by lightly blotting the powder puff over the epidermal surfaces. When using this method, care must be taken to avoid leaving excessive deposits of powder on the surface. It is necessary to remove all surplus powder from the powder puff before starting the application. This will prevent over-application and caking of the powder on the epidermal surface. After the application is completed, using a soft brush, lightly stipple and smooth out the powder over the epidermal surface.

Removal of Powder from Facial Hair

As a final treatment it is necessary to remove all powder from the facial hair. Special attention should be given to excess powder deposits in the corners of the eyes and mouth, nasal openings, and wings of the nose. This surplus powder is easily removed with cold water or the application of an aersol hair spray. Another method of removing powder is the use of the eyebrow pencil. Sharpen the end of the pencil into a wedge shape. To treat the eyelash, place the blade of a spatula under the lash, so the lash lies flat on the blade. Stroke the eyelash lightly with the flat edge of the pencil. This procedure removes the powder, darkens the lashes, and imparts a natural sheen to the hair of the lash. The eyebrows are treated by placing the flat edge of the pencil against the eyebrow then stroking very lightly from the inner corner to the distal edge of the brow.

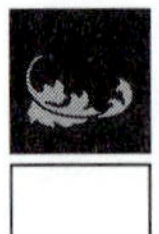

COSMETIZING THE HANDS

Cosmetic procedures used in treating the hands and fingers call for the same degree of cosmetic skill as that used in treating the face.

The hand during life and even in sleep is never rigidly extended. It invariably appears in a convex contour with the fingers bent slightly inward. This gives the hand a graceful semi-oval shape symbolic of peaceful rest, with thumb and forefinger in natural parallel contact. Before applying the cosmetics to the hands, the final cleansing and manicuring should be done.

Restoring the Fingernails

When it becomes necessary to restore the entire nail plate because of badly lacerated or fractured surfaces, the restoration can easily be accomplished by attaching artificial fingernails. These prosthetics, realistically molded from plastic, are available at any cosmetic counter. Some are offered in kit form complete with an adhesive. Super glue, an adhesive on hand in most preparation rooms, can be used for attaching artificial fingernails. The surface should be dry and free of all foreign substances. Trim away all broken nail and skin fragments and pack the fingertip in cotton saturated with a cauterant chemical. Allow this external pack to remain in place as long as possible, preferably overnight. After cauterization is completed, remove the cotton pack and clean the nailbed, removing any fibers that may have become attached to the surface. After cleansing treatments are completed, seal the surface with a clear liquid sealer. This will create a dry and firm foundation. Take a fine layer of premium-grade cotton and fit it over the nailbed so that it conforms perfectly to the contour of the nailbed surface. Apply two or three coats of liquid sealer over the cotton and allow to thoroughly dry. Trim the false nail to the correct contour, and attach it firmly with the super glue. Allow the adhesive to harder before applying nail lacquer and a cosmetic finish.

Dehydrated Fingertips

Troublesome problems concerning dehydration can easily be prevented by early recognition of warning signs which indicate incipient dehydration. One well-defined sign is the presence of abnormally soft tissue in the fingertips. It is an indication that these extremities have not received sufficient chemical preservation during the arterial injection and preventive measures should be taken immediately. It is too late to compensate for it after the fingertips have turned brown and the tips have hardened and leatherized. Immediately upon detection, hypodermically inject the fingertips with a preservative type feature builder or a 50/50 mixutre of cavity solution and humectant chemical until they attain their normal contour and firmness. The natural contour of the fingertips is marked by a smooth roundness with no trace of wrinkling or flattening. Even when there is no visible sign of dehydration in the fingertips, it is a sensible precaution to inject some preservative into them instead of wating for signs of dehydration to appear. These conditions frequently occur after the arterial injection, even under average conditions.

Feature Building the Hands

Feature building techniques compensate for tissue losses caused by wasting diseases before death. It takes only a few moments to inject feature builder into the emaciated areas of the hands and fingers, and it can substantially improve the overall natural appearance. Use of feature builder on the hands and fingers should be standard operating procedure.

▶ BASIC COLOR APPLICATION

The base cosmetic is applied to the hands and fingers as a background colorant, using the same method of application as that used for the face. For all normal applications the following types of cosmetics are used for the basic color application: (1) transparent liquid tint, (2) liquid powder tint, and (3) tinted emollient cream. When it is necessary to use masking-type cosmetics to cope with discolorations and to cover restorative media, the covering qualities of the semi-opaque emollient creams, opaque creams and opaque liquid cosmetics are preferred. The opaque creams and opaque liquids may also be used to create transparent effects when applied sparingly.

Surface Preparation Procedure

When using transparent (alcohol-based) liquid tints, liquid powder tint, or opaque liquid cosmetics, the epidermal surface should be thoroughly clean and free of all massage cream and oily substances. To cleanse and degrease the skin, saturate a gauze pad with mortuary solvent and remove all traces of massage cream from the face and hands. On female subjects make sure that the lower arms (if a short sleeved dress is to be used) are totally devoid of massage cream residue. Thoroughly cleanse and degrease the area around the fingernails, cuticles, knuckles, and lines on the backs of the hands and fingers. A grease-free skin surface is essential for the successful application of all liquid cosmetics. When applying emollient or opaque cream cosmetics, degreasing is not required. All that is necessary is to wipe off all excess massage cream with a gauze pad until a clean, smooth foundation is established. This type of epidermal surface will respond very well to all cream cosmetic media. Transparent liquid and powder tints are applied by using the brush application method and blotting the skin surface with a gauze pad. The liquid opaque medium is also brush applied, the only difference in use is after the liquid opaque is deposited it is stippled out over the skin surface using a stipple brush rather than blotted with a gauze pad to produce a smooth and uniform application.

Warm Color Application

Treating the warm-colored areas of the hands and fingers and re-establishing their natural lines and markings is a very important phase of mortuary cosmetology. The illustrations in Figures 14, 15, 16, and 17 show the specific areas of the hands and fingers subject to warm-color cosmetic application and the captions explain the reasons why these warm-color areas require special attention. The hands and fingers receive only minimal amounts of color through the arterial injection. The palms, fingertips, fingernails, cuticles and inner surfaces of the thumbs are all areas of warm color in the living body. After the arterial injection is completed these areas are usually devoid of this characteristic warm color. The skin around the thumb and forefinger and along the side of the hand usually appears unnaturally white in color with the waxy pallor indicative of embalmed tissue. A similar absence of natural color is also visible on dark-skinned Latins and Afro-Americans after embalming. These missing warm-color characteristics must be cosmetically restored if we wish to achieve a natural lifelike appearance in lifeless tissue.

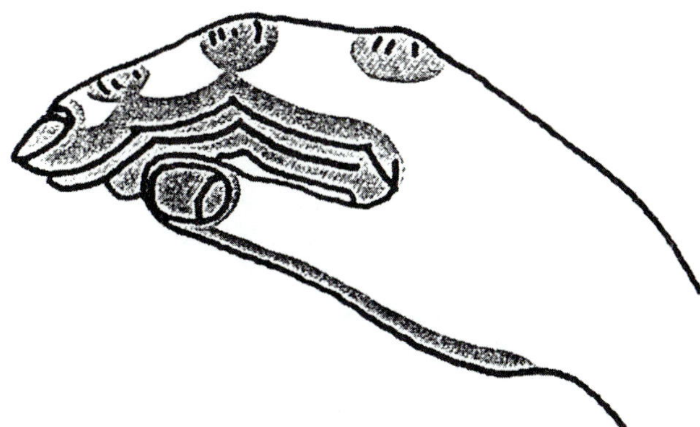

Figure 14. This lateral view of the hand and fingers seen with the thumb in the foreground shows warm color locations indicated by the shaded areas. Note that warm color starts in the palm of the hand and spreads to the underside of the fingers and thumb and appears along the outer contour of the thumb and forefinger. Warm color also extends to the fingertips, encircles the fingernails (cuticles) and leaves a glow of warm color at each finger joint. Color is carried slightly beyond the thumb pad at the base of the palm and blended into the wrist.

Cosmetic Treatment of Discolorations

Cosmetic treatments used to conceal tissue discolorations have a high priority in preparing the deceased human body for viewing. When we analyze the causes and effects of discoloration, we find that they are divided into two major categories: ante-mortem discolorations, and post-mortem discolorations. The professional embalmer/cosmetician should have a general knowledge of the basic anatomical and physiological structure of the epidermal tissues and be able to ascertain whether the discoloration is of a chemical, physi-

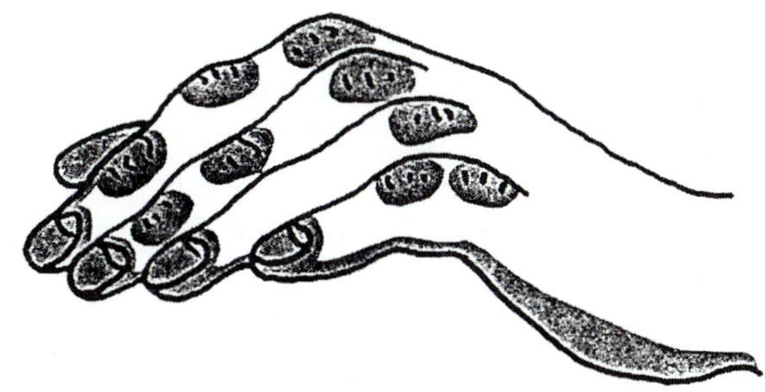

Figure 15. This side and top view of the hand is seen with the little finger in the foreground, showing the distribution of warm color rising upward from the palm and extending around the contour of the hand, fingers, and fingertips and encircling the fingernails. A glow of warm color appears on the knuckles. Color is carried toward the wrist from the palmar surface of the hand. All warm color areas must be blended into the basic complexion colorant so that no distinct lines of demarcation are visible.

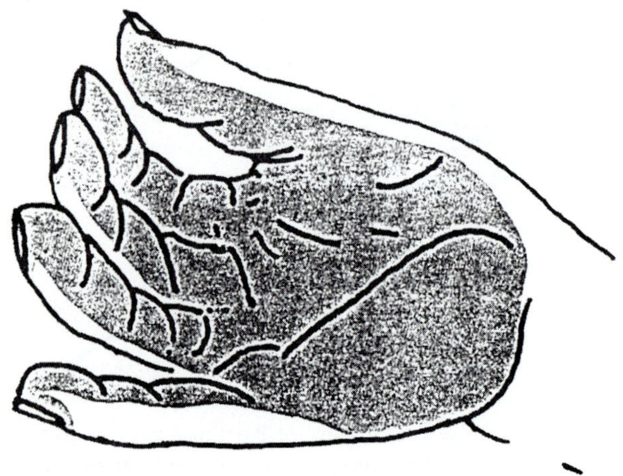

Figure 16. Here the upturned palm is seen from above to indicate the characteristic natural distribution of warm color. Note that the warm color of the palm radiates into the lower surfaces and sides of the thumb, small finger, forefinger, all fingertips, and the palm itself. Although we normally do not apply warm color to the invisible palms of the hands, the illustration serves to show how the color radiates into the visible areas of the hands and fingers, where it contributes greatly to natural-looking cosmetic results.

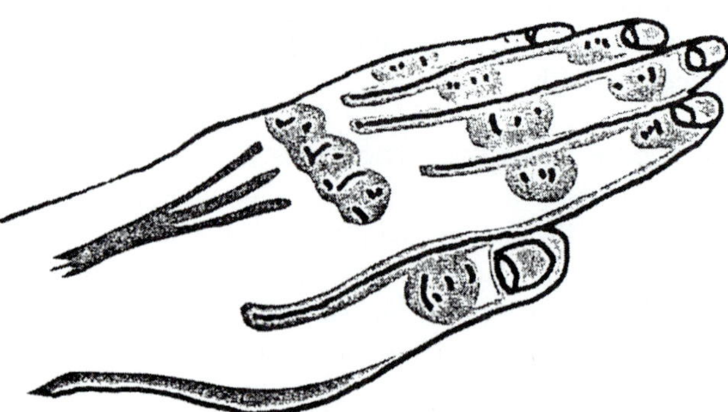

Figure 17. This view of the back of the hand shows how warm color radiates from the palmar surface around the contours of the fingers and thumb. The illustration also shows how warm color accents begin at the fingertips, and continue around the cuticles with a blush of color on the knuckles and tendons on the back of the hand. In some cases the tendons on the back of the hand appear more prominently than in others. The warm color in this area would vary according to the prominence of this feature in each individual case. All red colorant should be blended to a full vanishing point for a realistic natural effect.

cal, or mechanical nature. Unbroken skin surfaces and discolorations, other than discolored swollen tissues, are treated in post-embalming procedures and need no further attention prior to the cosmetic application. Broken skin surfaces and discolorations are subject to special pre-embalming and restorative treatments if a thoroughly professional result is to be expected.

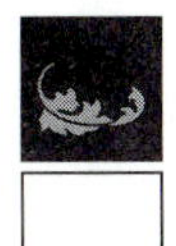

DISCOLORATIONS

▶ POST-EMBALMING TREATMENTS OF DISCOLORATIONS

Broken Skin Surfaces: The arterial injection will normally cause swelling and leakage in broken skin. A cauterant chemical can be injected into the affected area before the arterial injection is made, which prevents swelling, dries and seals the broken skin tissues, prevents leakage and, most important, establishes a stable restorative foundation. When it is not possible to treat the broken skin before the arterial injection and when delay is unavoidable, make sure that the subcutaneous injection of the cauterant is made at least one or preferably two hours before starting the restorative treatments. This will insure a stable foundation.

Unbroken Skin Surface: Evaluate the preservative stability and extent of the discoloration before starting the cosmetic treatments. Small discolorations where the tissues have been well preserved by the arterial solution will require no further treatment beyond masking with opaque cosmetics. Large discolorations usually do not readily respond to preservation via the arterial injection and therefore should be given supplementary hypodermic treatment. Prepare a solution consisting of 50% cavity solution and 50% humectant (some embalmers use 100% cavity chemical). Inject it subcutaneously throughout the entire discolored area using a 22 gauge hypodermic needle. Distribute the solution in the tissues by manual manipulation until spread uniformly throughout. Always keep in mind that tissue breakdown in the dermal layer tends to retard the chemical circulation and these areas should be treated independently by subcutaneous hypodermic injection. Properly executed, this procedure will produce a smooth, natural skin texture and contour. The humectant in the hypodermic solution inhibits dehydration and wrinkling. The cavity chemical preserves the tissues and helps dispel the discoloration by its bleaching action. Ecchymosis is characterized by an intense, purple-black discoloration of the skin, most commonly appearing on the back of the hand and in trauma to the eyes, and it is frequently accompanied by swelling. Correction of ecchymosis can be accomplished by subcutaneous hypodermic injection using a cauterant chemical.

Discoloration on Back of Hands: Swelling may be associated with ecchymosis in the back of the hand caused by hypodermic needle punctures. This swelling may be reduced by injecting a cauterant chemical into the affected area before the arterial injection. Massage the tissues with your fingertips until the swelling is visibly reduced. The bleaching action of the cauterant chemical also dispels most of the discolorations. After the arterial injection is completed, apply an external pack by saturating absorbent cotton (premium grade) with the cauterant and placing it over the discolored area. Allow the compress to remain on the surface until a noticeable reduction of color intensity results.

Discolored and Swollen Eyelids: Swelling and discoloration of the eyelids (black eye) may be reduced by two methods: hypodermic injection and the electrical reducing iron. Because the arterial injection normally increases swelling in traumatized eyelids, it is imperative that the reduction be made before injection, while the tissues are still pliable and the blood is in its natural liquid state and not coagulated.* Hypodermically injecting a cauterant chemical into the eyelids will reduce the swelling and bleach out most of the purple-black discoloration. Both the upper and lower eyelids are injected subcutaneously, and excess serous liquid is pressed out through the needle-entry puncture. Use a 20 cc syringe fitted with a 22 gauge x 2 inch hypodermic needle. Starting with an empty syringe, insert the needle at the distal end of the eyebrow, and channel underneath the eyelids by repeated back and forth movements. Upon completing the channeling, do not withdraw the hypodermic needle. Simply disengage the needle from the barrel of the syringe, fill the syringe with the cauterant chemical, and reattach it to the syringe. Inject both the upper and lower eyelids with the cauterant chemical. Inject the upper lid first, and move the hypodermic needle back and forth so the swollen tissue becomes completely saturated with the cauterant. Remove the syringe and needle. Massage the eyelids and press downward with very firm pressure using your fingertips and thumb. Apply pressure in an outward di-

* Some embalmers prefer to perform all invasive tissue corrections *after* arterial injection.

rection toward the needle-entry point. Apply a heavy coat of cosmetic massage cream before rubbing the eyelids. Continue the massage until swelling is visibly reduced. Massaging should always immediately follow hypodermic injection. Any delay will allow the tissues to harden and become set, making it impossible to reduce the swelling. The bleaching action of the cauterant chemical also lightens any eyelid discoloration.

The electric reducing iron can be used effectively to reduce slight eyelid swelling or excessive wrinkling when the tissues are soft and pliable, even when no hypodermic reduction has preceded its use. However, maximum performance results when subcutaneous injection and heat reduction treatments are combined.

The Electric Reducing Iron

The electric reducing iron is equipped with two interchangeable attachments. The heavy attachment retains maximum working temperature and is used for reducing and smoothing swollen tissues. The light attachment is designed with a tapered, semi-rounded tip for re-establishing natural character lines and wrinkles. The heavy attachment is used for reducing swollen eyelids with the iron heated to its maximum temperature level. Coat the eyelids with a heavy layer of cosmetic massage cream and keep the skin well lubricated with massage cream, because it melts from the heat of the iron. Repeat cream application and heat contact until swelling is reduced. Treat the upper eyelid first by placing the flat side of the heavy attachment on the surface of the lid, allowing contact with the skin for a mere fraction of a second. Start at the inner corner of the eyelid and slowly advance outward carefully to the distal corner. Avoid using an "ironing" motion because this will cause leatherization and browning of the delicate eyelid tissues. Caution should be used in treating the edges of the eyelids which tend to curl the eyelashes upward in an unnatural fashion when the hot iron is placed too close to the edge of the lid. Also, avoid contact with the eyelashes. If curling should occur in the upper eyelashes, insert the heavy attachment under the eyelid and apply pressure upward and outward in one movement, running the edge of the iron back and forth under the perimeter of the eyelid. Repeat this procedure until the eyelashes resume their natural alignment.

After reduction treatments are completed, replace the eye cap. Apply a small amount of adhesive stay cream on the contact surface of the eye cap and position the eyelids in their natural alignment. Seal the edges of the upper and lower eyelids together with super glue to prevent separation of the lids after establishing the natural closure.

Cosmetics Used in Treating Discolorations

In treating discolorations and restored skin surfaces, the combination of opaque liquid and opaque cream cosmetics is a very effective combination in establishing natural skin coloring. These cosmetics will mask virtually any type of discoloration or restored surface.

Liquid Opaque Cosmetic: This liquid opaque pigment is formulated to conceal difficult post-mortem discolorations. They are available in liquid and aerosol media. The liquid opaques are fast drying and impart a natural looking, non-caking translucent coloring with good stability to the skin surface and are used in all "undercoating" treatments.

Opaque Cream Pigments: The opaque cream pigments are widely used in cosmetic procedures involving the masking of skin discolorations, concealing minor blemishes and imparting natural color (basic complexion color) over surface restoration media.

Toning Creams: The toning cream cosmetic is very versatile and exceptionally well formulated for toning and color coordinating procedures when used over masked discolorations and restored skin surfaces. The following colors are used in toning treatments: light brown, dark brown, black, purple, blue, yellow, light rouge, and dark rouge.

Technical Procedure in Treating Discolorations

The following technical procedures are designed to treat discolored and restored skin surfaces and these techniques are used for masking unbroken skin conditions such as yellow jaundice, petechial hemorrhage, ecchymosis, and contusions. The following steps list the order of application in masking epidermal surfaces and restorative media.

1. Undercoat Application. Brush apply liquid opaque cosmetic (or spray the aerosol media) directly over the discoloration. The color should match the natural (untreated) skin surface. Carefully apply the liquid opaque cosmetic evenly over the surface allowing it to extend about $\frac{1}{4}$ inch beyond the margin of the area being treated. Stipple out all lines of demarcation and allow to thoroughly dry.

2. Basic Color Application. Apply the correct shade of basic complexion colorant over the normal skin surfaces, extending it very lightly over the undercoat previously applied in step 1. Stipple and blend the basic colorant softly into the undercoating deposit. Smooth out the basic complexion cosmetic, stippling the opaque pigment very lightly over the treated surface, adjusting the application to attain a translucent effect.

3. Toning Application. Select the correct shade of toning cream to match the individual's natural complexion color as closely as possible. Using a light stippling movement with a camel hair stippling brush, apply the toning cream very lightly over the basic complexion colorant. This treatment replaces the melanin pigmentation naturally present in all complexions. Use light brown toning cream for all light to medium complexions; dark brown toning cream on dark complexions ranging in the brown to black category; and black toning cream is used on dark complexions ranging in the ebony to black range. The toning cream is applied very lightly, so lightly that it is barely visible. This light application tones the opaque cosmetic into a natural translucent skin coloring with an undertone of natural lifelike color.

4. Drying and Finishing Powder Application. Apply white drying and finishing powder over the cosmetized epidermal surfaces, using the powder blower for uniform distribution. Allow the powder to remain on the cosmetized surface for at least five minutes so that it will dry and set the cosmetics properly. Remove the surplus powder with a powder brush.

5. Replacing Natural Facial Lines and Markings. After removing all surplus powder, use light brown or dark brown toning cream to duplicate the characteristic coloring of facial lines, wrinkles, and natural markings. As the color is deposited, gently blend the cosmetic into a natural color intensity by lightly stippling over the skin with a clean and dry brush.

Individual Minor Discolorations

Opaque cosmetics (liquid spray or cream) applied over small discolorations will create a contrasting line on the skin surface. When treating small discolorations, liquid opaque cosmetic is applied as an undercoat to permanently obscure the discolored area. It is essential that this undercoat be a close approximation of the natural skin coloring. The basic complexion cosmetic should be lightly blended over the undercoat application. Upon completion of the basic complexion application, stipple a very light, thin coat of opaque cream cosmetic (matching the basic color application) over the discolored surface. With the basic complexion colorant properly blended over the undercoat application, the treated area is now perfected with the application of the correct shade of toning cream. The application of the toning cream removes all marginal lines of demarcation and brings out the true complexion coloring, achieving undetectable masking of the discoloration.

Warm Color Discolorations

When discolorations extend to the warm color areas of the face and hands, red colorant should be added to the liquid opaque undercoat. Brush apply the liquid opaque cosmetic and let it dry thoroughly. Blend the correct basic complexion color over the undercoat application, leaving a red undertone of color. Make the usual warm color application, blending the colorant out so that no line of demarcation is apparent. Apply toning cream and accent natural lines and markings as indicated.

Complete Surface Discoloration

In some situations, such as yellow jaundice, carbon monoxide poisoning, and petechial hemorrhage, it becomes necessary to totally mask the entire skin surface. Liquid opaque pigment is applied as an undercoat or an aerosol spray undercoat can be applied. The liquid opaque is brush applied in a overall application on the face and hands masking the discolored skin surface. This procedure will undercoat and seal the epidermal surface masking the discoloration. After the liquid opaque has thoroughly dried, match the complexion colorant with opaque cream cosmetic. Apply uniformly as lightly as possible, blending the cream over the undercoat. The opaque cream bonds with the undercoat and establishes a translucent background color of living tissue. Apply the warm color (red) in a heavier deposit than normal because the soft texture of the opaque cream base will reduce and absorb the red colorant. A second application of red colorant may have to be applied over the warm color areas to produce a natural-looking effect. Blend the warm color into the basic complexion colorant until no line of demarcation can be seen. Apply the correct shade of eye shadow to the upper eyelid and apply purple colorant along the lash line. The muted purple is applied where the lash enters the ridge of the eyelid, producing a rounded contour and natural color. When masking cosmetics have been used, it is necessary to apply white drying powder before cosmetically treating the facial lines and natural markings. Because of the absorbent quality of the opaque cream medium it is nearly impossible to realistically duplicate the lines and markings. The skin surfaces must be completely dry and stable before these treatments can be accomplished. After the detailing treatments are completed, white drying powder is applied. Hairspray can be applied after excess powder is removed.

Cosmetically Treating Wax Surfaces

Epidermal surfaces restored with wax may be cosmetically treated by several different procedures to produce a natural texture and skin coloring. The three most commonly used methods are:

1. Surface Undercoating. Liquid opaque cosmetic is brush applied as an undercoat over the restored surface or an aerosol spray undercoat may be used. After the opaque undercoat has completely dried, surface restorer wax is applied over the undercoated surface. This will mask the restoration and any discoloration associated with the traumatized tissue around the restoration. Opaque cosmetic medium (cream or liquid) is then lightly applied over the wax surface, matching the opaque application with the basic complexion colorant.

2. Intermixing Wax Colors. This procedure is based on matching the surface restorer wax by coordinating the color of the wax with the complexion or warm color tone. Various shades of wax are intermixed (usually two or three shades) until a basic or warm color equivalent is attained. The opaque cosmetic medium (cream or liquid) is then lightly blended over the wax surface, matching the natural complexion or warm colorant.

3. Cosmetic Over Wax. Restorations should be completed, including duplication of natural lines and wrinkles and simulation of pore texture, before applying the opaque cosmetic medium over the waxed surface. It is essential that the waxed restoration surface be allowed to firmly re-set to its natural consistency before applying the opaque cosmetic medium. It usually takes about 20 minutes at room temperature for the wax to harden. After the wax has set, brush apply the opaque medium (cream or liquid) over the waxed surface. Very lightly stipple blend the opaque cosmetic over the wax surface. Avoid wax build-up on the bristles of the brush during this operation. Clean the brush frequently while working or the wax build-up on the bristles will damage and distort the restored surface.

History of Modern Restorative Art

Edward C. Johnson • Gail R. Johnson • Melissa J. Williams

SECTION III

The reader is advised to reread the section on Egyptian embalming procedures entitled Ancient Restorative Art found in the preceding section of this text.

To date, no record of a restorative art procedure applied during the anatomical or middle period of embalming history has been found. Virtually all documented reports of embalming in this period include the practice of enclosing the preserved body within a metal-lined, hermetically sealed coffin, which precluded viewing. To satisfy some medieval customs relating to funeral practices and chivalry, an imago or effigy of the decedent was created by preparing a death mask as the basis for the head. The features were painted to closely resemble the normal lifelike appearance, and effigies were often adorned with a wig. The completed head was attached to a torso, complete with arms and legs, proportional to the life size of the decedent. The effigy was dressed in the clothing or armor of the decedent and placed on the coffin containing the corpse, where it remained during the entire period preceding actual interment (Figure 1).

A few examples of effigies still remain in storage at Westminster Abbey, London, England.

During the U.S. Civil War a few, a very few, documents indicate that some effort was made to repair traumatic injuries. One such document in the Frank Hutton collection is a letter from the family of a Union Army soldier who was embalmed and sent home for burial. The family wrote in their letter to Hutton, that the corpse "looked pretty good for being dragged by mules."

By and large, however, it can be stated without fear of contradiction that very little of what is referred to today as restorative art was practiced until the second decade of the 20th century. There were exceptions occasionally, such as the treatment of the anarchist bomber's suicide in Chicago briefly described in the section on Felix Aloysius Sullivan (see the preceding section). Joseph H. Clarke briefly mentions the treatment of a tumor case in his book *Reminiscences of Early Embalming.*

What is termed restorative art today represents the greatest remaining challenge to the skill, the ability to improvise, and the courage of the practicing embalmer. It is the last frontier and poses problems to test those who choose to grapple with its manifest difficulties. Formerly known most commonly by several popular terms such as plastic surgery, demisurgery, and dermasurgery, it is today most commonly referred to as restorative art.

The term *restorative art,* not adopted until the early 1930s, is in reality a poorly contrived label for specialized postmortem treatment accorded those dying of trauma or debilitating disease, the practice of which is most often believed to have originated entirely in the United States in recent years. Such a premise is false inasmuch as the practice of restorative art is dependent on and inseparable from the embalming procedure. Thus, one realizes that restorative art has been practiced from the origin of embalming in Egypt and so it was (Figure 2).

The year 1912 marks the establishment of the modern era of what is today known as restorative art. The first articles appeared in the April 19, 1912, issue of *The Sunnyside. Demisurgery,* as it was to be termed by its founder, was "the art of building or creating parts of the body which have been destroyed by accident, disease, decomposition or discoloration, and making the body perfectly natural and lifelike."

The science of restorative art as known today was founded by one man, Joel E. Crandall, then an embalmer in New York City. Although many others made important contributions to this science through the years, no other one person can claim the honor of stimulating the interest of fellow embalmers in this most difficult technical subject area.

An editorial in the April 19, 1912 issue of *The Sunnyside* stated that "the photographs of before and after appearance of a mutilated body show what can and should be done. The originator of the new art of demisurgery is Joel E. Crandall of New York City and his first article on the new technique appears in the pages of this issue of *The Sunnyside*" (Figure 3).

An early acknowledgement of Crandall's primacy

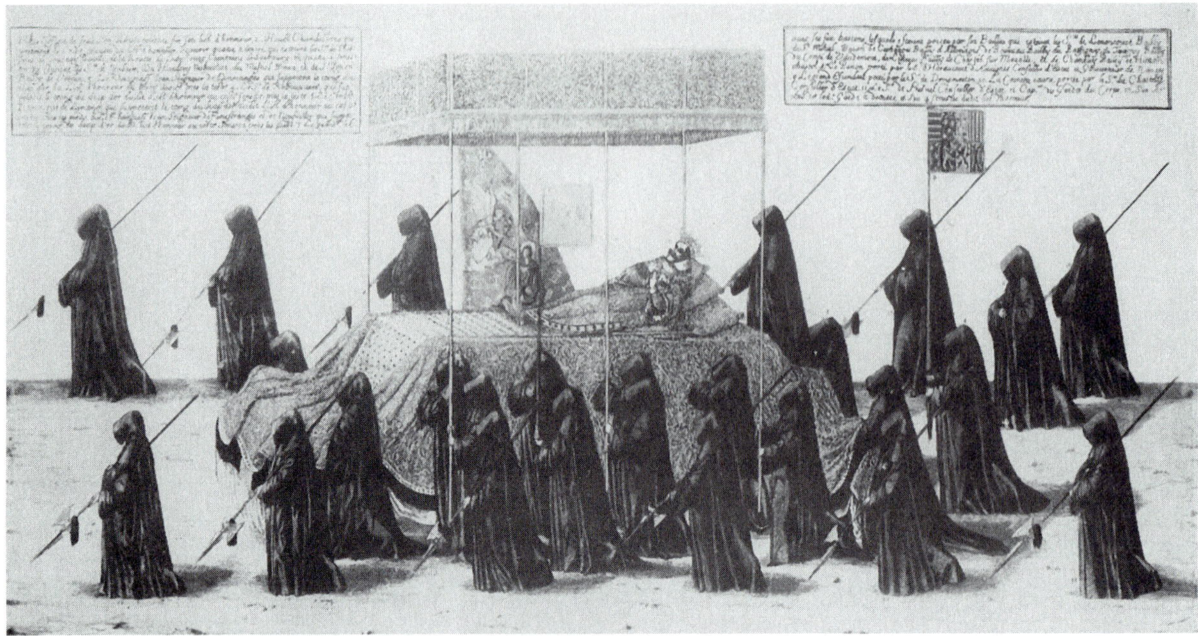

Figure 1. Medieval funeral procession. Note effigy of deceased.

in the field was made by Howard S. Eckels in a letter published in the May 14, 1914, issue of *The Sunnyside,* stating that the science of demisurgery was indeed founded by Joel E. Crandall.

A. Johnson Dodge quoted in the June 1, 1917, issue of *The Casket,*

> How to care for mutilated or postmortem cases, or bodies which from any cause have become unsightly and make them presentable, should constitute a part of the education of the embalmer. Thorough instruction in this difficult part of the art should be given by the instructors in our schools. But this part of the work requires special experience and some study either to practice or teach it successfully. It was first taught as a specialty by Mr. Joel E. Crandall of New York City, and to him belongs the credit of introducing it. We think Mr. Crandall is the only person who has attained any great degree of success in the practice of this art, and would recommend the student who wishes to attain a high degree of proficiency in this part of his profession to apply to Mr. Crandall for instruction, as he appears to be the only known person really competent to teach it.

Joel E. Crandall (1878–1942) was born on September 16, 1878, in Whitesville, New York, the son of Norris Crandall and Caroline Andrews Crandall. Fol-

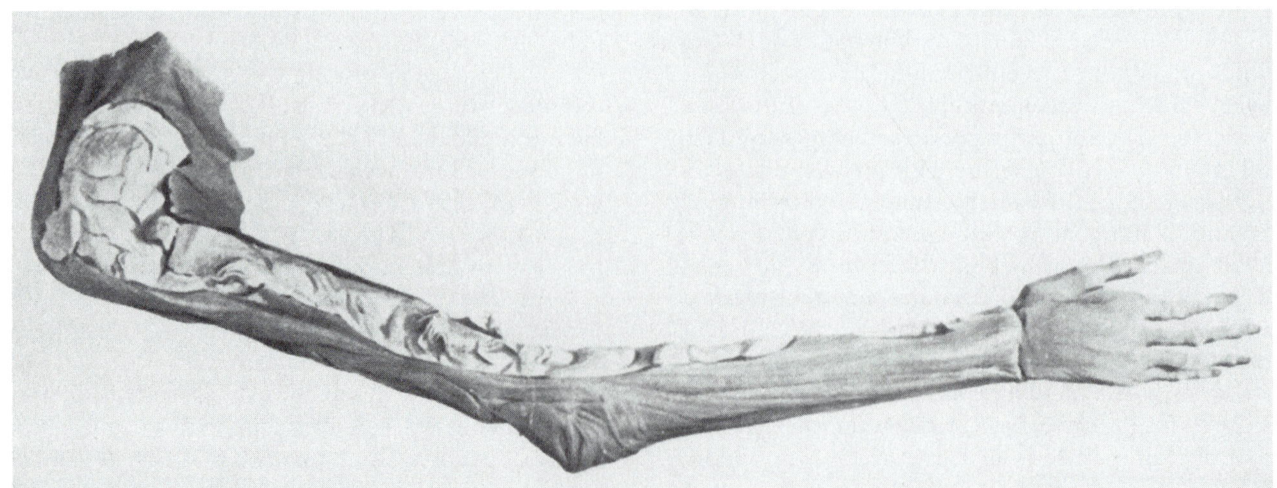

Figure 2. Arm of a mummy of Egypt's XXIst Dynasty, showing the packing material.

Wishing you a continuance of good health and success,
I beg to remain,

Respectfully yours,

Franklin F. Briggs

The following is the close of an article in the Hackensack paper:

The Board of Education has ordered the schools closed tomorrow.

On many buildings flags are already noticed at half mast.

The body of the deceased Mayor will be taken to his late home from the undertaking establishment of Demarest—Briggs, Hackensack, this evening, and despite all rumors to the contrary the remains will be viewed by the many friends who care to call, thanks to the skill of the undertakers.

The services will be conducted by the Masons.

REMEMBER

I guarantee satisfaction or no charge.

—

Can you ask for a more liberal offer?

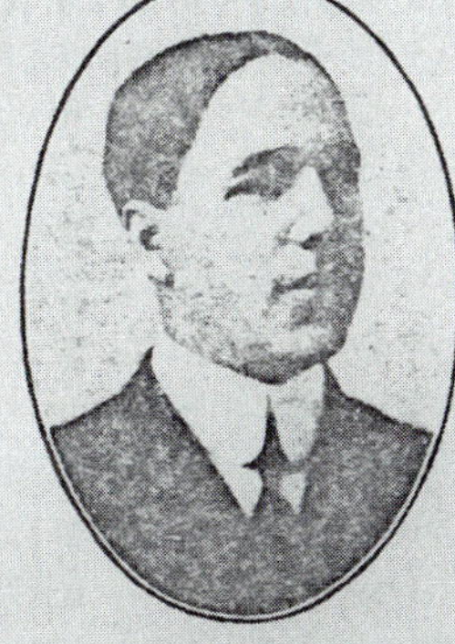

For REFERENCE

I will give the names of many undertakers to whom my work has been very satisfactory.

CALLS ANSWERED AT ANY TIME---ANY WHERE

Any questions regarding this work cheerfully answered upon request

J. E. CRANDALL

TELEPHONE
451 Chelsea

254 WEST 25th STREET
NEW YORK CITY

Figure 3. Crandall's advertisement for his services.

lowing the customary education available at the time, he worked at a variety of jobs. At about 20 years of age he began working for a New York City undertaker. Deeply interested in embalming and becoming increasingly skillful, his services were much in demand and he was employed by both the Frank E. Campbell and Stephen Merritt undertaking establishments as well as the National Casket Company.

Writing in 1912 about his efforts to repair mutilated cases, he stated that he had studied the problems over a period of 10 years. His early efforts to use conventional materials such as plaster of Paris were abandoned for any use except as an interior deep filler in contact with bone. He formulated covering cosmetics and a waxlike putty to fill in missing or damaged areas.

His earliest experiments were on severely mutilated bodies that neither the family nor the undertaker believed could be restored to viewability. Little by little over the years, by trial and error, he developed a successful system for treatment of mutilated cases that eventually embodied most present-day principles or techniques.

Among the requirements Crandall advocated were a recent photograph of the decedent as a reference for the restoration, hardening of the soft tissues of the face as a prerequisite to demisurgery, and enough working time to carry out the entire treatment. Crandall also made the earliest mention of the use of "concealed stitches" to close lacerations and "corrective surgery" to remove remnants of features or tissue impossible to incorporate into the restoration. For his early research he made use of plaster life-size heads that he mutilated and repaired: a procedure that was eventually adopted in one form or another by most embalming schools for laboratory practice and is generally used to this day.

Crandall began his career in demisurgery by offering his services anywhere within a 400-mile radius of New York City. Gradually, by demand, he was compelled to offer instruction in demisurgery. Each class was limited to 25 students for a 1-month period of instruction.

About the same time he manufactured and sold the first demisurgical grip containing all required instruments, cosmetics, brushes, prefabricated mustaches and eyelashes, and preformed facial features of wax.

The use of prefabricated features as a base for individual modification of the decedent's facial topography enabled the unskilled or untrained embalmer to perform a reasonable restoration otherwise impossible. Crandall's brilliant concept was to be duplicated by others a number of times over the ensuing years.

A report of a restoration in 1924 mentions the use of prefabricated eyes and nose. The manufacturer of the parts, William Collier of New York City, advertised a kit containing prefabricated features in 1929 and patented the same in 1931. The Eckels Company of Philadelphia offered a similar kit in October of 1930 (Figure 4), as did the Paasche Air Brush Company of Chicago in 1936. An interesting improvement on prefabricated features was developed by a dental plastic surgeon named C. J. Speas, who taught restorative art at Gupton–Jones College of Mortuary Science in Nashville, Tennessee, in the late 1940s. The basic con-

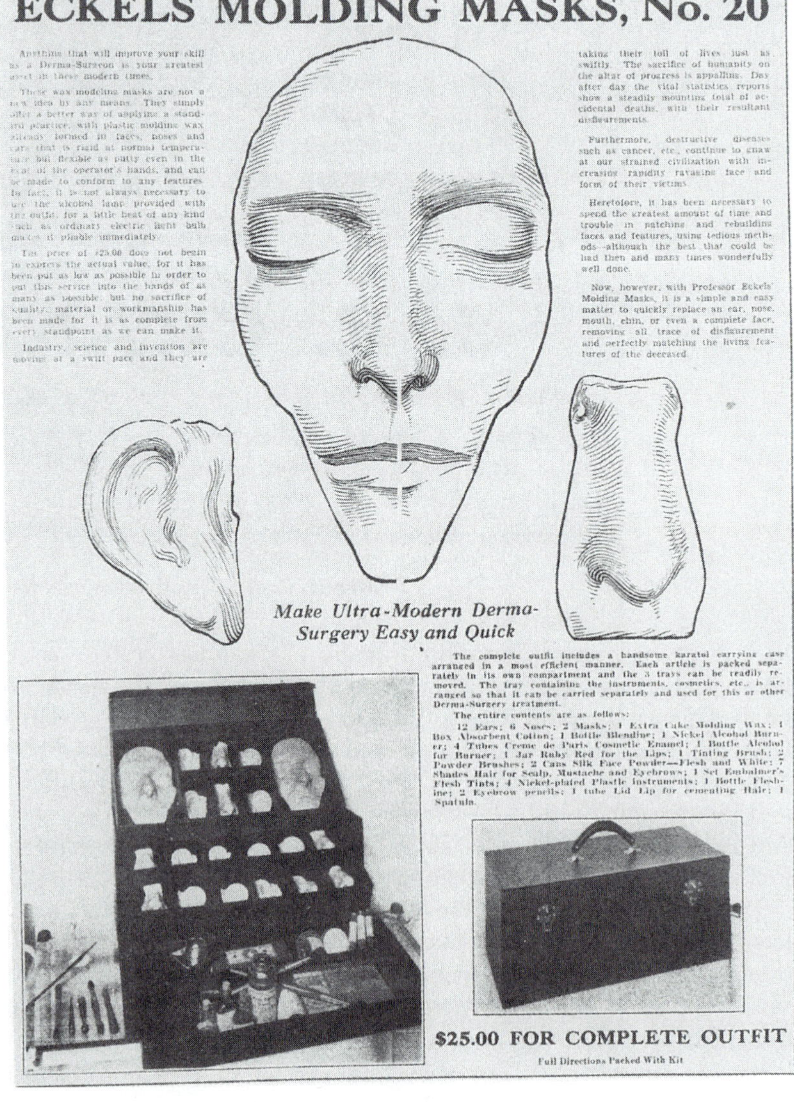

Figure 4. Advertisement for Eckels molding masks.

cept was the "family resemblance theory," that is, members of the same family frequently resemble one another very closely. Thus, for example, when a nose is destroyed, a mold is made of the nose of a family member most closely resembling the decedent, cast in wax, and fitted into the decedent's face. Thus, a custom-made prefabrication is created.

Crandall purchased the Clerihew Undertaking Company located at 133 Broadway, Paterson, New Jersey, in 1913, and continued to maintain premises in New York City for his demisurgical supply company and school. Crandall must have written at some length on the subject of demisurgery, because *The Funeral Director's Encyclopedia,* a proposed three-volume work, each volume supposed to contain about 600 pages, was described in *The Sunnyside* in 1916 as having 100 pages on the art of demisurgery by Joel E. Crandall. No copies of this three-volume encyclopedia are known to exist and it is suspected that it was never published. The 100 pages on demisurgery referred to were most likely the basic lectures used by Crandall in the resident course of instruction at the Demisurgical Institute of New York and as a teaching text in his correspondence course in 1918 (Figure 5). (The writers have never seen this material and would be most grateful to any member of our profession having a copy of same, making it available for inspection and study.)

The greatest impact of Crandall's influence on the embalmers of America resulted from his published photographs of mutilated cases taken before and after treatment, most of which were extremely difficult to restore even by today's standards. His work was exceptionally well done and was an inspiration to embalmers who desired to improve their skills, for he showed and proved that difficult cases could be restored to a viewable condition.

The effect of Crandall's announcement of the founding of the art of demisurgery on the embalming schools of the country varied. Some heads of schools such as Robbins of Boston, C. O. Dhonau of Cincinnati, and Thorton Barnes of New York were rather vocal in their protest concerning Crandall's claim to founding the science (Figure 6). All three claimed that their schools had taught the subject for years, though in truth no mention of the matter in advertising nor listing of the subject matter in the school curricula is noted prior to April 1912. Barnes' Schools began to advertise the teaching of DerMort-Ology, and the Cincinnati School added a course in demisurgery, whereas Robbins stated that his school taught artistic embalming, decoloration, and postmortem surgery. C. A. Renouard stated that he neither taught nor recommended the use of cosmetics and, further, that much of demisurgery was unnecessary and unwelcome.

DEMISURGERY

—OR—

THE NEW ART IN UNDERTAKING

WE WISH TO ANNOUNCE THE OPENING OF THE

DEMISURGICAL INSTITUTE

OF NEW YORK

On Feb. 18th, 1918, the Demisurgical Institute of New York will open its doors to the Profession with a complete course in the Art of Demisurgery.

The course will consist of Lectures, Experimental and Practical work and when completed every student will be able to restore nearly every mutilated case to its natural condition.

Each student will also receive a diploma, which will entitle him to the degree of "Demisurgeon," which name may be used in any way in connection with his business.

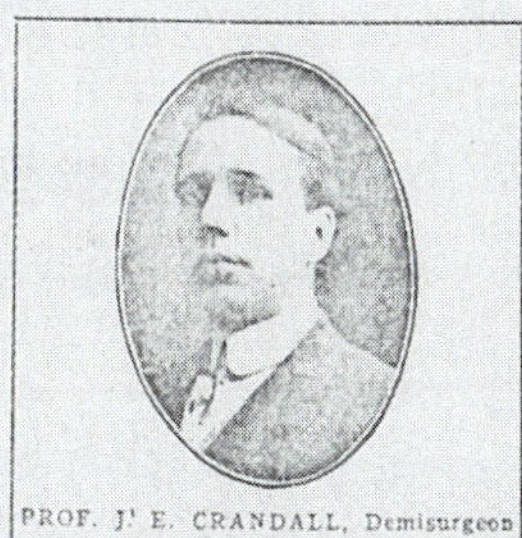

PROF. J. E. CRANDALL, Demisurgeon

The course will be given each month from Feb. 18th to June 18th, at which time the Institute will close to resume again on Sept. 18th.

As we have had many requests from prospective students, to be entered in the first class, we have decided that no applications will be considered until this announcement appears, and then each one accepted in turn, and as each class will be limited to 25 students, each applicant will be notified what month he may enter.

Write your application at once if you wish to enter one of the first classes and don't wait until your competitor forces you to do so.

ADDRESS ALL COMMUNICATIONS TO

DEMISURGICAL SUPPLY CO., 500 Fifth Avenue, New York City

Figure 5. Copy of the first ad for demisurgery in 1918.

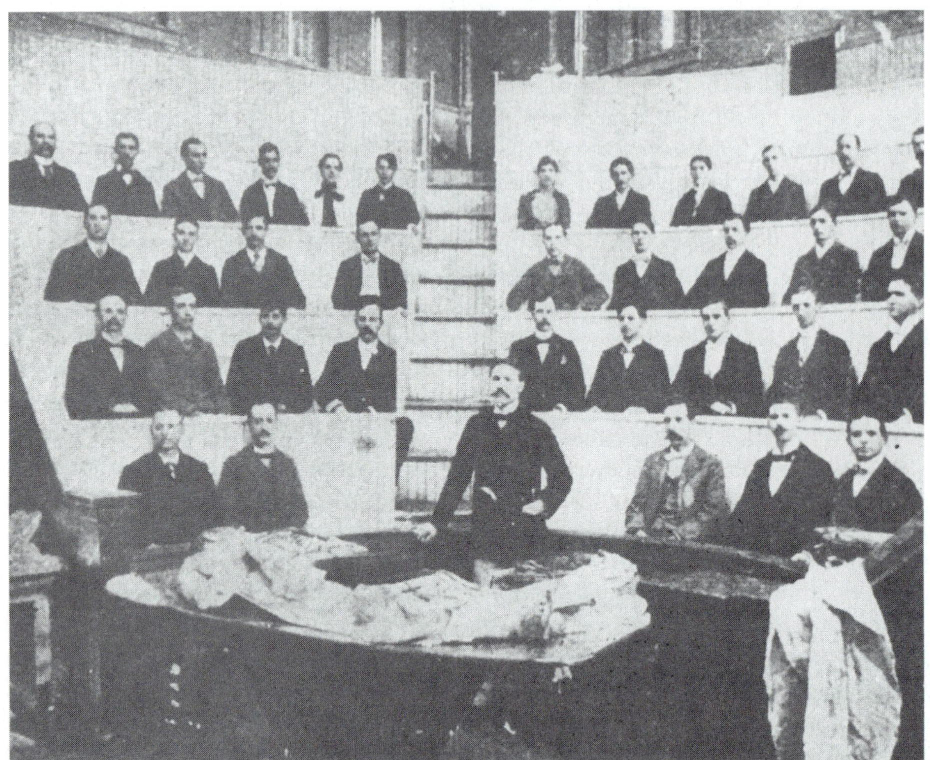

Figure 6. Carl L. Barnes (center) giving a demonstration in the Cook County Morgue, contiguous to the Barnes college building.

Before his death, in 1953, Renouard was to reverse his opinion to the extent of even providing special short-term courses in restorative art.

Dhonau additionally accused Crandall of publishing retouched photographs of his restored cases. This so incensed Crandall that he secured affidavits from every one concerned—the undertaker, the photographer, lawyers, and family representatives, who attested to the authenticity of his work as represented by the case photographs.

Lena Simmons composed a satirical account of a fictional Lemuel, the young embalmer at Burrywell & Company who "fixed him up." She skillfully concocted a case report using quotations from published articles on demisurgical procedures by Robbins and others, but curiously enough did not include any by Crandall.

The interest in the new art of demisurgery was immediate and has continued to the present day. The professional journals increasingly carried both photographs and case reports of successful treatment of mutilated cases, while advertisements multiplied for cosmetics, instruments, and demisurgical materials.

Crandall's career blossomed as he lectured on demisurgery at the New York State Embalmers Convention in the fall of 1912 and continued a busy demisurgical practice.

Among the cases Crandall treated was the famous Colonel Jacob Astor, who in 1912 as a passenger on the Titanic died at sea. His body, like hundreds of others, was taken from the sea near the site of the sinking and transported to Halifax, Nova Scotia, and from there returned to New York City for burial. Crandall was called by the New York undertaker in charge to treat Astor's badly discolored face. By means of Crandall's cosmetic skill, the casket was open for viewing of the body as it lay in state at the Astor estate near Rhinebeck, New York.

The February 1917 issue of *The Sunnyside* carried a notice that Crandall had motion pictures taken of a number of his demisurgical cases and that the films would be available for teaching purposes and presentation at conventions. Historically, this is the first known recording of any restorative procedures in motion pictures.

Crandall continued to be in demand to lecture before large crowds at state conventions on this new and intriguing subject, appearing on several state programs in New England in 1917. By 1918 the effect of World War I on the funeral profession was becoming evident and Crandall was interviewed by *The Sunnyside* for his views on the application of demisurgery to U.S. war casualties. He was most forthright in his conviction that all our war dead should be embalmed shortly after death and restored later at a convenient time and place.

Crandall's illustrated demisurgical case reports continued to be seen in professional journals through 1922. From 1923 on, however, Crandall fades in national note, though continuing to operate his Paterson, New Jersey, funeral home until death on July 19, 1942.

Joel E. Crandall demonstrated that any case, no matter how badly mutilated, could be restored to viewability. Further, he devised not only the materials for his newly created science of demisurgery, but the technical instructions to accomplish this new skill.

All practicing embalmers owe a debt of gratitude to Joel E. Crandall, demisurgeon and founder of demisurgery, known today as restorative art.

The sudden and unforeseen arrival of Joel E. Crandall on the educational scene as the founder of the new art of demisurgery created the problem of partial loss of educational leadership for the American embalming schools. Recovering quickly from this threat, most schools began to teach the subject, although some, out of pride or vanity, refused to give the new art Crandall's title: demisurgery.

The immediate exception was Cincinnati College, which called the subject demisurgery but insisted that the subject had been taught there for years. Eckels College used the term *demisurgery* and acknowledged Crandall as its founder. Boston College called the course *postmortem surgery and the art of decoloration,* and the Barnes School dubbed it *Der-Mort-Ology and dermasurgery.* An article describing Albert Worsham's demonstration of demisurgery calls it *plastic work.* The terms *dermasurgery* and *plastic surgery* also were noted as descriptive titles for the art, although one of the most original titles was used in 1917 by the New York School of Embalming (formerly Barnes School), which advertised derma sculpture taught by a sculptor and demisurgery taught by an embalmer. An advertisement for Dermatol Cosmetics in 1913 stated that it was not necessary to go to school to learn demisurgery or cosmetic application as everything one needed to know was in the pamphlet wrapped around each jar of cosmetics.

From 1912 onward the pages of our professional journals disclose early contributions to the science of what today is termed restorative art. More and more advertisements are seen for cosmetics, demisurgery kits, and equipment (Figure 7). Before-and-after case photos, pioneered by Crandall, appeared with some frequency in product advertisements as well as in articles. Demonstration of demisurgery at meetings and conventions became every bit as popular and as well attended as embalming demonstrations had been 30 years earlier.

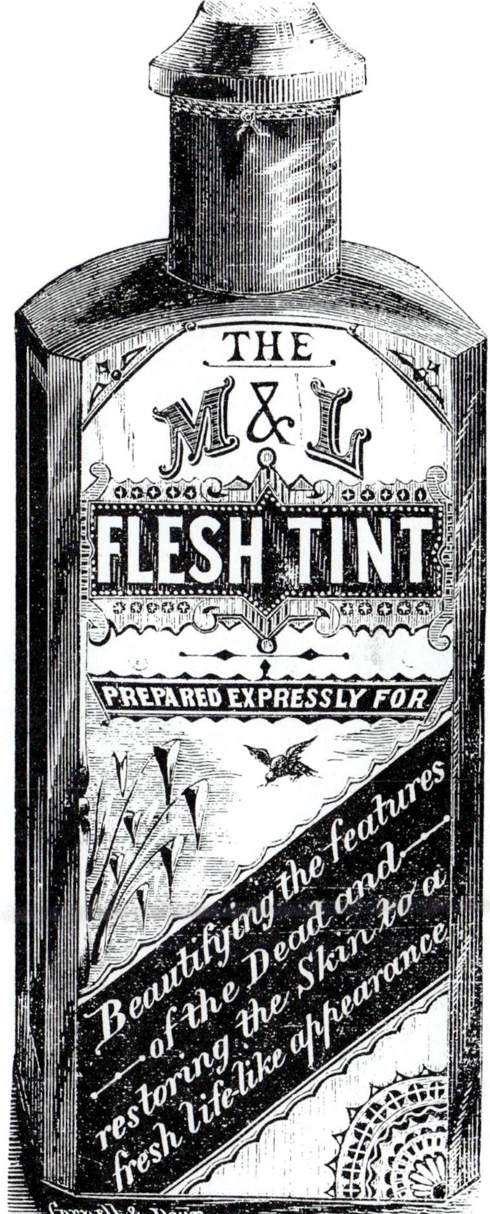

Figure 7. This preparation, though not a preservative, is a valuable aid to the embalmer's art.

Many prominent teachers and heads of embalming colleges wrote about the "new art." Some made first mention of standard basic procedures or techniques still employed today. Others advanced practices that were proven later to have little real value; for example, Robbins, in 1912, advocated the grafting of skin from another area of the body to replace damaged skin on the head. Such procedures were seldom very successful.

Robbins together with Lena Simmons, in 1912, mentions invisible or blind stitching (subcutaneous sutures), and C. O. Dhonau in the same year recommended baseball stitching with wax covering and concealing the sutured area, a rather unsatisfactory technique. Razorless shaving cream (a depilatory) made a brief but unsuccessful appearance in 1914, as it has a number of times since then.

Basic principles of demisurgery practice, such as using very concentrated fluid to produce firm tissue as ideal for final restoration and performing basic restoration to a near-normal anatomical relationship prior to arterial injection, were reiterated by C. O. Dhonau, Robbins, Worsham, Lena Simmons, and others. Some recommended removal of tumors and other surgical procedures prior to embalming, but Worsham and most modern authorities recommended that this be done after arterial injection. Most early authorities agreed that it was necessary to wait between completion of the arterial treatment and final application of wax and cosmetics. Most recommended a minimum of 6 to 10 hours' time-lapse to ensure drying and halting of leakage from torn tissues.

In 1915 Worsham mentions using cotton and Collodion as a cavity filler to within one-sixteenth of an inch of the normal surface, then covering this surface with wax. He also used the cotton and Collodion to form such basic features as lips, ears, nose, and eyelids.

Dhonau, writing at some length on demisurgery in 1915, called attention to the individuality of the human face, differences in the lateral halves, as well as cosmetic skin variations. His suggestion, noted for the first time, to do the "work in the same light as that in which the body will rest until its final disposition," is still heeded today. In 1915 he demonstrated modeling of the facial features on a plaster skull, a technique that is today fairly standard throughout the schools for the teaching of restorative art.

One of the more dramatic demisurgical cases of the era was that treated by Worsham in Chicago in mid-1917. A lion tamer was attacked, mangled, and killed while performing in the lions' cage. A Chicago undertaker, Lafayette C. Ball, who was present at the attack, ran to his nearby funeral home, secured several bottles of formalin-based cavity fluid, returned to the circus cage, and poured the contents of the bottles over the dead lion tamer's torn body. This ingenious technique stopped the lions from further mangling the body, and permitted the circus personnel to retrieve it. Worsham, called on to prepare the body, was confronted with the need to replace both ears, much of the face, and both arms, and to close the torn open abdomen from which some viscera had been devoured. Before and after photos disclose a reasonable restoration.

Practicing embalmers were stimulated to try to repair difficult cases, too. *The Sunnyside* issue of September 15, 1914, published a story and before-and-after photos of two cases, a murder and suicide by shotgun. In both, the skulls had been shattered by the 16-gauge shot. Mr. and Mrs. G. A. Rousevell of Lead, South Dakota, restored the bodies to a virtually normal appearance.

During the period 1910–1920 there was much preoccupation with the problem of jaundice. Every fluid manufacturer who made, as most did, a formalin-based arterial fluid received complaints about the change in color of a jaundiced body from yellow to green after embalming. Despite the manufacture of numerous new formulas by many companies through the intervening years, this problem remains not completely solved to the present day.

During 1924 J. H. De Normandie of New York City developed a treatment for jaundice. He injected a solvent (not specified) into the carotid artery without drainage and allowed it to remain for 20 minutes, during which time a special ointment was applied to the face and the face covered with hot moist towels. This was followed by the injection of about 3 gallons of arterial fluid and drainage from the jugular vein. The system was declared successful but chemical components were never fully disclosed.

Other individual embalmers experimented with the use of various bleaching solutions such as phenol, chlorine (laundry bleach), and hydrogen peroxide, none of which produced any measure of uniform results.

In 1917 C. O. Dhonau announced a new technique for treating swollen, blackened eyes. He incised the underside of the affected lid or lids, pressed out the accumulated blood and serum, and then applied 50% phenol solution to shrink and bleach the area.

At this time the schools, which conducted courses of instruction of quite varying lengths averaging 3 months' duration at most, allotted some instruction time to demisurgery. Some schools scheduled regular periods in the laboratory for learning to form facial features in wax or clay on a plaster skull. Unique among these courses was that taught by Worsham, whose class in demisurgery was most often given at the end of the entire course of instruction. By the 1930s it amounted to 25 to 40 total hours of laboratory work. The actual practice was carried out on mutilated human heads left over from the anatomy dissection classes. The heads were stored in preservative fluid between class sessions and were, of course, rather wet, distorted, and chemically malodorous. The actual practice, however, was realistic, as all suturing, cavity filling, feature forming, and cosmetizing were practiced just as on an actual case.

In 1948 at the Postgraduate Institute of Restorative Art of Chicago, the laboratory teaching system was modified by the recreation of dozens of mutilated heads in plastic and rubber, which permitted suturing, [illegible]ing, and cosmetizing. The school was headed by [illegible]rd C. Johnson.

[illegible]fter photos of a case handled by the [illegible] the Simmons School in 1921 in- [illegible] 1924 Cincinnati College fea- [illegible]tic surgery laboratory in an [illegible]me. In 1926 Dhonau criti- [illegible]or issuing diplomas in [illegible]lance at their free clin- [illegible]ars earlier when fluid [illegible] issuing diplomas to [illegible]linics.

[illegible]*nd Sunnyside* during [illegible]ature article about demisurgery, [illegible]ry, before-and-after photos, new products [illegible]isurgeon, or editorial praise and commendation for [illegible]e procedure. In 1925 an advertisement appeared announcing that Clyde E. Richardson of Paterson, New Jersey, was available for dermasurgical cases. It is believed he was trained by Joel E. Crandall. The April 1, 1925, issue of *Casket and Sunnyside* had a four-page insert by the Eckels Chemical Company of Philadelphia on dermasurgery. The copy was a combination of a sales pitch for the Eckels Company's cosmetics, instruments, and other materials and technical advice on case treatment.

Some American folk heroes were the subjects of restorative treatment. One of the earliest was Floyd Collins, who in 1925 was trapped in Sand Cave, Kentucky, where he died. Eighty-three days later, his body was recovered and removed to Bowling Green, Kentucky, where it was embalmed and the destroyed facial features (eyes, nose, and mouth) were replaced. His mother expressed satisfaction with his appearance in the casket.

Three notorious criminals—John Dillinger, Bonnie Parker, and Clyde Barrow—died at the hands of law enforcement agents in July 1934. Dillinger, dead from bullet wounds in a Chicago alley, was taken to the Cook County morgue, where a Worsham College of Mortuary Science instructor, Don Asheworth, was requested to make a death mask of Dillinger for the FBI. Asheworth related to the writers that he was visited by the FBI at 2 AM and that he was persuaded to hand over the extra mask.

Bonnie and Clyde were slain near Arcadia, Louisiana, and taken to a mortuary there. Both were embalmed in Louisiana, but Clyde was taken to the Sparkman–Holly–Brand Mortuary in Dallas, while Bonnie was taken to McKamy–Campbell Funeral Home, also in Dallas. Clyde, his head shattered, received more than 100 bullet or shotgun pellet wounds; Bonnie received more than 50 bullet wounds. Both bodies were restored and viewed in their respective caskets by an estimated 50,000 people.

In 1936 the convicted kidnapper and murderer of Charles A. Lindbergh's baby, Bruno Hauptmann, was executed by electrocution. Reports of his preparation state that restorative art procedures were required to repair burns on his face and head. Services were private, however, and followed by cremation.

In the December 1926 issue of *Casket and Sunnyside* appeared the first advertisement for the electric-heated spatula, manufactured by the Montez Manufacturing Company, of Addison, Michigan (Figure 8). This device, highly touted when first developed as an excellent spatula to smooth and model wax as well as to reduce swollen areas, was less effective than anticipated. The heat of the iron had a tendency to melt wax and leave an unnaturally shiny surface. When used to reduce swelling, the device produced only a very minor evident reduction after much effort. Perhaps its best use was to "iron" tissue.

In August 1927 during the Minnesota 37th State Convention at St. Paul, the term *restorative art* was first used. The Worsham College advertisement of December 1927 used the term *restorative art* but later reverted to the term *dermasurgery*. In 1929, the McAllister School listed Robert C. Harper as professor of restorative art. In November 1928 William G. Collier, Collier School, New York City, stated in an address, "Any man can be taught the principles of this restorative art." It was to take some years, however, before the term *restorative art* was adopted and uniformly applied to the subject area first termed demisurgery by Joel E. Crandall in 1912.

By the mid-1920s, articles by teachers and practitioners of embalming on restorative art appeared with frequency in most professional journals and house organs of chemical manufacturers and supply companies. One such writer and practitioner was William G. Collier, a trade embalmer of New York City who became a prolific author of articles on restorative art. Collier, scion of a well-established funeral service family, first appeared in print in *Casket and Sunnyside* in 1925 with an article on jaundice treatment. From that moment on he was a more or less regular contributor of articles dealing with treatment of facial cancer, decapitation, general demisurgical procedures, and cosmetics.

Collier founded both a school of embalming instruction and a shipping service in New York City, and was the holder of several patents for restorative wound fillers and preformed facial features. Collier is remembered as a patient teacher, excellent speaker, and excruciating writer.

The Champion Company in March 1929 introduced the subject area to the readers of its house organ, *Champion Expanding Encyclopedia of Mortuary Prac-*

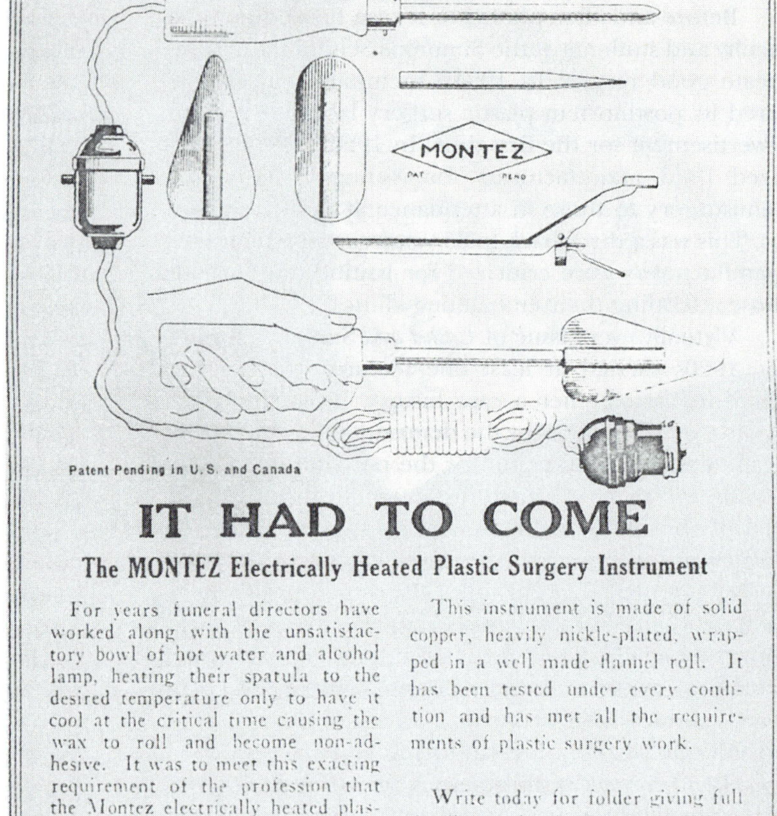

Figure 8. Early heated spatula used to smooth wax and reduce swollen facial tissues, circa 1926.

tice, with an article entitled The Art of Plastic Surgery. Such articles by the supervising chemist, A. O. Spriggs, on a variety of subjects (e.g., treatment of gunshot cases, subcutaneous suture, hypodermic injection of tissue filler cream) were assembled into a textbook in 1934 that is still available today under the title *Champion Restorative Art.*

As early as 1927, C. F. Callaway was lecturing, demonstrating, and writing on the subject of restorative art. Callaway became a special representative of the Undertaker's Supply Company of Chicago, and wrote many articles on plastic surgery for its house organ, as well as trade publications. Ten years later he was joined in these activities by Ralph Hensen, who later taught mortuary science subjects at the College of Mortuary Science at St. Louis, and by Clarence G. Strub (Figure 9), whose last years in a long and distinguished professional career in funeral service were spent with the University of Iowa as curator of the Anatomy Department of the Iowa Medical College eye enucleation training program. Strub's early contribution to restorative art was his publication in 1932 of a small textbook of 32 pages entitled *The Principles of Restorative Art As the Embalmer Should Know Them* (Figure 10). The little text was extremely well written in a simple and direct style with emphasis on the practical application of technique, though it did embody some elements of theory. Taken as a whole, the book can be recognized as the true prototype of the best contemporary restorative art textbook.

The Dodge Chemical Company, during this period, also had a team of talented writers, lecturers, and demonstrators in the persons of Frank Stallard, a voluminous writer whose articles appeared for years in trade publications and the Dodge Chemical Company house organ, and Ray Slocum, a most popular embalming and restorative art demonstrator on the Dodge "faculty." Both Stallard and Slocum produced pamphlets of instruction on the subject of embalming and restorative art, which were much

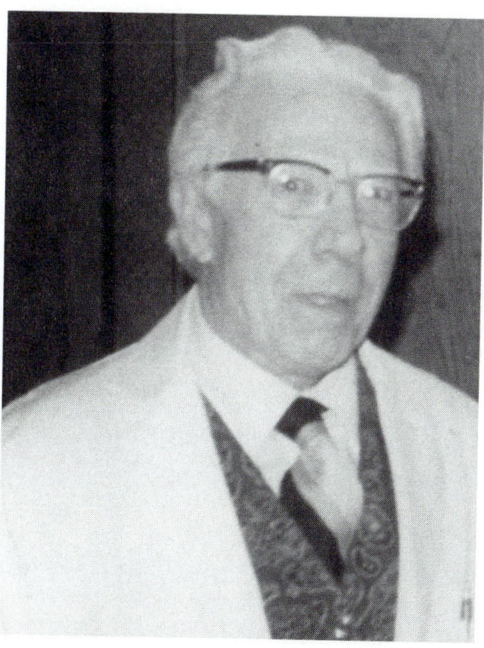

Figure 9. Photograph of Clarence G. Strub.

sought after and highly prized by practicing embalmers.

In 1945 *Casket and Sunnyside* inaugurated a monthly feature, Restoration Clinic by E. C. Johnson. Each monthly article described treatment for a particular type of case and was illustrated by before-and-after photographs of each case. The series continued monthly for more than 14 years.

The spring of 1931 was marked by the untimely death of one of the early full-time embalming college teachers of restorative art, Ivan P. Bowsher. Bowsher, dying at age 33, was a World War I veteran who had graduated from Cincinnati College in the class of 1921. While a student at the college he was recognized as a gifted artist and was invited to join the faculty, on graduation, as a teacher of restorative art. For 10 brief years he gave the students of Cincinnati College one of the best courses of instruction in restorative art available. On his death, the college instituted the Ivan P. Bowsher Medal for outstanding achievement in restorative art to be awarded to one member of each graduating class. Cincinnati College had another outstanding teacher of restorative art, G. Joseph Prager, who with Dean C. O. Dhonau wrote an excellent textbook entitled *Manual of Restorative Art,* published in 1934. Prager continued and expanded the restorative art curriculum inaugurated by Bowsher and in 1955 published another textbook entitled *Post Mortem Restorative Art.*

The post-World War II era witnessed the publication of a number of textbooks on restorative art, ranging in quality from poor to classic. An example is the *Technique of Restorative Art* by Maude Adams Adair published in 1948. The text is superficial, and has a conglomeration of nonrelevant subject matter ranging from flower arrangement, to hairdressing, to the National Funeral Directors Association's code of ethics, to committal services.

An excellent book that deals with a very limited area of the field of restorative art, written by Gladys P. Curry of Boston in 1947, is titled *A Textbook of Facial Reconstruction.* Gladys Curry was an internationally recognized authority on the identification of the dead, and her expertise was often requested in disasters such as the infamous Coconut Grove nightclub fire, which claimed more than 500 victims, and the recovery of de-

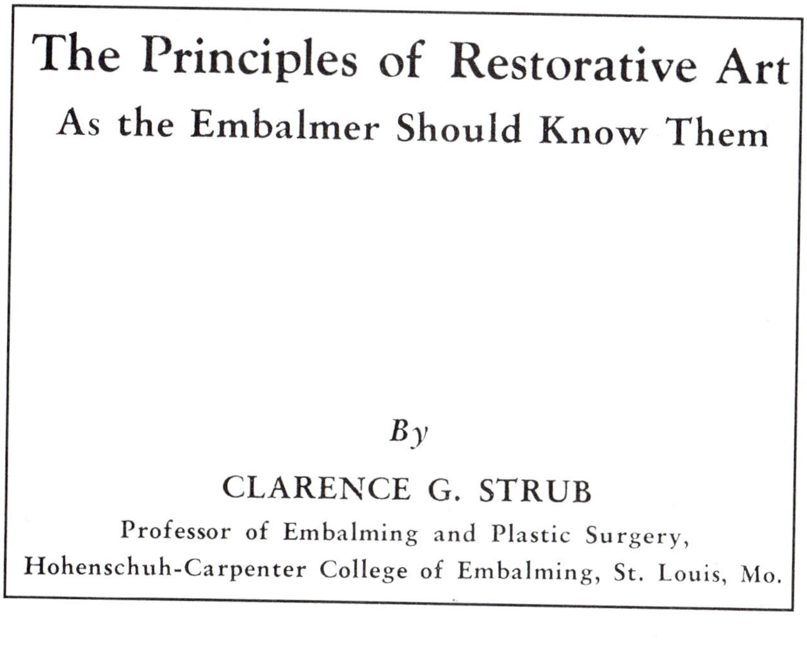

The Principles of Restorative Art

As the Embalmer Should Know Them

By

CLARENCE G. STRUB

Professor of Embalming and Plastic Surgery,

Hohenschuh-Carpenter College of Embalming, St. Louis, Mo.

Figure 10. Title page of Clarence G. Strub's book.

composing bodies of the crew members of the submarine Sqaulus lost in U.S. waters in 1939.

Her book is well illustrated with photographs depicting the step-by-step reconstruction or replacement on the bare skull of the soft tissues of the face and neck to the individual's normal appearance. The task is carried out logically and methodically by replacing the muscles in their normal position as to origin and insertion and finally sculpting the features and skin surface and adding the hair. The Curry system has been successfully employed by a number of embalmers who have assisted various law enforcement agencies in the identification of skeletal remains.

The Curry text is devoted solely to instruction in reconstruction of the soft tissues of the head and neck with clay or wax, and is devoid of any instruction on or concern with the ordinary restorative problems or embalming of such cases. This text is highly recommended as an invaluable addition to an embalmer's library for reference on modeling and identification techniques.

The contemporary standard textbook on restorative art was written by the late Sheridan Mayer (Figure 11), published as a lengthy treatise in 1940 and as a fully hardbound textbook in 1943 entitled simply *Restorative Art.* This work has gone through many revisions and is now used in most mortuary science college programs. Mayer also wrote the treatises *Workbook on Color* published in 1947 and *Mortuary Cosmetology* published in 1948. In 1973 he published the textbook *Color and Cosmetics,* which is in use in mortuary science college programs.

Mayer was born in a Philadelphia suburb in 1908 and was educated in primary schools in the area. He attended the University of Pennsylvania and a number of private schools where he enrolled in courses largely in the field of art, sculpture, and public speaking. His allied interests included the theater; he acted on stage and studied, taught, and was employed as a theatrical cosmetician and makeup specialist in the Philadelphia and New York City areas.

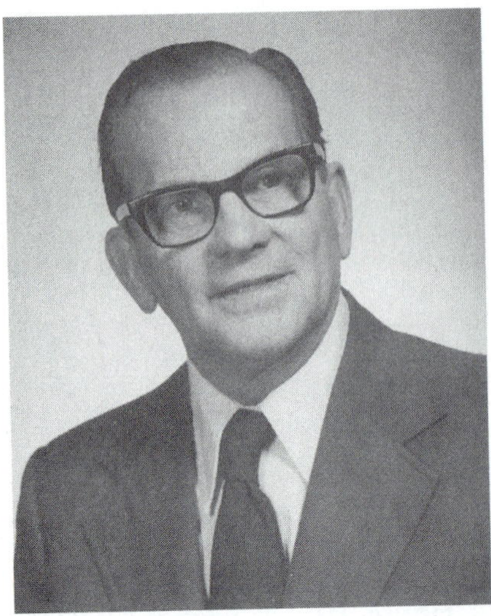

Figure 11. Photograph of J. Sheridan Mayer.

It is noteworthy and to his great credit that Mayer overcame the handicap of not being a practicing embalmer and yet was able to impart instruction intelligently. Mayer is one of the very few, if not the only, truly successful teachers who had never been a practicing embalmer.

His introduction to the teaching of restorative art was at a clinic at the Eckels College of Mortuary Science in Philadelphia, September 6–8, 1939, where he appeared on the program with the famed Covermark cosmetic formulator Lydia O'Leary. His dynamic and informative presentation was so well received by all in attendance that he was offered a position on the faculty, which he accepted and retained until 1947.

During 1943 to 1945 Mayer volunteered for duty in the U.S. Maritime Service and was assigned to the harbor antisubmarine net division. In 1947 he joined the faculty of the Pittsburgh Institute of Mortuary Science, where he met Otto S. Margolis and formed an admiration for him. In 1951 when Margolis assumed control of the American Academy of Mortuary Science in New York City, Mayer accompanied him there to strengthen the faculty. The American Academy merged with the McAllister Institute in 1964.

Mayer has written extensively on the subject of cosmetics and restorative art and has written articles for many professional journals. His greatest contribution to the subject of restorative art, however, has been his influence and steady guidance of mortuary colleges toward the development and acceptance of a uniform course of instruction, as well as the adoption of uniform standards of facilities for such instruction and relevant examination questions. He has been the chairman of the restorative art course content committee of mortuary science schools and colleges for many years, where he accomplished monumental tasks in curriculum studies and syllabus preparation and screening of a bank of examination questions on the subject of restorative art. Mayer taught until 1975. In December of 1993, he died in Cincinnati, Ohio, where he had retired.

Unfortunately, not all who have taught restorative art were as dedicated or qualified as Mayer. Some were individuals with basic training in art or sculpture, who had little interest or understanding of the problems involved in restorative art. Some examples come to mind. In one case an instructor had his students practice modeling each feature in supersize; ears, for example, were a foot long. Another instructor was most insistent that the students practice sculpturing of the eyes and mouth open! Surely such practices lack any semblance of relevance to normal professional procedures. The writers personally believe very strongly that the teaching of embalming and restorative art requires not only a background of practical experience in such areas, but, equally important, a continuing experience of practice while teaching.

The present-day requirement of the possession of a college degree to become a faculty member at colleges of mortuary science sharply limits the employment of many capable potential teachers with genuine expertise in embalming and restorative art. The words of A. Johnson Dodge, as so well stated in 1917, are still valid today: "How to care for mutilated bodies and make them presentable should constitute a part of the education of the embalmer. Thorough instruction in this difficult art should be given by instructors in our schools. But this part of the work required *special experience* and some study either to practice or teach it successfully."

One area of instruction in restorative art that has been recognized increasingly as a valuable practical working asset is the study of physical anthropology. Physical anthropology has been defined as a science that deals with the physical likenesses and differences of the races and sexes as well as the changes wrought by age and disease of humans. Such study has been most helpful in the practice of restorative art. It has been particularly invaluable in identification and reconstruction of skeletal remains. Study of skeletal remains can reveal sex, race, age, general height range, as well as individual characteristics such as right or left handedness, old trauma, (e.g., healed fractures), and diseases. Perhaps the most interesting use of such knowledge is the reconstruction of the face on a fleshless skull.

The technique used today by experts such as Betty Catliff, assistant to Clyde Snow, physical anthropologist, retired Chief of the Federal Aviation Authority, Physical Anthropology Unit, at Norman, Oklahoma, is virtually identical to the original system devised by Wilhelm His of Leipzig University in Germany.

In brief in 1895, His was compelled to devise a method of identifying a skull as to whether or not it and its associated bones were the remains of the renowned composer Johann Sebastian Bach. The bones had been disinterred from the church cemetery during enlargement of the church of St. John and a new more elaborate grave and monument for the remains, if indeed they were his, were planned. Proof of the identity was imperative.

His studied the bones in his anatomy laboratory and recognized the key to the solution. The bones of the face support the soft tissues, muscles, fat, and skin. The soft tissues vary in thickness at various points, for example, thin over the forehead, nose, and prominences of the temples, cheeks, lips, and chin. He also deduced that tissue thickness was fairly uniform at about 15 key points over the anterior and lateral skull surface of individuals of like sex, name, and age.

His began assembling measurements of the key points from the numerous undissected cadavers in his laboratory. He recorded each point thickness for each corpse, then averaged these measurements to secure a single working measurement for each such point. He had small metal markers constructed that were labeled A, B, and so on, to correspond with the tissue thickness at that point.

He secured the services of a well-known sculptor who agreed to undertake the project of reconstruction of the skull using the His technique. The metal markers were put in position on the skull, embedded in clay. When they were all correctly placed, strips of clay were applied connecting the points, and these in turn were interconnected. Finally the vacant spaces were filled in and the features formed. The reconstructed skull appearance obtained closely resembled contemporary portraits and sculptures of Bach and the committee for construction of the new tomb and monument was satisfied.

This technique has been updated from time to time by creating new tables, as His did, of females and other races. The technique has produced good results even by those using the procedure for the first time.

While the schools of mortuary science steadily increased the hours allotted to the teaching of restorative art, they recognized the fact that many practicing embalmers felt a distinct lack of ability in this field. Consequently, from time to time virtually all schools of mortuary science offered practicing embalmers special short courses varying in length from 1 to 7 days. Some featured actual demonstrations on mutilated bodies, whereas others offered only practice modeling of features.

Through the years special schools were founded to teach cosmetic application and restorative art. An example of such a school, unaffiliated with an existing school of mortuary science, was the Embalmers Graduate College formed in Chicago in 1937 by L. Roy Davenport and Honora D. Mannix, which offered 30 hours of instruction and practice in both cosmetology and restorative art.

In 1948 the Post Graduate Institute of Restorative Art was organized in Chicago. The curriculum included a short 2-week course and the standard 7-month course that offered 25 hours per week of instruction. When the school was merged into Worsham College in 1955, the course had been taken by 16 mortuary college restorative art instructors or their assistants.

Education of embalmers at all levels of skill in restorative art has been enhanced by the production of photographic records of actual restorative procedures. Some of these productions were in black and white, some in full color, some in motion, and others in still pictures. Most are silent and very few have either sound or voice accompaniment.

The earliest still photographs of restorative art cases taken before, during, and after restoration were, of course, those of cases treated by demisurgeon Joel E. Crandall dating no later than 1912. Crandall also bears the distinction of producing the first black and white motion pictures of restorative procedures made in the year 1917.

Other great early teachers such as C. A. Renouard and Albert Worsham made films prior to 1920 not only on the subject of restorative art but also on embalming technique and anatomical dissections.

The truly classic motion picture on restorative procedures was produced in color in the early 1930s by the late Earle K. Angstadt (Figure 12) of the Auman Funeral Home of Reading, Pennsylvania, who also performed all the actual restorative art techniques displayed in the film. The silent film has subtitles and is expertly photographed. It depicts classic technique, flawlessly performed, during the restoration of a surgically removed mandible, reduction of facial swelling, hypodermic tissue filling of face and hand, and replacement of eyelids and eyelashes damaged beyond salvage by an infection. This film, still available from either National Selected Morticians or National Funeral Directors Association headquarters, will never be improved on.

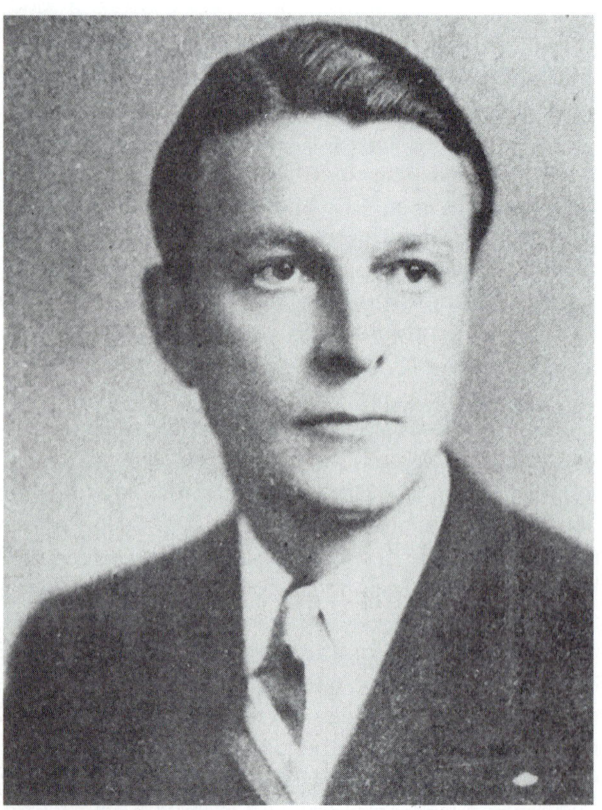

Figure 12. Photograph of Earle K. Angstadt.

Another much longer film recording many more cases of severe trauma was produced in the late 1930s by the late R. Victor Landig, founder of the Landig College of Mortuary Science at Houston. The photography of the 10 or 12 cases recorded on the film varies widely from poor to good, with respect to color fidelity, focus, and technique, where as restorative skill is uniformly good except for the handling of hair restorations.

The Los Angeles College of Mortuary Science produced a fine color motion picture complete with sound and voice in the late 1940s. The film depicts no actual cases but does show how to produce plaster practice masks and provides excellent modeling instruction for producing the individual facial features. The Champion Company of Ohio has a motion picture in color made in the 1940s by A. O. Spriggs, featuring his technique in treating a small group of actual restorative cases. E. C. Johnson has slides recording the treatment of several hundred cases, including virtually every conceivable problem requiring restorative art treatment.

Our profession desperately needs more visual aids such as the foregoing to provide wider exposure of our practitioners to successful techniques at conventions, meetings, seminars, and workshops.

While textbooks, films, and teachers were providing more instruction and training for every level of embalmer competence, skill, and capability, the chemical and embalming supply manufacturers were also active in providing better tools and materials for the embalmer to complete restorations more skillfully.

In 1933 the Hydrol Chemical Company made a most significant announcement in the trade journals concerning the patenting of liquid tissue builder that coagulated or jelled on being hypodermically introduced into the body tissue. This, of course, was a vast improvement over ordinary liquids such as glycerin, then in use for this purpose, as such liquids, remaining liquid, tended to settle away from the high point in response to the pull of gravity. This failure of the hypodermically deposited material to maintain its position obviously ultimately destroyed the effect of such treatment.

Another equally vexatious problem resulting from the use of such permanent-liquid-state tissue builders was the most disturbing occurrence of seepage from

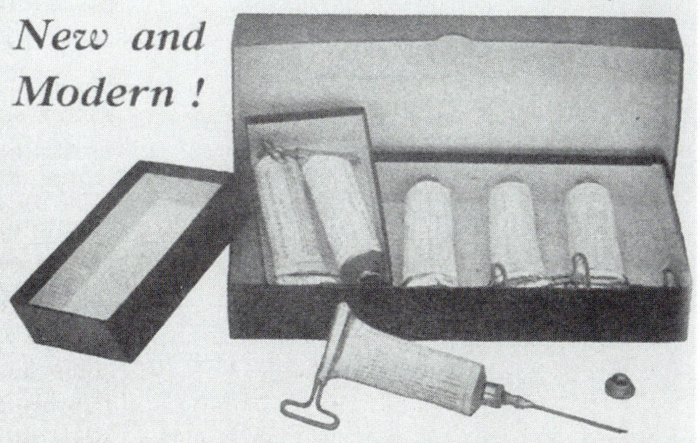

Figure 13. Tissue filler using cream, circa 1930.

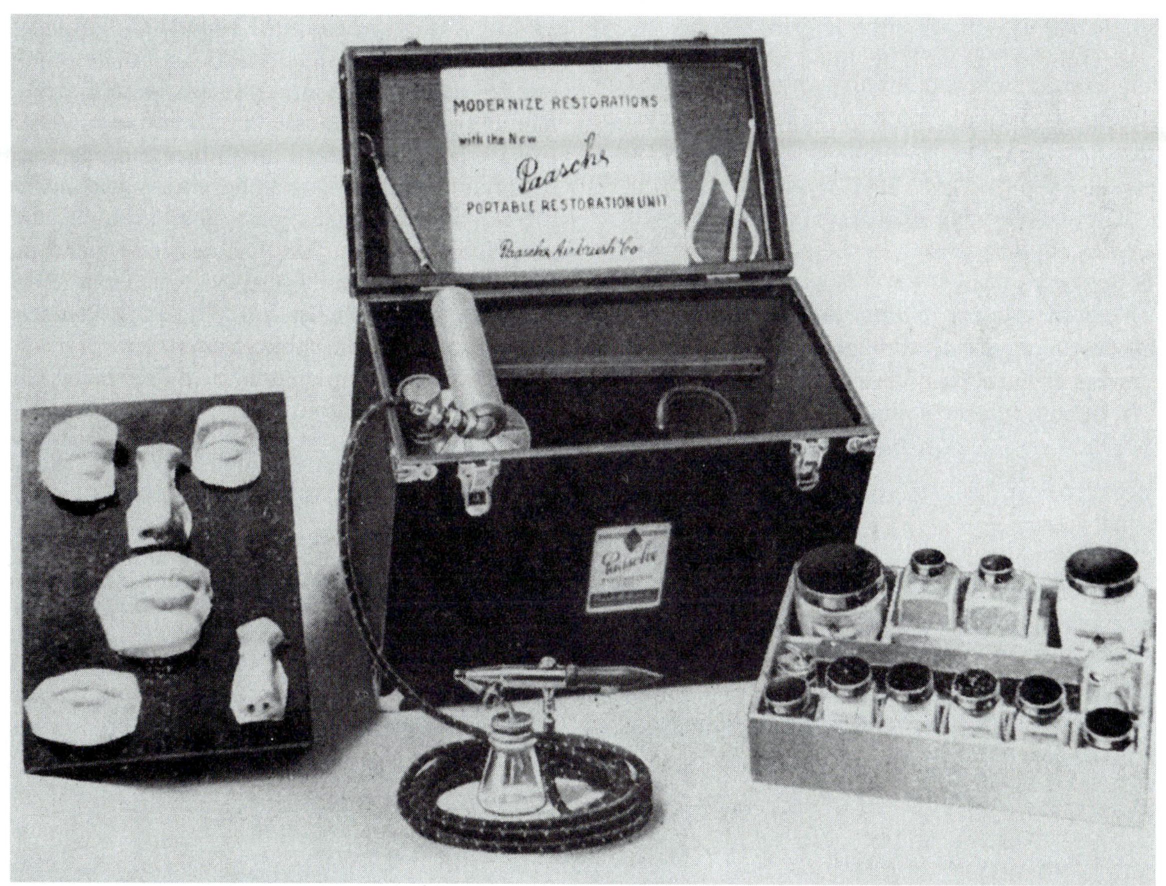

Figure 14. Paasche Company's restorative art air brush kit designed for embalmers' use.

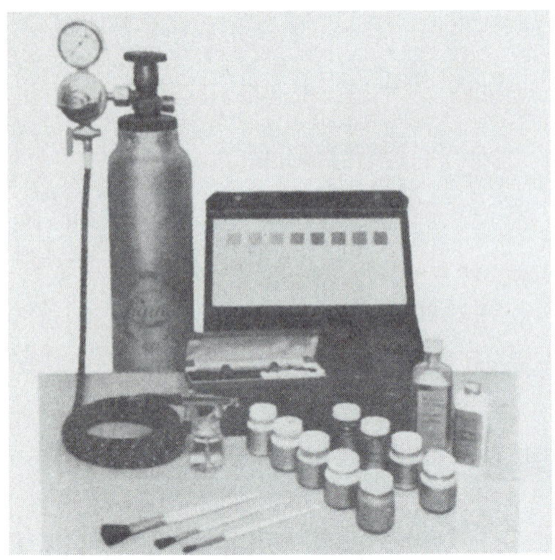

Figure 15. Master Nuance Aire-Tynt Unit.

the point of insertion of the hypodermic needle. Both of these problems were corrected by the new jelling tissue builder as it would neither seep nor shift its position due to the change in its structure from liquid to semisolid to solid.

An alternative material such as hand cream or petroleum jelly had been used, but the technique for successful use required that both the filled syringe and the large-diameter needle be kept warm to permit a free flow of the semisolid material. Special hypodermic syringes with screw-threaded plungers were devised to make the ejection of thick creams easier, but they never did become very popular, and after introduction of coagulable liquid filler, they virtually disappeared from the market (Figure 13).

In 1935 the Dodge Chemical Company introduced De-Ce-Co needle injector and needles as an improved means of securing mouth closure, and in 1937 offered a complete set of eight specially designed restorative art instruments. In addition the company, like many others, offered a complete range of cosmetics, waxes, and restorative art chemicals.

Methods of cosmetic application, but primarily application of highlight or accent cosmetics over waxed areas, had always required improvement. The difficulty in applying accent cosmetics evenly and naturally on waxed surfaces is a problem familiar to all experienced embalmers. The best solution is to apply the cosmetics with an air brush or power sprayer. By these means the cosmetics are literally floated into position, and disturbance of either the underlying base cosmetics or the wax surface is completely avoided.

As far back as 1911, spray applicators, powered by carbon dioxide cylinders, were available to the embalmer for cosmetic application, but it was not until the 1930s that the need and desire for sprayer-applied cosmetics became popular.

In 1934 the Undertaker's Supply Company announced the availability of the E-Z Way manually operated spray cosmetic applicator and a compatible cosmetic. The device was well received because it was most efficient and was generally conceded to be the best of the non-power-operated sprayers, many of which are still in use today.

In 1936 the Paasche Company of Chicago, a manufacturer of industrial and artistic air brush equipment, offered a restorative art air brush kit designed for embalmers' use (Figure 14). The kit contained an electric-powered air compressor, an air brush applicator of high quality, restorative art wax, cosmetic instruments, preformed features such as ears, nose, and lips, and an instruction pamphlet. The Nuance Aire-Tynt cosmetic applicator was advertised in 1937 by J. Horace Griggs of Amarillo, Texas (Figure 15). The air brush applicator could be adapted to apply cosmetics, whether powered by a manually operated pump, an electric-powered air compressor, or a carbonic gas cylinder.

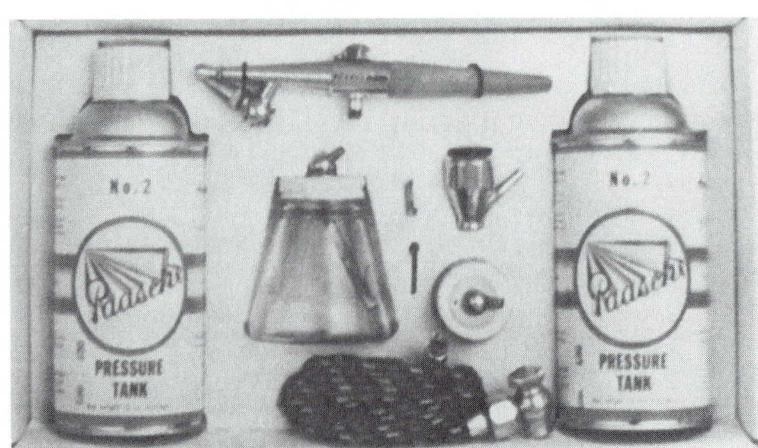

Figure 16. Hand-held model paint sprayer powered by small replaceable containers of freon gas.

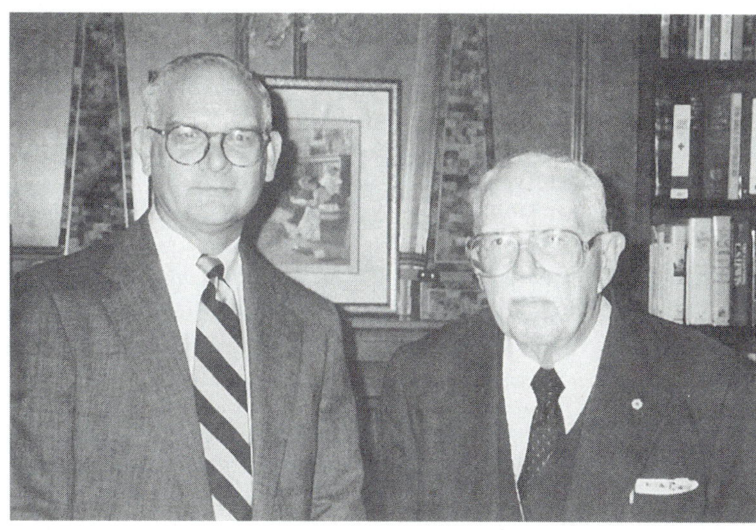

Figure 17. Robert G. Mayer (left) and Edward C. Johnson are instructors of embalming and restorative art. They are the primary authors of *Embalming: History, Theory, and Practice*.

Today many embalmers have been using, when the need arises, inexpensive easily available handheld model paint sprayers that are powered by small replaceable containers of freon gas. These units, readily available in hobby shops, hardware stores, or paint stores, serve the purpose equally as well as the more expensive air compressor-powered sprayers (Figure 16).

Restorative art was considered of sufficient importance in 1945 to have Richard G. Reichle, registrar of Worsham College, address the National Funeral Directors Association convention in Chicago on the continuing value and need for these procedures. The National Funeral Directors Association has recognized the importance of restorative art at several of its professional conferences in the past years.

American advances in restorative art over the years has been significant. We have ample supplies of materials and equipment, fine school laboratory teaching facilities, and dedicated teachers, yet the most important need of all remains unchanged. Now, as in the origin of the art, it is necessary for the individual embalmer, in charge of the case, to initiate the restoration of that case and to bring it to a successful conclusion. No amount of material, equipment, or training can substitute for the individual will and determination to overcome a most distressing case. The individual, now as always, is the key to success. The will to succeed and the ability to improvise are more often of value than any other asset.

Today, while you are reading this, the American way of funeral service is under attack by a variety of critics. It is therefore necessary that we in funeral service rededicate ourselves to the fulfillment, to the very best of our ability, of the American way—the funeral with the body present and viewable (Figure 17).

▶ BIBLIOGRAPHY

Benkard E. *Undying Faces* (a collection of death masks from the 15th century to the present). London: Hogurth Press; 1929.

Clarke CH. *Practical Embalming*. Cincinnati, OH: C. H. Clarke; 1917.

Crane EH. *Manual of Instruction to Undertakers,* 8th ed. Kalamazoo, MI: Kalamazoo; 1888.

Curry GP. *Facial Reconstruction.* Boston; 1947.

Dhonau CO, Prager GJ. *Manual of Restorative Art.* Cincinnati, OH: Embalming Book Co; 1932

Dodge AJ. *The Practical Embalmer.* Boston: A. Johnson Dodge; 1908.

Dutra FR. Identification of person and determination of cause of death. *Archives of Pathology* 1944; 38: 339.

Eckles HS. *Derma Surgery.* Philadelphia: H. S. Eckles.

Espy JB. *Espy's Embalmer.* Springfield, OH: Espy's Fluid Co.; 1895.

Gerasimov MM. *The Face Finder.* Philadelphia/New York: Lippincott; 1971.

Gradwohl RBH. *Legal Medicine.* St. Louis, MO: CV Mosby; 1954.

His W. *Anatomische Forschungen über Johann Sebastian Bach's Gegeine und Antlitz Nebst Bermerkungen über dessin Bilder.* Leipzig: S. Hirzel; 1895.

Hooten EA. *Up from the Ape.* New York; Macmillan; 1946.

Johnson EC. *Restorative Art.* Chicago: Worsham College; 1948.

Krogman W. *A Guide to the Identification of Human Skeletal Material.* Washington, DC: FBI Law Enforcement Bulletin.

Krogman W. *The Human Skeleton in Forensic Medicine.* Springfield, IL: C C Thomas; 1962.

Mayer JS. *Workbook on Color.* 1947.

Mayer JS. *Mortuary Cosmetology.* 1948.

Mayer JS. *Color and Cosmetics.* Bergenfield, NJ: Paul Publishing; 1973.

Mayer JS. *Restorative Art.* Dallas, TX: Professional Training Schools; 1993.

Michel G. *Scientific Embalmer.* Cleveland, OH; 1922.

Quiring DP. *Skeletal Identification.* Address to Ohio State Coroners Association; May 23, 1951.

Reichle RG. *Practical Problems in Restorative Art.* Chicago: Lecture—NFDA 63rd Convention; 1945.

Smith E, Dawson WR. *Egyptian Mummies.* New York; Dial Press; 1924.

Spriggs AO. *Plastic Surgery.* 4th ed. Springfield, OH: Champion Chemical; 1946.

Stewart TD. *Essentials of Forensic Anthropology.* Springfield, IL: Charles C Thomas; 1979.

Strub CG. The principles of restorative art. *Embalmer's Monthly.* 1932.

Wentworth B, Wilder HH. *Personal Identification.* Chicago: T.G. Cooke Fingerprint; 1932.

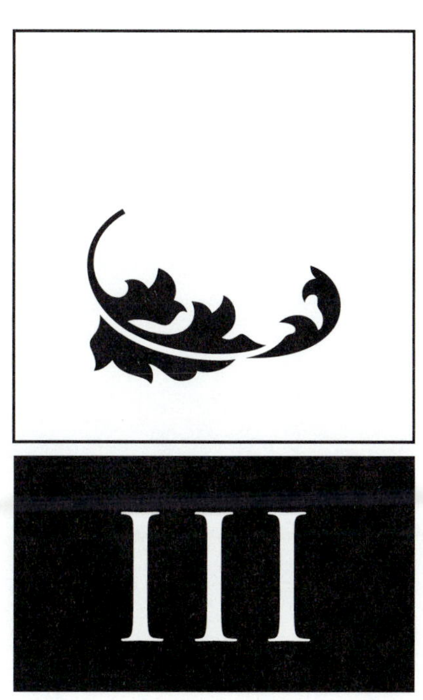

GLOSSARY AND SELECTED READINGS

Glossary

SECTION I

Prepared by the Embalming and Restorative Art Course Content Committees of the American Board of Funeral Service Education

Abdominal anatomical regions. (1) Nine regions of the abdomen as demarcated by four imaginary planes, two of which are horizontal (indicated by lines drawn across the right and left tenth ribs and across the right and left anterior superior iliac spines) and two sagittal (indicated by lines drawn from the midpoint of inguinal ligament to the nipples on the chest, right and left sides). Upper row: right hypochondriac, epigastric, left hypochondriac. Middle row: right lateral, umbilical, left lateral. Lower row: right inguinal, pubic, left inguinal. (2) Four regions of the abdomen as demarcated by two imaginary planes, one horizontal and the other midsagittal: upper right quadrant, upper left quadrant, lower right quadrant, lower left quadrant.

Abrasion. Antemortem injuries resulting from friction of the skin against a firm object and causing removal of the epidermis.

Abscess. Localized accumulation of pus.

Absorption. Process of taking in, as in a colored object which absorbs certain rays of light and reflects other rays giving the object its recognizable color (e.g., an apple is called red if the red rays are reflected and the other rays in the light are absorbed).

Abut. To touch or contact, as with the tarsal plates of the closed eyelids.

Accessory chemicals. Chemicals used in addition to vascular (arterial) and cavity embalming fluids. Include but are not limited to hardening compounds, preservative powders, sealing agents, mold-preventive agents, and compress application agents.

* 1996 Glossary of Terms for the Course Content in Embalming. Prepared by the American Board of Funeral Service Education.

* 1998 Glossary of Terms for the Course Content in Restorative Art. Prepared by the American Board of Funeral Service Education.

Acetone. Dimethylketone; a colorless liquid used to soften and remove scabs; a solvent for restorative wax; a stain remover.

Achromatic color. Color not found in the visible spectrum; a neutral color such as white, black, gray, silver, or gold (for decorative purposes).

Acquired facial markings. Facial markings that develop during one's lifetime, primarily as a result of repetitious use of certain muscles.

Acquired immunodeficiency syndrome (AIDS). Specific group of diseases or conditions that are indicative of severe immunosuppression related to infection with the human immunodeficiency virus (HIV). Persons who died with AIDS may exhibit conditions such as wasting syndrome, extrapulmonary tuberculosis, and Kaposi's sarcoma.

Action level (AL). Exposure limit usually one half of the Occupational Health and Safety Administration (OSHA) legal limit for a regulated substance. This level is established to ensure adequate protection of employees at exposures below the OSHA limits, but to minimize the compliance burdens for employers whose employees have exposures below the 8-hour permissible exposure limit (PEL). The AL for formaldehyde is 0.5 ppm.

Actual pressure. See Pressure.

Additive method. Process of mixing colored lights on a surface on which the wavelengths of each are combined; adding two or more colored lights together to create another color of light.

Adhesive. Sticking to or adhering closely; substances that may be applied in order to sustain contact of two surfaces.

Adipocere/Grave Wax. Soft, whitish, crumbly or greasy material that forms on postmortem hydrolysis and hydrogenation of body fats.

Adsorption. Assimilation of gas, vapor, or dissolved matter by the surface of a solid or liquid.

Aerobic. In the presence of free oxygen.

Aerosol. Colloidal solution dispensed as a mist.

Aerosolization. Dispersal as an aerosol. Minute particles of blood and water become atomized and suspended in air when water under pressure meets the blood drainage or when flushing an uncovered flush sink.

After-image. (psychological) Visual impression remaining after the stimulus has been removed.

Agglutination. Intravascular: increase in viscosity of blood brought about by the clumping of particulate formed elements in the blood vessels.

Agonal algor. Decrease in body temperature immediately before death.

Agonal coagulation. In reference to blood, a change from a fluid into a thickened mass.

Agonal dehydration. Loss of moisture from the living body during the agonal state.

Agonal edema. Escape of blood serum from an intravascular to an extravascular location immediately before death.

Agonal fever. Increase in body temperature immediately before death.

Agonal period. Period immediately before somatic death.

Agonal Translocation. See Translocation.

Airbrush. Pressured atomizer used for spraying liquid paint or cosmetic on a surface.

Algor Mortis. Postmortem cooling of the body to the surrounding temperature.

Alternate drainage. Method of injection-drainage in which embalming solution is injected and then injection is stopped while drainage is open.

Alveolar process. Bony ridge found on the inferior surface of the maxilla and the superior surface of the mandible that contains the sockets for the teeth.

Alveolar prognathism. Abnormal protrusion of the alveolar process(es).

Amino acids. Building blocks of which proteins are constructed, and the end products of protein digestion or hydrolysis. The basic formula is NH_2–CHR–COOH–amino group, an alpha carbon, any aliphatic or aromatic radical, and a carboxyl group.

Amputate. To cut off a limb; to dismember.

Anaerobic. In the absence of free oxygen.

Analogous. In color harmony, two or more hues that have the same hue in common.

Anasarca. Severe generalized edema.

Anatomical guides. Descriptive references for locating arteries and veins by means of the anatomical structures which are known.

Anatomical limits. Points of origin and points of termination in relation to adjacent structures. Used to designate the boundaries of arteries.

Anatomical position. The body is erect, feet together, palms facing forward, and thumbs pointed away from body.

Anchor. Material or technique employed to secure tissues or restorative materials in a fixed position; an armature.

Aneurysm. Localized abnormal dilation or outpocketing of a blood vessel resulting from a congenital defect or a weakness of the vessel wall.

Aneurysm hook. An embalming instrument that is used for blunt dissection and in raising vessels.

Aneurysm needle. An embalming instrument used for blunt dissection and in raising vessels that has an eye in the hook portion of the instrument for placing ligatures around the vessels.

Angle. Angulus; sharp turn formed by the meeting of two borders or surfaces.

Angle of the mandible. Body angle formed by the junction of the posterior edge of the ramus of the mandible and the inferior surface of the body of the mandible.

Angle of projection. Degree from vertical at which the surface(s) of a prominent feature projects.

Angular spring forceps. Multipurpose instrument (size can vary) used in the embalming process (e.g., as a drainage instrument).

Angulus oris eminence. Small, convex prominence found lateral to the end of the line of closure of the mouth; a natural facial marking.

Angulus oris sulcus. Groove found at each end of the line of closure of the mouth; a natural facial marking.

Anomaly. Deviation from the normal.

Antecubital. In front of the elbow/in the bend of the elbow.

Antemortem. Before death.

Anterior. Before or in front of; an anatomical term of position and direction which denotes the front or forward part.

Anterior nares. External nostril openings.

Anterior superior iliac spine. A bony protuberance that can be palpated topographically, found on the ilium, the superior broad portion of the hip bone; the origin of the inguinal ligament and the sartorius muscle.

Anticoagulant fluid. Ingredient of embalming fluids that retards the natural postmortem tendency of blood to become more viscous or prevents adverse reactions between blood and other embalming chemicals.

Antihelix. Inner rim of the ear.

Antiragus. Small eminence obliquely opposite the tragus on the superior border of the lobe of the ear.

Aperture. Opening.

Apparent death. Condition in which the manifestations of life are feebly maintained.

Aqueous. Watery; prepared with water as a solvent.

Aqueous humor. Clear, thin, alkaline fluid that fills the anterior chamber of the eyeball.

Aquiline. Curved, as the beak of an eagle; as viewed from the profile, a nose that exhibits a hook or convexity in its dorsum.

Arch. Structure exhibiting a curved or bow-like outline.

Arch of the wing. Inferior margin of the nasal wing that forms a distinct concave arc superiorly.

Areolar. Containing minute interspaces in a tissue.

Armature. Framework; a material, commonly of pliable metal or wood, employed to provide support for a wax restoration.

Arterial (solution) delivery. Movement of the vascular solution from its source (e.g., embalming machine tank) through the machine apparatus, connective tubing and arterial tube into an artery.

Arterial (vascular) fluid. Concentrated, preservative, embalming chemical that is diluted with water to form the arterial solution for injection into the arterial system during vascular embalming. Its purpose is to inactivate saprophytic bacteria and render the body tissues less susceptible to decomposition.

Arterial solution. Mixture of arterial (vascular) fluid and water used for the arterial injection. May include supplemental fluids.

Arterial tube. Tube used to inject embalming solution into the blood vascular system.

Arteriosclerosis. Term applied to a number of pathological conditions causing a thickening, hardening, and loss of elasticity of the walls of the arteries.

Articulation. Place of union between two or more bones.

Ascites. Accumulation of serous fluids in the peritoneal cavity.

Asepsis. Freedom from infection and from any form of life. Sterility.

Asphyxia. Insufficient intake of oxygen. Numerous causes.

Aspiration. Withdrawal of gas, fluids, and semisolids from body cavities and hollow viscera by means of suction with an aspirator and a trocar.

Asymmetry. Lack of symmetry, balance, or proportion.

Atheroma. Fatty degeneration or thickening of the walls of the larger arteries occurring in atherosclerosis.

Autoclave. Apparatus used for sterilization by steam pressure, usually at 250°F (121°C) for a specific time.

Autolysis. Self-destruction of cells. Decomposition of all tissues by enzymes that form without microbial assistance.

Autopsy. Postmortem examination of the organs and tissues of a body to determine cause of death or pathological condition. Necropsy.

Bactericidal agent. Agent that destroys bacteria.

Bacteriostatic agent. Agent that has the ability to inhibit or retard bacterial growth. No destruction of viability is implied.

Balsamic substance. Resin combined with oil. A fragrant, resinous, oily exudate from various trees and plants.

Base. (1) In cosmetology, the vehicle in a cosmetic (oil base); the initial application of cream or cosmetics. (2) The lower part of anything, the supporting part.

Base of the axillary space. Armpit.

- **Anterior boundary.** Established by drawing a line along the fold of skin that envelops the lateral border of the pectoralis major muscle.
- **Posterior boundary.** Established by drawing a line along the fold of skin that envelops the lateral border of the latissimus dorsi muscle.

- **Medial boundary.** Established by drawing a line that connects the two points where the pectoralis major and latissimus dorsi muscles blend into the chest wall.
- **Lateral boundary.** Established by drawing a line that connects the two points where the pectoralis major and latissimus dorsi muscles blend into the arm.

Basic pigment. White, yellow, red, and brown; four hues which correspond to the pigments of the skin.

Basket weave suture. (cross stitch) Network of stitches that cross the borders of a cavity or excision to anchor fillers and sustain tissues in their proper position.

Beard area. Areas of the fleshy lips, cheeks, chin, and neck that exhibit hair growth.

Bilateral. Having two sides.

Bilateral differences. Dissimilarities existing in the two sides or halves of an object.

Bilateral silhouette. The bilateral view; an inferior or superior viewpoint that permits the comparison of the two sides or halves of an object or facial feature.

Biohazard. Biological agent or condition that constitutes a hazard to humans.

Biological death. Irreversible somatic death.

Bischloromethyl ether (BCME). A carcinogen potentially produced when formaldehyde and sodium hypochlorite come into contact with each other. Normally occurs only in a controlled laboratory setting and requires a catalyst.

Black. Achromatic color; the absence of all color in pigmentation.

Blanch. To whiten by removing color; to make pale.

Bleach. Chemical that lightens or blanches skin discoloration.

Bleaching. Act of lightening a discoloration by hypodermic means or by surface compress.

Bleaching agent. A chemical that lightens a skin discoloration.

Bleed. Color that escapes at the edge of a mixture.

Blend. To mix or intermingle colors smoothly; to make a gradual change from one color to another.

Blister. Thin vesicle on the skin containing liquid matter.

Blood. Cell-containing fluid that circulates through the blood vascular system and is composed of approximately 22% solids and 78% water.

Bloodborne pathogens. See Bloodborne Pathogen Rule.

Bloodborne pathogen rule. Occupational Health and Safety Administration (OSHA) regulation concerning exposure of employees to blood and other body fluids. The following are OSHA definitions.

- **Blood.** Human blood, human blood components, and products made from human blood.
- **Bloodborne pathogens.** Pathogenic microorganisms that are present in human blood and can cause disease in humans. These pathogens include, but are not limited to, hepatitis B virus (HBV) and human immunodeficiency virus (HIV).
- **Contaminated.** Marked by the presence or reasonably anticipated presence of blood or other potentially infectious materials on an item or surface.
- **Contaminated laundry.** Laundry that has been soiled with blood or other potentially infectious materials or may contain sharps.
- **Contaminated sharps.** Any contaminated object that can penetrate the skin including, but not limited to, needles, scalpels, broken glass, and exposed ends of wires.
- **Engineering controls.** Controls (e.g., sharps disposal container, self-sheathing needles) that isolate or remove the bloodborne pathogen hazard from the workplace.
- **Exposure incident.** Specific eye, mouth, other mucous membrane, nonintact skin, or parenteral contact with blood or other potentially infectious materials that results from the performance of an employee's duties.
- **Occupational exposure.** Reasonably anticipated skin, eye, mucous membrane, or parenteral contact with blood or other potentially infectious materials that may result from the performance of an employee's duties.
- **Parenteral.** Introduced into the body by way of piercing the mucous membranes or the skin barrier, for example, by needlesticks, human bites, cuts, and abrasions.
- **Personal protective equipment (PPE).** Specialized clothing or equipment worn by an employee for protection against a hazard.
- **Universal precautions.** An approach to infection control in which all human blood and certain human body fluids are treated as if they are contaminated with HIV, HBV, and other bloodborne pathogens.
- **Work practice controls.** Controls that reduce

the likelihood of exposure by altering the manner in which a task is performed (e.g., prohibiting recapping of needles, not allowing blood splatter or aerosolization of blood while draining during the embalming process).

Blood discoloration. Discoloration resulting from changes in blood composition, content, or location, either intravascularly or extravascularly.

Blood pressure. Pressure exerted by the blood on the arterial wall in the living body and measured in millimeters of mercury.

Blood vascular system. Circulatory network composed of the heart, arteries, arterioles, capillaries, venules, and veins.

Blonde. Light yellow in coloration; a term commonly employed to describe hair color.

Blotched. Having relatively large patches of color somewhat different from the remainder of the coloring.

Blunt dissection. Separation and pushing aside of the superficial fascia leading to blood vessels and then the deep fascia surrounding blood vessels, using manual techniques or round-ended instruments that separate rather than cut the protective tissues.

Body of the mandible. Horizontal portion of the lower jaw.

Boil. Acute, deep-seated inflammation in the skin. Usually begins as a subcutaneous swelling in a hair follicle.

Bridge. Raised support; the arched portion of the nose which is supported by the nasal bones; a structure or span connecting two parts of a mutilated bone.

Bridge stitch. (interrupted suture) A temporary suture consisting of individually cut and tied stitches employed to sustain the proper position of tissues.

Bridge suture (temporary interrupted suture). Individual stitch knotted at the tissue edge. May be applied prior to embalming to align tissues.

Brilliance. Brightness; in colored illumination, the quantity of illumination passing through a color transparency.

Bronze. Brown or copper-like in coloration.

Brown. The color of tanned leather.

Bruise. (ecchymosis) An injury caused by a blow without laceration; a contusion.

Brunette. Dark brown in coloration; a term commonly employed to describe hair color.

Buccal cavity. The space between the lips and the gums and teeth; the vestibule of the oral cavity.

Buccal depressions. Natural, shallow concavities of the cheeks that extend obliquely downward from the medial or lateral margins of the cheekbones.

Buccinator. Principle muscle of the cheek that compresses the cheeks and forms the lateral wall of the mouth.

Bucco-facial sulcus. Vertical furrow of the cheek; an acquired facial marking.

Buffer. Embalming chemical that effects the stabilization of acid–base balance within embalming solutions and in embalmed tissues.

Bulb syringe. Self-contained, soft rubber manual pump designed to create pressure to deliver fluid as it passes through oneway valves located within the bulb. It is used only to deliver fluids; it cannot be used for aspiration.

Burn. To oxidize or to cause to be oxidized by fire or equivalent means; a tissue reaction or injury resulting from the application of heat, extreme cold, caustic material, radiation, friction, or electricity.

Cadaver. Dead human body used for medical purposes, including transplantation, anatomical dissection, and study.

Cadaveric lividity. Postmortem intravascular red–blue discoloration resulting from hypostasis of blood (livor mortis).

Cadaveric spasm. Prolongation of the last violent contraction of the muscles into the rigidity of death.

Cake. (cosmetology) Compressed powder.

Calvarium. Domelike superior portion of the cranium. That portion removed during cranial autopsy.

Calvarium clamp. Device used to fasten the calvarium to the cranium after a cranial autospy.

Canalization. Formation of new channels in a tissue.

Cancer. Any malignant neoplasm marked by uncontrolled growth and spread of abnormal cells.

Capillaries. Minute blood vessels, the walls of which comprise a single layer of endothelial cells. Capillaries connect the smallest arteries (arteriole) with the smallest veins (venule) and are where pressure filtration occurs.

Capillary permeability. Ability of substances to diffuse through capillary walls into the tissue spaces.

Carbohydrate. Compound containing hydrogen, carbon, and oxygen. Sugars, starches, and glycogen.

Carbuncle. Circumscribed inflammation of the skin and deeper tissues that ends in suppuration and is accompanied by systemic symptoms, such as fever and leukocytosis.

Carcinogen. Cancer-causing chemical or material.

Carmine. (crimson) Purple-red in coloration.

Carotene. The yellow pigment of the skin.

Cartilage. A specialized type of dense connective tissue; attached to the ends of bones and forming parts of structures, such as the nasal septum and the framework of the ear.

Cast. Casting; any object which has been made from a mold; the positive reproduction obtained from a negative impression.

Cauterizing agent. A chemical capable of drying tissues by searing; caustic.

Cavitation. Formation of cavities in an organ or tissue. Frequently seen in some forms of tuberculosis.

Cavity. Hollow place or area.

Cavity embalming. See Embalming.

Cavity fluid. Embalming chemical that is injected into a body cavity following aspiration in cavity embalming. Cavity fluid can also be used as the chemical in hypodermic and surface embalming.

Cellular death. Death of the individual cells of the body.

Cement. Substance used to promote the adhesion of two separated surfaces, such as the lips, eyelids, or margins of an incision.

Center of fluid distribution. Ascending aorta and/or arch of the aorta.

Center of venous drainage. Right atrium of the heart.

Centers for Disease Control and Prevention (CDCP, CDC). Major agency of the Department of Health and Human Services, with headquarters in Atlanta, Georgia, concerned with all phases of control of communicable, vectorborne, and occupational diseases.

Centrifugal force machine. Embalming machine that uses motorized force, pulsating and nonpulsating type.

Channeling. Restorative treatment usually accompanied by aspiration, gravitation, or external pressure to remove gasses or excess liquids from tissues; passages are made through the tissues with a scalpel, hypodermic needle, or trocar.

Charred. Reduced to carbon; the state of tissues destroyed by burning.

Chelate. Substances that bind metallic ions. Ethylenediaminetetracetic acid (EDTA) is used as an anticoagulant in embalming solutions.

Chemical postmortem change. Change in the body's chemical composition that occurs after death, for example, release of heme leading to postmortem staining.

Chemotherapy. Application of chemical reagents in the treatment of disease in humans. May cause an elevated preservation demand.

Chin. The prominence overlying the mental eminence; located at the medial-inferior part of the face; mentum.

Chin rest. One of several methods used for mouth closure (antiquated).

Chromatic color. Color having hue; color of the visible spectrum.

Cilia. Eyelashes.

Clinical death. Phase of somatic death lasting from 5 to 6 minutes in which life may be restored.

Closed drainage technique. A drainage procedure that limits the exposure of the embalmer to the drainage. Tubing is attached to a drain tube allowing drainage to flow directly from a vein into a sanitary disposal system; tubing may also be attached to a trocar and aspirator allowing drainage to be taken from the right atrium of the heart to the sanitary disposal system.

Clostridium perfringens. Anaerobic, saphrophytic, spore-forming bacterium, responsible for tissue gas. Referred to as a gas bacillus.

Coagulating agents. Chemical and physical agents that bring about coagulation.

Coagulation. Process of converting soluble protein into insoluble protein by heating or contact with a chemical such as an alcohol or an aldehyde. Solidification of a sol into a gelatinous mass. Agglutination is a specific form of coagulation.

Coinjection fluid. Supplemental fluid used primarily to enhance the action of vascular (arterial) solutions.

Collodion. Clear syrup-like liquid that evaporates, leaving a contractile, white film; a liquid sealer.

Colloid. Suspension of pigments in a liquid vehicle bound together in such a manner that there is no separation of particles.

Color. Visual sensation perceived by the eye and the mind due to the activity and vibration of light.

Colorant. (cosmetology) Substance used to impart color to an object; dye, pigment, ink, or paint.

Colored filter. Colored glass, gelatin, or other substances which transmit light of certain wave lengths while absorbing the others.

Colored light. Illumination of an identifiable hue.

Color wheel. Circle in which the primary, secondary, and intermediate hues are arranged in orderly intervals.

Columna nasi. Fleshy termination of the nasal septum at the base of the nose; located between the nostrils; the most inferior part of the mass of the nose.

Coma. Irreversible cessation of brain activity and loss of consciousness. Death beginning at the brain.

Communicable disease. Disease that may be transmitted either directly or indirectly between individuals by an infectious agent.

Complements. Directly opposite hues on the color wheel; any two pigmentary hues which, by their mixture in equal quantities, produce gray.

Complexion. Color and texture of the skin, especially that of the face.

Component. Forming a part or ingredient.

Compound fracture. A broken bone piercing the skin.

Compress. Gauze or absorbent cotton saturated with water or an appropriate chemical and placed under or upon tissues to preserve, bleach, dry, constrict, or reduce swelling.

Concave. Exhibiting a depressed or hollow surface; a concavity.

Concave-convex profile. Facial profile variation in which the forehead protrudes beyond the eyebrows while the chin recedes from the plane of the upper lip.

Concave nasal profile. Depressed profile form, which may dip concavely from root to tip.

Concave profile. (infantine, retrousse) Basic facial profile form in which the forehead protrudes beyond the eyebrows while the chin protrudes beyond the plane of the upper lip (least common).

Concave-vertical profile. Facial profile variation in which the forehead protrudes beyond the eyebrows while the upper lip and chin project equally to an imaginary vertical line.

Concha. Concave shell of the ear; the deepest depression of the ear.

Concurrent. Treatments of a restorative nature performed during the embalming operation.

Concurrent disinfection. Disinfection practices carried out during the embalming process.

Concurrent drainage. Method of drainage in which drainage occurs continuously during vascular (arterial) injection.

Condyle. Rounded articular process on a bone.

Cones of the eye. Sensory nerves in the retina of the eye having to do with color detection.

Congealing. See Coagulation and Agglutination.

Conjunctiva. Mucous membrane that lines the eyelid and covers the white portion of the eye.

Constrict. To contract or compress.

Contagious disease. Disease that may be transmitted between individuals, with reference to the organism that causes a disease.

Contaminated. See Bloodborne Pathogen Rule.

Contour. Outline or surface form.

Contusion. Bruise.

Conversion. Color of an object being converted or completely destroyed when one color of illumination strikes an object of a completely different color.

Convex. Curved evenly; resembling a segment of the outer edge of a sphere.

Convex-concave profile. A profile variation in which the forehead recedes from the eyebrows while the chin protrudes beyond the plane of the upper lip.

Convex nasal profile. (Roman, aquiline) Nasal profile that exhibits a hump in its linear form.

Convex profile. Basic profile form in which the forehead recedes from the eyebrows while the chin recedes from the plane of the upper lip (most common).

Convex-vertical profile. Profile variation in which the forehead recedes from the eyebrows while the chin and upper lip project equally to an imaginary vertical line.

Cool hue. Blue, green, purple, or any intermediate pigmentary hue in which they predominate; a receding hue which creates the illusion of distance from the observer; a color of short wavelengths.

Cords of the neck. Vertical prominences of the neck; an acquired facial marking.

Cornea. Transparent part of the tunic of the eyeball that covers the iris and pupil and admits light into the interior.

Corneal sclera button. That portion of the cornea recovered for transplantation in situ.

Coroner. Official of a local community who holds inquests concerning sudden, violent, and unexplained deaths.

Coronoid process. The anterior, nonarticulating process of the ramus of the mandible which serves as the insertion for the temporalis muscle.

Corpulence. Obesity.

Corrective shaping with cosmetics. (Corrective shaping) Cosmetic technique consisting of highlighting those parts of the face or individual features to enlarge or bring them forward or shadowing them to reduce the appearance of size or deepen a depression.

Corrugator. Pyramid-shaped muscle of facial expression that draws the eyebrows inferiorly and medially.

Cosmetic. Preparation for beautifying the complexion and skin, and so on.

Cosmetic base. Initial application of a cream or paste cosmetic to skin tissues.

Cosmetic compound. Cosmetic medium composed of two, three, or all four basic pigments.

Cosmetic fluid. Embalming fluid that contains active dyes and coloring agents intended to restore a more natural skin tone through the embalming process.

Cosmetizing. Process of applying cosmetics to a surface.

Cosmetologist. (beautician) Professional trained in the application of cosmetics and the styling of hair.

Cosmetology. Study of beautifying and improving the complexion, skin, hair, and nails.

Counterstaining compound. Dye that helps to cover internal discolorations such as jaundice or postmortem stain.

Coverall. Plastic garment designed to cover the body from the chest down to the upper thigh.

Cranial embalming. Method used to embalm the contents of the cranial cavity through aspiration and injection of the cranial chamber by passage of a trocar through the cribriform plate.

Cranium. That part of the human skull which encloses the brain.

Cream cosmetic. Semisolid cosmetic.

Cremated remains. Those elements remaining after cremation of a dead human body.

Crepitation. Crackling sensation produced when gases trapped in tissues are palpated, as in subcutaneous emphysema or tissue gas.

Crest. Top of a curve (as a wave) where the direction changes.

Creutzfeldt–Jakob disease. Disease of the central nervous system with unknown etiology, assumed to be a slow virus. Because etiology is unknown, caregivers using invasive procedures use extreme caution.

Cribriform plate. Thin, medial portion of the ethmoid bone of the skull.

Crimson. Deep purplish-red in coloration.

Cross-linkage of proteins. In embalming, the chemical joining of proteins brought about by the chemical reaction of aldehydes with different forms of nitrogen. Cross-linkage results in firmness of embalmed tissue.

Crown. (vertex) Topmost part of the head.

Crura of the antihelix. Superior and anterior bifurcating branches of the antihelix of the ear.

Crus of the helix. Origin of the helix, which is flattened in the concha.

Cuticle remover. Commercially prepared solvent used to remove dead cuticle from the nails and obstinate scabs.

Cyst. Closed sac, with a definite wall, that contains fluid, semifluid, or solid material.

Death. Irreversible cessation of all vital functions—non-legal definition.

Death rattle. Noise made by a moribund person caused by air passing through a residue of mucus in the trachea and posterior oral cavity.

Death struggle. Semiconvulsive twitches that often occur before death.

Decapitation. Separation of the head from the body; to decapitate is the act of such separation.

Decay. Decomposition of proteins by enzymes of aerobic bacteria.

Decomposition. Separation of compounds into simpler substances by the action of microbial and/or autolytic enzymes.

Deep filler. Material used to fill cavities or excisions and to serve as a foundation for the superficial wax restoration.

Dehydrated. Loss of water from the body or tissues.

Dehydration. Loss of moisture from body tissue that may occur antemortem or postmortem (antemortem: febrile disease, diarrhea, or emesis; postmortem: injection of embalming solution or through absorption by the air).

Denatured protein. Protein whose structure has been changed by physical or chemical agents.

Dense. Having component parts closely compacted together; relatively opaque.

Density. Thickness of the applied cosmetic.

Dental prognathism. (buck teeth) Oblique insertion of the teeth.

Dental tie. Ligature around the superior and inferior teeth employed to hold the mandible in a fixed position; antiquated method of mouth closure.

Dentures. Artificial teeth.

Depress. To lower inferiorly or to reduce projection.

Depression. Hollow or concave region; the lowering of a part.

Depressor anguli oris. Facial expression muscle that depresses the angle of the mouth.

Depressor labii inferioris. Facial expression muscle that draws the lower lip inferiorly and slightly lateral.

Depth. State or degree of being deep.

Derma. (dermis, skin) Corium, or true skin.

Desiccation. Process of drying out.

Desquamation (skin-slip). Sloughing off of the epidermis, wherein there is a separation of the epidermis from the underlying dermis.

Deviations. Variation from the common or established.

Dialysis. Separation of substances in solution by the difference in their rates of diffusion through a semipermeable membrane.

Diamond. Frontal view, geometric head shape which is widest across the cheekbones, narrowing in width in both the forehead and the jaws.

Differential pressure. See Pressure.

Diffusion. Movement of molecules or other particles in solution from an area of greater concentration to an area of lesser concentration until a uniform concentration is reached.

Diffusion (arterial solution). Passage of some components of the injected embalming solution from an intravascular to an extravascular location. Movement of the embalming solutions from the capillaries into the interstitial fluids.

Digastricus. Double-bellied muscle which draws the hyoid bone superiorly.

Digits. Fingers and toes. The thumb is the No. 1 digit for each hand and the large toe is No. 1 digit for each foot.

Dilution. Substance thinned or reduced in concentration; a cosmetic lessened in brilliance.

Dimples. Shallow depressions located on the cheek or chin in a rounded or vertical form; natural facial markings.

Disarticulate. Disjoining of bones.

Discoloration. Any abnormal color in or on the human body.

Disease. Any deviation from or interruption of the normal structure or function of a body part, organ, or system.

Disinfectant. An agent, usually chemical, applied to inanimate objects/surfaces to destroy disease-causing microbial agents, but usually not bacterial spores.

Disinfection. Destruction and/or inhibition of most pathogenic organisms and their products in or on the body.

Dissection. Act of cutting apart.

Distend. To expand or swell.

Distention. State of stretching out or becoming inflated.

Distortion. State of being twisted or pushed out of natural shape or position.

Distribution (fluid). Movement of embalming solutions from the point of injection throughout the arterial system and into the capillaries.

Dorsum. Top; the anterior protruding ridge of the nose from the root to the tip of the lobe.

Dowel. Wooden or metal rod used as an armature.

Drain tube. Embalming instrument used to aid the drainage of venous blood from the body.

Drainage. Discharge or withdrawal of blood, blood clots, interstitial and lymphatic fluid and embalming solution from the body during vascular embalming, usually through a vein.

Drench shower. Occupational Safety and Health Administration-required safety device for release of a copious amount of water in a short time.

Dry gangrene. See Gangrene.

Dry rouge. Compacted cake-type cosmetic of red coloration.

Drying powder. Non-preserving powder utilized in setting cosmetics and a wax firming agent. Examples include talcum powder, cosmetic powder, and cornstarch.

Dryness. Freedom from wetness; a condition of tissues necessary for the adhesion of cement, sealer, deep filler, or wax.

Dusky. (swarthy) Somewhat dark in color; when used to describe the complexion color.

Dye (coloring agent). Substances that, on being dissolved, impart a definite color to the embalming solution. Dyes are classified as to their capacity to permanently impart color to the tissue of the body into which they are injected.

Ear. (pinna) Organ of hearing.

Ecchymosis. (bruise) Discoloration of the skin caused by the escape of blood within the tissues and generally accompanied by swelling.

Edema. Abnormal accumulation of fluids in tissues or body cavities.

Electric aspirator. Device that uses a motor to create a suction for the purpose of aspiration.

Electric spatula. Electrically heated blade that may be used to dry moist tissue, reduce swollen tissue, and restore contour.

Electrocardiogram (ECG, EKG). Record of the electrical activity of the heart.

Electroencephalogram (EEG). Record of the electrical activity of the brain.

Elevation. Raised surface or part.

Elliptical curve. Relatively long and slightly dipping curve.

Emaciated. Excessive leanness; a wasted condition resulting in sunken surfaces of the face.

Embalming. Process of chemically treating the dead human body to reduce the presence and growth of microorganisms, to temporarily inhibit organic decomposition, and to restore an acceptable physical appearance.

- **Cavity embalming.** Direct treatment other than vascular (arterial) embalming of the contents of the body cavities and the lumina of the hollow viscera. Usually accomplished by aspiration and then injection of chemicals using a trocar.
- **Hypodermic embalming.** Injection of embalming chemicals directly into the tissues through the use of a syringe and needle or a trocar.
- **Surface embalming.** Direct contact of body tissues with embalming chemicals.
- **Vascular (arterial) embalming.** Use of the blood vascular system of the body for temporary preservation, disinfection, and restoration. Usually accomplished through injection of embalming solutions into the arteries and drainage from the veins.

Embalming analysis (case analysis). That consideration given to the dead body prior to, during, and after the embalming procedure is completed. Documentation is recommended.

Embed. To fix or fasten in place.

Eminence. Prominence or projection of a bone.

Emollient. Soothing agent having the ability to soften tissues; massage cream or a cosmetic possessing this characteristic.

Emphasis. Using the same color of light as the color of the object.

Emulsion. Permanent mixture of two or more immiscible substances (oil and water) which are united with the aid of a binder (gum) or emulsifier (soap).

Engineering controls. See Bloodborne Pathogen Rule.

Enucleation. Removal of an entire mass or part, especially a tumor, or the eyeball, without rupture.

Environment. Surroundings, conditions, or influences that affect an organism or the cells within an organism.

Environmental Protection Agency (EPA). Governmental agency with environmental protection regulatory and enforcement authority.

Enzyme. Organic catalyst produced by living cells and capable of autolytic decomposition.

Epidermis. Outermost layer of skin; cuticle or scarf skin.

Ether. Clear, volatile liquid used as a wax solvent or to remove grease, oil, and adhesive tape stains.

Evert. Turn outward.

Excise. To remove as by cutting out.

Excision. Area from which tissue has been removed.

Expert tests of death. Any procedure used to prove a sign of death, usually performed by medical personnel.

Exposed area. Any visible surface which is to remain uncovered or unclothed.

Exposure incident. See Bloodborne Pathogen Rule.

External auditory meatus. Opening or passageway of the ear.

External pressure. Weight applied to a surface.

Extraction. Drawn or pulled out.

Extravascular. Outside the blood vascular system.

Extravascular blood discoloration. Discoloration of the body outside the blood vascular system, for example, ecchymosis, petechia, hematoma, and postmortem stain.

Extrinsic. From outside the body.

Eye enucleation. Removal of the eye for tissue transplantation, research, and education.

Eye enucleation discoloration. Extravasation of blood as a result of eye enucleation.

Eye shadow. Cosmetic color applied to the upper eyelid; the cosmetic colorant so applied.

Eye socket. (orbit) Bony region containing the eyeball; the orbital cavity.

Eyebrows. (supercilium) Also the superficial hairs covering the superciliary arches.

Eyebrow pencil. Cosmetic in pencil form for coloring the hairs of the eyebrow, or creating an eyebrow where the hairs were removed.

Eyecap. Thin, dome-like shell made of hardened cloth, metal, or plastic placed beneath eyelids to restore natural curvature and to maintain the position of the closed eye.

Eyelids. (palpebrae) Two movable flaps of skin which cover and uncover each eyeball.

Eyelid overlap. Method of eye closure in which the upper lid is placed on top of the lower lid.

Eyewash station. Occupational Safety and Health Administration-required emergency safety device providing a steady stream of water for flushing the eye.

Face. Anatomically, the region from the eyes to the base of the chin; physiognomically, the region from the normal hairline to the base of the chin.

Facial markings. Character lines of the face and neck; wrinkles, grooves, cords, and dimples.

Facial profiles. Silhouettes of the face from the side view.

Facial proportions. Mathematical relationship of the facial features to one another and/or to the head and face.

Fat. Organic compound containing carbon, hydrogen, and oxygen. Chemically, fat is a triglyceride ester composed of glycerol and fatty acids.

Fatty acids. Product of decomposition of fats.

Feather. To reduce gradually to an indistinguishable edge; to taper.

Febrile. Characterized by a high fever, causing dehydration of the body.

Fermentation. Bacterial decomposition of carbohydrates.

Fever blisters. Lesions of the mucous membrane of the lip or mouth caused by herpes simplex type I or II virus or by dehydration of the mucous membrane in a febrile disease.

Filler. Material used to fill a large cavity (e.g., plaster of Paris and cotton; liquid sealer and cotton).

Firming. Rigidity of tissue due to chemical reaction.

Firmness. Degree of rigidity or stability; a condition of the tissues necessary for the application of wax.

Firm wax. (wound filler) The most viscous type of wax; a putty-like material used to fill large cavities or model features.

First degree burn. (hyperemia) Injury caused by heat which produces redness of the skin.

Fixation. Act of making tissue rigid. Solidification of a compound.

Fixative. Agent employed in the preparation of tissues, for the purpose of maintaining the existing form and structure. A large number of agents are used, the most important one being formalin.

Florid. Flushed with red, when describing a complexion; not as vivid as ruddy.

Fluorescent light. Illumination produced by a tubular electric discharge lamp; the fluorescence of phosphors coating the inside of a tube.

Flush (flushing). Intravascular blood discoloration that occurs when arterial solution enters an area (such as the face), but due to blockage, blood and embalming solution are unable to drain from the area.

Fold. Elongated prominence adjoining a surface.

Foramen magnum. Opening in the occipital bone through which the spinal cord passes from the brain.

Force. Quality of a color to draw attention by means of its intensity or advancing characteristics.

Forehead. That part of the face above the eyes.

Formaldehyde (HCHO). Colorless, strong-smelling gas that when used in solution is a powerful preservative and disinfectant. Potential occupational carcinogen.

Formaldehyde gray. Gray discoloration of the body caused by the reaction of formaldehyde from the embalming process with hemoglobin to form methyl-hemoglobin.

Formaldehyde rule. Occupational Safety and Health Administration regulation limiting the amount of occupational exposure to formaldehyde gas.

Fossa. Depression; concavity.

Foundation. Complexion cosmetic in ornamental cosmetology.

Fourth degree burn. Total evacuation (absence) of tissue.

Fracture. Broken bone.

Frenulum. Vertical restraining fold of mucous membrane on the midline of the inside of each lip connecting the lip with the gum.

Frontal. Anterior; anterior view of the face or features.

Frontal bone. Anterior third of the cranium, forming the forehead and the anterior portion of the roof of the skull.

Frontal eminences. Paired, rounded, unmargined prominences of the frontal bone found approximately 1 inch beneath the normal hairline.

Frontal process of the maxilla. Ascending part of the upper jaw that gradually protrudes as it rises beside the nasal bone to meet the frontal bone; the ascending process of the upper jaw.

Funeral lighting. Quality and quantity of illumination used for presentation of casketed or reposed remains.

Furrow. (wrinkle) Crevice in the skin accompanied by adjacent elevations.

Furuncle. See Boil.

Gangrene. Necrosis, death, of tissues of part of the body usually due to deficient or absent blood supply.

- **Dry gangrene.** Condition that results when the body part that dies had little blood and remains aseptic. The arteries but not the veins are obstructed.
- **Gas gangrene.** Necrosis in a wound infected by an anaerobic gas-forming bacillus, the most common etiologic agent being *Clostridium perfringens.*
- **Moist (wet) gangrene.** Necrotic tissue that is wet as a result of inadequate venous drainage. May be accompanied by bacterial infection.

Gauze. Light, open-mesh variety of muslin or similar material.

Geometric. Shape of a plane figure determined by its outline, such as rounded, oval, square, etc.

Germicide. Agent, usually chemical, applied either to inanimate objects/surfaces or to living tissues to destroy disease-causing microbial agents, but usually not bacterial spores.

Glabella. Single bony prominence of the frontal bone located between the superciliary arches in the inferior part of the frontal bone above the root of the nose.

Glycerin. Syrupy, colorless liquid obtained from fats or oils as a by-product of the manufacturing of soaps and fatty acids; used as a vehicle for some cosmetics.

Gooseneck. Rubber stopper containing two tubes, one to create vacuum or pressure and the other to deliver fluid or achieve aspiration. Possibly used in conjunction with a hand pump.

Grave wax. See Adipocere.

Gravity filtration. Extravascular settling of fluids by gravitational force to the dependent areas of the body.

Gravity injector. Apparatus used to inject arterial fluid during the vascular (arterial) phase of the embalming process. Relies on gravity to create the pressure required to deliver the fluid (0.43 pounds of pressure per 1 foot of elevation.)

Gray. Neutral, achromatic color resulting from the mixture of black and white pigments; color resulting from the mixture of complementary pigmentary hues in equal quantities.

Grecian. (straight nasal profile) Nasal profile form in which the dorsum exhibits a straight line from the root to the tip.

Green. Hue resulting from the mixture of yellow and blue pigments in equal quantities; one of three secondary pigmentary hues.

Groove. Elongated depression in a relatively level plane or surface.

Groove director. Instrument used to guide vein tubes into vessels.

Hairline. Outline of hair growth on the head or face; the lowest centrally located part of the hair of the cranium.

Hair patch. Grouping of hairs, affixed by suturing, utilized in hair restorations.

Hand pump. Historical instrument resembling a large hypodermic syringe attached to a bottle apparatus. Used to create either pressure for injection or vacuum for aspiration.

Hard palate. Anterior portion of the roof of the mouth.

Hard water. Water containing large amounts of mineral salts. These mineral salts must be removed from or sequestered in water (vehicle) to be used in mixing vascular embalming solutions.

Hardening compound. Chemical in powder form that has the ability to absorb and to disinfect. Often used in cavity treatment of autopsied cases.

Hazard Communication Standard (Rule). Occupational Safety and Health Administration regulation that deals with limiting exposure to occupational hazards.

Hazardous material. Agent or material exposing one to risk.

Headrest. Piece of equipment used to maintain the head in the proper position during the embalming process.

Head shape. Outline of the exterior margins of the head.

Height. Vertical measurement of a feature or part of a feature; the distance above the base.

Helix. Outer rim of the ear.

Hematemesis. Blood present in vomitus. Vomiting of blood.

Hematoma. A swelling or mass of clotted blood caused by a ruptured blood vessel and confined to an organ or space.

Heme. Nonprotein portion of hemoglobin. Red pigment.

Hemoglobin. Red respiratory portion of the red blood cells. Iron-containing pigment of red blood cells functioning to carry oxygen to the cells.

Hemolysis. Destruction of red blood cells that liberates hemoglobin.

Hepatitis. Inflammation of the liver that may be caused by a variety of agents, including viral infections, bacterial invasion, and physical or chemical agents. It is usually accompanied by fever, jaundice, and an enlarged liver.

Hepatitis B virus (HBV). Severe infectious bloodborne virus.

Herpes. Inflammatory skin disease marked by small vesicles in clusters, usually restricted to diseases caused by herpesvirus.

High-index fluids. Special vascular (arterial) fluid with a formaldehyde content of 25 to 36%.

Highlight. Surface lying at right angles to the source of illumination which reflects the maximum amount of light; the brighter part.

Highlighting and shadowing with cosmetics. Application of a color which is lighter or brighter than the complexion would highlight the complexion; application of a color darker than the complexion color would shadow the complexion.

Horseshoe curve. Roughly U-shaped, with the front being narrower than the sweep of the curve.

Household bleach. Five percent sodium hypochlorite solution. Mixing 12 ounces of household bleach with 116 ounces of water yields 1 gallon of a 10% household bleach solution (5000 ppm sodium hypochlorite).

Hue. Property of a color by which it is distinguished from other colors.

Human immunodeficiency virus (HIV). Retrovirus that causes acquired immunodeficiency syndrome (AIDS).

Human remains. Body of a deceased person, including cremated remains.

Humectant. Chemical that increases the ability of embalmed tissue to retain moisture.

Humor. Any liquid or semiliquid of the body, as the aqueous or vitreous humor of the eyeball.

Hunting bow. Shaped as a bent wood weapon with a central belly; resembling a cupid bow.

Hydroaspirator. Apparatus that is connected to the water supply. When the water is turned on, a suction is developed and is used to aspirate the contents of the body's cavities.

Hydrocele. Abnormal accumulation of fluids in a saclike structure, especially the scrotal sac.

Hydrocephalus. Abnormal accumulation of cerebrospinal fluids in the ventricles of the brain.

Hydrolysis. Reaction in which water is one of the reactants and compounds are often broken down. In the hydrolysis of proteins, the addition of water accompanied by the action of enzymes results in the breakdown of protein into amino acids.

Hydropericardium. Abnormal accumulation of fluid within the pericardial sac.

Hydrothorax. Abnormal accumulation of fluid in the thoracic cavity.

Hygroscopic. Absorbing moisture readily.

Hypertonic solution. Solution having a greater concentration of dissolved solute than the solution with which it is compared.

Hypodermic embalming. See Embalming.

Hypodermic injection. Injection of chemicals directly into the tissues through the use of a syringe and needle.

Hypodermic tissue building. Injection of special creams or liquids into the tissues through the use of a syringe and needle to restore natural contour.

Hypostasis. Settling of blood and/or other fluids to dependent portions of the body.

Hypotonic solution. Solution having a lesser concentration of dissolved solute than the solution with which it is compared.

Illumination. Giving or casting of light.

Imbibition. Absorption of the fluid portion of blood by the tissues after death, resulting in postmortem edema.

Incandescent light. (white light) Illumination resulting from the glowing of a heated filament.

Incision. A clean cut made with a sharp instrument. In embalming, a cut made with a scalpel to raise arteries and veins.

Incisive fossa. Depression between the mental eminence and the inferior incisor teeth.

Incisor teeth. Four teeth located anteriorly from the midline on each jaw, used for cutting.

Inclination. Slope; deviation from the horizontal or vertical; oblique.

Index. Strength of an embalming fluid, indicated by the number of grams of pure formaldehyde gas dissolved in 100 mL of water. Index usually refers to a percentage; an embalming fluid with an index of 25 usually contains 25% formaldehyde gas.

Indigo. Blue dye obtained from certain plants or made synthetically, usually from aniline dyes; a deep violet blue designated by Newton as one of the seven prismatic colors.

Infant. Child less than 1 year of age.

Infantine. Babyish, childlike in regard to much adipose tissue.

Infectious disease. Disease caused by the growth of a pathogenic microorganism in the body.

Infectious waste. See Biohazard.

Inferior. Beneath; lower in plane or position; the under surface of an organ or indicating a structure below another structure; toward the feet.

Inferior nasal conchae. Lowermost scroll-shaped bones on the sidewalls of the nasal cavity.

Inferior palpebral sulcus. Furrow of the lower attached border of the inferior palpebra; acquired facial marking.

Inflammation. Reaction of tissues to injurious agents, usually characterized by heat, redness, swelling, and pain.

Infranasal prognathism. Form of prognathism in which the base of the nasal cavity protrudes abnormally.

Infrared. Part of the invisible spectrum adjacent to the red end of the visible spectrum.

Inguinal ligament. Anatomical structure forming the base of the femoral triangle; Extends from the anterior superior iliac spine to the pubic tubercle.

Inhibit. To restrain, hinder, or retard.

Inject. To introduce forcibly into the circulatory system, tissues, etc. with a hypodermic syringe or the like.

Injection. Act or instance of forcing a fluid into the vascular system or directly into tissues.

Injection pressure. See Pressure.

Inner canthus. Eminence at the inner corner of the closed eyelids.

Instant tissue fixation. Embalming technique which uses a very strong arterial solution (often waterless). The solution is injected under high pressure in spurts into a body area. Very little solution is injected; the technique attempts to limit swelling; for example, bodies with facial trauma or early decomposition.

Instantaneous rigor mortis. Instantaneous stiffening of the muscles of a dead human body.

Integumentary lips. Superiorly, the skin portion of the

upper lip from the attached margin of the upper mucous membrane to the base of the nose; and inferiorly, the skin portion of the lower lip from the attached margin of the lower mucous membrane to the labiomental sulcus.

Intense. Existing in a high degree of brilliance; vivid.

Intensify. To become more brilliant or more vivid in color.

Intensity. (chroma) Brightness or dullness of a hue.

Intercellular. Between the cells of a structure.

Intercellular fluid. Fluid inside cells of the body (constituting about one half of the body weight).

Interciliary sulci. Vertical or transverse furrows between the eyebrows; acquired facial markings.

Intercostal space. Space between the ribs.

Intermediate hue. Pigmentary hue produced by mixing, in equal quantities, a primary hue with its adjacent secondary hue on the color wheel.

Intermittent drainage (restricted drainage). Method of drainage in which the drainage is stopped at intervals while the injection continues.

Interstitial fluid. Fluid in the supporting connective tissues surrounding body cells (about one fifth the body weight).

Intertragic notch. Notch or opening between the tragus and the antitragus of the ear.

Intradermal suture. (hidden suture) Type of suture used to close incisions in such a manner that the ligature remains entirely under the epidermis.

Intravascular. Within the blood vascular system.

Intravascular blood discoloration. Discoloration of the body within the blood vascular system, for example, hypostasis, carbon monoxide, and capillary congestion.

Intravascular fluid. Fluid contained within vascular channels (about one twentieth of the body weight).

Intrinsic. From within the body.

Inversion. Tissues turned in an opposite direction or folded inward.

Inversion suture. See worm suture.

Inverted triangle. Three-sided figure whose base is superior to its apex; when used to describe a frontal view geometric headshape, a head which is wide at the forehead and narrow at the jaw.

Isotonic solution. A solution having a concentration of dissolved solute equal to that of a standard of reference.

Jaundice. Conditions characterized by an excessive concentration of bilirubin in the skin and tissues and deposition of excessive bile pigment in the skin, cornea, body fluids, and mucous membranes with the resulting yellow appearance of the patient.

Jaundice fluid. Arterial fluid with special bleaching and coloring qualities for use on bodies with jaundice. Usually, formaldehyde content is low.

Jawline. Inferior border of the mandible.

Jugular drain tube. Tubular instrument of varying diameter and shape, preferably with a plunger, that is inserted into the jugular vein to aid in drainage.

Juxtaposition. (simultaneous contrast) Any two hues seen together that modify each other in the direction of their complements.

Labia. Lips.

Labial sulci. (furrows of age) Vertical furrows of each lip extending from within the mucous membranes into the integumentary lips; acquired facial markings.

Labiomental sulcus. Junction of the lower integumentary lip and the superior border of the chin, which may appear as a furrow; a natural facial marking.

Lacerated. Cut or torn into irregular segments.

Laceration. Wound characterized by irregular tearing of tissue.

Lanolin. Oil from sheep wool.

Lanugo. (peach fuzz) Downy hair of a fetus, children, or women.

Larvicide. Substance used to kill insect larvae.

Lateral. Away from the midline.

Leak. Escape of blood or fluid.

Legionnaires' disease. Severe, often fatal bacterial disease characterized by pneumonia, dry cough, and sometimes gastrointestinal symptoms (Legionella pneumophilia).

Length. Vertical dimension.

Leptorrhine. Nasal index common to individuals of Western European descent having a long, narrow, and high bridge.

Lesion. Any change in structure produced during the course of a disease or injury.

Levator anguli oris. Muscle of facial expression that elevates the angle of the mouth.

Levator labii superioris. Muscle of facial expression that elevates and extends the upper lip.

Levator labii superioris alaeque nasi. Muscle of facial expression that elevates the upper lip and dilates the nostril opening; the common elevator.

Levator palpebrae superioris. Muscle of facial expression that raises the upper eyelid.

Ligate. To tie off, as in ligating an artery and vein on completion of embalming or ligating the colon in autopsied bodies.

Ligature. Thread, cord, or wire used for tying vessels, tissues, or bones.

Light. To shine; form of electromagnetic radiation that acts on the retina of the eye to make sight possible.

Linear guide. Line drawn or visualized on the surface of the skin to represent the approximate location of some deeper lying structure.

Line of closure. Line that forms between two structures, such as the lips or the eyelids when in a closed position, which marks their place of contact with each other.

Linear sulci. Eyelid furrows which are short and broken, extending horizontally on the palpebrae themselves and which may fan from both the medial and lateral corners of the eyes.

Lip brush. Small flat brush having soft hairs of uniform length.

Lipolysis. Decomposition of fats.

Lip wax. Soft restorative wax, usually tinted, used to surface the mucous membranes or to correct lip separations.

Liquid cosmetic. Fluid, facial colorant in which pigments are dissolved or suspended.

Liquid sealer. Quick drying fluid adhesive.

Liquid suspension. Aqueous mixture or powder with a suspending agent.

Livor mortis. See Cadaveric Lividity.

Lobe. Fatty inferior third of the ear.

Loop stitch. Single, noose-like suture, not pulled taut before knotting, which stands from the skin and which anchors restorative materials.

Lumen. Cavity of a vein, artery, or intestine.

Lysin. Specific antibody acting destructively on cells and tissues.

Lysosome. Organelle that exists within a cell, but separate from the cell. Contains hydrolytic enzymes that break down proteins and certain carbohydrates.

Magenta. Red-purple or purplish-red, (e.g., a product of red and blue illumination projected on the same area).

Maggot. Larva of an insect, especially a flying insect.

Major restoration. Those requiring a long period of time, are extensive, require advanced technical skill, and expressed written consent to perform.

Make-up. Cosmetic material; the way in which one is painted; the process of application of a cosmetic.

Mandible. Horseshoe-shaped bone forming the inferior jaw.

Mandibular fossa. Glenoid fossa; the small oval depression on the zygomatic process of the temporal bone into which the condyle of the mandible articulates, just anterior to the external auditory meatus. Forms the temporal mandibular joint (TMJ).

Mandibular prognathism. Inferior jaw protrudes.

Mandibular sulcus. Furrow beneath the jawline which rises vertically on the cheek; an acquired facial marking.

Mandibular suture. Stitch used to hold the mouth closed; placed behind the lips, one part is passed through the inferior jaw at the median plane, while the other part extends through the nasal septum or the superior frenulum.

Manual aid. Those treatments or procedures that are applied by the use of hands. Scrubbing with soap and water to remove a surface discoloration; flexing, bending, rotating and massage of the limbs to stimulate the circulation of arterial solution and movement of blood and body fluids.

Margin. Boundary or edge.

Mascara. Cosmetic preparation used to darken the eyelashes.

Mask. (face mask) Anything that hides or conceals, as cosmetics.

Masking agent. See Perfuming Agents.

Massage. Manipulation of tissue in the course of preparation of the body.

Massage cream. Soft, white, oily preparation used as a protective coating for external tissues; a base for cream cosmetics and a wax softener; an emollient.

Masseter muscles. Muscles of mastication that close the mandible.

Mastic compound. Putty-like substance; an absorbent sealing adhesive that can be injected under the skin or applied to surface tissues to establish skin contour.

Mastoid process. The rounded projection on the inferior portion of the temporal bones just posterior to the lobe of the ear.

Material safety data sheet (MSDS). Form that must accompany a hazardous product. Requirement of the Department of Labor and Occupational Safety and Health Administration under the Hazard Communication Standard.

Matte. Having a dull finish; as afforded by the application of loose powder, lack of sheen.

Maxilla. Paired bone with several processes that form the skeletal base of most of the superior face, roof of the mouth, sides of the nasal cavity, and floor of the orbit.

Maxillary prognathism. Superior jaw protrudes.

Mechanical aid. The application of treatments or procedures which utilize machines or instruments. Adjustments of pressure and rate of flow on the embalming machine; utilization of properly sized arterial tubes and/or drainage instruments.

Medial. Toward the midline.

Medial lobe. Tiny prominence on the midline of the superior mucous membrane.

Medical examiner. Official elected or appointed to investigate suspicious or unnatural deaths.

Medium wax. Dermasurgery or restorative wax.

Melanin. The brown to black-brown pigment in the epidermis and hair.

Meningitis. Inflammation of the meninges.

Mental eminence. Bony triangular projection on the inferior portion of the anterior mandible.

Mentalis muscle. Elevates and protrudes the inferior lip, wrinkles the skin over the chin.

Mesorrhine. Nasal classification which is medium-broad and medium-low bridged; common to individuals of Asian descent.

Microbe (microorganism). Minute one-celled form of life not distinguishable as to vegetable or animal nature.

Midaxillary line. Vertical line drawn from the center of the medial border of the base of the axillary space.

Millicurie (mCi). That amount of radioactive material in which 37 million atoms disintegrate each second.

Minor restoration. Those requiring a minimum effort, skill, or time to complete.

Mixture. Composition of two or more substances that are not chemically bound to each other.

Modeling. Constructing a form with a pliable material such as wax or clay.

Modifying agents. Chemical components of vascular fluids which control the rate and degree of tissue firmness by the fluid (e.g., humectants, buffers); chemicals for which there may be greatly varying demands predicated on the type of embalming, the environment, and the embalming fluid used.

Mold-preventive agents. Agents that prohibit the growth of mold.

Monochromatic. Variations of one hue; tints, tones, and shades of one hue.

Mortuary mastic compound. See mastic compound.

Mottle. To diversify with spots or blotches of different color (or shade).

Moribund. In a dying state. In the agonal period.

Mouth former. Device used in the mouth to shape the contour of the lips.

Mucous membranes. The visible red surfaces of the lips; the lining membrane of body cavities that communicate with the exterior.

Multipoint injection (multisite). Vascular injection that utilizes two or more injection sites.

Musculature suture. Method of mouth closure in which a suture is passed through the septum of the nose and through the mentalis muscle of the chin.

Mute. To reduce the intensity of a color by the addition of another color.

Mutilated. Disfigured by a loss of a natural part by force.

Nasal bones. Directly inferior to the glabella and forming a dome over the superior portion of the nasal cavity.

Nasal cavity. Space between the roof of the mouth and the floor of the cranial cavity.

Nasal spine of the maxilla. Sharp, bony projection located medially at the inferior margin of the nasal cavity.

Nasal sulcus. Angular area between the posterior margin of the wing of the nose and the nasolabial fold; a natural facial marking.

Nasal tube aspirator. Embalming instrument used to aspirate the throat by means of the nostrils.

Nasolabial fold. The eminence of the cheek and adjacent to the mouth; extending from the superior part of the posterior margin of the wing of the nose to the side of the mouth; a natural facial marking.

Nasolabial sulcus. Furrow originating at the superior border of the wing of the nose and extending to the side of the mouth; acquired facial marking.

Naso-orbital fossa. Depression superior to the medial portion of the superior palpebrae.

Natural facial markings. Those that are present at birth, hereditary.

Natural shadows. Areas of color in the tissues normally darker than the adjacent areas.

Necrobiosis. Antemortem, physiological death of the cells of the body followed by their replacement.

Necropsy. See Autopsy.

Necrosis. Pathological death of a tissue still a part of the living organism.

Needle injector. Mechanical device used to impel specially designed metal pins into bone.

Neoplasm. New and abnormal formation of tissue, as a tumor or growth.

Nephritis. Inflammation of the kidneys.

Nevus. Birthmark; congenital skin blemish; any congenital anomaly, including various types of birthmarks and all types of moles.

Nitrogenous waste. Metabolic by-products that contain nitrogen, such as urea and uric acid. These compounds have a high affinity for formaldehyde and tend to neutralize embalming chemicals.

Noncosmetic fluid. Type of arterial fluid that contains inactive dyes that will not impart a color change on the body tissues of the deceased.

Norm. The most common characteristics of each feature; typical, common, average.

Notch. Relatively deep indentation, usually between two projections.

Obese. Having an abnormal amount of fat on the body. Corpulent.

Oblique. Slanting or inclined, neither perpendicular nor horizontal.

Oblique palpebral sulcus. Shallow, curving groove below the medial corner of the eyelids; natural facial marking.

Oblong. Frontal head form in which the head is long and narrow throughout.

Occipital bone. Lowest part of the back and base of the cranium, forming a cradle for the brain.

Occipital protuberance. The prominence at the center of the external surface of the occipital bone.

Occipitofrontalis muscle. Epicranius; draws the scalp posteriorly and anteriorly and raises the eyebrows.

Occupational exposure. See Bloodborne Pathogen Rule.

Occupational Safety and Health Administration (OSHA). A Governmental agency with the responsibility for regulation and enforcement of safety and health matters for most U.S. employees. An individual state OSHA agency may supercede the U.S. Department of Labor OSHA regulations.

Oil-base cosmetics. Coloring medium in which the pigments are combined with a petroleum product.

Olive. Yellow-tan of medium value with a greenish tinge.

One-point injection. Injection and drainage from one location.

Opacity. State of being opaque.

Opaque. Not transparent or translucent; not allowing light to pass through a concealing cosmetic.

Opaque cosmetic. A cosmetic medium able to cover or hide skin discolorations.

Operative aid. (corrections) Invasive treatments or procedures. Examples include channeling, incisions, and excisions.

Ophthalmoscope. Optical instrument with an accompanying light that makes it possible to examine the retina and to explore for blood circulation.

Optic facial sulci. (crow's feet) Furrows radiating from the lateral corner of the eye; acquired facial markings.

Optimum. Most favorable condition for functioning.

Oral cavity. Mouth and vestibule, or the opening to the throat.

Orange. Hue obtained from the mixture of red and yellow; a secondary color of pigments.

Orbicularis oculi muscles. Closes the eyelids; compresses the lacrimal sacs.

Orbicularis oris muscle. Closes the lips.

Orbital cavity (orbit). Eyesocket.

Orbital pouch. Bags under the eyes; the fullness between the inferior palpebrae and the oblique palpebral sulcus.

Orifice. Entrance or outlet of any body cavity; an opening.

Origin. Attachment of a muscle which moves least when the muscle contracts; the beginning.

Ornamental. Adornment or embellishment; a cosmetic material manufactured for street wear; the technique of cosmetic application to beautify the face.

Osmosis. Passage of solvent from a solution of lesser to one of greater solute concentration when the two solutions are separated by a semipermeable membrane.

Oval. Frontal head form in which the head is generally egg shaped, with the cranium slightly wider than the jaws; most common geometric head form.

Overtone. Coloring modified by an overlying color; color that visibly predominates more than general coloring; a wash.

Packing forceps. Embalming instrument used in closing the external orifices of the body.

Palatine bone. One of the bones forming the posterior part of the hard palate and lateral nasal wall between the interior pterygoid plate of the sphenoid bone and the maxilla.

Palpate. To examine by touch.

Palpebrae. Eyelids both superior and inferior; singular palpebra.

Pancake. Cosmetic face powder pressed into a flat cake.

Parallel incision. Incision on the surface of the skin to raise the common carotid arteries. It is made along the posterior border of the inferior one third of the sternocleidomastoid muscle.

Parenteral. See Bloodborne Pathogen Rule.

Parietal bones. Two bones that form the roof and part of the sides of the skull.

Parietal eminence. Rounded peak of the external convexity of the parietal bones; determines the widest part of the cranium.

Parts per million (ppm). In contaminated air, the parts of vapor or gas (formaldehyde) per million parts of air by volume. In solution, the parts of chemical per million parts of solution.

Passive transport system. Method by which solutes and/or solvents cross through a membrane with no energy provided by the cells of the membrane. In embalming, examples include pressure filtration, dialysis, diffusion, and osmosis.

Paste. Soft, moist opaque cosmetic with the consistency of dough and bound together with the aid of gum, starch, and water. If oils and fats are present, water is absent.

Patch of hair. Group of hairs of uniform length applied simultaneously as a method of hair replacement.

Pathological condition. Diseased; due to a disease.

Pathological discoloration. Antemortem discoloration that occurs during the course of certain diseases such as gangrene and jaundice.

Pediculicide. Substance able to destroy lice.

Penetrating wounds. Wounds entering the interior of an organ or cavity.

Percutaneous. Effected through unbroken skin.

Perfuming agents (masking agents). Chemicals found in embalming arterial formulations having the capability of displacing an unpleasant odor or of altering an unpleasant odor so that it is converted to a more pleasant one.

Perfusion. To force a fluid through (an organ or tissue), especially by way of the blood vessels. Injection during vascular (arterial) embalming.

Peritonitis. Inflammation of the peritoneum, the membranous coat lining the abdominal cavity and investing the viscera.

Permissible exposure limit (PEL). Maximum legal limit established by the Occupational Safety and Health Administration for a regulated substance. These are based on employee exposure and are time-weighted over an 8-hour work shift. When these limits are exceeded, employers must take proper steps to reduce employee exposure. For formaldehyde, the PEL is 0.75 ppm.

Perpendicular plate of the ethmoid bone. Superior portion of the bony nasal septum.

Personal protective equipment (PPE). See Bloodborne Pathogen Rule.

Petechia. Antemortem, pinpoint, extravascular blood discoloration visible as purplish hemorrhages of the skin.

Petroleum jelly. Semisolid, yellow mixture of hydrocarbons obtained from petroleum.

Pharmaceutical. Drug or medicine.

Phenol. (carbolic acid) Antiseptic/disinfectant employed to dry moist tissues and to bleach discolored tissues.

Philtrum. Vertical groove located medially on the superior lip; a natural facial marking.

Physiognomy. Study of the structures and surface markings of the face and features.

Pigment. Coloring matter which can be applied to an object, when combined with some type of vehicle.

Pigment powder. Powder (usually composed of dry, pulverized pigments and talcum) employed to impart color to the skin.

Pigment theory. The Prang system; the basis for mortuary cosmetology.

Pinna. (ear) Auricle or projected part of the exterior ear.

Pitting edema. Condition in which interstitial spaces contain such excessive amounts of fluid that the skin remains depressed after palpation.

Planes. Surfaces having very little curvature.

Plaster of Paris. Calcium sulfate; a white powdery substance which forms a quick-setting paste when mixed with water.

Platyrrhine. Nasal classification which is short and broad and has the minimum of projection; common to individuals of African descent.

Platysma muscle. Thin layer of muscle covering anterior aspect of neck.

Platysmal sulci. Transverse, dipping furrow of the neck; acquired facial marking.

Pledget. Small ball, cylinder, or tuft often made of cotton.

Plug. Any device as cotton, cloth, wood, etc. used to fill or close an opening.

Pneumonia. Acute infection or inflammation of the alveoli. The alveolar sacs fill up with fluid and dead white blood cells. Causes include bacteria, fungi, and viruses.

Point of entry. Place (usually invisible) at which access to inner positions may be had; a place at which a hypodermic needle may be inserted to pass into the same or another area.

Pores. Minute depressions in the surface of the skin, as in the openings of the sweat glands.

Positioning devices. Preparation room equipment for properly positioning bodies prior to, during, and after vascular embalming.

Postembalming. Treatments of restorative nature performed after the embalming operation.

Posterior. Toward the back.

Postmortem. Period that begins after somatic death.

Postmortem caloricity. Rise in body temperature after death due to continued cellular metabolism.

Postmortem chemical changes. Change in the body's chemical composition that occurs after death (e.g., decomposition, change in body pH, rigor mortis, postmortem stain, postmortem caloricity).

Postmortem examination. See autopsy.

Postmortem physical change. Change in the form or state of matter without any change in chemical composition, e.g., algor mortis, hypostasis, dehydration, livor mortis, increase in blood viscosity, translocation of microbes.

Postmortem stain. Extravascular color change that occurs when heme, released by hemolysis of red blood cells, seeps through the vessel walls and into the body tissues.

Potential of hydrogen (pH). Degree of acidity or alkalinity. The scale ranges from 0 to 14—0 being completely acid, 14 completely basic, and 7 neutral. Blood has a pH of 7.35 to 7.45.

Potential pressure. See pressure.

Powder. Any solid substance in the state of fine, loose particles as produced by crushing or grinding.

Powder atomizer. Device used to blow powder onto a surface.

Powder brush. Device containing hairs or bristles set in a handle; used to apply and/or remove powder.

Powder puff. Soft, circular pad for applying powder.

Precipitant. Substance bringing about precipitation. The oxilates formerly used in water conditioning chemicals are now illegal because of their poisonous nature.

Pre-embalming. Treatments (of a restorative nature) performed before the embalming operation.

Preinjection fluid. Fluid injected primarily to prepare

the vascular system and body tissues for the injection of the preservative vascular (arterial) solution. This solution is injected before the preservative vascular solution is injected.

Preparation room. That area or facility wherein embalming, dressing, cosmetizing, or other body preparation is effected.

Preservation. See Temporary Preservation.

Preservative. Chemicals that inactivate saprophytic bacteria, render unsuitable for nutrition the media upon which such bacteria thrive, and will arrest decomposition by altering enzymes and lysins of the body as well as converting the decomposable tissue to a form less susceptible to decomposition.

Preservative demand. Amount of preservative (formaldehyde) required to effectively preserve and disinfect remains. Depends on the condition of the tissues as determined in the embalming analysis.

Preservative powder. Chemical in powder form, typically used for surface embalming of the remains.

Pressure. Action of a force against an opposing force (a force applied or acting against resistance).

- **Actual pressure.** That pressure indicated by the injector gauge needle when the arterial tube is open and the arterial solution is flowing into the body.
- **Blood pressure.** Pressure exerted by the blood on the vessel walls measured in millimeters of mercury.
- **Differential pressure.** Difference between potential and actual pressures.
- **Injection pressure.** Amount of pressure produced by an injection device to overcome initial resistance within (intravascular) or on (extravascular) the vascular system (arterial or venous).
- **Intravascular pressure.** Pressure developed as the flow of embalming solution is established and the elastic arterial walls expand and then contract, resulting in filling of the capillary beds and development of pressure filtration.
- **Potential pressure.** Pressure indicated by the injector gauge needle when the injector motor is running and the arterial tubing is clamped off.

Pressure filtration. Passage of embalming solution through the capillary wall to diffuse with the interstitial fluids by application of positive intravascular pressure. Embalming solution passes from an intravascular to an extravascular position.

Primary dilution. Dilution attained as the embalming solution is mixed in the embalming machine.

Primary disinfection. Disinfection carried out prior to the embalming process.

Primary hue. Three pigmentary hues—red, yellow, and blue—which can be combined to make all other hues.

Procerus muscle. Draws the skin of the forehead inferiorly.

Procurement. Recovery of organs or tissues from a cadaver for transplantation.

Professional portrait. Photograph or painting in which the subject has been posed and lighted flatteringly by a professional photographer or artist.

Profile. Side view of the human head.

Prognathism. Projection of the jaw or jaws that may cause problems with mouth closure and alignment of the teeth.

Projection. Act of throwing forward; a part extending beyond the level of its surroundings.

Proportions. Relationships of the size of one feature as compared with another feature or with the width or length of the face.

Prosthetic device. Artificial device used to replace a limb, appendage, or other body part.

Protein. Organic compound found in plants and animals that can be broken down into amino acids.

Proteolysis. Decomposition of proteins.

Protruding lobe. Rounded, anterior projection of the tip of the nose.

Protrusion. State or condition of being thrust forward or projecting.

Ptomaine. Any one of a group of nitrogenous organic compounds formed by the action of putrefactive bacteria on proteins, for example, indole, skatole, cadaverine, and putrescine.

Pubic symphysis. Fibrocartilage that joins the two pubic bones in the median plane.

Puncture. Hole or slight wound resulting from piercing.

Purge. Postmortem evacuation of any substance from an external orifice of the body as a result of pressure.

Purple. Color between blue and red; a secondary hue of pigments.

Purse string suture. Suture made around the circumference of a circular opening or puncture to close it or to hold the margins in position.

Pus. Liquid product of inflammation containing various proteins and leukocytes.

Pustular lesion. Characteristic pus-filled wound of a disease, such as smallpox, syphilis, and acne.

Pustule. Small elevation of the skin with an inflamed base, containing pus.

Putrefaction. Decomposition of proteins by the action of enzymes from anaerobic bacteria.

Pyramid. Apparently solid structure having a square base and four triangular sides which meet at a central point.

Radiant energy. Energy traveling through space in the form of electromagnetic waves of various lengths.

Radiate. To spread out from a common point.

Radiation protection officer. Supervisor, in an institution licensed to use radionuclides, who has the responsibility to establish procedures and make recommendations in the use of all radioactive matter.

Radionuclide. Chemical element that is similar in chemical properties to another element, but differs in atomic weight and electric charge and emits radiation. An atom that disintegrates by emission of electromagnetic radiation.

Ramus. Vertical portion of the mandible.

Raspberry. Dark, purplish-red color.

Rate of flow. Speed at which fluid is injected, measured in ounces per minute.

Rat-tail comb. Comb with a long, thin handle employed in curling hair.

Razor burn (razor abrasion). Mark of desiccation.

Reaspiration. Repeated aspiration of a cavity.

Reblend. Redistribution of massage cream or cosmetics to insure a uniform density.

Recession. Withdrawal of a part from its normal position.

Rectangular. Shaped by four-sides and four right angles.

Reduce. To diminish in size, mass, or projection.

Reducing agent. Substance that easily loses electrons and thereby causes other substances to be reduced. Formaldehyde is a strong reducing agent.

Reflection. Return of light waves from surfaces; the bending or folding back of a part upon itself.

Resinous substance. Amorphous, nonvolatile solid or soft side substance, a natural exudation from plants. Any of a class of solid or soft organic compounds of natural or synthetic origin.

Respose. To lay at rest.

Restoration. Treatment of the deceased in the attempt to recreate natural form and color.

Restorative art. Care of the deceased to recreate natural form and color.

Restorative fluid (humectant). Supplemental fluid, used with the regular arterial solution, whose purpose is to retain body moisture and retard dehydration.

Restricted cervical injection. Method of injection wherein both common carotid arteries are raised.

Restricted drainage. See Intermittent Drainage and Alternate Drainage.

Retrousse. Nose which is turned up superiorly at its tip.

Right atrium. Chamber on the right side of the heart seen as the center of drainage. Used as a site of drainage via instruments from the right internal jugular vein and direct via the trocar or through the thoracic wall.

Rigor mortis. Postmortem stiffening of the body muscles by natural body processes.

Rim. Border, edge, or margin of a thing, usually of a circular or curving form, as the rim of the eye socket.

Risorius muscle. (laughing muscle) Narrow superficial band of muscle which pulls the angle of the mouth laterally.

Rods of the eye. Long, rod-shaped sensory bodies of the retina of the eye responsive to light but not color.

Roman. Aquiline profile of the nose.

Root. Apex (top) of the pyramidal mass of the nose which lies directly inferior to the forehead; the concave dip inferior to the forehead (profile view).

Round. (infantine) Frontal head from in which the head exhibits maximum curvature.

ROYGBIV. Acronym for red, orange, yellow, green, blue, indigo, and violet.

Ruddy. Red complexion; having a healthy reddish color, said of the complexion, more vivid than florid.

Saccharolysis. Decomposition of sugars.

Sallow. Yellowish, sickly color of the complexion.

Sanitation. Process to promote and establish conditions that minimize or eliminate biohazards.

Saturation. Visual aspect indicating the vividness of the hue in the degree of difference from gray of the same lightness.

Saponification. Process of soap formation. As related to decomposition, the conversion of fatty tissues of the body into a soapy waxy substance called adipocere or grave wax.

Saprophytic bacteria. Bacteria that derive their nutrition from dead organic matter.

Scab. Crust over a healing sore or wound.

Scalpel. Two-piece embalming instrument consisting of a handle and a blade used to make incisions and excisions.

Scapha. Fossa between the inner and outer rims of the ear; the shallowest depression of the ear.

Scarlet. Bright red color inclining toward orange.

Sealer. Quick-drying liquid which leaves a hard, thin transparent coat or layer through which moisture cannot pass.

Sealing agents. Agents that provide a barrier or seal against any leakage of fluid or blood.

Sear(ing). To cauterize tissues by heat or chemical in order to provide a dry foundation.

Second degree burn. Those resulting in acute inflammation of the skin and blisters.

Secondary dilution. Dilution of the embalming fluid by the fluids in the body, both vascular and interstitial.

Secondary hue. Equal mixture of two primary pigmentary hues (orange, green, and purple).

Sectional hypodermic embalming. Embalming of a large body area (e.g., hand or side of face) by the injection of embalming chemicals directly into the tissues through the use of a syringe and needle or a trocar.

Sectional vascular embalming. Embalming of a body area or region (e.g., arm or side of face) by the injection of an embalming solution into an artery which in life supplied blood to that particular body region.

Semilunar incision. Crescent shaped or flap-like incision.

Semi-opaque. Almost opaque; not transparent or translucent.

Sepsis. Pathologic state resulting from the presence of microorganisms or their products in the blood or other tissues.

Septicemia. Condition characterized by the multiplication of bacteria in blood.

Septum. Vertical cartilage dividing nasal cavity into two chambers, responsible for asymmetry of the nose.

Sequestering agent. Chemical agent that can "fence off" or "tie up" metal ions so they cannot react with other chemicals.

Serrated. Notched on the edge like a saw, as seen with forceps.

Severed. To have been cut or broken apart; disjoined.

Shade. Hue into which various quantities of black are mixed; the darkened hue.

Shadow. Surfaces that do not lie at right angles to the source of illumination or are obscured by other surfaces and which reflect little or no light.

Sharps. Hypodermic needles, suture needles, injector needles, scalpel blades, razor blades, pins, and other items sharp enough to cause percutaneous injury, penetration of unbroken skin. Many include other items normally not disposed of following use such as scissors, teeth, fingernails, and ribs.

Sharps container. Occupational Safety and Health Administration-required receptacle for proper disposal of sharps.

Sheen. Shine; as of the reflection of natural oils of the skin.

Short-term exposure limit (STEL). Legal limits established by the Occupational Health and Safety Administration to which workers can be exposed continuously for a short period without damage or injury. Exposures at the STEL should not be longer than 15 minutes and not repeated more than four times per workday.

Sideburns. Growth of hair located anterior of the ears.

Side of the nose. Lateral walls of the nose between the wings and the bridge.

Sign of death. Manifestation of death in the body.

Simple fracture. Fractured bone does not pierce the skin.

Singe. To burn superficially as the hair which shows partial destruction from scorching heat.

Six-point injection. A multipoint injection in the autopsied or unautopsied body in which six areas of the body are separately injected: right and left common carotid, axillary and femoral arteries are six arteries frequently used for a six-point injection.

Sodium hypochlorite. Unstable salt usually produced in an aqueous solution and used as a bleaching and disinfecting agent. (See Household bleach).

Soft wax. Surface restorer.

Solute. Substance that is dissolved in a solution.

Solution. Liquid containing dissolved substance.

Solvent. Liquid holding another substance in solution.

Somatic death. Death of the organism as a whole.

Spatula. Flat, blunt, knife-like instrument used for mixing cosmetics and modeling; a palette knife.

Spectrum. Visible band; the original standard of color; the progressive arrangement of colors (ROYGBIV) seen when a beam of white light is broken down into its component colors.

Splint. Appliance as of wood, metal, etc. used to keep in place or protect a displaced or movable part.

Split injection. Injection from one site and drainage from a separate site.

Sponge. Elastic, porous mass of interlacing horny fibers which are permanently attached; remarkable for its power of absorbing water and becoming soft when wet without losing its toughness.

Spray cosmetic. Liquid cosmetic so compounded that it can be atomized to provide a means of application to a surface.

Squama. Vertical surface of the temporal bone.

Square. (strong) Frontal head form in which the head is broad and exhibits very little curvature; the forehead is wide and the angles of the mandible are usually low as well as wide.

Stain. To discolor with foreign matter; an area so discolored.

Stain removers. Any substances or agents which will cause an external discoloration to be removed or lessened.

Starch. (cornstarch) Used as a dusting powder and an absorbent; used to firm wax.

Sterilization. Process that renders a substance free of all microorganisms.

Sterilizers. Oven or appliance for sterilizing. An autoclave that sterilizes by steam under pressure at temperatures above 100°C.

Sternocleidomastoideus muscle. Muscle of the neck that is attached to the mastoid process of the temporal bone and superior nuchal line and by separate heads to the sternum and clavicle. They function together to flex the head, form the lateral boundaries of the cervical triangle, and widest part of the neck.

Stethoscope. Delicate instrument used to detect almost inaudible sounds produced in the body.

Stillborn. Dead at birth. A product of conception either expelled or extracted dead.

Stipple brush. Small, rounded, stiff brush, all bristles the same length, used to simulate pores on wax; stencil brush.

Straight nasal profile. (Grecian) Nasal profile in which the dorsum exhibits a straight line from the root to the tip; the most common nasal profile.

Subcutaneous. Situated or occurring beneath the skin.

Subcutaneous emphysema. Distension of the tissues beneath the skin by gas or air. An antemortem condition brought about by a surgical procedure or trauma.

Subdued. Lowered in intensity or strength; reduced in fullness or color; muted.

Submandibular. Describing those portions which lie immediately inferior to the mandible.

Submental sulcus. Junction of the base of the chin and the submandibular area, which may appear as a furrow; a natural facial marking.

Subtractive method. Method of diminishing the wave lengths of light by superimposing two or more color transparencies over the same light source; the light is gradually reduced by absorption of colors in the light.

Sunken. Situated as a depression; concave.

Superciliary arches. Inferior part of the forehead just superior to the median ends of the eyebrows.

Supercilium. Eyebrows.

Superficial. Toward the surface.

Superior. Anatomically toward the head.

Superior palpebral sulcus. Furrow of the superior border of the upper eyelid; acquired facial marking.

Supplemental fluid. A fluid the embalmer injects prior

to the preservative solution (e.g., preinjection fluid) or adds to the preservative solution to enhance certain qualities of the preservative fluid (e.g., coinjection, dye, humectant, water conditioner).

Supraorbital area. Region between the supercilium and the superior palpebrae.

Supraorbital margins. Superior rim of the eye sockets.

Surface compress. An absorbent material (pack) saturated with an embalming chemical and placed in direct contact with the tissue.

Surface discoloration. Discoloration due to the deposit of matter on the skin surface. These discolorations may occur antemortem or during or after embalming of the body. Examples are adhesive tape, ink, iodine, paint, and tobacco stains.

Surface embalming. See Embalming.

Surface restorer. (surface filler) Wax used to fill shallow depressions; which is softer and more pliable than wound filler.

Surfactant (surface tension reducer; wetting, penetrating, or surface-active agent). Chemical that reduces the molecular cohesion of a liquid so it can flow through smaller apertures.

Surgical reduction. Restoration to a normal position or level through surgical excision.

Suspension. Substance in which particles of ground pigments are mixed with a fluid but are undissolved.

Sustain. To provide support for; to hold in a fixed position.

Suture. Act of sewing; also the completed stitch.

Swab. Bit of cotton or cloth used for removing moisture or discharges from mucous membranes as well as for applying bleaches or liquid disinfectants.

Swarthy. Dark-colored complexion, as a face made swarthy by the tropical sun.

Symmetry. Correspondence in size, shape, and relative position of parts that are on opposite sides of the face.

Taper. Form that receded away from a given point; form that becomes gradually smaller toward one end; to reduce gradually from the center.

Temporal bones. Inferior portion of the sides and base of the cranium, inferior to the parietal bones and anterior to the occipital bone.

Temporal cavity. Concave surface of the head overlying the temporal bones.

Temporalis muscles. Muscle of mastication which helps to close the mandible (the strongest chewing muscles).

Temporary preservation. Science of treating the body chemically so as to temporarily inhibit decomposition.

Tenacity. Property of holding fast; adhesiveness.

Terminal disinfection. Institution of disinfection and decontamination measures after preparation of the remains.

Termination/terminal. Limit; end; the part which terminates.

Tertiary hue. Hue which results from the mixture of two secondary pigmentary hues or an unbalanced proportion of complements with the warm hue or cool hue predominating.

Test of death. Any procedure used to prove a sign of death.

Texturizing brush. Brush with a relatively large tuft of good quality, fine bristles, such as black sable or finch; used to blend and stipple cosmetics or powder into the applied (cream) cosmetic, and clean out deposits impacted in pores.

Thanatology. Study of death.

Third-degree burns. Burns that result in destruction of cutaneous and subcutaneous tissues (seared, charred, or roasted tissue).

Three-quarter view. In reference to a photograph, a view revealing the fullness of the cheeks.

Time-weighted average (TWA). Exposure that is time-weighted over an established period. It allows the exposure levels to be averaged generally over an 8-hour period.

Tint. Hue into which various quantities of white are mixed.

Tinted powders. Powder that is lightly colored with non–moisture-absorbing pigments.

Tip. Extremity of anything that tapers (e.g., the tip of the nose; the termination of the forward projection of the nose).

Tissue builder. Substance used to elevate sunken (emaciated) tissues to normal level by hypodermic injection.

Tissue coagulation. See Coagulation.

Tissue gas. Postmortem accumulation of gas in tissues or cavities brought about by an anaerobic gas-forming bacillus, *Clostridium perfringens.*

Tobacco tar. Yellow/brown discoloration of the fingernails and fingers from excessive use of cigarettes.

Tone. Hue mixed with either a small quantity of gray or the complement of the hue, resulting in dulling the hue.

Topical disinfection. Disinfection of the surface of the body or an object.

Toupée. Small wig or patch of false hair covering a bald spot; a hairpiece.

Tragus. Elevation protecting the ear passage (external auditory meatus).

Translocation. Agonal or postmortem redistribution of host microflora on a hostwide basis.

Translucent. Transmitting light but causing sufficient diffusion to eliminate perception of distinct images; somewhat transparent.

Transparent. Having the property of transmitting rays of light through its substance so that bodies situated beyond or behind can be distinctly seen.

Transplantation. Grafting of living tissue from its normal position to another site or of an organ or tissue from one person to another.

Transverse. Lying at right angles to the long axis of the body.

Transverse frontal sulci. Furrows which cross the forehead; acquired facial markings.

Trauma. Physical injury or wound caused by external force or violence.

Triangular. Frontal head form in which the face is wider between the angles of the mandible than it is at the forehead; representing a triangle in shape; formed by three lines and having three angles (least common geometric head form).

Triangular fossa. Depression between the crura of the ear; the second deepest depression of the ear.

Trocar. Sharply pointed surgical instrument used in cavity embalming to aspirate the cavities and inject cavity fluid. The trocar may also be used for supplemental hypodermic embalming.

Trocar button. Plastic, threaded screwlike device for sealing punctures and small round trocar openings.

Trocar guide. Line drawn or visualized on the surface of the body or a prominent anatomic structure used to locate internal structures during cavity embalming, from a point of reference 2 inches to the left of and 2 inches superior to the umbilicus.

Tumor. Spontaneous new growth of tissue forming an abnormal mass.

Turbid. In liquids, muddy with particles of extraneous matter, not clear or transparent.

Ultraviolet. Invisible rays of the spectrum lying outside the violet end of the visible spectrum.

Undercoat. Coloring (opaque) applied to an area which, when dry, will be covered with wax or another colorant.

Undercut. Angled cut of the borders of an excision, made so that the skin surface will overhang the deeper tissues.

Unexposed area. Part that is, or will be, hidden from view.

Unionall. Plastic garment designed to cover the entire body from the neck down to and including the feet.

Universal precautions. See Bloodborne Pathogen Rule.

Vacuum breaker. Apparatus that prevents the backsiphoning of contaminated liquids into potable water supply lines or plumbing cross-connections within the preparation room.

Value. Lightness or darkness of a hue.

Variation. Changes in form, extended, etc.; things somewhat different from another of the same kind.

Vascular (arterial) embalming. See Embalming.

Vehicle. Liquid that serves as a solvent for the numerous ingredients incorporated into embalming fluids.

Vertex. Top of the head.

Vertical. Perpendicular to the plane of the horizon, balanced.

Vertical-concave profile. One in which the forehead and the eyebrows project equally to a vertical line and the chin protrudes more than the superior mucous membrane.

Vertical-convex profile. One in which the forehead and the eyebrows project equally to a vertical line and the chin recedes less than the superior mucous membrane.

Vertical profile. (balanced) One in which the forehead, upper lip and chin project equally to an imaginary vertical line.

Viral hepatitis. Inflammation of the liver caused by a virus (possibly as many as seven in number) capable of causing acute or chronic hepatitis illness. The transmission can be oral-fecal, parenteral, or sexual.

Viscosity. Resistance to the flow of a liquid. Thickness of a liquid.

Vitreous humor. Semifluid, transparent substance which lies between the retina and lens of the eyeball.

Vivid. Brilliance; intensely bright color(s).

Vividity. Degree of brilliance.

Vomer bone. Bone of the nasal cavity situated between the nasal passages on the median plane; forms the inferior and posterior portion of the septum of the nose.

Warm color areas. Areas of the skin surface which, during life, are naturally reddened; places where cosmetics will be applied to restore the warmth that red will give.

Warm hue. Color that appears in the spectral band, characterized by long wavelengths; color that makes an object appear closer and larger; color that reflects warmth (red, orange, yellow, and other colors in which they predominate).

Water conditioner. Complexing agent used to remove chemical constituents from municipal water supplies that could interfere with arterial formulations.

Water hardness. Quality of water containing certain substances, especially soluble salts of calcium and magnesium.

Waterless embalming. Arterial injection of an embalming solution composed of arterial fluid, humectant, and co-injection fluid. No water is added to the solution.

Waterlogged. Condition resulting from the use of an embalming solution containing an insufficient amount of preservative to meet the preservative demand of the tissues. The interstitial spaces are overly filled, engorged with water.

Wax. Restorative modeling or surfacing material composed of beeswax, spermaceti, paraffin, starch, etc. and a coloring pigment which will soften at body temperature and will reflect light in a manner similar to normal skin.

Weather line. Line of color change at the junction of the wet and dry portions of each mucous membrane.

Weight. Aspect of physical heaviness associated with different colors; i.e. warm, light, or grayed hues do not appear as heavy as cold, dark, or pure hues respectively; the size of the colored object will also create the illusion of greater or lesser weight.

Wet gangrene. See Gangrene.

Wetting agent. See Surfactant.

White. Color of pure snow; color reflecting to the eye all of the rays of the spectrum combined; opposite of black; achromatic color.

White light. Ray of light containing all the hues of the visible spectrum, in such proportion that the light appears colorless or natural; as daylight or sunlight.

Wicking. Operative or mechanical aid where an absorbent material, such as webbed cotton, is inserted into a body area where moisture is present, the absorbent material draws the moisture to the outside of the body.

Width. Dimension of an object measured across from side to side.

Wings of the nose. Lateral lobes of the nose.

Wire bridging. Length of wire used to connect two structures which are undamaged such as remaining parts of a bone; wire mesh placed within an aperture to hold other restorative fillers.

Work practice controls. See Bloodborne Pathogen Rule.

Worm suture. (inversion, draw stitch) Method of sewing an incision along the edges without entering the opening whereby the suture becomes invisible and the line of suture becomes depressed, which lends it ease of concealment by waxing.

Zygomatic arch. Processes on the temporal and zygomatic bones; determines the widest part of the face.

Zygomatic arch depression. One of the lesser concavities of the face located on the lateral portion of the cheek inferior to the zygomatic arch.

Zygomatic bones. Small bones of the cheeks; widest part of the cheek.

Zygomaticofrontal process. Lateral rim of the eye socket formed by a process of the frontal bone and a process of the zygomatic bone.

Zygomaticus major muscles. Muscles of the face that draw the superior lip posteriorly, superiorly, and anteriorly.

Zygomaticus minor muscles. Muscles of the face that draw the superior lip superiorly and anteriorly.

▶ ACRONYMS

ACGIH	American Congress of Governmental Industrial Hygienists
AIDS	Acquired immunodeficiency syndrome
AL	Action level
BCME	Bischloromethyl ether
CDCP	Centers for Disease Control and Prevention
ECG	Electrocardiogram (also EKG)
EEG	Electroencephalogram
EPA	Environmental Protection Agency
FTC	Federal Trade Commission
HBV	Hepatitis B virus
HIV	Human immunodeficiency virus
IVP	Intravascular pressure
mCi	Millicurie
MRSA	Methicillin-resistant *Staphylococcus aureus*
MSDS	Material Safety Data Sheet
NIOSH	National Institute for Occupational Safety and Health
OSHA	Occupational Safety and Health Administration
PEL	Permissible exposure limit
pH	Potential of hydrogen
PPE	Personal protective equipment
ppm	Parts per million
STEL	Short-term exposure limit
TLV	Threshold limit value
TWA	Time-weighted average

▶ REFERENCES

Benenson AS. *Control of Communicable Diseases in Man.* 15th ed. Baltimore: Victor Graphics; 1990.

Embalming Course Content Syllabus. American Board of Funeral Service Education; 1996.

Frederick LG, Strub CG. *The Principles and Practices of Embalming.* 5th ed. Dallas: Professional Training Schools; 1989.

Mayer JS. *Color and Cosmetics.* Dallas: Professional Training Schools; 1991.

Mayer JS. *Restorative Art.* 13th ed., Dallas: Professional Training Schools; 1993.

Mayer RG. *Embalming: Theory, Practices, and History,* Norwalk, CT: Appleton & Lange; 1996.

Merriam Webster's Collegiate Dictionary. 10th ed. Springfield, MA: Merriam-Webster; 1993.

Restorative Art Course Content Syllabus. American Board of Funeral Service Education; 1998.

Thomas CL. *Taber's Cyclopedic Medical Dictionary.* 18th ed. Philadelphia: F.A. Davis; 1997.

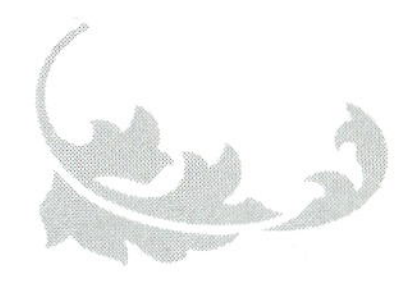

Selected Readings

The following articles have been reprinted for extra research and information:

1. Summary of Guidelines Submitted to OSHA from the National Funeral Directors Association Committee on Infectious Disease (Summer, 1989)
2. Armed Services Specification for Mortuary Services (Care of Remains of Deceased Personnel and Regular and Port of Entry Requirements for Caskets and Shipping Cases). Appendix D Federal Acquisition Regulation AR 638-2.9, February 1996
3. *The Mathematics of Embalming Chemistry: Part I. A Critical Evaluation of "One Bottle" Embalming Claims,* by Jerome F. Frederick (1968)
4. *The Measurement of Formaldehyde Retention In the Tissues of Embalmed Bodies,* by John Kroshus, Joseph McConnell, Jay Bardole (1983)
5. *The Two Year Fix: Long-Term Preservation for Delayed Viewing,* by Kerry Don Peterson (1992)
6. *Occupational Exposure to Formaldehyde in Mortuaries,* by L. Lamont Moore and Eugene C. Ogrodnik (1986)
7. *Formaldehyde Vapor Emission Study in Embalming Rooms,* by Edward J. Kerfoot (1975)
8. *Reported Studies on Effects of Formaldehyde Exposure,* by Leandro Rendon (1983)
9. *Final Report on Literature Search on the Infectious Nature of Dead Bodies for the Embalming Chemical Manufacturers Association,* September 1, 1968, by Maude R. Hinson (1968)
10. *Dangers of Infection,* by Leandro Rendon (1980)
11. *Creutzfeldt-Jakob Disease,* by Edward C. Johnson and Melissa Johnson (1996)
12. *In-Use Evaluation of Glutaraldehyde as a Preservative-Disinfectant in Embalming,* by Robert N. Hockett, Leandro Rendon, and Gordon W. Rose (1973)
13. *The Antimicrobial Activity of Embalming Chemicals and Topical Disinfectants on the Microbial Flora of Human Remains,* by Peter A. Burke and A. L. Sheffner (1976)
14. *The Microbiologic Evaluation and Enumeration of Postmortem Specimens from Human Remains,* by Gordon W. Rose and Robert N. Hockett (1970)
15. *Recommendations for Prevention of HIV Transmission in Health-Care Settings* (1987)
16. *Can Magnesium Sulfate Be Safely Used to Rid the Body of Fluid in the Lower Extremities?,* by Murray Shor (1965)

Summary of Guidelines Submitted to OSHA from the National Funeral Directors Association Committee on Infectious Disease (Summer, 1989)

PUBLIC HEALTH PRECAUTIONARY REQUIREMENTS AND STANDARDS

I. Background. Prevention of the transmission of recognized classical and/or opportunistic pathogens from human remains to the embalmer, from the embalmer to his or her family, and to the families and friends of the deceased is a reasonable public health expectation.

Many of the infectious agents associated with medical and paramedical environments are classified as "opportunistic" pathogens or microbial agents considered to be of lower or reduced virulence. The increasing association of "opportunistic" pathogens with symptomatic infectious diseases has all but eliminated the reference to the category "nonpathogen."

The implementation of minimum professional practice standards in embalming is necessary to provide a standard of quality control and quality assurance in the preservation and disinfection of human remains. It is important that when embalming is performed, a significant measure of uniformity of professional skills will be employed by all funeral service practitioners.

Following somatic or functional death, normally structurally intact epithelial, facial, and other tissue barriers undergo a loss of structural integrity and permit the bodywide translocation and distribution of systemic microflora and create alternate body fluid and body tissue reservoir sites of host contamination.

During life, the body fluids or body secretions most frequently associated with the transmission of potentially infectious doses or densities are quite definable. After death, this is no longer true. All body fluids and body tissues may become reservoirs of infectious agents within a relatively short postmortem interval.

Cellular death may not be complete for up to 12 hours after somatic or functional death. During this postmortem interval, the viability and potential infectivity of bloodborne viruses, e.g., HIV and hepatitis B, may persist and the exiting of the agents from any body opening, natural or artificial, may occur.

Funeral service practitioners normally have more than casual contact with parenteral (including open wound) and mucous membrane exposure to blood and body tissues. Such individuals occupationally exposed to blood, body fluid, or tissues can be protected from the recognized risks of bloodborne agents such as HIV and HBV [hepatitis B virus] by imposing barriers in the form of engineering controls, work practices, in-service training, and protective equipment and attire.

II. Recommendations. It is recommended that every funeral service firm/facility in the United States adopt the following policies and guidelines for implementation: (1) public health guidelines; (2) personnel health precautions for the prevention of bloodborne microbial agent(s) and infections; (3) minimum standards for the embalming and disinfection of human remains. The recommendations and guidelines within each of the three categories described above are as follows.

1. PUBLIC HEALTH GUIDELINES

A. Care of the Human Remains. Thoroughly cleanse and disinfect the body surface and natural or artificial body orifices/body openings with a suitable EPA-registered, hospital or health care facility-acceptable agent, e.g., tuberculocidal, germicidal detergent. The tuberculocidal germicidal detergent, e.g., a phenylphenol or a third-generation quaternary ammonium compound complex, should be an EPA-registered product offering confirmatory evidence of all label claims, including the recommended use dilution. The disinfected body surfaces should be thoroughly rinsed following a minimum of a 10-minute exposure interval.

Injection and drainage procedures should include (a) multisite injection and drainage procedures, (b) intermittent or restricted drainage, (c) the use of a 3.0% v/v formaldehyde-base arterial injection solution or a 2.0% glutaraldehyde-base solution, and (d) the use of 1 pint of concentrated cavity chemical per major or primary body cavity, e.g., abdominal, pelvic, and thoracic, or 1 pint of concentrated cavity chemical per 50 pounds of body weight.

B. The Embalmer (Universal Precautions). This category of barrier attire utilization and precautions has replaced the health care facility category of Blood and Body Fluid Precautions. The category requires the *minimum* barrier attire utilization of a whole body gown or apron and gloves. The wraparound, moisture-repellent or moistureproof gown or apron of rubber, plastic, or impregnated fabric is considered to be disposable or a single-use barrier attire item. The same is true for the gloves. Double rubber or plastic gloves are recommended for funeral service personnel.

This minimum standard of barrier attire protection is to be employed in the preparation of *all* human remains, no matter what the indicated cause of death reported. The risk of blood and body fluid exposure is significantly high for all funeral service personnel and frequently the infectious disease status of the deceased is unknown. Therefore, it is recommended that all persons performing postmortem procedures consider the use of additional barrier attire items such as protective eyewear, oral–nasal masks, and shoe and head covers.

Hands should be thoroughly scrubbed, using an EPA-registered* medicated liquid soap, before and after gloving. If a glove is penetrated by a sharp or the uneven edge of a bone, the glove is to be removed and replaced as soon as possible.

All instruments employed during the embalming should be sterilized or disinfected prior to reuse. A high-level disinfecting liquid immersant may be employed in lieu of a steam sterilizer if the latter is not available. Chemical germicidal detergents registered with EPA as "cold chemical sterilants" can be used either for sterilization or for high-level disinfection, depending on the interval or contact.

C. Air Handling Within the Environment "at Risk." An efficient air supply and air exhaust system or an air purification system must be operative within the embalming environment. The air handling system should protect the embalmer from a hazardous airborne density of biologic particulates as well as from the accumulation of formaldehyde monomers exceeding 1.0 ppm, the permissible exposure limit or 8-hour time-weighted average (TWA) concentration. The TWA "action level" is 0.5 ppm of formaldehyde monomer concentration.

---

* For example, *para*-Chloro-*meta*-xylenol (PCMX) or chlorhexidene gluconate (CHG) biocidal additive.

D. Terminal Disinfection and Decontamination. All instruments, horizontal surfaces such as floor, operating table, sink, and countertop, waste receptacles, and any other surface in direct or indirect contact with the preparation site must be cleansed and disinfected upon removal of the human remains from the preparation environment.

All instruments, including trocars and venous drainage tubes, must either be steam sterilized or immersed in a suitable cold chemical sterilant. Note: the use of a hypochlorite, 1000 to 5000 ppm, may be used for the "spot" disinfection of body fluid spills on hard, nonporous surfaces. However, immediate rinsing is necessary to prevent the formation of BCME (bischloromethyl ether), a confirmed carcinogen, in the presence of formaldehyde monomers.

E. Solid Waste Management. Potentially infective, contaminated solid wastes associated with the preparation of human remains should be placed in "alert" colored plastic bags, e.g., red, the bag twist-closed and securely tied prior to ultimate disposition. Local codes permitting, bulk blood and suctioned/aspirated fluids may be carefully drained into the sanitary sewer system and vacuum breakers must be installed on all involved water lines to prevent the back-siphoning of contaminated liquids into potable water supply lines.

F. Hearse/First Call Vehicles. Cleanse and disinfect all mortuary cots or trays following exposure to the unembalmed human remains. Employ cleansed and disinfected cot or tray covers for each transfer of unembalmed human remains from the home or from the health care facility to the preparation room. Cleanse and sanitize the internal horizontal surfaces of the hearse/first call vehicle following the transfer of the remains to the preparation room.

G. Funeral Service Personnel Health Recommendations.

1. Annual physical examination
2. Annual TB skin testing
3. Immunizations—annual influenza, single dose/single series Pneumovax, hepatitis B. Rubella vaccine is recommended for all women of pregnancy age if not protected and for all male employees because they can transmit to the female employee.

2. PERSONNEL HEALTH PRECAUTIONS FOR PREVENTION OF BLOODBORNE AGENT(S) AND INFECTIONS

A. Removal/Transfer of Human Remains.

1. Removal personnel (licensees, resident trainees, nonlicensees, and nonresident trainees)—disposable whole-body barrier attire and plastic or rubber gloves.
2. Avoid contact with covering of remains at sites of body fluid or exudative contamination. Place the remains in an impervious plastic whole-body pouch and effect zipper closure.
3. Sanitize the transfer vehicle following the transfer of remains to the preparation room.

B. Transfer of the Remains to the Preparation Room, Using a Team of Two Employees. Transfer the pouched remains to the preparation room table, open pouch, and loosen body coverings. Allow the body coverings to fall into the pouch. Carefully position the remains from side to side for the careful removal of the pouch and contents. Dispose of the pouch and contents as contaminated solid wastes.

C. Terminal Disinfection

1. Disinfect all horizontal inanimate surfaces in direct or indirect contact with preparation site.
2. Sterilize or disinfect all instruments by cold chemical sterilizer immersion or by steam sterilization.
3. Remove all barrier attire items, place in plastic bag, and treat as contaminated solid wastes in terms of final disposition.
4. Scrub ungloved hands and wrists with a medicated liquid soap preparation, preferably one that is recommended as a health care personnel handwash.
5. Complete whole-body bathing or showering and shampooing prior to return to home or office.

3. MINIMUM STANDARDS FOR THE EMBALMING AND DISINFECTION OF HUMAN REMAINS. The following professional profile of standards for embalming practices and procedures is based on laboratory evaluations and postembalming observations.

A. Multiple-Site Injection and Drainage. Multiple-site (two or more) injection and drainage procedures assure a more consistent distribution and ultimate diffusion of the disinfection and preservation chemicals to all receptive tissue sites, deep and superficial. This will more consistently provide public health protection as expected from the thorough preparation of human remains for ultimate disposition.

B. Rate of Flow of Arterial Injection Chemicals. A moderate rate of flow, 12 to 15 minutes per gallon of arterial injection solution, accompanied by a sufficient arterial injection pressure to maintain the desired rate of flow, 2 to 10 psi, are recommended for the assurance of distribution and diffusion of the arterial injection chemicals.

C. Intermittent or Restricted Drainage. This method of venous drainage should produce maximum preservation and disinfection. It is considered to be one of the most effective procedures for the assurance of adequate distribution of arterial injection solution(s). It is especially recommended following the removal of surface discolorations.

D. Total Volume of Arterial Injection Solution Employed. Consideration should be given to the use of a minimum of 3 to 4 gallons of arterial injection solution in adult remains weighing 125 to 175 pounds. Injection and drainage procedures may involve the removal of 4 to 6 quarts of body fluids. To properly restore the loss of body fluids and overcome the loss, through drainage, of arterial injection chemicals, it becomes necessary to employ the recommended volume of arterial injection solution, e.g., 1 gallon per 50 pounds of body weight, exclusive of the primary injection solution(s) volume.

E. Use of Supplemental Injection Chemicals. The enhancement of the arterial distribution of the arterial injection solution may often require the use of supplemental additives, e.g., modifying and surface tension-reducing additives, water softeners, etc. The use of such additives may increase the efficacy of injection solution distribution as well as the efficacy of venous drainage.

F. Concentration (%) of Preservative/Disinfecting Chemicals in the Arterial Injection Solution. Laboratory investigative data indicate that the percent of formaldehyde v/v in the formaldehyde-base arterial injection solution should not be less than 2.0. Formaldehyde concentrations ranging from 2.3 to 3.0% v/v will inactivate resident bacterial densities 95% or more. Formaldehyde concentrations less than 2.0%, e.g., 1.0% v/v, may produce expected tissue fixation, but may not produce the desired level of microbial inactivation. Significant reduction in the endogenous microbial populations should always exceed 70% if public health expectations are to be fulfilled on a consistent basis.

Formaldehyde is categorized as an "intermediate" to a "high-level" chemical disinfectant when employed in concentrations ranging from 3.0 to 8.0% v/v. The recommended use of a minimum 2.0% v/v concentration of formaldehyde is based on this categorization as well as investigative data.

G. Cavity Chemical Utilization. Following the thorough treatment of the thoracic, abdominal, and pelvic cavities, including the aspiration of liquids and semisolids from nonautopsied remains, the injection of 1 pint (16 ounces) of undiluted cavity chemical into each of the three trocar-prepared cavities is recommended. In remains weighing in excess of 150 to 200 pounds, it is recommended that the embalmer use 1 pint of concentrated cavity chemical per 50 pounds of body weight. The weight of the body viscera may approximate 15% of the total body weight. The chemically targeted hollow and solid organ tissues require maximal chemical contact following the trocar penetration and separation to ensure the prevention of the microbial generation of putrefactive activity, including body opening purge.

III. Administration. The funeral home owner/manager/employer should establish formal policies and procedures to ensure that all job-related tasks that involve an inherent potential for mucous membrane or skin contact with blood, body fluids, or tissues, or a potential for spills or splashes of blood or body fluids, will require appropriate preventive/protective measures. These preventive measures would be applicable to licensed, nonlicensed, resident trainee, and nonresident trainee personnel. Engineering controls, work practices, and protective barrier attire are critical to minimize exposure to HBV, HIV, and other blood and body fluid transmitted microbial agents and to prevent infection(s). It is essential that the funeral home employee be fully aware of the reasons for the required preventive measures. Therefore, employee education programs must be implemented to assure familiarity with applicable work practices.

The employer should establish the following formal policies:

1. Develop and provide in-service training programs for all employees whose responsibilities include the direct or indirect exposure(s) to blood, body fluids, or tissues.
2. Document the attendance of employees at all scheduled and announced in-service training programs. The in-service training course content should include the approved Standard Operating Procedures (SOPs) for embalming practices and the required items of protective equipment and personnel barrier attire items.
3. Assure the convenient availability of all items of protective equipment and barrier attire items.
4. Surveillance of the workplace to ensure that the required work practices are being observed and that the protective barrier attire items and equipment are conveniently available and properly used.
5. Investigation of known or suspected parenteral exposures to body fluids or tissues to establish the conditions associated with the exposure and to improve training, work prac-

tices, or preventive equipment to prevent a recurrence.

IV. Training and Education. As recommended under the heading "Administration," the employer must establish an initial and periodic training program for all employees who may sustain direct or indirect exposure to blood, body fluids, or tissues. The employee must understand the following as a result of adequate in-service training:

1. Modes of transmission of HBV, HIV, and other blood and body fluid transmitted microbial agents.
2. The basis for the employment of the types of protective equipment and items of barrier attire.
3. The location of protective equipment and items of barrier attire, the procedures for the proper use of same and for the removal, decontamination, and disposition of contaminated barrier attire items or equipment.
4. The corrective actions necessary to disinfect blood and body fluid spills or splashes.
5. Concurrent and terminal disinfection and decontamination procedures. Disposable, puncture-resistant containers are to be employed for used needles, blades, etc.

V. Work Practices

1. Work practices should be developed on the assumption that all body fluids and tissues are infectious.
2. Provision must be made for the safe removal, handling, decontamination, and disposition of protective clothing items, equipment, soiled linens, etc.
3. Work practices and SOPs should provide guidance on procedures to follow in the event of spills or personal exposure to fluids or tissues.

VI. Personal Protective Equipment. A required minimum of choice of barrier attire items or protective equipment should be specified by the firm's SOPs. As more departments of public health require the reporting of infectious disease causes of death by category of precautions implemented by the health care facility, it becomes increasingly important for the funeral service firm to be aware of the infectious diseases included in a given category or patient isolation precautions. The following is a recommended listing of barrier attire items that should be employed for a reported category of health care patient isolation precautions:

Category-Specific Health Care Facility Precautions	Recommended Funeral Service Personnel Barrier Attire Precautions
1. Strict precautions	Masks (face covers), gowns, gloves (double plastic or rubber gloves are recommended), head covers, shoe covers, eye protectors
2. Contact precautions	Gowns, gloves, shoe covers
3. Respiratory precautions	Masks, gowns, gloves, head covers, shoe covers
4. Enteric precautions	Gowns, gloves, shoe covers
5. Blood and body fluid or **universal precautions**	Gowns, gloves, masks, head covers, shoe covers, eye protectors

VII. Medical. The employer should make available, at no cost to the employee, the voluntary HBV immunization for all employees whose responsibilities involve the direct or indirect exposure to blood, body fluids, or tissues. The employer should also provide for the monitoring, at the request of the employee, for HBV or HIV antibodies following known or suspected parenteral exposure to blood, body fluids, or tissues.

VIII. Record Keeping. The employer should require the completion of a case report for the preparation of all remains. Each case report should include (1) health care facility reporting of category of patient isolation precautions implemented, if applicable, (2) sites of injection and drainage employed, (3) volumes and concentrations of arterial injection and cavity treatment chemicals, (4) protective equipment and barrier attire items employed, (5) preembalming appearance and condition of the remains, and (6) any other observations or procedure relating to the public health status of the remains.

Armed Services Specification for Mortuary Services (Care of Remains of Deceased Personnel and Regular and Port of Entry Requirements for Caskets and Shipping Cases). Appendix D, Federal Acquisition Regulation AR 638-2.9, February 1996.

D-1. (1) Scope. (1.1.) This specification (in two parts) establishes minimum standards for the care and handling of deceased personnel. It encompasses professional services and requirements, caskets and shipping cases, transportation and hygienic practices. This specification is applicable to regular and port of entry requirements.

SECTION I REMAINS

D-2. (2) Classification. a. (2.1) Remains defined. Autopsied (partial or complete) or unautopsied remains are defined as one of the following types.

b. (2.1.1) Nonviewable. Any remains where there exists extreme mutilation, advanced stages of decomposition, or severe burn wounds or charring and restoration of viewable exposed tissue surfaces to the known antemortem appearance of the deceased by restorative art is not possible, for example, floater, homicidal, suicidal, and major trauma cases.

c. (2.1.2) Viewable. Any remains (1) undamaged by trauma or disease or (2) remains damaged by trauma or disease but the viewable tissue surfaces are restored to the known antemortem appearance of the deceased by restorative art work.

d. (2.1.3) Casket. The standard and oversize 18-gauge metal, sealer, cut-top casket shall be used for viewable and nonviewable adult remains.

D-3. (3) Applicable Documents. (3.1) There are no applicable documents to this part of this specification.

D-4. (4) Services. a. (4.1) General. The contractor shall be responsible for providing professional services of the highest quality to assure viewing of the remains under optimal conditions. The contractor shall practice hygienic measures that will assure complete and satisfactory disinfection and sanitation of the funeral establishment.

b. (4.2) Processing or reprocessing remains. See the following paragraphs.

c. (4.2.1) Processing of remains. The complete preservation (embalming) and disinfection, application of restorative art techniques and/or cosmetics, dressing and/or wrapping, casketing, and transportation of remains as directed by the contracting officer or his designee.

d. (4.2.2) Reprocessing of remains. The inspection and correction of all discrepancies noted in preservation (embalming). Application of restorative art techniques and cosmetics, dressing and wrapping, casketing, and transportation of remains as directed by the contracting officer or his designee.

e. (4.2.3) Unidentified remains. If identification of the remains is not officially established, the remains shall be placed under refrigeration at 38–40° Fahrenheit (3.3–4.4° Celsius). If mechanical refrigeration is not available within a reasonable distance, ice chests or ice packs shall be used in lieu of the mechanical refrigeration. Processing (embalming) shall not be accomplished until the remains are released by a responsible official as identified.

f. (4.2.4) Restorative art. Major restorative art is an integral part of the processing and/or reprocessing of remains. It shall include, but not be limited to, rebuilding a large wound; rebuilding of facial features such as ear, nose, eye, mouth, chin, and so forth; removal of damaged tissue followed by restoration; restoration of scalp hair; and the application of cosmetics to render restored surfaces undetectable. Restorative art shall be accomplished in accordance with the highest professional standards.

g. (4.2.5) Chemical preservative preparations. Under this armed services specification, arterial, cavity, and other embalming chemicals used in the treatment of all remains shall effect the maximum preservation and disinfection of all body tissue, including that associated with body cavities (organs).

h. (4.2.6) Standards and techniques. The contractor shall provide high quality service and a sufficient number of licensed embalmers to process (embalm) or reprocess any remains under this armed services specification on a timely basis. Interns (apprentices) may be used to assist the licensed embalmer in accordance with applicable state regulations. All supplies and technical procedures shall conform to standards, and professional techniques acceptable to the funeral service industry. Embalmers shall utilize any and all optional techniques available to assure complete and adequate treatment of remains.

D-5. (5) Treatment of Remains. a. (5.1) General. Frequently, final disposition of processed or reprocessed remains may not be effected for a period of 10 days or more; remains may be transported over long distances or subjected to hot, humid conditions. At all times the remains must be free of putrefaction and infectious agents. This requires the thorough disinfection and uniform preservation of all body tissues. Employment of continuous injection and intermittent drainage will enhance chemical distribution and penetration. Use of humectants (moisture retention chemicals) in the arterial injection solution will help to achieve greater tissue penetration and to restore normal body moisture content.

b. (5.1.1) Pre-embalming procedures. The following basic steps shall be accomplished in the course of processing or reprocessing of all viewable remains and, to the extent possible, nonviewable remains.

c. (5.1.2) Washing and grooming. When possible, remains shall be bathed; male facial and scalp hair shall be washed and groomed to conform to military standards (suitable hair preparations shall be accomplished on females). Fingernails shall be cleaned and trimmed. The mouth shall be securely closed to form a natural expression and proper attention given to the eyes to prevent wrinkling of the eyelids and sunken appearance of the eyes. Cosmetics shall be applied only in the amount necessary to produce natural color and texture.

d. (5.1.3) Wounds and stains. All lacerations, abrasions, incisions, excisions and burn wounds shall be sutured or sealed to prevent leakage. Swollen or distorted features shall be reduced to the normal contours enjoyed during life. Postmortem stains shall be chemically bleached by applying packs and/or needle injection. On viewable areas, further treatment shall consist of the use of masking cosmetics to render stains nondetectable.

e. (5.1.4) Body orifices and injured tissue. All body orifices shall be treated with a disinfectant non-astringent chemical (generic categories such as phenylphenols and iodophors) and then packed with cotton. Bedsores and ulcerated, burned, and necrotic tissue shall be treated either by hypodermic injection or pack application of a deodorizing and preserving chemical.

f. (5.1.5) Insecticide treatment. Maggots and other insect larvae shall be destroyed and their breeding sites in or on the remains thoroughly treated with an insecticide chemical.

g. (5.1.6) Contractor's performance. The contractor's performance shall be such that all remains are effectively disinfected and uniformly preserved and that all offensive odors are eliminated before the remains are casketed.

D-6. (6) Preparation of Remains. *a. (6.1) General.* The military services require that all remains be processed or reprocessed in a manner reflecting the highest standards of the funeral service profession. Each remains, viewable and nonviewable, requires variation in the embalming treatment to accomplish the optimum results. A recommended procedure to achieve these goals is the injection of the solution at a moderate rate. The addition of a humectant to the solutions is also helpful in reducing overdehydration effects.

b. (6.1.1) Processing nonviewable remains. In all instances multisite injection and drainage technique shall be attempted. When arterial injection is possible, each gallon of arterial fluid shall have a minimum concentration of 5 percent by volume aldehyde or aldehyde derivative preservative agents. The total volume of arterial solution injected shall be not less than 1 gallon per 50 pounds of body weight. All body areas shall be further treated by means of a trocar using undiluted cavity chemicals having a 30-index (percent) or greater. In addition, packs, special gel, and dry sanitizers shall be used, as required, to assure preservation, prevent leakage, and eliminate all offensive odor. Cranial, thoracic, and abdominal cavities, when present, shall be relieved of gases and distention. The cavities shall then be treated by injecting a minimum of 32 ounces of a concentrated cavity chemical, having a 30-index (percent) or greater. When arterial injection or cavity treatment is impossible, all articulated and disarticulated anatomical portions shall be thoroughly disinfected and preserved via accessory chemical embalming techniques. Non-injectable intact remains and disarticulated anatomical portions shall be immersed or hypo injected with trocar or syringe and needle, using full strength cavity chemicals of 30-index (percent) or greater. Surface application of liquid, gel, or dry sanitizers and preservatives is also required to supplement primary needle or hypo injection techniques.

c. (6.1.2) Processing viewable remains. A thorough pre-embalming case analysis shall be made in order to determine the best embalming techniques to be used to obtain optimum results. The technique of arterial injection and venous drainage is of utmost importance as well as the need for adding humectants (moisture retention chemicals) to the arterial solution injected. Whenever possible, a six-point arterial injection with multi-site drainage shall be accomplished. The arterial chemical injection solution shall contain a 2 to 3 percent concentration, by volume, of aldehyde or aldehyde derivative preservative agents, with equal parts of a humectant chemical also being added to the injection solution. The thoracic, abdominal and pelvic cavities shall be thoroughly aspirated and injected with full strength cavity chemicals having a 30-index (percent) or greater, using a minimum of 16 ounces for each cavity. In addition, needle injections, packs, or other special treatment shall be accomplished, as required, to assure the preservation and disinfection of all body tissues including those associated with body cavities (organs). A lanolin-base (or comparable) massage cream shall be applied on the face and hands.

d. (6.1.3) Autopsied remains. If a partial or complete autopsy has been performed, a six-point injection with multi-site drainage shall be accomplished, using arterial chemical injection solutions as specified for processing viewable remains. Thoracic and abdominal walls shall be hypo-injected using the same strength solution as injected arterially. On thoracic and abdominal autopsies, the viscera shall be removed and immersed in concentrated cavity chemical having a 30-index (percent) or greater. When a cranial autopsy has been performed, the calvarium shall be replaced and securely stabilized. The scalp shall be replaced over the calvarium and neatly sutured to avoid an unnatural appearance and the hair shall be washed. The inner surfaces of the body cavities shall be given a liberal application of gel preservative, the organs replaced within the cavities in normal anatomical location and liberally covered with hardening compound.

e. (6.1.4) Treatment of scalp (viewable remains). When the scalp has been shaved because of medical treatment or surgery, processing or reprocessing shall be accomplished as specified for viewable remains, after which the head shall then be wrapped with gauze or equivalent in a neat and professional manner.

f. (6.1.5) Mutilated hands (viewable remains). When the hands are mutilated so that restoration is not possible, the hands shall be treated in a manner that shall render all tissue firm, dry, and thoroughly preserved. The hands will then be covered by either wrapping with gauze or equivalent in a neat and professional manner or by placing surgical gloves on the hands followed by white (military) gloves.

g. (6.1.6) Dressing remains, including intact nonviewable. Remains shall be dressed in the clothing provided by the contracting officer. Nonviewable remains that cannot be dressed shall be wrapped in the rubber or polyethylene sheeting and blanket furnished by the contracting officer. Wrapping shall be accomplished as follows: A blanket, furnished by the contracting officer, shall be spread on the dressing table with opposing corners at the head and foot ends of the table. The blanket is then covered with a white cotton sheet followed by a sheet of polyethylene. Two strips of cotton are laid down the center of the plastic sheet and liberally sprinkled with hardening compound. The remains are then laid on the cotton strips, coated with hardening compound and covered with additional cotton strips. The polyethylene sheet is then wrapped around the remains. The white cotton sheet is then wrapped around the plastic sheathed remains followed by the blanket which shall have as few creases as possible, and be secured with large safety pins placed no more than 8 inches apart.

h. (6.1.7) Embalmer Evaluation. The embalmer (contractor's agent) processing or reprocessing the remains shall critically evaluate the completed treatment to ensure that any remains cared for under this contract are effectively disinfected, uniformly preserved, and shall arrive at destination in a satisfactory condition. The contracting officer or designate will authorize delivery or shipment of remains when he is assured that the services and supplies furnished by the contractor meet this specification. The contractor shall state on a certificate (Preparation Room History) furnished by the contracting officer that the services and supplies meet this specification in its entirety.

i. (6.1.8) Placement in casket. Remains shall be placed in the casket in a manner that will create an appearance of rest and composure and to ensure maintenance of position during transit. When remains are to be shipped, pads will be placed around the remains to prevent shifting. The pillow shall be turned over and a clean piece of cloth placed over the face. The casket shall be of sufficient size to prevent the appearance of crowding and cramping the remains.

j. (6.1.9) Quality assurance evaluation. Failure to pass inspector's evaluation after placement of remains in a casket and before delivery will require the contractor to remove remains from the casket and perform one or more of the following services as directed by the contracting officer or his designate: (1) Additional disinfective or preservative treatment; (2) re-dressing; (3) change or add decorations or insignia; (4) place remains in new casket. When services under this paragraph are performed, services as set forth in paragraphs 6.1.6, 6.1.8, and 6.1.10 shall again be performed by the contractor.

k. (6.1.10) Encasing casket. The casket shall be carefully and professionally placed in the protective *outer* container, as directed by the contracting officer. All shipping documents will be affixed or enclosed.

l. (6.1.11) Loading remains. The remains shall be carefully and professionally placed in the type of vehicle designated by the contracting officer for the delivery of remains.

D-7. Transportation of Remains. *a. (7.1) Removal of remains.* Transport remains in a suitable funeral coach, ambulance, or service car to the place where processing or reprocessing is performed. This transportation shall include calling at the place where death occurs or remains are located when such place is on the activity(ies) or any place designated by the contracting officer or his designate.

b. (7.2) Escorted delivery. Delivery of remains, including escort in:

(1) (*a*) Contractor's funeral coach to a place of religious service and then to a common carrier, another funeral home, or to a Government or non-Government cemetery.

(2) (*b*) Contractor's funeral coach shall arrive at any location at the time specified by the contracting officer.

c. (7.3) Rail or air delivery. Remains being shipped by common carrier shall be delivered to airport or rail terminal not later than 2 hours before scheduled departure of aircraft or train.

d. (7.4) Escort attire. Personnel used in transportation of the remains or escort, off the installation, shall be dressed in a seasonal suit with shirt and tie. Other vehicle operators may wear clean cotton twill matching shirt and trousers in dark or neutral colors.

D-8. Cremation. *a. (8.1) Cremation.* This paragraph provides for services, supplies, and transportation for local cremation when called for by the contracting officer or designated representative. Remains shall be prepared, dressed, and cosmetized as prescribed in these specifications. The casket provided shall meet or exceed the armed services hardwood casket specification. Transportation of the remains (including escort and escort's return) shall be provided to the crematory engaged under contract by the Government and return of cremated remains to the Government facility. The contracting officer or designated representative shall specify whether a bronze or hardwood urn is to be provided. The contractor shall provide an urn that meets or exceeds the applicable urn specification. The urn shall be engraved (the urn itself shall be engraved if a bronze urn or if a hardwood urn, the specified engraving plate shall be engraved) with the name, rank, date of birth, and date of death of the deceased. The contractor will place all the cremated remains received from the crematory in the urn.

Note: Cremation charges will be paid by the Government directly to the crematory engaged by the Government.

b. (8.2) Processing procedure. Following the preparation, dressing, and cosmetizing of the remains according to these specifications, the contractor shall attach to the right ankle of the deceased or to the top of the blanket, when remains are wrapped, and to the casket handle at the head end of the casket a tag exhibiting the decedent's name, rank, social security number, and date of death. The contractor shall deliver the casketed remains to the crematory in sufficient time to ensure cremation is accomplished and completed on the same day as delivery to the crematory. The contractor shall return the cremated remains to the funeral service establishment or port mortuary facility not later than the day following cremation for inurnment in the designated urn. The cremated remains shall be inurned promptly upon return to the contractor's facility or port mortuary facility.

D-9. Hygienic Practices. *a. Concurrent and terminal disinfection and decontamination.* The contractor shall employ protective, precautionary hygienic measures and techniques designated to accomplish concurrent and terminal disinfection and decontamination of the entire funeral service establishment or port of entry mortuary preparation room and shipping area environment. The application of appropriate in-use concentrations of chemical disinfectants (such generic categories as phenyphenols or iodophors) to body surfaces and orifices, instruments, preparation room, floor, walls, and equipment surfaces and general sanitation of public visitation areas (as applicable) will help prevent the transmission of actual and potential pathogens to personnel.

b. Inhalation protection. Also recommended is the wearing of a protective surgical-type oral-nasal mask designed to prevent the inhalation of infectious particles originating from the surface, orifices, and cavities of human remains.

D-10. Additional Requirement—Port of Entry (POE) Mortuary. *a. (10.1) Processed remains (embalmed).* The contractor (responsible licensed embalmer) shall remove remains from the transfer case or casket and with the contracting officer or designate determine:

(1) (*a*) Whether remains are viewable or nonviewable.

(2) (*b*) Effectiveness of disinfection, uniformity of preservation, and any additional disinfective and preservative treatment and restorative art work and cosmetic work required.

(3) (*c*) Size casket to be used.

b. (10.2) Unembalmed remains. The contractor (responsible licensed embalmer) shall remove the remains from the transfer case or casket and with the contracting officer or designate determine:

(1) (*a*) Whether the remains are viewable or nonviewable.

(2) (*b*) The treatment to effectively disinfect and uniformly preserve the remains and also eliminate all offensive odors emanating from the remains.

(3) (*c*) Restorative art and cosmetic work required.

(4) (*d*) Size casket to be used.

c. (10.3) Reprocessing viewable remains. Tissue areas requiring further or special attention shall be treated to assure that the remains are effectively disinfected and uniformly preserved. The treatment shall be accomplished by one or more of the following: trocar or hypodermic injection and external pack application using full strength cavity chemicals having a 30-index (percent) or greater. Thoracic, abdominal, and pelvic cavities shall be relieved of gases and distention and reinjected with a minimum of 32 ounces of concentrated cavity chemical having a 30-index (percent) or greater.

d. (10.4) Reprocessing nonviewable remains. Those tissues requiring further or special attention shall be treated to assure the remains are effectively disinfected and uniformly preserved. This treatment shall be accomplished by means of one or more of the following: trocar or hypodermic injection and external pack application using full strength cavity chemicals have a 30-index (percent) or greater. Thoracic and abdominal cavities, when present, shall be relieved of gases and distension and reinjected with a minimum of 32 ounces of concentrated cavity chemicals having a 30-index (percent) or greater.

e. (10.5) Processing unembalmed adult remains. The contractor shall perform those requirements enunciated in paragraph 6 of this armed services specification for preparation of remains.

f. (10.6) Infant and child remains. Treatment of infant and child remains—neonatal, infant, and child remains (birth through 60 months)—follows.

g. (10.6.1) Viewable and injectable remains.

h. (10.6.2) Nonviewable and non-injectable remains. Nonviewable and non-injectable remains shall be disinfected and preserved by means of accessory embalming techniques. Superficial and deep tissues shall be injected by infant trocar or syringe and needle. The arterial injection solution shall have a minimum concentration of 3 percent by volume aldehyde or aldehyde derivative preservative agents. The supplemental use of liquid (packs), gel, or dry sanitizers for the confirmed disinfection and preservation of superficial tissue shall also be accomplished. The cranial, thoracic, abdominal, and pelvic cavities shall be thoroughly aspirated. The cavities shall then be injected by means of trocar and sufficient amount of cavity fluid (having a 30-index or greater) to thoroughly saturate the organs and contents.

i. (10.6.3) Autopsied remains. If a partial or complete autopsy has been performed, a six-point arterial injection with multi-site drainage shall be accomplished. The arterial chemical injection concentration solution requirements indicated in paragraph 10.6.1, as applicable, shall also apply. Following the arterial injection, the thoracic and abdominal walls shall be hypo-injected by means of a trocar or syringe with an arterial solution of the same strength as injected arterially. Treatment for organs or portions of organs that have become separated during autopsy investigation shall be removed from the cavities and immersed in concentrated cavity chemical having a 30-index (percent) or greater. Inner surfaces of body cavities shall be treated with a liberal application of a gel preservative, then the organs or portions of organs returned to the cavities in their normal anatomical location and covered with hardening compound. The calvarium shall be replaced, scalp sutured, and hair treated as indicated for adult autopsied remains.

j. (10.6.4) Treatment of scalp (viewable). When scalp has been shaved, procedures indicated in paragraph 6.1.4 shall apply.

k. (10.6.5) Mutilated hands (viewable). Procedures indicated in paragraph 6.1.5 shall apply.

l. (10.6.6) Dressing remains. Procedures indicated in paragraph 6.1.6 shall apply.

m. (10.6.7) Embalmer evaluation. Procedures indicated in paragraph 6.1.7 shall apply.

n. (10.6.8) Placement in casket. Procedures indicated in paragraph 6.1.8 shall apply.

o. (10.6.9) Quality assurance. Procedures indicated in paragraph 6.1.9 shall apply.

p. (10.6.10) Encasing casket. Procedures indicated in paragraph 6.1.10 shall apply.

q. (10.6.11) Loading remains. Procedures indicated in paragraph 6.1.11 shall apply.

The Mathematics of Embalming Chemistry*: Part I. A Critical Evaluation of "One-Bottle" Embalming Chemical Claims

Jerome F. Frederick, Ph.D
Director of Chemical Research, Dodge Chemical Company.

Few concepts can be more misleading and destructive to the professional future of the modern embalmer than the belief that "one-bottle embalming" is technically possible or even ethically admissible. The faulty reasoning behind this kind of wishful thinking is predicated on the premise that one single 16-ounce bottle of embalming chemical can be made to contain *all* of the essential chemical components required for the complete embalming of the "average" case, regardless of the condition-variables present in such a case.

Certain unscrupulous "fluid merchants," who are actually not bonafide embalming chemical manufacturers at all, have good reason to foster this misleading and unrealistic view. They do so with an obvious ulterior motive in mind. To put it plainly, they hope to win favor in the profession on the strength of a sensational economy appeal by claiming that embalming can be accomplished far more inexpensively with just one bottle of their super-duper elixir. Nothing could be further from the truth. To those who really understand the science of tissue preservation, such a claim smacks strongly of the chicanery and flim-flam of the old-time "medicine men" who in earlier days ranged the frontiers in their flashy horse-drawn vans and sold cure-alls "good for man or beast" to the trusting pioneer folk in the far-flung outposts of expanding America. Times have changed, but credulity, it seems, remains a dominant factor of human nature even in this enlightened day and age. Although stemming more from trustfulness than ignorance, unquestioning belief in the impossible and impractical still threatens the success of the misguided individual, but even more important, tends to undermine the very foundation of funeral service itself.

Misleading, illogical, and technically faulty, the "one-bottle" concept must be explored in depth before its pitfalls can be made clear to all ethical embalming practitioners, for if allowed to gain momentum unopposed, such a trend can only give the critics and detractors of funeral service valid evidence to win public suport for their destructive efforts.

* Reprinted from the *De-Ce-Co Magazine* 1968;60(5).

In order to guide our readers toward a true and realistic evaluation of the hazards inherent in the "one-bottle" concept, we will divide discussion of the subject into two parts. In the first portion we will center our analysis upon a hypothetically "perfect case"—one in which no type of chemotherapy had been administered prior to death and where no problems other than those met within the normal course of tissue preservation face the embalmer. We must realize, of course, that no such case actually exists. But it gives us the unbiased starting point needed to expose the fallacies of the "one-bottle" embalming chemical concept and so reveal its hidden threat to the profession.

In cases where modern chemotherapy has been brought into play prior to death—and this encompasses some 90% of the cases treated by embalmers nowadays—the calculations for the analysis and critical evaluation must be revised. For here the hazards of "one-bottle embalming" take a sharp upward turn—and its inadequacy becomes greatly intensified.

We know, for instance, that cases in which the new antibiotic *kanamycin* has been used for some time prior to death require a much greater concentration of the arterial chemical than that indicated for cases which have not been treated with this drug. Expressed in its simplest terms, this requirement stems from the fact that the antibiotic causes changes in the kidneys. In consequence, the kidney tissues accumulate large concentrations of nitrogenous and ammoniacal wastes. And, as every embalmer knows, there is no more effective way to neutralize formaldehyde than reacting it with ammonia.

This part of our discussion, however, we shall take up at a later date and for the present confine ourselves to an analysis of the "perfect case," keeping in mind that it is purely hypothetical—for nowhere in our present chemotherapeutic era will the professional embalmer ever encounter such a case! Remember also that in any discussion concerning a topic such as this one, it is necessary to establish and accept certain basic scientific assumptions. While these may not apply directly to 100% of our cases in actual practice—"perfect" or otherwise—they do take into consideration the most common variables and so hypothesize a truly realistic and typical "specimen" case. For example, an *average* adult cadaver weighing 65.3 *kilograms* (or 65,300 grams) has been shown to contain a *total protein* content of 10.7 kilograms (or 10,700 grams of protein), by Brozek et al. (*Ann NY Acad Sci* 1963;110:123).

When formaldehyde reacts with protein, and *only* protein—and here again, we simplify the discussion by deliberately overlooking the fact that formaldehyde will also react with *other* components of the human body besides protein—it requires about 4.0 to 4.8 grams (or 4.4 *grams* average) of formaldehyde to totally react with and fix exactly *100 grams of a soluble protein.* Nonsoluble proteins require even more preservative.

Now, as pointed out by J. F. Walker in his treatise (*Formaldehyde,* 2nd ed., New York: Rheinhold; 1953: 315), the 4.4 grams of formaldehyde are required to totally fix and preserve, for "all times," the 100 grams of soluble protein.

The average cadaver has about 10,700 grams of protein. To totally and "forever" preserve *all* the protein present in this average cadaver, we would need

$$10{,}700/100 \times 4.4 = \textit{470.8 grams of formaldehyde}$$

Let us consider, then, an average 16-ounce bottle of arterial fluid. If it contains only 30% formaldehyde (most modern arterials contain other preservatives in addition to formaldehyde) it would be technically defined as a "firming" or "high-index" fluid. Its formaldehyde content is computed as follows:

1 U.S. fluid ounce = 29.6 ml

16 fl oz = 473.6 ml of fluid, of which 30% is formaldehyde,

hence $0.30 \times 473.6 =$ *142.08 grams of formaldehyde.*

If we require 470.8 grams of formaldehyde to totally preserve all the protein in an average body, then that amount of this chemical in a 30% fluid will contain only enough formaldehyde to preserve

$142.08/470.8 = 0.3$ or 30% of all the protein in that average cadaver.

These calculations, as we pointed out earlier in this article, are necessarily predicated upon assumptions which must be accepted in order to establish a basis for computation. But even allowing the most liberal margin of error, it can be readily seen that *no single 16-ounce bottle of fluid* could possibly deliver the minimal acceptable degree of preservation—even in a "high-index" formulation! And this, remember, is calculated on the conditions of an *average* case!

Yet, as theoretical figures, these must not be construed as applicable to every like instance. There are many truly capable and excellent embalmers whose professional standards demand the most critical technical perfection who can point to instances where they have achieved adequate preservation with as little as $1\frac{1}{2}$ or 2 bottles of arterial fluid.

But none among them would rightfully claim that he uses *only one* bottle of arterial per case as *standard operating procedure,* for to do so would reflect unfavorably upon his professional judgment. Even the most ingenious and careful practitioners must admit that they are compelled to vary the concentrations of arterial chemical to meet the exigencies and special conditions present in each specific case. Most conscientious embalmers, in fact, use the full complement of "adjunct" chemical when the need for them is indicated—restorative humectants when there's evidence of emaciation or dehydration, water conditioners to neutralize chemical conflict in their solutions, modifiers, preinjections, coinjections, and vascular conditioning expedients. It is their familiarity with these "tools of the trade" which sets them apart as an elite professional class, where attitude and course of action are closely patterned on that of the medical man who employs every pharmaceutical and surgical expedient available to him as the need becomes apparent and modifies his treatment according to the conditional factors present in the case at hand. Imagine, if you can, a doctor who would be content to use the *same drug* in the *same concentration* on every case he treats! The analogy is very close to "one-bottle embalming."

But even if it were possible to produce a reasonably acceptable, if not perfect, embalming result with the "one-bottle" tactic, the embalmer who chose to place such paltry economy above the true objectives of his profession would indeed be asking for trouble. For the value of his reputation can scarcely be counted in fluid ounces of arterial chemical. Sensibly enough, few are ready to risk so much for so little in return—and the profession can well spare those who fall by the wayside with "one-bottle embalming."

Now, back to the hard facts of embalming chemistry:

Even if it were technically possible to increase the amount of formaldehyde in a 16-ounce bottle of arterial chemical to an absolute 100%, we'd have barely enough to "fix" the total protein present in the "average perfect case." This, of course, is not feasible because of the intrinsic chemical–physical nature of formaldehyde. But mere "fixation" or stabilization of the body proteins does not constitute total embalming. The result of using such an arterial would be a rock-hard, ghastly gray cadaver—a far cry indeed from the lofty standards of modern embalming! And where would we put our diffusion-stimulating constituents in a 100% formaldehyde fluid? Our cosmetic modifiers, blood solvents, and vascular conditioning components? Without these, could this super-duper 100% formaldehyde arterial do the job we want it to do? Could it penetrate and preserve *all* the proteins in our hypothetical "average" case? Could it get past the "average" number of circulatory obstacles we'd be almost certain to encounter in such a case? Lacking its normal complement of supporting constituents, it's hardly likely that this 100% formaldehyde fluid would win any applause from experienced professionals.

It should be plainly apparent at this point in our discussion that the "one-bottle" technique offers more danger to embalming results and professional reputation than the earnest, ethical embalmer is willing to risk. But our analysis and evaluation would not be quite complete if we did not take a moment to quiet the suspicion that "one-bottle" embalming might become valid through technical advances in injection equipment. We refer specifically to the use of high-pressure embalming. Although embalming under such pressures may *appear* to use only one bottle of arterial chemical to achieve preservation, the technique merits the most critical scientific scrutiny. There is now evidence that high-pressure embalming actually causes the preservation to be "blown" to the superficial areas of the body. The result is a "taut skin" appearance which gives the *impression* of true preservative firming, but actually fails to embalm the deep underlying tissues, creating a condition which can obviously cause the embalmer a great deal of trouble.

In any event—no matter which technique is employed—we must face the incontrovertible mathematical truths of embalming. Knowing the way proteins react with preservatives leaves no illusions that one-bottle embalming will ever become a practical reality. Claims to the contrary should be viewed with cautious skepticism, for there is every indication that they will prove wholly false and unworthy of acceptance by the ethical professional.

The Measurement of Formaldehyde Retention In the Tissues of Embalmed Bodies*

John Kroshus • Joseph McConnell • Jay Bardole

Editor's Note: John Kroshus is Chairman of the Funeral Service Education Program and Jay Bardole is Chairman of the Chemistry Department at Vincennes University. Joseph McConnell is an Evansville (Indiana) Funeral Director.

INTRODUCTION

As a result of tests conducted jointly by the Funeral Service Education Program and Chemistry Department at Vincennes (Indiana) University, a procedure has been developed by which the amount of formaldehyde re-

* Reprinted from *The Director*, Vol. 54, No. 3, Milwaukee, WI: National Funeral Directors Association, NFDA Publications Inc., 1983, with permission.

tained in the tissues of a dead human body can be measured. It appears as though this project, which can provide a quantitative analysis of formaldehyde retention, might be used to evaluate the efficiency of new embalming techniques or products, and thereby create the possibility of reducing the material expenditures in embalming.

In addition, improved techniques may also upgrade the quality of embalming results. Reducing material expenditures means that costs can be reduced, and if this can be accomplished without sacrificing results it will constitute a significant advance for funeral service.

Embalmers have long suspected that a substantial amount of chemicals injected into a body during arterial embalming simply pass through the blood vascular system and are lost with the other fluids that drain from the body. Other tests have indicated that this was perhaps true. Now it is possible to measure quite accurately just how much chemical is lost, and how much remains in the body.

The research project has indicated that approximately 50 to 55 percent of the arterial fluid injected into a body is lost along with the venous drainage. It seems evident that funeral service needs to examine ways by which embalming can be made more efficient and thereby reduce the waste of arterial fluid. Again, this procedure can be used to evaluate the efficiency with which embalmers are operating.

The procedure for measuring formaldehyde retention in the tissue of embalmed bodies has been adopted from a quantitative analysis experiment used to determine the amount of formaldehyde in pesticides.[1] Basically the formaldehyde retention experiment involves reacting a sample of the venous drainage with sodium hydroxide and hydrogen peroxide.

The ratio of sodium hydroxide to formaldehyde is one to one in the reaction. This means that for every mole of formaldehyde present, one mole of sodium hydroxide will be used up in the reaction. Thus, by determining how much sodium hydroxide is used the amount of formaldehyde present in the venous drainage can be calculated. That amount is then subtracted from the amount of formaldehyde originally injected into the body, and the amount of formaldehyde retained in the body is known.

The hydrogen peroxide is reduced during the reaction and provides hydroxide ions to the formaldehyde, which oxidizes to formic acid. The formic acid reacts with the sodium hydroxide to produce a sodium salt and water.

That solution is then titrated with sulfuric acid and the data gathered is used to calculate how much sodium hydroxide reacted with the formaldehyde in the venous drainage sample.

METHODOLOGY OF THE STUDY

Standardization of Chemicals. The sodium hydroxide and sulfuric acid used in the experiment must be standardized before being used. The procedure for the standardization of these chemicals is similar to that used in most elementary chemistry courses, and in this instance the object is to make solutions which have a Normality of one. What this means basically, is that the acid and the base will react in such a way that they will neutralize one another if mixed in equal amounts.

Practice Titration. Once the chemicals have been standardized, it is also necessary to test them in laboratory conditions. For this reason, the solutions of sodium hydroxide and sulfuric acid were tested against a solution where the amount of formaldehyde was known. This allowed for a comparison of the calculations based on data gathered by titrations with predictable results.

PROCEDURE. Embalming chemicals were mixed with water to produce 150 milliliters of one percent formaldehyde solution. This was possible because of the standard "index" of arterial fluids, which states that index is the amount of formaldehyde present in 100 milliliters of solution. By using the formula: Volume one times Concentration one is equal to Volume two times Concentration two, the formaldehyde solution was mixed to contain one percent formaldehyde. Since the experiment used a thirty index fluid, five milliliters of the arterial fluid was mixed with 145 milliliters of water to produce the solution.

Using a volumetric flask, the 150 milliliters of formaldehyde solution was divided into three 50 milliliter portions, each of which was poured into separate 500 milliliter flasks.

Fifty milliliters of the sodium hydroxide was then added to each of the flasks.

Fifty milliliters of hydrogen peroxide was then added to each of the flasks.

Heat was then added to each of the 500 milliliter flasks to stimulate the reaction. The heat was continued until the bubbles of the reaction stopped, and then for about ten minutes longer.

When the reaction was completed, the flasks were cooled.

Next, a 50 milliliter burette was thoroughly cleaned and rinsed and filled with sulfuric acid. The amount was recorded on a data sheet.

Indicator was then added to the now cool "basic" solution, and the titration was begun. This procedure was repeated for each of the 50 milliliter portions of the formaldehyde solution with the initial and final burette readings recorded on the data sheet.

OBSERVATION. The titration is a back titration. The amount of acid delivered to reach the point of equilibrium was inversely proportional to the amount of formaldehyde that was present in the original solution. Therefore, the greater the amount of sulfuric acid delivered, the less the amount of formaldehyde present.

At the end point of the titration, the equivalents of the base and the equivalents of the acid should be equal. The difference between the equivalents in the calculations indicates that a certain amount of the sodium hydroxide was used up as formaldehyde was oxidized. As previously mentioned, the formaldehyde and the sodium hydroxide react on a one to one basis. The amount of sodium hydroxide absent from the original 50 milliliters is therefore directly proportional to the amount of formaldehyde that is in the drainage taken from a body, or in this case, to the amount of formaldehyde mixed to create the one percent solution.

TITRATION DATA. The burette readings indicate the amount of acid delivered in the titrations. The amounts are averaged, and the average is used to calculate the amount of base that reacted with formaldehyde.

CALCULATIONS. The difference of the equivalents of acid and base will determine the amount of base equivalents that react with formaldehyde. That figure is then multiplied by the formula weight of formaldehyde (which equals one equivalent of formaldehyde) which has as its product the grams of formaldehyde that reacted with the sodium hydroxide.

The Embalming Procedure. The embalming procedure in the experiment was done using the legs of a dead human body as subjects in obtaining samples. This was done for two main reasons. One, to insure that there was no adverse effects from the embalming that would distort the normally exposed portions of the body, namely the face, neck and hands. Two, it allowed the experimenter to strike a comparison on tissue that was very similar in nature.

The researcher made every effort to keep the procedures identical for the injection of each limb. It should also be pointed out there is no deviation from normal embalming procedure.

Femoral arteries and veins were raised and ligated on both the left and right legs of the deceased.

Two gallons of pre-injection was then mixed in one gallon quantities. Six ounces to the gallon of a formaldehyde-free pre-injection chemical was added to each gallon. The embalming machines were then filled and set for pressure and rate of flow.

One machine was set to a pressure gauge reading of six pounds per square inch, with a rate of flow of one gallon per five minutes. The other machine was set to a pressure gauge reading of 60 pounds per square inch, with pulsation, and a rate of flow of one gallon per five minutes.

Arterial injection tubes and venous drain tubes were then inserted into the arteries and veins respectively.

The embalming machines were then started and the legs were injected simultaneously.

During the pre-injection, the drainage was not saved. The object of the pre-injection was to "flush" out the vascular system, and replace the blood and tissue fluids with the pre-injection solution. This is a very important point because the pre-injection solution was composed of known elements, while the embalmer could not be sure what was in the blood and tissue fluids of the body.

Once the pre-injection was completed, hoses were placed on the venous drain tubes, and collection containers were installed to collect the drainage from the preservative injection.

The preservative solution was mixed in a one gallon container with a dilution of six ounces of arterial fluid per gallon. The arterial fluid used was 30 index. The solution was then divided into one-half gallon portions, and each machine was filled with a half-gallon of the arterial solution.

Again the limbs were injected simultaneously, and this time the drainage was saved from the beginning to the end of the injection of the half-gallon portions. By saving the drainage throughout the injection it was felt that the samples saved constituted a representative sample of the drainage total.

It should be pointed out that the independent variable in this experiment was a variation in pressure gauge readings on the embalming machines being used. As mentioned previously, the independent variable could be changed to include a new technique, new product or new solution mixture. Whatever the independent variable being tested happens to be, the remainder of the experiment stays the same.

Titration of Drainage Samples. The drainage samples saved from the embalming were kept in separate containers. Care was taken throughout the titration to make sure the samples were not mixed.

A 150 milliliter portion of the "low pressure" sample was divided into three 50 milliliter portions and placed into three 500 milliliter flasks.

To each flask, 50 milliliters of sodium hydroxide was added.

To each flask, 50 milliliters of hydrogen peroxide was added.

The flasks were then placed over heat. The heat served to speed up the reaction, and was maintained until the tiny bubbles of the reaction ceased. As the reaction was in full progress during heating, the mixture in the flasks tended to foam over. Toward the end of the reaction the foam would gradually disappear.

The same procedure was then followed for a 150 milliliter portion of the "high pressure" sample.

All flasks were carefully labeled and observed during the course of the reaction. It should be pointed out that heat has no adverse effect on the final results. The solutions cannot be overheated.

When all reactions were complete the flasks were placed in an ice bath until they were cool.

The contents of a flask was then placed into a clean 250 milliliter beaker. A magnetic stirring rod was placed in the beaker, and the beaker was placed on an automatic magnetic stirring device.

An electrode was then placed into the beaker, and the pH of the solution was registered on a pH meter connected to the electrode. The pH reading was recorded on a graph sheet. The graph sheet was contained in a grapher which was connected to the pH meter. The grapher would make a graph of the pH changes during the titration.

To begin the titration, an Automatic Constant Rate Burette and the grapher were turned on simultaneously. The Automatic Burette would deliver sulfuric acid into the 250 milliliter beaker of drainage sample. The automatic stirring device would mix the solution as the titration progressed.

The researcher was able to monitor the titration through the end-point, and until it could be determined that the basic solution present at the outset of the titration had become an acid solution.

The final pH reading was recorded on the end of the graph, and the amount of sulfuric acid delivered by the Automatic Burette was also recorded on the end of the graph. The initial and final pH and burette readings were used to calculate the amount of sulfuric acid needed to reach equilibrium in the solution.

That amount would help determine the amount of sodium hydroxide which had reacted with formaldehyde in the solution. That figure, in turn, was used to determine the amount of formaldehyde in the drainage sample. The difference of the amount of formaldehyde in the drainage sample and the amount of formaldehyde injected was the amount of formaldehyde retained in the tissues.

This entire experiment was repeated over ten times during the course of about two and one-half years. The object was to find a pattern that would indicate proof of the superiority of either "high" or "low" pressure in embalming. At no time was any direct comparison made between bodies. Direct comparisons were made between legs of the same body until an overall pattern was established. In this case, the experiment showed that there was very little difference in formaldehyde retention in bodies embalmed with "high" pressure as compared to bodies embalmed with "low" pressure. It has already been pointed out that an independent variable of pressure could be switched for any number of variables that would warrant testing.

The procedure is precise and accurate. It would seem to open countless possibilities for improvement of presently accepted arterial embalming techniques, as well as for the testing of newly developed techniques. It may also provide definitive answers to questions about the value of the multitude of pre-injects, co-injects, water correctives and supplemental chemicals that are on the market today.

REFERENCE

1. Frank J. Welcher, Ph.D., Editor. *Standard Methods of Chemical Analysis.* Sixth Edition, Volume Two—Industrial and Natural Products and Non-instrumental Methods. Part B., (D. Van Nostrand Company, Inc., Princeton, New Jersey, 1963), pp. 1878 and 1879.

The Two Year Fix: Long-Term Preservation for Delayed Viewing*

by Kerry Don Peterson

This article is taken from excerpts of a workshop presented at NFDA's 1991 annual convention by Kerry Don Peterson, Director of the Body Donor Program–University of Utah School of Medicine.

Operating a body donor program is in many ways an enlightening experience, and I have found a number of similarities exist between funeral service and anatomic science. Just one of these similarities is the practice of embalming.

The history of funeral service and anatomic science merged for a brief period at the close of the Civil War as a result of the work of Anatomist Thomas Holmes who developed a method to preserve dead human bodies to elongate and enhance the dissection process. Holmes capitalized on the idea after the war by offering his embalming services to Washington, D.C., funeral homes and from this embalming evolved into what it is today.

Anatomic embalming is unique when compared to mortuary embalming as we in the anatomic sciences

* Reprinted from *The Director*, Vol. 63, No. 4, Milwaukee, WI: National Funeral Directors Association, NFDA Publications Inc., 1992, with permission.

have the opportunity to view our embalming successes or failures over a period of two years. As a result, we must learn the necessary techniques for long-term preservation or suffer the consequences.

One of the last cases I embalmed while a full-time employee of a funeral home eight years ago was the body of a 39 year old woman who had been stabbed 109 times. The family desired a traditional funeral with embalming followed by cremation. Being a homicide, the body was autopsied and couldn't be cremated until the county attorney cleared the case because cremation would have destroyed potential unfound evidence. It was going to be six to nine months until the cremation could be performed, yet the family indicated a desire to see the body just prior to cremation for a final goodbye. So here I was, presented with an autopsied body carrying 109 stab wounds on every part of the body, including the face. It was the beginning of summer and the family wanted a final viewing in six to nine months.

I embalmed the woman as thoroughly as I knew possible by using a higher volume of more concentrated arterial fluid, hypoed the autopsy flaps, quadruple bagged the viscera and treated it with three bottles of cavity chemical, packed pledgets of cotton soaked in insecticide and cavity chemical in the body's orifices, and used an inordinant amount of drying compound in the abdominal and thoracic cavities. At the time of the funeral, the body looked great. Afterward, it was stored in the coolest room in the funeral home, which usually stayed between 60 and 70 degrees. Application of stone oil and lanolin cream were applied to the face and hands throughout this time. Over the storage period of seven months, the body manifested increasing signs of dehydration and tissue shrinkage, some graying and darkening of the tissues, and development of a slight odor.

All in all, I didn't feel too bad about the results given the circumstances. With deodorant powder in the casket and some opaque makeup and wax, the body looked okay. The family didn't sing praises at the final viewing, but they seemed happy. Again, this all took place about eight years ago and since then, I found I could have done a much better job.

Over the last five years I have experimented with normal mortuary supplies and chemicals on 135 cadavers (these cadavers exhibited a full compliment of physical and pathologic conditions including edema, ascites, jaundice, chemotherapy, obesity, skin slip, etc.; there were even a few "normal" cases) and through trial and error have devised what I consider to be the best method to preserve and store a body for extended periods of time. Each of these 135 cadavers was held and observed for two years. The majority of them exhibited minute dehydration, no discoloration, no blebs, no odor, and no mold. Using this method, I have also reinjected cases that were embalmed a week prior and it has not affected the end result, provided cavity work was not performed. I would like to mention the method was derived on the prep room table, not on a computer or through chemical equations on paper.

I have arbitrarily broken the long-term preservation process into three steps: 1) pre-injection details, 2) application of chemicals, and 3) method of storage. Most of the steps covered are no doubt part and parcel of your normal routine, but it is the sum of all these steps that leads to long-term embalming success. Negligence in one or two of the procedures can lead to partial or total embalming failure.

PRE-INJECTION

To achieve long-term preservation, the embalmer must employ all known and accepted techniques of thorough embalming; shortcuts will cause future headaches. The body should be thoroughly disinfected using a reputable disinfectant and warm water, and the body's orifices should be sprayed or swabbed. *Rigor mortis* should be broken up. Elevate the body above the preparation table with positioning devices under the buttocks, shoulders, and ankle bones. This will take the weight off of most tissues on the back of the body, allowing for better fluid distribution to the area. Prior to the use of positioning devices, I had some bodies exhibit fluid distribution failure on only the weight-bearing posterior portions of the body. Once positioned, the face can be shaved and the facial and body features posed. In setting the facial features, I suggest you restore as much natural contour to the cheeks and eyelids as possible because the arterial fluid recommended will set the facial features firmer than you may be used to. Hypoing of tissue builder will still be an option after the injection of the arterial chemical but, once again, the tissues will be more rigid and less susceptible to tissue builder distension.

An embalmed body is like a petri dish for mold to grow on when stored for long periods of time. Since cotton and absorbent paper products (tissues and paper towels) are likely to harbor mold spores, they should be treated with a sporicide, such as phenol, prior to contact with the body during all three steps of the process.

APPLICATION OF CHEMICALS

To begin step two, select the vessel to be raised. I have had success with both the femoral artery and the carotid arteries, although I personally prefer the latter because it allows for better draining of the internal jugular vein. Most important is that you use the vessel you are most familiar working with. Be advised that venous drainage is of the utmost importance for cosmetic effect, but is of no consequence for preservation; in fact, many medical schools do not drain a drop of blood when injecting their cadavers.

After you have raised the selected vessel, make a "T" incision in the artery with the base of the "T" pointing the direction of cannula insertion. This should be part of your normal embalming routine. When a cannula is inserted in the "T" incision, it is less likely that the tunica intima or tunica media will separate from the tunica adventitia. Ligature compression will also do less damage to the arterial layers when the "T" incision is used, which is very important in those cases you reinject. I generally insert a closing drain tube in the vein as it seems a superior way to regulate venous drainage and resistance, when it works! About 60 percent of the time I replace the drain tube with drainage forceps at some point during the injection process.

Chemical selection and storage techniques are the crux of long-term preservation. In mixing your chemicals, you want a sufficient amount of preservatives, antidehydrants, mold retardants, and accessory chemicals to break up clots, lubricate the vessels, and reduce surface tension. Water has none of these qualities. If you only have arterial and cavity chemicals on your shelves, your success will be no better than what I had with the stab victim. Every reputable manufacturer of embalming chemicals has an array of chemicals which preserve, break up clots, lubricate vessels, reduce surface tension, act as an antidehydrant, and contain phenol or specific retardants. The truth of the matter is you *do not* need most of these chemicals to inject the average case, but you *do* need all of them to inject a case you are going to keep around the funeral home for a couple of years unless you want to deal with dehydration, blebs, mold, odor, discoloration, etc.

The minimum amount of chemical I've injected with 100 percent satisfactory results is two tanks of the following:

First Injection. *Formaldehyde:* 64 ounces (four 16-ounce bottles) with an index range of 21–27 percent. I have tried using less, but some of those cases failed.

Water corrective: Use 64 ounces, even if your morgue has soft water. Water corrective has an array of qualities that enhance the injection process, some of which include: 1) it inactivates the minerals in body fluids just as it inactivates minerals in the water supply, 2) it extracts inert gases from the water supply and the body, 3) it defibrinates the blood, 4) it maintains a proper acid base relationship between chemicals and the body, 5) it intensifies permeability of arterial solutions, and 6) it maintains the potency of formaldehyde and co-injectants against the body's natural chemical barriers.

Vascular lubricant/clot dispenser: 64 ounces, which not only aids in drainage but protects the capillaries from searing when using harsher chemicals and makes the tissues more receptive.

Mold retardant: 32 ounces of mold retardant or eight ounces of phenol-containing cauterant *or* 16 ounces of phenol-containing cavity fluid. *Note:* To avoid jelling, this chemical is usually best when premixed with your vascular lubricant or clot disperser prior to adding it to the embalming machine tank. When mixing new chemicals, it is a good idea to test mix a small batch.

Dye: More or less than normally added, but the amount of time you hold a body will be the main factor in determining how much dye to use if you choose to dye at all.

Water: Add enough water to make a solution totaling no more than 16 ounces over two gallons.

Second Injection. The second injection is the same as the first *unless* you are using an arterial formaldehyde that does not contain a humectant, or if one of the accessory chemicals does not contain a glycol (such as ethylene or propylene glycol) which acts as a humectant. If you have not injected a humectant in the first injection, add humectant to the second injection by reducing the water corrective and vascular lubricant by 16 ounces each (a total of 32 ounces) and replacing it with 32 ounces of humectant. If you do not keep a humectant in stock, add 32 ounces of Downy fabric softener instead.

Usually two injections of this chemical mixture will suffice, but at times I have had to mix and inject subsequent batches. Don't be tempted to shortcut chemicals on subsequent batches and remember that other rules of embalming apply, so do what you always do when you successfully embalm a case. Sometimes you will need to inject multiple points, and sometimes you will need to hypo an area to get adequate fluid to the tissues. Contrary to what I was told in mortuary science school, I have found hypoing to be a very effective treatment for any tissues not receptive to arterial injection. Hypoing the flaps of an autopsy with the same chemical is a must. Also on autopsy, a liberal application of external preservation cream on the underside of the scalp is warranted.

I do not recommend a pre-injection prior to the injection of this arterial formula. Pre-injection was part of my normal routine in the funeral home and I tried to incorporate it into the anatomical routine, but my results were less than satisfactory. Tissues only have the capacity to absorb limited amounts of fluid and when embalming for long-term preservation you want the more stringent fluid absorbed by the tissues.

Particular items to be aware of during the injection procedure include:

- *Manifestations of the chemical:* While embalming, you may note the skin manifesting what I call an orange peel demarcation. The skin sometimes takes on the color and texture of a dehydrated orange peel. This demarcation is normal and passes in 24 to 48 hours. When using phenol, you might also note one-eighth to one-fourth inch white patches; this is also normal and goes away shortly after embalming.
- *Drainage:* When phenol is used, your drainage may become gritty. But regardless of whether or not phenol is used, the more stringent chemicals inherently lead to poor drainage late in the embalming process. It is also a good practice to tie off the vein while injecting the last quart or two of chemicals.
- *Swelling considerations:* Weigh the variables. If you see swelling of facial features occurring and the body is well perfused except the feet, stop injecting and hypo the feet. If the face starts swelling and the body is a long way from being embalmed, lower the pressure or flow, raise and clamp both carotids, and open the jugulars. Be aware that when the body is in storage, swelling diminishes to near normal contours naturally within a month's period of time.
- *Purge:* The more stringent fluids often lead to copious purge. This purge is often the same color as the fluid you are injecting and seems to run out as fast as it is injected, but most of the time fluid distribution is unaffected.
- *Pressure and flow considerations:* I find the pressure versus flow debate to be one of the most confusing issues of embalming science. With the flow closed on my machine, I set the pressure gauge at 25 pounds and open the flow until the pressure drops to 18–20 pounds; on my machine this is an unencumbered rate of flow of 22 ounces per minute. I do adjust the pressure down when injecting those bodies which appear prone to swell and often increase the rate of flow later in the embalming process when the body is taking fluid well and not swelling. If your normal pressure and flow settings give you good results, I advise you to continue using these settings. **Always use the pulse**—studies prove the slight pause in fluid movement increases the amount of fluid absorbed into the tissues. If your machine does not have a pulse feature, turn the machine off for five minutes at each quarter tank interval; also wait 10 minutes between the first and second injection as the rest periods give the tissues a chance to absorb the fluid and offer you a chance to evaluate your progress.
- *Bright dye effect:* The accessory chemicals you mix in this arterial formula not only make the tissues more receptive to formaldehyde but also make the tissues more receptive to dyes. The catch here, however, is that over a period of two months the dye starts to bleach or wash out. When embalming, if you know how long you will have to hold the body, add dye accordingly. What appears bright red at the conclusion of embalming will be very light red in a year. Take this into consideration.
- *Monitor body features for displacement during embalming.*
- *Chemistry:* Provided you have injected two tanks of formula and feel you have adequately preserved the body, you have actually injected twice as much formaldehyde as embalming chemistry tells us is necessary to react with and preserve the soluble proteins of a 160-pound person. Considering you lose arterial formula during drainage and that there are other factors to consider when embalming besides soluble proteins, it should become apparent that this dilution of fluid is in line with the accepted chemical principles of embalming.

When the body has received enough fluid, ligate the arteries and veins, treat the internal incision, suture, and apply incision sealer to the outside of the incision.

Using a 30 cc syringe and your longest hypo needle, inject the brain. Direct the needle through the medial canthus of the eye (pretty much straight back, but you may have to feel around a bit to locate the superior orbital fissure), through the superior orbital fissure, and into the cranial cavity. Inject 30 ccs of formaldehyde slowly through each eye socket into the cranial cavity, drawing the needle outward. Avoid swelling the eye sockets by injecting the bulk of fluid well within the cranial cavity.

At this point, I suggest you do any hypo tissue building or restorative work necessary. Then apply a liberal amount of cream to the face, neck, hands, and wrists.

If the body does not warrant immediate cavity treatment, delay cavity work for 12 to 24 hours and then perform the work in the usual manner followed by an injection of 16 to 32 ounces of cavity chemical.

METHOD OF STORAGE

In storage you want to create an environment for the body that 1) maintains an osmotic balance of moisture between the body and its environment to prevent dehydration, 2) protects the body from mold growth, and

3) provides a preservative buffer between the body and its external environment. The storage technique is easily accomplished and requires five minutes a week, at most, to maintain. The required supplies include:

1. A thick, plastic sheet large enough to loosely wrap the body with excess to tuck beneath.
2. A hospital gown or cloth shroud.
3. A spray bottle.
4. A chemical wetting agent consisting of two-thirds of a gallon of humectant (glycol or antifreeze), four ounces of mold retardant (thymol or phenol), and one gallon of water.
5. A body rest or wooden two-by-fours or four-by-fours.

PROCEDURE

1. Lay the large plastic sheet on a table surface.
2. Place the body rest or cut wood on the plastic sheet (body rests should be high enough to keep all parts of the body off of the table surface).
3. Semi-saturate the hospital gown or shroud with the wetting agent. Dress or wrap the body in the gown or shroud but do not cover the face or feet. Put the rest of the wetting agent in a spray bottle.
4. Place the draped body on the body rests and wrap the plastic sheet loosely around the body. Tuck the free ends of the plastic snugly under the body, trapping a moderate amount of air in with the body (do not wrap the body tightly in the plastic sheet).
5. Place the body in a cool spot. Refrigeration is not necessary but it does help.

Check the body every three or four days for the first couple of weeks. Aspirate or sponge out free liquids in the bag (it is quite normal for some bodies to precipitate two gallons of fluid), keep the cloth shroud moist with the spray bottle, and apply cream to the face and hands as necessary. The plastic wrapping normally creates a rain garden environment.

After the first two weeks have passed, weekly maintenance consisting of spraying the shroud with wetting agent, draining pooled liquids, and reapplying cream to the face and hands is more than sufficient to maintain the body in its environment. Mix more wetting agent when necessary. If a part of the body seems to be going soft (which I have never had happen), hypo treatment is still an option.

Prior to final viewing, remove the body from the wraps, wash thoroughly with an ample amount of soap, and proceed with the normal cosmetic routines.

I do not suggest this method of preparation for every case as the method is costly and time consuming. As embalmers, we know it is not our charge to preserve artifacts for future centuries, but to disinfect and prepare bodies of the dead for therapeutic funeralization of the presently living. I do, however, suggest this method for long-term preservation or when a firm base is required for reconstruction or restoration.

Occupational Exposure to Formaldehyde in Mortuaries*

L. Lamont Moore, CIH CSP
Safety Sciences Department, Indiana University of Pennysylvania, Indiana, Pennsylvania

Eugene C. Ogrodnik, MS
Dean, Pittsburgh Institute of Mortuary Science, Pittsburgh, Pennsylvania

---

A short-term project was conducted to evaluate occupational exposure to formaldehyde in mortuaries. The study group consisted of 23 mortuaries located in Allegheny County, Pennsylvania. These establishments had business volumes ranging from 35 to 500 embalmings per year. On-site surveys were conducted at each location to examine ventilation systems and review work practices. Breathing zone and room air samples were subsequently collected during actual embalming procedures in a number of the smaller facilities with less well designed ventilation systems. One of the primary objectives of the project was to educate participating mortuary directors about the potential health hazards associated with occupational exposure to formaldehyde. An extensive literature review was completed to summarize related epidemiological and environmental studies for participants. Additionally, the monitoring data were compared to previous observations and exposure estimates. Results of this study did not reveal employee exposures which approached existing limits established by the Occupational Safety and Health Administration (OSHA).

Formaldehyde is a colorless, pungent, irritant gas that is water soluble and most frequently marketed as 37–56% aqueous solutions, commonly known as formalin. Formaldehyde vapor is very irritating to the respiratory tract, eyes, and exposed surfaces of the skin. Inhalation of high concentrations can cause laryngitis, bronchitis, and bronchopneumonia. Liquid formaldehyde solutions may cause severe burns on contact with the eye. Formaldehyde will act as a primary skin irritant, causing an erythematous or eczematous dermatitis reaction.

* Reprinted from the *J Environ Health* 1986;49(1), with permission.

Formaldehyde solutions do not have a high degree of systemic toxicity, and acute and chronic exposures generally result in varying degrees of irritation which are usually localized. Symptoms commonly experienced by the general population are nonspecific, transient, exposure dependent, and usually mild. In some cases, however, formaldehyde may act as an allergic (immunologically mediated) skin sensitizer, and it may also exacerbate respiratory distress in individuals with preexisting or formaldehyde-induced bronchial hyperactivity. It may not be feasible for sensitized persons to work in an area where there is any possibility of exposure, even at very low levels.

Formaldehyde has an odor threshold far below 1 part per million (ppm). Stern[1] reported the lower limit for odor detection to be 0.05 ppm with throat irritation first occurring at 0.5 ppm. Bourne and Seferman[2] established the threshold for eye irritation at 0.13 to 0.45 ppm. The experience of numerous investigators has been that rapid inurement to such concentrations develops and there is a general absence of complaints from most workers exposed below 2 or 3 ppm.[3] According to existing OSHA regulations, the permissible limit for 8-hour time-weighted average exposure to formaldehyde is 3 ppm. The acceptable ceiling concentration is 5 ppm and the acceptable maximum peak is 10 ppm for 30 minutes. This standard was adopted in the mid-70s based on the irritant properties of formaldehyde.

The American Conference of Governmental Industrial Hygienists[3] has listed formaldehyde as a substance suspect of carcinogenic potential for man. In 1983 they proposed an 8-hour time-weighted average exposure limit of 1 ppm with a short-term exposure limit of 2 ppm for a maximum of 15 minutes. They point out that these concentrations may not be sufficient to prevent sensitized persons from suffering irritation but should be adequate to avoid development of persistent adverse effects.

In 1976 the National Institute for Occupational Safety and Health[4] recommended to OSHA that occupational exposure to formaldehyde be limited so that no employee is exposed at concentrations which exceed 1 ppm during any 30-minute period. This recommendation presumably was designed to protect the health of employees over their working lifetime, but may not be adequate to protect sensitized or hypersensitive individuals.

Plunkett and Barbela[5] completed a mail survey of 57 embalmers in 20 California funeral homes during 1976. Nine had symptoms compatible with acute bronchitis, and 17 were considered to have chronic bronchitis. No data on formaldehyde exposure levels, work practices, ventilation, or frequency of exposure was gathered. Nevertheless, there was enough evidence to suggest that more in-depth studies of this profession should be considered.

Levine et al[6] studied nearly 100 West Virginia morticians who were attending an educational program during 1978. Standardized respiratory disease questionnaires and pulmonary function tests were administered to the group. The pulmonary function of morticians compared favorably with that of residential populations in Oregon and Michigan. Among the study group, those who had presumably embalmed the largest number of bodies did not demonstrate a higher than expected incidence of chronic bronchitis or pulmonary function deficits. The authors concluded that long-term intermittent exposure to low levels of formaldehyde had exerted no meaningful chronic effect on respiratory health. No actual data on formaldehyde exposures, ventilation, or work practices were gathered as part of this study.

Williams et al[7] recently published the results of exposure studies conducted in seven West Virginia funeral homes. Area and personal samples were used to evaluate the embalmers' exposure to formaldehyde, phenol, and 23 organic solvents and particulates. Twenty-five personal samples revealed time-weighted average formaldehyde concentrations which ranged from 0.1 to 0.4 ppm during the embalming of intact bodies, and ranging between 0.5 and 1.2 ppm during preparation of autopsied cases. The overall average exposures were 0.3 ppm and 0.9 ppm, respectively. Concentrations of other airborne chemicals and of particulates were negligible. Time-weighted averages were calculated over the length of time actually required for the embalming. Embalming technique and condition of the body appeared to be the major determinants of formaldehyde exposure in preparing autopsied bodies. The importance of room air exchange rate could not be determined from this study. Overall, exhaust ventilation appeared to reduce formaldehyde concentrations in general room air but had little effect on the embalmer's personal exposure.

Kerfoot and Mooney[8] completed an extensive study of six funeral homes in the Detroit area, collecting 187 air samples under a variety of conditions. The vapor concentrations encompassed a range between 0.09 and 5.26 ppm. The average formaldehyde concentrations ranged between 0.25 and 1.30 ppm under normal working conditions with an overall average of 0.74 ppm.

It was not clear whether personal or area samples were obtained. Ventilation systems were evaluated in terms of air changes per hour and compared with average concentrations of formaldehyde found in each facility. The largest number of air changes did not always correspond to the lowest concentration of vapors. The authors concluded that the location of the fan and size of the room were also significant factors. They also pointed out that all six establishments were above average facilities and inferred that formaldehyde concentrations in smaller, less well designed funeral homes might be markedly higher.

In 1979, NIOSH[9] conducted a health hazard evaluation of the embalming laboratory at the Cincinnati College of Mortuary Science. The request had been prompted by the early disability retirement of an embalming instructor who had developed asthmatic bronchitis after 5 years of laboratory exposure. Air samples were collected via general area and personal breathing zone sampling during actual work conditions and simulated accidents involving spillage of embalming fluids. Formaldehyde concentrations exceeded the proposed ACGIH threshold limit value of 1 ppm in 7 of 13 samples collected. All of the excessive concentrations were detected during simulated (worst case) situations, or during one afternoon when the ventilation system was inoperable.

A study of mortality among undertakers licensed in Ontario, Canada, was completed by R. J. Levine[10] in late 1982. He selected a cohort of 1477 embalmers licensed between 1928 and 1957 and examined the cause of death in 337 men who had died prior to 1978. The ratio of observed to expected deaths from each cause was expressed as a percentage or standard mortality ratio. No significant increase in mortality was detected for any form of cancer. Deaths from cancers at sites of potential contact with formaldehyde—skin, nose, oropharynx, larynx, and esophagus—were less than expected, as were deaths from cancer of the lung.

Walrath and Fraumeni[11] of the National Cancer Institute published a study in 1983 which investigated whether embalmers in New York State, compared with the general population, had a greater proportion of cancer deaths that might be associated with exposure to formaldehyde. The study group consisted of approximately 1132 deceased embalmers who had been licensed to practice in New York State between 1902 and 1979. The difference between observed and expected numbers of deaths from malignant neoplasms was elevated, but not significantly. Skin cancer mortality was significantly elevated, primarily among those licensed for more than 35 years. Mortality was slightly elevated for kidney cancer, leukemia, and brain cancer. No excess mortality was observed for cancers of the respiratory tract and no deaths ascribed to nasal cancer.

Walrath and Fraumeni[12] published the results of a similar study of California embalmers in 1984. The authors examined the death certificates of 1007 embalmers and calculated proportionate mortality ratios for the major causes of death. Mortality was significantly elevated for total cancer, arteriosclerotic heart disease, leukemia, as well as cancers of the colon, brain, and prostate. There were no deaths from nasal cancer and the pattern of lung cancer mortality was unremarkable. One of the inherent weaknesses of both the California and New York studies is that sample sizes were of insufficient size to detect rare conditions such as nasal cancer. Although the respiratory tract would presumably be the prime target site for formaldehyde carcinogenicity, the authors conclude that available epidemiological evidence suggests attention should be given to possible cancer risks at other sites, including the brain, bone marrow, and colon. It may be of significance to note that the Ontario study[10] did not indicate an elevated risk of cancer based on a study of 300+ death certificates. However, larger studies performed in New York[11] and California[12] both showed excess deaths from leukemia and brain cancer.

Patty's text[13] suggests that aldehydes cannot be regarded as potent carcinogens. The irritant properties of the compounds preclude substantial worker exposure under normal conditions. The extreme reactivity of formaldehyde, acrolein, and chloroacetaldehyde, for example, produces reactions at epithelial surfaces which tend to limit their absorption into the body. The rapid metabolic conversion to innocuous materials also may limit those critical reactions necessary to initiate systemic tumorigenesis. However, formaldehyde-induced tissue irritation may promote tumor formation initiated by another compound. Therefore, caution is warranted, and certainly further epidemiologic studies must be performed to define any hazard that may exist.

Since 1979, there have been several research reports linking formaldehyde exposure to cancer. These studies were based on exposure of rats and mice to concentrations of 2, 6, and 15 ppm for 30 hours per week over a period exceeding 2 years.[14] Based on these findings, NIOSH recommended in 1981 that as a prudent measure, occupational exposure be reduced to the lowest feasible limit.

MATERIALS AND METHODS

On-site surveys were conducted at each facility to interview the funeral director about work procedures, evaluate the overall floor plan, calculate room volume, and record air flow measurements where appropriate. Subsequently, air sampling was conducted in a number of the funeral homes with poorly designed ventilation systems. Where feasible, samples were collected from the breathing zone of the embalmer during the entire period required for the embalming, usually 45–75 minutes.

Air was drawn through a liquid sampling medium using MSA Model G pumps set at a flow rate of 500 cubic centimeters per minute. Calibration was accomplished prior to the surveys using a primary standard (soap-bubble meter) as suggested by the manufacturer. Pumps were adjusted as necessary to maintain the desired flow rate throughout the sampling period. A midget impinger with fitted glass bubbler containing 15 ml of a 10% aqueous methanol solution was used to collect air samples to be analyzed for formaldehyde. At the conclusion of the sampling period, samples were transferred to polyethylene bottles, sealed, labeled, and shipped to an approved industrial hygiene laboratory.

At the laboratory, samples are reacted with hydrazine reagent to form a hydrazone derivative, then analyzed by differential pulses polarography. This sampling and analytical technique (ID-102) was developed at OSHA's Analytical Laboratory in Salt Lake City, Utah. The coefficient of variation (CY_T) for the total sampling and analytical technique is 0.08. This value corresponds to a standard deviation of 1 mg/m^3 at the OSHA permissible exposure limit of 3 ppm.

RESULTS AND DISCUSSION

The embalming rooms examined as part of this study varied significantly in terms of their size, layout, and the effectiveness of the ventilation system. Preparation rooms were equipped with ventilation systems which produced from 0 to 20 air changes per hour with a mean of 7.6 air changes per hour. Three facilities had exhaust systems which produced no measurable air movement at all. Only 17% of these rooms had an exhaust grate or fan which was positioned to prevent fumes from being drawn through the breathing zone of the employee.

The size of embalming rooms ranged from 735 to 5000 ft^3 with a mean of 1950 ft^3. Less than 10% of the establishments had any provisions for the introduction of makeup air into the work area. The only source of makeup air would have been leakage around doors or windows throughout the structure.

Eight personal samples were collected from the breathing zone of funeral directors during separate embalming procedures in six different funeral homes. None of these establishments had ventilation systems which would be considered above the norm described above. Exposure concentrations summarized in Table 1 show a range of 0.03 to 3.15 ppm with an overall average of 1.1 ppm during the period required for the embalming. Embalming procedures typically last 45–75 minutes depending on the condition of the subject. When we assumed zero exposure during the unsampled portion of the shift, 8-hour time-weighted average exposures ranged from 0.01 to 0.49 ppm, with an overall mean of 0.16 ppm.

TABLE 1. SUMMARY OF FORMALDEHYDE EXPOSURE MEASUREMENTS BASED ON PERSONAL SAMPLING

	Low	High	Average
Time-weighted average exposure during the period required for the embalming procedure	0.03 ppm	3.15 ppm	1.1 ppm
Exposure estimate for the full workshift, an 8-hour time-weighted average	0.01 ppm	0.49 ppm	0.16 ppm

Note. Calculation of 8-hour time-weighted averages was completed making the assumption that exposure would have been zero during the unsampled portion of the workshift.

The data summarized in Table 2 provide a comparison of our limited data with that of more extensive studies by Kerfoot and Mooney[8] and Williams et al.[7] Allegheny County exposure estimates reflect slightly higher formaldehyde concentrations which may be associated with the smaller, poorly designed preparation rooms where sampling was conducted. Plans for a longer term study were abandoned when our initial monitoring revealed 8-hour time-weighted average exposures to be well below the OSHA permissible exposure limit of 3 ppm.

Six area samples were also collected from general workroom air in proximity to preparation tables, usually in conjunction with personal sampling. Results

TABLE 2. COMPARISON OF ALLEGHENY COUNTY EXPOSURE DATA WITH PREVIOUS STUDIES

	Estimated Formaldehyde Exposure During Embalming (in ppm)		
	Low	High	Average
Kerfoot/Mooney (1975)[8]	0.25 ppm	1.39 ppm	0.74 ppm
Williams/Levine/Blunden (1984)[7]			
Intact cases	0.10 ppm	0.40 ppm	0.30 ppm
Autopsied cases	0.50 ppm	1.20 ppm	0.90 ppm
Allegheny County (1984)	0.03 ppm	3.15 ppm	1.10 ppm

TABLE 3. COMPARISON OF FORMALDEHYDE CONCENTRATIONS DETECTED IN WORKROOM AIR DURING EMBALMING PROCEDURES—AREA VS PERSONAL SAMPLING

	Low	High	Average
Area samples taken in proximity to preparation tables	N.D.[a]	0.84 ppm	0.45 ppm
Personal samples collected from the breathing zone of embalmers	0.03 ppm	3.15 ppm	1.1 ppm

[a] N.D. signifies "not detected."

summarized in Table 3 suggest that area sampling is not representative of the embalmers' actual exposure. Where concurrent sampling was carried out, concentrations found in the employee's breathing zone were up to twice as high as measurements taken from general workroom air several feet away.

There are a number of conclusions to be drawn from this study, despite its limited scope. First, the authors found many funeral directors to be largely unaware or poorly informed about the continuing controversy over the carcinogenic potential of long-term exposure to formaldehyde. Second, it was clear that most funeral homes in this study had ventilation systems or floor plans which were largely ineffective in controlling exposure during embalming procedures. The position of the exhaust grate commonly draws contaminants through the embalmer's breathing zone. Third, the authors' data suggest that personal breathing zone samples are likely to provide the most accurate indicator of employee exposure in the embalming room.

Occupational exposure to formaldehyde in funeral homes should rarely exceed permissible exposure limits established by OSHA. These limits were adopted in the early 1970s to protect employees against the irritant properties of formaldehyde, and may not be sufficiently stringent in view of the chemical's suspected carcinogenic potential. It is reasonable to assume, however, that there are regular occasions where embalmers' exposures exceed the short-term exposure limits of 2 ppm during any 15-minute period recommended by ACGIH in 1983 and the NIOSH recommendation of 1981 which suggests exposure be kept at the lowest feasible limit.

More extensive epidemiological and laboratory studies will be carried out before the issue of formaldehyde carcinogenicity is resolved. Funeral directors or embalmers represent a profession which should be of continuing interest to epidemiological researchers studying the long-term exposure to formaldehyde. Should more definitive evidence be developed with regard to the carcinogenic effects of formaldehyde, large-scale education efforts and installation of improved engineering controls will become priority within the funeral home industry.

REFERENCES

1. Stern AC. *Air Pollution.* New York: Academic Press; 1968; Vol. 1, p. 484.
2. Bourne HG, Seferman S. Wrinkle proofed clothing may liberate toxic quantities of formaldehyde. *Ind Med Surg* 1959;28:232.
3. American Conference of Governmental Industrial Hygienists. *Documentation of the Threshold Limit Values.* Cincinnati, OH: ACGIH; 1983:197.1.
4. National Institute of Occupational Safety and Health. *Criteria for a Recommended Standard. . . . Occupational Exposure to Formaldehyde.* Baltimore, MD: NIOSH; 1976:P.B. 76-273805.
5. Plunkett ER, Barbela T. Are embalmers at risk? *Am Ind Hyg Assoc J* 1977;38:61–62.
6. Levine RJ, DalCorso RD, Blunder PB, Battigelli MC. The effects of occupational exposure on the respiratory health of West Virginia morticians. *J Occup Med* 1984;26:91–98.
7. Williams TM, Levine RJ, Blunden RB. Exposure of embalmers to formaldehyde and other chemicals. *Am Ind Hyg Assoc J* 1984;45:172–176.
8. Kerfoot EJ, Mooney TF. Formaldehyde and paraformaldehyde study in funeral homes. *Am Ind Hyg Assoc J* 1975;36:533–537.
9. National Institute of Occupational Safety and Health. *Health Hazard Evaluation.* Cincinnati: College of Mortuary Science Embalming Laboratory; 1980:HHE 79-146-670, NTIS Pub. PB80-192099.
10. Levine RJ. Mortality of Ontario undertakers. In: *C.I.I.T. Activities.* Research Triangle Park, NC: Chemical Industry Institute of Toxicology; 1982.
11. Walrath J, Fraumeni JF. Mortality patterns among New York embalmers. *Int J Cancer* 1983;31:407–411.
12. Walrath J, Fraumeni JF. Cancer and other causes of death among California embalmers. *Cancer Res* 1984;44:4638–4641.
13. Clayton GD, Clayton FE (Eds). *Patty's Industrial Hygiene and Toxicology.* 3rd ed. New York: John Wiley & Sons; 1981:Vol 2A.
14. National Institute of Occupational Safety and Health. *Intelligence Bulletin 34: Formaldehyde: Evidence of Carcinogenicity,* Baltimore, MD: NIOSH; 1981.

Formaldehyde Vapor Emission Study in Embalming Rooms

Edward J. Kerfoot, Ph.D. Applicant

Department of Physiology, Department of Occupational and Environmental Health, College of Medicine, Wayne State University (Graduate of Department of Mortuary Science, Wayne State University), Detroit, Michigan

Most funeral service licensees are familiar with the physical properties and uses of formaldehyde, but few are fully aware of its toxic properties. Industries that use formaldehyde, as permanent-press fabric and paper processing, show concern about this gas and its effect on their workers. Investigation revealed that no experimentation had ever been done to determine the concentrations of formaldehyde to which funeral licensees are exposed.

It seemed that some study in this area was needed—not only to determine if the concentrations of formaldehyde during embalming were within accepted "safe" levels, but also to evaluate the effectiveness of controls on the formaldehyde concentrations and to consider some possible adverse effects of this gas.

It may be worthwhile here to describe some of the properties of formaldehyde that are important to this particular study. Formaldehyde is a toxic gas and classified as an upper respiratory irritant because it has a high solubility in water and is held by the moisture covering the upper respiratory tract. Gases that dissolve more slowly in water travel more deeply into the respiratory tract before they are dissolved. So, under ordinary circumstances, formaldehyde, though toxic, doesn't cause any damage. Formaldehyde possesses distinctive physiological properties causing symptoms very familiar to all funeral licensees such as burning of the eyes, lacrimation, and irritation of the upper respiratory passages. These symptoms allow formaldehyde to act as its own warning agent as other gases like ammonia do.

The main purpose of this research was to determine the concentration of formaldehyde vapors that embalmers inhale while embalming. In six Detroit area funeral home preparation rooms the formaldehyde content during embalming procedures was determined chemically. These establishments were not representative of a general cross section of all funeral homes but were actually better than average. The concentration of formaldehyde vapors for the total 187 samples taken ranged from 0.09 to 5.26 ppm (parts per million). At the higher levels of this range, the fumes caused such severe upper respiratory distress that the licensees and sampler were unable to remain in the room.

Ventilation systems in the preparation rooms were evaluated in two ways. First, samples of formaldehyde concentrations were taken with the fan off (with an average of 1.34 ppm), then with the fan on (with an average of 0.74 ppm), indicating that use of a fan reduces the vapors by about half. Secondly, the fans were evaluated in terms of air changes per hour. The larger number of air changes did not always correspond to the lower concentration of formaldehyde vapors, indicating the probability that other factors, specifically the location of the fan and size of the room, were also significant in the efficiency of the ventilation systems.

At one funeral home, still another factor was evaluated. A surgical cloth mask was placed in the sample holder and the concentration of formaldehyde after being filtered through the mask again determined. Here the samples showed average values of 2.50 ppm with no ventilation or mask, 1.21 ppm with ventilation but without a mask, and 0.78 ppm using both the ventilation system and mask. This indicated that as the use of the fan reduced the formaldehyde concentrations by half, the further use of a mask reduced the concentrations by nearly half again. Masks are not commonly used during embalming but concerned licensees should be aware of the efficiency of a mask in reducing the amount of formaldehyde vapors inhaled.

Air samples containing embalming powders and hardening compounds were taken with a thermal precipitator and then sized microscopically; the mean particle size was found to be 1.6 microns. This finding was of definite importance because particles between 1 and 2 microns are respirable, deposited, and, most importantly, retained in the lung depths. Larger particles could not penetrate as deeply and smaller particles, which could penetrate deeply, are too small to be retained but would be exhaled. Also, the particles of paraformaldehyde powders have the ability to absorb formaldehyde vapors in the air, so that not only the particles of paraformaldehyde but the attached formaldehyde vapors (which normally affect only the upper respiratory tract) may be carried into the lower respiratory tract of the licensee.

A small-scale toxicity survey was done among the licensees at these funeral homes; they filled out questionnaires concerning the known toxic effects of formaldehyde. This study clearly demonstrated that formaldehyde is mainly an upper respiratory irritant causing eye and nose burns, sneezing, coughing, and headaches: It is interesting that 3 out of 7 men suffered from asthma or sinus problems, which is a somewhat higher proportion than in the general population.

The workers who were bothered more by the irritant action of formaldehyde were exposed to the higher concentrations and those who spent more of their work time embalming also experienced more severe symptoms. Keep in mind that these symptoms were experienced by workers who spend only part of their work day exposed to formaldehyde and at concentrations well below the present limit.

The study, then, showed several facts of importance. For one thing, it found the formaldehyde vapor concentrations to which licensees who embalm are exposed to be within the levels of the present TLV (threshold limit value). This means that if the concentrations exceed 5 ppm they pose a possible health hazard to the worker but under this level the worker is "safe." It must be mentioned here that the current TLV of 5 ppm is being challenged and proposals have been made (by OSHA) to lower it to 2 ppm. If this happens it would mean that some licensees would be working in concentrations of formaldehyde far above the accepted "safe" limit.

The results of the toxicity survey verified the fact that formaldehyde is mainly an upper respiratory irritant because all involved experienced, to some degree, the symptoms of upper respiratory irritation. The possibility that more serious damage could occur, however, was evident with the determination of paraformaldehyde particle size. Because it's known that these powders can absorb formaldehyde, the fact that their size makes them able to be carried deep into the lungs and retained there becomes a finding of much importance. It means that these powders and compounds, as well as the attached formaldehyde vapors, can reach an area where they may cause serious lung damage.

This research also showed that ventilation systems reduce the vapor concentration roughly by half and also showed that great variations in the effectiveness of ventilation systems existed. The importance of several factors, namely the size of the fan, the size of the room, and the location of the fan, in influencing the effectiveness of a good ventilation system was shown. Further, it showed that these concentrations can be reduced by almost half again by the use of a mask.

From these results some conclusions may be drawn:

There definitely is a need for further study in this area, particularly concerning the paraformaldehyde powders and their ability to penetrate the lung depths.

The need for lowering the TLV to 2 ppm (as has been proposed) seems quite evident. As previously mentioned, when the formaldehyde concentrations approached the present TLV of 5 ppm, the licensee and sampler were too distressed to remain in the embalming room, and the irritating effects experienced by those involved in the toxicity survey at much lower levels seem to back this up.

There certainly is good reason for licensees to be well educated in the known and even possible effects of formaldehyde as well as in the effectiveness of the controls available to them. This knowledge might make more licensees responsible in protecting themselves as well as they can, even to employing the annoyance of a mask, especially when the embalming powders and hardening compounds are used.

Finally, there is a real need for setting up definite standards regarding formaldehyde exposure. Definite regulations should be set up regarding size of embalming rooms, size of fans, and their locations in the embalming rooms to insure good ventilation systems. Perhaps even the number of hours that one embalmer could be exposed in a given amount of time should be limited. Whether such standards will be determined will depend, in large part, on the interest of funeral service licensees themselves.

Reported Studies on Effects of Formaldehyde Exposure*

Leandro Rendon
Director of Research and Educational Programs,
Champion Chemical Company, Springfield, Ohio

The general effects related to human exposure to formaldehyde appear to include many different symptoms and conditions. Perhaps, the most frequently mentioned effects are those associated with the pungent, irritating properties of formaldehyde involving the eyes, nose, and throat. The degree of response will vary depending upon the amount of formaldehyde present and from individual to individual.

It has long been known that high concentrations of formaldehyde are irritating to man and that it can cause skin sensitization. Because of formaldehyde's importance, the Chemical Industry Institute of Toxicology (CIIT) sponsored a conference in November 1980, in which current research on formaldehyde was presented. The event brought scientists and government regulators together to hear and discuss the wide variety of then-current research.

Issue no. 517, May 1981, of the *Expanding Encyclopedia* discussed some of the available data regarding "Health Risk From Formaldehyde." Since then, more information has become available and it is the purpose of this discussion to update what is known regarding effects of formaldehyde exposure.

In his presentation at the November 1980 conference, Richard J. Levine et al[1] distinguished two impor-

* Reprinted from the *Expanding Encyclopedia*, No. 542, Springfield, OH: Champion Chemical Co.; 1983, with permission.

tant categories of embalming practice in relation to exposure: the embalming of "normal" (nonautopsied) and of autopsied remains. In their studies, the group found time-weighted-average formaldehyde concentrations to be 0.3 ppm during the embalming of nonautopsied cases and 0.9 ppm for autopsied remains. The highest concentrations were 0.4 ppm and 2.1 ppm, respectively. The investigator commented that while exposures found in embalming autopsied bodies are more intense, autopsied bodies usually comprise only a minority of total bodies embalmed. He further stated:

> In a summary, pulmonary function of West Virginia (where the study was performed) morticians compared favorably to that of residential populations in Oregon and Michigan. Among morticians, high exposure was linked neither to chronic bronchitis nor to pulmonary function deficits. The results suggest that intermittent exposure to low levels of formaldehyde gas over the long term exerts no meaningful chronic effect on respiratory health.

At the same CIIT conference on November 1980, Walrath et al[2] presented a preliminary study that investigated whether embalmers, compared with the general population, have a greater proportion of cancer deaths that might be associated with exposure to formaldehyde. The study group consisted of deceased embalmers licensed to practice embalming in New York State between 1902 and 1979. The death certificates revealed data indicating that the embalmers in that group experienced a slightly elevated mortality from cancer, a significant excess of arteriosclerotic heart disease, and a very low incidence of pneumonia deaths. Skin cancer mortality was significantly elevated as well as kidney and brain cancers. On the other hand, there was no excess mortality from cancer of the respiratory tract, including the nasal passages. The investigators point out, however, "that embalming fluids contain a mixture of other chemicals that are partly intended to offset the adverse reactions of formaldehyde."

It should be pointed out that commercially available fluids from 1902 to approximately the late 1930s tended to be rather harsh and astringent compositions. The embalmer did not often use or wear gloves when working with embalming compositions as happens today. It is possible to assume that prolonged contact of the embalming fluids with the skin could produce adverse effects. Also, it is possible that adequate ventilation and exhaust systems were not available in preparation rooms in the "early" days.

On November 3, 1982, the Formaldehyde Institute sponsored a formaldehyde toxicology conference as a means of continuing the open dialogue between interested parties that was initiated at the November 1980 meeting. Another important paper was presented at that meeting by Dr. Richard J. Levine et al.[3]

The investigators made a study of the mortality of Ontario undertakers during the period between 1928 and 1957. As was the purpose in the study among West Virginia funeral licensees, Dr. Levine was interested in learning more about possible effects of formaldehyde among groups of workers who are known to work with the compound possibly to a greater extent than others and over a longer period of time.

The sites felt to be of particular interest as being of a special risk for cancer from exposure to formaldehyde were skin, nasal passages, buccal cavity, pharynx, and larnyx. Among the Canadian funeral licensees no deaths due to nasal cancer were observed. Mortality attributed to cancers of the buccal cavity, pharynx, and respiratory system exclusive of trachea, bronchus, and lung was less than expected.

Cirrhosis of the liver was the only cause of death found to be significantly in excess. The investigators felt that perhaps this might be due to a higher consumption of alcoholic beverages by this group than the general population. They believed this might account for the increases in mortality from liver cancer, disease of the circulatory system, and acute respiratory diseases, which are characteristically elevated among alcoholics. The preliminary conclusion is that formaldehyde exposure among Ontario's funeral licensees has had no effect on cancer mortality.

A new British epidemiology study released in August 1983 contains some interesting information. Dr. E. A. Acheson, Director of the British Medical Research Council's Environmental Epidemiology Unit, Southampton General Hospital, in the United Kingdom, presented a report based on a study of more than 7700 chemical workers from six factories among the country's chemical industry where formaldehyde has been manufactured or used for more than 15 years. The study sought to find an increase in the incidence of cancer types among long-term employees exposed to formaldehyde. The levels workers were exposed to over the period studied were as much as three times higher than those allowed under present regulations.

Results of the Acheson study show no excessive risk for formaldehyde workers of contracting nasal, lung, prostate, brain, skin, kidney, or bladder cancers. The report, according to the Formaldehyde Institute, brings the total number of epidemiology studies performed to 12, all revealing no excess cancer types in persons exposed to formaldehyde. In this country, the major manufacturers of formaldehyde have accomplished similar studies among their workers and report data similar to those of Acheson.

In Iowa, a study was accomplished jointly by the Iowa State Department of Health and the University

Hygienic Laboratory. The study was carried out with the endorsement of the Board of Mortuary Science Examiners and the Iowa Funeral Directors Association. The first phase of the two-part study determined formaldehyde exposure during embalmings. The second part examined cancer death rates among funeral directors as compared to the general population.

During the study, personnel from the Iowa State Department of Health visited 44 funeral homes that had been randomly selected throughout the state. At each place, two samples of formaldehyde gas were collected during embalming procedures—one at the operator's breathing zone and one ambient room air sample. According to the Iowa State Department of Health, the following determinations were found as a result of the study, June 1983;

Formaldehyde concentrations measured in breathing zone samples ranged from nondetectable to 3.5 ppm. The *average* detectable level of formaldehyde in the breathing zone was 0.84 ppm. Ambient room sample concentrations ranged from nondetectable to 1.99 ppm, with an *average* reading of 0.23 ppm determined.

The Iowa State Department of Health reported its findings to the Iowa Funeral Directors Association and listed the following measures that should be followed to reduce exposure whenever practicable *although none of the reported levels were in excess of federal standards:*

1. Local exhaust ventilation should be used whenever persons are working in the preparation room, particularly during embalming procedures. Significantly higher concentrations of formaldehyde would be expected when no local exhaust ventilation is used during embalming procedures. Ventilation systems should be properly designed with consideration for room volume, embalming workload, and avoidance of dead air spaces.
2. During embalming procedures, personnel should avoid working in locations between the exhaust vent and sources of formaldehyde (for example, embalming tank, mixing tank, etc.).
3. Situations in which formaldehyde is exposed to room air (for example, spills, open tanks, open bottles, etc.) should be minimized. In situations where opportunities for volatilizing formaldehyde into the room air cannot be avoided, the length of exposure should be maintained at as short an interval as is practicable.
4. Direct skin contact with formaldehyde should be avoided. Use of protective equipment, such as rubber gloves and aprons, will reduce the chances of skin exposure. In this study, at least one instance of contact dermatitis was reported to occur from embalming fluid.

ACKNOWLEDGMENT

Acknowledgment is hereby extended to the Iowa Funeral Directors Association for making available the preceding information which should be of immense interest to all funeral licensees.

REFERENCES

1. Levine RJ, et al. The effects of occupational exposure on the respiratory health of West Virginia morticians. In: *Formaldehyde Toxicity*. New York: Hemisphere Pub. Corp.; 1983:212–226.
2. Walrath J, et al. Proportionate mortality among New York embalmers. In: *Formaldehyde Toxicity*. New York: Hemisphere Pub. Corp.; 1983:227–236.
3. Levine RJ, et al. Mortality of Ontario undertakers: A first report. In: *Formaldehyde Toxicology–Epidemiology–Mechanisms*. New York: Marcel Dekker; 1983: 127–140.

Final Report on Literature Search on the Infectious Nature of Dead Bodies for the Embalming Chemical Manufacturers Association, September 1, 1968*

Maude R. Hinson

Medical Research Librarian, Downers Grove, Illinois

INTRODUCTION

In recent years, critics of American funeral practices and customs have charged that embalming is an economic waste and that it serves no useful purpose in protecting the public health. This claim is based on the theory that "the germ dies with the host." Therefore, it is argued, the unembalmed dead human body is harmless and not a source of possible infection and disease. Although such statements have sometimes been credited to men who would be expected to be knowledgeable in the field (in one notable instance, a pathologist), no scientific, documented facts have been offered to substantiate the statements.

* Literature search conducted by Maude R. Hinson, Medical Research Librarian, Bibliographic Service, 4912 Wallbank Avenue, Downers Grove, IL 60515.

To disprove this theory, or to prove that the dead human body does harbor infectious organisms, that it can be a public hazard, and that modern embalming lessens that hazard, the Embalming Chemical Manufacturers Association (ECMA) sponsored this literature research project. The principal guidelines for the search were to avoid any literature published by an embalming chemical manufacturer, a college of embalming, or any related "interest." The search was to be centered in literature in the fields of medicine, pathology, biology, and related sciences.

THE SEARCH

The search began with a review of *Index Medicus* for the years 1963, 1964, 1965, and part of 1966, from which 265 references were selected. Eighty-eight book references were taken from the 1966 *Subject Guide to Books in Print,* published by R. R. Bowker. These lists were submitted to a committee of ECMA to select the articles to be photocopied at the National Library of Medicine in Bethesda, Maryland, and the books to be purchased. Photocopies were not ordered of all 265 reference articles, nor were all 88 books purchased. Some were passed over because they seemed too general to have direct bearing on the subject under investigation; others were passed because they appeared too similar to others already ordered. Twenty-one foreign language articles were translated to English. Not all of the articles photocopied will be cited in this report, again because of similarities among several of the articles. To include them would serve only to lengthen the report, without substantially increasing the weight of documentation.

DISCUSSION

To reasonably maintain the proposition that embalming has a real public health value, two questions must be answered. The first question concerns the validity of the claim that an infectious organism will invariably die when its host organism dies. If this theory has basis in fact, it must be conceded that the dead human body is harmless and does not present a public health hazard. If, on the other hand, we find this theory in error, we are led to another question. Can these organisms endanger public health?

Since the second question is somewhat rhetorical, perhaps it can be dealt with most simply. Establishing the reality of contact infection is an integral part of the proof that dead bodies can support living organisms. Establishing the validity of airborne infection may be even more pertinent, since it would be a hazard only to a small circle of mourners, funeral home personnel, pathologists, medical students, etc.

In "Airborne Infection: How Important for Public Health?" Alexander Langmuir maintains the reality and danger of airborne infection based upon systematic epidemiological studies, supported by extensive laboratory studies in experimental animals and human subjects. He lists psittacosis, Q fever, histoplasmosis, coccidioidomycosis, anthrax, brucellosis, primary tuberculosis, and primary mycosis as only a few diseases which are "intrinsically and exclusively airborne infections."[1]

Having broken order to eliminate a fairly straightforward question, we now turn back to question number one, which is perhaps the crux of this investigation. Do infectious organisms live on in a dead human body? There may be differing opinions on this question among laymen, but little variance of opinion can be found at the scientific level. In his article Virulence of Some Organisms in Cadavers, Giuseppe Fiorito says "Obviously, not all bacteria die in a cadaver."[2] He points out that even the process of putrefaction itself "is largely bacterial." He continues, "The high and rapid toxicity of cultures from cadavers indicates that restraining influences in living humans cease with death."[2] Fiorito injected one group of guinea pigs with *E. coli* from cadavers. The bacteria were 100% lethal in 9 to 55 hours. In a second group innoculated with *E. coli* from living humans, some guinea pigs survived completely and none lived less than 9 days. As is most often the case in recent articles, the article by Carpenter and Wilkins, Autopsy Bacteriology: Review of 2,033 Cases,[3] takes for granted the proposition that bacteria live in cadaver. If infectious organisms die with the host, the phrase "autopsy bacteriology" would have no meaning. In this article, the researchers show that length of postmortem and number of bacteriological organisms were positively correlated. That is, the longer the dead body is untreated, the higher the bacteria count.

In a study by J. Putnoky,[4] it was discovered that 68.5% of a sample of 400 cadavers "had bacteria in their internal organs." An article entitled Growth Conditions for Pathogenic Organisms in Dead Tissues[5] lists dermatomycetes, trichophyton fungi, *Anchorion quinckeana,* staphylococci, and *B. anthracis* as a few of the many organisms that linger on after death of the host. Vincenzo Mario Palmieri[6] has determined the life span of many organisms in dead, untreated tissue. For example, tetanus lives 234 days and typhus, 90 days. The supply of such articles is unending. Five others[7–11] are listed in the References.

Up to this point, we have mentioned only articles documenting the life of infectious organisms, in general, after the death of the host. There is an abundance of scientific literature which deals with specific infectious organisms and demonstrates their ability to survive in dead tissue. Perhaps the greatest number of articles have been written on tuberculosis. In The

Dissemination of Tubercle Bacilli from Fresh Autopsy Material,[12] Ruell A. Sloan concludes: "First, methods of examination which make use of a compression technique contaminate the atmosphere in the vicinity of the autopsy. Second, within the limitations of this study, fresh tuberculosis lungs are decidedly dangerous and are a potent source of atmospheric contamination against which methods of proper protection should be devised."

A statement from a paper by Hans Popper and colleagues[13] is rather convincing: "Blood from living tuberculosis patients gave no conclusive results in culturing tuberculosis bacilli. That is, the tests failed to prove the existence of bacillemia. Yet 85–90% of blood samples, arterial and venous, from tubercular cadavers yielded viable cultures after miliary or pulmonary tuberculosis." We have found a great number of additional papers dealing with tuberculosis in dead tissue.[14–21]

Studies of tuberculosis, while numerous, are by no means the only such studies of disease existing in a dead host. A. Tjoschkoff and others, in Further Studies of the Causes of Easy Infection During the Postmortem Examinations of Septic Cadavers,[22] concentrate on the problem caused by staph and strep in these circumstances. We learn, "staphylococci multiply 10–100 times and even more in the blood and tissues of corpses kept at room temperatures." They maintain that the danger is compounded by the fact that after death "there is an increase not only in the number of microbe cells," but also "of their virulence (infectious potency) and to an exceptionally high degree." In a paper by Erich Hoffman[23] we find, "the dangerous teaching that syphilis cannot be transmitted from cadavers to autopsy workers is refuted." Among 38 previous case histories, such transmission was proved in 20 and was probable in 14. In cases involving animal cadavers known to be infected with *B. anthracis,* P. Begnescu[24] has found, "Burial in animal cemeteries and throwing into dry wells do not suffice." Rather than fill this report with quotation after quotation other articles on this subject will simply be listed in the References.[25–28]

SUMMARY

In the light of several references cited here, it seems that there is no sound, scientific basis for the "germ dies with the host" theory. Secondly, we have established the fact that these infectious organisms can be spread by physical contact or may be airborne. Laboratory studies indicate that compounds such as aldehydes, phenols, alcohols, etc., are effective disinfectants and preservatives. Since these compounds and similar ones are incorporated in modern embalming formulations, it can be predicted that such chemicals, when injected and used according to present-day embalming techniques, will also be effective in killing and reducing bacterial flora.

REFERENCES

1. Langmuir AD. Airborne infection: How important for public health? *Am J Public Health* 1964; 54(10):1666–1668.
2. Fiorito G. Virulence of some organisms in cadavers. *Riforma Med* 1924;40:270–273.
3. Carpenter HM, Wilkins RM. Autopsy bacteriology: Review of 2,033 cases. *Arch Pathol* 1964;77:73–81.
4. Putnoky J. Bacteriological test results from 400 autopsies. *Zentralbl Bakteriol Parasitenkunde Infectionskrankheiten Hyg* 1932;126:248–252.
5. Truffi G. Growth conditions for pathogenic organisms in dead tissues. *G. Ital Dermatol Sifilol* 1932; 73:839–857.
6. Palmieri YM. Resistance of pathogenic organisms to putrefaction and biological reactions in cadavers. *Rasseqna Int Clin Ter* 1930;11:648–653.
7. Wood WH, Oldstone M, Schultz RB. A re-evaluation of blood culture as an autopsy procedure. *Am J Clin Pathol* 1965;43(43):241–247.
8. Branch A, Lo M. Occurrence of bacteremia in one hundred consecutive autopsy cases. *Med Services J Canada* 1964;20:232–234.
9. Sulkin ES, Pike RM. Survey of laboratory acquired infections. *Am J Public Health* 1951;41(7):769–781.
10. Hunt HF, et al. A bacteriologic study of 567 postmortem examinations. *J Lab Clin Med* 1929; 14(10):907–912.
11. Epstein EZ, Kugel MA. The significance of postmortem examination. *J Infect Dis* 1929;44:327–334.
12. Sloan RA. The dissemination of tubercle bacilli from fresh autopsy material. *NY State J Med* 1942;42:133–134.
13. Popper H, et al. Culturing tuberculosis bacilli from cadaver blood. *Virchow's Arch Pathol Anat Physiol Klin Med* 1932;285:789–802.
14. Reid DD. Incidence of tuberculosis among workers in medical laboratories. *Br Med J* 1957;July:10–14.
15. Morris SI. Tuberculosis as an occupational hazard during medical training. *Am Rev Tuberculosis* 1946;54:140–158.
16. Woringer F. Dissection tuberculosis in an autopsy orderly, a case of pulmonary bacillosis. *Bull Soc Fr Dermatol Syphilogr* 1933;40:204–206.
17. Hein J. Tubercles in cadavers and autopsy lesions followed by general tubercular infection. *Beitrage Klin Tuberkulose* 1933;82:682–696.
18. Neuhaus C. Culturing tubercle bacilli from ca-

davers. *Zentralbl Allg Pathol Pathol Anat* 1928; 42:337–344.
19. Purrman W. Tuberculosis as an occupational disease. *Dtsch Gesundheit* 1964;19:2389–2390.
20. Hedvall E. The incidence of tuberculosis among students at Lund University. *Am Rev Tuberculosis* 1940;41:770–780.
21. Alderson HE. Tuberculosis from direct inoculation with autopsy knife. *Arch Dermatol Syphilol* 1931;24:98–100.
22. Tjoschkoff A, et al. Further studies of the causes of easy infection during the postmortem examinations of septic cadavers. *Dokl Bolq Akad Nauk Tome* 1965;18(2):179–181.
23. Hoffman E. Occupational syphilitic infection from cadavers. *Dermatol Wochenschr* 1929;88:284–286.
24. Begnescu P. Local excharizing in combating zoonoses microbiologia. *Parazitol Epidemiol* 1964; 9(1):73.
25. Weilbaecher JO, Moss ES. Tularemia following injury while performing postmortem examination on human case. *J Lab Clin Med* 1938;24:34–38.
26. Zurhelle E, Stempil R. Studies on viability & virulence retention in *Spirochaeta pallida* in dead tissue. *Arch Dermatol Syphilis* 1927;153:219–266.
27. Mgaloblischwili P. Syphilis infection from cadavers. *Dermatol Z* 1927;51:167–189.
28. Balbi E. Development of pathogenic bacteria in dead tissue. *Pathologica* 1931;23:351–354.

Dangers of Infection*

Leandro Rendon
Director of Research and Educational Programs, Champion Chemical Company, Springfield, Ohio.

The possibility of acquiring disease as the result of handling and caring for human remains is very real and is of concern to funeral licensees. Unfortunately, there are those who do not seem to be aware of the potential risks involved or who do not seem to believe such danger exists or that it is even possible. Such individuals, in and out of funeral service, seem to minimize the existence of disease-producing organisms in dead human remains.

At the Continuing Education program sponsored April 18, 1980, by the faculty of San Antonio College, San Antonio, Texas, Dr. Kendall O. Smith, Professor of Microbiology, University of Texas Health Science Center at San Antonio, was one of the participants. He presented information about some of the biological hazards that should be of concern to the funeral licensee. The following discussion is based on some of the information presented by Dr. Smith. It is hoped this discussion serves to further stress the potential dangers of infection that the licensee does encounter in his or her work and the need, therefore, to follow prescribed hygienic practices and certain procedures of disinfection and decontamination to protect himself or herself against infection.

The most often reported infections associated with handling of human remains are tuberculosis and infectious hepatitis. In the survey among funeral licensees made by this Department some time ago, of those who sustained one or more infections, about 14% said they had contracted tuberculosis and 12.7%, infectious hepatitis. The medical literature makes reference to similar and other incidences of infection (*Proc Roy Soc Med* 1973:66;25).

Causes of death in cancer patients for the year 1970 were studied in New York (*J Med* 1975;6:61) at a hospital on the basis of clinical and pathology reports of 506 cases. The single major cause of death was infection (36%), which also was a contributory factor in an additional 68% of the cases. The organisms causing the infection were mostly gram-negative, antibiotic-resistant bacteria. Other important causes of death were hemorrhagic and thromboembolic phenomena (18%) which also were contributory factors in an additional 43%.

In a study performed by personnel of the M. D. Anderson Hospital and Tumor Institute, Houston, Texas (*Am J Med Sci* 1974;268:97), the causes of death in patients with malignant lymphoma were reviewed. The records of some 206 patients over an 8-year period were used for the report. The commonest cause of death in those patients was infection which accounted for 51% of the deaths. These infections were primarily caused by gram-negative bacilli.

Toxoplasmosis is a disease caused by infection with the protozoan *Toxoplasma.* In infants and children, the disease usually is characterized by an encephalomyelitis. In adults, a form clinically resembling a spotted fever has been reported.

Five patients with lethal disseminated toxoplasmosis were seen within a 2-year period at the Swedish Hospital Medical Center and the University of Washington Hospital (*Arch Intern Med* 1974;134:1059). In all patients, there was a severe underlying disease treated with various chemotherapeutic agents, corticosteroids,

* Reprinted from the *Expanding Encyclopedia,* No. 508. Springfield, OH: Champion Chemical Co.; 1980, with permission.

splenectomy, or irradiation. Although the clinical symptoms were variable and masked by the underlying illness, therapeutic measures, or concomitant infectious processes, or both, the autopsy findings were strikingly uniform in that the brain, myocardium, and lungs were invariably affected. Reports in the literature and the experience of the investigators indicate that disseminated toxoplasmosis in compromised hosts is being recognized with increasing frequency.

One episode has been reported (*JAMA* 1967; 202:284) in which toxoplasmosis was transmitted during postmortem examination. The occurrence of lymphadenitis in human toxoplasmosis is well recorded. However, the mode of transmission and time course of the disease remain far from clear.

Most of the knowledge of acquired toxoplasmosis is based on infections in laboratory workers and on occasional cases of accidental inoculation. A case is recorded where a pathologist became acutely ill with toxoplasmosis 2 *months* after the autopsy of a patient who died with Hodgkins's disease and toxoplasmic ventriculitis.

Personnel from the National Institute of Neurological Diseases and Stroke, National Institutes of Health, call attention to another type of potential infection (*J Neurosurg* 1974;41:394). Precautions are mentioned in conducting biopsies and autopsies on patients with pre-senile dementia.

The report mentions that such patients may have Creutzfeldt–Jakob disease, a disease transmissible by a virus likely to be extremely resistant to inactivation. It is recommended:

1. That instruments used in any surgical or autopsy procedures on patients with presenile dementia be autoclaved for at least 30 minutes
2. That all organs, including those fixed in formalin, be treated as infectious materials
3. That floors and other surfaces in contact with tissues from such patients be decontaminated with a solution known to inactivate the scrapie agent, for instance, 0.5% NaOCl solution. The fact that the agent is susceptible to sodium hypochlorite but not to the well-known disinfectants tells us something about the newly emerging pathogens that seemingly are highly resistant to the commonly used chemical sterilants.

The literature references many instances of cross-infections among patients in hospitals. The May 1980 issue (No. 507) of this *Encyclopedia* alludes to infections of this type among hospitalized populations. A typical situation found in the literature is the following case. Serological evidence of cross-infection in a dialysis unit hepatitis B epidemic has been reported (*Kidney Int* 1974;6:118).

It is of interest to call this report to the attention of the reader because it points to the ease with which personnel can acquire infections. If this can happen in a hospital, consider the possibility of such occurrence in the preparation room while handling the remains of individuals who have been in a dialysis unit. There were 74 patients and staff who developed HB-Ag-positive hepatitis during a 28-month surveillance period. Twenty-six (26) of these cases were intimately related to the dialysis unit (21 dialysis/transplant patients and 5 hospital staff) and 48 were not. Representative sera from each group of cases were further tested for HB-Ag subtype specificity. Thirteen (13) of fourteen (14) dialysis/transplant patients had subtype *ay* whereas 10 of 15 general hospital patients had the alternate pheonotype *ad.*

All four staff individuals who had probably acquired their infection from dialysis/transplant patients were *ay* subtype. Eight of the dialysis/transplant patients had never received blood. Transfusion rate in the infected dialysis patients was one third that of leukemic patients but the hepatitis rate was higher. The bacteriological procedures are mentioned in detail simply to illustrate the thoroughness of establishing proof of cross-contamination. There is little doubt as to the source of the infection.

An interesting incident is found in the literature (*Am J Clin Pathol* 1969;51:260) that should be of pertinent interest to funeral licensees—tubercular infection. Inoculation tuberculosis of the skin, occurring in physicians and medical students engaged in performing postmortem examinations, has been referred to by a variety of names among which "prosector's wart" appears to be a particularly appropriate term. A medical student–prosector developed typical primary cutaneous tuberculosis of the hand despite having practiced most currently accepted precautionary methods in performing an autopsy on a patient who had harbored active turberculosis. The nature of the infection was established by culture as well as by demonstration of acid-fast bacilli in the surgically excised lesion of the hand.

In a study to establish the incidence of tuberculosis among workers in medical laboratories, an investigator (*Br Med J* 1957;5035:10–14) at the London School of Hygiene and Tropical Medicine made a survey among personnel of the National Health Service and the Public Health Laboratory Service. There was a large number of incidences of infection among individuals employed in laboratory and mortuary tasks which exposed them to the risk of contact with infected pathological material. The incidence was highest in the second and third years of such employment.

Tuberculosis as an occupational disease among workers in pathology institutes is the subject of a report from West Germany (*Dtsch Gesundheit* 1964; 19:2389–2390). Incidence of tuberculosis among pathologists was found to be 20-fold greater in one study, and 25-fold greater in another, than in the general population.

Investigators in Europe (*Dokl Bolg Akad Nauk* 1965;18:179–181) have shown that streptococci and staphylococci multiply 10–100 times and even more in the blood and tissues of corpses kept at room temperatures. Additional investigations have also shown that there is an increase not only of the number of septicemic agents (Pasteurellae, the erysipelosis, and *Bact. pyocyaneum*), but also in their virulence. The virulence of the strains isolated from dead remains held at room temperatures rises immediately after death and reaches maximum at the 5th to the 7th hours for the streptococci and the 10th to the 12th hours for the staphylococci after which it may gradually decrease.

The newly emerging pathogens that are frequently arriving on the scene seem to be "unconventional" types. They are difficult to isolate in some cases and present problems in classification. Some seem to be able to change their structure, i.e., mutate, and thereby become resistant to commonly used drugs.

Often, infections are acquired and the host is unaware of the infection. The organisms may not indicate their presence for days, weeks, months, and even years. As can be seen from the very brief overview of the literature, there is ample scientific evidence for the need to practice effective measures in the preparation room to reduce, as much as possible, the risk factors of such an environment.

Creutzfeldt-Jakob Disease*

Edward C. Johnson and Melissa Johnson

Recently, the media in the United States and Britain have been reporting almost daily on "Mad Cow Disease." The reports were prompted by two new cases of Creutzfeldt-Jakob Disease (CJD) diagnosed in adolescents and the recent disclosure that four dairy farmers died from CJD in the past three years.

There is a suspected connection between CJD in humans and Mad Cow Disease. CJD is a concern for embalmers, because it resists the most common forms of disinfection and because so little is known about the modes of transmission. In 1993, a medical journal reported that at least 24 health care workers have contacted CJD, or their diagnosis is highly suspicious for it.[1]

The first part of this article will discuss the medical and scientific literature regarding Creutzfeldt-Jakob Disease, and the second part will look at the implications for the embalmer.

In the overall incidence of CJD, the two new cases of the disease and the four deaths in the past three years are not overwhelming numbers of new cases. About 0.5 to 1 new case per 1 million population can be expected in a one-year period. The usual onset of CJD is between 60 and 70 years, and onset before age 30 is rare. However, the age of these recent patients is younger and hence a greater reason for concern than in the past.

Creutzfeldt-Jakob Disease was first observed in the 1920s. It is described as a rare, rapidly fatal (one estimate is that 90% of those with the disease will die within one year of its diagnosis) neurologically degenerative disease probably with a long onset.

TECHNICAL PLAN

Our experience has indicated that there is no technical difference between preparation of a deceased from CJD and one from a non-contagious disease.

- **Thorough washing**
- **Disinfect orifices**
- **Set features in customary manner**
- **Selection of vessels for injection/drainage is up to embalmer**
- **Normal fluid dilutions used**
- **Normal cavity aspiration**
- **Incision closed in usual manner**

Many of its symptoms appear similar to Alzheimer's disease and other degenerative neurological disorders.[2] Scientists in the United States and United Kingdom have for several decades been looking into the cause of this disease.

There is still a debate in the medical community as to the correct pathological designation of CJD. Although some have called it a virus, it is an unconventional virus because of its lack of nucleic acid. Many scientists include CJD in a family of diseases called prions, designated for both humans and animals. Prions are defined as small biological entities with at least one protein, but no demonstrable acids.[3]

Prions cause "spongiform encephalopathy" in both humans and animals. In humans it can cause

* Reprinted from *The American Funeral Director*, Vol. 119, No. 7, Iselin, NJ : Kates-Boylston Publications, Inc..; 1996, with permission.

CJD, kuru, fatal familial insomnia, and Gertsmann-Straussler-Scheiner disease. Similar diseases in animals include scrapie in sheep, bovine spongiform encephalopathy (Mad Cow Disease), and feline and mink encephalopathy.

There are three types of CJD: sporadic, iatrogenic, and familial. Sporadic CJD is designated as such because there is no ability to identify a causal event. These patients have no family history of CJD, nor do they have any other risk factors for exposure.

Iatrogenic CJD ("iatrogenic" is the medical term for "therapeutic misadventure" or any medical/surgical treatment that results in an unfavorable response) is found in patients who have had cornea transplants, human pituitary growth factor treatments, neurosurgical procedures, cadaveric dura mater homografts, and occupational exposure (dairy farmers, pathologists, histopathology technicians, etc.).

Included in this group of iatrogenic CJD patients are health care workers who have been diagnosed with CJD.[5]

An aberrant chromosome 20 is believed to cause familial CJD and is responsible for about 15% of the diagnosed cases.

No laboratory tests are diagnostic for CJD. Magnetic resonance imaging of the brains of CJD patients reveals degenerative changes normal in older patients.[6] The most reliable method of diagnosing CJD prior to death is a brain biopsy. Biopsy specimens show the small "sponge" appearing vacuoles along with degenerative and cerebral atrophy.[4, 7, 8]

Initial symptoms include memory loss, noncoordination of extremities, spastic weakness, drowsiness, irritability, unusual behavior, visual and auditory hallucinations, and other neurological symptoms.[2, 4, 7, 8]

How does "Mad Cow Disease" fit into the picture? Scientists are not sure. For a human to become infected with an "animal disease." the infecting agent has to be able to cross certain species boundaries and the "human" has to be susceptible.

From 1963 to 1993, the National Institutes of Health conducted experiments to determine whether trans-species infection could occur. These experiments consisted of inoculating a variety of laboratory animals (a total of 3,418 were inoculated) with different types (and levels of infectivity) of autopsy-proven spongiform encephalopathies from the brains of deceased humans (a total of 1,113).

In 300 cases, these scientists were able successfully to transmit a spongiform encephalopathy to a laboratory animal. Inoculation was directly into the brain tissue.

The highest transmission percentage—100%—was from individuals with iatrogenic CJD. This is suggestive that this form of CJD is more virulent.

As for the theory that "Mad Cow Disease" causes CJD, there is little in the medical literature to suggest that intragastric or oral inoculation is an efficient and effective means of transmitting this virus.[6, 9, 10, 11] In fact, the only known cases of intragastric human-to-human transmission of a spongiform encephalopathy are in countries such as New Guinea and Zaire, where ritualistic cannibalism is still practiced.

All this leaves us asking the question, What implications does CJD have for embalmers?

We should consider ourselves in the category of health care workers, which means we are at risk for possible occupational transmission of the disease. Medical journal articles vary on what body organs, tissues, and secretions are capable of infectivity and to what degree.[2, 9, 13, 15]

Creutzfeldt-Jakob Disease has been found at varying levels in the brain, cerebrospinal fluid, corneas, blood, urine, lymph nodes, liver, and other organs. As embalmers, we come into contact with some or all of these during the normal course of embalming. We have become familiar with universal precautions and, it is hoped, practice them regularly.

What makes this disease so troublesome is the inability of the most common disinfectants to kill this virus. Ionizing radiation, ultraviolet light, formaldehyde, iodine, and phenol at standard disinfection recommendations do not kill this virus.[16]

Household bleach (sodium hypochlorite) at 0.5% solution for one hour will successfully render the CJD inactive. Autoclaving at 121 degrees Fahrenheit for one hour is the preferred method for instruments.[17] Where this is concerned, we need to practice rigorously infection control and universal precautions.

EMBALMING PREPARATION

In view of the limited available research data concerning the risk of transmission of CJD, it is essential to regard the embalming and handling of an individual dead of CJD as a highly communicable operation—far more so than AIDS.

Some general observations include the fact that most, if not all, cases seem to have died in a hospital and autopsies currently are infrequently performed. It is highly recommended that highest level of universal precautions be observed.

The body will in all probability be in a plastic pouch. It is suggested that as a precaution a pouch be brought along at the time of removal in the event the body is not in a pouch, or the hospital-provided pouch is torn. All gloves and other paraphernalia used during the removal should be bagged and disposed of by medical waste handling agencies.

The embalming procedure (provided by embalmers in suitably clad protective gear) should follow the normal pattern of embalming for the funeral home.

Our technical plan includes the following:

1. A thorough washing of the body/hair with a disinfectant soap.
2. The eyes, nose, mouth are thoroughly swabbed with cotton saturated in a disinfectant.
3. Setting of the features in the usual/customary manner.
4. Selection of vessels for injection/draining are left to the discretion of the embalmer. However, no medical journal articles suggest that significant enlargement of the lymph nodes of the neck preclude use of the carotid/jugular. There are two alternatives for drainage from the jugular: using the femoral vein raised at the femoral/iliac junction and not draining at all. The latter is now commonly used for persons who died from AIDS.

   If drainage is performed, it is recommended that the embalmer use a drainage tube that can be inserted into the hole at the foot end of the table for femoral drainage. If no drainage tube is used, it is recommended that the area be covered with plastic sheeting to reduce/prevent airborne contamination. Additionally, the hydroaspirator can be connected to the drainage tube and a low rate of suction applied.
5. Since formaldehyde does not kill this virus, normal embalming fluid dilutions can be used to preserve and produce a firm, clear body. Hypodermic injection of any areas not treated satisfactorily by normal arterial injection can be treated through the usual methods.
6. Normal cavity aspiration followed by up to two 16-ounce bottles of cavity fluid complete with standard embalming treatment.
7. Incisions are closed in the usual manner. The body and hair are rewashed. Lips and eyelids can be closed with a cynoacrylic glue with the hands in their final position. A massage cream is applied to the face and hands. Eight to 12 hours after embalming, the body is inspected for appearance and preservation. Reaspiration and reinjection are completed as required.

In summation, our experience has indicated that there is no technical difference between preparation of a deceased from CJD and one from a non-contagious disease.

Acknowledgment. The authors would like to thank Dr. Gregory Gruener, associate professor of neurology, at Loyola University Medical Center in Maywood, Ill, for his assistance in reviewing this manuscript for accuracy.

REFERENCES

1. Berger JR, David NJ. Creutzfeldt-Jakob Disease in a Physician: A Review of the Disorder in Health Care Workers. *Neurology* 1993;43:205–206.
2. Infections of the Nervous System, *Merritt's Textbook of Neurology*. Rowland LP, editor. Williams & Wilkins, Media, Pa., 1995.
3. *Stedman's Medical Dictionary;* 1258. Hensyl WR, editor. Williams & Wilkins, Baltimore. 25th Edition, 1990.
4. Tabrizia SJ. Creutzfeldt-Jakob Disease in a Young Woman. *Lancet* 1992;347:945–948.
5. Brown P, Preece MA, Will RG, "Friendly Fire" in Medicine: Hormones, Homografts, and Creutzfeldt-Jakob Disease. *Lancet* 1992;340:24–27.
6. Brown P. Bovine Spongiform Encephalopathy and Creutzfeldt-Jakob Disease. *British Medical Journal* 1996;312:790–791.
7. Miller DC. Creutzfeldt-Jakob Disease in Histopathology Technicians. *New England Journal of Medicine* 1985;318:853.
8. Sitwell L, Lach B, Atack E, et al. Creutzfeldt-Jakob Disease in Histopathology Technicians. *New England Journal of Medicine* 1985;318:854.
9. Brown P, Gibbs CJ, Rodgers-Johnson P, et al. Human Spongiform Encephalopathy: The National Institutes of Health Series of 300 Cases Experimentally Transmitted Disease. *Annals of Neurology* 1994; 35:315–529.
10. Ridely RM, Baker HF. Who Gets Creutzfeldt-Jakob Disease? *British Medical Journal* 1995;35:513–529.
11. Tyler KL. Risk of Human Exposure to Bovine Spongiform Encephalopathy. *British Medical Journal* 1995;311:1420–1421.
12. Prusiner SB, DeArmond SJ. Prion Diseases and Neurodegeneration. *Annual Reviews of Neuroscience* 1994;17:311–339.
13. Committee on Health Care Issues, American Neurological Association. Precautions in Handling Tissues, Fluids, and Other Contaminated Materials From Patients With Documented or Suspected Creutzfeldt-Jakob Disease. *Annals of Neurology* 1986;19:75–77.
14. Gajdusek DC. Unconventional Viruses and the Origin and Disappearance of Kuru. *Science* 1977; 197:943–960.
15. Tateoshi J. Transmission of Creutzfeldt-Jakob Disease From Human Blood and Urine Into Mice. *Lancet* 1985;2:1074.
16. Brown P, Gajdusek D, et al. Transmission of Creutzfeldt-Jakob Disease From Formalin-Fixed Paraffin-Embedded Human Brain Tissue. *New England Journal of Medicine* 1986;315:1614–1615.
17. Brown P, Gibbs C, Amyx H, et al. Chemical Disinfection of Creutzfeldt-Jakob Disease Virus. *New England Journal of Medicine* 1982;306:1279–1282.

In-Use Evaluation of Glutaraldehyde as a Preservative–Disinfectant in Embalming*

Robert N. Hockett, M.S.
Research Associate, School of Dentistry, University of Michigan, Ann Arbor, Michigan

Leandro Rendon, M.S.
Director of Research and Educational Programs, Champion Chemical Company, Springfield, Ohio

Gordon W. Rose, Ph.D.
Associate Director, Department of Mortuary Science, Wayne State University, Detroit, Michigan

INTRODUCTION

The use of formaldehyde as a disinfectant has been described by Walker,[1] Lawrence and Block,[2] and Spaulding.[3] Walker states that its commercial importance as a fungicide is probably greater than as a bactericide, and that a 4.0% solution will destroy all vegetative and many spore-forming bacteria "in less than 30 minutes."

The three "high-level" germicides described by Spaulding are 3 to 8% formaldehyde (7.5–20% formalin), 2.0% alkalinized glutaraldehyde, and gaseous ethylene oxide. He reports that in order for formaldehyde to exert a "high level of disinfection" or destruction of large numbers of bacterial and fungal spores, tubercle bacilli, and enteric viruses, including the hepatitis viruses, it should be used in a concentration of 8.0% (20% formalin). The indicated exposure time for formaldehyde (8.0%) plus alcohol (60–70%) was 12 hours in situations calling for high-demand disinfection.

The concentration of formaldehyde solution used as a preservative-disinfectant in funeral service and other areas of biologic preservation seldom exceeds 2.0% (5.0% formalin).[4] Inasmuch as 2.0% alkalinized glutaraldehyde possesses "high-level" disinfection properties equal to or surpassing those of 8.0% formaldehyde, it was decided that an in-use evaluation of glutaraldehyde as a preservative–disinfectant in the embalming of human remains should be conducted. Further, this study and similar unpublished investigations were suggested by earlier reports from pathologists that several etiologic agents of infection are recoverable from human remains embalmed with conventional formaldehyde-base chemicals. *Klebsiella pneumoniae, Haemophilus influenzae, Mycobacterium tuberculosis, Nocardia asteroides, Histoplasma capsulatum,* and other recognized pathogens were recovered from human remains embalmed for extended periods of time.[5–7]

Rubbo et al,[8] Pepper and Lieberman,[9] and Stonehill et al[10] reported that buffered aqueous solutions of glutaraldehyde may be employed without loss of effectiveness for up to 3 weeks. The consensus from available reports indicates that the most effective use-concentration of glutaraldehyde for rapid sporicidal effect, with or without alcohol, is 2.0% by weight and buffered to a pH of 7.4–8.5. Concentrations as low as 0.05% are equally effective against some vegetative bacteria. The use of 2.0% alkalinized glutaraldehyde for the sterilization of urological instruments[11] and anesthesia equipment[12] in the medical care area fulfilled many of the criteria of an "ideal" cold sterilizing agent. Also of particular interest were the reports of low toxicity for the user. No toxicity or tissue irritation were reported after extensive use. Buffered glutaraldehyde was so highly regarded as a broad-spectrum disinfectant that it was one of the three disinfectants used in the Apollo space program's post-recovery operation of the spaceships that had landed on the moon.

MATERIALS AND METHODS

A. Sampling. The microbial sampling protocol employed in this study was the same as previously reported. Additional postembalming sampling was performed to comparatively evaluate the microbial effectiveness of the test chemicals. Preembalming body fluid and tissue aspirate samples were withdrawn from test cases (human remains) that had been dead for from 6 to 11 hours. These postmortem time intervals were selected as a result of previous temporal indications that the postmortem microbial populations were in a state of exponential growth.[13]

B. Embalming Procedures

1. Injections and drainage procedures always involved multipoint selections, such as the carotid artery/jugular vein and the femoral artery/femoral vein sites.
2. The arterial "test" injection solution was administered using a moderate rate of flow (10–12 minutes to inject each gallon) and sufficient pressure (2–10 pounds) to maintain that rate of injection.

* Reprinted from abstracts of the annual meeting of the American Public Health Association, Session 449. Contributed papers: Microbiology–Immunology, November 1973.

3. After visible discolorations were removed, the intermittent and/or restricted type of drainage was used for the remainder of the operation.
4. Following arterial injection, the contents of the abdominal and thoracic cavities were chemically treated with 32 ounces of "test" cavity chemicals per cavity.

All test cases were professionally embalmed at the Wayne State University Department of Mortuary Science by a licensed member of the embalming teaching staff. Medical certifications indicated the primary cause of death to be other than an infectious disease. *All cases were evaluated and deemed completely suitable for normal funeral service viewing purposes* following completion of investigational handling.

C. Test Chemical Solutions

1. "TEST" ARTERIAL SOLUTIONS. *Solution "A"*—Prepared by diluting concentrated, commercially available, formaldehyde–glutaraldehyde products so that each gallon contained 2.0% formaldehyde and 2.0% glutaraldehyde, plus 4 ounces EDTA-base chemical water conditioner.

Solution "B"—Prepared by diluting concentrated, commercially available, formaldehyde–glutaraldehyde products so that each gallon contained 3.3% formaldehyde and 2.0% glutaraldehyde, plus 4 ounces EDTA-base chemical water conditioner.

Solution "C"—Prepared by diluting concentrated, commercially available, formaldehyde–glutaraldehyde products so that each gallon contained 2.8% formaldehyde and 2.37% glutaraldehyde, plus 4 ounces EDTA-base chemical water conditioner.

2. "TEST" CAVITY SOLUTION. Concentrated, commercially available biologic preservative–disinfectant containing 10% formaldehyde, 2.0% glutaraldehyde, and 8.5% phenol in an alcohol base.

D. Microbial Identification and Enumeration. All samples were initially diluted 1:10 in phosphate-buffered saline (PBS) and 0.1 ml of each diluted sample was impinged onto a 0.45-μm Millipore (Millipore Corp., Bedford, MA) membrane filter (MF), washed once with 10 ml of PBS and then with 10 ml of Dey–Engley universal neutralizing medium (broth) for antimicrobial chemicals.[14] The Dey–Engley antimicrobial neutralizer contains chemicals selective for the neutralization of formaldehyde and glutaraldehyde. A 6-place manifold with sterile funnels and accessory items (Millipore) was utilized throughout the study to standardize sample handling and microbial quantitation. The MFs, with impinged, washed, and neutralized samples, were rolled onto primary isolation media (MacConkey and Blood Agar plates) and incubated at 35–37°C for 24 to 48 hours. Colonial isolates were subcultured and characterized by pertinent methods.[15] The gram-negative and the gram-positive aerobic and facultatively aerobic "indicator" isolates were previously reported by Rose and Hockett.[13]

RESULTS

In test cases II, IV, and V, the quantitative postembalming reduction of microbial densities exceeded 95% within 20 to 24 hours (Table 4). The total volume of arterial injection solution used in these three test cases was 3.5 to 4.0 gallons. In test case 1 *only 2 gallons* of arterial injection solution were used and the microbial populations increased progressively throughout the postembalming sampling period of 22 hours. This indicated to the investigators that both the volume of solution and the concentration of active ingredients employed were insufficient. While tissue fixation in terms of normal in-state preparation and appearance was adequate, the microbial effects were unsatisfactory.

In case III, no microbial agents were recoverable

TABLE 4. MICROBICIDAL EFFECTS OF "TEST" EMBALMING SOLUTIONS

Case No.	Body Weight (lbs)	Interval Between Death and Embalming (hr)	Injection Solution		Microbial Densities[b]		Percent Reduction
			Type[a]	*Volume (gal)*	*Preembalming*	*Postembalming*	
I	180	8	A	2.0	1,000	10,000–100,000	Densities inc.[c]
II	90	11	B	4.0	100,000–1,000,000	0–100	> 95
III	105	8	C	4.0	0	0	No change[c]
IV	160	6	C	4.0	1,000–10,000	0–400	> 95
V	150	10	C	3.5	100,000–1,000,000	0–50	> 95

[a]See "Test" chemicals.
[b]Average, all sampling sites.
[c]See text (Results section).

from the unembalmed body. The investigators believe that the extensive antemortem administration of therapeutic antimicrobial agents was responsible for the negative baseline or control densities. It is interesting to note, however, that throughout the postembalming period of 25 hours there was no evidence of microbial colonization or recolonization from exogenous or other sources. The embalming chemicals effectively prevented the possible resumption of microbial growth and proliferation.

The volume of arterial injection solution and the concentrations of active arterial and cavity chemical ingredients used in cases II, IV, and V produced irreversible or cidal reductions of the control or preembalming microbial densities.

DISCUSSION

While internal anatomic sterilization may be neither chemically achievable nor environmentally necessary, the postembalming production of a nonhazardous index of hygienic safety is a reasonable and essential public health expectation of modern embalming chemistry and techniques. The investigators feel that the microbial inactivation properties of embalming chemicals should assure an 80% or greater reduction in the postmortem microbial flora. Such a reduction would help to reduce the possible transmission of infectious doses of microbial agents within a variety of environments associated with the presence of embalmed human remains. These environments might well include areas or sites of earth interment, above-ground facilities such as mausoleums and storage or receiving vaults, refrigerated and nonrefrigerated storage facilities in medical and paramedical science programs, schools of funeral service education, and funeral homes. It is reasonable to expect that the postembalming microbial survivors or persisters might exit via one or more of the body orifices and contaminate environmental surfaces adjacent to the temporary or permanent location of the embalmed human remains.

The investigators concluded that the use of arterial and cavity chemicals containing an in-use concentration of 2.0% alkalinized glutaraldehyde in conjunction with formaldehyde and/or formaldehyde derivatives will effectively accomplish both the preservation and the disinfection functions of embalming.

ACKNOWLEDGMENT

Support for this study was provided by the Champion Company, Springfield, Ohio. The commercial products employed in the study were PLX, FAX, Di-San, and Searine compounded by the Champion Company.

REFERENCES

1. Walker JF. *Formaldehyde.* 3rd ed. American Chemical Society Monograph Series. New York: Reinhold 1964.
2. Lawrence CA, Block SS. *Disinfection, Sterilization and Preservation.* Philadelphia: Lea & Febiger; 1968.
3. Spaulding EH. Role of chemical disinfection in the prevention of nosocomial infections. In: *Proceedings of the International Conference on Nosocomial Infections.* Atlanta: Centers for Disease Control; August 1970.
4. Pervier NC. *Textbook of Chemistry for Embalmers.* rev. ed. Minneapolis: University of Minnesota Bookstores; 1956:131.
5. Meade GM, Steenken W. Viability of tubercle bacilli in embalmed human lung tissue. *Am Rev Tuberculosis* 1949;59:429.
6. Weed LA, Baggerstoss AH. The isolation of pathogens from tissues of embalmed human bodies. *Am J Clin Pathol* 1951;21:1114.
7. Weed LA, Baggerstoss AH. The isolation of pathogens from embalmed tissues. *Proc Soc Mayo Clin* 1952;27:124.
8. Rubbo S, Gardner J, Webb R. Biocidal activities of glutaraldehyde and related compounds. *J Appl Bacteriol* 1967;30(1):78–87.
9. Pepper R, Lieberman E. Dialdehyde alcoholic sporicidal composition. U.S. Patent 3,016,328 to Ethicon, Inc., 1962.
10. Stonehill A, Krop S, Borick P. Buffered glutaraldehyde—A new chemical sterilizing solution. *Am J Hosp Pharm.* 1963;20:458–465.
11. O'Brien HA, Mitchell JD, Haberman S, Rowan DF, Winford TE, Pellet J. The use of activated glutaraldehyde as a cold sterilizing agent for urological instruments. *J Urol* 1966;95.
12. Haselhuhn DH, Brason FW, Borick PM. "In use" study of buffered glutaraldehyde for cold sterilization of anesthesia equipment. *Anesth Analg Curr Res* 1967;46.
13. Rose GW, Hockett RN. The microbiologic evaluation and enumeration of postmortem specimens from human remains. *Health Lab Sci* 1971;8:75–78.
14. Engley FB, Dey BP. A universal neutralizing medium for antimicrobial chemicals. In: *Proceedings of the 56th Mid-year Meeting, Chemical Specialities Manufacturers Association,* May 1970.
15. Blair JF, Lennette EH, Truant JP. *Manual of Clinical Microbiology.* Bethesda, MD: American Society for Microbiology; 1970.

The Antimicrobial Activity of Embalming Chemicals and Topical Disinfectants on the Microbial Flora of Human Remains*

Peter A. Burke and A.L. Sheffner
Department of Microbiology, Foster D. Snell, Inc.,
Florham Park, New Jersey

The antimicrobial activity of embalming chemicals and topical disinfectants was evaluated to determine the degree of disinfection achieved during the embalming of human remains. The administration of arterial and cavity embalming chemicals resulted in a 99% reduction of the postmortem microbial population after 2 hours of contact. This level of disinfection was maintained for the 24-hour test period. Topical disinfection of the body orifices was also observed. Therefore, it is probable that present embalming practices reduce the hazard from transmission of potentially infectious microbial agents within the immediate environment of embalmed human remains.

INTRODUCTION

For many years embalming chemicals have been utilized to preserve and disinfect biological tissues for anatomical studies, environmental storage, and hygienic safety. The majority of these embalming chemicals are formaldehyde-based products, whose disinfectant properties have been described by Walker,[1] Lawrence and Block,[2] and Spaulding.[3] It has been reported that pathogenic organisms, such as *K. pneumoniae, H. influenzae, M. tuberculosis,* and *H. capsulatum,* are recoverable from embalmed human remains.[4–6] Thus, conceivably, infection could occur from contact with postembalming microbial fluids and swabs of areas around orifices from cadavers to determine if commercially available embalming chemicals produce a significant reduction in the microbial flora.

MATERIALS AND METHODS

Samples of biological fluids and swabs of the area around orifices were taken from eight cadavers to determine the antimicrobial activity of embalming fluids in vivo as a function of time. Four of the bodies were embalmed while the other four cadavers were not and served as controls. The primary cause of death of the subjects was diagnosed to be other than an infectious disease (i.e., coronary thrombosis, cerebrovascular accident, arteriosclerosis).

Embalming Procedure. The bodies were embalmed by a professional licensed mortician using the following procedure: The body was washed with an antiseptic soap containing 0.75% hexachlorophene and thoroughly rinsed. The cadaver was sprayed with a topical embalming disinfectant and the orifices swabbed with the same disinfectant. This disinfectant was a solution of 1.0% (w/v) formaldehyde and 0.5% (w/v) quaternary ammonium compounds in a base of isopropanol and ethylene dichloride.

Prior to dilution of the arterial embalming chemical, the tap water was treated with a water conditioning mixture formulated specifically for embalming use. This conditioner is a complexing agent that removes chemical constituents found in municipal water supplies which could interfere with the preservative and disinfecting properties of the arterial solutions. This conditioner is basically a mixture of trisodium ethylenediaminetetraacetate and polyvinylpyrrolidone in a base of various glycols.

The arterial embalming chemical consisted of 29.8% (w/v) formaldehyde, 3.8% (w/v) anionic detergents, 4.0% (w/v) borate and germicides, 9.6% (w/v) alcohol, and various inert ingredients in a water base. The arterial embalming chemical was then diluted 6 ounces to a half gallon of water. An equal amount of coinjection chemical for the purpose of stimulating drainage and inducing penetration was added to the solution. This chemical consisted of 8.9% (w/v) chelating agents, 0.1% (w/v) reducing agents, 0.7% (w/v) preservatives, 2.0% (w/v) plasticizers, 9.9% (w/v) humectants, and various inert ingredients in a water base.

The total amount of solution injected into the body was approximately 2 to $3\frac{1}{2}$ gallons, depending on the body size and weight. Two pints of cavity embalming chemical (24–28% [w/v] formaldehyde) were injected into each subject, one into the thoracic cavity and the other into the abdominal cavity. All products used in the study were commercially available embalming chemicals.

Sample Collection. Samples were drawn from superior and inferior anatomical sites, with sterile 18-gauge needles and 30-ml syringes. Needle puncture sites were topically disinfected with 95% ethanol. Swab samples were taken with sterile polyester swabs which just prior to swabbing were immersed in sterile phosphate-buffered saline.* Biological fluids and swab cultures were taken from the following areas:

* Reprinted from *Health Lab Sci* 1976;13(2):267–270, with permission from the American Public Health Association.

* Phosphate-buffered saline prepared by diluting 0.25 M phosphate buffer 1/1000 in physiological saline (0.9% NaCl).

FLUID SAMPLES

- **Lung:** The needle was inserted 3 inches to the right of the midline, through the fifth intercostal space. Pulmonary fluids or aspirates were extracted from the middle lobe of the right lung.
- **Heart blood:** The needle was inserted 1 inch to the left of the midline, through the fifth intercostal space.
- **Descending colon:** A longitudinal incision 3 inches long was made midway between the tip to the 12th rib and the anterior iliac spine; the descending colon was identified and the fecal extracted from the lumen of the colon.
- **Urinary bladder:** The needle was inserted through the external urethral orifice and the urine extracted from the lumen of the bladder.

Dehydrated or coagulated sample sites were injected with sterile phosphate-buffered saline.

Swabs of Orifices

- **Oral cavity:** Samples were taken from the buccal furrow between the mucous membrane of the upper lip and the gingiva.
- **Nasal cavity:** Swabs were made from the vestibule of the left half of the nasal cavity.
- **Anus:** Swabs were taken from the terminal inch of the anal canal.

Immediately after taking samples, the swabs were placed in Stuart's transport medium.

Samples were taken prior to embalming and then 2, 4, 8, and 24 h after embalming. The bodies were covered with plastic sheeting while sampling procedure was not in process. All samples were packed in dry ice during transportation to the laboratories of Foster D. Snell, Inc., where they were immediately plated.

Quantitative Measurement of Microbiological Flora. Immediately following receipt in the laboratory, the biological fluids were serially diluted in thiotone peptone water blanks and subsequently plated on MacConkey and Heart Infusion Agar with 5% defribrinated sheep blood. Into both agar preparations, 0.5% Tween-80 and 0.1% lecithin were incorporated to neutralize residual microbial activity from the embalming fluids. The plates were incubated at 35–37°C for 48 h following which a colony count was performed.

Microbial Identification. Isolates were identified using standard morphological and biochemical tests with the general outline utilized for identification as defined in *Bergey's Manual of Determinative Bacteriology,* eighth edition,[7] and Skerman's *Identification of the Genera of Bacteria,* second edition.[8]

TABLE 5. ANTIMICROBIAL ACTIVITY OF EMBALMING CHEMICALS AND TOPICAL DISINFECTANTS ON MICROFLORA OF HUMAN REMAINS

Treatment	Anatomical Site	Pre-embalming	Treatment Period (hours) 2	4	8	24	% Reduction After 24 Hours
			Mean Microbial Poulations[a]				
Embalmed	Heart	8.0×10^5	1.8×10^2	1.6×10^2	2.0×10^2	70	> 99%
Embalmed	Lung	2.5×10^1	< 10	< 10	< 10	< 10	> 99%
Embalmed	Colon	7.4×10^1	80	< 10	< 10	< 10	> 99%
Embalmed	Bladder	1.3×10^5	3.8×10^2	< 10	< 10	< 10	> 99%
Embalmed	Oral cavity	++[b]	0	0	0	0	–
Embalmed	Nasal cavity	+	0	0	+	0	–
Embalmed	Anus	+++	0	+	0	0	–
Unembalmed	Heart	2.8×10^5	7.2×10^5	7.8×10^5	7.5×10^5	9.0×10^5	–
Unembalmed	Lung	2.5×10^5	3.2×10^5	3.0×10^5	2.4×10^5	3.8×10^5	–
Unembalmed	Colon	1.5×10^6	1.6×10^6	1.7×10^6	1.5×10^6	2.2×10^6	–
Unembalmed	Bladder	2.9×10^6	2.3×10^6	2.3×10^6	2.4×10^6	2.5×10^6	–
Unembalmed	Oral cavity	+	+	+	+	+	–
Unembalmed	Nasal cavity	+	+	+	+	+	–
Unembalmed	Anus	+++	+++	++	++	+++	–

[a]Organism ml (mean of 4 subjects per group).
[b]Scale of growth from swab cultures: 0 = none, + = slight, + + = moderate, + + + = heavy.

TABLE 6. ISOLATION AND DISTRIBUTION OF MICROFLORA ASSOCIATED WITH HUMAN REMAINS: ANATOMICAL SITES

Heart	Lung	Colon	Bladder
Proteus mirabilis	*Escherichia coli*	*Escherichia coli*	*Escherichia coli*
Pseudomonas sp.	*Pseudomonas aeruginosa*	*Micrococcus* sp.	*Klebsiella aerogenes*
Staphylococcus aureus	*Staphylococcus aureus*	*Proteus mirabilis*	*Proteus vulgaris*
Staphylococcus epidermidis	*Staphylococcus epidermidis*	*Proteus vulgaris*	*Proteus morganii*
Streplococcus	*Streptococcus* sp.	*Pseudomonas aeruginosa*	*Pseudomonas aeruginosa*
Bacillus sp.	*Alcaligenes faecalis*	*Staphylococcus aureus*	*Staphylococcus aureus*
Escherichia coli		*Staphylococcus epidermidis*	*Staphylococcus epidermidis*
		Streptococcus sp.	*Bacillus* sp.
		Bacillus sp.	
		Klebsiella aerogenes	

RESULTS AND DISCUSSION

In vitro, germicidal activity of formaldehyde has been established and documented for many years.[2] However, the amount of microbiological data concerning the in vivo efficacy of embalming chemicals on human remains is scant. In the present study, formaldehyde-based embalming fluids were found to be highly active in reducing the microbial flora in human remains. The microbial population was reduced greater than 99% at every site 2 hours after embalming; with control bodies, as anticipated, a continuous microbial growth pattern was observed (Table 5). The antimicrobial action of formaldehyde-based embalming chemicals was apparently not limited or adversely affected by the proteinaceous material or other macromolecules present in the biological fluids and tissues.

Following topical disinfection of the areas around the orifices, no growth or limited growth could be detected after 24 h of exposure. Disinfection of the orifices occurred within 2 h of contact. Random positive results after disinfection, however, were seen because the bodies were not protected from the environment with the exception of a nonsterile plastic cloth.

Differential monitoring of the microbial population revealed that microorganisms translocate across anatomical barriers which during life prevent penetration and translocation. These body defenses are as follows: epithelial and mucous membrane coverings, reticuloendothelial system, blood drainer barrier.

The organisms which were isolated from the human remains are listed in Table 6.

Comparison of the microbial flora prior to and after embalming produced no pattern or general trend. Specific microbial resistance to the antimicrobial action of formaldehyde-based embalming chemicals was not observed. No pathogenic bacteria were found following embalming.

In conclusion, it was found that the use of formaldehyde-based embalming chemicals is a satisfactory disinfectant when applied as a public health measure to reduce microbial hazards when human remains are handled.

ACKNOWLEDGMENTS

We thank J. B. Christensen of the George Washington School of Medicine, Department of Anatomy, Washington, D.C., and R. Swaminathan, Foster D. Snell, Inc., for their professional assistance. This study was supported by the Embalming Chemical Manufacturers Association.

REFERENCES

1. Walker JF. *Formaldehyde.* American Chemical Society Monograph Series. 3rd ed. New York: Reinhold; 1964.
2. Lawrence CA, Block SS. *Disinfection, Sterilization, and Preservation.* Philadelphia: Lea & Febiger; 1968.
3. Spaulding EH. Role of chemical disinfection in the prevention of nosocomial infection. In: *Proceedings of the International Conference on Nosocomial Infections.* Atlanta: Centers for Disease Control; 1970.
4. Meade GM, Steenken W. Viability of tubercle bacilli in embalmed human lung tissue. *Am Rev Tuberculosis* 1949;59:429.
5. Weed LA, Baggerstoss AH. The isolation of pathogens from tissues of embalmed human bodies. *Am J Clin Pathol* 1951;21:1114.
6. Weed LA, Baggerstoss AH. The isolation of pathogens from embalmed tissues. *Proc Soc Exp Biol Med* 1952;27:124.
7. Buchanan RE, Gibbons NE (Eds). *Bergey's Manual of Determinative Bacteriology.* 7th ed. 1957.
8. Skerman VK. *Identification of the Genera of Bacteria.* 2nd ed. 1967.

The Microbiologic Evaluation and Enumeration of Postmortem Specimens from Human Remains*

Gordon W. Rose, Ph.D.
Associate Director, Department of Mortuary Science, Wayne State University, Detroit, Michigan

Robert N. Hockett, M.S.
Research Associate, School of Dentistry, University of Michigan, Ann Arbor, Michigan

Several recognized and potential pathogens, both bacterial and mycotic, were recovered consistently from body fluids and/or aspirates withdrawn from human cases certified to have died from causes other than an infectious disease. Samples were taken from 5 anatomic sites of varying postmortem time intervals. Filter membrane culture techniques were used for primary isolation and enumeration. Some isolates seemed to imitate classical growth curve indications of exponential increase at the 6–8 hr postmortem interval. Densities reached a level of 3.0–3.5 million organisms per milliliter or gram of sample at the 12–14 hr interval, the time period of maximal microbiologic translocation and proliferation. These studies indicate that unembalmed human remains are capable of contributing a multitude of infectious doses of microbial agents to a body handler, the body storage area, or to the environment adjacent to the body storage area.

INTRODUCTION

Research in postmortem microbiology is not new; Achard and Phulpin presented data on the recovery of microorganisms from human remains in 1895.[1] Sampling has generally followed the opening of body cavities.[2–4] One improvement in technique was the use of animal model systems[5] as an investigational tool. The amount of scientific data originating from this area of microbiologic investigation remains scant. The bibliography of the Embalming Chemical Manufacturers Association[6] is to be recommended for background.

The study utilized the application of the relatively new technique of membrane filtration (MF) to the qualitative and quantitative microbiological evaluation of body fluids and/or aspirates. Winn et al. reported the use of this technique in postmortem studies in 1966.[7] They described two advantages of the MF technique: (1) the MF method provides a three-dimensional approach to the cultivation of microoganisms; (2) it yields more accurate and reproducible quantitative results.

METHOD

Death certifications on all human remains sampled indicated the primary cause of death to be other than an infectious disease (e.g., coronary thrombosis, cerebrovascular accident, arteriosclerotic disease). Samples were secured from refrigerated cases over a postmortem period of 72 hr for temporal profile purposes. Samples were withdrawn from upper or superior to lower or inferior anatomic sites, with 18-gauge needles and 25-ml Luer syringes. Dehydration or coagulation of some samplings required aspirates of injected sterile phosphate-buffered saline (PBS). Topical disinfection of needle puncture sites was effected with an iodophore (Hi-Sine (R), Huntington Laboratories, Huntington, IN). The sampling needle was directed into the cisterna magna (cisterna cerebellomedullaris) at the base of the cerebellum via the foramen magnum for the withdrawal of cerebrospinal fluid. Heart blood samples were taken from the left ventricle by directing the needle to the upper border of the fifth rib just to the left of the sternum. Pulmonary fluids and/or aspirates were taken from the lungs for the third sampling. The needle was directed into the tranverse colon at the level of the umbilicus to sample the lumen contents. Finally, urinary bladder needle taps were made from a site marking the intersection of the median line and the pubic bone.

All samples were initially diluted 1:3 or 1:4 in PBS, and 0.1 ml of each diluted sample impinged on 0.45-μm MF, and then washed with 10.0 ml of PBS. The MFs with impinged organisms were rolled onto primary isolation agar plates of MacConkey, phenylethyl alcohol/blood, and chocolate blood. Aerobic incubation at 35–37°C for 24–48 hr and preliminary picking of isolates were routinely practiced. Isolates were characterized by pertinent methods.[8, 9]

RESULTS AND DISCUSSION

Table 7 lists the bacterial isolates from the five anatomical areas sampled.

The selection of sampling sites was based on anatomic considerations of the normal microbial flora associated with specific anatomic areas during life. The epithelial and mucous membrane coverings and linings

* Reprinted from *Health Lab Sci* 971;8(2), with permission from the American Public Health Association. Presented before the laboratory section at the Ninety-eighth Annual Meeting of the American Public Health Association, Houston, TX, Oct. 29, 1970.

TABLE 7. BACTERIAL ISOLATES FROM FIVE ANATOMICAL SITES

Organism	Cerebrospinal Fluid	Lung	Heart Blood	Transverse Colon	Bladder Urine
Alcaligenes faecolis	×	×		×	×
Bacillus sp.			×	×	
Corynebacterium diphtheriae[a]	×	×		×	
Escherichia coli	×	×	×	×	×
E. coli (A–D)					×
Klebsiella aerogenes	×	×	×	×	×
Micrococcus sp.	×	×	×	×	×
Proteus mirabilis			×	×	×
Proteus vulgaris				×	
Providencia				×	
Pseudomonas aeruginosa	×	×	×	×	×
Shigella flexneri		×		×	
Staphylococcus aureus	×	×	×	×	×
Staphylococcus epidermidis	×	×	×	×	×
Streptococcus (Group D)	×	×	×	×	×
Streptococcus pneumoniae		×		×	×

[a]Not a typical isolate.

are normally during life intact anatomic barriers to bacterial penetration and translocation. The reticuloendothelial system is a second nonselective barrier which helps to deter translocation during life. The blood–brain barrier is probably the last line of anatomic defense against many potential microbial invaders. The cerebrospinal fluid, a filtrate of circulating blood, maintains its biologic integrity in a closed system of circulation.

All of the selected sampling sites were easily accessible and, with the exception of the colon, yielded essentially liquid specimens. The colon contents occasionally required a presampling injection of sterile PBS. Needle penetration of the selected sites involved minimal manipulation of the body areas and permitted the rapid procurement of specimens in a state best suited for MF processing.

Thorough washing of each impinged MF reduced or removed the possible effects of specific and nonspecific inhibitors that might have been associated with the specimens. Each MF was quickly transferred to the basic group of primary isolation agars. The direct rolling of the MFs onto the agar surfaces facilitated contact between the matrix- and surface-oriented microorganisms and growth substrates.

The MF allowed the impingement of a standardized volume (0.1 ml) of diluted specimen which gave total plate colony counts that were mathematically referable to densities per milliliter or per gram of original sample. Gridded MFs improved the accuracy of

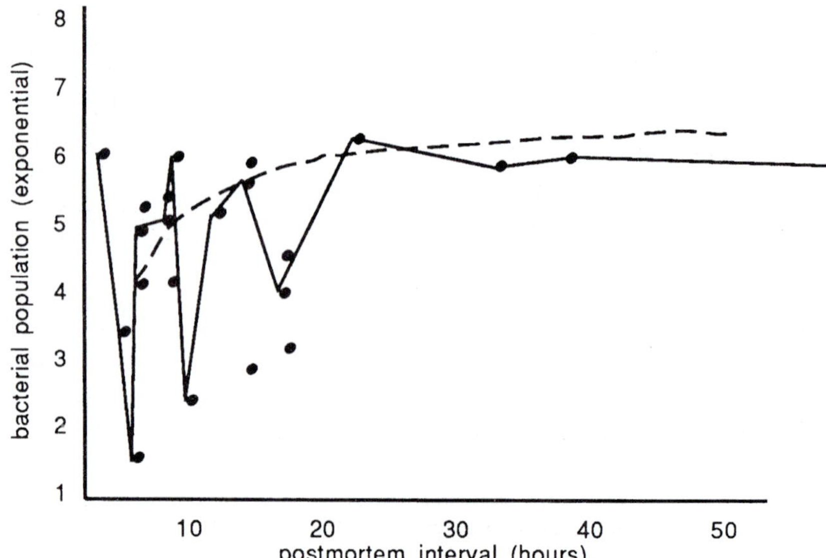

Figure 1. Bacterial population versus postmortem interval.

colony counting; plate counts in excess of 200 per plate were not recorded. Processed MFs were sterilized with ethylene oxide and stored for possible future serotaxonomic or other studies.

Bacteria *normally* associated with the transverse colon during life, with the exception of clinically opportunistic conditions, do not translocate. They are, by description of the U.S. Public Health Service Ad Hoc Committee on the Safe Shipment and Handling of Etiological Agents,[10] "Agents of no . . . [to] ordinary potential hazard." This general statement assumes a knowledge of infectious disease and immunology. There might well be logical disagreement originating from those who have attempted the treatment of infections from enteric "commensals."

The colon was chosen as the translocation reference baseline for indicator organisms isolated from other sampling sites. The brain, lung, and heart samples frequently yielded recognized pathogens in addition to the indicator commensals and opportunists. Many of the same indicator organisms were isolated from all 5 sampling sites. This is indicative of the extent to which bacteria, both pathogenic and nonpathogenic, can be translocated within a period of 6–8 hr after death.

The quantitative results (Fig. 1) of the study indicate that a postmortem multiplication of the isolates begins approximately 4 hr after death and assumes a logarithmic-like increase between 6 and 8 hr after death. The bacterial cell densities reach a peak of approximately 3 to $3\frac{1}{2}$ million organisms/ml or g of fluid or tissue within 24–30 hr after death.

Within a postmortem interval of 4–6 hr there is a body-wide redistribution of endogenous flora. Postmortem chemical changes in and manual manipulation of human remains may cause these organisms to exit from any of the body orifices and contribute contamination to adjacent environments. This places the body handlers and other personnel in or near the body storage area at higher risk.

ACKNOWLEDGMENT

Support for this study was received from the National Funeral Directors Association.

REFERENCES

1. Achard C, Phulpin E. Contribution a l'etude de l'envahissement des organes par les microbes pendant l'agonie et apres le mort. *Arch Med Expert Anat Pathol* 1895;7:25–47.
2. Burn CG. Experimental studies of postmortem bacterial invasion in animals. *J Infect Dis* 1934;54: 388–394.
3. Carpenter HM, Wilkins RM. Autopsy bacteriology: Review of 2,033 cases. *Arch Pathol* 1964;77:73–81.
4. De Jongh D, Lottis JW, Green GS, Shinely JA, Minckler TM. Postmortem bacteriology. *Am J Clin Pathol* 1968;49:424–428.
5. Burn CG. Postmortem bacteriology. *J Infect Dis* 1934;54:395–403.
6. Hinson MR. Final report on literature search on the infectious nature of dead bodies for the Embalming Chemical Manufacturers Association. Mimeo, 1968.
7. Winn WR, White ML, Carter WT, Miller AB, Finegold SM. Rapid diagnosis of bacteremia with quantitative differential membrane filtration culture. *JAMA* 1966;197:539–548.
8. Cowan ST, Steel KJ. *Manual for the Identification of Medical Bacteria.* London: Cambridge University Press; 1966.
9. Harris AH, Coleman MB. *Diagnostic Procedures and Reagents.* Washington, DC: American Public Health Association; 1963.
10. Anonymous. *Classification of Etiologic Agents on the Basis of Hazard.* Atlanta: Centers for Disease Control (U.S. DHEW, USPHS); 1970.

Recommendations for Prevention of HIV Transmission in Health-Care Settings*

INTRODUCTION

Human immunodeficiency virus (HIV), the virus that causes acquired immunodeficiency syndrome (AIDS), is transmitted through sexual contact and exposure to infected blood or blood components and perinatally from mother to neonate. HIV has been isolated from blood, semen, vaginal secretions, saliva, tears, breast milk, cerebrospinal fluid, amniotic fluid, and urine and is likely to be isolated from other body fluids, secretions, and excretions. However, epidemiologic evidence has implicated only blood, semen, vaginal secretions, and possibly breast milk in transmission.

The increasing prevalence of HIV increases the risk that health-care workers will be exposed to blood from patients infected with HIV, especially when blood and body fluid precautions are not followed for all patients. Thus, this document emphasizes the need for health-care workers to consider **all** patients as potentially infected with HIV and/or other bloodborne pathogens and to adhere rigorously to infection-

* Reprinted from *MMWR* 1987;38(25).

control precautions for minimizing the risk of exposure to blood and body fluids of all patients.

The recommendations contained in this document consolidate and update CDC recommendations published earlier for preventing HIV transmission in health-care settings; precautions for clinical and laboratory staffs[1] and precautions for health-care workers and allied professionals[2]; recommendations for preventing HIV transmission in the workplace[3] and during invasive procedures[4]; recommendations for preventing possible transmission of HIV from tears[5]; and recommendations for providing dialysis treatment for HIV-infected patients.[6] These recommendations also update portions of the "Guideline for Isolation Precautions in Hospitals"[7] and reemphasize some of the recommendations contained in "Infection Control Practices for Dentistry."[8] The recommendations contained in this document have been developed for use in health-care settings and emphasize the need to treat blood and other body fluids from **all** patients as potentially infective. These same prudent precautions also should be taken in other settings in which persons may be exposed to blood or other body fluids.

DEFINITION OF HEALTH-CARE WORKERS AND HEALTH-CARE WORKERS WITH AIDS

Health-care workers are defined as persons, including students and trainees, whose activities involve contact with patients or with blood or other body fluids from patients in a health-care setting.

As of July 10, 1987, a total of 1875 (5.8%) of 32,395 adults with AIDS, who had been reported to the CDC national surveillance system and for whom occupational information was available, reported being employed in a health-care or clinical laboratory setting. In comparison, 6.8 million persons—representing 5.6% of the U.S. labor force—were employed in health services. Of the health-care workers with AIDS, 95% have been reported to exhibit high-risk behavior; for the remaining 5%, the means of HIV acquisition was undetermined. Health-care workers with AIDS were significantly more likely than other workers to have an undetermined risk (5% versus 3% respectively). For both health-care workers and non–health-care workers with AIDS, the proportion with an undetermined risk has not increased since 1982.

AIDS patients initially reported as not belonging to recognized risk groups are investigated by state and local health departments to determine whether possible risk factors exist. Of all health-care workers with AIDS reported to CDC who were initially characterized as not having an identified risk and for whom follow-up information was available, 66% have been reclassified because risk factors were identified or because the patient was found not to meet the surveillance case definition for AIDS. Of the 87 health-care workers currently categorized as having no identifiable risk, information is incomplete on 16 (18%) because of death or refusal to be interviewed; 38 (44%) are still being investigated. The remaining 33 (38%) health-care workers were interviewed or had other follow-up information available. The occupations of these 33 were as follows: five physicians (15%), three of whom were surgeons; one dentist (3%); three nurses (9%); nine nursing assistants (27%); seven housekeeping or maintenance workers (21%); three clinical laboratory technicians (9%); one therapist (3%); and four others who did not have contact with patients (12%). Although 15 of these 33 health-care workers reported parenteral and/or other nonneedlestick exposure to blood or body fluids from patients in the 10 years preceding their diagnosis of AIDS, none of these exposures involved a patient with AIDS or known HIV infection.

RISK TO HEALTH-CARE WORKERS OF ACQUIRING HIV IN HEALTH-CARE SETTINGS

Health-care workers with documented percutaneous or mucous-membrane exposures to blood or body fluids of HIV-infected patients have been prospectively evaluated to determine the risk of infection after such exposures. As of June 30, 1987, 883 health-care workers have been tested for antibody to HIV in an ongoing surveillance project conducted by CDC.[9] Of these, 708 (80%) had percutaneous exposures to blood, and 175 (20%) had a mucous membrane or an open wound contaminated by blood or body fluid. Of 396 health-care workers, each of whom had only a convalescent-phase serum sample obtained and tested $>$ 90 days postexposure, one—for whom heterosexual transmission could not be ruled out—was seropositive for HIV antibody. For 425 additional health-care workers, both acute- and convalescent-phase serum samples were obtained and tested; none of 74 health-care workers with nonpercutaneous exposures seroconverted, and 3 (0.9%) of 351 with percutaneous exposures seroconverted. None of these 3 health-care workers had other documented risk factors for infection.

Two other prospective studies to assess the risk of nosocomial acquisition of HIV infection for health-care workers are ongoing in the United States. As of April 30, 1987, 332 health-care workers with a total of 453 needle-stick or mucous-membrane exposures to the blood or other body fluids of HIV-infected patients were tested for HIV antibody at the National Institutes of Health.[10] These exposed workers included 103 with needlestick injuries and 229 with mucous-membrane exposures; none had seroconverted. A similar study at the University of California of 129 health-care workers with documented needlestick injuries or mucous-membrane exposures to blood or other body fluids from patients with HIV infection has not identified any seroconversions.[11] Results of a prospective study in the United Kingdom identified no evidence of transmission among 150 health-care workers with parenteral or mucous-membrane exposures to blood or other body fluids, secretions, or excretions from patients with HIV infection.[12]

In addition to health-care workers enrolled in prospective studies, eight persons who provided care to infected patients and denied other risk factors have been reported to have acquired HIV infection. Three of these health-care workers had needlestick exposures to blood from infected patients.[13–15] Two were persons who provided nursing care to infected persons; although neither sustained a needlestick, both had extensive contact with blood or other body fluids, and neither observed recommended barrier precautions.[16,17] The other three were health-care workers with non-needlestick exposures to blood from infected patients.[18] Although the exact route of transmission for these last three infections is not known, all three persons had direct contact of their skin with blood from infected patients, all had skin lesions that may have been contaminated by blood, and one also had a mucous-membrane exposure.

A total of 1231 dentists and hygienists, many of whom practiced in areas with many AIDS cases, participated in a study to determine the prevalence of antibody to HIV; one dentist (0.1%) had HIV antibody. Although no exposure to a known HIV-infected person could be documented, epidemiologic investigation did not identify any other risk factor for infection. The infected dentist, who also had a history of sustaining needlestick injuries and trauma to his hands, did not routinely wear gloves when providing dental care.[19]

PRECAUTIONS TO PREVENT TRANSMISSION OF HIV (UNIVERSAL PRECAUTIONS)

Since medical history and examination cannot reliably identify all patients infected with HIV or other blood-borne pathogens, blood and body-fluid precautions should be consistently used for **all** patients. This approach, previously recommended by CDC,[3,4] and referred to as "universal blood and body-fluid precautions" or "universal precautions," should be used in the care of **all** patients, especially including those in emergency-care settings in which the risk of blood exposure is increased and the infection status of the patient is usually unknown.[20]

1. All health-care workers should routinely use appropriate barrier precautions to prevent skin and mucous-membrane exposure when contact with blood or other body fluids of any patient is anticipated. Gloves should be worn for touching blood and body fluids, mucous membranes, or nonintact skin of all patients, for handling items or surfaces soiled with blood or body fluids, and for performing venipuncture and other vascular access procedures. Gloves should be changed after contact with each patient. Masks and protective eyewear or face shields should be worn during procedures that are likely to generate droplets of blood or other body fluids to prevent exposure of mucous membranes of the mouth, nose, and eyes. Gowns or aprons should be worn during procedures that are likely to generate splashes of blood or other body fluids.
2. Hands and other skin surfaces should be washed immediately and thoroughly if contaminated with blood or other body fluids. Hands should be washed immediately after gloves are removed.
3. All health-care workers should take precautions to prevent injuries caused by needles, scalpels, and other sharp instruments or devices during procedures; when cleaning used instruments; during disposal of used needles; and when handling sharp instruments after procedures. To prevent needlestick injuries, needles should not be recapped, purposely bent or broken by hand, removed from disposable syringes, or otherwise manipulated by hand. After they are used, disposable syringes and needles, scalpel blades, and other sharp items should be placed in puncture-resistant containers for disposal; the puncture-resistant containers should be located as close as practical to the use area. Large-bore reusable needles should be placed in a puncture-resistant container for transport to the reprocessing area.
4. Although saliva has not been implicated in HIV transmission, to minimize the need for emergency mouth-to-mouth resuscitation, mouthpieces, resuscitation bags, or other ventilation devices should be available for use in areas in which the need for resuscitation is predictable.
5. Health-care workers who have exudative lesions or weeping dermatitis should refrain from all direct patient care and from handling patient-care equipment until the condition resolves.
6. Pregnant health-care workers are not known to be at greater risk of contracting HIV infection than health-care workers who are not pregnant; however, if a health-care worker develops HIV

infection during pregnancy, the infant is at risk of infection resulting from perinatal transmission. Because of this risk, pregnant health-care workers should be especially familiar with and strictly adhere to precautions to minimize the risk of HIV transmission.

Implementation of universal blood and body-fluid precautions for **all** patients eliminates the need for use of the isolation category of "Blood and Body Fluid Precautions" previously recommended by CDC[7] for patients known or suspected to be infected with bloodborne pathogens. Isolation precautions (e.g., enteric, "AFB"[7]) should be used as necessary if associated conditions, such as infectious diarrhea or tuberculosis, are diagnosed or suspected.

PRECAUTIONS FOR INVASIVE PROCEDURES

In this document, an invasive procedure is defined as surgical entry into tissues, cavities, or organs or repair of major traumatic injuries in (1) an operating or delivery room, emergency department, or outpatient setting, including both physicians' and dentists' offices; (2) cardiac catheterization and angiographic procedures; (3) a vaginal or caesarean delivery or other invasive obstetric procedure during which bleeding may occur; or (4) the manipulation, cutting, or removal of any oral or perioral tissues, including tooth structure, during which bleeding occurs or the potential for bleeding exists. The universal blood and body-fluid precautions listed above, combined with the precautions listed below, should be the minimum precautions for **all** such invasive procedures.

1. All health-care workers who participate in invasive procedures must routinely use appropriate barrier precautions to prevent skin and mucous-membrane contact with blood and other body fluids of all patients. Gloves and surgical masks must be worn for all invasive procedures. Protective eyewear or face shields should be worn for procedures that commonly result in the generation of droplets, splashing of blood or other body fluids, or the generation of bone chips. Gowns or aprons made of materials that provide an effective barrier should be worn during invasive procedures that are likely to result in the splashing of blood or other body fluids. All health-care workers who perform or assist in vaginal or caesarean deliveries should wear gloves and gowns when handling the placenta or the infant until blood and amniotic fluid have been removed from the infant's skin and should wear gloves during the postdelivery care of the umbilical cord.
2. If a glove is torn or a needlestick or other injury occurs, the glove should be removed and a new glove used as promptly as patient safety permits; the needle or instrument involved in the incident should also be removed from the sterile field.

PRECAUTIONS FOR DENTISTRY*

Blood, saliva, and gingival fluid from **all** dental patients should be considered infective. Special emphasis should be placed on the following precautions for preventing transmission of bloodborne pathogens in dental practice in both institutional and noninstitutional settings.

1. In addition to wearing gloves for contact with oral mucous membranes of all patients, all dental workers should wear surgical masks and protective eyewear or chin-length plastic face shields during dental procedures in which splashing or spattering of blood, saliva, or gingival fluids is likely. Rubber dams, high-speed evacuation, and proper patient positioning, when appropriate, should be utilized to minimize generation of droplets and spatter.
2. Handpieces should be sterilized after use with each patient, since blood, saliva, or gingival fluid of patients may be aspirated into the handpiece or waterline. Handpieces that cannot be sterilized should at least be flushed, the outside surface cleaned and wiped with a suitable chemical germicide, and then rinsed. Handpieces should be flushed at the beginning of the day and after use with each patient. Manufacturers' recommendations should be followed for use and maintenance of waterlines and check valves and for flushing of handpieces. The same precautions should be used for ultrasonic scalers and air/water syringes.
3. Blood and saliva should be thoroughly and carefully cleaned from material that has been used in the mouth (e.g., impression materials, bite registration), especially before polishing and grinding intraoral devices. Contaminated materials, impressions, and intraoral devices should also be cleaned and disinfected before being handled in the dental laboratory and before they are placed in the patient's mouth. Because of the increasing variety of dental materials

* General infection-control precautions are more specifically addressed in previous recommendations for infection-control practices for dentistry.

used intraorally, dental workers should consult with manufacturers as to the stability of specific materials when using disinfection procedures.

4. Dental equipment and surfaces that are difficult to disinfect (e.g., light handles or x-ray unit heads) and that may become contaminated should be wrapped with impervious-backed paper, aluminum foil, or clear plastic wrap. The coverings should be removed and discarded, and clean coverings should be put in place after use with each patient.

PRECAUTIONS FOR AUTOPSIES OR MORTICIANS' SERVICES

In addition to the universal blood and body-fluid precautions listed above, the following precautions should be used by persons performing postmortem procedures:

1. All persons performing or assisting in postmortem procedures should wear gloves, masks, protective eyewear, gowns, and waterproof aprons.
2. Instruments and surfaces contaminated during postmortem procedures should be decontaminated with an appropriate chemical germicide.

ENVIRONMENTAL CONSIDERATIONS FOR HIV TRANSMISSION, STERILIZATION, AND DISINFECTION

Standard sterilization and disinfection procedures for patient-care equipment currently recommended for use[25,26] in a variety of health-care settings—including hospitals, medical and dental clinics and offices, hemodialysis centers, emergency-care facilities, and long-term nursing-care facilities—are adequate to sterilize or disinfect instruments, devices, or other items contaminated with blood or other body fluids from persons infected with bloodborne pathogens including HIV.[21,23]

Instruments or devices that enter sterile tissue or the vascular system of any patient or through which blood flows should be sterilized before reuse. Devices or items that contact intact mucous membranes should be sterilized or receive high-level disinfection, a procedure that kills vegetative organisms and viruses but not necessarily large numbers of bacterial spores. Chemical germicides that are registered with the U.S. Environmental Protection Agency (EPA) as "sterilants" may be used either for sterilization or for high-level disinfection depending on contact time.

Contact lenses used in trial fittings should be disinfected after each fitting by using a hydrogen peroxide contact lens disinfecting system or, if compatible, with heat (78–80°C [172.4–176.0°F]) for 10 minutes.

Medical devices or instruments that require sterilization or disinfection should be thoroughly cleaned before being exposed to the germicide, and the manufacturer's instructions for the use of the germicide should be followed. Further, it is important that the manufacturer's specification for compatibility of the medical device with chemical germicides be closely followed. Information on specific label claims of commercial germicides can be obtained by writing to the Disinfectants Branch, Office of Pesticides, Environmental Protection Agency, 401 M Street, SW, Washington, DC 20460.

Studies have shown that HIV is inactivated rapidly after being exposed to commonly used chemical germicides at concentrations that are much lower than used in practice.[27–30] Embalming fluids are similar to the types of chemical germicides that have been tested and found to completely inactivate HIV. In addition to commercially available chemical germicides, a solution of sodium hypochlorite (household bleach) prepared daily is an inexpensive and effective germicide. Concentrations ranging from approximately 500 ppm (1:100 dilution of household bleach) sodium hypochlorite to 5000 ppm (1:10 dilution of household bleach) are effective depending on the amount of organic material (e.g., blood, mucus) present on the surface to be cleaned and disinfected. Commercially available chemical germicides may be more compatible with certain medical devices that might be corroded by repeated exposure to sodium hypochlorite, especially to the 1:10 dilution.

SURVIVAL OF HIV IN THE ENVIRONMENT

The most extensive study on the survival of HIV after drying involved greatly concentrated HIV samples, i.e., 10 million tissue-culture infectious doses per milliliter.[31] This concentration is at least 100,000 times greater than that typically found in the blood or serum of patients with HIV infection. HIV was detectable by tissue-culture techniques 1–3 days after drying, but the rate of inactivation was rapid. Studies performed at CDC have also shown that drying HIV causes a rapid (within several hours) 1–2 log (90–99%) reduction in HIV concentration. In tissue-culture fluid, cell-free HIV could be detected up to 15 days at room temperature, up to 11 days at 37°C (98.6°F), and up to 1 day if the HIV was cell-associated.

When considered in the context of environmental conditions in health-care facilities, these results do not require any changes in currently recommended sterilization, disinfection, or housekeeping strategies. When medical devices are contaminated with blood or other body fluids, existing recommendations include the cleaning of these instruments, followed by disinfection or sterilization, depending on the type of medical device. These protocols assume "worst-case" conditions of extreme virologic and microbiologic contamination, and whether viruses have been inactivated after drying plays no role in formulating these strategies. Consequently, no changes in published procedures for cleaning, disinfecting, or sterilizing need to be made.

HOUSEKEEPING

Environmental surfaces such as walls, floors, and other surfaces are not associated with transmission of infections to patients or health-care workers. Therefore, extraordinary attempts to disinfect or sterilize these environmental surfaces are not necessary. However, cleaning and removal of soil should be done routinely.

Cleaning schedules and methods vary according to the area of the hospital or institution, type of surface to be cleaned, and the amount and type of soil present. Horizontal surfaces (e.g., bedside tables and hard-surfaced flooring) in patient-care areas are usually cleaned on a regular basis, when soiling or spills occur, and when a patient is discharged. Cleaning of walls, blinds, and curtains is recommended only if they are visibly soiled. Disinfectant fogging is an unsatisfactory method of decontaminating air and surfaces and is not recommended.

Disinfectant–detergent formulations registered by EPA can be used for cleaning environmental surfaces, but the actual physical removal of microorganisms by scrubbing is probably at least as important as any antimicrobial effect of the cleaning agent used. Therefore, cost, safety, and acceptability by housekeepers can be the main criteria for selecting any such registered agent. The manufacturers' instructions for appropriate use should be followed.

CLEANING AND DECONTAMINATING SPILLS OF BLOOD OR OTHER BODY FLUIDS

Chemical germicides that are approved for use as "hospital disinfectants" and are tuberculocidal when used at recommended dilutions can be used to decontaminate spills of blood and other body fluids. Strategies for decontaminating spills of blood and other body fluids in a patient-care setting are different than for spills of cultures or other materials in clinical, public health, or research laboratories. In patient-care areas, visible material should first be removed and then the area should be decontaminated. With large spills of cultured or concentrated infectious agents in the laboratory, the contaminated area should be flooded with a liquid germicide before cleaning, then decontaminated with fresh germicidal chemical. In both settings, gloves should be worn during the cleaning and decontaminating procedures.

LAUNDRY

Although soiled linen has been identified as a source of large numbers of certain pathogenic microorganisms, the risk of actual disease transmission is negligible. Rather than rigid procedures and specifications, hygienic and commonsense storage and processing of clean and soiled linen are recommended.[26] Soiled linen should be handled as little as possible and with minimum agitation to prevent gross microbial contamination of the air and of persons handling the linen. All soiled linen should be bagged at the location where it was used; it should not be sorted or rinsed in patient-care areas. Linen soiled with blood or body fluids should be placed and transported in bags that prevent leakage. If hot water is used, linen should be washed with detergent in water at least 71°C (160°F) for 25 minutes. If low-temperature (< 70°C [158°F]) laundry cycles are used, chemicals suitable for low-temperature washing at proper use-concentration should be used.

INFECTIVE WASTE

There is no epidemiologic evidence to suggest that most hospital waste is any more infective than residential waste. Moreover, there is no epidemiologic evidence that most hospital waste has caused disease in the community as a result of improper disposal. Therefore, identifying wastes for which special precautions are indicated is largely a matter of judgment about the relative risk of disease transmission. The most practical approach to the management of infective waste is to identify those wastes with the potential for causing infection during handling and disposal and for which some special precautions appear prudent. Hospital wastes for which special precautions appear prudent include microbiology laboratory waste, pathology waste, and blood specimens or blood products. While any item that has had contact with blood, exudates, or secretions may be potentially infective, it is not usually considered practical or necessary to treat all such waste as infective.[23,26] Infective waste, in general, should either be incinerated or should be autoclaved before disposal in an sanitary landfill. Bulk blood, suctioned fluids, excretions, and secretions may be carefully poured down a drain connected to a sanitary sewer. Sanitary sewers may also be used to dispose of other infectious wastes capable of being ground and flushed into the sewer.

IMPLEMENTATION OF RECOMMENDED PRECAUTIONS

Employers of health-care workers should ensure that policies exist for:

1. Initial orientation and continuing education and training of all health-care workers—including students and trainees—on the epidemiology, modes of transmission, and prevention of HIV and other bloodborne infections and the need for routine use of universal blood and body-fluid precautions for **all** patients
2. Provision of equipment and supplies necessary to minimize the risk of infection with HIV and other bloodborne pathogens
3. Monitoring adherence to recommended protective measures. When monitoring reveals a failure to follow recommended precautions, counseling, education, and/or retraining should be provided, and, if necessary, appropriate disciplinary action should be considered. Professional associations and labor organizations, through continuing education efforts, should emphasize the need for health-care workers to follow recommended precautions.

REFERENCES

1. Centers for Disease Control. Acquired immunodeficiency syndrome (AIDS): Precautions for clinical and laboratory staffs. *MMWR* 1982;31:577–580.
2. Centers for Disease Control. Acquired immunodeficiency syndrome (AIDS): Precautions for health-care workers and allied professionals. *MMWR* 1983;32:450–451.
3. Centers for Disease Control. Recommendations for preventing transmission of infection with human T-lymphotropic virus type III/lymphadenopathy-associated virus in the workplace. *MMWR* 1985; 34:681–686, 691–695.
4. Centers for Disease Control. Recommendations for preventing transmission of infection with human T-lymphotropic virus type III/lymphadenopathy-associated virus during invasive procedures. *MMWR* 1986;35:221–223.
5. Centers for Disease Control. Recommendations for preventing possible transmission of human T-lymphotropic virus type III/lymphadenopathy-associated virus from tears. *MMWR* 1985;34:533–534.
6. Centers for Disease Control. Recommendations for providing dialysis treatment to patients infected with human T-lymphotropic virus type III/lymphadenopathy-associated virus infection. *MMWR* 1986;35:376–378, 383.
7. Garner JS, Simmons BP. Guideline for isolation precautions in hospitals. *Infect Control* 1983; 4(suppl):245–325.
8. Centers for Disease Control. Recommended infection control practices for dentistry. *MMWR* 1986; 35:237–242.
9. McCray E. The Cooperative Needlestick Surveillance Group. Occupational risk of the acquired immunodeficiency syndrome among health care workers. *N Engl J Med* 1986;314:1127–1132.
10. Henderson DK, Saah AJ, Zak BJ, et al. Risk of nosocomial infection with human T-cell lymphotropic virus type III/lymphadenopathy-associated virus in a large cohort of intensively exposed health care workers. *Ann Intern Med* 1986;104:644–647.
11. Gerberding JL, Bryant-LeBlanc CE, Nelson K, et al. Risk of transmitting the human immunodeficiency virus, cytomegalovirus, and hepatitis B virus to health care workers exposed to patients with AIDS and AIDS-related conditions. *J Infect Dis* 1987; 156:1–8.
12. McEvoy M, Porter K, Mortimer P, Simmons N, Shanson D. Prospective study of clinical, laboratory, and ancillary staff with accidental exposures to blood or other body fluids from patients infected with HIV. *Br Med J* 1987;294:1595–1597.
13. Anonymous. Needlestick transmission of HTLV-III from a patient infected in Africa. *Lancet* 1984; 2:1376–1377.
14. Oksenhendler E, Harzic M, Le Roux JM, Rabian C, Clauvel JP. HIV infection with seroconversion after a superficial needlestick injury to the finger. *N Engl J Med* 1986;315:582.
15. Neisson-Vernant C, Arfi S, Mathez D, Leibowitch J, Monplaisir N. Needlestick HIV seroconversion in a nurse. *Lancet* 1986;2:814.
16. Grint P, McEvoy M. Two associated cases of the acquired immune deficiency syndrome (AIDS). *PHLS Commun Dis Rep* 1985;42:4.
17. Centers for Disease Control. Apparent transmission of human T-lymphotropic-associated virus type III/lymphadenopathy-associated virus from a child to a mother providing health care. *MMWR* 1986;35:76–79.
18. Centers for Disease Control. Update: Human immunodeficiency virus infections in health-care workers exposed to blood of infected patients. *MMWR* 1987;36:285–289.
19. Kline RS, Phelan J, Friedland GH, et al. Low occuptional risk for HIV infection for dental professionals (Abstract). In: *Abstracts from the III International Conference on AIDS, 1–5 June 1985, Washington, DC,* p. 155.
20. Baker JL, Kelen GD, Sivertson KT, Quinn TC. Unsuspected human immunodeficiency virus in criti-

cally ill emergency patients. *JAMA* 1987;257:2609–2611.
21. Favero MS. Dialysis-associated diseases and their control. In: Bennett JV, Brachman PS (eds): *Hospital Infections.* Boston: Little, Brown; 1985;267–284.
22. Richardson JH, Barkley WE (eds). *Biosafety in Microbiological and Biomedical Laboratories.* Washington, DC: U.S. Department of Health and Human Services, Public Health Service; 1984: HHS Pub. No. (CDC) 84–8395.
23. Centers for Disease Control. Human T-lymphotropic virus type III/lymphadenopathy-associated virus: Agent summary statement. *MMWR* 1986;35:540–542, 547–549.
24. Environmental Protection Agency. *EPA Guide for Infectious Waste Management.* Washington, DC: U.S. Environmental Protection Agency; May 1986: Pub. No. EPA/530-SW-86-014.
25. Favero MS. Sterilization, disinfection, and antisepsis in the hospital. In: *Manual of Clinical Microbiology.* 4th ed. Washington, DC: American Society for Microbiology; 1985;129–137.
26. Garner JS, Favero MS. *Guideline for Handwashing and Hospital Environmental Control.* Atlanta: Public Health Service, Centers for Disease Control: 1985:HHS Pub. No. 99–1117.
27. Spire B, Montagnier L, Barre-Sinoussi F, Chermann JC. Inactivation of lymphadenopathy associated virus by chemical disinfectants. *Lancet* 1984; 2:899–901.
28. Martin LS, McDougal JS, Loskoski SL. Disinfection and inactivation of the human T lymphotropic virus type III/lymphadenopathy-associated virus. *J Infect Dis* 1985;152:400–403.
29. McDougal JS, Martin LS, Cort SP, et al. Thermal inactivation of the acquired immunodeficiency syndrome virus-III/lymphadenopathy-associated virus, with special reference to antihemophilic factor. *J Clin Invest* 1985;76:875–877.
30. Spire B, Barre-Sinoussi F, Dormont D, Montagnier L, Chermann JC. Inactivation of lymphadenopathy-associated virus by heat, gamma rays, and ultraviolet light. *Lancet* 1985;1:188–189.
31. Resnik L, Veren K, Salahuddin SZ, Tondreau S, Markham PD. Stability and inactivation of HTLV-III/LAV under clinical and laboratory environments. *JAMA* 1986;255:1887–1891.
32. Centers for Disease Control. Public Health Service (PHS) guidelines for counseling and antibody testing to prevent HIV infection and AIDS. *MMWR* 1987;3:509–515.
33. Kane MA, Lettau LA. Transmission of HBV from dental personnel to patients. *J Am Dent Assoc* 1985;110:634–636.
34. Lettau LA, Smith JD, Williams D, et al. Transmission of hepatitis B, with resultant restriction of surgical practice. *JAMA* 1986;255:934–937.
35. Williams WW. Guideline for infection control in hospital personnel. *Infect Control* 1983;4(suppl): 326–349.
36. Centers for Disease Control. Prevention of acquired immune deficiency syndrome (AIDS): Report of interagency recommendations. *MMWR* 1983;32:101–103.
37. Centers for Disease Control. Provisional Public Health Service inter-agency recommendations for screening donated blood and plasma for antibody to the virus causing acquired immunodeficiency syndrome. *MMWR* 1985;34:1–5.

Can Magnesium Sulfate Be Safely Used to Rid the Body of Fluid in the Lower Extremities?

Murray Shor
Instructor, American Academy, McAllister Institute, New York, New York

Considering the wide distribution of news media, the public in general and basic medical science students in particular are surely aware that the major causes of death in both the preceding and current decade are neoplasms and cardiovascular diseases. This is of special interest to the embalmer because these different pathologies, vascular disorders and malignancies, may lead to edema. Considering that the combined deaths from these causes combined account for about 90% of the mortalities in this country, a large number of the bodies received by the embalmer have edema.

Generally, lymph, the fluid of the tissue spaces, is derived from the blood plasma by filtration. If more lymph enters the interstitial spaces than is carried off by the lymphatic vessels, edema results. Therefore, any abdominal neoplasm at the level of the second lumbar vertebra or higher could press against the thoracic duct, obstruct it, and cause lymphatic fluid to gather in the lower extremities. Because such tumors are involved in a large percentage of deaths, edema of the lower extremities is a common finding in bodies received by the mortician.

PRESSURE FROM HEART DISEASES

Many diseases of the heart have a similar effect on the fluid content of the lower extremities and the abdomen. If, for example, the right atrium remained filled after systole because of an inefficient right atrioventricular valve, blood attempting to enter the right atrium from the inferior vena cava during diastole would be prevented from doing so. A high intravenous pressure would result, preventing the reentry of fluid into the venous end of the capillary, and edema would ensue.

Complicating the problems of patients in the terminal stages of severe gastrointestinal or cardiac disease is the fact that they are unable to chew or swallow or retain protein foods such as meat. This reduces the protein content of the blood and, in turn, renders it hypotonic to the fluids of the surrounding tissues. Consequently, the outpouring of fluid from the capillary bed to the intercellular spaces is increased. The result is nutritional edema.

In addition to the disease just described, myriad circulatory disorders and infectious diseases can result in edema. So, without belaboring the point, I submit that edema is an embalming problem of some significance.

Now, let's get to the treatment.

Some embalmers treat edema of the lower extremities simply by elevating those parts. Others treat the condition by wrapping a spiral bandage from the ankle to the hip. These are tried and accepted methods. Were it not for still another, controversial technique, I would not feel compelled to write this article.

Most qualified operators agree that addition of magnesium sulfate to arterial fluid solution helps dehydrate the affected parts. Some, however, argue that the solution reaches the features and overdehydrates them. I believe this treatment can be applied with impunity.

We know that fluids pass through a membrane by osmosis and filtration. If pressure within the vascular system is kept high, it would favor the passage of fluids into the interstices by filtration. If fluids within the small blood vessels are hypotonic to extravascular fluids, again the condition would favor flow into the extravascular spaces.

USE OF SOLUTION AT LOW PRESSURE

Therefore, prudence dictates that we use a hypertonic solution at low pressure to encourage flow in the direction of the capillaries and eventually out of the body via venous drainage. According to Professor Pervier, a 6.77% solution exerts the same osmotic pressure as the human circulatory system. Because the extent of edema and the volume of fluids that can be tolerated vary in each case, it is impossible to recommend a specific concentration or volume. If, however, 6.77% solution exerts the same osmotic pressure as human circulatory tissue, 10% would be a good concentration at which to start.

To arrive at the volume of Epsom salt required to make a 10% solution, multiply the volume of solution required by the percentage desired. For use in a lower extremity, where 2 quarts of solution seems a reasonable quantity, multiply 64 ounces by 10%. The result is 6.4. Weigh out 6.4 ounces of Epsom salt and add it to enough arterial fluid solution to make 2 quarts. This gives you 2 quarts of 10% solution.

To overcome the possibility that the strong salt solution will reach the face and cause undue dehydration of the features, it is imperative that the embalmer raise and open both the femoral vein and the great saphenous vein. It must be remembered that the great saphenous vein enters the femoral vein about an inch and a half below the inguinal ligament. The embalmer usually raises the femoral vessels distal to this point, so that drainage from the lower extremity bypasses the femoral drainage point and reaches the face via the superficial return. In view of the fact that more return is accomplished by the superficial return than the deep return, failure to open the great saphenous vein would result in passage of the salt solution to the features by vascular channels too numerous to describe here.

Still another benefit derived by opening both the femoral and great saphenous vessels is the low intravenous pressure achieved by this procedure. With both major vessels of return wide open, it is obvious that pressure in the veins will not be high. If intracellular fluid pressure is high, due to accumulation of excess fluids, flow into the capillaries is favored, promoting drainage.

Removal of edematous fluids from the extremities is only one of the problems posed by the degenerative diseases of older members of the population. In the future, we shall discuss edema of other areas.

REFERENCE

Pervier NC. *Textbook of Chemistry for Embalmers.* Minneapolis: University of Minnesota; 1961.

INDEX

Page numbers followed by *f* indicate figures; page numbers followed by *t* indicate tables.

ISBN 0-8385-2187-8